MW01014987

ANESTHESIA OUTSIDE THE OPERATING ROOM

ANESTHESIA OUTSIDE THE OPERATING ROOM

SECOND EDITION

EDITED BY Richard D. Urman, MD, MBA

ASSOCIATE PROFESSOR OF ANESTHESIA
HARVARD MEDICAL SCHOOL
DIRECTOR, ANESTHESIA SERVICE, BWH HEALTHCARE CENTER—CHESTNUT HILL
MEDICAL DIRECTOR, PROCEDURAL SEDATION FOR INTERVENTIONAL MEDICINE
DIRECTOR (ANESTHESIA), CENTER FOR PERIOPERATIVE RESEARCH
FELLOWSHIP DIRECTOR, PERIOPERATIVE MEDICINE
BRIGHAM AND WOMEN'S HOSPITAL, BOSTON, MA

Wendy L. Gross, MD, MHCM

ASSISTANT PROFESSOR OF ANESTHESIA
HARVARD MEDICAL SCHOOL
VICE CHAIR, PLANNING AND ANALYTICS
DIRECTOR, NON-OR SERVICES
FACULTY, DIVISION OF CARDIAC ANESTHESIA
BRIGHAM AND WOMEN'S HOSPITAL, BOSTON, MA

Beverly K. Philip, MD

PROFESSOR OF ANESTHESIA
HARVARD MEDICAL SCHOOL
FOUNDING DIRECTOR, DAY SURGERY UNIT
BRIGHAM AND WOMEN'S HOSPITAL, BOSTON, MA

OXFORD
UNIVERSITY PRESS

OXFORD
UNIVERSITY PRESS

Oxford University Press is a department of the University of Oxford. It furthers the University's objective of excellence in research, scholarship, and education by publishing worldwide. Oxford is a registered trade mark of Oxford University Press in the UK and certain other countries.

Published in the United States of America by Oxford University Press
198 Madison Avenue, New York, NY 10016, United States of America.

© Oxford University Press 2018

First edition published in 2009

All rights reserved. No part of this publication may be reproduced, stored in a retrieval system, or transmitted, in any form or by any means, without the prior permission in writing of Oxford University Press, or as expressly permitted by law, by license, or under terms agreed with the appropriate reproduction rights organization. Inquiries concerning reproduction outside the scope of the above should be sent to the Rights Department, Oxford University Press, at the address above.

You must not circulate this work in any other form
and you must impose this same condition on any acquirer.

CIP data is on file at the Library of Congress
ISBN 978-0-19-049575-6

9 8 7 6 5 4 3 2 1
Printed by Sheridan Books, Inc., United States of America

To my parents, my wife, Zina Matlyuk, MD, and my daughters, Abigail and Isabelle

—R. D. U.

To my family and my colleagues who make every day a learning experience

—W. L. G.

To the outstanding physician, scientist, and husband, James H. Philip, MD

—B. K. P.

CONTENTS

FOREWORD TO THE FIRST EDITION

In the years since the publication of the first edition of this book, its predictions about the explosive pace of growth in anesthesia practice outside-of-the-operating room [OOOR] have been borne out in the full range of healthcare facilities. Fortunately, as this second edition demonstrates, practitioners of OOOR anesthesia have been diligent in studying and sharing their experiences. The editors have done a superb job of assembling these observations and the guidance emerging from them in this second edition.

The unifying thread throughout the content of these chapters is the imperative to achieve levels of efficiency and safety in the diverse settings described that are comparable to those seen in the traditional operating room setting. There is an inherent tension between the natural desire to recreate the traditional operating everywhere anesthetics are administered and adapting design and systems for the specific locale and clinical care delivered. In large facilities with large staffs, the benefits of concentrating staff experience (and thereby promoting familiarity) in OOOR settings can stress the capacity to efficiently schedule personnel for the larger enterprise. Indeed, a deliberate approach to adapting the scheduling of procedures and staff to a much more complex scope of service will be one of the most important investments in a successful OOOR anesthesia program.

The vexing problem we face—and will increasingly face as systems develop to deliver OOOR services more and more effectively—is that the demand for our services can easily grow beyond the capacity of the anesthesia workforce to deliver them. As an OOOR proceduralist, why wouldn't you seek anesthesiology support for all your procedures requiring sedation? The involvement of a team of anesthesia specialists boosts efficiency, increases capacity and throughput, reduces professional liability, and diminishes the burden of managing a dimension of patient care for which the proceduralists' training is probably minimal. Today's dominant fee-for-service payment models provide no incentive to do otherwise, although this is rapidly changing. As bundled and prospective payment systems come to include professional services, the true cost of utilizing anesthesia staff will be borne by the physicians themselves. When demand exceeds capacity, we will need to know when to say "no" and effectively triage the limited resources available and understand the full range of options for patient management. Great caution is warranted in considering the financial incentives at work for both users and providers of anesthesia services. There are dangerous potential conflicts of interest when economic interests are superimposed on judgments of necessity.

A role for anesthesiologists in the training and monitoring of personnel delivering sedation will inevitably emerge. Reflex reluctance and fear of empowering one's competition must be overcome and the rightful place of the anesthesiologist as the expert authority in such care should be embraced. Doing so strengthens, not weakens, the stature of the specialty across many disciplines and professions and will be a necessary ingredient to insure both quality and efficiency in the delivery of care in a health system strained to meet the needs of an aging population.

The reader will find useful guidance in defining the institutional investments that must be made in support of OOOR care. Physical distance from the mass of support (people and equipment) available in traditional settings is a challenge that must be overcome. First-rate equipment and, especially, communication tools will be critical and are justifiably identified as a prerequisite for establishing OOOR services. Detailed and ongoing discussions with the anesthesia "customers" (proceduralists) are vital to establish a shared vision of the day-to-day clinical collaboration in a rapidly changing patient care environment. Consider these chapters fair warning that failure to insist on these investments will produce regret (or worse) later.

You have in your hands a built-for-purpose toolkit for success in managing your OOOR anesthesia practice. Use it well !

Alexander A. Hannenberg, MD
Faculty, Safe Surgery Program, Ariadne Labs at Harvard
T.H. Chan School of Public Health and
Brigham & Women's Hospital
Chief Quality Officer and Past President
American Society of Anesthesiologists
Clinical Professor of Anesthesiology
Tufts University School of Medicine

FOREWORD TO THE SECOND EDITION

In the years since the publication of the first edition of this book, its predictions about the explosive pace of growth in anesthesia practice outside-of-the-operating room [OOOR] have been borne out in the full range of healthcare facilities. Fortunately, as this second edition demonstrates, practitioners of OOOR anesthesia have been diligent in studying and sharing their experiences. The editors have done a superb job of assembling these observations and the guidance emerging from them in this second edition.

The unifying thread throughout the content of these chapters is the imperative to achieve levels of efficiency and safety in the diverse settings described that are comparable to those seen in the traditional operating room setting. There is an inherent tension between the natural desire to recreate the traditional operating everywhere anesthetics are administered and adapting design and systems for the specific locale and clinical care delivered. In large facilities with large staffs, the benefits of concentrating staff experience (and thereby promoting familiarity) in OOOR settings can stress the capacity to efficiently schedule personnel for the larger enterprise. Indeed, a deliberate approach to adapting the scheduling of procedures and staff to a much more complex scope of service will be one of the most important investments in a successful OOOR anesthesia program.

The vexing problem we face—and will increasingly face as systems develop to deliver OOOR services more and more effectively—is that the demand for our services can easily grow beyond the capacity of the anesthesia workforce to deliver them. As an OOOR proceduralist, why wouldn't you seek anesthesiology support for all your procedures requiring sedation? The involvement of a team of anesthesia specialists boosts efficiency, increases capacity and throughput, reduces professional liability, and diminishes the burden of managing a dimension of patient care for which the proceduralists' training is probably minimal. Today's dominant fee-for-service payment models provide no incentive to do otherwise, although this is rapidly changing. As bundled and prospective payment systems come to include professional services, the true cost of utilizing anesthesia staff will be borne by the physicians themselves. When demand exceeds capacity, we will need to know when to say "no" and effectively triage the limited resources available and understand the full range of options for patient management. Great caution is warranted in considering the financial incentives at work for both users and providers of anesthesia services. There are dangerous potential conflicts of interest when economic interests are superimposed on judgments of necessity.

A role for anesthesiologists in the training and monitoring of personnel delivering sedation will inevitably emerge. Reflex reluctance and fear of empowering one's competition must be overcome and the rightful place of the anesthesiologist as the expert authority in such care should be embraced. Doing so strengthens, not weakens, the stature of the specialty across many disciplines and professions and will be a necessary ingredient to insure both quality and efficiency in the delivery of care in a health system strained to meet the needs of an aging population.

The reader will find useful guidance in defining the institutional investments that must be made in support of OOOR care. Physical distance from the mass of support (people and equipment) available in traditional settings is a challenge that must be overcome. First-rate equipment and, especially, communication tools will be critical and are justifiably identified as a prerequisite for establishing OOOR services. Detailed and ongoing discussions with the anesthesia "customers" (proceduralists) are vital to establish a shared vision of the day-to-day clinical collaboration in a rapidly changing patient care environment. Consider these chapters fair warning that failure to insist on these investments will produce regret (or worse) later.

You have in your hands a built-for-purpose toolkit for success in managing your OOOR anesthesia practice. Use it well!

Alexander A. Hannenberg, MD
Faculty, Safe Surgery Program, Ariadne Labs at Harvard T.H. Chan School of Public Health and Brigham & Women's Hospital
Chief Quality Officer and Past President, American Society of Anesthesiologists
Clinical Professor of Anesthesiology
Tufts University School of Medicine

CONTRIBUTORS

Basem Abdelmalak, MD
Professor of Anesthesiology
Cleveland Clinic Lerner College of Medicine
Cleveland, Ohio

Hairil R. Abdullah, MBBS, MMED
Associate Consultant
Department of Anesthesiology
Singapore General Hospital
Singapore

Kevin Abnet, MD
Associate Professor
Department of Anesthesiology and Pediatrics
University of Vermont College of Medicine
Burlington, Vermont

Annie Amin, MD
Department of Anesthesia
University of Chicago Medicine
Chicago, Illinois

James E. Andruchow, MD, MSc, FRCPC, ABEM
Emergency Physician, Department of Emergency Medicine
Clinical Assistant Professor, University of Calgary
Clinician Scientist, Alberta Health Services
Calgary, Alberta, Canada

Lori Kral Barton, MD
Assistant Professor of Anesthesiology
UK HealthCare
University of Kentucky
Lexington, Kentucky

Yasmeen Beg, MD
Clinical Instructor, Department of Anesthesiology
Northwestern University, Feinberg School of Medicine
Chicago, Illinois

Benjamin W. Berg, MD
Professor of Medicine
Director of Simulation: SimTiki
John A. Burns School of Medicine
University of Hawaii
Honolulu, Hawaii

Sharath K. Bhagavatula, MD
Resident in Radiology
Brigham and Women's Hospital/Harvard Medical School
Boston, Massachusetts

Steven Boggs, MD, MBA
Director of the OR and Chief of the Anesthesia Service
James J. Peters VA Medical Center
Associate Professor, Anesthesiology
The Icahn School of Medicine at Mount Sinai
New York, New York

Robert H. Burch III, MD

Keith Candiotti, MD
Professor, Executive Vice Chair, and Chief Operating Officer
Department of Anesthesiology, Perioperative Medicine, and Pain Management
University of Miami Miller School of Medicine
Miami, Florida

Frances Chung, MBBS, FRCPC
Professor of Anesthesia
University of Toronto Faculty of Medicine
Toronto, Ontario, Canada

Christopher Connor, MD, PhD
Department of Anesthesiology and Biomedical Engineering
Boston University School of Medicine
Boston, Massachusetts

Lebron Cooper, MD
Chair of Anesthesiology
University of Tennessee Health Science Center College of Medicine
Memphis, Tennessee

Thomas W. Cutter, MD, MAEd
Professor of Anesthesia & Critical Care
Professor, Department of Surgery
Medical Director for Perioperative Services
University of Chicago Medicine
Chicago, Illinois

Suanne M. Daves, MD
Associate Professor, Departments of Anesthesiology and Pediatrics
Vanderbilt University Medical Center
Nashville, Tennessee

Karen B. Domino, MD, MPH
Professor and Vice Chair for Clinical Research
Department of Anesthesiology and Pain Medicine
University of Washington School of Medicine
Seattle, Washington

Benjamin Easter, MD
Assistant Professor, Emergency Medicine
Assistant Medical Director, Emergency Department
University of Colorado School of Medicine
Denver, Colorado

Robert T. Faillace, MD, ScM
Chair, Department of Medicine for the North Bronx Healthcare Network
Professor, Department of Medicine
Albert Einstein College of Medicine
Bronx, New York

Benjamin T. Fedeles, MD
Department of Anesthesiology
University of Maryland School of Medicine
Baltimore, Maryland

Milana Flusberg, MD
Assistant Professor in Radiology
Department of Abdominal Imaging
Montefiore Medical Center/Albert Einstein College of Medicine
Bronx, New York

Regina Y. Fragneto, MD
Chief, Division of Obstetric Anesthesia
UK Health Care
University of Kentucky
Lexington, Kentucky

Kai U. Frerichs, MD
Director of Interventional Neuroradiology
Director of Endovascular Neurosurgery
Assistant Professor
Harvard Medical School
Brigham and Women's Hospital
Boston, Massachusetts

Elizabeth Frost, MD
Clinical Professor
Anesthesiology, Perioperative, & Pain Medicine
Mount Sinai Hospital
New York, New York

Samuel M. Galvagno Jr., DO, PhD, FCCM
Associate Professor
Associate Director of Critical Care Services, University of Maryland Medical Center
Chief, Division of Critical Care Medicine
Department of Anesthesiology
University of Maryland School of Medicine
Baltimore, Maryland

Clifford M. Gevirtz, MD, MPH
Department of Anesthesiology
School of Medicine
LSU Health New Orleans
New Orleans, Louisiana

Ori Gottlieb, MD
Associate Professor
Department of Anesthesia and Critical Care
University of Chicago
Chicago, Illinois

Dennis Grech, MD
Assistant Professor of Anesthesiology
Section Chief and Director of Ambulatory Anesthesia
American University of the Caribbean School of Medicine
Cupecoy, St. Maarten

Mark A. Gromski, MD
Assistant Professor of Clinical Medicine
Indiana University School of Medicine
Indianapolis, Indiana

Wendy L. Gross, MD, MHCM
Assistant Professor of Anesthesia
Harvard Medical School
Vice Chair, Planning and Analytics
Director, Non-OR Services
Faculty, Division of Cardiac Anesthesia
Brigham and Women's Hospital
Boston, Massachusetts

Lynda Harhad, DDS
Assistant Professor
Assistant Director, General Practice Residency Clinic
Baton Rouge, Louisiana
Department of Comprehensive Dentistry and Biomaterials
LSUHSC School of Dentistry
New Orleans, Louisiana

Eric A. Harris, MD, MBA
Associate Professor, Department of Anesthesiology
Perioperative Medicine, and Pain Management
University of Miami Miller School of Medicine
Miami, Florida

Laurence M. Hausman, MD
Professor of Anesthesiology Vice-Chair
Academic Affiliations Director
Ambulatory Anesthesia Assistant Director
Perioperative Services Department of Anesthesiology
Perioperative and Pain Medicine Icahn School of Medicine
New York, New York

Gabriel Hernandez, DDS
Assistant Professor
Assistant Director, General Practice Residency Clinic
New Orleans, Louisiana
Department of Comprehensive Dentistry and Biomaterials
LSUHSC School of Dentistry
New Orleans, Louisiana

Robert S. Holzman, MD
Clinical Professor, Department of Medicine
Professor Emeritus of Medicine and Environmental Medicine
NYU Langone Health
New York University
New York, New York

Gaelen Horne, DO

Shawn S. Jackson, MD, PhD
Resident in Anesthesiology
Department of Anesthesiology, Perioperative and Pain Medicine
Brigham and Women's Hospital
Boston, Massachusetts

Alan D. Kaye, MD, PhD
Professor and Chair
Department of Anesthesiology
Louisiana State University
New Orleans, Louisiana

Bhavani Kodali, MD
Associate Professor
Department of Anesthesiology, Pain and Perioperative Medicine
Brigham and Woman's Hospital/Harvard Medical School
Boston, Massachusetts

Vesela Kovacheva, MD, PhD
Attending Anesthesiologist
Brigham and Women's Hospital
Boston, Massachusetts

Edward M. Lopez, MD, LT COL, US Army
Anesthesiology, Fort Sam Houston, Texas

Christopher V. Maani, MD
Attending Anesthesiologist
SAMMC Department of Anesthesia & Operative Services
Associate Program Director for Research
SAUSHEC Anesthesiology Residency
San Antonio, Texas

Alex Macario, MD, MBA
Vice-Chair for Education
Professor, Department of Anesthesiology, Perioperative and Pain Medicine
Professor, Department of Health Research and Policy
Program Director, Anesthesiology Residency
Stanford University School of Medicine
Stanford, California

Erin M. Maddy, MD
Anesthesiology Resident
University of Vermont College of Medicine
Burlington, Vermont

Mohamed Mahmoud, MD
Associate Professor, Department of Anesthesiology
Cincinnati Children's Hospital
University of Cincinnati
Cincinnati, Ohio

Keira P. Mason, MD
Director, Radiology Anesthesia
Senior Associate in Perioperative Anesthesia
Associate Professor of Anesthesia
Boston Children's Hospital
Harvard Medical School
Boston, Massachusetts

Kai Matthes, MD, PhD
The Anesthesia Medical Group, Inc.
Maui, Hawaii

Donald M. Matthews, MD
Professor and Chair
Department of Anesthesiology
University of Vermont College of Medicine
Burlington, Vermont

Craig McFarland, MD
Department of Anesthesiology
Uniformed Services University for the Health Sciences
Fort Sam Houston, Texas

Julia Metzner, MD
Associate Professor
Education Director of UWMC
Department of Anesthesiology and Pain Medicine
University of Washington Medical Center
Seattle, Washington

Daniel M. Moseley, MD

W. Bosseau Murray, MD
Professor of Anesthesiology
Penn State University, Hershey Medical Center
Hershey, Pennsylvania

Ben O'Brien, MD, PhD (Habil), FRCA, FFICM, MHBA, ATPL
Department of Perioperative Medicine
St. Barthlolomew's Hospital
London, United Kingdom

Bijal Patel, MD
Assistant Professor
University of Calgary and University of Saskatchewan
Staff Radiologist, Mayfair Diagnostics
Calgary, Alberta, Canada

Robert Perelmut, MD

Ernesto A. Pretto Jr., MD, MPH
University of Miami Health System
Miami, Florida

Matthew Read, MD
Anesthesiology, Brooke Army Medical Center
Fort Sam Houston, Texas

Lisa Ross, MD, MBA
Director, Department of Anesthesia
NYC Health + Hospitals/Harlem
Associate Clinical Professor of Anesthesia
Columbia University Medical Center
New York, New York

Keith J. Ruskin, MD
Department of Anesthesia and Critical Care
University of Chicago
Chicago, Illinois

Robert M. Savage, MD, FACC

Leslie B. Scorza, MD, FSIR
Associate Professor of Radiology, Surgery, and Medicine
Cardiovascular and Interventional Radiology
Penn State Hershey Heart and Vascular Institute
Penn State Milton S. Hershey Medical Center
Hershey, Pennsylvania

Geoffrey Scriver
Assistant Professor of Interventional Radiology
University of Vermont College of Medicine
Burlington, Vermont

Patricia M. Sequeira

Deepak Sharma, MD, MBA

Douglas C. Shook, MD
Department of Anesthesiology, Perioperative and Pain Medicine
Brigham and Women's Hospital
Boston, Massachusetts

Mrinal Shukla
Vascular Surgery Fellow
University of Vermont College of Medicine
Burlington, Vermont

Paul B. Shyn, MD
Assistant Professor of Radiology
Director of Cross-Sectional Interventional Radiology
Department of Abdominal Imaging and Intervention
Brigham and Women's Hospital/Harvard Medical School
Boston, Massachusetts

Stuart G. Silverman, MD
Professor in Radiology
Director of Abdominal Imaging and Intervention
Brigham and Women's Hospital/Harvard Medical School
Boston, Massachusetts

Daniel A. T. Souza, MD
Instructor in Radiology
Department of Abdominal Imaging and Intervention
Brigham and Women's Hospital/Harvard Medical School
Boston, Massachusetts

Francis Spaulding, MD

BobbieJean Sweitzer, MD
Professor, Department of Anesthesiology
Director, Perioperative Medicine
Northwestern University, Feinberg School of Medicine
Chicago, Illinois

Ruth Thiex, MD, PhD

Janice A. Townsend, DDS, MS
Associate Professor and Chair of the Division of Pediatric Dentistry
The Ohio State University College of Dentistry
Department Chief of Dentistry and Section Chief of Pediatric Dentistry
Nationwide Children's Hospital
Columbus, Ohio

Kemal Tuncali, MD
Instructor of Radiology
Department of Abdominal Imaging and Intervention
Brigham and Women's Hospital/Harvard Medical School
Boston, Massachusetts

Sorin Vaduva, MBA

Sanjana Vig, MD, MBA
Assistant Clinical Professor
Director of Preoperative Evaluation Clinic
Department of Anesthesiology
University of California, San Diego
San Diego, California

1 | CHALLENGES OF ANESTHESIA OUTSIDE OF THE OPERATING ROOM

WENDY L. GROSS, MD, MHCM, RICHARD D. URMAN, MD, MBA

The increase in volume and scope of procedures performed outside of the operating room (OOOR), both with and without the involvement of the anesthesia provider is incontrovertible. As health care adjusts to simultaneous rapid technological development and increasing financial constraints, diagnostic and therapeutic interventions are performed more frequently OOOR by a broad spectrum of medical practitioners. The broadening scope and complexity of noninvasive procedures as well as the increasing acuity of patients undergoing them often make deeper sedation, general anesthesia, and robust hemodynamic monitoring necessary and challenging. Anesthesiologists are more frequently needed to provide care for medically complex patients (American Society of Anesthesiologists [ASA] physical status ≥ 3) undergoing novel, unfamiliar procedures in nontraditional locations. As technology advances, the number of procedural areas and the need for anesthesia services proliferate. The expansion of OOOR cases has changed the boundaries of anesthesiology practice as new challenges and opportunities emerge.

The OOOR environment confronts the anesthesiologist with considerable and diverse clinical situations. The proliferation of practitioners and the variety of service environments (Table 1.1) expand the professional relationship beyond that characterized by the traditional anesthesiologist–surgeon interface. Evolving concerns encompass clinical, financial, safety, and political questions.

ASSESSMENT AND DESIGN OF OOOR PROCEDURE LOCATIONS

The provision of anesthesia care for cases performed OOOR requires flexibility (both physical and intellectual) and good communication skills on the part of the anesthesiologist. For the most part, OOOR locations are not built with anesthesiologists in mind. It is often necessary to rearrange equipment, particularly monitors, anesthesia machines, airway equipment, and pumps, so that they are close to the patient. Many suites are located in the most remote parts of the hospital. They are often small, crowded, and not conducive to the introduction of anesthesia machines or monitoring devices. For example, radiology suites designed and built to house complex, heat-sensitive computers, and magnetic resonance imaging (MRI) facilities expose personnel and equipment to high-level magnetic fields. Radiotherapy suites require delivery of anesthesia in heavily shielded radiation-proof rooms where only remote surveillance of the patient via a video camera and a vital signs monitor is possible. It may be difficult for the anesthesiologist to see the progress of the procedure, talk to the proceduralist, or even observe the patient's vital signs in such circumstances.

Many items routinely utilized in traditional operating rooms (ORs) may not be present in procedural areas, and the individuals performing the procedure may be unaware of the importance of such equipment. Gas scavenging may be unavailable, oxygen or suction sources may be limited, and thermostats may be fixed to accommodate imaging equipment while increasing a risk of hypothermia in the patient under anesthesia. In addition, ancillary caregivers may have

TABLE 1.1. OOOR Anesthetizing Locations (Sites and Physicians Involved)

Radiology suites (radiologists, urologists, neurosurgeons)
Interventional radiology (neuroradiology and angiography)
Magnetic resonance imaging
Computed tomography
Ultrasound
Cardiac catheterization and electrophysiology (EP) laboratory (cardiologists)
Endoscopy suite (gastroenterologists, surgeons)
Family planning and obstetrics unit (obstetricians, gynecologists)
Emergency room (ER physicians, surgeons, internal medicine physicians)
Lithotripsy suite (urologists)
Outpatient procedure rooms (dermatologists, surgeons, dentists, podiatrists)
Electroconvulsive therapy unit (psychiatrists)
Critical care units (surgeons, cardiologists, neonatologists) Interventional pulmonology (pulmonologists, surgeons)

OOOR, outside of the operating room.

SOURCE: Adapted from Russell GB. *Alternate-Site Anesthesia*. Oxford, England: Butterworth-Heinemann; 1997.

limited understanding of what constitutes an airway or anesthetic emergency and what the response to such a situation should be.

Regardless of the unusual physical parameters of the OOOR environment, anesthesiologists must be sure that their practice conforms to the same standards adhered to in the main OR. The ASA has established guidelines designed to improve the safety of OOOR anesthetic practice. The "ASA Statement on Non-Operating Room Anesthetizing Locations"[1] is summarized in Table 1.2. It is important to note that these are minimum standards recommended for all OOOR locations. This is a dynamic situation however, as procedural suites evolve these guidelines will as well.

NEW SITE EVALUATION

When evaluating new sites, it is important to consider both the needs of anesthesiologists and the context of the available and necessary technical and procedural priorities of the specialty requiring anesthesiology support. Ideally, the anesthesia service should be involved with the design and site selection in the planning phase so that all anesthesia-specific requirements are taken into consideration before the new site is constructed. This ultimately allows for better case management and resource utilization. Table 1.3 outlines questions to be asked during site evaluation for potential OOOR anesthesia.

TABLE 1.2. Summary of the ASA Statement on Non–Operating Room Anesthetizing Locations

1. A reliable source of oxygen.
2. An adequate and reliable source of suction.
3. An adequate and reliable system for scavenging waste anesthetic gases.
4. A self-inflating hand resuscitator bag capable of administering at least 90% oxygen as a means to deliver positive pressure ventilation; adequate anesthesia drugs, supplies, and equipment for the intended anesthesia care; adequate monitoring equipment to allow adherence to the "Standards for Basic Anesthetic Monitoring." If inhalation anesthesia is to be administered, there should be an anesthesia machine maintained to current operating room standards.
5. Sufficient electrical outlets.
6. Adequate illumination of the patient, anesthesia machine, and monitoring equipment.
7. Sufficient space to accommodate necessary equipment and personnel and to allow expeditious access to patient, anesthesia machine, and monitoring equipment.
8. An emergency cart with a defibrillator, emergency drugs, and other equipment needed to provide cardiopulmonary resuscitation.
9. Adequate staff trained to support the anesthesiologist.
10. All applicable building and safety codes and facility standards should be observed.
11. Appropriate postanesthesia management should be provided.

ASA, American Society of Anesthesiologists.

SOURCE: Based on "Statement on Non-Operating Room Anesthetizing Locations of the American Society of Anesthesiologists." A copy of the full text can be obtained from ASA, 520 N. Northwest Highway, Park Ridge, Illinois 60068-2573.

MONITORING AND EQUIPMENT CONSIDERATIONS

Equipment and monitoring considerations are critical when assessing and designing new OOOR locations. Many anesthesiologists bring portable equipment to the site, whereas some locations routinely stock anesthesiology equipment at the site. Sometimes delivery of a safe anesthetic OOOR requires more equipment than it is typically needed in the OR. Depending on the patient's condition, more advanced monitoring may be needed if the OOOR site is distant from the OR or isolated from the main part of the hospital. Frequently, the specific procedures performed dictate the need for unusual monitoring. Some procedures may require cerebral oximetry, whereas others may require echocardiography equipment. Defibrillators should be uniformly present at all procedure sites, just as they are in the OR. Whatever monitoring is utilized, it should be accessible by, and visible to, the anesthesiologist delivering the anesthetic. For example, electrocardiogram (ECG) equipment visible only to the cardiologist in the cardiac catheterization lab is essentially not available to the anesthesiologist. Special equipment may be needed for specific sites, such as MRI-compatible equipment for the magnetic resonance tomography (MRT) suite. Smaller, more portable, anesthesia machines are readily available and are more practical for some sites.[2,3]

TABLE 1.3. Considerations During OOOR Site Evaluation

1. Where will anesthesia be induced (procedure bed, stretcher, in another room), and where will the patient recover?
2. Are oxygen and suction close enough to the patient and dedicated to anesthesia utilization, or are they shared?
3. Are lighting and temperature controls adequate?
4. Is it possible to monitor the patient and vital signs outside of the procedure room if the anesthesia provider needs to step outside (i.e., due to significant radiation exposure)?
5. How can additional help be obtained if needed urgently?
6. Are monitors in place and adequate, or is it necessary to transport additional equipment?
7. Where is the code cart? Does every care team member know where it is and how to call a code?
8. Are the personnel on site aware of what constitutes an anesthetic emergency and how to address it?
9. Is there enough physical space dedicated to anesthesia personnel and all the required or potentially required anesthesia equipment?

OOOR, outside of the operating room.

SOURCE: Adapted from Russell GB. *Alternate-Site Anesthesia*. Oxford, England: Butterworth-Heinemann; 1997.

No matter the physical or financial constraints imposed by the procedure area itself, standard essential monitors for the safe delivery of anesthetic care must be present. Because all regional or local anesthesia can require conversion to a general anesthetic, the standards of care practiced in the OR must be followed in OOOR areas: An anesthesia machine should be readily available and/or present in all OOOR anesthetizing locations.

Proper patient monitoring is key to improving patient safety in any OR location. The ASA has published "Standards for Basic Anesthetic Monitoring,"[4] which specifically state the following:

1. Qualified anesthesia personnel must be present in the room throughout the conduct of all anesthetics.
2. The patient's oxygenation, ventilation, circulation, and temperature must be continually evaluated.

A more detailed discussion on patient monitoring is found in Chapter 3 (Patient Monitoring). Many investigators have written about the capability of monitors to reduce morbidity and mortality. Several closed claims analyses[5,6] suggested that appropriate monitoring leads to more timely rectification of potentially deleterious states and therefore prevention of untoward events. Because sicker patients are being cared for OOOR and more complex procedures are evolving, there may be less room for error than ever before. OOOR sites are usually removed from core locations of anesthesia care delivery, and the availability of backup equipment and extra staff is therefore reduced. Anesthesiologists, who have achieved tremendous success advancing safety in the OR with the use of appropriate monitoring, must maintain monitoring and other practice standards in OOOR sites. *Since every minimal-moderate sedation case OOOR can potentially devolve into a deep sedation or general anesthesia case*, appropriate patient monitoring is truly critical.

ORGANIZATION AND INTEGRATION OF ANESTHESIA AND PATIENT CARE TEAMS

The patient care team in the OOOR environment includes medical practitioners and consultants who may not be familiar with the scope and practice of anesthesiology. This team includes ancillary personnel such as radiology technicians, nurses, and other technical and physician (nonanesthesia) staff. In addition, anesthesiologists dispatched to OOOR sites may be unfamiliar with the procedures that they are supporting. It is any lack of understanding of the unique requirements of a particular OOOR site or case on the part of either the procedure suite staff or the anesthesia team that can adversely affect outcome. In addition, the priorities of anesthesiologists may be challenged by the flow of cases in procedural areas. Uninformed ancillary personnel may obstruct the normal flow of anesthetic delivery; at the same time, uninformed anesthesiologists may obstruct the flow of a procedure. Communication among the procedure site staff and the anesthesia care team is therefore essential.

The "ASA Statement on the Anesthesia Care Team"[7] addresses the structure of the anesthesia team performing the anesthetic. However, structure does not always dictate function, and the goal is to integrate services, include nonanesthesia staff in decision-making, and plan responsibility. An emphasis on teamwork and communication in the context of patient safety is imperative in OOOR locations, and interdisciplinary collaboration is necessary. Team leadership, situational awareness, and establishment of an environment where continued learning is supported are all critical features of an arena in which integrated patient care teams can develop and operate optimally.[8] Goals must be clarified and broadened to include those of proceduralists, anesthesiologists, and all members of the patient care team.

In some circumstances, the anesthesiologist essentially becomes a consultant; communication and resolution of conflict are therefore critical. Just as these are essential in the OR [9–11] the same need exists OOOR. In the case of the latter, the process is potentially more complicated. Conflict resolution is more difficult in an environment where the equipment of one specialty imposes physical constraints on the capacity of another to work and where the vocabulary of one discipline does not necessarily include the vocabulary of another.

Preoperative assessment must be clearly addressed and discussed by both the proceduralist and the anesthesiologist because it affects the delivery and type of anesthetic as well as the course of the procedure. Proceduralists may not be aware of the results of preoperative assessments or the potential limitations these might impose on the performance of procedures or the postprocedure care of patients. Although preoperative visits and checklists are standard in many hospitals with respect to OR cases, this may not be so with respect to procedures performed OOOR. Because many such interventions are "noninvasive," the perception is that they are less dangerous or less risky. However, this is often not the case. OOOR procedures are frequently undertaken simply because the patient population is deemed "too sick" for the OR. Despite all efforts, conflict can be hard to avoid in medical settings where multiple specialties interact. Overlapping areas of expertise, tradition, culture, and vocabulary may contribute to this environment. However, inclusion and negotiation are critical to optimal outcome.

SAFETY GUIDELINES

Anesthesiologists enhance safety in the OR by standardizing and utilizing protocols for many procedures. Algorithms abound in the OR. Characteristic room setup, equipment maintenance, preprocedure setup and checklists, and postprocedure care priorities all contribute to a smooth process. OOOR, anesthesiologists often find themselves outside of their comfort zone in environments that lack rigor and standardization. Unfamiliar equipment may be in place OOOR, variation in physical setup is common, patient records may be unavailable, the procedure may be new, and proceduralists may not understand the nuances of anesthetic management. The OOOR location may be quite a distance from the OR itself so that support is less available when an emergency arises. For all of these reasons, consistent safety standards and guidelines must be in place.

Site evaluation, assessment of space and equipment needs, and monitoring requirements must be standardized across locations if consistent patient safety is to be realized.[8,12] Although anesthesiology has dramatically moved OR safety forward in the past 10 years, anesthesia providers must continue to drive this theme further as the perimeter of practice extends outward to include OOOR venues. Although economic and political pressures may interfere with this process, it is the anesthesiologist's responsibility to maintain the priorities of the specialty in order to practice quality medicine and achieve optimal results while pursuing medical practice at the cutting edge. Strong leadership by the anesthesia provider is a key feature of success in OOOR environments. The procedures performed are often complex, as are the patients. Procedural equipment may be new, sophisticated, and outside of the realm of anesthesiology practice.

PREPROCEDURAL EVALUATION OF PATIENTS AND POSTPROCEDURE CARE

Anesthetics performed OOOR pose many challenges. The most significant of these is that the concept of an "anesthetic" is unclear to medical proceduralists, who may be under the impression that anything that does not include an endotracheal tube and an anesthesia machine is simply "sedation." Because the procedures as well as the patients are often complex, consistent and effective preprocedure evaluation is critical to both optimization of outcome and operational efficiency OOOR. The ASA "Basic Standards for Preanesthesia Care"[13] apply to all patients who receive care from an anesthesiologist *regardless of location or approach.* It is the responsibility of the anesthesia provider to review the available medical record, interview the patient, perform a focused examination, order and review pertinent available tests and consultations, prescribe appropriate preoperative medications, and obtain anesthesia consent. It is also imperative that the anesthesiologist discuss these findings with the proceduralist involved because preprocedure assessment must be accomplished in the context of a clear understanding of the technical demands and goals of the procedure itself. Specific limitations of the procedure suite may also be important to consider.

Because any procedure performed OOOR may develop into a situation requiring urgent patient transfer to the OR, good communication and a thorough appreciation of the patient's comorbidities are imperative. Complications OOOR as well as in the OR are associated with extremes of age, increasing ASA status, and obesity.[14] Although the patient population for elective procedures may include relatively healthy individuals, it also includes patients with multisystem disease who either need urgent procedures or who are deemed high risk for surgery. For some patients, anesthesia preprocedure workups take place right before the procedure, whereas for others a separate preprocedure appointment is needed.[15] The decision to involve an anesthesiologist may be a function of the patient's physical status, the technical complexity of the procedure, or both. Appropriate triage pathways must be developed so that anesthesiologists are made aware of patients who will require their attention as early as possible. A more detailed discussion of preanesthesia patient assessment can be found in Chapter 2.

As OOOR sites evolve, additional postanesthesia care units (PACUs) for patient recovery are needed. Many significant complications occur in the postoperative period, with respiratory depression and aspiration being the most common. Therefore, it is imperative that properly trained staff be available to care for the postprocedure patient in an appropriate environment. Concise and consistent handoff from one caregiver to another is imperative. This is a focus of the goals published by The Joint Commission. Having PACUs that specialize in caring for patients undergoing a subset of OOOR procedures encourages both specialization and standardization of protocols. This can improve efficiency and care while minimizing burdens on postsurgical PACU capacity. The principles of patient recovery are the same whether care is delivered by PACU nurses, recovery area nurses in a radiology suite, or the anesthesiologist in an office-based setting. Guidelines established by the American Society of PeriAnesthesia Nurses (ASPAN) describe recommended nurse–patient ratios relative to patient characteristics. Patients requiring life-supportive care such as mechanical ventilation or vasopressor support need 1:1 nursing, whereas patients who have undergone a major procedure but are stable require a 1:2 nursing ratio.

The ASA and other professional organizations offer guidelines that standardize practices that affect quality of care and patient safety. For example, the ASA has published "Standards for Post-anesthesia Care"[16] that apply to all locations. These standards emphasize the need for the following:

1. Appropriate postanesthesia management for all patients who receive general anesthesia, regional anesthesia, or monitored anesthesia care (MAC)
2. A member of the anesthesia care team to accompany the patient to the PACU
3. A verbal report to the responsible PACU nurse by the member of the anesthesia care team
4. Continued evaluation of the patient's condition while in the PACU
5. A physician to be present and responsible for the discharge of the patient from the PACU

However, publication of guidelines alone is not a substitute for collaborative, interdisciplinary discussion among involved caregivers. Recovery room practice often dictates case turnover time, for example; therefore, it is critical that all involved understand the goals to be accomplished by each unit. The existence of infrastructure alone does not guarantee that "the parts" will all move at the right time or in the right direction.

ADMINISTRATION OF SEDATION BY NONANESTHESIA PROVIDERS

The inclusion of an anesthesiologist in an OOOR case is often at the request of the evaluating or treating physician. After the consulting anesthesiologist evaluates the patient's medical status and the nature of the planned procedure, he or she should make a recommendation regarding whether the need for anesthesiology involvement. Many OOOR cases do not require the presence of an anesthesiologist. Most institutions have developed their own anesthesia consult criteria and have policies in place that govern the administration of conscious sedation by nonanesthesiologists. Again, timely communication among the patient's care team members is essential. The ASA recently issued two statements that address the administration of moderate and deep sedation by nonanesthesiologists. The ASA "Statement on Granting Privileges for Administration of Moderate Sedation to Practitioners Who Are Not Anesthesia Professionals" states that only physicians, dentists, or podiatrists who are qualified by education, training, and licensure to administer moderate sedation should supervise the administration of moderate sedation.[17] The ASA "Statement on Granting Privileges to Nonanesthesiologist Practitioners for Personally Administering Deep Sedation or Supervising Deep Sedation by Individuals Who Are Not Anesthesia Professionals" states that due to a significant risk that patients who receive deep sedation may enter a state of general anesthesia, privileges to administer deep sedation should be granted only to practitioners who are qualified to administer general anesthesia or to appropriately supervised anesthesia professionals.[18] This last statement emphasizes the fact that sedation is essentially a "continuum," and that each patient may respond differently to the sedation being administered: That is, what is intended as "moderate" sedation can quickly evolve into "general" anesthesia. Consequently, the ASA, in its statement on "Continuum of Depth of Sedation: Definition of General Anesthesia and Levels of Sedation/Analgesia," emphasized the need for practitioners intending to produce a given level of sedation to be able to rescue patients whose level of sedation becomes deeper than initially intended.[19] The topic of sedation administration under the supervision of nonanesthesia providers is discussed in Chapter 9 (Procedural Sedation by Nonanesthesia Providers).

QUALITY ASSURANCE AND IMPROVEMENT

The transition to OOOR practice must build on the collective experience and standards of anesthesiology practice, which has provided a foundation for notable improvements in OR patient safety and quality of care over the past 20 years. The same attention to rigor and detail exercised in traditional OR practice must be ensured in remote anesthesia locations. Unfortunately, there are limited data available regarding patient safety and outcomes in the OOOR. One recent analysis[14] examined data from 63,000 patients undergoing diagnostic or therapeutic procedures under sedation or anesthesia in OOOR locations; 41% of patients were sedated by nonanesthesiologists. The data suggested that the use of capnography allowed for faster detection of apnea and respiratory compromise. The results point to a need for robust quality assurance systems that can accurately track adverse events associated with procedural sedation and anesthesia in order to improve clinical practice and patient safety.[20,21]

A recent ASA closed claims analysis of 87 cases[22] performed under anesthesia in remote locations found that, compared to OR claims, remote location claims involved older and sicker patients, and they demonstrated an increased incidence of death and significant respiratory events that were judged as potentially preventable with better monitoring. These data suggest that remote anesthetizing locations pose a significant risk to patients and that a large fraction of adverse outcomes is associated with oversedation, inadequate ventilation, and inadequate oxygenation during MAC. Another study examined patient complications in various non-OR locations.[23] The study found that the most common minor complications were postoperative nausea and vomiting, inadequate pain control, and hemodynamic instability, with increased complication rates in interventional cardiology and radiology suites. Such findings emphasize the need for institution of the same monitoring and anesthesia standards in OOOR locations as in the traditional OR settings. However, in reality the imposition of new rules and culture in medical procedure suites can be difficult.

COMMON PROBLEMS IN OOOR ANESTHETIZING LOCATIONS

Anything that can go wrong inside the OR can go wrong OOOR. Remote locations are far from OR supplies, equipment, and anesthesia colleagues. Rapid-response assistance may be anything but "rapid." What is easy to deal with in the OR may be difficult in the hinterlands of the hospital. Careful planning and readiness for possible problems are critical. The problems discussed next are unique to OOOR locations.

PATIENT TRANSPORT: SAFETY PARAMETERS

Frequently, OOOR anesthesia involves patient transport and may require moving hemodynamically unstable or intubated patients to radiology or cardiac catheterization suites usually found in remote locations within the hospital. The same is true when the patient needs to be transported to the intensive care unit (ICU) or the PACU after the procedure, and critically ill or intubated patients will require ventilatory support. These patients need to be continuously monitored, in which case a portable monitor capable of displaying ECG, pulse oximetry, blood pressure (invasive or noninvasive), and capnography is needed.

Patients who are intubated will need ventilatory support via a resuscitation bag connected to appropriate oxygen flows or a portable mobile ventilator machine. It is important to ensure adequate oxygen supply. If the patient is awake, then ascertaining that the patient is stable and cooperative before transport is preferable. However, some patients are best transported intubated and sedated to and from an ICU or the PACU. It is important to have an adequate supply of drugs such as propofol, thiopental, or fentanyl in case the patient needs to be anesthetized or further sedated during transport. The anesthesia provider should also have access to a neuromuscular blocker (succinylcholine), vasopressors (ephedrine, phenylephrine), and antihypertensives (labetalol, hydralazine). One also should consider bringing an appropriate size endotracheal tube, a functioning laryngoscope, a resuscitation bag (even if the patient is not intubated), oral and nasal airways, and a laryngeal mask airway (LMA). A member of the patient's care team must accompany the anesthesiologist during transport and handoff.

CARDIAC ARREST/AIRWAY EMERGENCY

Cardiac arrest or an airway emergency can occur at any stage; this includes the preoperative holding area, the procedural area, the recovery room, or en route to or from the procedure area. All patient care personnel must be familiar with the location of essential emergency equipment, such as the defibrillator and the emergency airway cart. They must also be able to call for help and properly describe the location of the patient in distress. It is important that all patient care staff familiarize themselves with the basic life support (BLS) or advanced cardiac life support (ACLS) protocols (see Appendix 4), according to their specialty and hospital policy requirements. Periodic team training of the OOOR personal and "mock codes" may be of significant benefit.

OTHER POTENTIAL ADVERSE EVENTS

Additional problems sometimes encountered in the OOOR settings include adverse reactions to drugs and materials. These include anaphylactic reactions to antibiotics, latex, or iodinated contrast dye, which require immediate treatment for their potentially life-threatening effects, such as bronchospasm, airway edema, or hypotension.[24] Malignant hyperthermia (MH) is a rare but serious condition that can be caused by potent inhalation anesthetics or depolarizing neuromuscular blockers such as succinylcholine. Prompt recognition and initiation of resuscitative measures can significantly improve patient outcome.[25] Familiarity with the MH treatment protocol and the necessary equipment by the OOOR staff is necessary. The MH protocol is outlined in Appendix 2. Familiarity with the treatment of local anesthetic toxicity is important as well. Significant cardiovascular side effects are more likely to occur with the repeated infiltration of large volumes of local anesthetic.

FINANCIAL CONSIDERATIONS

Important financial considerations continue to drive the practice of anesthesiology as it expands its perimeter. The need to at least maintain budget neutrality in the face of increasing demand, the cost of technological innovation, the cost of poorly integrated care, and the financial implications of potential modifications to resource management in the OR (i.e., changes in staffing models, use of certified registered nurse anesthetists [CRNAs], creation of "shifts") are all relevant to the future of anesthesiology as a specialty. Financial silos tend to drive the benefits of efficient staffing toward proceduralists and away from anesthesiologists; bundling of fees and poor reimbursement reinforce this trend. Budget inspection often fails to reveal costly practices because the analyses are fragmented across departments. In the current environment, anesthesia service provided OOOR for routine cases is not well reimbursed. Newer, high-tech procedures tend to be well reimbursed, at least initially. Opportunity costs for anesthesia departments are enormous because coverage OOOR often requires a ratio of 1:1 staffing. Scheduling is often poorly organized. As a result, anesthesiologists cover non-OR cases in an ad hoc manner, which is expensive. The demand for comprehensive and reliable anesthesiology services OOOR is growing, but the benefits commonly accrue to other departments and to hospitals as a whole. Just as surgical procedures in the OR often require an integrative and interdisciplinary approach to patient care and strategic management of reimbursements, so do many of the emerging minimally invasive procedures performed OOOR. Creative financing and alternative staffing models may need to be considered, as well as further development of process and outcomes measures and appropriate efficiency metrics.[26,27]

The future promises to be even more complex: Medicare (Acute Care Episode demonstration project[28]) is considering bundled payments that lump together institutional and provider payments for certain procedures. In this model, the providers themselves, rather than Medicare fee schedules, will make decisions about the value of each provider's contribution to the care of the patient. Bundled payments and shift of financial risk from insurers to providers will provoke discussions among providers about the value of anesthesia services. Most recently, with the passing of the Medicare Access and CHIP Reauthorization Act (MACRA), the Centers for Medicare and Medicaid Services (CMS) will base payments on quality and value metrics. The CMS has proposed payments to physicians through the Quality Payment Program (QPP), and they will have an option of reimbursement through either a Merit-Based Incentive Payment System (MIPS) or advanced Alternative Payment Models (APMs).[29]

In the present financial model, enlisting the services of an anesthesiologist increases efficiency, reduces risk, lowers the patient care burden, and costs the facility nothing (unless the insurance company refuses to pay for anesthesia services; this occurred when Aetna tried to impose limitations on payment for anesthesia services during endoscopy).[30] Financial integration of providers in a bundled payment model turns this arrangement on its head because the cost of anesthesia services comes from a fixed budget—as do all services. The debate about who pays for health care might best be focused on what (and how) health care is paid for, and this may determine our practice parameters more profoundly than anything else.[31]

CONSIDERATIONS FOR THE FUTURE

As anesthesiologists adjust to the expanding perimeter of anesthesiology practice, new problems and opportunities emerge. Drivers include new environments, complex technologies, new procedures and high acuity patients. We must summon all of our abilities as perioperative physicians to deal with these new issues and the exponential growth of OOOR procedures.[32] As anesthesiologists, we will clearly need to improve our communication skills, assume leadership positions, and encourage teamwork among our colleagues. In the process, we will have to leave behind some cultural boundaries and prejudices. While economic and political pressure may temporarily reshape our environment, we must be vigilant in ensuring that our practice standards are not degraded or driven by financial constraints or the politics of resource allocation.

REFERENCES

1. American Society of Anesthesiologists. Statement on non-operating room anesthetizing locations, last amended 2013. Available at: https://www.asahq.org/quality-and-practice-management/standards-guidelines-and-related-resources-search. Accessed on March 1, 2018.
2. Cote C, Wilson S, Work Group on Sedation, et al. Guidelines for monitoring and management of pediatric patients during and after sedation for diagnostic and therapeutic procedures. *Pediatrics*. 2006;118:2587–2602.
3. Galvano S, Kodali B. Critical monitoring issues outside the operating room. *Anesthesiol Clin*. 2009;27:141–156.
4. American Society of Anesthesiologists. Standards for basic anesthetic monitoring, last amended 2015. Available at: https://www.asahq.org/quality-and-practice-management/standards-guidelines-and-related-resources-search. Accessed on March 1, 2018.
5. Bhananker SM, Posner KL, Cheney FW, Caplan RA, Lee LA, Domino KB. Injury and liability associated with monitored anesthesia care: a closed claims analysis. *Anesthesiology*. 2006;104:228–234.
6. Caplan R, Posner KL, Ward RJ, Cheney FW. Adverse respiratory events in anesthesia: a closed claims analysis. *Anesthesiology*. 1990;72:828–833.
7. American Society of Anesthesiologists. Statement on the anesthesia care team, last amended 2013. Available at: https://www.asahq.org/quality-and-practice-management/standards-guidelines-and-related-resources-search. Accessed on March 1, 2018.
8. Frankel A. Patient safety: anesthesia in remote locations. *Anesthesiol Clin*. 2009;27:127–139.
9. Lingard L, Reznick R, Espin S, Regehr G, DeVito L. Team communications in the OR: talk patterns, sites of tension and implications for novices. *Acad Med*. 2002;77(3):232–237.
10. Lingard L, Regehr G, Orser B, et al. Evaluation of a preoperative checklist and team briefing among surgeons, nurse and anesthesiologists to reduce failures in communication. *Arch Surg*. 2008;143(1):12–17.
11. Booij LH. Conflicts in the operating theatre. *JAMA*. 2007;20(2):152–156.
12. Eichorn JH, Cooper JB, Cullen DJ, et al. Anesthesia practice standards at Harvard: a review. *J Clin Anesth*. 1988;1:55–65.
13. American Society of Anesthesiologists. Basic standards for preanesthesia care, last amended 2015. Available at: https://www.asahq.org/quality-and-practice-management/standards-guidelines-and-related-resources-search. Accessed on March 1, 2018.
14. Pino RM. The nature of anesthesia and procedural sedation outside of the operating room. *Curr Opin Anaesthesiol*. 2007;20:347–351.
15. Chang B, Urman RD. Non-operating room anesthesia: the principles of patient assessment and preparation. *Anesthesiol Clin*. 2016;34(1):223–240. doi:10.1016/j.anclin.2015.10.017.
16. American Society of Anesthesiologists. Practice guidelines for postanesthetic care: An updated report by the American Society of Anesthesiologists Task Force on postanesthetic care. *Anesthesiology*. 2013;118(2):291–307.
17. American Society of Anesthesiologists. Statement of Granting Privileges for Administration of Moderate Sedation to Practitioners. 2016. Available at: https://www.asahq.org/quality-and-practice-management/standards-guidelines-and-related-resources-search. Accessed on March 1, 2018.
18. American Society of Anesthesiologists. Statement on Granting Privileges to Non-Anesthesiologist Physicians* for Personally Administering or Supervising Deep Sedation. 2017. Available at: https://www.asahq.org/quality-and-practice-management/standards-guidelines-and-related-resources-search. Accessed on March 1, 2018.
19. American Society of Anesthesiologists. Continuum of depth of sedation: definition of general anesthesia and levels of sedation/analgesia, last amended 2014. Available at: https://www.asahq.org/quality-and-practice-management/standards-guidelines-and-related-resources-search. Accessed on March 1, 2018.
20. Kodali BS, Urman RD. Capnography during cardiopulmonary resuscitation: current evidence and future directions. *J Emerg Trauma Shock*. 2014;7(4):332–40. doi:10.4103/0974-2700.142778.
21. Karamnov S, Sarkisian N, Grammer R, Gross WL, Urman RD. Analysis of adverse events associated with adult moderate procedural sedation outside the operating room. *J Patient Saf*. 2017;13(3):111–121.
22. Metzner J., Posner KL, Domino KB. The risk and safety of anesthesia at remote locations: the US closed claims analysis. *Curr Opin Anaesthesiol*. 2009;22:502–508.
23. Chang B, Kaye AD, Diaz JH, Westlake B, Dutton RP, Urman RD. Interventional procedures outside of the operating room: results. *J Patient Saf*. 2018;14(1):9–16.
24. Russell GB. *Alternate-Site Anesthesia: Clinical Practice Outside of the Operating Room*. Oxford, England: Butterworth-Heinemann; 1997.
25. Joshi GP, Desai MS, Gayer S, Vila H Jr; Society for Ambulatory Anesthesia (SAMBA). Succinylcholine for emergency airway rescue in class b ambulatory facilities: the Society for Ambulatory Anesthesia position statement. *Anesth Analg*. 2017;124(5):1447–1449. doi:10.1213/ANE.0000000000001682.
26. Peccora CD, Gimlich R, Cornell RP, Vacanti CA, Ehrenfeld JM, Urman RD. Anesthesia report card—a customizable tool for performance improvement. *J Med Syst*. 2014;38(9):105. doi:10.1007/s10916-014-0105-2. Epub 2014 Jul 20.
27. Gabriel RA, Gimlich R, Ehrenfeld JM, Urman RD. Operating room metrics score card-creating a prototype for individualized feedback. *J Med Syst*. 2014;38(11):144. doi:10.1007/s10916-014-0144-8. Epub 2014 Oct 15.
28. Medicare Acute Care Episode demonstration. Available at: https://innovation.cms.gov/initiatives/ACE. Accessed March 10, 2018.
29. Rosenkrantz AB, Hirsch JA, Allen B Jr, Wang W, Hughes DR, Nicola GN. The proposed MACRA/MIPS threshold for patient-facing encounters: what it means for radiologists. *J Am Coll Radiol*. 2017;14(3):308–315. doi:10.1016/j.jacr.2016.10.014. Epub 2016 Dec 22.
30. Feder BJ. Aetna to end payment for a drug in colonoscopies. *NY Times*. December 28, 2007. Available at: http://www.nytimes.com/2007/12/28/business/28colon.html. Accessed March 10, 2010.
31. Hannenberg AA. Introduction to section 1: financial considerations. *Anesthesiology Clin*. 2009;27:5–6.
32. Nagrebetsky A, Gabriel RA, Dutton RP, Urman RD. Growth of nonoperating room anesthesia care in the United States: a contemporary trends analysis. *Anesth Analg*. 2017;124(4):1261–1267.

2 | PREOPERATIVE PATIENT EVALUATION FOR ANESTHESIA CARE OUTSIDE OF THE OPERATING ROOM

YASMEEN BEG, MD, BOBBIEJEAN SWEITZER, MD

Preoperative evaluation and medical optimization of patients are important components of anesthesia practice. Increasing numbers of patients with serious comorbidities undergo procedures that require anesthesia services outside of the operating room (OOOR). [1,2] Often, the location alters the challenges of caring for these patients. Surgical, anesthesia, or nursing personnel who can assist with airway and resuscitation management may not be available; equipment and medications may be limited. Many OOOR locations will not have the support of an intensive care unit (ICU), skilled postanesthesia recovery personnel, respiratory therapy, or ready access to an inpatient bed, blood banking, interventional cardiology, or diagnostic services. Many of the patients are elderly, ill, and even unlikely candidates for conventional surgery (e.g., transmucosal resection of gastric tumors, transjugular intrahepatic portosystemic shunts). Yet, patients or providers may be reluctant to expend time and energy in extensive preoperative evaluation before a seemingly minor procedure. This chapter outlines the basics of preprocedure preparation of patients scheduled to receive anesthesia in OOOR settings.

The preanesthesia evaluation is a basic, essential component of anesthesia care. The American Society of Anesthesiologists (ASA) indicates that, at minimum, a preanesthesia visit includes the following[3]:

- An evaluation of pertinent medical records
- An interview with the patient or guardian to review medical, anesthesia, and medication history
- A pertinent physical examination, which at minimum includes an airway, cardiovascular, and pulmonary examination
- Review of diagnostic data (laboratory, electrocardiogram [ECG], radiographs, consultations)
- Assignment of ASA physical status (ASA-PS) score
- A formulation and discussion of anesthesia plans with the patient or a responsible adult

Many anesthesiologists rely on screening batteries of tests to evaluate patients. This practice may be based on institutional policies or on the mistaken belief that tests can substitute for taking a history or performing a physical examination. Preoperative tests without specific indications lack utility and may lead to patient injury because they prompt further testing to evaluate abnormal results, or they may lead to unnecessary interventions, delay of surgery, anxiety, and even inappropriate therapies. Studies have shown that elimination of routine testing during preoperative clinical evaluation does not increase perioperative risk.[4,5] Selective preoperative testing should only be done if indicated based on a patient's medical history or physical examination.[3] Complete and thorough histories not only assist in planning appropriate and safe anesthesia care but are more accurate and cost effective than screening laboratory tests for establishing diagnoses.[6] The task of gathering the necessary information and sharing it among the various providers can be challenging.

The important components of the anesthesia history are shown in Figure 2.1. The form can be completed by the patient in person (paper or electronic version), via Internet-based programs, by a telephone interview, or by medical staff. In Figure 2.1, the bold may predict patients who are at a higher risk of complications. Evaluating these patients or having a mechanism to gather notes and tests ahead of time may facilitate care. The patient's medical problems, medications, allergies, past operations, and use of tobacco, alcohol, or illicit drugs are documented. Cardiovascular, pulmonary, or neurologic symptoms are noted. Equally important as identifying the presence of disease is establishing its severity, stability, current or recent exacerbations, treatment of the condition, or planned interventions. A determination of the patient's cardiorespiratory fitness or functional capacity is useful in guiding evaluation and predicting outcome and perioperative complications.[7,8] Better fitness improves cardiorespiratory reserve, and decreases morbidity through improved lipid and glucose profiles and reductions in blood pressure and obesity. Conversely, an inability to exercise may be a result of cardiopulmonary disease. An inability to perform average levels of exercise (4–5 metabolic equivalents [METs] or the ability to walk four blocks or go up two flights of stairs) identifies patients at risk of perioperative complications.[8] A personal or family history of adverse events related to anesthesia is always important, but severe postoperative nausea or vomiting, prolonged emergence or delirium, or susceptibility to malignant hyperthermia or pseudocholinesterase deficiency have added significance given the often-limited resources, as previously described.

PATIENT PREOPERATIVE HISTORY

Name ______________________________ **DOB** ________________ **Phone #**__________________

Planned surgery ____ **Today's Date** _____________

Surgeon _______________**Primary Care Physician** _______________**PCP Phone #**_____________

Please list all previous surgeries (and approximate dates)

Please list any allergies to medications, latex, food or other (and your reactions to them)

Please list all medications you have taken in the last month (include over-the-counter drugs, inhalers, herbals, dietary supplements and aspirin)

Drug Name	Dose and How Often?	Drug Name	Dose and How Often?
1.		7.	
2.		8.	
3.		9.	
4.		10.	
5.		11.	
6.		12.	

Weight: (lbs or kg) __________ Height: (inches or cm) __________ (Circle the measurement units you use)

Please check any of the following that apply to your health:

☐ Heart attack at any time	☐ Irregular or rapid heartbeat	☐ LVAD
☐ Heart failure	☐ Atrial fibrillation	☐ Heart device
☐ Chest pain or pressure with activity	☐ Arrhythmia	☐ Pacemaker
☐ Heart attack within past 60 days	☐ Valve disorder	☐ Defibrillator
☐ Angina	☐ Murmur	☐ Fainted in the last year
☐ Heart surgery	☐ Abnormal EKG	☐ Congenital heart disease
☐ Heart stent in the last 6 months	☐ Heart Stent at any time	☐ Any heart condition
☐ Have to stop while climbing 2 flights of stairs or walking 2 city blocks because of chest pain or trouble breathing		

☐ Oxygen at home	☐ Asthma	☐ Abnormal chest x-ray
☐ Pulmonary hypertension	☐ COPD	☐ Any problems with your lungs
☐ Bronchitis	☐ Severe cough	☐ Trouble breathing
☐ Emphysema	☐ Pneumonia in last 2 months	☐ Hospitalized within last 30 days

☐ Face, arm or leg weakness	☐ Dementia	☐ Spinal cord injury
☐ Stroke/TIA within past 60 days	☐ Parkinson's	☐ Brain tumor
☐ Difficulty Speaking	☐ Myasthenia gravis	☐ Brain aneurysm or AVM
☐ Paralysis	☐ Muscular dystrophy	☐ Epilepsy, blackouts or seizures

☐ Anemia	☐ Liver disease	☐ Lupus
☐ Sickle cell disease	☐ Cirrhosis	☐ Rheumatoid arthritis
☐ Blood transfusion in last 3 months	☐ Hepatitis B/C	☐ Scleroderma
☐ Blood clots	☐ Jaundice	☐ Sjogren's
☐ Pulmonary embolus	☐ Hyperthyroidism	☐ Jehovah's Witness
☐ Diabetes	☐ Hypothyroidism	☐ Use illegal drugs (excluding marijuana)
☐ Take insulin	☐ Adrenal disorder	☐ Kidney failure
☐ HIV	☐ Pituitary disorder	☐ Dialysis
☐ Blood thinners or anticoagulants other than aspirin		☐ Kidney disease other than stones

Figure 2.1. Example of a patient health history form. AVM, arteriovenous malformation; COPD, chronic obstructive pulmonary disease; CPAP, continuous positive airway pressure; DOB, date of birth; LVAD, left ventricular assist device; PCP, primary care provider; TIA, transient ischemic attack.

☐ **Severe nose bleeds** ☐ **Hemophilia** ☐ **Known bleeding disorder**
☐ **Bleeding with surgery or tooth extractions** ☐ **Von Willebrands**
☐ **Malignant hyperthermia (in blood relatives or self) with anesthesia**

☐ **Cancer: What type?** ☐ **Need assistance with eating**
☐ **Chemotherapy or radiation last 3 months** ☐ **Need assistance with bathing**
☐ ***Unintentional weight loss >10 lbs** ☐ **Need assistance with getting dressed**
☐ **Severe nausea or vomiting from anesthesia** ☐ **Difficult airway with anesthesia**

☐ **Tired/fall asleep frequently during the day** ☐ **Very loud snoring**
☐ **Observed to stop breathing during sleep** ☐ **Sleep apnea**
☐ **High blood pressure/Hypertension** ☐ **Use CPAP**

☐ **Cramping pain in legs while walking** ☐ **Cannot lie flat for 45 min** ☐ **Deaf**
☐ **Problems opening your mouth** ☐ **Speak and understand English** ☐ **Blind**
☐ **Your physical abilities limit your daily activities** ☐ **Fallen in the last 6 months:____times** ☐ **Dentures**
☐ **Currently pregnant. Last menstrual period began:______** ☐ **Loose teeth**
☐ **Smoker (current or past) Indicate: _____ packs/day for _____years. Quit date_______**
☐ **Drink alcohol. How much each day? _____ beers _____ glasses of wine ______shots of hard alcohol**
☐ **Cold, fever or flu within last month** ☐ **Taking antibiotics for any reason**
☐ ***Feel that everything you did was an effort: _____days in the last week**
***What is the most strenuous physical activity (work or pleasure) that you have done in the past month?**

Please list any medical illness or medications not noted already:

Figure 2.1. (Cond)

At a minimum, the preanesthetic examination includes the airway, heart and lungs, vital signs, oxygen saturation, height, and weight. Examination of the airway, always a necessary assessment before anesthesia, has special significance. When challenging airways are identified, advanced planning is needed for equipment and skilled personnel. Auscultation of the heart and inspection of the pulses, peripheral veins, and extremities for the presence of edema are important diagnostically and in development of care plans. The pulmonary examination includes auscultation for wheezing and decreased or abnormal breath sounds. Cyanosis or clubbing and the effort of breathing are noted. For patients with deficits or disease or those undergoing neurologic procedures or regional anesthesia, a neurologic examination is performed to document abnormalities that may aid in diagnosis or interfere with positioning and to establish a baseline. The following section discusses the most important conditions that are likely to affect the administration of anesthesia in OOOR locations.

Coronary artery disease (CAD) varies from mild, stable disease with little impact on perioperative outcome to severe disease accounting for significant complications during anesthesia and surgery. The basis of cardiac assessment includes the history and the physical examination. Review of medical records and previous diagnostic studies, especially stress tests and catheterization results, is necessary. Often, a phone call to the primary care physician or cardiologist will yield important information and obviate the need for further testing or consultation.

Major adverse cardiac events (MACE) after noncardiac surgery are often associated with prior CAD events. Perioperative morbidity and mortality is impacted by the timing of surgery as well as the stability of patients' CAD. Data suggest that at least 60 days should elapse after a myocardial infarction (MI) before noncardiac surgery/procedures.[8,9]

The most recent American College of Cardiology/American Heart Association (ACC/AHA) guidelines for cardiovascular evaluation for noncardiac surgery have decreased recommendations for testing or revascularization.[8] The guidelines have an algorithm to be followed in stepwise fashion, stopping at the first point that applies to the patient (Figure 2.2). Step 1 considers the urgency of the procedure. If emergency procedures are needed, the focus is perioperative surveillance (e.g., serial ECGs, enzymes, monitoring) and risk reduction with guideline-directed medical therapy (GDMT). Step 2 considers active cardiac conditions such as MI within 60 days, unstable or severe angina, decompensated heart failure (HF), severe valvular disease (severe aortic stenosis [AS] or symptomatic mitral stenosis), or significant arrhythmias (new-onset ventricular tachycardia, symptomatic bradycardia, supraventricular arrhythmia such as atrial fibrillation (AF) with rapid ventricular rates, and high-grade conduction abnormalities such as third degree or Mobitz, type 2 atrioventricular block). Active cardiac conditions warrant postponement for all except life-saving emergency procedures. Step 3 considers the perioperative risk of MACE. Patients without active cardiac conditions (see step 2) with a risk of MACE less than 1% can proceed to surgery without further testing. Risk can be determined by using tools such as the American College of Surgeons National Surgical Quality Improvement Program (NSQIP) risk calculator (http://www.riskcalculator.facs.org/RiskCalculator/) or the American College of Surgeons NSQIP MICA Surgical Risk Calculator (http://www.surgicalriskcalculator.com/miorcardiacarrest) or the Revised Cardiac Risk Index (RCRI) in Table 2.1.[10] Those with two or more RCRI or 1% or higher risk of MACE using a calculator proceed to step 5 to assess functional capacity as defined by METs.[7] Patients with average functional capacity (4–5 METs) without symptoms can proceed to surgery.

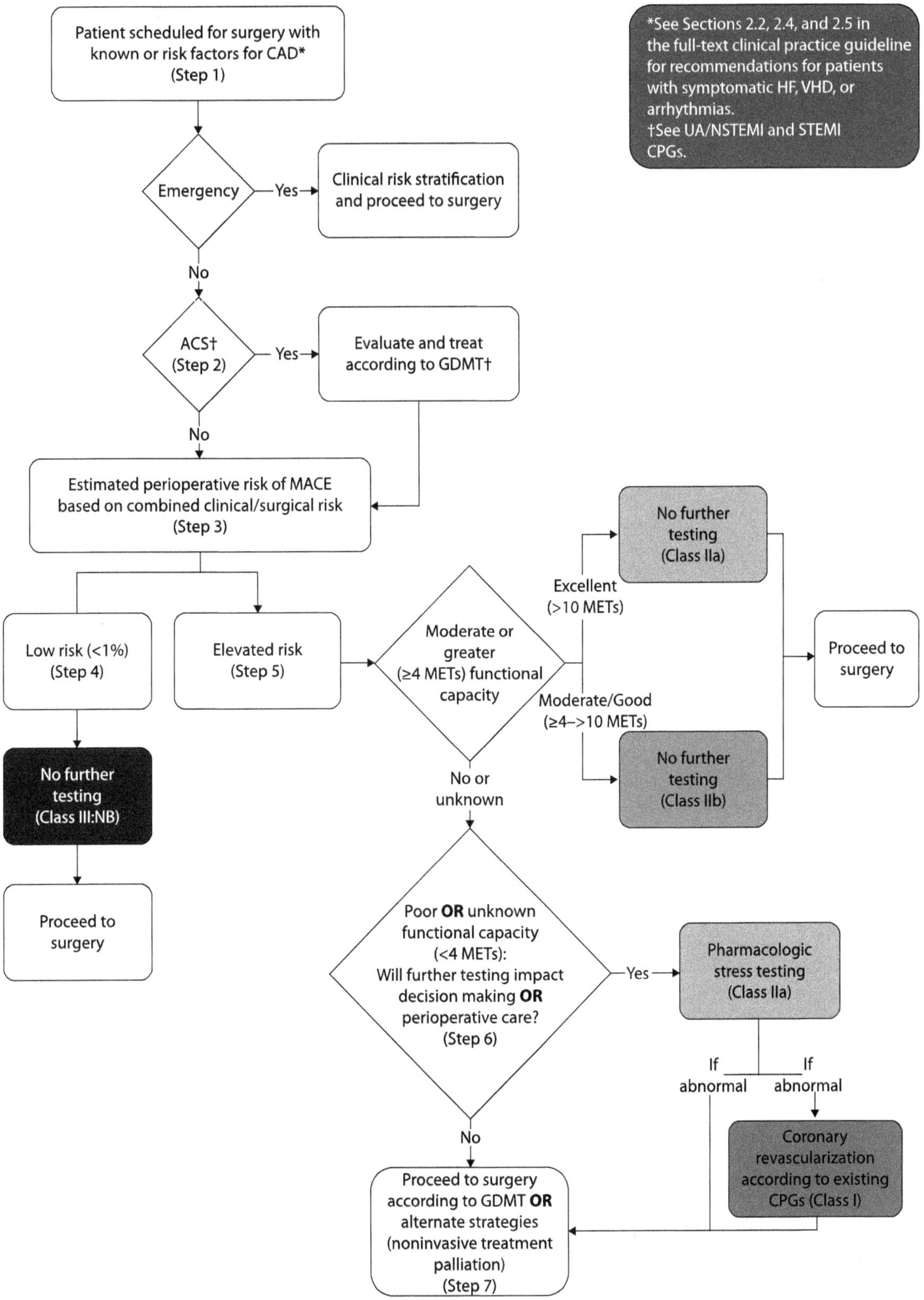

Figure 2.2. *Stepwise approach to perioperative cardiac assessment for noncardiac surgery.*

American College of Cardiology/American Heart Association stepwise approach to perioperative cardiac assessment algorithm. ACS, acute coronary syndromes; CAD, coronary artery disease; GDMT, guideline-directed medical therapy; HF, heart failure; MACE, major adverse cardiac events; MET, metabolic equivalent task; STEMI, ST-segment elevation myocardial infarction; UA/NSTEMI, unstable angina/non-ST elevation myocardial infarction. (Reprinted with permission 2014 American Heart Association. Guideline on perioperative cardiovascular evaluation and management of patients undergoing noncardiac surgery. J Am Coll Cardiol. 2014;64:e(77)–(e)137. © 2014 American Heart Association, Inc.)

TABLE 2.1. Revised Cardiac Risk Index

RISK FACTORS[a]
1. Ischemic heart disease
2. Congestive heart failure
3. Cerebrovascular disease
4. Diabetes mellitus requiring insulin
5. Chronic kidney disease with creatinine > 2.0 mg/dL
6. Intraperitoneal, intrathoracic, or suprainguinal vascular surgery
Risk of Major Cardiac Event (cardiac death, acute myocardial infarction, ventricular fibrillation/cardiac arrest, complete heart block, pulmonary edema)

POINTS	CLASS	RISK
0	I	0.4%
1	II	0.9%
2	III	6.6%
3 or more	IV	11%

[a] Each risk factor is assigned 1 point.

SOURCE: Adapted from Lee TH, Marcantonio ER, Mangione CM, et al. Derivation and prospective validation of a simple index for prediction of cardiac risk of major noncardiac surgery. Circulation. 1999;100:1043–1049.

Step 6 considers patients with poor or indeterminate functional capacity, who may benefit from further testing but only if the results will alter management. The traditional risk factors for CAD such as smoking, hypertension, older age, male gender, hypercholesterolemia, and family history have not been shown to predict perioperative risk.

The benefits versus the risks of coronary revascularization before noncardiac surgery are controversial. The largest randomized prospective study of preoperative revascularization (coronary artery bypass graft [CABG] or percutaneous coronary intervention [PCI]) versus medical management failed to show a difference in outcome, with the exception of those with left main disease, a left ventricular ejection fraction (LVEF) less than 20%, or severe AS.[11] Noncardiac surgery soon after revascularization is associated with high rates of morbidity and mortality.[12–14] Patients who have had a PCI, especially with a drug-eluting stent (DES), require months, if not a lifetime, of antiplatelet therapy to prevent restenosis or acute thromboses.[13–15] Identifying whether there is a DES or bare metal stent (BMS) is important. Antiplatelet agents are not withdrawn without consultation with a cardiologist familiar with coronary stents and an in-depth discussion with the patient regarding the risks of stopping these drugs.[15] Elective procedures that necessitate interrupting dual-antiplatelet therapy (DAPT) should be delayed during the high-risk period. The most recent ACC/AHA guideline on duration of DAPT recommends that elective noncardiac surgery/procedures be delayed 30 days after BMS implantation and optimally 6 months after DES implantation.[16] Figure 2.3 illustrates the suggested treatment algorithm for the timing of noncardiac surgery/procedures in patients with coronary stents. For patients for whom the $P2Y_{12}$ inhibitor (typically clopidogrel) will need to be discontinued perioperatively, elective noncardiac procedures can be considered after 3 months post-DES implantation if the risk of further delay of procedures is greater than the expected risks of stent thrombosis.[16] For patients treated with DAPT who must have their $P2Y_{12}$ inhibitor therapy withheld for a procedure, it is recommended that aspirin be continued. The $P2Y_{12}$ inhibitor is restarted as soon after surgery as possible. Evidence supports the low risk of bleeding complications with continued aspirin during most procedures.[17,18]

Premature discontinuation of DAPT can cause catastrophic stent thrombosis, MI, or death. Noncardiac surgery and most invasive procedures increase the risk of stent thrombosis, which is associated with high mortality.[12–14] Stent thrombosis is best treated with PCI, which can be performed safely even in the immediate postoperative period.[19] High-risk patients may best be managed in facilities with immediate access to interventional cardiology.[11]

Heart failure is a significant risk factor for perioperative adverse events. There is an increasing prevalence of HF due to the increasing age of the general population as well as the improved treatments and increased survival in patients with HF and ischemic heart disease. Patients with compensated HF have a 5%–7% risk of cardiac complications; however, those with decompensated failure have a 20%–30% incidence. There is also an increased incidence of perioperative death in those with HF versus those with CAD without HF.[20] HF may be due to systolic dysfunction (decreased ejection fraction [EF] from abnormal contractility), diastolic dysfunction (elevated filling pressures with abnormal relaxation but normal contractility and EF), or a combination. Diastolic HF accounts for almost half of all cases, but there is little science to guide perioperative care. Hypertension can cause diastolic dysfunction, and left ventricular hypertrophy on an ECG raises suspicion of hypertension and diastolic dysfunction. Ischemic heart disease is a common cause of systolic dysfunction (50%–75% of cases). Recent weight gain, complaints of shortness of breath, fatigue, orthopnea, paroxysmal nocturnal dyspnea, nocturnal cough, peripheral edema, hospitalizations, and recent changes in management are significant. Elective surgery needs to be deferred for patients with decompensated HF.[8] Patients with a preserved EF (>40%) have lower perioperative mortality when compared to those with reduced EF; however, their mortality rate is increased when compared to patients without HF.[21] Measurement of LVEF and diastolic function with echocardiography may be helpful. Patients with class IV failure (symptoms at rest) are best evaluated by a cardiologist before undergoing anesthesia.

Cardiac murmurs can be clinically unimportant or caused by significant valvular abnormalities. Functional murmurs from turbulent flow across the aortic or pulmonic outflow tracts are found with high-outflow states (hyperthyroidism, pregnancy, anemia). Elderly patients, those with risk factors for CAD, a history of rheumatic fever, volume overload, pulmonary disease, cardiomegaly, or an abnormal ECG are likely to have valvular pathology. Echocardiography is recommended in patients where moderate or greater degrees of valvular

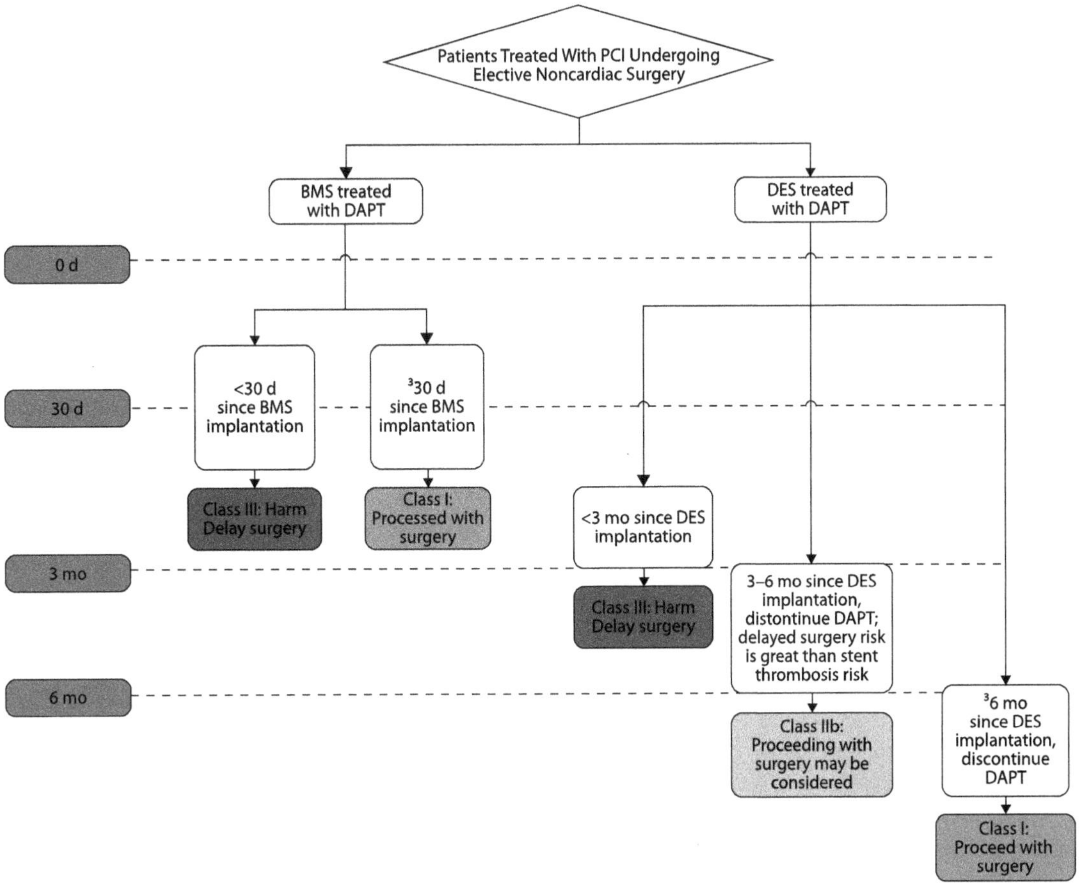

Figure 2.3. *Algorithm for antiplatelet management in patients with PCI and noncardiac surgery.*

American College of Cardiology/American Heart Association treatment algorithm for the timing of elective noncardiac surgery in patients with coronary stents. BMS, bare metal stent; DAPT, dual-antiplatelet therapy; DES, drug-eluting stent; PCI, percutaneous coronary intervention. (Reprinted with permission 2016 American Heart Association. A guideline focused update on the duration of dual antiplatelet therapy in patients with coronary artery disease. J Am Coll Cardiol. 2016;68:1082–1115. © 2016 American Heart Association, Inc.)

pathology is suspected if there has been no echocardiography done within a year or where a significant change in clinical status or physical examination is noted.[8] This information is especially beneficial if general or spinal anesthesia is planned. Diastolic murmurs are always pathologic and require evaluation. Regurgitant disease is tolerated perioperatively better than stenotic disease. AS is the most common valvular lesion in the United States (2%–4% of adults > 65 years); severe AS is associated with a high risk of perioperative complications. Aortic sclerosis, present in 25% of people 65–74 years of age and 50% of those more than 84 years old, causes a systolic ejection murmur similar to that of AS, but it has no hemodynamic compromise.[22] Elevated-risk elective procedures are reasonable to perform in patients with asymptomatic severe AS with appropriate hemodynamic monitoring.[8] Patients with symptomatic severe or critical AS should not have anesthesia (unless an emergency and life-saving) without a cardiology evaluation. Antibiotic prophylaxis to prevent infective endocarditis (IE) is no longer recommended for patients with valvular abnormalities except for patients with heart transplants who develop cardiac valvulopathy, those with a prosthetic cardiac valve or prosthetic material used in valve repair, unrepaired cyanotic congenital heart defect (CHD), repaired CHD with prosthetic material, repaired CHD with residual defects, or prior history of IE. Prophylaxis in these cases is limited to certain dental procedures as well as procedures in the presence of infections of the respiratory tract, infected skin, or infected musculoskeletal tissue.[23] Prophylaxis is not recommended for routine gastrointestinal endoscopy.[18]

Pacemakers and implantable cardioverter-defibrillators (ICDs) can be affected by electrical/magnetic interference. Consultation with the device manufacturer or cardiologist may be needed. Patients usually have a wallet card with important device information and phone numbers. Patients with ICDs invariably have HF, ischemic or valvular disease, cardiomyopathies, or potentially lethal arrhythmias. Some monitors, ventilators, vibrations, or chest prepping may fool the sensors into increasing pacing, leading to ischemia or inappropriate treatment. Electromagnetic interference from electrocautery can occur; therefore, bipolar cautery is preferred over monopolar cautery. Special features, such as rate-adaptive mechanisms in some pacemakers are disabled or the device is reprogrammed to asynchronous pacing to prevent interference. The pacemaker should have been interrogated or checked within the past 6 months (this can be increased to 12 months if the patient has had a stable history).[24] Anti-tachyarrhythmia functions are disabled before procedures if interference or unexpected patient movement is undesirable. During delicate intracranial, spinal, or ocular procedures, an unexpected discharge with patient movement can be catastrophic. Central line placement can trigger cardioversion. ICDs are deactivated only after arrival to a facility with monitoring and external defibrillation devices. Magnets affect the anti-arrhythmia function, not the pacing function, of an ICD. If a pacemaker or ICD is reprogrammed, the device needs to be re-enabled before the patient leaves a monitored setting.

Hypertension severity and duration correlate with the degree of end-organ damage, morbidity, and mortality. Ischemic heart disease, HF, renal insufficiency, and cerebrovascular disease are common in hypertensive patients. However, there is little evidence of an association between preoperative blood pressure (BP) less than 180/110 mm Hg and perioperative cardiac risk. It is generally recommended that elective procedures be delayed for patients with severe hypertension (diastolic blood pressure (BP) > 115 mm Hg; systolic BP > 200 mm Hg) until BP is less than 180/110 mm Hg. If severe end-organ damage is present, the goal is to normalize BP as much as possible before surgery.[25] Effective lowering of risk may require weeks of therapy for regression of vascular changes, and too rapid or extreme lowering of BP may increase cerebral and coronary ischemia. Studies suggest that intraoperative hypotension is far more dangerous than hypertension.[25] For BP less than 180/110 mm Hg, there is no evidence to justify cancellation of anesthesia, although if time allows, preoperative interventions are appropriate.

Atrial fibrillation is the most common arrhythmia in the population. It is increasing and is present in 1% of individuals more than 60 years old and in 10% of individuals more than 75 years old.[26] Many patients have asymptomatic AF, and often a complication associated with AF, such as stroke, is the first presentation of the disease. Over half of new-onset AF can be attributed to common cardiovascular risk factors such as hypertension, obesity, diabetes mellitus, and smoking.[27]

Mainstays of AF treatment involve the assessment of thromboembolic risk, appropriate thromboprophylaxis, rate and rhythm control, treatment of underlying disease, and associated therapy (e.g., angiotensin-converting enzyme inhibitors, angiotensin-receptor blockers).[28] AF is an independent risk factor for stroke and thromboembolism, which leads to increased morbidity and mortality and prolonged hospitalizations. Patients with AF can be risk stratified into low, moderate, and high risk for stroke with an annual estimate of stroke using the $CHADS_2$ or the CHA_2DS_2-VASc score (Table 2.2).[28] These scores are used for appropriate anticoagulation with AF: oral anticoagulation for high- and moderate-risk patients, aspirin for low-risk patients. Historically, high-risk patients have been treated with warfarin, which requires regular international normalized ratio (INR) monitoring. Many new oral anticoagulants are increasingly being used for thromboprophylaxis in patients with AF. These include direct thrombin inhibitors such as dabigatran etexilate and factor Xa inhibitors such as apixaban and rivaroxaban. These drugs have been shown to be as efficacious as warfarin with significantly less major bleeding and intracranial hemorrhage.[29–31]

TABLE 2.2 CHA_2DS_2-VASc Score

1. (Congestive) Heart failure-1 point
2. Hypertension-1 point
3. Age (65–74 yrs)-1 point; (> 75 years)-2 points
4. Diabetes-1 point
5. Stroke, transient ischemic attack (TIA), thromboembolism-2 points
6. Vascular disease (Myocardial infarction, peripheral arterial disease, aortic or carotid plaque)-1 point
7. Female Sex-1 point

Before elective procedures, oral anticoagulants are appropriately and timely discontinued. A prospective trial illustrated that discontinuing warfarin alone was not inferior to bridging anticoagulation for the prevention of arterial thromboembolism. With less major bleeding in the nonbridging group, a net clinical benefit in favor of forgoing bridging with low-molecular-weight heparin (LMWH) was shown.[32]

Stroke can be a devastating outcome for patients and their families in the perioperative setting. For patients having noncardiac, noncarotid, nonneurologic surgery, a *perioperative stroke* is defined as an ischemic or hemorrhagic infarct occurring during or within 30 days after surgery.[33] Various risk factors for perioperative stroke have been identified, with advanced age, renal failure, and a previous history of stroke or transient ischemic attack (TIA) most consistent.[34] Recent stroke causes impaired cerebral autoregulation and places patients at increased risk for cerebral hypoperfusion during general anesthesia and surgery. It is therefore recommended that elective surgery in a patient with a recent stroke is delayed 1 to 3 months to prevent a secondary event.[35] A Danish study indicated that this period of increased risk may be as long as 9 months after stroke.[36] Appropriate bridging strategies in patients at high risk for stroke are important. Continuing antiplatelet therapy is considered for procedures with a low risk of bleeding. The POISE trial showed that high doses of metoprolol started on the day of surgery increase the risk of nonfatal strokes.[37] Patients taking β-blockers and statins should continue them perioperatively.[34]

Pulmonary disease increases both pulmonary and nonpulmonary perioperative complications. Postoperative pulmonary complications (PPCs) occur frequently and increase costs, morbidity, and mortality. Predictors of PPCs are advanced age, HF, chronic obstructive pulmonary disease (COPD), smoking, general health status (including impaired sensorium and functional dependency), and obstructive sleep apnea (OSA).[38,39] Well-controlled asthma does not appear to increase perioperative complications.[40] However, patients whose asthma is poorly controlled, as evidenced by wheezing at the time of anesthesia induction, have a higher risk of complications.[40] Unlike asthma, COPD does increase the risk of PPC, and the more severe the COPD, the greater the risk, but there is no prohibitive degree of severity that precludes surgery. Surprisingly, the risk with COPD is less than that with HF, advanced age, and poor general health.

Preoperative corticosteroids and inhaled β-agonists markedly decrease the incidence of bronchospasm after tracheal intubation, and they may shorten hospital and ICU stays.[40,41] Recovery time, pain, and reduction in lung volumes are less after laparoscopic procedures, but it is unclear whether this lowers PPC rates.[38] PPC risk is lower for percutaneous interventions; in a study of endovascular versus open abdominal aortic aneurysm repair, PPC rates were 3% and 16%, respectively.[38] General anesthesia carries greater risk than peripheral nerve blocks. Two large meta-analyses, and retrospective and randomized trials, suggested that PPC rates are lower for patients who have spinal or epidural anesthesia or epidural analgesia postoperatively.[38,41]

Routine pulmonary function tests, chest radiography, or arterial blood gases do not predict PPC risk and offer little more than can be determined by clinical evaluation.[41] Maximizing airflow in obstructive disease, treating infections and HF, and using lung expansion maneuvers (including cough, deep breathing, incentive spirometry, positive end-expiratory pressure [PEEP], and positive airway pressure [PAP]) reduce PPC rates.

Obstructive sleep apnea is caused by intermittent airway obstruction. It affects up to 9% of women and 24% of men, and most are unaware of the diagnosis.[42] Snoring, daytime sleepiness, hypertension, obesity, and a family history of OSA are risk factors for OSA.[42] A large neck circumference (>17 inches in men, > 16 inches in women) predicts a greater chance of OSA.[43] Patients with OSA have increased rates of diabetes, hypertension, AF, bradyarrhythmias, ventricular ectopy, stroke, HF, pulmonary hypertension, dilated cardiomyopathy, and CAD.[44] Mask ventilation, direct laryngoscopy, endotracheal intubation, and fiberoptic visualization of the airway are more difficult in patients with OSA. Airway obstruction, hypoxemia, atelectasis, ischemia, pneumonia, and prolonged hospitalizations occur in patients with OSA.[39] Patients should be advised to bring their PAP device on the day of the procedure. The Society for Ambulatory Anesthesia (SAMBA) has published recommendations for the perioperative care of patients with OSA, including a scoring system to predict perioperative risk.[45]

Renal disease is associated with hypertension, cardiovascular disease, volume overload, electrolyte disturbances, metabolic acidosis, and a need for modification of anesthetic drugs; it is also a risk factor for CAD. In elective procedures, it is recommended that dialysis be performed within 24 hours, but not immediately before procedures, due to acute volume depletion and electrolyte alterations. It may not be necessary to correct chronic hyperkalemia if potassium is less than 6 mEq/dL and within a range of a given patient's established levels. Radiocontrast media transiently decrease the glomerular filtration rate (GFR) in almost all patients, but patients with diabetes or renal insufficiency are at highest risk. For patients with a GFR below 60 $mL/kg^{-1}/min^{-1}$, alkalinizing renal tubular fluid with sodium bicarbonate or simple hydration may reduce injury.

Diabetic patients are at risk for multiorgan dysfunction, with renal insufficiency, strokes, peripheral neuropathies, and cardiovascular disease most prevalent. Tight glucose control in stroke or critically ill individuals may improve outcomes, but it is controversial.[46] It has not been proven that tight control in the immediate perioperative period for noncardiac procedures confers benefit. It may simply increase the risk of hypoglycemia. Chronically poor control increases comorbid conditions such as vascular disease, HF, CAD, and infections and the risk of surgery. It is unlikely that simply targeting perioperative glucose control will have a substantial impact on outcomes in diabetics having low-risk procedures. No data exist that support cancellation of procedures for any level of elevation of blood glucose or even treatment of such. Diabetic ketoacidosis and hypoglycemia (glucose < 50 g/dL) are the only conditions that absolutely warrant perioperative intervention. Preoperative goals are to prevent hypoglycemia during fasting and extreme hyperglycemia and ketosis.

Extreme obesity is defined by a body mass index (BMI) of 40 kg/m^2 or more, and these patients may have OSA, HF, diabetes, hypertension, pulmonary hypertension, a difficult airway, decreased arterial oxygenation, and increased gastric volume. Special equipment is needed, such as blood pressure cuffs, airway management devices, procedure tables, and gurneys to support the additional weight. A recent systematic review found that the superobese patient (BMI > 50 kg/m^2) was at an increased risk for perioperative complications.[47] Those with lower BMIs were not shown to be at increased risk unless they had multiple other comorbidities or comorbidities were not optimized prior to their procedure.[47]

Anemia is common preoperatively, is a marker of increased perioperative mortality, and is a predictor of short- and long-term outcomes in the general population.[48] Preoperative anemia is the strongest predictor of the need for transfusions, which increase morbidity and mortality.[48] If patients have a hemoglobin greater than 6 g/dL, are asymptomatic, and have no history of CAD, the minimal physiologic perturbations with a well-conducted anesthetic and a low-risk procedure are unlikely to pose enough risk to warrant transfusion. However, if time allows treating anemia preoperatively with nontransfusion practices, lowers risks, costs of care, and transfusions.

Pregnant patients with a viable fetus may require fetal monitoring. Plans to manage preterm labor or delivery should be made. The American College of Obstetricians and Gynecologists has recommendations to guide care.[49] General guidelines for fetal monitoring include the following:

- For a previable fetus, it is generally sufficient to confirm the fetal heart rate (FHR) by Doppler before and after the procedure.
- Intraoperative fetal monitoring may be considered for previable fetuses to facilitate positioning or hemodynamic optimization.
- At a minimum, for a viable fetus simultaneous electronic FHR and contractions are monitored before and after the procedure to assess the absence of contractions.
- Electronic fetal monitoring during procedures may be appropriate when all of the following apply:
  - The fetus is viable.
  - It is physically possible to allow intraoperative monitoring.

- A provider with obstetric surgery privileges is available and willing to intervene.
- The woman has given informed consent for emergency cesarean delivery.
- The planned procedure can be altered to allow emergency delivery.

Extremes of age may affect the selection of patients for procedures in OOOR locations. An ex-premature infant less than 60 weeks postconceptual age needs overnight observation to monitor for postanesthetic apnea. Patients more than 85 years of age with a history of hospital admission within the previous 6 months have a high risk of postoperative admission after ambulatory surgery.[50]

Diagnostic testing done routinely versus disease-indicated testing shows that few abnormalities detected by nonspecific testing result in changes in management, and rarely such changes have a beneficial patient effect.[51,52] On average, 1 in 2000 preoperative tests result in patient harm from pursuit of abnormalities detected by those tests.[6] It has been suggested that not following up on an abnormal result is a greater medicolegal risk than not identifying the abnormality to begin with.

In a pilot study by Chung and coworkers involving over 1000 patients undergoing ambulatory surgery, no increase in adverse perioperative events occurred in patients who had no preoperative testing.[4] There was no increase in operating room delays or cancellations or differences in outcome from lack of testing. Similarly, Schein et al. showed that routine medical testing in patients having cataract surgery did not offer benefit.[5] Several studies indicated that preoperative resting 12-lead ECGs do not add value to the care of ambulatory surgical patients.[8,53] The specificity of an ECG abnormality in predicting postoperative cardiac adverse events is only 26%, and a normal ECG does not exclude cardiac disease.[52] An ECG should not be done simply because the patient is of advanced age. Recommendations for age-based testing were derived from the high incidence of abnormalities found on ECGs of elderly patients. A prospective observational study in patients aged 50 years or older having noncardiac surgery found abnormalities in 45% of the preoperative ECGs, and bundle branch blocks were associated with postoperative MI and death but had no added predictive value over clinical risk factors.[54] The Centers for Medicare and Medicaid Services (CMS) do not reimburse for "preoperative" or age-based ECGs. There must be a medical necessity with a supporting International *Classification of Diseases, Tenth Revision* (*ICD-10*) code.[55] The ASA Preoperative Evaluation Practice Advisory recognized that ECG did not improve prediction beyond risk factors identified by patient history.[3] The ACC/AHA guidelines state that ECGs are not indicated in asymptomatic persons undergoing low-risk surgical procedures.[8] Chest radiographs have not been shown to predict PPCs.[39]

Healthy patients of any age and patients with known, stable, chronic diseases undergoing low-risk procedures are unlikely to benefit from any "routine" tests. A test should be ordered only if the results will affect the decision to proceed with the planned procedure or alter the care plans. Discovering abnormalities by laboratory tests or on ECGs and chest x-rays does not impact outcomes for patients receiving anesthesia for low-risk procedures. Eliciting a history of increased dyspnea on exertion, new-onset chest pain, or syncope and providing patients with appropriate preoperative medication instructions are of greater benefit than ordering ECGs or blood tests.

According to the ASA preoperative evaluation practice advisory, the literature "is insufficient to inform patients or physicians whether anesthesia causes harmful effects on early pregnancy," (p. 528) and pregnancy testing may be offered to women if the test result would alter patient management.[3] Some practices and facilities provide patients with information about the potential risks of anesthesia and surgery on pregnancy but allow them to decline testing. Other practices mandate that all females of childbearing age undergo a preoperative pregnancy test. It has been suggested that if a mandatory testing policy is utilized that patients be informed that consent for surgery or anesthesia includes consent for pregnancy testing. Recommended testing guidelines are in Table 2.3.

Medication instructions that advise patients to continue or discontinue drugs will likely improve outcomes more than perioperative testing. The patient's comorbidities and the nature of the procedure are considered when managing medications preoperatively. Continuing medications may be beneficial or detrimental, and in some cases suddenly stopping them has a negative effect. A summary of recommendations for perioperative administration of medications is in Table 2.4. Several drug classes and emerging controversies deserve special mention.

Generally, cardiac medications and antihypertensive agents are continued preoperatively. Selectively continuing or discontinuing these drugs depends on the volume and hemodynamic status of the patient, the degree of cardiac dysfunction, the adequacy of blood pressure control, and the anticipated anesthetic and volume challenges. Continuing all medications for patients with severe

TABLE 2.3. Preoperative Testing Guidelines for Patients Outside of the Operating Room

PROCEDURE/PATIENT TYPE	TESTS
Injection of contrast dye	**Creatinine**[a]
Potential for significant blood loss	Hemoglobin/hematocrit[a]
Likelihood of transfusion requirement	Type and screen
Possibility of pregnancy	Pregnancy test[b]
End-stage renal disease	Potassium level[c]
Diabetes	Glucose level on day of surgery[c]
Active cardiac condition (e.g., decompensated heart failure, arrhythmia, chest pain, murmur)	Electrocardiogram

[a]Results from laboratory tests within 3 months of surgery are acceptable unless major abnormalities are present or a patient's condition has changed.

[b]A routine pregnancy test before surgery is not recommended *before* the day of surgery. A careful history and local practice determine whether a pregnancy test is indicated.

[c]There is no absolute level of either potassium or glucose that precludes surgery and anesthesia. The benefits of the procedure must be balanced against the risk of proceeding in a patient with abnormal results.

TABLE 2.4. Summary of Common Medication Instructions

CONTINUE ON DAY OF SURGERY	DISCONTINUE ON DAY OF SURGERY UNLESS OTHERWISE INDICATED
Antidepressants, anxiolytics and psychiatric medications (including monoamine oxidase inhibitors)	
Antihypertensives	Antihypertensives
Generally to be continued	Consider discontinuing angiotensin-converting enzyme inhibitors or angiotensin receptor blockers 12–24 h before surgery, especially if
	Procedures: lengthy, significant blood loss or fluid shifts, use of general anesthesia
	Patients: taking multiple antihypertensive medications, well-controlled blood pressure, for whom hypotension is dangerous
Aspirin	Aspirin
Patients with known vascular disease	Discontinue 5–7 days before surgery:
Patients with drug-eluting stents < 6 months	If risk of bleeding is greater than risk of thrombosis
Patients with bare metal stents < 1 month	For procedures with serious consequences from bleeding
Before routine endoscopic procedures or cataract surgery	Taken only for primary prophylaxis (no known vascular disease)
Before vascular surgery	
Taken for secondary prophylaxis (known vascular disease)	
Asthma medications	
Autoimmune medications	Autoimmune (best to check with prescribing physician)
Methotrexate (if no risk of renal failure)	Methotrexate (if risk of renal failure)
	Entanercept (Enbral) 2 weeks before surgery
	Infliximab (Remicade) 6 weeks before surgery
	Adalimumab (Humira) 8 weeks before surgery
Birth control pills	
Cardiac medications	
Clopidogrel (Plavix)	Clopidogrel (Plavix)
Patients with drug-eluting stents < 6 months	Patients not included in group recommended for continuation
Patients with bare metal stents < 1 month	
Before cataract surgery	
Cyclooxygenase 2 inhibitors	Cyclooxygenase 2 inhibitors
	If surgeon concerned about bone healing
Diuretics	Diuretics
Triamterene, hydrochlorothiazide	Potent loop diuretics
Eye drops	
Estrogen compounds	Estrogen compounds
When used for birth control or cancer therapy	When used to control menopause symptoms or for osteoporosis
Gastrointestinal reflux medications (Prilosec, Zantac)	Gastrointestinal reflux medications (Tums)
	Herbals and nonvitamin supplements

(continued)

TABLE 2.4. *(Cont'd.)*

CONTINUE ON DAY OF SURGERY	DISCONTINUE ON DAY OF SURGERY UNLESS OTHERWISE INDICATED
	7–14 days before surgery
	Hypoglycemic agents, oral
Insulin	Insulin
Type 1 diabetes: take ~ one-third of intermediate to long-acting insulin (NPH, lente) Type 2 diabetes: up to half long-acting (NPH) or combination (70/30) preparations	Regular insulin (exception insulin pump: continue lowest basal rate—generally nighttime dose) Discontinue if blood sugar level < 100
Glargine (Lantus)	
If insulin pump delivery, continue lowest basal rate	
Opioids for pain or addiction	Nonsteroidal anti-inflammatory drugs
	48 h before day of surgery
Seizure medications	
Statins (Zocor, simvastatin, others)	Topical creams and ointments
Steroids (oral or inhaled)	Viagra or similar medications
	Discontinue 24 h before surgery
Thyroid medications	Vitamins, minerals, iron
Warfarin	Warfarin
Cataract surgery Routine endoscopy, low bleeding risk	Discontinue 5 days before surgery

disease having minor procedures is likely best. Angiotensin-converting enzyme inhibitors (ACEIs) and angiotensin receptor blockers (ARBs) may cause refractory hypotension. A suggested approach is to continue these drugs and alter the anesthetic plan, especially induction dosages and drugs, and have vasopressin available to prevent or mitigate significant hypotension.[56] Patients with a high risk of stroke or adverse effects from hypotension, undergoing a general anesthetic or presenting in a hypovolemic state may be best advised to hold ACEIs and ARBs for 24 hours. The potential for refractory hypotension must be balanced against the positive therapeutic impact of continuing these agents perioperatively on a case-by-case basis. Holding potent diuretics on the day of surgery is likely best as furosemide can be administered intravenously after induction of anesthesia if needed.

Aspirin is ubiquitously used to lower the risk of events in patients with known vascular disease, diabetes, renal insufficiency, or simply advanced age. Traditionally, aspirin has been withdrawn in the perioperative period because of concern of increased bleeding. However, this practice has come under scrutiny. A meta-analysis involving almost 50,000 patients undergoing a variety of noncardiac surgeries (30% on perioperative aspirin) found that aspirin increased bleeding complications by a factor of 1.5, but not the severity of bleeding complications except in patients undergoing intracranial surgery and possibly transurethral resection of the prostate.[17] When surgeons are blinded to aspirin administration, they cannot identify patients taking or not taking aspirin based on bleeding.[19] There is an increased risk of vascular events when aspirin is stopped perioperatively in patients who take it regularly.[57] A rebound hypercoagulable state may result.[58] Acute coronary syndromes occurred 8.5 ± 3.6 days and acute cerebral events 14.3 ± 11.3 days after aspirin cessation, the typical duration of cessation before surgery. Events were twice as common in patients who had stopped aspirin in the previous 3 weeks than in those who had not.[17]

Stopping aspirin for 3–4 days should be sufficient, if aspirin is stopped at all, and dosing is resumed as soon as possible. New platelets formed after aspirin (half-life of ~ 15 minutes) is stopped will not be affected. Normally functioning platelets greater than 50,000/mm^3 are adequate to control surgical bleeding. For many minor, superficial procedures such as cataract extraction, endoscopies, and peripheral procedures, the risk of withdrawing aspirin in at-risk patients is greater than the risk of bleeding.[18] An algorithm for the management of dual-antiplatelet therapy in patients with coronary artery stenting is shown in Figure 2.3.[16]

Consideration may be given to discontinuing aspirin perioperatively if taken only for primary prevention (no history of stents, strokes, MI).[42] Continuing aspirin, if taken for secondary prevention (history of stents, vascular disease), is recommended except for procedures with a risk of bleeding in closed spaces (e.g., intracranial, intraspinal, posterior chamber of the eye). Neuraxial or peripheral anesthesia is safe for patients taking aspirin.[59] The risk of spinal hematoma with clopidogrel is unknown. Based on labeling and guidelines of the American Society of Regional Anesthesia, clopidogrel is discontinued 7 days before planned neuraxial blockade.[59] Table 2.5 provides an approach to patients being considered for regional anesthesia who take antiplatelet, anticoagulant, or antifibrinolytic agents.

TABLE 2.5. An Approach to Antiplatelet, Anticoagulant, and Antifibrinolytic Medications for Regional Anesthesia

DRUG	NUMBER OF DAYS TO DISCONTINUE
Abciximab	2–5 days
Alteplase	10 days
Apixaban	3 days
Argatroban	8–10 hours
Aspirin and aspirin combinations	No need to stop
Cilostazol	2 days
Clopidogrel	7 days
Dabigatran (CrCl ≥ 30)	5 days
Dabigatran (CrCl < 30)	7 days
Dipyridamole	2 days
Enoxaparin	24 hours
Eptifibatide	8–24 hours
Fondaparinux	4 days
Heparin, unfractionated SQ 5000 units (twice or three times daily dosing)	Avoid peak effect 20 minutes to 4 hours
Heparin, unfractionated intravenous	4 hours
Nonsteroidal anti-inflammatories	No need to stop[a]
Prasugrel	7–10 days
Reteplase	10 days
Rivaroxaban	3 days
Streptokinase	10 days
Tenecteplase	10 days
Ticagrelor	5–7 days
Tirofiban	8–24 hours
Urokinase	10 days
Warfarin	5 days, INR normalized

[a]Surgeon/proceduralist may have different guidelines.

Low-molecular-weight heparin (LMWH) is discontinued 24 hours before procedures with a risk of bleeding or planned neuraxial block.[59] Warfarin may increase bleeding except for minor procedures, such as cataract surgery or diagnostic endoscopy.[18] The usual recommendation is to withhold four or five doses of warfarin before the procedure date if the INR is 2–3, until the INR decreases to less than 1.5, a level considered safe for procedures and neuraxial blockade.[59] If the INR is greater than 3.0, it is necessary to withhold warfarin longer. If the INR is measured the day before a procedure and is more than 1.8, a small dose of vitamin K (1–5 mg orally or subcutaneously) can reverse anticoagulation.[60] Substitution with shorter-acting anticoagulants such as unfractionated or LMWH, referred to as bridging, is controversial. Kearon and Hirsh recommended preoperative bridging only for patients who have had an acute arterial or venous thromboembolism within 1 month before a procedure that cannot be postponed.[60]

Type 1 diabetics have an absolute insulin deficiency and require insulin to prevent ketoacidosis even if they are not hyperglycemic. Type 2 diabetics are often insulin resistant and prone to extreme hyperglycemia. Both type 1 and 2 diabetics should discontinue short-acting insulins. An exception is for patients with insulin pumps who continue their lowest basal rate, typically a nighttime rate. Type 1 diabetics should take a small amount (usually a third to half) of their usual morning dose of intermediate to long-acting insulin (e.g., lente or NPH) the day of surgery to avoid ketoacidosis. Type 2 diabetics should take none or up to a half dose of intermediate to long-acting insulin (e.g., lente or NPH) or a combination (e.g., 70/30) insulin on the day of the procedure. Taking half of the usual dose of intermediate, long-acting, or combination insulins on the day of surgery improves perioperative glycemia compared to taking no insulin.[61] Glargine (e.g., Lantus) or other ultra–long-acting insulin can be taken as scheduled.

Metformin does not need to be discontinued *before* the day of surgery. Metformin will not cause hypoglycemia during fasting periods of 1–2 days, and there is no risk of lactic acidosis with metformin except in cases of renal or hepatic failure. Do not restart this drug postoperatively until any risk of organ failure has passed. Procedures should not be cancelled if patients continue metformin. There are no data to support the recommendation to stop metformin 24–48 hours before surgery, which increases the risk of hyperglycemia. Sulfonylurea agents with long half-lives (e.g., chlorpropamide) can cause hypoglycemia in fasting patients. Newer oral agents (acarbose, pioglitazone) used as single-agent therapy do not cause hypoglycemia during fasting. However, to avoid confusion, oral hypoglycemic agents are generally held the day of procedures.

Patients who are taking steroids should take their usual dose on the day of procedures. Stress-associated adrenal insufficiency is possible in some patients unless additional steroids are given. A normal daily adrenal output of cortisol (30 mg) is equivalent to 5–7.5 mg of prednisone. The hypothalamic-pituitary axis (HPA) is not suppressed with 5 mg/day or less of prednisone or its equivalent. In patients who have taken more than 5–20 mg/day of prednisone or its equivalent for 3 weeks or longer, the HPA may be suppressed. The HPA is suppressed with more than 20 mg/day of prednisone or its equivalent taken for 3 or more weeks. The risk of adrenal insufficiency remains for up to 1 year after the cessation of high-dose steroids. Surgery, trauma, or infection may be stressful, and an intact HPA will respond by increasing output of glucocorticoids. The known secretory rate of cortisol for most major surgeries is in the 75 to 150 mg/day range.[62] Most OOOR procedures will induce minimal physiologic stress, and nothing more than the patient's usual daily dose of steroid is required. Supplementation depends on the amount of stress, duration and severity of the procedure, and the daily dose of steroid (Table 2.6). Infections, psychosis, decreased wound healing, and hyperglycemia increase with high doses of perioperative steroids, which are rarely necessary.[62]

It is generally recommended to discontinue herbals and supplements 7–14 days before surgery. The exception is valerian, a central nervous system depressant that may cause a benzodiazepine-like withdrawal when abruptly discontinued. If possible, valerian consumption is tapered. Mandatory discontinuation of supplements, or cancellation of anesthesia when these compounds have been continued, is not supported by available data. Historically, monoamine oxidase inhibitors (MAOIs) are discontinued before surgery, but because of their long duration of action, they must be stopped at least 3 weeks beforehand. Suicides or severe depression can occur when patients discontinue an MAOI. The safest approach is to continue these drugs and adjust the anesthetic plan.

Patients can continue narcotic pain medications to prevent withdrawal symptoms and discomfort. Drugs used to treat addiction such as methadone and nicotine-replacement therapies are continued as scheduled.[63] Inhalers and long-term medications for asthma or COPD are continued and taken on the day of procedures.[41]

Current guidelines for the adult patient recommend fasting for 6 hours after a light meal (toast and clear liquids) or nonhuman milk and 8 hours after meals containing fried or fatty foods or meat before general or regional anesthesia or sedation.[64] Clear liquids up to 2 hours before anesthesia are acceptable for patients without conditions that may increase the risk of aspiration, such as gastroesophageal reflux disease, symptomatic hiatal hernia, poorly controlled diabetes mellitus, gastric motility disorders, intra-abdominal masses (including the gravid uterus), and bowel obstruction.[64]

TABLE 2.6. Perioperative Steroid Therapy Recommendations for Adults

No supplemental steroids	Minor/intermediate-risk surgical procedure
	Prednisone < 10 mg daily (or equivalent)
	Every other day steroid dosing
	Topical steroids
Hydrocortisone 50 mg IV intraoperatively and every 8 hours after surgery for 24–48 hours	Major surgical procedures
	Volume refractory hypotension
	Patients receiving physiologic replacement therapy[a]

[a] Patients with Addison disease (primary adrenal failure), congenital adrenal hyperplasia, secondary adrenal failure due to hypopituitarism.

SOURCE: Adapted from MacKenzie CR, Goodman SM Stress dose steroids: myths and perioperative medicine. *Curr Rheumatol Rep.* 2016;18:1–5.

CONCLUSION

Preparation to lower the risk of complications and improve outcomes during and after procedures requiring anesthesia is the most important goal. Traditionally, surgical risk has been considered more important than the anesthetic risk. However, a general anesthetic requiring instrumentation of the airway with associated significant physiologic perturbations may pose a greater risk than many procedures typically performed in OOOR settings. Identification and modification of risk require fundamentally good medicine, systems of care, clinical assessment, and experienced, knowledgeable, and dedicated health care providers. As the numbers of patients having anesthesia in OOOR locations increase, anesthesiologists must continue to innovate to provide patients with the best preoperative services.

REFERENCES

1. Chang B, Urman RD. Non-operating room anesthesia: the principles of patient assessment and preparation. *Anesthesiol Clin.* 2016;34(1):223–240.
2. Nagrebetsky A, Gabriel RA, Dutton RP, Urman RD. Growth of nonoperating room anesthesia care in the United States: a contemporary trends analysis. Anesth *Analg.* 2017;124(4):1261–1267.
3. American Society of Anesthesiologists Task Force on Preanesthesia Evaluation. Practice advisory for preanesthesia evaluation: an updated report by the American Society of Anesthesiologists Task Force on Preanesthesia Evaluation. *Anesthesiology.* 2012;116:522–538.
4. Chung F, Yuan H, Yin L, et al. Elimination of preoperative testing in ambulatory surgery. *Anesth Analg.* 2009;108:467–475.
5. Schein OD, Katz J, Bass EB, et al. The value of routine preoperative medical testing before cataract surgery. Study of medical testing for cataract surgery. *N Engl J Med.* 2000;342:168–175.
6. Apfelbaum JL. Preoperative evaluation, laboratory screening, and selection of adult surgical outpatients in the 1990s. *Anesth Rev.* 1990;17(suppl 2):4–12.
7. Hlatky MA, Boineau RE, Higginbotham MB, et al. A brief self-administered questionnaire to determine functional capacity (the Duke Activity Status Index). *Am J Cardiol.* 1989;64:651–654.
8. Fleisher LA, Fleischmann KE, Auerbach AD, et al. ACC/AHA 2014 guideline on perioperative cardiovascular evaluation and management of patients undergoing noncardiac surgery. *J Am Coll Cardiol.* 2014;64:(e)77–(e)137.
9. Livhits M, Ko CY, Leonardi MJ, et al. Risk of surgery following recent myocardial infarction. *Ann Surg.* 2011;253:857–864.
10. Lee TH, Marcantonio ER, Mangione CM, et al. Derivation and prospective validation of a simple index for prediction of cardiac risk of major noncardiac surgery. *Circulation.* 1999;100:1043–1049
11. McFalls EO, Ward HB, Moritz TE, et al. Coronary artery revascularization before elective major vascular surgery. *N Engl J Med.* 2004;351:2795–804.
12. Breen P, Lee JW, Pomposelli F, et al. Timing of high-risk vascular surgery following coronary artery bypass surgery: a 10-year experience from an academic medical centre. *Anaesthesia.* 2004;59:422–427.
13. Newsome LT, Weller RS, Gerancher JC, et al. Coronary artery stents: II. Perioperative considerations and management. *Anesth Analg.* 2008;107:570–590.

14. Rabbitts JA, Nuttall GA, Brown MJ, et al. Cardiac risk of non-cardiac surgery after percutaneous coronary intervention with drug-eluting stents. *Anesthesiology.* 2008;109:596–604.
15. Grines CL, Bonow RD, Casey DE, et al. Prevention of premature discontinuation of dual antiplatelet therapy in patients with coronary artery stents: a science advisory from the American Heart Association American College of Cardiology, Society for Cardiovascular Angiography and Interventions, American College of Surgeons, and American Dental Association with representation from the American College of Physicians. *J Am Coll Cardiol.* 2007;49:734–739.
16. Levine GN, Bates ER, Bittl JA, et al. 2016 ACC/AHA guideline focused update on duration of dual antiplatelet therapy in patients with coronary artery disease. *J Am Coll Cardiol.* 2016;68:1082–1115.
17. Burger W, Chemnitius JM, Kneissl GD, et al. Low-dose aspirin for secondary cardiovascular prevention–cardiovascular risks after its perioperative withdrawal versus bleeding risks with its continuation—review and meta-analysis. *J Intern Med.* 2005;257:399–414.
18. Anderson MA, Ben-Menachem T, Gan SI, et al. Management of antithrombotic agents for endoscopic procedures. *Gastrointest Endosc.* 2009;70:1060–1070.
19. Berger PB, Bellot V, Bell MR, et al. An immediate invasive strategy for the treatment of acute myocardial infarction early after noncardiac surgery. *Am J Cardiol.* 2001;87:1100–1112.
20. Van Diepen S, Bakal JA, McAlister FA, et al. Mortality and readmission of patients with heart failure, atrial fibrillation, or coronary artery disease undergoing noncardiac surgery: an analysis of 38,047 patients. *Circulation.* 2011;124:289–296.
21. Meta-analysis Global Group in Chronic Heart Failure (MAGGIC). The survival of patients with heart failure with preserved or reduced left ventricular ejection fraction: an individual patient data meta-analysis. *Eur Heart J.* 2012;33:1750–1757.
22. Otto CM, Lind BK, Kitzman DW, et al. Association of aortic-valve sclerosis with cardiovascular mortality and morbidity in the elderly. *N Engl J Med.* 1999;341:142–147.
23. Wilson W, Taubert KA, Gewitz M, et al. Prevention of infective endocarditis. Guidelines from the American Heart Association. *Circulation.* 2007;116:1736–1754.
24. Crossley GH, Poole JE, Rozner MA, et al. The Heart Rhythm Society/American Society of Anesthesiologists expert consensus statement on the perioperative management of patients with implantable defibrillators, pacemakers and arrhythmia monitors. *Heart Rhythm.* 2011;8:e1–e18.
25. Howell SJ, Sear JW, Foex P. Hypertension, hypertensive heart disease and perioperative cardiac risk. *Br J Anaesth.* 2004;92:570–583.
26. Miyasaka Y, Barnes ME, Gersh BJ, et al. Secular trends in incidence of atrial fibrillation in Olmsted County, Minnesota, 1980–2000, and implications on the projections for future prevalence. *Circulation.* 2006;114:119–125.
27. Huxley RR, Lopez FL, Folsom AR, et al. Absolute and attributable risks of atrial fibrillation in relation to optimal and borderline risk factors: the Atherosclerosis Risk in Communities (ARIC) study. *Circulation.* 2011;123:1501–1508.
28. Lip GY, Tse HF, Lane DA. Atrial fibrillation. *Lancet.* 2012;379:648–661.
29. Connolly SJ, Ezekowitz MD, Yusuf S, et al, for the RE-LY Steering Committee and Investigators. Dabigatran versus warfarin in patients with atrial fibrillation. *N Engl J Med.* 2009;361:1139–1151.
30. Connolly SJ, Eikelboom J, Joyner C, et al, for the AVERROES Steering Committee and Investigators. Apixaban in patients with atrial fibrillation. *N Engl J Med.* 2011;364:806–817.
31. Granger CB, Alexander JH, McMurray JJ, et al for the ARISTOTLE Committees and Investigators. Apixaban versus warfarin in patients with atrial fibrillation. *N Engl J Med.* 2011;365:981–992.
32. Douketis JD, Spyropoulos AC, Kaatz S, et al. Perioperative bridging anticoagulation in patients with atrial fibrillation. *N Engl J Med.* 2015;373:823–833.
33. Sacco RL, Kasner SE, Broderick JP, et al. An updated definition of stroke for the 21st century: A statement for healthcare professionals from the American Heart Association/American Stroke Association. *Stroke.* 2013;44:2064–2089.
34. Mashour GA, Moore LE, Lele AV, et al. Perioperative care of patients at high risk for stroke during or after non-cardiac, non-neurologic surgery: consensus statement from the society for neuroscience in anesthesiology and critical care. *J Neurosurg Anesthesiol.* 2014;26:273–285.
35. Blacker DJ, Flemming KD, Link MJ, et al. The preoperative cerebrovascular consultation: common cerebrovascular questions before general or cardiac surgery. *Mayo Clin Proc.* 2004;79:223–229.
36. Jorgensen ME, Torp-Pedersen C, Gislason G, et al. Time elapsed after ischemic stroke and risk of adverse cardiovascular events and mortality following elective noncardiac surgery. *JAMA.* 2014;312:269–277.
37. Devereaux PJ, Yang H, Yusuf S, et al. Effects of extended-release metoprolol succinate in patients undergoing non-cardiac surgery (POISE trial): a randomized controlled trial. *Lancet.* 2008;371:1839–1847.
38. Smetana GW, Lawrence VA, Cornell JE. Preoperative pulmonary risk stratification for noncardiothoracic surgery: systematic review for the American College of Physicians. *Ann Intern Med.* 2006;144:581–595.
39. Hwang D, Shakir N, Limann B, et al. Association of sleep-disordered breathing with postoperative complications. *Chest.* 2008;133:1128–1134.
40. Warner DO, Warner MA, Barnes RD, et al. Perioperative respiratory complications in patients with asthma. *Anesthesiology.* 1996;85:460–467.
41. Lawrence VA, Cornell JE, Smetana GW. Strategies to reduce postoperative complications after noncardiothoracic surgery: systematic review for the American College of Physicians. *Ann Intern Med.* 2006;144:596–608.
42. Young T, Skatrud J, Peppard PE. Risk factors for obstructive sleep apnea in adults. *JAMA.* 2004;291:2013–2016.
43. Chung F, Yegneswaran B, Liao P, et al. STOP questionnaire. A tool to screen patients for obstructive sleep apnea. *Anesthesiology.* 2008;108:812–821.
44. Caples SM, Gami AS, Somers VK. Obstructive sleep apnea. *Ann Intern Med.* 2005;142:187–197.
45. Joshi GP, Ankichetty SP, Gan TJ, et al. Society for Ambulatory Anesthesia consensus statement on preoperative selection of adult patients with obstructive sleep apnea scheduled for ambulatory surgery. *Anesth Analg.* 2012;115:1060–1068.
46. Lipshutz AK, Gropper MA. Perioperative glycemic control. *Anesthesiology.* 2009;110:408–4021.
47. Joshi GP, Ahmad S, Riad W, et al. Selection of obese patients undergoing ambulatory surgery: a systematic review of the literature. *Anesth Analg.* 2013;117:1082–1091.
48. Beattie WS, Karkouti K, Wijeysundera DN, et al. Risk associated with preoperative anemia in noncardiac surgery. *Anesthesiology.* 2009;110:574–581.
49. American College of Obstetricians and Gynecologists Committee Opinion: Nonobstetric surgery during pregnancy. *Obstet Gynecol.* 2011;117:420–421.
50. Fleisher LA, Pasternak LR, Herbert R, et al. Inpatient hospital admission and death after outpatient surgery in elderly patients: importance of patient and system characteristics and location of care. *Arch Surg.* 2004;139:67–72.
51. Narr BJ, Hansen TR, Warner MA. Preoperative laboratory screening in healthy Mayo patients: cost-effective elimination of tests and unchanged outcomes. *Mayo Clin Proc.* 1991;66:155–159.
52. Liu LL, Dzankic S, Leung JM. Preoperative electrocardiogram abnormalities do not predict postoperative cardiac complications in geriatric surgical patients. *J Am Geriatr Soc.* 2002;50:1186–1191.
53. Gold BS, Young ML, Kinman JL, et al. The utility of preoperative electrocardiograms in the ambulatory surgical patient. *Arch Intern Med.* 1992;152:301–305.
54. van Klei WA, Bryson GL, Yang H, et al. The value of routine preoperative electrocardiography in predicting myocardial infarction after noncardiac surgery. *Ann Surg.* 2007;246:165–170.
55. Centers for Medicare and Medicaid Services. Available at: http://www.cms.gov/. Accessed November 22, 2016.
56. Comfere T, Sprung J, Kumar MM, et al. Angiotensin system inhibitors in a general surgical population. *Anesth Analg.* 2005;100:636–644.
57. Chassot PG, Delabays A, Spahn DR. Perioperative antiplatelet therapy: the case for continuing therapy in patients at risk of myocardial infarction. *Br J Anaesth.* 2007;99:316–328.
58. Senior K. Aspirin withdrawal increases risk of heart problems. *Lancet.* 2003;362:1558.
59. Horlocker TT, Wedel DJ, Rowlingson JC, et al. Regional anesthesia in the patient receiving antithrombotic or thrombolytic therapy: American Society of Regional Anesthesia and Pain Medicine evidence-based guidelines (third edition). *Reg Anesth Pain Med.* 2010;35:64–101.
60. Kearon C, Hirsh J. Management of anticoagulation before and after elective surgery. *N Engl J Med.* 1997;336:1506–1511.
61. Likavec A, Moitra V, Greenberg J, Drum M, Sweitzer B. Comparison of preoperative blood glucose levels in patients receiving different insulin regimens. *Anesthesiology.* 2006;105:A567.
62. MacKenzie CR, Goodman SM. Stress dose steroids: myths and perioperative medicine. *Curr Rheumatol Rep.* 2016;18:1–5.
63. Spell NO III. Stopping and restarting medications in the perioperative period. *Med Clin North Am.* 2001;85:1117–1128.
64. American Society of Anesthesiologists. Practice guidelines for preoperative fasting and the use of pharmacologic agents to reduce the risk of pulmonary aspiration: application to healthy patients undergoing elective procedures: a report by the American Society of Anesthesiologists Task Force on Preoperative Fasting. *Anesthesiology.* 2011;114:495–511.

3 | PATIENT MONITORING

BENJAMIN T. FEDELES, MD, SAMUEL M. GALVAGNO JR., DO, PHD, FCCM,
BHAVANI KODALI, MD

INTRODUCTION

The expertise and skill of the modern anesthesiologist is increasingly required when anesthesia is administered for procedures performed outside of the operating room (OOOR). The OOOR environment is fraught with challenges and often requires a great deal of flexibility without compromising patient care. In the practice of anesthesiology, physiological monitoring of patients is imperative and is recognized as a standard of care; this is reflected in the American Society of Anesthesiologists' (ASA's) "Statement on Nonoperating Room Anesthetizing Locations," which requires, at a minimum, adequate monitoring equipment be available to adhere to the "standards for basic anesthesia monitoring."[1] Although definitive data are lacking, some studies have suggested that adverse events occurring in the OOOR environment have a higher severity of injury and may result from substandard care, including lack of adherence to minimum monitoring guidelines.[2,3] This chapter focuses on the physics, physiology, limitations, and recommendations for standard physiological monitors that should be utilized in the OOOR environment. A special emphasis is placed on pulse oximetry and capnography.

MONITORS

PULSE OXIMETRY

Numerous studies have demonstrated significant knowledge deficits among clinicians regarding the limitations and interpretation of pulse oximetry results.[2,4–7] An understanding of pulse oximetry is obligatory for all providers of OOOR anesthesia because this technology is employed as the principal means of ensuring adequate oxygenation in a sedated or anesthetized patient.

Dr. Takuo Aoyagi, a Japanese bioengineer, is credited with developing and marketing the first functional pulse oximeter in 1972.[8] Based on a century of experimental antecedents, Aoyagi recognized that the absorbency ratios of pulsatile variations varied with oxygen saturation at different wavelengths. By the early 1980s, use of the pulse oximeter rapidly expanded, eventually becoming integrated into the clinical practice of anesthesiologists and clinicians working in operating room and critical care settings.

Pulse oximetry relies on the spectral analysis of oxygenated and reduced hemoglobin and is explained by the Beer-Lambert law.[9,10] This law describes how the concentration of a substance in solution can be determined by transmitting a known intensity of light through a solution. With pulse oximetry, the Pao_2 is approximated by transmitting light of a specific wavelength across tissue and measuring its intensity on the other side. Red and near-infrared (near-IR) light readily penetrates tissue, whereas other wavelengths of light tend to be absorbed (Figure 3.1).

Light-emitting diodes (LEDs) are used to emit red light (660 nm) and near-IR light (940 nm) because these two wavelengths have known absorption qualities when directed at hemoglobin (Hb). Specifically, 660-nm red light is absorbed by reduced Hb, while 940 nm is absorbed preferentially by oxygenated Hb. When these wavelengths are emitted through tissue and a vascular bed such as a finger, nostril, or earlobe or even through a neonatal hand or foot, a photodiode detector on the opposite side measures the amount of light transmitted. The red/near-IR ratio is calculated by the oximeter and compared to reference values for Pao_2 derived from healthy human subjects. The Pao_2 is further discriminated from venous blood or connective tissue by measuring the pulse-added component of the signal. This signal comprises alternating current, representing pulsatile arterial blood, and direct current, which corresponds to tissue, venous blood, and nonpulsatile arterial blood.[11] By cancelling out the static

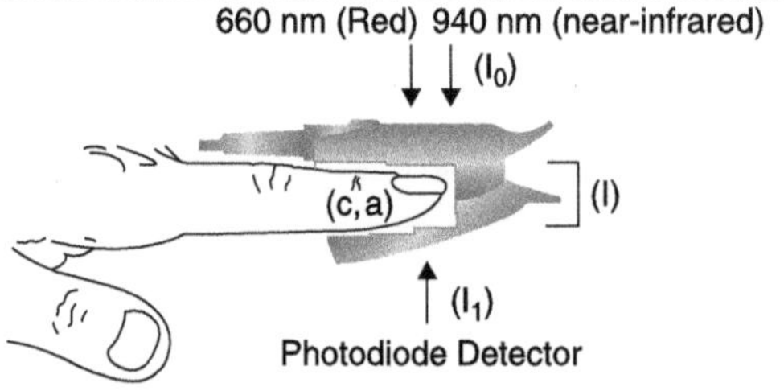

$$T = \frac{I_0}{I_1} = 10^{-A} = 10^{-elc}$$

T-Transmittance
I_0 -Intensity of incident light
I_1 -Intensity of light after passing through material
A- Absorbance of sample
l- Distance the light travels
a- Absorption coefficient of the absorber
e- Molar absorptivity of the absorber
c- Concentration of the absorbing species

Figure 3.1. Pulse oximetry: application of the Beer-Lambert law.

components, the pulsatile component can be isolated and the Pao_2 estimated; this is called *photoplethysmography*.

The pulsatile waveform can provide useful information, albeit limited and indirect, to clinicians in the absence of more advanced monitoring. For example, an irregular heart rhythm such as atrial fibrillation can be observed on the waveform monitor. Changes in waveform amplitude and during the respiratory cycle may reflect a change in vascular volume (e.g., hypovolemia from hemorrhage) and has been observed in healthy patients who underwent removal of 10% of their blood volume and subsequent reinfusion.[12] In the absence of intra-arterial cannulation to measure pulse pressure, pulse oximetry can serve as a gross surrogate and can also be used to predict fluid responsiveness in the operating room.[13,14] These concepts can be applied in situations OOOR, especially in emergent situations, where resources may be more limited.

Pulse oximetry has several limitations. Nail polish and dark skin may cause a variable degree of interference; the physical obstruction to light transmittance appears to be related to darker skin pigmentation and dark-opaque nail polish.[15–17] In critically ill patients, a low signal-to-noise ratio may exist due to hypovolemia, peripheral vasoconstriction, or peripheral vascular disease.[18] Extra "noise" in the form of ambient light, deflection of light around and not through the vascular bed (optical shunt), and motion artifact may cause false readings.[19–21] Shivering is considered a common source of motion artifact, but normal pulse oximetry readings have been recorded in patients with tonic-clonic seizures.[22]

Dyshemoglobinemias represent a well-known cause of optical interference with pulse oximetry. Both carboxyhemoglobin (COHb) and methemoglobin (MetHb) absorb light within the red and near-IR wavelength ranges utilized in pulse oximetry; standard pulse oximeters are unable to distinguish COHb and MetHb from normal oxyhemoglobin (O_2Hb). Hence, COHb will falsely absorb red light, and the pulse oximeter will display a falsely high saturation reading.[23] With MetHb, standard oximeters falsely detect a greater degree of absorption of both Hb and O_2Hb, increasing the absorbance ratio. When the absorbance ratio reaches 1, the calibrated saturation level approaches a plateau of approximately 85%.[24] Co-oximetry offers a multiwavelength analysis that takes into account the absorption of O_2Hb, MetHb, and COHb and should be used to determine an accurate saturation reading if these dyshemoglobins are suspected to be present. Intravenous dyes such as methylene blue and indigo carmine cause reliable spurious decreases in oximetry readings.[25,26] Fetal hemoglobin, hyperbilirubinemia, and anemia have not been found to yield inaccurate oximetry readings in most cases.[27–29]

CAPNOGRAPHY

Over the last three decades, capnography has become a standard for monitoring in anesthesia practice.[30] The measurement of carbon dioxide (CO_2) in expired air directly indicates changes in the elimination of CO_2 from the lungs. Indirectly, it indicates changes in the production of CO_2 at the tissue level and in the delivery of CO_2 to the lungs by the circulatory system. Capnography is a noninvasive monitoring technique that allows fast and reliable insight into ventilation, circulation, and metabolism.[31] While the technique is used primarily for confirmation of successful endotracheal intubation, it is also useful for assessing the quality of cardiopulmonary resuscitation (CPR).[30,32] Numerous national organizations, including the American Heart Association, endorse capnography and capnographic methods for confirming endotracheal tube placement.[33] Despite these recommendations, capnography is not always widely available or consistently applied.[34]

Capnometry refers to the measurement and display of CO_2 on a digital or analog monitor. Maximum inspiratory and expiratory CO_2 concentrations during a respiratory cycle are displayed. *Capnography* refers to the graphic display of instantaneous CO_2 concentration (FCO_2) versus time or expired volume during a respiratory cycle (CO_2 waveform or capnogram). CO_2 waveforms are displayed as two types: FCO_2 can be plotted against expired volume or against time during a respiratory cycle.

Infrared spectrographs are the most compact and least expensive means to measure end-tidal CO_2 ($ETCO_2$). The wavelength of IR rays exceeds 1.0 μm, whereas the visible spectrum is between 0.4 and 0.8 μm.[35] The IR rays are absorbed by polyatomic gases such as nitrous oxide, carbon dioxide, and water vapor. Carbon dioxide selectively absorbs specific wavelengths (4.3 μm) of IR light (Figure 3.2).

Because the amount of light absorbed is proportional to the concentration of the absorbing molecules, the concentration of a gas can be determined by comparing the measured absorbance with the absorbance of a known standard. The CO_2 concentration measured by the monitor is usually expressed as partial pressure in millimeters of mercury, although some units display percentage CO_2, obtained by dividing the partial pressure of CO_2 by the atmospheric pressure. Other techniques used to measure $ETCO_2$ include Raman spectography, molecular correlation spectography, mass spectography, and photoacoustic spectography.

A time capnogram can be divided into inspiratory (phase 0) and expiratory segments (Figure 3.3).

Standard terminology for capnography has been adopted.[36] The expiratory segment, similar to a single-breath nitrogen

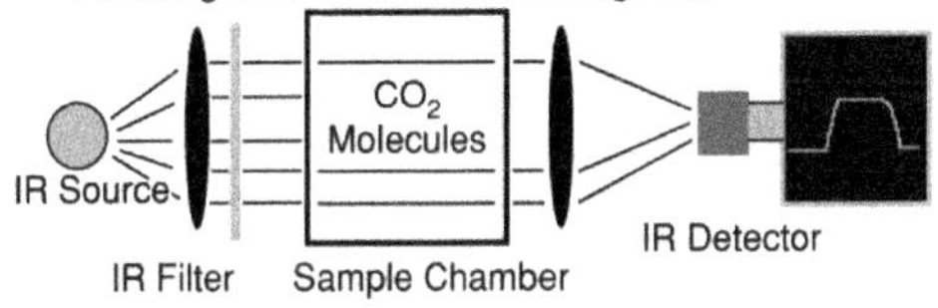

Figure 3.2. Infrared (IR) spectrography.

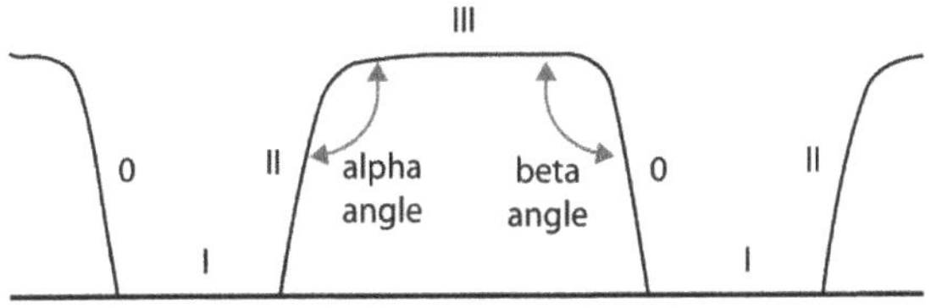

Figure 3.3. Current terminology for components of a time capnogram.

curve or single-breath CO_2 curve, is divided into three phases. The angle between phase II and phase III is the alpha angle. The nearly 90° angle between phase III and the descending limb is the beta angle.

Causes of increased or decreased CO_2 are listed in Table 3.1.

Under normal circumstances, the end-tidal Pco_2 ($ETPCO_2$) is lower than $Paco_2$ by 2–5 mm Hg in adults.[37–38] The Pco_2 gradient is due to the ventilation–perfusion (V/Q) mismatch in the lungs as a result of temporal, spatial, and alveolar mixing defects.[39,40] The arterial-to-end-tidal (a-ET) Pco_2/$Paco_2$ fraction is a measure of alveolar dead space, and changes in alveolar dead space correlate well with changes in (a-ET) Pco_2.[35] An increase in (a-ET) Pco_2 suggests an increase in dead space ventilation; hence, (a-ET) Pco_2 can provide an indirect estimate of V/Q mismatching of the lung. Nevertheless, (a-ET) Pco_2 does not correlate with alveolar dead space in all circumstances. Changes in alveolar dead space correlate with (a-ET) Pco_2 only when phase III is flat or has a minimal slope. If phase III has a steeper slope, the terminal portion of phase III may intercept the line representing $Paco_2$, resulting in either zero or negative (a-ET) Pco_2, even in the presence of alveolar dead space. Therefore, the (a-ET) Pco_2 is dependent on both alveolar dead space and factors that influence the slope of phase III. This implies that an increase in the alveolar dead space need not always be associated with an increase in the (a-ET) Pco_2. The (a-ET) Pco_2 may remain the same if there is an associated increase in the slope of phase III.

A reduction in cardiac output and pulmonary blood flow results in a decrease in $ETCO_2$ and an increase in (a-ET) Pco_2. Increases in cardiac output and pulmonary blood flow result in better perfusion of the alveoli and a rise in $ETCO_2$.[41] The decrease in (a-ET) Pco_2 is due to an increase in the alveolar CO_2 with a relatively unchanged arterial CO_2 concentration, suggesting better excretion of CO_2 into the lungs. The improved CO_2 excretion is due to better perfusion of upper parts of the lung. There is an inverse linear correlation between pulmonary artery pressure and (a-ET) Pco_2.[42] Thus, under conditions of constant lung ventilation, $ETCO_2$ monitoring can be used as a monitor of pulmonary blood flow.

In one study of 17 elderly patients, transcutaneous monitoring of Pco_2 provided a more accurate estimation of arterial CO_2 partial pressure than $PETCO_2$ monitoring[43]; however, it is not widely practiced or widely available in clinical settings at this time.

$ETCO_2$ monitoring can be utilized in nonintubated spontaneously breathing patients. When applied in this manner, capnography waveforms can be distorted by the dilution of air or oxygen; $ETCO_2$ readings are typically decreased. Numerous devices are commercially available to provide capnography for nonintubated patients. While not quantitatively accurate, many of these devices provide baseline measurements, and the presence of waveforms can be used to confirm ventilation.

TABLE 3.1. Causes of Changes in End-Tidal Carbon Dioxide as Measured by Capnography

CAUSES OF INCREASED CO_2	CAUSES OF DECREASED CO_2
- Hypoventilation	- Hyperventilation
- Hyperthyroidism/thyroid storm	- Hypothermia
- Malignant hyperthermia	- Venous air embolism
- Fever/sepsis	- Pulmonary embolism
- Rebreathing	- Decreased cardiac output
- Other hypermetabolic states	- Hypoperfusion

BLOOD PRESSURE MEASUREMENT

Blood pressure in OOOR locations is commonly measured with noninvasive oscillometric devices. An electronic pressure transducer detects oscillating blood flow as the cuff is deflated. Assuming the upper extremity is used, the compressed brachial artery oscillates as restricted blood flows through it, and the systolic, diastolic, and mean pressures are determined. The reader is referred to an excellent in-depth review by Polanco and Pinsky.[44]

ELECTROCARDIOGRAPHY

Both transmural and subendocardial ischemia can be detected when electrocardiography (ECG) leads are properly positioned.[45] Lead V_5, the precordial lead originally described in Kaplan and King's classic paper on intraoperative ischemia, has been validated and found to detect up to 75% of ischemic changes seen in all 12 leads.[46,47] The combination of leads II, V_2, V_3, V_4, and V_5 has a sensitivity of 100% for detecting intraoperative ischemia.[45] The reader is directed to an exceptional review of perioperative electrocardiography previously published in *Anesthesiology Clinics*.[48]

TEMPERATURE MONITORING

Perioperative hypothermia increases the incidence of adverse myocardial outcomes, increases blood loss, and increases wound infection.[49–51] Mild hypothermia also changes the kinetics of various anesthetics and may delay postoperative recovery.[51] Intraoperative hypothermia usually develops in three phases. The first phase is caused by redistribution of heat from the core thermal compartment to the outer shell of the body. A slower, linear reduction in the core temperature follows and may last several hours.[51] In the last phase, the core temperature plateaus and may remain unchanged throughout the remainder of the perioperative period as thermoregulatory control is impaired during general or regional anesthesia. Numerous temperature-monitoring devices are available, but it is the site of temperature monitoring rather than the type of temperature probe that is most important. Core temperature can be estimated from accessible sites, such as the nasopharynx, bladder, esophageal, or rectal sites.[51] Clinicians should be aware that the ambient temperature in many OOOR locations is deliberately kept lower to protect sensitive equipment. As temperature monitoring is a standard of care, anesthesiologists are expected to be proactive in maintaining normothermia and preventing temperature derangements throughout the perioperative period.

SPONTANEOUS ELECTROENCEPHALOGRAPHIC ACTIVITY MONITORS

Depth of anesthesia monitoring with the bispectral index (BIS) monitor has been shown to reduce, but not eliminate, the incidence of awareness under anesthesia.[52] Actual patterns of intraoperative use of BIS by anesthesia professionals vary, depending on procedure anesthesia type, as well as other factors.[53] In the neurocritcal care setting, BIS monitoring has been shown to provide a more objective means of sedation assessment that may lead to a decrease in overall rates of propofol administration and fewer incidences of oversedation.[54] A Cochrane review concluded that anesthesia guided by BIS monitoring within the recommended range (40 to 60) could improve anesthetic delivery and postoperative recovery from relatively deep anesthesia while reducing the incidence of intraoperative recall in surgical patients with high risk of awareness.[55] The Patient State Index (PSI) is another monitor for awareness that has not been studied as thoroughly as the BIS monitor but has been shown to provide indications that correlate with unconsciousness.[56] For a detailed review of the state of monitors for preventing intraoperative awareness, the reader is encouraged to review the ASA's 2006 practice advisory.[57]

IMPEDANCE-BASED RESPIRATORY VOLUME MONITORING

Surveillance of respiratory status is a critical component of patient care in any clinical setting. Unfortunately, current clinical practice relies on secondary indicators of respiratory status, usually oxygen saturation (SpO_2) measured by pulse oximetry, in lieu of monitoring ventilation. Early identification of respiratory insufficiency using real-time respiratory volume monitoring has the potential to allow clinicians to alter treatments in time to prevent more serious complications.

A noninvasive bioimpedance-based respiratory volume monitor (RVM; ExSpiron, Respiratory Motion, Inc., Waltham MA) approved by the Food and Drug Administration has become available and provides real-time respiratory data with continuous trends of minute ventilation (MV), tidal volume (TV), and respiratory rate (RR) in nonintubated patients.[91–93] The device uses bioelectrical impedance, which involves measurement of electrical current flow through the chest wall and lung tissue. A small electrical current is passed between electrodes, and the voltage is measured. With the advent of complex waveform analysis and improved computing, impedance-based methods have demonstrated strong correlation (mean of 0.96, 95% CI from 0.93 to 0.99) for regular and erratic breathing and clinically relevant accuracy (average error accuracy of 9.3% for MV, 9.0% for TV, and 1.8% for RR) between an RVM and spirometric measurements.[90] RVM and ventilator volume measurements during mechanical ventilation or spontaneous breathing demonstrated an average MV and TV accuracy of more than 90% and RR accuracy greater than 95%.[92] Continuous monitoring with an RVM identified opioid-induced respiratory depression and postoperative apnea in a cohort of adults undergoing elective joint replacement therapy.[94] Such a monitor may have utility in OOOR settings where respiratory status may be challenging to observe and quantitate. Such a device may prove to be useful for the early detection of deterioration in respiratory function.

CONSIDERATIONS FOR OOOR ENVIRONMENTS

THE MAGNETIC RESONANCE IMAGING SUITE

Anesthesia in the magnetic resonance imaging (MRI) suite is hazardous for a variety of reasons: an extremely strong static magnetic field, high-frequency electromagnetic (radio-frequency) waves, and a time-variable magnetic field. Secondary dangers are also present in the form of acoustic noise, systemic and local heating, and the potential for projectiles.[58] These inherent risks, combined with the fact that the anesthesiologist is physically removed from the patient during the study, compounded by noise, a dimly lit environment, the lengthy time it requires to complete the study, an obstructed line of sight, and competing environmental distractions, transform a seemingly benign procedure (e.g., diagnostic imaging) into one rife with risks. The ASA released an updated practice advisory report in 2015 to provide guidelines and support to clinicians.[58]

The MRI suite poses a profound risk to patients with implanted ferromagnetic material because the high magnetic field may dislodge pacemakers, implants, cardiac valves, or other prostheses. Before entering the MRI suite, all ferromagnetic items need to be removed to prevent injury; an MRI-compatible anesthesia machine and equipment are compulsory (Figure 3.4).[59]

The intense radio-frequency waves may cause surface heating on the patient's body, and the lead wires from the ECG also pose a potential burn hazard.[60] The ECG monitor is subject to considerable artifact from the background static magnetic field and radio-frequency impulses as well as the electronics within the device that create magnetic fields.[61] Modern devices minimize these limitations, and a variety of commercial devices for ECG monitoring in the MRI suite are available (Figure 3.5).

Blood pressure monitoring by the oscillometric method is most commonly utilized and provides reliable readings. Pulse oximetry may be difficult in the MRI suite because the signal may become degraded due to currents in the oximetry cable and a decreased signal-to-noise ratio.[62] Capnography may be utilized; a decrease in the phase II slope of the capnogram may be observed due to a long circuit pathway. Remote monitoring via a closed-circuit monitor—preferably with zoom lens magnification capability—may be necessary.

COMPUTED TOMOGRAPHY

An anesthetized patient in the computed tomography (CT) scanner presents logistical problems similar to those

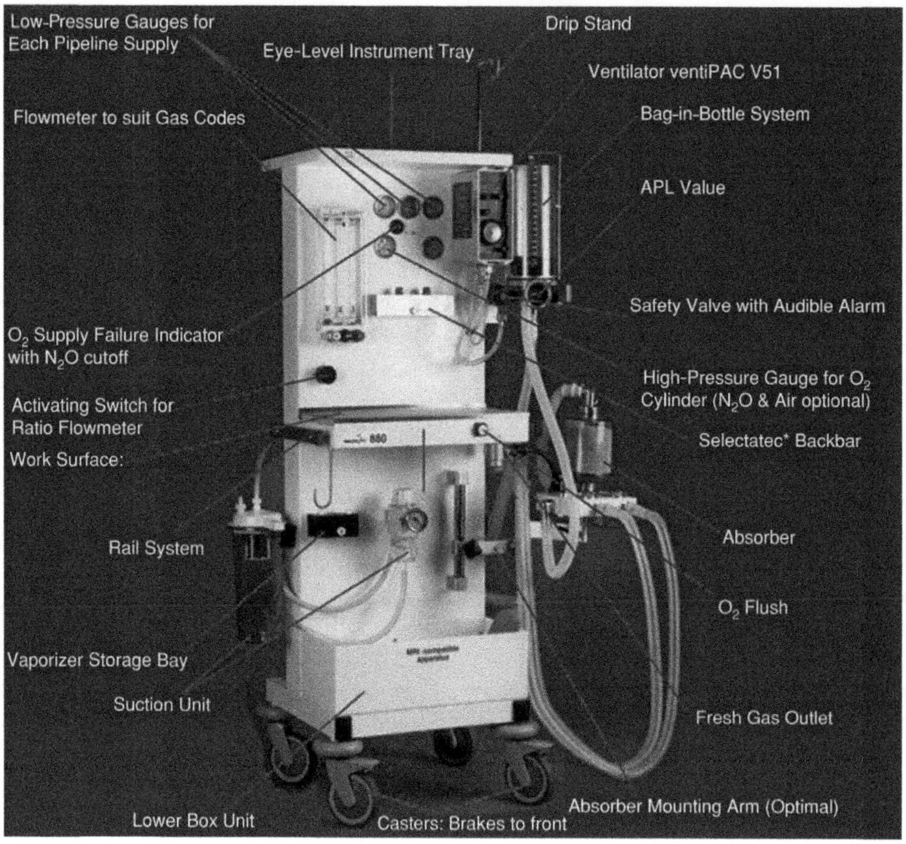

Figure 3.4. *A magnetic resonance imaging (MRI)–compatible anesthesia machine.*

encountered in the MRI suite; however, the impact on interference with standard monitors is not as profound. Blood pressure should be monitored at relatively short intervals because radiocontrast media reactions may lead to a precipitous loss of systemic vascular resistance. Standard monitors such as the ECG, temperature probe, pulse oximetry, and capnography should be utilized. As with procedures done in the MRI suite and elsewhere, remote monitoring may be required. Special attention should be given to patients in trauma situations undergoing stat imaging where proper preanesthesia evaluation is often limited or nonexistent and situations are often complicated by unstable patient hemodynamics (Figure 3.4 Figure 3.5).

ELECTROCONVULSIVE THERAPY

Electroconvulsive therapy (ECT) is used for treatment of severe psychiatric disorders as well as depression, complex regional pain syndrome, and chronic pain.[63] ECT involves provocation of a generalized epileptic seizure by electrical stimulation of the brain. The procedure is usually performed under general anesthesia with muscle relaxation. Excessive alterations in heart rate, blood pressure, and cardiac functions are prevented by anticholinergic and antihypertensive agents; hence, blood pressure and ECG monitoring is mandatory.[64] Train-of-four monitoring for neuromuscular blockade and BIS monitoring should also be considered. Capnography is essential for safe and effective anesthetic management of patients undergoing

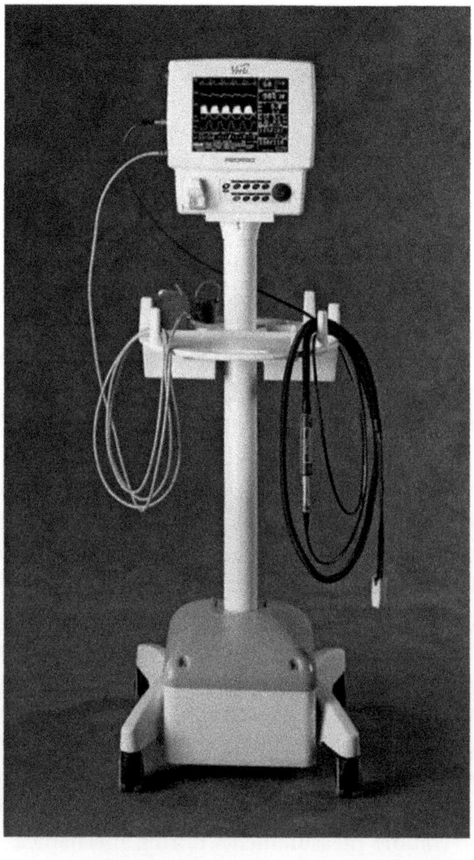

Figure 3.5. *The Veris Medrad magnetic resonance imaging (MRI)–compatible monitor.*

ECT, especially patients with intracranial disorders or coronary artery disease.[65] ECT may be used in pregnant women with refractory depression, bipolar disorders, or significant psychiatric disorders as its potential risks are minimal compared to pharmacologic therapy. In these situations, the normal changes in physiology brought on by pregnancy, rather than the procedure itself, may present a challenge. Procedural anesthesia in the pregnant population is outside the scope of this chapter but is widely available.

THE ENDOSCOPY SUITE

Most endoscopic procedures are performed in an OOOR environment, and in many cases, these procedures may be accomplished with moderate or deep sedation. Capnography should be utilized in view of the fact that significant delays in detecting respiratory compromise have been demonstrated in its absence.[66] In addition to blood pressure and ECG monitoring, pulse oximetry and capnography should be considered standard monitors to ensure adequate ventilation and oxygenation during endoscopic procedures, whether they are performed under general anesthesia or varying degrees of sedation.[67]

INTERVENTIONAL ANGIOGRAPHY

Electrocardiogram, blood pressure, pulse oximetry, and capnography are standard monitors for procedures in interventional angiography. In addition, intracranial pressure (ICP) monitoring and invasive arterial blood pressure monitoring are frequently employed. In some instances, central venous pressure monitoring and monitoring of evoked potentials may be necessary. In recent years, the endovascular treatment of diseases of intracranial and spinal vessels has become widely accepted; invasive monitoring is frequently required based on the usual underlying pathophysiology and severity of these disorders.[68]

CONTROVERSIES IN MONITORING

Numerous investigators have focused a critical eye on the ability of monitors to prevent morbidity and mortality. In a well-known randomized controlled trial by Watkinson et al., the authors concluded that mandated electronic vital sign monitoring in high-risk medical and surgical patients had no effect on adverse events or mortality.[69] While this study had numerous limitations that may have led to type II error, the "number needed to monitor" to alter outcomes was estimated to be large.[70] In a systematic review of randomized controlled trials examining the role of pulse oximetry, there was no evidence of a significant difference between groups regarding duration of postoperative mechanical ventilation, duration of intensive care unit stay, or postoperative complications; the authors were unable to find reliable evidence that pulse oximetry affects the outcome of anesthesia.[71] Moller's landmark studies in 1993, based on a design that was similar to both a randomized controlled trial and a cluster randomized trial that included 20,802 patients, concluded that pulse oximetry did not have a significant impact on mortality or hospital stay.[71–73] In a review of clinical trials on monitoring, the authors acknowledged that pulse oximetry may enable clinicians to detect desaturation episodes more readily, and that this technology may be beneficial, but to prevent one adverse event, a large number of patients must be monitored.[74] The findings of these and other related studies were summarized in a Cochrane review that concluded that the value of perioperative monitoring with pulse oximetry is unproven.[75]

Earlier studies, including a closed claims analysis, suggested that pulse oximetry was an invaluable modality for preventing adverse outcomes in anesthesia, and that improvements in monitoring—specifically pulse oximetry—may have helped reduce serious mishaps over the last several decades by at least 35%.[76] Two additional studies suggested that monitoring with pulse oximetry facilitates prompt detection of arterial hypoxemia, allowing earlier and potentially lifesaving treatment.[73,77,78] Oversedation with ensuing respiratory depression is an important contributor to adverse events that have occurred under monitored anesthesia care (MAC), and appropriate use of monitoring has been cited as a crucial preventive measure that is often neglected.[79] Studies based on analyses of closed claims data suggested that better monitoring may lead to earlier correction of potentially harmful perioperative events.[77,79,80]

Despite numerous national guidelines and recommendations, there seems to be a paucity of data to support the use of monitors in preventing mortality OOOR. In a 2006 study by Watkinson et al., monitoring of heart rate, noninvasive blood pressure, oxygen saturation, RR by impedance pneumography, and skin temperature did not separate groups with adverse outcomes from beneficial interventions in a heterogeneous population of 402 high-risk medical and surgical ward patients.[69] Similarly, when a medical emergency team was tasked with closely following vital signs in an effort to rapidly recognize critical threshold patterns suggestive of potential adverse events, no benefit was found.[81] While each of these studies had significant limitations, they helped promulgate the idea that mandatory monitoring, even with a high incidence of abnormal vital signs, does not confer a mortality benefit. Nevertheless, other investigators determined that improved monitoring might have prevented a significant number of adverse outcomes identified in the ASA closed claims database.[82]

Initial studies utilizing capnography as a supplement during procedures requiring sedation suggested that this practice might serve as an early warning mechanism for impending respiratory embarrassment.[83,84] Capnography may have an advantage over pulse oximetry because capnography is a better measure of ventilation. With capnography, providers are able to institute early stimulation for nonbreathing patients, thereby preventing arterial oxygen desaturation. Lightdale et al. demonstrated that microstream capnography significantly prevented arterial oxygen desaturation in children undergoing sedation for procedures.[85] This was an important finding because most critical adverse events during sedation occur secondary to hypoventilation and respiratory failure.[86]

RECOMMENDATIONS

Although data to support a mortality benefit appear to be lacking, numerous organizations, including the ASA, strongly endorse monitoring in OOOR environments.[87,88] For OOOR anesthetizing locations, the ASA recommends adhering to the standards for basic anesthetic monitoring (Table 3.2).[89]

At the Brigham and Woman's Hospital, the University of Maryland Medical Center (UMMC), large tertiary care teaching hospitals, and the R. Adams Cowley Shock Trauma, in addition to the ASA standards, continuous capnography is employed. Table 3.3 lists recommended monitoring practices for procedural sedation.

CONCLUSION

Technological advances notwithstanding, the most critical monitor is the provider of anesthesia. It is likely that the dramatic decrease in anesthetic-related mortality over the past several years is as much the result of improved drugs and technology as the result of improved training of providers of anesthesia. While the true rate of complications from anesthesia in the OOOR environment is currently unknown, by implementing standards for monitoring that are similar to standards used in the operating room, the safe delivery of an anesthetic for procedures in the OOOR environment can be consistently achieved.

TABLE 3.2. American Society of Anesthesiologists (ASA) Standards for Basic Anesthetic Monitoring

PARAMETER	METHODS
Oxygenation	Inspired gas oxygen analyzer
	Pulse oximetry (with audible tone)
	Illumination to assess the patient's color
Ventilation	$PETCO_2$ monitoring: capnography, capnometry, or mass spectroscopy with audible CO_2 alarm to detect correct placement of endotracheal tube
	Utilization of a device capable of detecting disconnection of the components of the breathing system
Circulation	Continuous electrocardiogram
	Blood pressure and heart rate determination no less than every 5 minutes
	Assessment by at least one: palpation of a pulse, intra-arterial tracing of blood pressure, ultrasound peripheral pulse monitoring, pulse plethysmography or oximetry
Body temperature	Indicated when clinically significant changes in body temperature are intended, anticipated, or suspected

SOURCE: Based on "Standards for Basic Anesthetic Monitoring" of the American Society of Anesthesiologists. A copy of the full text can be obtained from ASA, 520 N. Northwest Highway, Park Ridge, IL 60068-2573.

TABLE 3.3. Recommended Monitoring for Procedural Sedation

PARAMETER	METHODS
Training	Providers must pass a procedural sedation course.
Establishment of protocols	All OOOR sites should have uniform protocols with an emphasis on ease of implementation.
Oxygenation	Pulse oximetry with an audible tone should be employed. Adequate lighting should be available to assess skin color.
Ventilation	$ETCO_2$ monitoring is recommended with an audible CO_2 alarm to detect hypoventilation and apnea.
Circulation	A continuous electrocardiogram should be available. Blood pressure and heart rate should be determined no less than every 5 minutes.
Body temperature	Continuous temperature monitoring is strongly recommended, especially during long noninvasive procedures.
Protocol review/process improvement	Periodic reviews should be conducted with appropriate amendments made to protocols to ensure that problems do not recur.

REFERENCES

1. American Society of Anesthesiologists. Statement on nonoperating room anesthetizing locations, standards and practice parameters, last amended October 16, 2013. Available at: http://www.asahq.org/~/media/sites/asahq/files/public/resources/standards-guidelines/statement-on-nonoperating-room-anesthetizing-locations.pdf. Accessed on October 1, 2016.
2. Robbertze R, Posner K, Domino K. Closed claims review of anesthesia for procedures outside the operating room. *Curr Opin Anaesthesiol.* 2006;19:436–442.
3. Galvagno S, Kodali B. Critical monitoring issues outside the operating room. *Anesthesiology Clin.* 2009;27:141–156.
4. Sinex J. Pulse oximetry: principles and limitations. *Am J Emerg Med.* 1999;17:59–67.
5. Elliott M, Tate R, Page K. Do clinicians know how to use pulse oximetry? A literature review and clinical implications. *Aust Crit Care.* 2006;19:139–144.
6. Rodriguez L, Kotin N, Lowenthal D, Kattan M. A study of pediatric house staff's knowledge of pulse oximetry. *Pediatrics.* 1994;93:810–813.
7. Stoneham M, Saville G, Wilson I. Knowledge about pulse oximetry among medical and nursing staff. *Lancet.* 1994;344:1339–1342.
8. Kelleher J. Pulse oximetry. *J Clin Monit.* 1989;5:37–62.
9. Tremper K, Barker S. Pulse oximetry. *Anesthesiology.* 1989;70:98–108.
10. Salyer J. Neonatal and pediatric pulse oximetry. *Respir Care.* 2003;48:386–396.
11. Wukitsch M, Petterson M, Pologe J. Pulse oximetry: analysis of theory, technology, and practice. *J Clin Monit.* 1988;4:290–301.
12. Shamir M, Eidelman LA, Floman Y, Kaplan L, Pizov R. Pulse oximetry plethysmographic waveform during changes in blood volume. *Br J Anaesth.* 1999;82(2):178–181.
13. Cannesson M, Besnard C, Durand PG, Bohé J, Jacques D. Relation between respiratory variations in pulse oximetry plethysmographic waveform amplitude and arterial pulse pressure in ventilated patients. *Crit Care.* 2005;9:R562. doi:10.1186/cc3799.
14. Cannesson M, Attof Y, Rosamel P, et al. Respiratory variations in pulse oximetry plethysmographic waveform amplitude to predict fluid responsiveness in the operating room. *Anesthesiology.* 2007;106(6):1105–1111. doi:10.1097/01.anes.0000267593.72744.20.

15. Volgyesi G, Spahr-Schopfer I. Does skin pigmentation affect the accuracy of pulse oximetry? An in vitro study. *Anesthesiology*. 1991;75:A406.
16. Cote C, Goldstein E, Fuchsman W, Hoaglin D. The effect of nail polish on pulse oximetry. *Anesth Analg*. 1988;67:683–686.
17. Ries A, Prewitt L, Johnson J. Skin color and ear oximetry. *Chest*. 1989;96:287–290.
18. Severinghaus J, Spellman M. Pulse oximeter failure thresholds in hypotension and vasoconstriction. *Anesthesiology*. 1990;73:532–537.
19. Hanowell L, Eisele JH Jr, Downs D. Ambient light affects pulse oximeters. *Anesthesiology*. 1987;67:864–865.
20. Costarino A, Davis D, Keon T. Falsely normal saturation reading with the pulse oximeter. *Anesthesiology*. 1987;67:830–831.
21. Severinghaus J, Kelleher J. Recent developments in pulse oximetry. *Anesthesiology*. 1992;76:1018–1038.
22. James M, Marshall H, Carew-McColl M. Pulse oximetry during apparent tonic-clonic seizures. *Lancet*. 1991;337:394–395.
23. Buckley R, Aks S, Eshom J, et al. The pulse oximetry gap in carbon monoxide intoxication. *Ann Emerg Med*. 1994;24:252–255.
24. Barker SJ, Tremper KK, Hyatt J. Effects of methemoglobinemia on pulse oximetry and mixed venous oximetry. *Anesthesiology*. 1989;70:112–117.
25. Kessler M, Eide T, Humayan B, Poppers P. Spurious pulse oximeter desaturaion with methylene blue injection. *Anesthesiology*. 1986;65:435–436.
26. Scheller M, Unger R, Kelner M. Effects of intravenously administered dyes on pulse oximetry readings. *Anesthesiology*. 1986;65:550–552.
27. Severinghaus J, Koh S. Effect of anemia on pulse oximeter accuracy at low saturation. *J Clin Monit*. 1990;6:85–88.
28. Harris A, Sendak M, Donham R, et al. Absorption characteristics of human fetal hemoglobin at wavelengths used in pulse oximetry. *J Clin Monit*. 1988;4:175–177.
29. Ramanathan R, Durand M, Larrazabal C. Pulse oximetry in very low birth weight infants with acute and chronic disease. *Pediatrics*. 1987;79:612–617.
30. Kodali B, Moseley H, Kumar A, Delph Y. Capnography and anaesthesia: review article. *Can J Anaesth*. 1992;39:617–632.
31. Kupnik D, Skok P. Capnometry in the prehospital setting: are we using its potential? *J Emerg Med*. 2007;24:614–617.
32. Kodali BS, Urman RD. Capnography during cardiopulmonary resuscitation: current evidence and future directions. *J Emerg Trauma Shock*. 2014;7(4):332–340.
33. American Heart Association. 2005 American Heart Association guidelines for cardiopulmonary resuscitation and emergency cardiovascular care. Part 7.1: adjuncts for airway control and ventilation. *Circulation*. 2005;112:IV-51–IV-57.
34. Deiorio M. Continuous end-tidal carbon dioxide monitoring for confirmation of endotracheal tube placement is neither widely available nor consistently applied by emergency physicians. *J Emerg Med*. 2005;22:490–493.
35. Colman Y, Krauss B. Microstream capnography technology: a new approach to an old problem. *J Clin Monit*. 1999;15:403–409.
36. Kodali B, Kumar A, Moseley H, Ahyee-Hallsworth R. Terminology and the current limitations of time capography: a brief review. *J Clin Monit*. 1995;11:175–182.
37. Nunn J, Hill D. Respiratory dead space and arterial to end-tidal CO_2 tension difference in anesthetized man. *J Appl Physiol*. 1960;15:383–389.
38. Fletcher R, Jonson B. Deadspace and the single breath test carbon dioxide during anaesthesia and artificial ventilation. *Br J Anaesth*. 1984;56:109–119.
39. Kodali B, Moseley H, Kumar Y, Vemula V. Arterial to end-tidal carbon dioxide tension difference during caesarean section anaesthesia. *Anaesthesia*. 1986;41:698–702.
40. Fletcher R, Jonson B, Cumming G, Brew J. The concept of dead space with special reference to the single breath test for carbon dioxide. *Br J Anaesth*. 1981;53:77–88.
41. Leigh M, Jones J, Motley H. The expired carbon dioxide as a continuous guide of the pulmonary and circulatory systems during anesthesia and surgery. *J Thoracic Cardiovasc Surg*. 1961;41:597–610.
42. Askrog V. Changes in a-ACO_2 difference and pulmonary artery pressure in anesthetized man. *J Appl Physiol*. 1966;21:1299–1305.
43. Casati A, Squicciarini G, Malagutti G, et al. Transcutaneous monitoring of partial pressure of carbon dioxide in the elderly patient: a prospective, clinical comparison with end-tidal monitoring. *J Clin Anesth*. 2006;18:436–440.
44. Polanco P, Pinsky M. Practical issues of hemodynamic monitoring at the bedside. *Surg Clin N Am*. 2006;86:1431–1456.
45. Fuchs R, Achuff S, Grunwald L, Yin F, Griffith L. Electrocardiographic localization of coronary artery narrowings: studies during myocardial ischemia and infarction in patients with one-vessel disease. *Circulation*. 1982;66:1168–1176.
46. Kaplan J, King S. The precordial electrocardiographic lead V5 in patients who have coronary-artery disease. *Anesthesiology*. 1976;45:570–574.
47. London M, Hollenberg M, Wong W, et al. Intraoperative myocardial ischemia: localization by continuous 12-lead electrocardiography. *Anesthesiology*. 1988;69:232–241.
48. John A, Fleisher L. Electrocardiography: the ECG. *Anesthesiol Clin*. 2006;24:697–715, v–vi.
49. Kurz A, Sessler D, Lenhardt R. Perioperative normothermia to reduce the incidence of surgical-wound infection and shorten hospitalization. Study of Wound Infection and Temperature Group. *N Engl J Med*. 1996;334:1209–1215.
50. Pestel G, Kurz A. Hypothermia—it's more than a toy. *Curr Opin Anaesthesiol*. 2005;18:151–156.
51. Insler S, Sessler D. Perioperative thermoregulation and temperature monitoring. *Anesthesiol Clin*. 2006;24:823–837.
52. Bruhn J, Myles P, Sneyd R, Struys M. Depth of anaesthesia monitoring: what's available, what's validated and what's next? *Br J Anaesth*. 2006;97:85–94.
53. Gelfand ME, Gabriel RA, Gimlich R, Beutler SS, Urman RD. Practice patterns in the intraoperative use of bispectral index monitoring. *J Clin Monit Comput*. 2017;31(2):281–289.
54. Olson D, Cheek D, Morgenlander J. The impact of bispectral index monitoring on rates of propofol administration. *AACN Clin Issues*. 2004;1:63–73.
55. Punjasawadwong Y, Boonjeungmonkol N, Phongchiewboon A. Bispectral index for improving anaesthetic delivery and postoperative recovery. *Cochrane Database Syst Rev*. 2007;4:CD003843.
56. Chen X, Tang J, White P, et al. A comparison of patient state index and bispectral index values during the perioperative period. *Anesth Analg*. 2002;95:1669–1674.
57. Apfelbaum J, Arens J, Cole D, American Society of Anesthesiologists Task Force on Intraoperative Awareness. Practice advisory for intraoperative awareness and brain function monitoring. *Anesthesiology*. 2006;104:847–864.
58. Practice advisory on anesthetic care for magnetic resonance imaging. *Anesthesiology*. 2015;122(3):495–520. doi:10.1097/aln.0000000000000458.
59. Deckert D, Zecha-Stallinger A, Haas T, et al. Anesthesia outside the core operating area [in German]. *Anaesthesist*. 2007;56:1028–1030, 1032–1037.
60. Rejger V, Cohn B, Vielvoye G, Raadt F. A simple anaesthetic and monitoring system for magnetic resonance imaging. *Eur J Anaesthesiol*. 1989;6:373–378.
61. Patterson S, Chesney J. Anesthetic management for magnetic resonance imaging: problems and solutions. *Anesth Analg*. 1992;74:123.
62. Peden C, Menon D, Hall A, et al. Magnetic resonance for the anaesthetist. *Anesthesia*. 1992;47:515.
63. Grundmann U, Oest M. Anaesthesiological aspects of electro-convulsive therapy [in German. *Anaesthesist*. 2007;56:202–204, 206–211.
64. Saito S. Anesthesia management for electroconvulsive therapy: hemodynamic and respiratory management. *J Anesth*. 2005;19:142–149.
65. Saito S, Kadoi Y, Nihishara F, et al. End-tidal carbon dioxide monitoring stabilized hemodynamic changes during ECT. *J ECT*. 2003;19:26–30.
66. Pino R. The nature of anesthesia and procedural sedation outside of the operating room. *Curr Opin Anaestheiol*. 2007;20:347–351.
67. Melloni C. Anesthesia and sedation outside the operating room: how to prevent risk and maintain good quality. *Curr Opin Anaesthesiol*. 2007;20:513–519.
68. Preiss H, Reinartz J, Lowens S, Henkes H. Anesthesiological management of neuroendovascular interventions [in German]. *Anaesthesist*. 2006;55:679–692.
69. Watkinson P, Barber V, Price J, Hann A, Tarassenko L, Young J. A randomised controlled trial of the effect of continuous electronic physiological monitoring on the adverse event rate in high risk medical and surgical patients. *Anesthesia*. 2006;61:1031–1039.
70. Pedersen T, Moller A, Pedersen B. Pulse oximetry for perioperative monitoring: systematic review of randomized, controlled trials. *Anesth Analg*. 2003;96:426–431.
71. Moller J, Johannessen N, Espersen K, et al. Randomized evaluation of pulse oximetry in 20,802 patients: II. Perioperative events and postoperative complications. *Anesthesiology*. 1993;78:445–453.
72. Moller J, Pedersen T, Rasmussen L, et al. Randomized evaluation of pulse oximetry in 20,802 patients: I. Design, demography, pulse oximetry failure rate, and overall complication rate. *Anesthesiology*. 1993;78:436–444.
73. Moller J, Wittrup M, Johansen S. Hypoxemia in the postanesthesia care unit: an observer study. *Anesthesiology*. 1990;73:890–895.
74. Young D, Griffiths J. Clinical trials of monitoring in anaesthesia, critical care and acute ward care: a review. *Br J Anaesth*. 2006;97:39–45.

75. Pedersen T, Pedersen B, Moller A. Pulse oximetry for perioperative monitoring. *Cochrane Database Syst Rev*. 2003;4:CD002013.
76. Tinker J, Dull D, Caplan R, et al. Role of monitoring devices in prevention of anesthetic mishaps: a closed claims analysis. *Anesthesiology* 1989;71:541–546.
77. Cote C, Rolf N, Liu L, et al. A single-blind study of combined pulse oximetry and capnography in children. *Anesthesiology*. 1991;74:980–987.
78. Cooper J, Cullen D, Nemeskal R, et al. Effects of information feedback and pulse oximetry on the incidence of anesthesia complications. *Anesthesiology*. 1987;67:686–694.
79. Bhananker S, Posner K, Cheney F, et al. Injury and liability associated with monitored anesthesia care: a closed claims analysis. *Anesthesiology*. 2006;104:228–234.
80. Cooper J, Newbower R, Kitz R. An analysis of major errors and equipment failures in anesthesia management: considerations for prevention and detection. *Anesthesiology*. 1984;60:34–42.
81. Hillman K, Chen J, Cretikos M, et al. Introduction of the medical emergency team MET system: a cluster-randomized controlled trial. *Lancet*. 2005;365:2091–2097.
82. Caplan R, Posner K, Ward R, et al. Adverse respiratory events in anesthesia: a closed claims analysis. *Anesthesiology*. 1990;72:828–833.
83. Soto R, Fu E, Vila H, Miguel R. Capnography accurately detects apnea during monitored anesthesia care. *Anesth Analg*. 2004;99:379–382.
84. Vargo J, Zuccaro G, Dumot J, et al. Automated graphic assessment of respiratory activity is superior to pulse oximetry and visual assessment for the detection of early respiratory depression during therapeutic upper endoscopy. *Gastrointest Endosc*. 2002;55:826–831.
85. Lightdale J, Goldmann D, Feldman H, et al. Microstream capnography improves patient monitoring during moderate sedation: a randomized, controlled trial. *Pediatrics*. 2006;117:e1170–e1178.
86. Cote C, Notterman D, Karl H. Adverse sedation events in pediatrics: a critical incident analysis of contributing factors. *Pediatrics*. 2000;105:805–814.
87. American Association of Anesthesiologists. Statement on nonoperating room anesthetizing locations. Last amended on October 16, 2013. Available at: http://www.asahq.org/quality-and-practice-management/standards-guidelines-and-related-resources/statement-on-nonoperating-room-anesthetizing-locations. Accessed on April 30, 2018.
88. Cote C, Wilson S, Work Group on Sedation. Guidelines for monitoring and management of pediatric patients during and after sedation for diagnostic and therapeutic procedures. *Pediatrics*. 2006;118:2587–2602.
89. American Society of Anesthesiologists. Standards for basic anesthetic monitoring. Available at: http://www.asahq.org/quality-and-practice-management/standards-guidelines-and-related-resources/standards-for-basic-anesthetic-monitoring. Accessed on April 30, 2018.
90. Voscopoulos C, Brayanov J, Ladd D, Lalli M, Panasyuk A, Freeman J. Special article: evaluation of a novel noninvasive respiration monitor providing continuous measurement of minute ventilation in ambulatory subjects in a variety of clinical scenarios. *Anesth Analg*. 2013;117(1):91–100.
91. Voscopoulos CJ, MacNabb CM, Brayanov J, et al. The evaluation of a non-invasive respiratory volume monitor in surgical patients undergoing elective surgery with general anesthesia. *J Clin Monit Comput*. 2015;29(2):223–30.
92. Galvagno SM Jr, Duke PG, Eversole DS, George EE. Evaluation of respiratory volume monitoring (RVM) to detect respiratory compromise in advance of pulse oximetry and help minimize false desaturation alarms. *J Trauma Acute Care Surg*. 2016;81(5 suppl 2 Proceedings of the 2015 Military Health System Research Symposium):S162–S170.
93. Voscopoulos CJ, MacNabb CM, Freeman J, Galvagno SM Jr, Ladd D, George E. Continuous noninvasive respiratory volume monitoring for the identification of patients at risk for opioid-induced respiratory depression and obstructive breathing patterns. *J Trauma Acute Care Surg*. 2014;77(3 suppl 2):S208–S215.
94. Voscopoulos C, Theos K, Tillmann Hein HA, George E. A risk stratification algorithm using non-invasive respiratory volume monitoring to improve safety when using post-operative opioids in the PACU. *J Clin Monit Comput*. 2017;31(2):417–426.

4 | ANESTHETIC TECHNIQUES

DENNIS GRECH, MD, LAURENCE M. HAUSMAN, MD

INTRODUCTION

Anesthetic techniques for procedures performed outside the traditional operating room (OOOR) are as varied as the surgeries themselves and wholly dependent on the equipment available at each specific location as well as any patient comorbidities that may exist. General anesthesia (GA) may be delivered with or without an anesthesia machine, monitored anesthesia care (MAC) with or without infusion pumps, and regional anesthesia (RA) with or without a nerve stimulator (NS) or ultrasound (US). Whichever technique is chosen, safety considerations are paramount, and perioperative monitoring must always be consistent with American Society of Anesthesiologists (ASA) guidelines (see Appendix 3 for a list of useful ASA documents).

The OOOR procedures are widely varied and include elective office-based anesthetics and emergency room ones, endoscopic retrograde cholangiopancreatographies (ERCPs) in the gastroenterology suite, and emergency interventions in the invasive radiology department. Most of these locations have limited postanesthesia care unit (PACU) capabilities, so both rapid return to baseline functioning and the ability to discharge a comfortable patient are important goals with rare exceptions, which are discussed in this chapter. This chapter focuses on the many anesthetic options available to the OOOR anesthesiology practitioner.

There are some important caveats concerning any anesthetic provided OOOR setting. If a non-GA technique is planned, the anesthesia professional must be ready for conversion to GA at any time. The proceduralist may need the patient to follow commands one minute, and then need the patient promptly to be unresponsive for the next procedural stimulation. The anesthesia provider should be prepared to provide a rapid change in depth of anesthesia. This is complicated by the fact that many of the OOOR procedures are new and evolving, and the anesthetic requirements may not be known. Furthermore, some proceduralists may not yet be used to working with an anesthesia professional and may not communicate effectively about the procedure and how it is progressing.

DEPTH OF SEDATION

It must be appreciated that sedation, as defined by the ASA, exists as a continuum from minimal, moderate, and deep sedation through GA (Table 4.1).[1] Minimal sedation is characterized by anxiolysis. The minimally sedated patient should maintain a normal response to verbal stimulation. The patient's airway should remain unaffected, as should both the patient's cardiovascular function and the patient's ability to spontaneously ventilate. Moderate sedation, formerly known as conscious sedation, is characterized by a sedated patient who retains *purposeful* response to both verbal and tactile stimulation. It is important to understand that reflex withdrawal from a painful stimulus is *not* considered a purposeful response, but rather a purposeful

TABLE 4.1. Continuum of Depth of Sedation Definition of General Anesthesia and Levels of Sedation/Analgesia

	MINIMAL SEDATION (ANXIOLYSIS)	MODERATE SEDATION/ ("CONSCIOUS SEDATION")	DEEP SEDATION/ ANALGESIA	GENERAL ANESTHESIA
Responsiveness	Normal response to verbal stimulation	Purposeful[a] response to verbal or tactile stimulation	Purposeful[a] response following repeated or painful stimulation	Unarousable even with painful stimulation
Airway	Unaffected	No intervention required	Intervention may be required	Intervention often required
Spontaneous ventilation	Unaffected	Adequate	May be inadequate	Frequently inadequate
Cardiovascular function	Unaffected	Usually maintained	Usually maintained	May be impaired

[a]Reflex withdrawal from a painful stimulus is *not* considered a purposeful response.

SOURCE: Based on "Continuum of Depth of Sedation" of the American Society of Anesthesiologists. A copy of the full text can be obtained from the ASA, 520 N. Northwest Highway, Park Ridge, IL 60068-2573.

response occurs when the patient is asked to raise an arm and is able to perform the appropriate action. Similarly, the patient can answer yes/no questions. Typically, the patient will be lying still with eyes closed. As with minimal sedation, no interventions should be required to assist the patient in maintaining a patent airway. Spontaneous ventilation should remain adequate, and cardiovascular function is usually maintained.

Similar to the moderately sedated patient, a deeply sedated one also displays *purposeful* responses to repeated or painful stimulation. However, he or she may require an intervention to maintain a patent airway. Spontaneous ventilation may be inadequate, but cardiovascular function is usually maintained. GA is characterized by a patient who is unconscious and is unresponsive, even to noxious stimulation. Maintaining a patent airway will often, but not necessarily, require an intervention. Spontaneous ventilation is frequently inadequate. Cardiovascular function may also be impaired in the patient undergoing GA. "If the patient loses consciousness and the ability to respond purposefully, the anesthesia care is a general anesthetic, irrespective of whether airway instrumentation is required."[1]

MONITORED ANESTHESIA CARE

Monitored anesthesia care does not correlate to depth of sedation. It simply refers to sedation that is delivered or supervised by a qualified anesthesia professional. It can range from minimal to deep sedation but does not include RA or GA. Many procedures performed OOOR are amenable to MAC with the use of supplemental local anesthesia, often provided by the surgeon. Other procedures can be performed under MAC without the use of supplemental local anesthesia. Such procedures include colonoscopies, upper gastrointestinal endoscopies, and magnetic resonance imaging (MRI) or computerized tomographic (CT) studies.

When selecting a depth of sedation for a particular procedure, it is vital that the anesthesia provider have the proper training, licensing, credentials, as well as supplies and equipment to rescue the patient from the next deeper level of sedation than what is planned. This is important because patients often drift from one anesthetic depth to another. Movement along the sedation continuum is usually a desirable condition because the patient will need to be more deeply sedated during painful parts of the procedure (i.e., injection of local anesthesia) and less deeply sedated during others. There is no particular dose of any medication that can reliably predict a specific anesthetic depth. Each patient will have a unique response to a given dose of a drug. Therefore, vigilance by the anesthesia provider is critical in maintaining the patient at the desired depth of sedation.

Providing a patient with MAC is truly a balancing act—attempting to provide the perfect depth of sedation to meet the ever-changing level of surgical stimulation. On one end of the spectrum is the patient who is oversedated, who may become disinhibited and uncooperative. This disinhibited state may actually mislead the anesthesia provider to further deepen the level of sedation (thinking that the patient may be inadequately sedated) and may ultimately result in the delivery of GA. Unrecognized oversedation can lead to hypoxia, hypercarbia, and cardiovascular instability. On the other end of the spectrum is the undersedated patient. Similar to the oversedated patient, the undersedated one may also become uncooperative. This patient's behavior may be due to pain from the surgical procedure. Pain when left untreated will often lead to tachycardia, hypertension, and myocardial ischemia. Uncontrolled sudden movements by the undersedated patient may lead to intraoperative motion, making the surgeon frustrated and the surgical procedure impossible.

Is MAC safer than GA? The answer to this question is not certain. A recent review of the ASA closed claims database revealed several important points regarding the relative safety of MAC.[2] Although MAC claims were fewer than GA claims (121 vs. 1519), 40% of the MAC claims were for death or permanent brain injury. This percentage is similar to that for GA. Most patient injuries during MAC arose from patient oversedation, which resulted in respiratory depression and hypoxic injury. The median payout from a MAC injury was $254,000 as compared to $140,000 for GA. The authors concluded that perioperative physiologic monitoring, vigilance, and early resuscitation during MAC can prevent many of the perioperative injuries.

There are potential benefits to using MAC when appropriate. By using fewer medications, such as muscle relaxants, neuromuscular reversal agents, and inhalational anesthetics, the incidence of postoperative nausea and vomiting (PONV) will decrease. Recovery time can be shorter after a sedation case than after GA, and patients undergoing MAC may be able to bypass the phase 1 PACU and proceed to either a phase 2 PACU or, in the case of an inpatient, their hospital room immediately following the procedure.[3]

Utilizing MAC over GA may shorten the average patient throughput time as anesthesia ready time (time to deliver anesthetic), emergence time (time to recover from anesthetic), and PACU time (time to meet discharge criteria) are all accelerated.[4]

A study released in 2016 compared GA and MAC. The authors focused on PACU arrival time, time until oral intake, hemodynamic parameters, and discharge from the PACU. The times from PACU admission to fluid intake (mean ± SD; 79 ± 34 vs. 99 ± 33 minutes, $p = .034$) and ambulation (77 ± 45 vs. 109 ± 45 minutes, $p = .013$) were significantly shorter in the MAC group ($n = 29$) than in the GA group ($n = 29$). Average systolic blood pressure (SBP) was significantly lower (89 ± 11 vs. 99 ± 16 mm Hg, $p = .011$), and the incidence of hypotension (SBP < 70 mm Hg) was higher (52 vs. 21%, $p = .014$) in the GA group than in the MAC group during anesthesia. In the PACU, there was no difference in pain visual analog scale (VAS) score between the GA and MAC groups. The percentages of patients with nausea and sore throat were significantly higher in the GA group than in the MAC group.[5]

THE PHARMACOLOGY OF MONITORED ANESTHESIA CARE

There are many classes of drugs that can be used in the delivery of MAC. The ideal MAC drug would be associated with fast onset and a short duration of action, would have no side effects, and would be inexpensive. Unfortunately, no such individual drug exists. Commonly used drugs include hypnotics (propofol); benzodiazepines (midazolam and diazepam); α_2-agonists (clonidine and dexmedetomidine); opioids (fentanyl and remifentanil); and ketamine. Most anesthesia providers will use these agents in a combination that will work synergistically and limit the negative side effects of each. Specific dose recommendations appear in Table 4.2. Newer medications such as intravenous acetaminophen and intravenous ibuprofen give practitioners a wider choice of medications when avoiding traditional opioid-based pain regimens. Remimazolam, an ultrashort-acting benzodiazepine, is awaiting approval by the Food and Drug Administration (FDA).[6]

Propofol, a diisopropyl phenol molecule, has long been a mainstay of ambulatory anesthesia because of its desirable pharmacokinetics and pharmacodynamics. It has a rapid onset (approximately one arm-brain circulation time) and, because of rapid redistribution, has a short clinical duration of action (approximately 15 minutes).[7] Even after long infusions, the context-sensitive half-time of propofol remains shorter than other intravenous drugs (except remifentanil).[8] In addition to its hypnotic properties, propofol has an intrinsic antiemetic effect. Propofol may cause a burning sensation on injection or elicit an allergic reaction. It is also associated with bradycardia and respiratory depression and supports microbial growth. This drug can be used alone or in combination with other agents by intermittent boluses or continuous infusion.

Unfortunately, OOOR delivery of anesthesia opens the door to diversion. Working alone and being far from colleagues creates an environment favorable for diversion. Additionally, most remote locations lack the protocols or devices for controlled substance containment or reconciliation. Diversion can be deterred by using Pyxis machines, qualitative waste sinks, and trained nursing staff who assist in reconciliation and wasting of medications with abuse potential.

Originally, propofol was not categorized as an addictive medication.[9] Recent animal study findings, however, supported propofol as having abuse potential.[10] A subanesthetic propofol dose has induced paradoxical excitement. The nucleus accumbens, located in the basal forebrain, is often implicated in addiction and the processes that lead to addiction. It is well known that the nucleus accumbens is activated by ethanol and nicotine.[11] In 2011, a landmark discovery was made that established propofol as an activator of the nucleus accumbens, just like ethanol and nicotine. Therefore, propofol can be considered habit forming.[10]

Reconciliation of propofol inventory and the use of Pyxis machines or other devices should be implemented to protect health care workers with access to this and other habit-forming medications.

Midazolam has replaced the older benzodiazepines in clinical practice because of its superior pharmacokinetics and pharmacodynamics. It has a rapid onset of action (1–3 minutes), and although its elimination half-life is 3.4–11 hours,[12] its clinical duration of action at small doses is short (approximately 30 minutes). These times provide a significant clinical improvement over the older benzodiazepines, which possess both longer onsets and longer half-lives. Benzodiazepines are used for their ability to provide anxiolysis and anterograde amnesia. All can cause respiratory depression, especially when used in combination with opioids, and can be associated with prolonged recovery when used in large doses.

Remimazolam is an ultrashort-acting benzodiazepine.[13,14] The ultrashort duration of action is achieved by adding a carboxylic ester linkage. This type of linkage is degraded in the serum by nonspecific blood esterases.[15] This property makes it ideal for conscious sedation for procedures of short duration. Remimazolam was found to be faster acting and to degrade more rapidly than midazolam.[16,17] Additionally, phase Ib dose-finding studies for procedural sedation demonstrated patients recovered faster from remimazolam than midazolam.[6]

Ketamine is a phencyclidine derivative that, in addition to its anesthetic properties, is a potent analgesic.[18] However, it is associated with increased saliva production and thus requires the concomitant administration of an antisialogogue agent. A significant benefit of ketamine is that it does not cause PONV or respiratory depression. Common side effects of ketamine include hallucinations and dysphoria, which can be ameliorated with the administration of a benzodiazepine or propofol.[19,20] This drug combination has been reported in both pediatric and adult anesthesia literature.[21–23] Other side effects of ketamine include increase in intracranial pressure, tachycardia, and hypertension.

TABLE 4.2. Reference for Induction, Bolus, and Infusion Rates of Commonly Used MAC and GA Anesthetics in Adults

AGENT	INDUCTION FOR GA	BOLUS DOSES FOR MAC	INFUSION (MAC OR GA)
Dexmedetomidine	0.5–1 μg/kg (over 10 min)		0.2–0.7 μg/kg/h, not to exceed 24 h
Fentanyl	50–100 μg/kg for single-agent GA	1–2 μg/kg for sedation	1–3 μg/kg/h
Ketamine	1–2 mg/kg	0.25–1 mg/kg for sedation	1–2 mg/kg/h
Midazolam	0.3–0.35 mg/kg for single-agent GA	10–20 μg/kg	0.02–0.1 mg/kg/h
Propofol	1.5–2.5 mg/kg for single-agent GA	0.25–0.5 mg/kg	25–200 μg/kg/min
Remifentanil		0.5–1 μg/kg	0.02–0.3 μg/kg min

GA, general anesthesia; MAC, monitored anesthesia care.

Ketamine can be used by intermittent boluses or as an infusion. Friedberg described a regimen for facial resurfacing using a laser that begins with a midazolam bolus of 2–4 mg IV, followed by a propofol infusion. After the patient is anesthetized (loss of both lid reflex and response to verbal command), a bolus of ketamine (50 mg) is given. After waiting 2 minutes, the surgeon can inject the local anesthetic while the patient remains immobile and amnestic.[24] Once the local anesthetic has been injected, the propofol infusion can be decreased. The patient will likely maintain spontaneous respiration, so supplemental oxygen can be avoided. Supplemental oxygen is problematic because it will support combustion and poses a risk of fire with the use of electrocautery.[25]

Dexmedetomidine, the dextroenantiomer of medetomidine, is a selective α_2-agonist drug that was originally approved for use by the FDA in 1999 for short-term sedation of patients in the intensive care unit. Its application for MAC has also been widely reported.[26–29] It works at the presynaptic α_2-receptors, inhibiting the release of norepinephrine in a negative-feedback mechanism.[30] Because of the presence of α_2-receptors in the central nervous system, dexmedetomidine possesses anxiolytic, sedative, and amnestic qualities with minimal respiratory depression and no PONV. These α_2-receptors are also present in the dorsal horn of the spinal cord, conferring analgesic properties to dexmedetomidine. The effects on the sympathetic nervous system can cause a decrease in cardiac output, with bradycardia and hypotension, most commonly after rapid administration.[31] Vasoconstriction at high or rapid doses has also been reported. It has a relatively short half-life of approximately 2–3 hours.

In a study by Candiotti et al.,[26] dexmedetomidine was used in conjunction with midazolam and fentanyl for MAC. Patients were randomized into one of three treatment groups. One group received dexmedetomidine, 0.1 μg/kg; the second group was given dexmedetomidine at 0.5 μg/kg; and the final group was given a placebo. All groups received midazolam titrated to a level of sedation as measured by the Observer's Assessment of Alertness/Sedation Scale (OAA/S). The reported dosages of both supplemental drugs (midazolam and fentanyl) were markedly decreased by the use of dexmedetomidine. In this study, patients who had received 1 μg/kg of dexmedetomidine had less respiratory depression and anxiety and less need for postoperative analgesics, while having higher patient satisfaction scores than did the placebo group.[26]

The use of local anesthesia and RA should always be considered for postoperative analgesia, either alone or in conjunction with GA. The use of local anesthesia or RA in addition to GA minimizes the amount of anesthetic required, thus hastening patient recovery and minimizing the need for opioid and its associated PONV.

Nonsteroidal anti-inflammatory drugs (NSAIDs), specifically including cyclooxygenase 2 (COX-2) drugs such as celecoxib, are another important component of postoperative analgesia. It must however be appreciated that NSAIDs may not always be able to provide enough pain relief.

Perioperative use of NSAIDs for pain and control of inflammation has increased. Their place in multimodal pain management is advantageous, as NSAIDs do not cause sedation or PONV.[32] Recent data support the use of intravenous ibuprofen perioperatively as coagulation disorders and nephrotoxicity have not been associated with its use.[33] Additionally, analysis of its use in elderly patients suggests no dose adjustment is needed.[33] A subsequent multicenter study has shown that intravenous ibuprofen increases quality of recovery, decreases postsurgical fatigue, and has an attenuated surgical stress response.[34]

Although intravenous acetaminophen is relatively new in the United States, the same formulation has been used extensively since 2002 in over 80 countries.[35] Evidence from randomized clinical trials has found intravenous acetaminophen to be a safe, effective, and well-tolerated analgesic for acute postoperative pain after a variety of surgical procedures.[36,37]

The popularity and acceptance of acetaminophen are attributed to its relative safety and effectiveness.[38] Acetaminophen is not associated with postoperative bleeding, gastric mucosal damage, dyspepsia, or renal injury, as seen with many NSAIDs. It does not cause the respiratory depression, nausea, vomiting, constipation, urinary retention, or sedation seen with opioids.[39,40] The most important safety concern with acetaminophen is the potential for hepatotoxicity when it is used at higher than recommended doses (>4000 mg/d for adult patients).[39,41] Compared to oral acetaminophen, intravenous acetaminophen reduces initial hepatic exposure by approximately 2-fold because of the lack of first-pass metabolism,[39,42] Reduced hepatic exposure of intravenous acetaminophen thus improves its safety profile However, intravenous acetaminophen is contraindicated in patients with a history of moderate-to-severe liver disease, such as active hepatitis, chronic hepatitis B or C, or severe active liver disease.[41]

As it lacks the commonly experienced side effects of NSAID or opioid medications, intravenous acetaminophen is an important part of a best practice multimodal, nonopioid basis pain management plan.[43–45] Side effects from intravenous acetaminophen are *rare*. When present, the most common are nausea, headache, and insomnia.[41] Because of its more favorable risk/benefit profile, acetaminophen may be considered as a foundation analgesic in multimodal pain management.[43–45]

A study compared intravenous and orally administered acetaminophen concentrations in the blood at a fixed point after surgery. The authors determined that therapeutic levels were achieved in 96% with the group receiving intravenous acetaminophen and in 67% in the oral group.[39,45] (Consistent serum levels will increase the number of patients who can completely avoid opioid administration for therapeutic pain management. This will lead to earlier discharge from the PACU for same-day surgery patients, as more patients will have their pain controlled after surgery.)

Remifentanil is an ultrashort-acting opioid that can be used as an infusion or as a bolus. This synthetic drug is quickly hydrolyzed by tissue esterases. Because of this and its very short context-sensitive half-time, remifentanil does not accumulate and redistribute within the body, leading to a short duration of action (approximately 5 to 6 minutes), even after long infusion times (up to 8 hours).[46] The benefit of these pharmacokinetics and pharmacodynamics is that remifentanil can be used to provide intense analgesia for the painful parts of the procedure and its effect will be eliminated quickly thereafter. Remifentanil is associated with respiratory depression, skeletal muscle rigidity, nausea, and vomiting.

Fentanyl, an older synthetic opioid, also has a rapid onset of 1–3 minutes; it has a peak effect of 5–10 minutes and an alpha elimination half-life of 18 minutes.[47] Fentanyl is highly lipophilic and redistributes quickly. Like all opioids, fentanyl can cause respiratory depression as well as PONV and itching. Like remifentanil, fentanyl can also be used as an infusion. Unlike remifentanil, fentanyl has a long context-sensitive half-time. Thus, long infusion times are associated with significant accumulation within the body and prolonged recovery times.[8]

When selecting which drugs to use, the non-operating room practitioner must determine the needs of the particular surgery, the location of the surgery both inside and outside the hospital, and the profile and cost of the individual drugs. No anesthetic technique for providing MAC is ideal or devoid of risk. Regardless of drug(s) utilized, the patient may at any point during the anesthetic inadvertently move along the sedation continuum into a deeper-than-intended depth of sedation. The practitioner must always be prepared to rescue the patient from a deeper level of sedation and to alter the anesthetic plan intraoperatively should the clinical situation change.

GENERAL ANESTHESIA

General anesthesia is frequently the technique of choice for an OOOR procedure.[48] The decision to perform GA is based on a number of factors, including the patient preference, the procedure, and the surgeon. There are some patients who are not amenable to anything other than GA. They might be severely "needle phobic" and may require an inhalation induction to secure an intravenous line. Others may be uncooperative or unable to lie still secondary to chronic pain syndromes, and others may desire complete amnesia for the surgical event. Although amnesia under GA can never be guaranteed (incidence of awareness of 0.1%–0.2%),[23,24] it is intuitive that the chance of successful amnesia is higher with GA than with MAC. In addition to patient-specific factors, there are some procedures that may not be amenable to anything other than GA. Finally, there are surgeon-specific issues. The surgeon may request a GA, or a particular surgeon may not be proficient in the use of local anesthesia.

When selecting a type of GA for an OOOR procedure, similar factors used to make a decision regarding drug selection for a MAC case must be considered. The induction of anesthesia (either intravenous or inhalational) should be rapid, and the patients should awaken quickly at the termination of surgery; there should be minimal postoperative pain, nausea, or vomiting; and the patient should be discharge ready quickly, to home or inpatient bed, using objective discharge criteria. Furthermore, cost is always an issue.

Wherever anesthetics that trigger malignant hyperthermia (MH) or depolarizing muscle relaxants are administered, dantrolene, and other supplies necessary for the treatment of MH, should readily available.[49] Dantrolene should be stored at room temperature. It is to be reconstituted with sterile water that is stored in a warming cabinet at 35°C–40°C. Current standards of care state that dantrolene should be administered within 10 minutes. This is extended from the 5-minute recommendation as medical facilities often have several scattered procedure rooms. Therefore, it is impractical to maintain dantrolene and the required supplies at each OOOR location.[49]

An alternative to the flushing technique has become available to clear triggering agents from an anesthesia machine. Activated charcoal canisters, placed in the inspiratory and expiratory limbs of the breathing circuit, absorb all anesthetic gases. This prevents residual triggering agents from reaching the patient. The charcoal filter system reduces the machine's volatile anesthetic concentrations to less than 5 parts per million (ppm) in less than 2 minutes. The charcoal canisters can maintain triggering gas levels to less than 5 ppm for 12 hours.[50,51]

Total intravenous anesthesia (TIVA) is a popular choice for OOOR procedures. This usually consists of propofol as the hypnotic component, often used in conjunction with fentanyl or remifentanil as the analgesic component. All three of these drugs can be given by intermittent bolus or infusion. Mathews and coworkers found that remifentinil 0.085 μg/kg per minute can substitute for nitrous oxide 66%.[52] Advantages of TIVA over inhalation anesthesia include avoidance of the need for gas scavenging and a reduced incidence of PONV. Since the availability of the newer less-soluble inhalation agents (e.g., desflurane and sevoflurane), many authors have compared recovery times from these agents with the recovery time after TIVA using a propofol infusion.[53,54]

Recently, Gupta et al.[55] conducted a meta-analysis of all publications looking at this and reported an overall faster recovery from desflurane when compared to either isoflurane- or propofol-based anesthetics. Recovery was also found to be faster from sevoflurane when compared to isoflurane. However, there was more PONV as well as postdischarge nausea and vomiting in the isoflurane groups compared to the propofol ones; isoflurane may not be the best choice of inhalation agent in OOOR locations for these considerations. Overall, the inhalation agent groups required more antiemetic treatment than did the propofol groups.[55]

The issue of PONV is quite important in any anesthetic practice, and those procedures performed in the OOOR setting are no exception. PONV may lead to delayed discharge or even result in unplanned admission to a hospital for the ambulatory patient. More than just an annoyance, PONV is often feared more by the patient than postoperative pain.[56] From a patient safety standpoint, uncontrolled retching postoperatively, often associated with nausea, can cause a precipitous increase in central venous pressure. This could lead to bleeding, especially after facial cosmetic surgery, and may even necessitate an emergency reoperation. There are many well-known surgical, anesthetic, and patient risk factors for the development of PONV, such as young age, female gender, nonsmoking, history of motion sickness or previous PONV, breast or laparoscopic or plastic procedures, and duration of surgery.[57] Risk factors must be considered preoperatively, and the use of prophylactic antiemetics, such as dexamethasone, ondansetron, or transdermal scopolamine, should be considered. Combination therapy has been consistently found to be more effective than single-medication regimens.[58,59]

The ASA Task Force on Acute Pain Management advocates that unless contraindicated, patients should receive an around-the-clock regimen of nonopioid analgesics as first-line agents and for opioids to be used as adjunctive agents.[60] In fact, there are many combinations of non-opioid analgesics in the anesthesiologist's armamentarium, and different pre-, intra- and post-procedure strategies and protocols can be implemented to encourage multimodal approaches to pain management.[61]

Health systems across the United States and Europe have identified certain treatment protocols that improve patient outcomes following surgery. The protocols vary and include measures like maintaining normothermia during surgery, avoiding opioid use, and providing early postoperative ambulation. When available, many hospitals and anesthesia groups incorporated the protocols into their practice.

The enhanced recovery after surgery (ERAS) pathway was designed to improve the quality of recovery and overall outcome of patients undergoing colorectal surgery. ERAS includes administering medications 2 hours before surgery to limit inflammation, PONV, and pain. The goal is to enable early ambulation, which enables the patient to return to daily premorbid activities faster.[62] Although designed for major high-risk surgeries, the ERAS protocols can be modified and applied to any surgical intervention.[63,64] Having patients drink a carbohydrate-rich clear liquid 2 hours prior to surgery and administering gabapentin, acetaminophen, and scopolamine patch are designed to prevent PONV, avoid postoperative pain, eliminate perioperative dehydration, and avoid the catabolic state.[65]

LARYNGEAL MASK AIRWAY VERSUS TRACHEAL TUBE

When performing GA, one may choose between securing the airway with a tracheal tube (TT) or placing a laryngeal mask airway (LMA). The TT is the classic standard for airway security and protection; however, the LMA confers several advantages. Its placement is relatively simple and does not require direct laryngoscopy, thus eliminating the sympathetic response associated with this maneuver. There is minimal risk of damage to the teeth and oropharynx as there is with the insertion of a rigid laryngoscope. Because the LMA is much better tolerated by the patient emerging from anesthesia than a TT, emergence can be smoother, and opioid requirements are often less.

The LMA has become more commonly used even during surgeries that cause blood accumulation in the oropharynx, such as adenotonsillectomies and rhinoplasties.[66] Although some believe that an LMA is helpful in preventing copious amounts of blood in the oropharynx from entering the stomach, it still must be appreciated that it may not prevent aspiration of blood into the lungs. An LMA should not be used in patients who are at risk for aspiration. Although patients at such a risk should not be considered an appropriate candidate for an office-based procedure[67] (a subset of the OOOR locations), these patients will likely present to other OOOR anesthetizing venues. An LMA should also not be used if it obscures the surgical field, as in the case of intraoral surgery. It should be appreciated that a conventional LMA may become dislodged intraoperatively if the patient becomes "light," if the surgeon moves the patient's head or changes the patient's body position during the case, or if surgery around the head and neck is planned. The concern about dislodgement is much less with the flexible (armored-tube) LMAs.

Monitoring depth of anesthesia can be considered, particularly if a total intravenous technique is planned. One such depth of anesthesia monitor is the BIS (bispectral index) monitor (BIS Aspect Medical Systems). On a scale of 1–100, an awake patient typically has a score of 100. As the patient becomes sedated, the BIS value decreases, and a score of 40–60 represents a patient under GA. In a recent meta-analysis of the existing clinical trials involving BIS monitoring, Punjasawadwong reported that utilizing the monitor during GA resulted in the intraoperative use of somewhat less propofol and volatile agents, 1.3 mg/kg per hour and 0.17 minimal alveolar concentration equivalents, respectively. Recovery times were decreased as well, with time to eye opening by 2.43 minutes, time to response to verbal command by 2.28 minutes, and time to extubation by 3.05 minutes. However, there was no improvement in the time to home discharge readiness. In addition, the BIS decreased the incidence of intraoperative awareness in the high-risk patient subset.[68] When analyzing whether this additional monitor will improve both patient care and efficiency of the OOOR anesthetic, cost of the monitor (approximately $10,000) as well as of the disposable head electrode (approximately $12–$15) must be considered. Also, for some procedures, the placement of the head electrode may be in the surgical field, thus limiting its utility.

THE REALITY OF GENERAL ANESTHESIA IN THE NON–OPERATING ROOM LOCATION

In a hospital operating room, many anesthetic agents and a variety of technologies are readily available. However, in the non–operating room setting, space (size), use of non–purpose-built locations, as well as cost may limit the technology readily available. An off-site location may not have state-of-the-art equipment. Although the anesthesia machine must not be obsolete,[69] it may not have vaporizers for newer inhalational agents. If there is no built-in gas-scavenging system, activated charcoal canisters can be considered for volatile agent scavenging. Alternatively, suction may be used for scavenging. In the absence of a reliable scavenging system, TIVA becomes the best alternative for the delivery of GA. If an infusion pump is not available, an inhalation-based anesthetic may be preferable. The anesthesia provider must be adept at performing GA under a variety of conditions.

REGIONAL ANESTHESIA

There is little written about the use of RA in OOOR locations. Hausman et al. described 123 peripheral nerve blocks (PNBs) and 2 neuraxial blocks, among 242 anesthetics administered in an orthopedic surgical office-based practice. The office was equipped with a separate procedure room, the standard ASA monitors, an anesthesia machine, and a resuscitation cart with a defibrillator. Blocks utilized included interscalene, femoral/three-in-one, popliteal, and infraclavicular. All blocks were performed with NS techniques, except axillary blocks, which were accomplished using the transarterial approach, and ankle blocks, which were placed by identifying superficial anatomic landmarks. In this study, there was one persistent paresthesia and one femoral neuropathy, both of which resolved. There were no episodes of dyspnea, local anesthetic toxicity, or unplanned admissions for pain or PONV.[70] This study was conducted in conjunction with an academic medical center, and each attending physician performing the blocks was accompanied by a clinical anesthesiology level 3 (CA-3) resident. This senior resident was able to expedite the process by performing a history and physical and placing an intravenous line and monitors so that as soon as the patient was brought to the PACU, the attending could immediately either place or supervise the placement of the next block. This staffing model minimized turnover and maximized the time available for the block to begin to work. Extrapolating to other practice models, this study underscores that when RA is performed in a OOOR location, it is important to have staff that supports this effort and is willing to both help expedite turnovers and lend a hand to inject agents, if necessary.

Since the mastery of PNBs frequently does not occur during residency, the successful incorporation of blocks into practice in any anesthetizing location requires that the anesthesiologist critically evaluate the practice, looking for blocks that fill specific needs and choosing techniques that offer a high likelihood of success. Moreover, the recent trend has been toward the use of US in placing blocks. The development of proficiency in US-guided blocks requires an entirely new skill set for practitioners. First, one must learn to operate the US machine and then use it to identify anatomy. Second, one must be able to use both hands simultaneously (one holding the US transducer and the other holding the block needle), while watching the display screen, and manipulate the needle into the nerve sheath. Third, it is necessary to learn to identify patterns of local anesthetic spread that are associated with the optimal plexus blockade. This process requires both a financial commitment for the cost of equipment as well as a time commitment to learn the techniques, which may require attendance in both lectures and workshops. Several websites are available with instructions, diagrams, and videos that serve as excellent guides to both US and NS techniques (http://www.usra.ca, http://www.nysora.com).

Local anesthetics should be chosen to minimize onset times and prevent procedure delays and complications. The desired duration of action and degree of motor blockade required should also be considered. For example, a patient undergoing a neuroplasty at the wrist (carpal tunnel) requires dense anesthesia. This can be accomplished rapidly with an intravenous regional anesthetic (IVRA). If a brachial plexus block is chosen, one must remember that an insensate extremity may place the patient at unnecessary risk for injury secondary to the loss of protective reflex of pain or proprioception, especially after a procedure that does not cause much postoperative discomfort. Combining local anesthetics to decrease onset and increase duration of analgesia results in unpredictable blockade characteristics.[71] The effect of alkalinization of agents on the speed of onset of the block is variable. It has been shown to offer no advantage in perivascular blocks with 0.5% bupivacaine[72] but improves both onset and quality of analgesia in axillary blocks with 1.25% mepivacaine[73] and in femoral and sciatic blocks with 2% mepivacaine.[74]

Adding sodium bicarbonate to lidocaine has been shown to have no effect on the onset of axillary block,[75] and in rats it has been shown to decrease both the intensity and the duration of the block.[76]

Practitioners who are using amide local anesthetics should consider having a 20% lipid infusion available, as it has been shown to reverse local anesthetic systemic toxicity (now referred to as LAST) associated with the intravascular injection of amide agents.[76–78] Directions for the administration of lipid infusion in the advent of a local anesthetic-induced cardiac arrest appear in Box 4.1.[79]

BOX 4.1 PRACTICE ADVISORY ON TREATMENT OF LOCAL ANESTHETIC SYSTEMIC TOXICITY

For Patients Experiencing Signs or Symptoms of Local Anesthetic Systemic Toxicity (LAST)

- Get help
- Initial focus
  - *Airway management*: ventilate with 100% oxygen
  - *Seizure suppression*: benzodiazepines are preferred
  - *Basic and advanced cardiac life support (BLS/ACLS)* may require prolonged effort
- Infuse 20% lipid emulsion (values in parentheses are for a 70-kg patient)
  - *Bolus 1.5 mL/kg (lead body mass) IV over 1 min (~100 mL)*
  - *Continuous infusion at 0.25 mL/kg/min (~18 mL/min; adjust by roller clamp)*
  - *Repeat bolus once or twice for persistent cardiovascular collapse*
  - *Double the infusion rate to 0.5 mL/kg/min if blood pressure remains low*
  - *Continue infusion for at least 10 min after attaining circulatory stability*
  - *Recommend upper limit: approximately 10 mL/kg lipid emulsion over the first 30 min*
- Avoid vasopressin, calcium channel blockers, β-blockers, or local anesthetic
- Alert the nearest facility having cardiopulmonary bypass capability
- Avoid propofol in patients having signs of cardiovascular instability
- Post LAST events at http://www.lipidrescue.org

SOURCE: Reprinted with permission from Neal JM, Bernards CM, Butterworth JF, et al. American Society of Regional Anesthesia and Pain Medicine practice advisory on local anesthetic systemic toxicity. *Reg Anesth Pain Med.* 2010;35:152–161.

Several blocks that are useful in the OOOR setting are discussed next. These blocks may be performed in locations as diverse as the office-based setting to the emergency department or even the radiology suite. The use of NS or US techniques is discussed; for specific descriptions to perform each block, please consult RA sources.

MIDTARSAL ANKLE BLOCK

First described in 1986 by Sharrock et al.,[80] the midtarsal ankle block technique blocks the five nerves to the forefoot where they are most superficial, thus requiring a small total volume of local anesthetic (10–15 mL) and offering a high degree of success. It is particularly useful for podiatric procedures and has the advantage over a traditional ankle block in that the posterior tibial nerve is anesthetized. It is possible to use US to locate the posterior tibial artery in patients where palpation is difficult.[81]

POPLITEAL BLOCK

The block of the sciatic nerve in the popliteal fossa provides excellent anesthesia for foot and ankle surgeries, including repair of a ruptured Achilles tendon. The saphenous nerve must be blocked to provide complete anesthesia below the knee. The intertendinous approach described by Hadzic et al. uses an NS.[82] US-guided techniques can be performed from the posterior or lateral approaches. The use of US guidance has been associated with a significantly higher success rate of block over NS techniques at 30 minutes.[83]

To supply complete anesthesia below the knee, it is necessary to add a saphenous nerve block. We do not recommend performing a femoral block with a popliteal block in patients undergoing office-based or ambulatory procedures. This combination of blocks renders the leg flail and will put the patient at risk of falling.

FEMORAL BLOCK

The lumbar plexus gives rise to the femoral, lateral femoral cutaneous (LFC), and obturator nerves, which provide sensory and motor innervation to the leg above the knee. Using an NS technique, the femoral nerve (including saphenous) can be blocked with as little as 10 mL of local anesthetic. By increasing the volume, one can encourage the spread of local anesthesia along the psoas muscle and block the LFC and obturator nerves, creating a "three-in-one" block. With 20–25 mL of a long-acting local anesthetic, a superior postoperative analgesia for anterior cruciate ligament repair has been seen, when compared to the use of intra-articular local anesthetics.[84,85] A US approach to the femoral nerve can also be used.

FASCIA ILIACA BLOCK

The fascia iliaca block provides a more consistent block of the LFC nerve than the three-in-one block. There is a reported increase in the successful blocking of the LFC from 62% to 90%,[86] although the obturator nerve is not reliably anesthetized. This block requires neither NS nor elicitation of a paresthesia and can therefore be performed postoperatively to provide analgesia to a patient whose surgical site is encased in a bulky dressing or knee immobilizer.

AXILLARY BLOCK

Axillary blocks are indicated for surgeries of the hand and forearm. A transarterial approach to the axillary blockade is technically simple and usually quick to perform. When large volumes (50–60 mL) of anesthetic are used, this block is associated with a high success rate.[87] Supplemental blocks at the elbow or wrist can convert a partial block into a successful one. The use of US guidance has improved axillary block success and was associated with fewer complications (intravascular injection, transient neuropathy).[88]

INFRACLAVICULAR BLOCK

Infraclavicular block of the brachial plexus provides anesthesia for surgery of the forearm, wrist, hand, and elbow. An advantage of this block is that it can usually be performed with the patient's arm in any position, and it does not require abduction. A motor response of the wrist or hand at a current of less than 0.5 mA has been associated with reliable anesthesia with minimal complications or side effects.[89–91]

SUPRACLAVICULAR BLOCK

Supraclavicular blocks are performed at the level of the divisions where the nerves of the brachial plexus are closely approximated and prior to branching of nerves supplying the forearm, hand, and elbow. Anatomic techniques have resulted in up to 6% rates of pneumothorax, as they require walking posteriorly off the first rib until a paresthesia or response to NS is achieved. The use of US has brought this block back into favor, with two large case series reporting more than 94% success rate.[90,91]

INTERSCALENE BLOCK

Surgery of the shoulder is easily performed with interscalene block anesthesia. Multiple studies have reported that interscalene anesthesia provides excellent surgical conditions (analgesia and muscle relaxation), and patients experience less PONV and shorter nonsurgical intraoperative and PACU times than those who have GA.[92,93] In a study of 25 patients who had previous shoulder surgery with GA and who chose interscalene block for a second operation, 24 reported that they would prefer the regional technique if they required any subsequent procedures.[94] Although many practitioners choose GA with an LMA as the primary anesthetic for shoulder surgery, then perform an interscalene block with a lower concentration of amide anesthesia for postoperative analgesia, surgery of the shoulder can be successfully performed with an interscalene block and MAC sedation.[95]

INTRAVENOUS REGIONAL ANESTHESIA

For procedures of short duration below the elbow, IVRA remains an excellent anesthetic because it has a quick onset and is easy to perform. Lidocaine 0.5% remains the agent of choice because of its low toxicity, although ropivacaine 0.2% may provide brief postanesthetic analgesia.[96] A cost analysis study of anesthetic techniques for outpatient hand surgery found that IVRA conferred an approximately 30% cost savings over GA and brachial plexus blocks, which was secondary to shorter induction times, and lower anesthetic drug and equipment costs.[97]

NEURAXIAL ANESTHETICS FOR NON-OPERATING ROOM USE

Anorectal and urologic procedures are now being performed in offices and OOOR locations, and occasionally spinal anesthesia may be indicated. Spinal anesthetics with pencil-point atraumatic needles have led to a reduction in postdural puncture headaches, but the optimum local anesthetic with a favorable recovery profile and low incidence of transient neurologic symptoms (TNSs) has not been identified. Hyperbaric bupivacaine 7.5 mg has resulted in a 161 ± 12 minute time until out of bed and 186 ± 14 minutes to micturition.[98] The use of 45 mg of isobaric mepivacaine yielded similar results but a 7.4% incidence of TNSs.[99] Procaine 5% 75–100 mg (approved for spinal anesthesia) or 30- to 40-mg doses of intrathecal 2-chloroprocaine have been used for intrathecal anesthesia for procedures lasting approximately an hour.[100] Epidural anesthesia with 2-chlorprocaine provided similar discharge times to GA.[101]

Liposomal bupivacaine (Exparel) is long-acting bupivacaine enclosed in multivesicular liposomes.[102,103,104] The liposomes form a barrier, which prevents bupivacaine from immediate release after injection. A recent meta-analysis reviewed eight studies on liposomal bupivacaine for postoperative pain. Liposomal bupivacaine use showed adequate safety and tolerability and, compared to traditional protocols, was equivalent or more effective in postoperative pain management.[105] It has been approved for use in treatment of postoperative pain by local infiltration. Although the duration of action varied according to which study is referenced, most authors indicated that liposomal bupivacaine provided analgesia from 18 to 36 hours.[106]

PATIENT INSTRUCTIONS AND FOLLOW-UP

Whenever RA is performed, detailed instructions must be given to the patient, offering an expectation of the duration and extent of their block, the requirement to protect the insensate limb, the need to begin analgesic medications as sensation returns, prior to the experience of severe pain. Timely follow-up must be conducted to determine complete block resolution. Should any persistent neurologic deficit be discovered during a postoperative call, the patient should be reassured that it will likely resolve, and that the anesthesiologist's participation in the follow-up is ensured. Discussion of a postblock deficit with the surgeon should include a plan for neurologic evaluation. Regardless of the anesthetic technique used, a responsible escort must be present if the patient is to be discharged home.

CONCLUSION

Any type of anesthetic used in a freestanding ambulatory surgery center or hospital operating room can be used successfully in an OOOR location, but to do so safely, the anesthesiology provider must be aware of the risks and benefits of each technique and agent employed. Although cost will play a significant role in decision-making, patient safety should always be the driving force for every clinical decision. Anesthetics should be associated with rapid onset and recovery and minimal risk for the development of PONV and should allow the patient to be comfortably discharged home or back to the hospital room soon after the termination of the procedure. Current agents and techniques available to provide GA, RA, and MAC allow for the safe delivery of anesthesia care in all OOOR environments.

REFERENCES

1. American Society of Anesthesiologists. Continuum of Depth of Sedation: Definition of General Anesthesia and Levels of Sedation/Analgesia. Available at: http://www.asahq.org/quality-and-practice-management/standards-guidelines-and-related-resources/continuum-of-depth-of-sedation-definition-of-general-anesthesia-and-levels-of-sedation-analgesia. Last Amended 2014. Last accessed March 1, 2018.
2. Bhanaker SM, Posner KL, Cheney FW, et al. Injury and liability associated with monitored anesthesia care: a closed claims analysis. *Anesthesiology.* 2006;104:228–234.
3. Sato M, Shirakami G, Fukuda KJ. Comparison of general anesthesia and monitored anesthesia care in patients undergoing breast cancer surgery using a combination of ultrasound-guided thoracic paravertebral block and local infiltration anesthesia: a retrospective study *Anesthesiology.* 2016;30(2):244–251. doi:10.1007/s00540-015-2111-z.
4. White PF, Rawal S, Ngueyn J, Watkins A. PACU fast-tracking: an alternative to "bypassing" the PACU for facilitating the recovery process after ambulatory surgery. *J Perianesth Nurs.* 2003;18:247–253.
5. Sato M, Shirakami G, Fukuda KJ. Comparison of general anesthesia and monitored anesthesia care in patients undergoing breast cancer surgery using a combination of ultrasound-guided thoracic paravertebral block and local infiltration anesthesia: a retrospective study. *J Anesth.* 2016;302:244–251. doi:10.1007/s00540-015-2111.
6. Worthington MT, Antonik LJ, Goldwater DR, et al. A phase Ib, dose-finding study of multiple doses of remimazolam (CNS 7056) in volunteers undergoing colonoscopy. *Anesth Analg.* 2013;117:1093–100. doi:10.1213/ANE.0b013e3182a705ae.
7. Johnson KB, Egan TD. Principles of pharmacokinetics and pharmacodynamics: applied clinical pharmacology for the practitioner. In: Longnecker DE, Brown DL, Newman MF, et al., eds. *Anesthesiology.* New York, NY: McGraw-Hill; 2007:821–848.
8. Hughes MA, Glass PS, Jacobs JR. Context sensitive half-time in multicompartment pharmacokinetic models for intravenous anesthetic drugs. *Anesthesiology.* 1992;76:334–341.
9. Li KY, Xiao C, Xiong M, Delphin E, Ye JH. Nanomolar propofol stimulates glutamate transmission to dopamine neurons: a possible mechanism of abuse potential? *Pharmacol Exp Ther.* 2008;325(1):165–174. doi:10.1124/jpet.107.132472.
10. Xiong M, Li J, Ye JH, Zhang C. Upregulation of DeltaFosB by propofol in rat nucleus accumbens. *Anesth Analg.* 2011;113(2):259–264. doi:10.1213/ANE.0b013e318222af17.
11. Volman S, Lammel S, Margolis E, et al. New insights into the specificity and plasticity of reward and aversion encoding in the mesolimbic system. *J Neurosci.* 2013;33(45):17569–17576. doi:10.1523/JNEUROSCI.3250-13.2013.

12. Wagner BK, O'Hara DA. Pharmacokinetics and pharmacodynamics of sedatives and analgesics in the treatment of agitated and critically ill patients. *Clin Pharmacokinet.* 1997;33:426–453.
13. Tanious MK, Beutler SS, Kaye AD, Urman RD. New hypnotic drug development and pharmacologic considerations for clinical anesthesia. *Anesthesiol Clin.* 2017;35(2):e95–e113.
14. Wesolowski AM, Zaccagnino MP, Malapero RJ, Kaye AD, Urman RD. Remimazolam: pharmacologic considerations and clinical role in anesthesiology. *Pharmacotherapy.* 2016;36(9):1021–1027.
15. Goudra BG, Singhl PM. Remimazolam: the future of its sedative potential. *Saudi J Anaesth.* 2014;83:388–391. doi:10.4103/1658-354X.136627.
16. Rogers WK, McDowell TS. Remimazolam, a short-acting GABA (A) receptor agonist for intravenous sedation and/or anesthesia in day-case surgical and non-surgical procedures. *IDrugs.* 2010;13(12):929–937.
17. Saari TI, Uusi-Oukari M, Ahonen J, Olkkola KT. Enhancement of GABAergic activity: neuropharmacological effects of benzodiazepines and therapeutic use in anesthesiology. *Pharmacol Rev.* 2011;63(1):243–267. doi:10.1124/pr.110.002717.
18. Vadivelu N, Schermer E, Kodumudi V, Belani K, Urman RD, Kaye AD. Role of ketamine for analgesia in adults and children. *J Anaesthesiol Clin Pharmacol.* 2016;32(3):298–306.
19. Friedberg BL. Hypnotic doses of propofol block ketamine-induced hallucinations. *Plast Reconstr Surg.* 1993;91:96.
20. Vinnik CA. An intravenous dissociation technique for outpatient plastic surgery: tranquility in the office-surgical facility. *Plast Reconstr Surg.* 1981;67:799.
21. Friedberg BL. Propofol ketamine anesthesia for cosmetic surgery in the office suite. *Anesthesiol Clin.* 2003;41:39–50.
22. Tosun Z, Esmaoglu A, Coruh A. Propofol-ketamine vs. propofol-fentanyl combinations for deep sedation and analgesia in pediatric patients undergoing burn dressing changes. *Paediatr Anaesth.* 2008;18:43–47.
23. Sun MY, Canete JJ, Friel JC, et al. Combination propofol/ketamine is a safe an efficient anesthetic approach to anorectal surgery. *Dis Colon Rectum.* 2006;49:1059–1065.
24. Friedberg BL. Facial laser resurfacing with the propofol-ketamine technique: room air, spontaneous ventilation (RASV) anesthesia. *Dermatol Surg.* 1999;25:269.
25. The American Society of Anesthesiologists Taskforce on Operating Room Fires. Practice advisory for the prevention and management of operating room fires. *Anesthesiology.* 2008;108:786–801.
26. Candiotti K, Bekker A, Feldman M, et al. Safety and efficacy of dexmedetomidine for sedation during MAC anesthesia: a multi-center trial. *Anesthesiology.* 2008;109:A1202.
27. Busick T, Kussman M, Scheidt T, Tobias JD. Preliminary experience with dexmedetomidine for monitored anesthesia care during ENT surgical procedures. *Am J Therapeut.* 2008;15:520–527.
28. Alhashemi JA. Dexmedetomidine vs midazolam for monitored anesthesia care during cataract surgery. *Br J Anesth.* 2006;96:722–726.
29. Taghinia AH, Shapiro FE, Slavin SS. Dexmedetomidine in aesthetic facial surgery: improving anesthetic safety and efficacy. *Plast Reconstr Surg.* 2008;121:269–276.
30. Correa-Sales C, Rabin BC, Maze M. A hypnotic response to dexmedetomidine, an alpha 2 agonist is mediated in the locus ceruleus of the rat. *Anesthesiology.* 1994;81:1527–1534.
31. Ingersoll WE, Manecke GR, Thislethwaite PA. Dexmedetomidine and cardiac arrest. *Anesthesiology.* 2004;100:738–739.
32. Vadivelu N, Gowda AM, Urman RD, Jolly S, Kodumudi V, Maria M, Taylor R Jr, Pergolizzi JV Jr. Ketorolac tromethamine—routes and clinical implications. *Pain Pract.* 2015 Feb;15(2):175–193.
33. Southworth SR, Woodward EJ, Peng, A., et al. An integrated safety analysis of intravenous ibuprofen (Caldolor®) in adults. *J Pain Res.* 2015;8:753–765. http://doi.org/10.2147/JPR.S93547
34. Le V, Kurnutala L, SchianodiCola J, et al. Premedication with intravenous ibuprofen improves recovery characteristics and stress response in adults undergoing laparoscopic cholecystectomy: a randomized controlled trial. *Pain Med.* 2016;17:1163–1173.
35. Smith HS. Perioperative intravenous acetaminophen and NSAIDs. *Pain Med.* 2011;12:961–981. doi:10.1111/j.1526-4637.2011.01141.x.
36. Macario A, Royal MA. A literature review of randomized clinical trials of intravenous acetaminophen (paracetamol) for acute postoperative pain. *Pain Pract.* 2011;11:290–296.
37. McNicol ED, Tzortzopoulou A, Cepeda MS, Fracia MB, Farhat T, Schumann R. Single-dose intravenous paracetamol or propacetamol for prevention or treatment of postoperative pain: a systematic review and meta-analysis. *Br J Anaesth.* 2011;106:292–297.
38. Pahr JS, Lee VK. Intravenous acetaminophen. *Anesthesiol Clin.* 2010;28:619–645.
39. Pasero C, Stannard D. Role of IV acetaminophen in acute pain management: a case-illustrated review. *Pain Manag Nurs.* 2012;13:107–124.
40. Cadence Pharmaceuticals, Inc. *OFIRMEV (Acetaminophen) Injection Prescribing Information.* San Diego, CA: Cadence Pharmaceuticals, Inc.; 2010.
41. McNicol ED, Tzortzopoulou A, Cepeda MS, Fracia MB, Farhat T, Schumann R. Single-dose intravenous paracetamol or propacetamol for prevention or treatment of postoperative pain: a systematic review and meta-analysis. *Br J Anaesth.* 2011;106:292–297.
42. Haas DA. An update on analgesics for the management of acute postoperative dental pain. *J Can Dent Assoc.* 2002;68:476–482.
43. Duggan ST, Scott LJ. Intravenous paracetamol (acetaminophen). *Drugs.* 2009;69:101–113.
44. Fletcher MC, Spera JF. Management of acute postoperative pain after oral surgery. *Dent Clin N Am.* 2012;56:95–111.
45. Van der Westhuizen J, Kuo PY, Reed PW, Holder K. Randomised controlled trial comparing oral and intravenous paracetamol (acetaminophen) plasma levels when given as preoperative analgesia. *Anaesth Intensive Care.* 2011;39:242–246.
46. Sebel PS, Bowdle TA, Ghoneim MM, et al. The incidence of awareness during anesthesia: a multicenter United States study. *Anesth Analg.* 2004;99:833–839.
47. Elbaridi N, Kaye AD, Choi S, Urman RD. Current concepts of phenylpiperidine derivatives use in the treatment of acute and chronic pain. *Pain Physician.* 2017;20(2S):SE23–SE31.
48. Myles PS, Williams DL, Hendrata M, Anderson H, Weeks AM. Patient satisfaction after anaesthesia and surgery: results of a prospective survey of 10,811 patients. *Br J Anaesth.* 2000;84:6–10.
49. Malignant Hyperthermia Association of the United States. *MHAUS Recommendations.* December 14, 2016. Available at: https://www.mhaus.org/healthcare-professionals/managing-a-crisis/. Accessed April 8, 2018.
50. Bilmen JG, Gillies RL. Clarifying the role of activated charcoal filters in preparing an anaesthetic workstation for malignant hyperthermia-susceptible patients. *Anaesth Intensive Care.* 2014;42:51–58.
51. Birgenheier N, Stoker R, Westenskow D, Orr J. Activated charcoal effectively removes inhaled anesthetics from modern anesthesia machines. *Anesth Analg.* 2011;112:1363–1370.
52. Mathews DM, Gaba V, Zaku B, Neuman GG. Can remifentanil replace nitrous oxide during anesthesia for ambulatory orthopedic surgery with desflurane and fentanyl? *Anesth Analg.* 2008;106:101–108.
53. Nathan N, Peyclit A, Lahrimi A, Feiss P. Comparison of sevoflurane and propofol for ambulatory anaesthesia in gynaecological surgery. *Can J Anaesth.* 1998;45:1148–1150.
54. Song D, Joshi GP, White PF. Fast-track eligibility after ambulatory anesthesia: a comparison of desflurane, sevoflurane and propofol. *Anesth Analg.* 1998;86:267–273.
55. Gupta A, Stierer T, Zuckerman R, Sakima N. Comparison of recovery profile after ambulatory anesthesia with propofol, isoflurane, sevoflurane and desflurane: a systematic review. *Anesth Analg.* 2004;98:632–641.
56. Orkin FK. What do patients want? Preferences for immediate postoperative recovery. *Anesth Analg.* 1992;74:S225.
57. Gan TJ, Meyer TA, Apfel CC, et al. Society for ambulatory anesthesia guidelines for the management of postoperative nausea and vomiting. *Anesth Analg.* 2007;105:1615–1628.
58. Gan TJ, Sinha AC, Kovac AL, et al. A randomized, double-blind, multicenter trial comparing transdermal scopolamine plus ondansetron to ondansetron alone for the prevention of postoperative nausea and vomiting in the outpatient setting. *Anesth Analg.* 2009;108:1498–1504.
59. White PF. Prevention of postoperative nausea and vomiting-a multimodal solution to a persistent problem. *N Engl J Med.* 2004;350:2511–2512.
60. American Society of Anesthesiologists Task Force on Acute Pain Management. Practice guidelines for acute pain management in the perioperative setting: an updated report by the American Society of Anesthesiologists Task Force on Acute Pain Management. *Anesthesiology.* 2012;111:248–273.
61. Prabhakar A, Cefalu JN, Rowe JS, Kaye AD, Urman RD. Techniques to optimize multimodal analgesia in ambulatory surgery. *Curr Pain Headache Rep.* 2017;21(5):24.
62. Feldheiser A, Aziz O, Baldini G, et al. Enhanced recovery after surgery (ERAS) for gastrointestinal surgery, part 2: consensus statement for anaesthesia practice. *Acta Anaesthesiol Scand.* 2016;60:289–334.
63. Beverly A, Kaye AD, Ljungqvist O, Urman RD. Essential elements of multimodal analgesia in Enhanced Recovery After Surgery (ERAS) guidelines. *Anesthesiol Clin.* 2017;35(2):e115–e143.
64. Helander EM, Billeaud CB, Kline RJ, Emelife PI, Harmon CM, Prabhakar A, Urman RD, Kaye AD. Multimodal approaches to analgesia in enhanced recovery after surgery pathways. *Int Anesthesiol Clin.* 2017;55(4):51–69.

65. Sarin A. Successful implementation of an enhanced recovery after surgery program shortens length of stay and improves postoperative pain, and bowel and bladder function after colorectal surgery. *BMC Anesthesiol.* 2016;16:55.
66. Gravningsbraten R, Nicklasson B, Raeder J. Safety of laryngeal mask airway and short-stay practice in office-based adenotonsillectomy. *Acta Anaesthesiol Scand.* 2009;53:218–222.
67. American Society of Anesthesiologists. *Office-Based Anesthesia: Considerations for Anesthesiologists in Setting Up and Maintaining a Safe Office Environment.* 2nd ed. Parkridge, IL: American Society of Anesthesiologists; 2009.
68. Punjasawadwong Y, Boonjeungmonkol N, Phongchiewboon A. Bispectral index for improving anesthetic delivery and postoperative recovery. *Anesth Analg.* 2008;106:1326.
69. American Society of Anesthesiologists. Guidelines for determining anesthesia machine obsolescence, 2004. Available at: https://www.google.com/url?sa=t&rct=j&q=&esrc=s&source=web&cd=1&cad=rja&uact=8&ved=0ahUKEwj77_O6gKzaAhXRct8KHSMYC3kQFggnMAA&url=https%3A%2F%2Fwww.asahq.org%2F~%2Fmedia%2Fsites%2Fasahq%2Ffiles%2Fpublic%2Fresources%2Fasa%2520committees%2Fasa%2520publications%2520anesthesia%2520machine%2520obsolescence%252020041.pdf%3Fla%3Den&usg=AOvVaw2Ox2SSEYQAZqYrgxt0rI-Z. Accessed April 8, 2018.
70. Hausman LM, Eisenkraft JB, Rosenblatt MA. The safety and efficacy of regional anesthesia in an office-based setting. *J Clin Anesth.* 2008;22:271–275.
71. Galindo A, Witcher T. Mixtures of local anesthesthetics: bupivacaine-chloroprocaine. *Anesth Analg.* 1980;59:683–685.
72. Bedder MD, Kozody R, Craig DB. Comparison of bupivacaine and alkalinized bupivacaine in brachial plexus anesthesia. *Anesth Analg.* 1988;67:48–52.
73. Quinlan JJ, Oleksey K, Murphy FL. Alkalinization of mepivacaine for axillary block. *Anesth Analg.* 1992;74:371–374.
74. Capogna G, Celleno D, Laudano D, Giunta F. Alkalinization of local anesthetics. Which block, which local anesthetic? *Reg Anesth.* 1995;20:369–377.
75. Chow MY, Sia ATH, Koay CK, Chan YW. Alkalinization of lidocaine does not hasten the onset of axillary brachial plexus block. *Anesth Analg.* 1998;86:566–568.
76. Sinnott CJ, Garfield JM, Thalhammer JG, Strichartz GR. Addition of sodium bicarbonate to lidocaine decreases the duration of peripheral nerve block in the rat. *Anesthesiology.* 2000;93:1045–1052.
77. Rosenblatt MA, Abel M, Fischer GW, Itzkovich CJ, Eisenkraft JB. Successful use of a 20% lipid emulsion to resuscitate a patient after a presumed bupivacaine-related cardiac arrest. *Anesthesiology.* 2006;105:217–218.
78. Litz RJ, Popp M, Stehr SN, Koch T. Successful resuscitation of a patient with ropivacaine-induced asystole after axillary plexus block using lipid infusion. *Anaesthesia.* 2006;61:800–801.
79. Foxall G, McCahon R, Lamb J, Hardman JG, Bedforth NM. Levobupivacaine induced seizures and cardiovascular collapse treated with intralipid. *Anaesthesia.* 2007;62:516–518.
80. Sharrock NE, Waller JF, Fierro LE. Midtarsal block for surgery of the forefoot. *Br J Anaesth.* 1986;58:37–40.
81. Redborg KE, Antonakakis JG, Beach ML, et al. Ultrasound improves the success rate of a tibial nerve block at the ankle. *Reg Anesth Pain Med.* 2009;34:256–260.
82. Hadzic A, Vloka JD, Singson R, et al. A comparison of intertendinous and classical approaches to popliteal nerve block using magnetic resonance imaging simulation. *Anesth Analg.* 2002;94:1321–1324.
83. Perlas A, Brull R, Chan VWA, et al. Ultrasound guidance improves the success of sciatic nerve block at the popliteal fossa. *Reg Anesth Pain Med.* 2008;33:259–265.
84. Mulroy MF, Larkin KL, Batra MS, et al. Femoral nerve block with 0.25% or 0.5% bupivacaine improves postoperative analgesia following outpatient arthroscopic anterior cruciate ligament repair. *Reg Anesth Pain Med.* 2001;26:24–29.
85. Iskandar H, Benard A, Ruel-Raymond J, et al. Femoral block provides superior analgesia compared with intra-articular ropivacaine after anterior cruciate ligament reconstruction. *Reg Anesth Pain Med.* 2003;28:29–32.
86. Capdevila X, Biboulet P, Bouregba M, et al. Comparison of the three-in-one and fascia iliaca compartment blocks in adults: clinical and radiographic analysis. *Anesth Analg.* 1998;86:1039–1044.
87. Aantaa R, Kirvela O, Lahdenpera A, Nieminen S. Transarterial brachial plexus anesthesia for hand surgery: a retrospective analysis of 346 cases. *J Clin Anesth.* 1994;6:189–192.
88. Lo N, Brull R, Perlas A, et al. Evolution of ultrasound guided axillary brachial plexus blockade: retrospective analysis of 662 blocks. *Can J Anesth.* 2008;55:408–413.
89. Salazar CH, Spinosa W. Infraclavicular brachial plexus block: variation in approach and results in 360 cases. *Reg Anesth Pain Med.* 1999;24:411–416.
90. Perlas A, Lobo G, Lo N, et al. Ultrasound guided supraclavicular block: outcome in 510 consecutive cases. *Reg Anesth Pain Med.* 2009;34:171–176.
91. Tsui BC, Doyle K, Chu K, et al. Case series: ultrasound-guided supraclavicular block using a curvilinear probe in 104 day-case hand surgery patients. *Can J Anaesth.* 2009;56:46–51.
92. Brown AR, Weiss R, Greenberg C, et al. Interscalene block for shoulder arthroscopy: comparison with general anesthesia. *Arthroscopy.* 1993;9:295–300.
93. D'Alessio JG, Rosenblum M, Shea KP, Freitas DG. A retrospective comparison of interscalene block and general anesthesia for ambulatory surgery shoulder arthroscopy. *Reg Anesth.* 1995;20:62–68.
94. Tetzlaff JE, Yoon HJ, Brems J. Patient acceptance of interscalene block for shoulder surgery. *Reg Anesth.* 1993;18:30–33.
95. Bishop JY, Sprague M, Gelber J, et al. Interscalene regional anesthesia for arthroscopic surgery: a safe and effective technique. *J Shoulder Elbow Surg.* 2006;15:567–570.
96. Atanassoff PG, Ocampo CA, Bande MC, et al. Ropivacaine 0.2% and lidocaine 0.5% for intravenous regional anesthesia in outpatient surgery. *Anesthesiology.* 2001;95:627–631.
97. Chan VWS, Peng PWH, Kaszas Z, et al. A comparative study of general anesthesia, intravenous regional anesthesia, and axillary block for outpatient hand surgery: clinical outcome and cost analysis. *Anesth Analg.* 2001;93:1181–1184.
98. Ben-David B, Levin H, Soloman E. Spinal bupivacaine in ambulatory surgery: the effect of saline dilution. *Anesth Analg.* 1996;83:716–720.
99. Zayas VM, Liguori GA, Chisholm MF, et al. Dose response relationships for isobaric spinal mepivacaine using the combined spinal epidural technique. *Anesth Analg.* 1999;89:1167–1171.
100. Yoos JR, Kopacz DJ. Spinal 2-chloroprocaine for surgery: an initial 10-month experience. *Anesth Analg.* 2004;99:553–558.
101. Mulroy MF, Larkin KL, Hodgson PS, et al. A comparison of spinal, epidural, and general anesthesia for outpatient knee arthroscopy. *Anesth Analg.* 2000;91:860–864.
102. Malik O, Kaye AD, Kaye A, Belani K, Urman RD. Emerging roles of liposomal bupivacaine in anesthesia practice. *J Anaesthesiol Clin Pharmacol.* 2017;33(2):151–156.
103. King CH, Beutler SS, Kaye AD, Urman RD. Pharmacologic properties of novel local anesthetic agents in anesthesia practice. *Anesthesiol Clin.* 2017;35(2):315–325.
104. Tong YC, Kaye AD, Urman RD. Liposomal bupivacaine and clinical outcomes. *Best Pract Res Clin Anaesthesiol.* 2014;28(1):15–27.
105. Vyas KS, Rajendran S, Morrison SD, et al. Systematic review of liposomal bupivacaine (Exparel) for postoperative analgesia. *Plast Reconstr Surg.* 2016;138(4):748e–756e.
106. Chahar P, Cummings KC. Liposomal bupivacaine: a review of a new bupivacaine formulation. *J Pain Res.* 2012;5:257–264.

5 | RECOVERY AND DISCHARGE FOR PROCEDURES CONDUCTED OUTSIDE OF THE OPERATING ROOM

HAIRIL R. ABDULLAH, MBBS, MMED, FRANCES CHUNG, MBBS, FRCPC

INTRODUCTION

Continued advances in procedural techniques, anesthetic pharmacology, and regional anesthesia allow more prolonged diagnostic and therapeutic interventions to be conducted at an increasing variety of locations outside of the operating room (OOOR). However, the recovery and discharge process may vary according to the patient's condition and the specifics of the procedure. Generally, most patients are sent to the postanesthesia care unit (PACU) and ambulatory surgery unit (ASU) or a medical postprocedure recovery unit not staffed by an anesthesiologist, while some patients receive special postoperative care in a step-down or intensive care unit. Therefore, ensuring rapid postoperative recovery and safe discharge are important components following these OOOR procedures.

In this chapter, we review contemporary perspectives on the issues of recovery assessment and monitoring, and we provide an overview of the criteria related to transport and discharge following anesthesia. The standards and guidelines mentioned in this chapter apply not only to the anesthesiologists but also to other physicians who supervise the recovery of patients in the different units.

DEFINITION OF RECOVERY

Recovery is an ongoing process that begins from the end of intraoperative care until the patient returns to his or her preoperative physiological state.[1] This process is divided into three phases (Table 5.1).

At most institutions, phase I recovery occurs in the inpatient or ambulatory surgery PACU. Once phase I recovery is completed, homeostasis has been regained. Phase II recovery usually occurs in the ASU, medical unit, or step-down unit; it is judged to be complete when the patient is ready for discharge home. Phase III recovery continues at home until the patient returns to preoperative psychological and physical function.

TABLE 5.1. Three Phases of Postoperative Recovery

• Early recovery (phase I), from the discontinuation of anesthetic agents until recovery of protective reflexes and motor function
• Intermediate recovery (phase II), when the patient achieves criteria for discharge
• Late recovery (phase III), when the patient returns to his or her preoperative physiological state

MONITORING DURING THE RECOVERY PERIOD

Few published data are available on OOOR anesthesia-related mortality and morbidity. Analysis of data from the National Anesthesia Clinical Outcomes Registry (NACOR), the largest anesthesia registry in the United States, demonstrated serious hemodynamic instability (0.10%, p = .0001) and upgrade of care (0.10%, $p < .0001$) as the most common major complication for OOOR anesthesia, followed by respiratory complications (0.9%, $p < .0001$) and resuscitation (0.03%, $p < .0001$).[2] Moreover, the 2009 closed claims database analysis by the American Society of Anesthesiologists (ASA) revealed that severe respiratory depression, due to oversedation, was responsible for the majority of sedation-/analgesia-related adverse outcomes claims of OOOR procedures.[3] Claims associated with inadequate oxygenation occurred seven times more frequently outside of the operating room (OR) than the OR (21% vs. 3%, $p < .001$).[3]

Appropriate monitoring is essential in the ongoing recovery process after OOOR anesthesia. Nonanesthesia personnel involved in postanesthetic care in an area remote from the OR may be less familiar with the overall management of patients after anesthesia. In addition, many locations are often unfamiliar for the anesthesiologist, with similarly unaccustomed equipment and personnel. Periodic assessment and monitoring of the OOOR patients should include assessing respiratory and cardiovascular function, neuromuscular function, mental status, temperature, pain, nausea and vomiting, drainage and bleeding, and urine output (Table 5.2).[4] Postanesthesia care should be documented in the medical records.

TRANSPORTATION

Because most of the OOOR procedures are conducted at some distance from the PACU and inpatient beds, issues

TABLE 5.2. Recommendations for Assessment and Monitoring

ROUTINE	SELECTED PATIENTS
Respiratory	
Respiratory rate	
Airway patency	
Oxygen saturation	
Cardiovascular	
Pulse rate	Electrocardiogram
Blood pressure	
Neuromuscular	
Physical examination	Neuromuscular blockade
Nerve stimulator	
Mental status	
	Temperature
Pain	
Nausea and vomiting	
	Urine
	Voiding
	Output
	Drainage and bleeding

SOURCE: Reprinted with permission from American Society of Anesthesiologists Task Force on Postanesthetic Care. Practice guidelines for postanesthetic care. A report by the American Society of Anesthesiologists Task Force on Postanesthetic Care. *Anesthesiology.* 2002;96:742–752.

related to the transport of patients should be addressed. This is particularly important in the cases of patients who are critically ill, ASA physical status 3 or 4, the elderly, and the morbidly obese. It is suggested that a minimum of two people, one of them a registered nurse, should accompany the patient during the transport.[5] A physician is required for a patient with an unstable condition who may require acute interventions. It is also recommended that personnel attending the transportation of patients be trained in basic and advanced life support.

During transportation, all the equipment and monitors necessary for a safe journey should be available immediately. Items and monitoring including the following should be available immediately: sufficient oxygen supplies; airway management equipment and a resuscitation bag (to allow for manual ventilation via mask or tube); continuous electrocardiographic and pulse oximetry monitoring; regular measurement of blood pressure; standard resuscitation drugs and intravenous fluids; as well as specific essential medications required by the patient's medical condition.[5]

DISCHARGE SCORING SYSTEMS

Various scoring systems have been devised to guide the process of discharge and home readiness. To avoid inappropriate or premature discharge, physicians must ensure that the patient is "home ready" prior to discharge, that there is appropriate documentation of recovery, and that specified discharge criteria are met. If a physician does not perform the discharge assessment, it must be undertaken according to a strict policy.

For any scoring system to be useful, it must be practical, simple, easy to remember, and applicable to most or all postanesthesia settings. Using commonly observed physical signs avoids additional burden to the recovery personnel. Furthermore, by assigning numerical values to criteria indicating patient recovery, the assessment of progress becomes more objective.

DISCHARGE FROM THE POSTANESTHESIA CARE UNIT

The Aldrete scoring system, a modification of the Apgar scoring system used to assess newborns, has been used in many PACUs since its introduction 35 years ago.[6] The system utilizes numeric scores of 0, 1, or 2 assigned to motor function, respiration, circulation, consciousness, and color, with a maximum total score of 10. More recently, oxygen saturation assessed by pulse oximetry replaced the color parameter (Table 5.3).[7] According to this scoring system, when patients achieve a score of 9 or more, they are considered fit for discharge from the PACU to a step-down unit, ASU, or medical unit.

DISCHARGE CRITERIA FROM THE AMBULATORY SURGERY UNIT OR MEDICAL UNIT

Discharge of patients from the ASU or medical unit requires strict adherence to predetermined criteria to ensure patient safety. This responsibility is generally delegated to nurses in the ASU or medical unit, who adhere to a written protocol for patient discharge that includes specific discharge criteria or a discharge scoring system. Chung et al. devised the postanesthesia discharge score (PADS) (Table 5.4).[8,9] This discharge score is a simple method for providing a uniform assessment, which may facilitate assessment of home readiness. It also establishes a routine of repeated evaluation, which may result in improved patient supervision. The PADS was modified to eliminate requirements for oral fluid intake and documentation of urinary output prior to discharge.

Alternatively, outcome-based discharge criteria may be used. All parameters of an outcome-based system need to be met before discharge; typically, they include the following:

- Patient alert and oriented to time and place
- Stable vital signs
- Pain controlled by oral analgesics

TABLE 5.3. The Modified Aldrete Scoring System

Activity (able to move voluntarily or on command)	
Four extremities	2
Two extremities	1
Zero extremities	0
Respiration	
Able to deep breathe and cough freely	2
Dyspnea, shallow or limited breathing	1
Apneic	0
Circulation	
Blood pressure ± 20% of preanesthetic level	2
Blood pressure ± 20%–49% of preanesthetic level	1
Blood pressure ± 50% of preanesthetic level	0
Consciousness	
Fully awake	2
Arousable on calling	1
Not responding	0
O2 saturation	
Able to maintain O_2 saturation > 92% on room air	2
Needs O_2 inhalation to maintain O_2 saturation > 90%	1
O_2 saturation < 90% even with O_2 supplementation	0
A score ≥ 9 was required for discharge.	

SOURCE: Reprinted from Aldrete JA. The post-anesthesia recovery score revisited. *J Clin Anesth.* 1995;7:89–91 with permission from Elsevier.

TABLE 5.4 Postanesthetic Discharge Scoring (PADS) System

Vital signs	
Within 20% of preoperative baseline	2
20%–40% of preoperative baseline	1
40% of preoperative baseline	0
Activity level	
Steady gait, no dizziness, consistent with preoperative level	2
Requires assistance	1
Unable to ambulate/assess	0
Nausea and vomiting	
Minimal: mild, no treatment needed	2
Moderate: treatment effective	1
Severe: treatment not effective	0
Pain	
VAS = 0–3; the patient has minimal or no pain	2
VAS = 4–6; the patient has moderate pain	1
VAS = 7–10; the patient has severe pain	0
Surgical bleeding	
Minimal: does not require dressing change	2
Moderate: required up to two dressing changes with no further bleeding	1
Severe: required three or more dressing changes and continues to bleed	0
Patients scoring ≥ 9 are fit for discharge	

VAS, visual analog scale.

SOURCE: Reprinted with permission from Chung F. Recovery pattern and home-readiness after ambulatory surgery. *Anesth Analg.* 1995;80:896–902.

- Nausea or emesis controlled
- Ability to walk without dizziness
- No unexpected bleeding from the operative site
- Discharge instructions and prescriptions received from procedural physician and anesthesiologist
- Patient accepts readiness for discharge
- Responsible adult present to accompany patient home

Every ASU or medical unit should adopt either the PADS or the outcome-based discharge criteria as part of the protocol for patient discharge after an OOOR procedure. Discharge score or criteria should be met and documented before patients can be safely discharged home.

FACTORS AFFECTING RECOVERY AND DISCHARGE

POSTOPERATIVE NAUSEA AND VOMITING

After anesthesia, studies indicated approximately 30% of patients experienced vomiting and about 50% experienced nausea.[10–12] Many of them do not experience postoperative nausea and vomiting (PONV) until after discharge.[10] Hence, postdischarge nausea and vomiting (PDNV) is a major concern in OOOR anesthesia. Among the risk factors for PONV and PDNV are female sex, history of PONV or motion sickness, nonsmoking, younger age, general versus regional anesthesia, use of volatile anesthetics and nitrous oxide, postoperative opioids, and duration of anesthesia.

Certain types of surgeries (cholecystectomy, laparoscopic, gynecological) were found to increase the risk of PONV.[10,11]

Furthermore, opioid use in the PACU and presence of nausea in the PACU were also found to be predictive of PDNV.

By knowing and identifying these risk factors, strategies to reduce the baseline risk could be employed. Patients at moderate risk could be given prophylaxis (single agent or in combination with another), and those deemed to be at high risk of PONV should be considered for a combination therapy.[10] Among medications that could be of use are dexamethasone, 5-HT_3 antagonist, neurokinin 1 receptor antagonist, scopolamine, haloperidol, and dimenhydranate.[10] If nausea and vomiting occur in recovery, treatment should be initiated, and, at the same time, an evaluation should be performed to exclude an inciting medication or mechanical factor for nausea or vomiting, such as opioid use, blood draining down the throat, or abdominal distension after gastroscopy or colonoscopy. Treatment should be administered with an antiemetic from a pharmacologic class that is different from the prophylactic drug initially given, or if no prophylaxis was given, the recommended treatment is a low-dose 5-HT_3 antagonist.[10] Repeating the same medication given for PONV prophylaxis within the first 6 hours after the initial dose conferred no additional benefit.[10,13]

PAIN

Due to the nature of the diagnostic and therapeutic interventions OOOR, severe postoperative pain is rare. However, inadequate analgesia after these procedures could still prolong the postoperative stay and delay a return to normal daily living function.

Postoperative pain management should be started intraoperatively by supplementing general anesthesia with short-acting opioids, paracetamol, nonsteroidal anti-inflammatory drugs (NSAIDs), or regional anesthesia; this should facilitate a smoother recovery.[14] When opioids are used in the recovery period, rapid and short-acting drugs should be administered and titrated to the desired effect.

Combinations of analgesics that act by different mechanisms result in additive or synergistic analgesia. This helps to lower the total doses of each drug and consequently reduces individual side effects.

HYPOTHERMIA

Many of the remote anesthetizing locations, such as magnetic resonance imaging (MRI) or computed tomography (CT) suites, are air-conditioned to avoid overheating of equipment. However, this may result in serious hypothermia if precautions are not taken.[15] It is especially important in the cases of pediatric and elderly patients due to their less-effective thermal response mechanisms. Hypothermia is associated with delayed postanesthetic recovery. Accordingly, temperature monitoring and an active warming device should be used in the procedural and recovery rooms to prevent or treat hypothermia to minimize adverse outcomes.

ORAL FLUID INTAKE PRIOR TO DISCHARGE

Mandatory oral intake is not necessary and may provoke nausea and vomiting and delay discharge.[4] Drinking oral fluids is not a requirement before discharge from the ASU or medical unit.[4,16] Mandating oral fluid intake prior to discharge should be done only for selected patients on a case-by-case basis, such as insulin-dependent diabetics.

VOIDING PRIOR TO DISCHARGE

Requiring patients to void before discharge is not a standard of care, and this is reflected in practice guidelines.[4,16] The type and duration of the procedure, old age, male sex, spinal/epidural anesthesia, and administered fluid volume are risk factors for postoperative urinary retention.[17] In the current practice, low-risk patients can be discharged home without voiding. They should be instructed to return to the hospital if they are unable to void within 6 to 8 hours. Patients at high risk of urinary retention should be required to void prior to discharge and display a residual volume less than 300 mL as measured by ultrasound. If the bladder volume is more than 500–600 mL, catheterization should be performed prior to discharge.[18]

PATIENT ESCORT

The ASA requires a responsible adult escort to accompany patients home after procedures involving any sedation or anesthesia.[4] Significant psychomotor and cognitive impairment exists after general anesthesia and monitored anesthesia care. In a prospective study conducted over a period of 38 months, the incidence of patients with no escort was found to be 0.2% (60/28,391 patients).[19]

In a 10-year review of litigations in ambulatory surgery in Canada, there were three malpractice cases of car accidents after ambulatory surgery in patients without an escort. Sedation with as little as 1 mg lorazepam as a premedication could result in a clinician being deemed negligent for allowing the patient to drive home.[20] Hospitals should implement policies to prevent discharge of patients without an escort. This should be a fundamental issue of patient safety in relation to OOOR anesthesia.

Patients should be advised not to drink alcohol, operate machinery, or drive for 24 hours after a general anesthetic or sedation. Those who have had regional anesthesia should also refrain from driving if they have an insensate limb.[21]

CONCLUSION

Procedures conducted OOOR will continue to grow and expand. Understanding potential complications during the recovery process, using discharge scores to facilitate discharge, updating patient information and clinical pathways based on current best evidence, and ensuring the availability of a patient escort will contribute to the safe recovery and discharge of patients following their procedures.

REFERENCES

1. Marshall SI, Chung F. Discharge criteria and complications after ambulatory surgery. *Anesth Analg.* 1999;88:508–517.

2. Chang B, Kaye AD, Diaz JH, Westlake B, Dutton RP, Urman RD. Complications of non-operating room procedures: outcomes from the National Anesthesia Clinical Outcomes Registry. *J Patient Saf.* 2015. doi:10.1097/PTS.0000000000000156.
3. Metzner J, Posner KL, Domino KB. The risk and safety of anesthesia at remote locations: the US closed claims analysis. *Curr Opin Anaesthesiol.* 2009;22:502–508.
4. Apfelbaum J, Silverstein J, Chung F, et al. Practice guidelines for postanesthetic care: an updated report by the American Society of Anesthesiologists Task Force on Postanesthetic Care. *Anesthesiology.* 2013;118:291–307.
5. Warren J, Fromm RE Jr, Orr RA, et al. Guidelines for the inter- and intrahospital transport of critically ill patients. *Crit Care Med.* 2004;32:305–306.
6. Suddarth B. *Textbook of Medical-Surgical Nursing.* Philadelphia, PA: Lippincott, William & Wilkins; 2004:303–306.
7. Aldrete JA. The post-anesthetic recovery score revisited. *J Clin Anesth.* 1995;7:89–91.
8. Chung F, Chan VW, Ong D. A post-anesthetic discharge scoring system for home readiness after ambulatory surgery. *J Clin Anesth.* 1995;7:500–506.
9. Chung F. Recovery pattern and home-readiness after ambulatory surgery. *Anesth Analg.* 1995;80:896–902.
10. Gan TJ, Diemunsch P, Habib AS, et al. Consensus guidelines for the management of postoperative nausea and vomiting. *Anesth Analg.* 2014;118: 85–113.
11. Apfel CC, Philip BK, Cakmakkaya OS, et al. Who is at risk for postdischarge nausea and vomiting after ambulatory surgery? *Anesthesiology.* 2012;117:475–486.
12. Apfel CC, Heidrich FM, Jukar-Rao S, et al. Evidence-based analysis of risk factors for postoperative nausea and vomiting. *Br J Anaesth.* 2012;109:742–5314.
13. Kovac AL, O'Connor TA, Pearman MH, et al. Efficacy of repeat intravenous dosing of ondansetron in controlling postoperative nausea and vomiting: a randomized, double-blind, placebo-controlled multicenter trial. *J Clin Anesth.* 1999;11:453–459.
14. Chou R, Gordon DB, de Leon-Casasola OA, et al. Management of postoperative pain: a clinical practice guideline from the American Pain Society, the American Society of Regional Anesthesia and Pain Medicine, and the American Society of Anesthesiologists' Committee on Regional Anesthesia, Executive Committee, and Administrative Council. *J Pain.* 2016;17:131–157.
15. Van De Velde M, Roofthooft E, Kuypers M. Risk and safety of anaesthesia outside the operating room. *Minerva Anestesiol.* 2009;75:345–348.
16. Verma R, Alladi R, Jackson I, et al. Guidelines: day case and short stay surgery: Association of Anaesthetists of Great Britain and Ireland, British Association of Day Surgery. *Anaesthesia.* 2011;66:417–434.
17. Awad IT, Chung F. Factors affecting recovery and discharge following ambulatory surgery. *Can J Anesth.* 2006;53:858–872.
18. Joshi GP. The Society for Ambulatory Anesthesia: 19th annual meeting report. *Anesth Analg.* 2005;100:982–986.
19. Chung F, Imasogie N. Frequency and implications of ambulatory surgery without a patient escort. *Can J Anesth.* 2005;52:1022–1026.
20. Chung F, Assmann N. Car accidents after ambulatory surgery in patients without an escort. *Anesth Analg.* 2008;106:817–820.
21. Abdullah HR, Chung F. Postoperative issues: discharge criteria. *Anesthesiol Clin.* 2014;32:487–493.

6 | MANAGEMENT OF STAFFING AND CASE SCHEDULING FOR ANESTHESIA OUTSIDE OF THE OPERATING ROOM

ALEX MACARIO, MD, MBA, DEEPAK SHARMA, MD, MBA

INTRODUCTION

"We'd like anesthesia coverage for our cases in OOOR [outside of the operating room] location XYZ. Can you help us out?" A good first step in answering this question is to look at your group's service contract with the hospital to see what language exists for covering elective cases OOOR. If this is the first time the anesthesia group has been asked to cover off-site cases, then discussion with the hospital is in order to negotiate an arrangement for anesthesia coverage.

Theoretically, anesthesia groups could arrange that off-site cases will be covered by an anesthesiologist at the convenience of the OOOR proceduralists. This approach requires obtaining financial support, sometimes referred to as a service agreement, from the hospital to subsidize the anesthesia group so it can deliver anesthesia care as requested to cover these often poorly scheduled OOOR locations. A good first step in this dialogue is for the hospital administration to identify the anesthetizing locations and hospital services that need anesthesia services.

According to a survey of hospital contracts by the Medical Group Management Association, 75% of hospitals provided some kind of subsidy to anesthesiologists in 2015, up from approximately 50% in 2000. The stipend associated with a service agreement may be expensive for the hospital, and it is at risk of disappearing if hospital finances deteriorate sufficiently. As a result, many anesthesia groups are working with the hospital and the multiple OOOR services to schedule cases in a way that is economically viable to both the anesthesia group and the hospital.

An anesthesia group has several important groups of people to which it provides service, including patients, surgeons, nurses, and hospital managers. Properly managing the relationship with the hospital manager customer, such as on issues related to OOOR cases, is an important goal. Otherwise, the anesthesia group runs the risk of losing the right to be the exclusive provider of anesthesia services at that facility. Many conflicts between the hospital and the anesthesia group have been reported where the relationship has deteriorated to the point that the anesthesia group leaves en masse. Perhaps one factor in such a separation is opposing views on the anesthesia service. For example, a view commonly held by anesthesiologists may be that there is endless demand for anesthesia support, with minimal professional compensation. In contrast, the administrator view may be that the hospital is an extremely valuable franchise for an anesthesia group to have as exclusive provider: "They ought to be paying us for the constant flow of business they get."[1]

Hence, a proactive approach to staffing and case scheduling for OOOR cases is optimal to maintain a positive working relationship in the hospital. A functional anesthesia service OOOR will generate operational and financial advantages for the hospital that are multiples of the anesthesia revenues. The goal for the anesthesia group is to work with hospital and the multiple OOOR services to schedule cases in a way that is economically viable to all parties. This reflects the hospital's desire to retain and grow physicians' practices, to enhance market share and reputation, and to fulfill community-service missions.

Optimizing OOOR scheduling is financially important to anesthesia groups (e.g., so anesthetists can do consecutive cases at the same location). Some anesthesia groups manage this uneven demand by assigning an anesthesiologist daily to do "utility infielder" work for OOOR cases Monday through Friday, with hours of 7:30 AM until 4:00 PM, for example. The list of their responsibilities goes throughout the hospital, but it may consist of electroconvulsive therapy (ECT), bone marrow biopsy, and cardiology catheterization lab duties, with either cardioversions or implantable cardioverter-defibrillator (ICD) testing. In such practices, outside this structure and timeline, the referring OOOR physician needs to declare an emergency to obtain anesthesia support on a particular day. Sometimes, OOOR cases are simply added to the surgery waiting list, but this is unsatisfactory to everyone involved. OOOR anesthetics can be challenging not only because the environment is not what the anesthesiologist is used to in the operating room (OR) but also because scheduling staff for these cases brings about problems.

With proper management weeks to months ahead of time, the groundwork for an efficient (well-functioning) OOOR elective schedule should be in place. This chapter's aims are as follows:

1. Reinforcing that OOOR case scheduling should aim to reduce overutilized time.
2. Recommending the reorganization of OOOR workflow processes such that activities are done in parallel rather than serial.

3. Identifying challenges of scheduling anesthesia services OOOR.
4. Explaining that *Current Procedural Terminology* (*CPT*) codes for OOOR cases are not predictive of anesthesia times.
5. Recommending that an OOOR service requesting anesthesia coverage receive a block of allocated time provided the service averages at least 10 hours of cases, including turnovers, every 2 weeks. The 10-hour threshold is set high to ensure that the allocated "block" remains filled. Two weeks is a reasonable length of time from the perspective of patient waiting times. An "overflow block" (i.e., first come, first scheduled time) is made available for any spillover cases or services that have less than 10 hours of cases per week.
6. Recommending the use of alternative metrics as tools to evaluate OOOR efficiency.
7. Encouraging the use of computer-based enterprise-wide scheduling so that control of scheduling of OOOR cases is distributed to each OOOR service.

OOOR CASELOAD WILL GROW

There is much pent-up demand for OOOR anesthesia services. The shift to non-OR settings will continue to expand, driven by cost savings (e.g., the office has lower overhead than the OR), convenience for patients and providers, desire by hospitals to avoid sedation mishaps by nonanesthesiologists, and availability of new treatments that are not dependent on a full-fledged OR. Although these increasing requests are burdensome in the short term to manage, they do indicate that anesthesia services are valued in a growing number of health care venues. This is a major positive move for the specialty in the long term.

TABLE 6.1. Differences Between the Surgical Suite and OOOR Anesthetizing Locations

• OOOR locations are not as interchangeable as normal ORs. For example, a pediatric electrophysiologist cannot "split out" and perform his or her next case in the CT suite. Similarly, an MRI cannot be done in another location as there is typically only one MRI machine and MRI-compatible equipment in one location.
• In contrast to the surgical suite, non-OR services are often small, composed of only one or two physicians. Depending on how time is allocated and cases scheduled, variation in workload at each location on any day will be larger (e.g., due to physicians' absences due to vacations/meetings, which will be more noticeable with a physician group that is small than with a bigger group).
• Whereas OR turnovers aim to be as low as 20–30 minutes, OOOR turnovers can be 1 hour or more. This is especially true when the change involves switching from one geographical area to another. Factors affecting turnover include transporting a patient to the PACU through a maze of halls and elevators, returning to the initial site to collect equipment, and moving the equipment to a new location.
• The distance between NORA locations is often larger, creating a safety issue that prevents the use of medical direction. An anesthesiologist can cover only one site at a time OOOR. For example, an anesthesiologist supervising CRNAs/residents may do a preoperative evaluation on his or her OR's next patient during the current case. This is difficult, if not impossible, when the next OOOR case will be done at a separate site.
• Diagnostic radiology cases (CT/MRI) that require anesthesia are often single cases, in the middle of a list of other cases not needing anesthesia. As a result, most facilities do not assign anesthesia blocks exclusively for CT/MRI cases requiring anesthesia. The challenge then is to predict a single case's duration.
• Unlike CT or MRI cases, interventional radiology cases requiring anesthesia are often scheduled sequentially in one room, so the management challenge is to estimate when the workday will end, not just the duration of one case.

CRNA, certified registered nurse anesthetist; CT, computed tomography; MRI, magnetic resonance imaging; NORA, non–operating room anesthesia; OOOR, outside of the operating room; OR, operating room; PACU, postanesthesia care unit.

CHALLENGES OF SCHEDULING ANESTHESIA SERVICES OUTSIDE OF THE OPERATING ROOM

"Horizontalization" of anesthesia locations that need to be covered first thing in the morning can stretch the anesthesia group's ability to promptly provide staff.[2] Scheduling and arranging for anesthesia coverage of an OOOR case can be complex (Figure 6.1). OOOR cases have different characteristics than OR surgical cases, and this affects their management (Table 6.1).[3–5]

If anesthesia groups primarily engage in medical direction of nurse anesthetists, then they need to be mindful of physical distances between anesthetizing locations. In many cases, medical direction of certified registered nurse anesthetists (CRNAs) is not possible due to such geographic restrictions. Patient safety issues trump the use of medical direction because distances between anesthetic locations in the OOOR setting are much further than in the OR. For example, in one OR suite, if two cases are running late, one MD could cover two residents/CRNAs. But, if there is one case running late in the main OR suite and one in the gastroenterology lab that is far away, then two anesthesiologists are needed. The longer distance may also necessitate adding another call position for nights at the OOOR location if procedures are consistently running late.[6]

The OOOR medical direction may be possible if the sites are located close to each other on the same floor. For example, an anesthesiologist could cover an electrophysiology case in the cardiac cath lab and a case in the interventional radiology suite without increasing risk to patient safety as long as the two procedure rooms are within a short distance.

OOOR SCHEDULING SHOULD AIM TO REDUCE OVERUTILIZED TIME

The OOOR caseload may be inconsistent and of varying duration (Figure 6.2). Nothing is more important in OOOR case

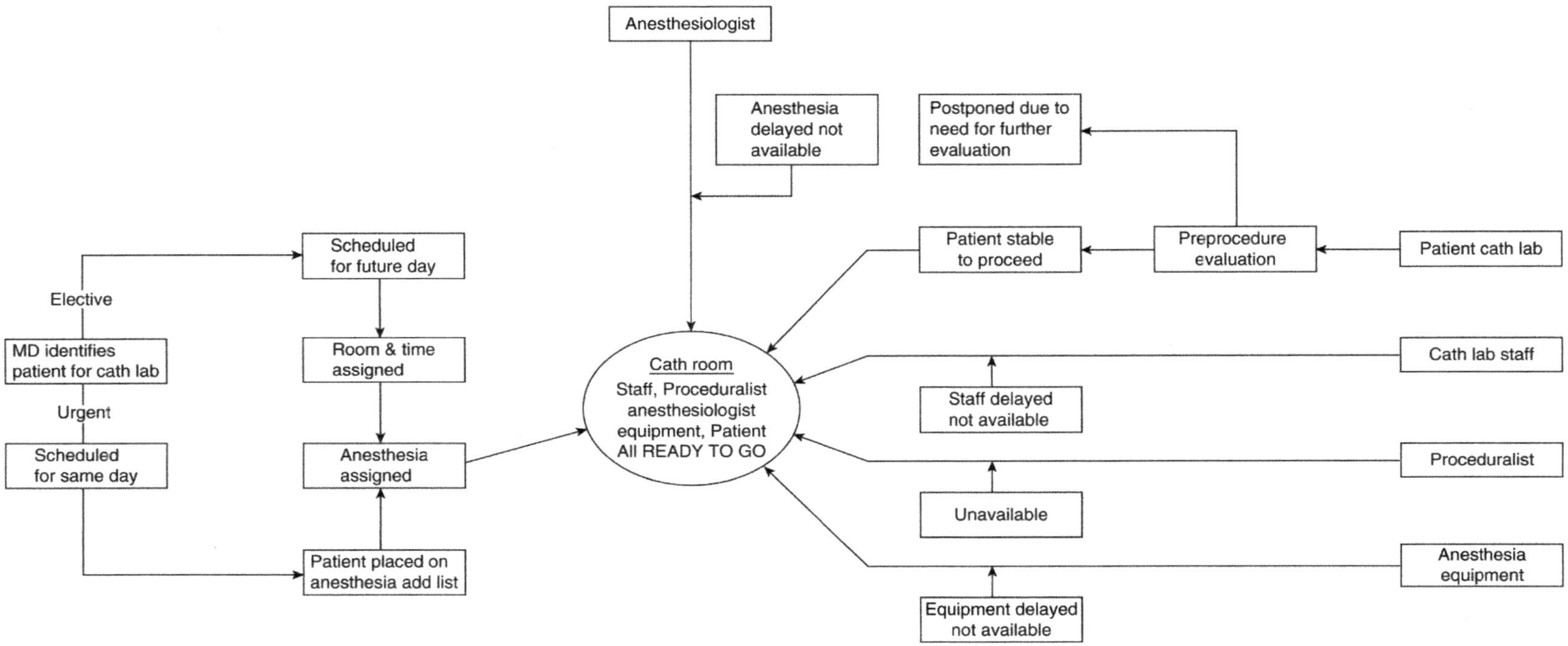

Figure 6.1. *Process map for scheduling a case in the catheterization lab. (Figure courtesy of Dr. Cliff Schmiesing.)*

scheduling than to first allocate the right amount of time to each OOOR service on each day of the week.[7]

To illustrate, we schedule two cerebral angiogram cases, each lasting 2.5 hours, into the Radiology Suite Room 1 (Figure 6.3). The radiology suite nurses and one anesthesiologist are scheduled to work a 9-hour day. The matching of workload to staffing has not been optimized. Little can be done on the day of the procedures to increase the efficiency of use of the nurses and anesthesiologists.

Neither awakening patients more quickly nor reducing the turnover time, for example, will compensate for management's poor initial choice of staffing for Radiology Suite Room 1 or how the cases were scheduled into Room 1.

Underutilized hours reflect how early the room finishes. In Scenario 1, if an anesthesiologist and a radiology nurse were scheduled to work from 8 AM to 5 PM and instead the room finished at 2 PM (including 1-hour turnover), then there would be 3 hours of underutilized time. The excess staffing cost would be 33% (3 hours/9 hours). In contrast, for Scenario 2, the 11 hours of OOOR cases are performed in the OOOR location with staff scheduled to work 9 hours.

The optimal amount of OOOR time that needs to be allocated to a particular service, sometimes referred to as a "block," should minimize the amount of underutilized time and the more expensive overutilized time.[8]

On the other hand, if 11 hours of OOOR cases are performed in an OOOR location with staff scheduled to work 9 hours, then the excess staffing cost is 44% (Scenario 2).[9] Overutilized hours are the hours that rooms run longer than the regularly scheduled end time, 2 hours in this example (2 hours/9 hours = 22%, which we then multiply by a "fudge" factor of 2 to include the additional cost of staff staying late). One component of this is the monetary time-and-a-half overtime cost paid to staff, and the second is the recruitment and retention costs related to disgruntled staff unexpectedly forced to work extra hours.

If the key is to allocate appropriate time to each OOOR service based on historical use, how do you deal with OOOR locations consistently running late? The answer is to make the allocated anesthesia OOOR blocks longer. For example, if the interventional radiologist performs 12 hours worth of cases needing anesthesia on 1 day every 2 weeks, do not assign 9 hours of interventional radiology block time (8 AM to 5 PM) and have the anesthesiologist and interventional radiology nurses frustrated by having to stay late. Rather, assign 12 hours of block time (8 AM to 8 PM); by doing so, anesthesia and nursing staff know they will be there 12 hours when they arrive to work, and overtime costs (both financial and morale) will be reduced.

The common response to this approach is, "No one wants to be in the interventional radiology room until 8 PM." The answer to that is, "You are there now until 8 PM, so why not make scheduled interventional radiology time 12 hours and have a more predictable workday duration?"

Optimizing staffing costs is finding the best balance between overtime and finishing early. Involvement by a high-level member of the facilities administrative staff (vice president or above) is essential to successfully bringing together the budget, staffing, and leadership to allocate such anesthesia time blocks for OOOR work.

SAVE TIME BY ARRANGING WORKFLOW PROCESSES TO BE DONE IN PARALLEL

Many institutions struggle to fit in more OOOR cases during the day without sacrificing overutilized time because they have arranged their workflows serially. Each process strictly follows the previous process sequentially without any overlap. To optimize the number of cases done within a block and reduce costs per case, the goal of an OOOR director should be to identify ways to run multiple processes simultaneously in parallel.

For example, a serial workflow for an anesthesia provider in pediatric OOOR cases, such as magnetic resonance imaging (MRI), would be to perform a mask induction followed by placing an intravenous line. However, an institution can employ a different workflow in which the intravenous line is placed by a skilled nurse using topical local anesthetic. This workflow is done simultaneously while the anesthesia provider is overseeing the emergence of the previous patient. This not only saves time with intravenous line placement but also allows for a faster induction via intravenous means as opposed to inhalational induction.

Parallel workflows have also enabled the creation of alternative anesthetic models to reduce total sedation time. At one institution performing cataract surgeries, anesthesia providers give enough sedation for the first few minutes of the procedure while a retrobulbar block is being placed. They then monitor the patient until the patient is alert and oriented. Care is then handed off midprocedure to a sedation nurse so the anesthesia provider can begin preparing the next patient in the holding area.[10]

CURRENT PROCEDURAL TERMINOLOGY CODES FOR OOOR CASES ARE NOT PREDICTIVE OF ANESTHESIA TIMES

Computed tomography (CT)/ MRI anesthesia time estimates based on historical *CPT* codes are strikingly inaccurate. They are not as predictive of OOOR anesthesia times as they are for surgery cases. For OOOR cases, one study found that for CT and MRI cases (with overall average duration of 2 hours), the mean absolute percentage error in case duration estimate equaled 45%, which was less accurate than the 27% error for OR cases of comparable durations.[11]

Cases involving CT and MRI have many different *CPT* codes, and most are rare. The most common *CPT* (70553, MRI brain without contrast) accounted for 31% of MRI anesthetics, and the most common three *CPT*s accounted for 44% of MRI anesthetics.

Using *International Classification of Diseases, Ninth Revision, Clinical Modification* (ICD-9-CM) procedure

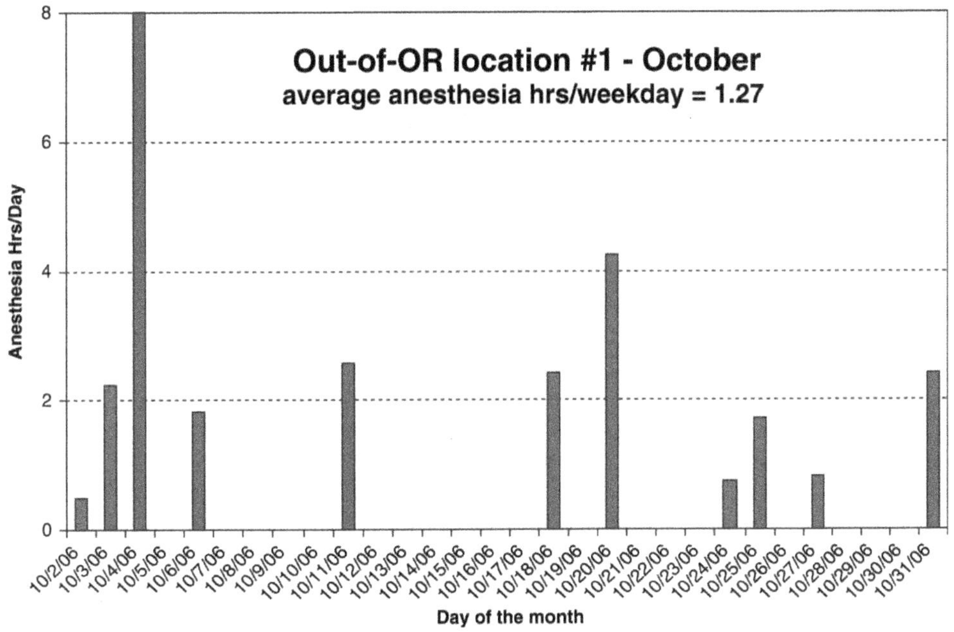

Figure 6.2. Anesthesia hours per day vary from day to day, from 0 hours to more than 8 hours for this outside of the operating room (OOOR) location. This prompted the anesthesia group to create a team that included the hospital administrator, scheduling personnel, OOOR proceduralist, and anesthesia group representative to better coordinate case scheduling.

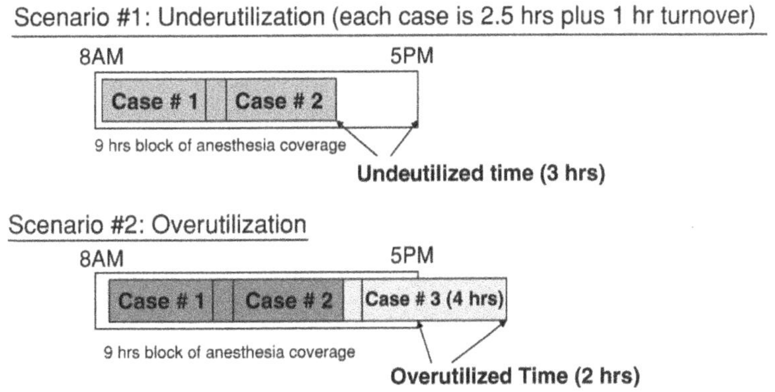

Figure 6.3. Scenario 1: Underutilization (each case is 2.5 hours plus 1-hour turnover). Scenario 2: Overutilization.

codes instead of *CPT*s yields even more inaccuracy. One cause of this inaccuracy is that procedure codes reflect organs imaged, not scanning times. For example, *ICD-9-CM* 88.38 could either be CT of the sinuses or CT of pelvis, which can differ by 10 minutes of scanning time. As a second example, *ICD-9-CM* 88.97 could be either an abdomen MRI or an orbit MRI, which also differ in scan duration. Differences in scanning times also arise depending on the type of machine used for imaging. Consider taking the estimates for individual cases provided by the chief radiology technologist as a best guess.

Similarly, diverse scheduled procedures also exist for pediatric cardiac catheterization. It is even more difficult to schedule anesthetic times for interventional radiology cases. Again, the *CPT*s are nonpredictive, and the anesthetics administered are usually long (average duration slightly less than 4 hours). The three most common interventional radiology *CPT*s accounted for 77% of interventional radiology anesthetics. The interventional radiology *CPT* (61624) accounted for 63% of anesthetics. This *CPT* encompasses a multitude of procedures and does not specify the size of the lesion—"transcatheter permanent occlusion or embolization [e.g., for tumor destruction, to achieve hemostasis, to occlude a vascular malformation], percutaneous, or any method" that involves the "central nervous system (intracranial, spinal cord)."

Because interventional radiology often schedules elective cases into allocated time, the necessary endpoint that would be nice to predict with some accuracy is the finish time for the day's entire list of cases, including turnovers. Methods have been published to determine the time (e.g., 4 PM) up to when interventional radiology could schedule, so that there is an 80% chance that the anesthesia team finishes no later than a specified time (e.g., 6 PM).

PROVIDE ENOUGH OPEN ACCESS ANESTHESIA TIME SO THAT EACH SPECIALTY CAN ACCOMMODATE MOST OF ITS OOOR CASES WITHIN TWO WEEKS

For OOOR cases, a reasonable approach is to provide anesthesia coverage of elective OOOR patients within a reasonable number of days. This length of time can be discussed with hospital management to meet hospital needs, but 50% of patients stated that 2 weeks is the longest acceptable wait time for a procedure, 75% stated 4 weeks was the longest acceptable wait time, and 90% stated that 8 weeks or less was the longest acceptable wait time.[12] The optimal reasonable number of days from the perspective of patient expectations of waiting times will vary by country and by medical system.

If the anesthesia department normally plans 10-hour workdays (from 7 AM to 5 PM) for their anesthetists, then an OOOR service requesting anesthesia coverage should receive a block of allocated time provided they average at least 10 hours of cases including turnovers every 2 weeks.[13] The threshold of 10 hours is set high to ensure that the allocated time remains filled. The anesthesia time commitment needs to be a fixed time to reduce OOOR physicians from wandering off (e.g., to do consultations, etc.).

If the OOOR service has a new elective case that needs to be scheduled and all the allocated time (block) is filled for the next 2 weeks, then additional "overflow" time (i.e., first come, first scheduled "unblocked" time) is made available on another day of the week for the extra case.[14] In this way, the new case can be performed within 2 weeks, but not by extending the duration of the original 10-hour staffed workday. A service guarantee of a maximum patient waiting time removes the argument that the anesthesia department is causing patients to wait for an unnecessarily long time. The service guarantee is no longer a commitment to a particular block (e.g., 10 hours) of anesthesia coverage, but that the case will be performed within 2 weeks or whatever time period is mutually agreed on.

One goal for the anesthesia group could be to generate 8 hours of anesthesia billing time per day and to be finished by 5 PM (Table 6.2).

By letting professional practices grow, open-access scheduling increases revenues for the hospital and anesthesia group. Planning for future staffing can potentially be more accurate because the total hours of anesthesia time performed in the past can then be used to forecast future anesthesia needs.[15]

TABLE 6.2. Example: Allocations of Two Ten-Hour Blocks per Day for Elective OOOR Cases During Each Two-Week Cycle for One Hospital

Monday: Adult cardiology; pediatric cardiac catheterization
Tuesday: Neuroradiology; MRI/CT
Wednesday: Adult cardiology; open overflow time
Thursday: Interventional radiology; MRI/CT
Friday: Adult cardiology: pediatric cardiac catheterization

CT, computed tomography; MRI, magnetic resonance imaging; OOOR, outside of the operating room.

Example XYZ: Data analysis for OOOR location XYZ is summarized in Table 6.3. On Mondays, how much anesthesia time (e.g., 8, 10, 12, or 13 hours) should be allocated to XYZ?

When you run the numbers for this example using this efficiency formula, it computes that 8 hours are the optimal allocation on Mondays because this amount mathematically minimizes underutilized and the more expensive overutilized time.

In this particular situation, with an 8-hour allocation and 6, 6, 8, and 10 hours of work on successive Mondays, there would be 2, 2, and 0 hours of underutilized time, respectively, for the first three Mondays and 2 hours of overutilized time, multiplied by 2, for the fourth Monday, for a total of 8 inefficiency hours. No other OR allocation (e.g., 7, 10, or 13 hours) gives fewer inefficiency hours. This efficiency hour analysis would be repeated to calculate optimal allocated time duration for each day of the week. Any additional caseload can be covered by the overflow anesthesia time.

CONSIDER USING ALTERNATIVE METRICS TO EVALUATE EFFICIENCY AT OOOR SITES

Measuring utilization by site is commonly used to assess efficiency in the OR as it is simple to calculate. For each OR, the amount of time spent performing surgical procedures, including turnover time, is divided by the total time allocated. However, this metric may not always provide a complete picture of efficiency in the OOOR setting. Many times, anesthesia providers spend part of their shift in one OOOR site and end their day in another location. For example, an anesthesiologist might start the day providing sedation for ECT and then finish the rest of the day in the endoscopy suite. By measuring efficiency by provider or minutes when assessing utilization by site, it may appear that ECT and endoscopy have low utilization because procedures are only being performed for part of the day. However, only one anesthesia provider is required to provide sedation for both sites, so physician efficiency is actually high. When faced with horizontal expansion of services, practice managers can leverage this metric to show that staffing requirements may not necessarily need to be increased. Efforts should be placed on facilitating collaboration between multiple OOOR sites so that the provider efficiency metric can be optimized.

ENTERPRISE-WIDE SCHEDULING ENABLES CONTROL OF OOOR SCHEDULING TO BE DISTRIBUTED TO EACH OOOR SERVICE

Inherent problems of OOOR scheduling include that OOOR cases are often written on a paper calendar, whereas OR cases are typically scheduled electronically, so it is difficult to assess demands for anesthesia staff. Also, rebookings/cancellations for OOOR anesthetics may not be passed on to the anesthesia scheduler if a paper scheduling system is used.

TABLE 6.3. Dates and Number of Anesthesia Hours, Including Turnovers, for OOOR Location XYZ

Mondays	4/2/2007	6	4/9/2007	6	4/16/2007	8	4/23/2007	10
Tuesdays	4/3/2007	4.5	4/10/2007	8.67	4/17/2007	18.94	4/24/2007	7.25
Wednesdays	4/4/2007	7.75	4/11/2007	11.02	4/18/2007	6.13	4/25/2007	5.8
Thursdays	4/5/2007	9.42	4/12/2007	0	4/19/2007	4.48	4/26/2007	0
Fridays	4/6/2007	6.32	4/13/2007	8.37	4/20/2007	0	4/27/2007	0.67

Computer-based, enterprise-wide patient scheduling systems permit clerks, nurses, physicians, or patients (e.g., via the Internet) to schedule patient appointments throughout a multiple-specialty physician group or health care system. An application of these systems is to coordinate patient scheduling in surgeons' clinics with patient scheduling in surgical suites or with OOOR areas. Better synchronization of such schedules is an important objective. Just as some radiology departments allow clerks at physicians' offices to schedule radiological procedures via a web browser and some clinics allow patients to schedule their own appointments, the anesthesia department can allow clerks and nurses in other departments to schedule directly into OOOR anesthesia time.

Advantages to scheduling OOOR anesthetics using an enterprise-wide scheduling system include the following:

- Clinic nurses and radiology schedulers do not have to phone the anesthesia department and wait to see if someone answers.
- Anesthetics can be coordinated with other appointments the patient may have on the same date. For example, a patient's schedule for the day might include preanesthesia evaluation at 9 AM, anesthetic administration starting at 11 AM, CT evaluation at 11:30 AM, and oncology clinic visit at 3:00 *International Classification of Diseases, Ninth Revision, Clinical Modification*

Deciding when patients should arrive for their OOOR case is also a major challenge. If patients are told to arrive too early in the morning for a procedure scheduled in the afternoon, they risk waiting several hours and the unpleasantness of remaining taking nothing by mouth (nil per os, npo) for most of the day. On the other hand, if patients do not arrive early enough, they may not be ready in the event an earlier case is canceled or finishes early.

Asking patients to arrive a fixed number of hours, such as 2 hours, before their scheduled OOOR procedure should be replaced by statistical methods that compute the earliest time that their scheduled case could begin. Patient waiting times must be balanced against patient availability and staff waiting times. A good general rule is that if the preceding case is canceled or finishes early, the patient should be ready and waiting 19 times out of 20. Thus, OR staff should wait only 5% of the time. Mathematically, the earliest possible start time is calculated from the scheduled and actual start times of historical cases performed by the same suite, service, and day of the week. While 99 historical cases by the same suite, service, and day of the week are desirable, a minimum of 19 suffices.

Knowledge of "the earliest possible start time" for each case, in conjunction with revised guidelines for patients consuming nothing by mouth, allows some patients to eat or drink on the morning of a procedure with little chance their case would have to be postponed because of food consumption.

Normally, the minimum amount of data to make this determination would be 2–3 months' worth of Mondays, with 9 months preferred. Efficiency of use of OOOR time = [Hours of underutilized time] + [Hours of overutilized time multiplied by a fudge factor (usually assumed to be 2) to account for overtime/staff morale].

CONCLUSION

Many anesthesia groups face large increases in demand for anesthesia OOOR. Unfortunately, it is often difficult to keep an anesthesiologist working all day without gaps in his or her schedule. Providing a functional anesthesia service outside the security of the traditional OR is part of the reason that more and more hospitals have service agreements with anesthesia groups, usually including a stipend.

Involvement by a high-level member of the facility (e.g., hospital vice president) is essential to bring together the budget, data analysis, staffing, and scheduling for OOOR cases. Interpersonal skill and flexibility are needed by the anesthesiologist to work as part of a team in the ambiguity and stresses OOOR.

Staffing and case scheduling for OOOR anesthesia differ from that of ORs. From the start, anesthesia departments should establish a goal to provide coverage of OOOR patients within a reasonable number of days (e.g., 2 weeks) by providing their procedural colleagues with open access to anesthesia-staffed OOOR time. This may require the direct input of the specialists because it is difficult to predict the duration of OOOR cases.

When an anesthesia group is perceived by surgeons, hospital managers, and OOOR proceduralists as "service oriented," the anesthesia group will have an easier time negotiating hospital support.

REFERENCES

1. Bierstein K. Negotiating with hospital administrators. *ASA Newsletter*. 2004;68:1.
2. Dexter F, Macario A, Cowen DS. Staffing and case scheduling for anesthesia in geographically dispersed locations outside of operating rooms. *Curr Opin Anaesthesiol*. 2006;19:453–458.

3. Gabriel RA, Burton BN, Tsai MH, Ehrenfeld JM, Dutton RP, Urman RD. After-hour versus daytime shifts in non-operating room anesthesia environments: national distribution of case volume, patient characteristics, and procedures. *J Med Syst.* 2017;41(9):140.
4. Wu A, Sanford JA, Tsai MH, O'Donnell SE, Tran BK, Urman RD. Analysis to establish differences in efficiency metrics between operating room and non-operating room anesthesia cases. *J Med Syst.* 2017;41(8):120.
5. Tsai MH, Huynh TT, Breidenstein MW, O'Donnell SE, Ehrenfeld JM, Urman RD. A system-wide approach to physician efficiency and utilization rates for non-operating room anesthesia sites. *J Med Syst.* 2017;41(7):112.
6. Martin R. Scheduling anesthesia services outside the operating room. In: Weiss MS, Fleisher LA, eds. *Non-Operating Room Anesthesia.* Philadelphia, PA: Elsevier Saunders; 2015:178–182.
7. Macario A. Are your hospital operating rooms "efficient"? A scoring system with eight performance indicators. *Anesthesiology.* 2006;105:237–240.
8. Strum DP, Vargas LG, May JH. Surgical subspecialty block utilization and capacity planning. A minimal cost analysis model. *Anesthesiology.* 1999;90:1176–1185.
9. Abouleish AE, Dexter F, Epstein RH, Lubarsky DA, Whitten CW, Prough DS. Labor costs incurred by anesthesiology groups because of operating rooms not being allocated and cases not being scheduled to maximize operating room efficiency. *Anesth Analg.* 2003;96:1109–1113.
10. Warner ME, Warner LL, Warner NS. Novel staffing coverage for anesthesia outside the operating room. In: Weiss MS, Fleisher LA, eds. *Non-Operating Room Anesthesia.* Philadelphia, PA: Elsevier Saunders; 2015:205–209.
11. Dexter F, Yue JC, Dow AJ. Predicting anesthesia times for diagnostic and interventional radiological procedures. *Anesth Analg.* 2006;102:1491–1500.
12. Dexter F, Macario A, Traub RD, Hopwood M, Lubarsky DA. An operating room scheduling strategy to maximize the use of operating room block time: computer simulation of patient scheduling and survey of patients' preferences for surgical waiting time. *Anesth Analg.* 1999;89:7–20.
13. Dexter F, Macario A. Changing allocations of operating room time from a system based on historical utilization to one where the aim is to schedule as many surgical cases as possible. *Anesth Analg.* 2002;94:272–1279.
14. Dexter F, Macario A, O'Neill L. Scheduling surgical cases into overflow block time–computer simulation of the effects of scheduling strategies on operating room labor costs. *Anesth Analg.* 2000;90:980–986.
15. Dexter F, Macario A, Qian F, Traub RD. Forecasting surgical groups' total hours of elective cases for allocation of block time Application of time series analysis to operating room management. *Anesthesiology.* 1999;91:1501–1508.

7 | FINANCIAL ANALYSIS AND COMPETITIVE STRATEGIES FOR NORA

SANJANA VIG, MD, MBA, STEVEN BOGGS, MD, MBA

INTRODUCTION

All of us, as both patients and professionals, are witness to the breathtaking progress in procedural medicine. Many interventions that previously would have required hospital admissions and major surgery are now performed outside of traditional operating rooms (ORs). Procedures are accomplished in a minimally invasive manner, and patients are discharged within hours, instead of days, following an intervention. These changes have turned many assumptions on their head. The foremost of these is that the true home of the anesthesiologist is in the OR. While the specialty of anesthesiology has naturally developed in association with surgery, the scientific and technical principles that form the basis of anesthesia practice are transferrable to any location where patients require monitoring, analgesia, and hypnosis.

If current trends remain as they have for the past two decades, surgical caseload in ORs will remain static, while growth in gastrointestinal (GI) suites, electrophysiological rooms, interventional and traditional radiology centers, and other non–operating room anesthesia (NORA) locations will continue to increase.[1] The advantages for patients include minimal or no surgical incisions, shorter hospital stays, lower infection risk, decreased costs, and increased patient convenience. These factors serve to drive more and more procedures out of the OR and to develop these offsite areas. Consequently, it behooves anesthesiologists to understand some basic managerial principles to better serve as leaders who promote efficiency, improve utilization, and reduce costs. Anesthesiologists can then advocate for their patients, and themselves, in a constrained reimbursement environment where all parties must demonstrate their value contribution for their share of bundled payments.

ACCOUNTING

Anyone who has mastered pharmacokinetics is fully capable of developing a basic understanding of the language of commerce, that is, accounting. Understanding the information that accounting statements provide is essential for analyzing the performance of a NORA unit and improving profitability.

The three fundamental accounting statements are the balance sheet, the income statement, and the statement of cash flows. The *balance sheet* is a *quantitative* snapshot of a company's financial condition at a given moment.[2] It is analogous to an x-ray and is defined by a company's assets and liabilities (Figure 7.1). The difference between the two is net assets, as seen in the following equation:

$$\text{Net assets} = \text{Assets} - \text{Liabilities}$$

For not-for-profit entities (e.g., hospitals and health care organizations), net, or shareholders', equity is typically listed as net assets. Assets and liabilities are broken down in current assets (C/A) and current liabilities (C/L). The ratio between the two is called the current ratio (CR). The goal of any entity is to keep this ratio at 2:1; in other words, maintaining high spending power is ensured. The current ratio indicates that the enterprise, or unit, can pay its bills promptly. If the current ratio falls below 2.0, then it is important to scrutinize the balance sheet for areas where intelligent paring of expenditures can be made.

The *income statement* or *statement of activities*, also referred to as the profit-and-loss statement, reports how an entity incurs its revenues and expenses through both operating and nonoperating activities. Company or unit performance is illustrated over a given period of time, analogous to the ongoing presentation of information seen in an anesthetic record (Figure 7.2). This statement comprises operating revenue, operating expenses, and then a class of other items that do not fit neatly into these categories (Table 7.1).

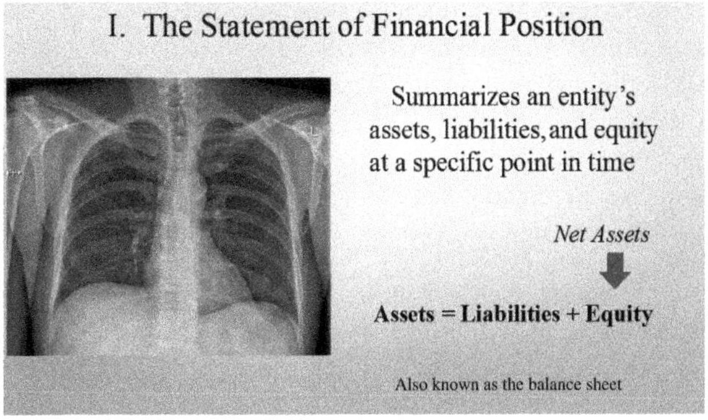

Figure 7.1. Balance sheet.

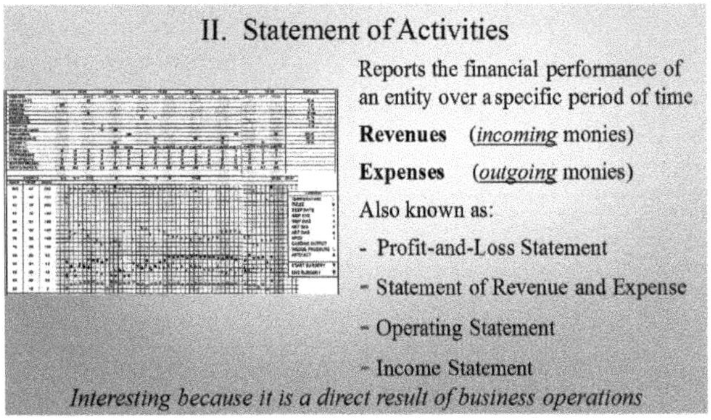

Figure 7.2. Statement of activities.

TABLE 7.1. Other Line Items in Profit/Loss Statement and Item Description

OTHER LINE ITEMS IN PROFIT/LOSS STATEMENT

ITEM	DESCRIPTION
Revenue	From patients, research/academic, investments
Expenses	Salaries/benefits, supplies/outside services
Operating gain and loss	Income earned after expenses are paid, or the bottom line
Excess of revenues over expenses	The money actually earned from all parts of the business or operating room
Operating gain/loss	Operating revenues—operating expenses

SOURCE: Adapted from Bragg SM. *Budgeting: The Comprehensive Guide*. 3rd ed. Centennial, CO: Accounting Tools; 2013.

This statement can also allow a manager to drill down to see where revenues are increasing or decreasing and where expenses are doing the same. It is a useful statement for optimizing financial performance on an ongoing basis.

The third major accounting statement is the *statement of cash flows*. This statement documents incoming and outgoing cash and cash equivalents and separates these activities into operating, investing, and financing activities.[2] To continue the medical analogy, this statement is similar to an input/output graph (Figure 7.3). In the same way that fluid output will decline without adequate input, a company's, or unit's, condition will decline without enough cash inflow. This will occur regardless of the health of the company or patient. For instance, a triathlete can expire in a desert marathon without fluid; in the same way, a company that has a strong balance sheet can fail without adequate cash reserves.

BUDGETS

All of this information is used not only in making operating decisions for an enterprise but also in determining future departmental budgets and financial planning. There are many budget types, of which the revenue budget is most central to the ongoing viability of a business. It reflects revenue expectations for the upcoming year. This budget has two parts, income and expenditure. With changing health care regulations and reimbursements, it is imperative that all assumptions made and conclusions drawn are appropriately described and appended to the budget.[2] Within an anesthesia department, a revenue budget can be broken down by location or specialty and corresponding line items can thus be viewed in multiple ways. Overall, the goal is to allocate resources appropriately and to cut back on waste and excess.

The largest budget to create for anesthesia departments, or groups, is the compensation budget, which accounts for salary and related expenses, social security, Medicare taxes, and federal unemployment taxes. Health insurance benefit, dental, and pension costs are also included. Differences in pay between salaried and hourly workers (plus any overtime costs) must also be considered.

The administration budget includes those support functions that are not accounted for elsewhere. This would include budgets for the executive, accounting, human resources, treasury, information technology, and legal departments.[2] Multiple factors are considered here, including compensation, historical bias (using numbers from the prior year), step costs (i.e., extra OR staff during a time of need), and zero-base analysis (justify each line item expense). While administrative costs generally fall within a fixed range, they must be reexamined often as changes in other budgets can affect administrative costs.

BUDGET CREATION

Budgets can be made using the quicker, but less comprehensive, top-down approach or the more detailed, but slower, bottom-up approach.[2]

Incremental budgeting utilizes historical data, and while it is not as labor intensive to create, the use of past data means that little review is conducted during each new budgeting period. As a result, any existing inefficiencies or budgetary slack are carried forward.

With zero-based budgeting, a bottom-up approach is used, and each line requires specific justification. Thus, historical data are not carried forward; each budgetary period receives a fresh update in regard to departmental fiscal needs. This detailed approach to budgeting requires several factors, as denoted in Table 7.2.

Performance-based budgets are another method that links inputs to outcomes. While this has traditionally been used in the public sector, it is also useful in health care by directly linking strategy and planning to outcomes.

NONBUDGET OPERATIONS; ROLLING FORECASTS

Traditional budgeting processes can be time consuming to create, communicate, and implement across organizations. As a result, many health care entities have begun to operate without a budget. Funds previously used to create budgets

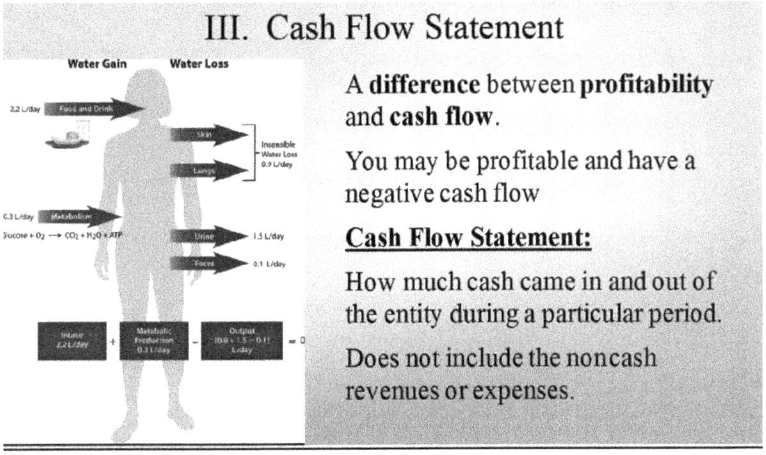

Figure 7.3. Statement of cash flows.

TABLE 7.2. Elements to Consider When Using Zero-Based Budgeting

FACTOR	INFORMATION NEEDED
Develop decision packages	Purpose of activity Business consequence of not performing it Alternatives to activity Costs and benefits of activity Performance metrics of activity
Rank decision packages	From most to least important Preliminarily done by lower-level managers Senior management uses ranking when allocating funds

are now being allocated into rolling forecasts.[2–6] This technique provides continuous feedback between operations and finance, improves efficiency, emphasizes continued performance improvement, and allows for last-minute changes as needed. Creating a rolling forecast is outlined in Table 7.3.[7]

TABLE 7.3. Creating a Rolling Forecast

TO DO	DESCRIPTION
Create strategic plan	Define capital allocations Create operating margins, volume, cost, and profitability targets Consider what-if scenarios: • Reimbursement and patient volume, payer mix changes • Loss of specialty groups
Determine organizational breakdown (i.e., service lines versus clinical specialty)	Identify key performance indicators for each subcategory Delivery information appropriately • Directors receive consolidated results, outliers, explanations • Managers receive detailed reports, and so on

ECONOMICS

The term *cost* may not connote something positive, but costs are critical for management decision-making, resource allocation, and reimbursement justification and can allow income and asset measurement for external parties to satisfy their fiduciary responsibilities. Costs are categorized as fixed or variable.

Fixed costs include

1. Clinical staff:
   - Nurses in preop, OR, postanesthesia care unit (PACU)
   - Ancillary staff
   - Housekeeping
   - Staff in central sterilization (sterile processing)
   - Salaried physicians
2. Administration
   - Accounting
   - Schedulers
   - Chief executive officer compensation
3. Equipment
   - Preop
   - OR
   - PACU
   - Central sterilization
4. Building costs
5. Depreciation of all facilities

However, fixed costs are not always "fixed." If you expand a NORA location from four to six rooms, the fixed costs of the additional salaries needed to staff the location, the overhead, the space, the equipment and depreciation all increase in a stepwise manner. Thus, fixed costs are generally considered to be fixed over a given *range* (Figure 7.4).

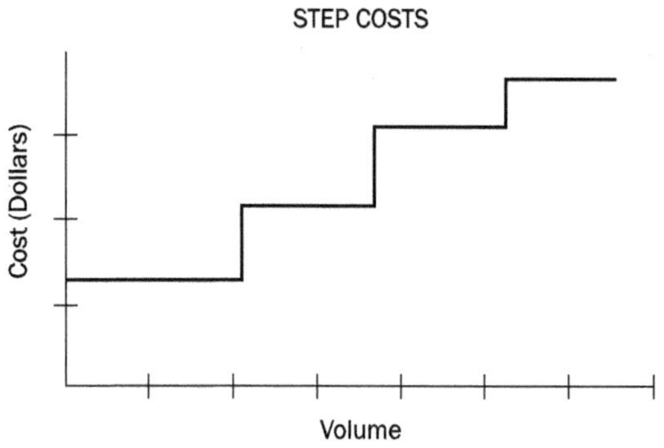

Figure 7.4. Incrementally increased costs as volume increases.

Variable costs, in contrast, vary directly with the number of procedures performed or output achieved. Variable costs in a NORA unit would include anesthetic supplies per case, medications used for each case, catheters used for an interventional radiology case, stents used in advanced endoscopy, and other incrementally increasing costs.

These costs together allow the calculation of the profit and contribution margin. Most hospitals have operating margins that are small, but typically positive. From a hospital's perspective (and likewise for a NORA unit), all revenue generated beyond the break-even point will go directly to profit. As long as a unit remains above the break-even point, the contribution margin may be assessed. This is why—typically—there is such pressure to perform additional cases in these units (Figure 7.5).

The cost of an OR minute is the fixed cost of that unit divided by the scheduled minutes in that unit. For example, if the overhead for a hybrid OR is $5.8 million per year and the unit is staffed 50 weeks × 5 days/week × 8 hours/day × 60 minutes/hour, then the cost per minute of this space would be $48.33. However, the average cost of a case in this unit would be the cost of an OR minute times the average duration of a case plus the variable costs of materials for the case. In other words, the cost would be case specific.

A corollary of this is that improving efficiency may or may not have a direct impact on financial performance. For example, if you improve first-time starts or decrease turnover, but the unit's payroll does not change, there may be no improvement in revenue. However, if these changes allow the performance of additional procedure(s) in the same amount of time without changing the physical space or staffing, then the performance improvements may have a positive financial impact.

SWOT ANALYSIS

SWOT is an acronym for strengths, weaknesses, opportunities, and threats. Strengths and weaknesses are internal factors, while opportunities and threats are external factors. As a planning tool, a SWOT analysis allows the organization to assess who is matching its resources and capabilities with the opportunities in the external environment.

For a NORA location, internal factors that would have to be analyzed include human resources, physical resources, reimbursement, and the way programs are organized. External factors involve both general economic trends and changes in the overall medical marketplace. Locally, the demographic of your patient population would be critical.

An example of a SWOT analysis for a GI center in a hospital would be as follows:

STRENGTHS	WEAKNESSES
• Brand new facility • 6 suites • State-of-the-art endoscopy scopes • High-definition monitors • Major GI group in town employed	• New *freestanding* GI ambulatory center just opened • New center pays better salaries and benefits, thus attracting better staff • New center is recruiting the major GI group by offering part equity stake and anesthesia billings • High efficiency of new center due to nonunionized staff
OPPORTUNITIES	**THREATS**
• Hospital can improve patient flow through the GI center • Valet parking can be offered • Improved convenience for GI services allows "brand association" with the hospital • Routine endoscopy *and* advanced endoscopy can be offered	• Loss of market share will impact the hospital and anesthesia group's bottom line • Market trend to boutique, outpatient facilities • Hospital's physical plant needs architectural redesign to make it more aesthetically pleasing • Possibility of degradation of payer mix if insured patients are not retained

Table 7.4 further analyzes the SWOT of an OR facility overall.

MARKETING

Anesthesiologists working in ORs have historically not needed to market their services.[8-11] It is a given that, in the OR, anesthesia is required. With the emergence of more novel and complex interventional procedures, anesthesiologists are now required to educate both patients and interventionists about the unique skills they provide to increase patient safety and comfort and, in many cases, to allow the procedure to be accomplished at all.

In NORA locations, anesthesiologists are critical to a well-functioning unit. By partnering with proceduralists they can demonstrate that case cancellations and delays can be minimized, that throughput and unit efficiency can increase, and with metrics such as Press Ganey® scores, and patients' satisfaction can improve. All of these factors, when presented in a comprehensive strategic plan can offer demonstrable clinical and financial reasons for the unit to incorporate anesthesia services.

Proceduralists and their units frequently do not have the infrastructure for what anesthesiologists consider to be

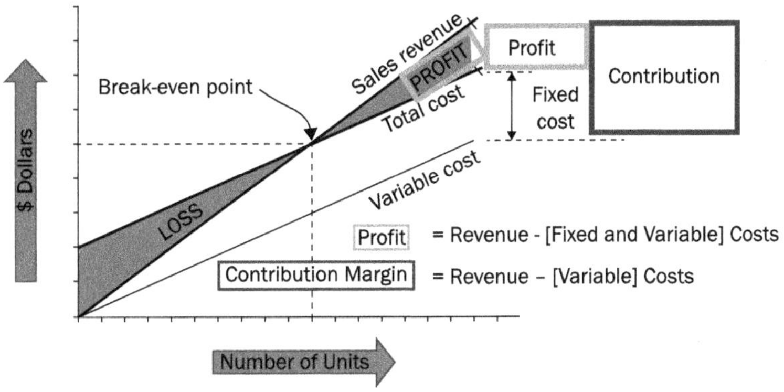

Figure 7.5. *Break-even point: revenues equal costs at a given volume. Profits: all revenues generated above the break-even point, less total costs. Contribution margin: revenues above the break-even point, less variable costs.*

TABLE 7.4. SWOT Analysis of Operating Room

STRENGTHS	WEAKNESSES
• Quick scheduling of cases into preset block times • Relatively quick turnovers • Advanced planning done for equipment needs	• Emergencies and unanticipated changes can drastically alter scheduling • Staffing shortages can limit the number of ORs running at any given time • PACU and ICU bottlenecks can cause backed-up schedules
OPPORTUNITIES	THREATS
• Changing reimbursements are leading to operational changes to improve overall OR efficiency and patient care • Preoperative clinic evaluations are becoming the norm (if not already) in many places • Increased OOOR procedures open up new areas for anesthesia to get involved	• Changing reimbursements also threaten to decrease patient quality of care (increased throughput, unchanged staffing) • Nonphysician providers are rapidly becoming the norm • Includes CRNA, NP, PA, for example • Cost less than having an actual MD

CRNA, certified registered nurse anesthetist; ICU, intensive care unit; NP, nurse practitioner; OOOR, out of the operating room; PA, physician assistant; PACU, postanesthesia care unit.

adequate preoperative assessment. By helping design the preoperative assessment process, anesthesiologists can ensure that patients arriving for a NORA procedure will be optimally assessed, thus allowing proceduralists to maintain focus on the procedure. In addition, it is imperative that anesthesiologists recognize that evidence-based literature of what constitutes a necessary workup for NORA procedures is quite different from that for a patient going to the OR for a major procedure.

Another contribution that anesthesia team members can make is to design the entire care map for a NORA unit.[12] Frequently, the order of cases is changed due to clinical criteria or proceduralist availability. The anesthesiologist can work with nursing colleagues to minimize frustration on the part of patients whose case is delayed.

Finally, as NORA locations grow, anesthesiologists will be called on more and more to design recovery and discharge protocols for these units. Frequently, there is minimal space in these locations, and decisions must be made about whether to transport the patients to a distant PACU (frequently unpopular with both patients and proceduralists) or to observe in a NORA location until discharge criteria are met. As NORA units continue to evolve, these recovery locations will be built into the design, but in the interim period, creativity will be called for.

STAFFING

The majority of hospital expenses involve fixed staffing costs. OR managers are thus incentivized to maximize labor productivity by matching staffing and OR scheduling as closely as possible. NORA cases, however, have some unique challenges[13,14]:

1. Miscommunication of rescheduling/cancellations.
2. Attending staffing of NORA cases may require that those faculty members remain in those off-site areas—this decreases their ability to help cover main OR rooms or even other off-site locations.
3. NORA locations are not interchangeable. For instance, if the GI suite finishes early, leftover electrophysiology cases cannot be moved there in hopes of running extra rooms or finishing early.
4. Longer turnovers (off-site locations may not be as tightly managed or regulated). As a result, while fewer cases may be scheduled during a NORA block, completing them may still take as long, or even longer, than the allotted staffing time available. In addition, patient transport

to the PACU, or other recovery locations, can increase turnover times.

Accurate staffing goes hand in hand with case scheduling. One technique to do this well is to allow open access. In other words, NORA staff can schedule cases ahead of time, thus allowing the anesthesia department advanced notice for coverage requirements. There are five advantages to allowing open access[14]:

1. A service guarantee of maximum patient waiting time allows cases to be done within a reasonable time frame and eliminates the blame factor that anesthesia is causing patients to wait unnecessarily.
2. Open access allows growth of OOOR procedure practices, thus making money for the hospital and anesthesia group.
3. Over time, historical data can be used to better predict future staffing needs.
4. With more accurate staffing predictions, there is a concomitant decrease in costs as NORA utilization is improved. For instance, within an EP department running two rooms, any overutilization in one room can be easily transferred to another, underutilized room, given that adequate staffing is already available to continue coverage.

Increasing NORA case numbers have also increased the overall patient load that PACU and intensive care units (ICUs) must handle. When managing these off-site locations and growing those practices, then, it is imperative to keep in mind the staffing needs of those units. Without appropriate coverage, bottlenecks may develop, which can lead to PACU delays and prolonged OR wait times for ICU beds.

UTILIZATION AND PRODUCTIVITY

Productivity is output *per unit* of input, while efficiency is output as a *percentage* of input. We focus on efficiency to reduce waste.[15] One significant factor to consider in the management of all anesthesia locations is the utilization rate. Depending on the case mix in a NORA unit, the utilization rate will vary. EGD (esophagogastroduodenoscopy) and colonoscopy procedures are much shorter than advanced endoscopy procedures. Therefore, multiple procedures can be performed in the same room in the same day, making rapid turnover essential for maximal efficiency. In contrast, an electrophysiological study may take several hours, increasing the importance of scheduling accuracy to avoid overutilization of resources.

As can be seen in Figure 7.6, 100% utilization is extremely difficult to achieve. It requires that a case begin exactly when schedule indicates it is planned to start (Example A) and conclude exactly at the end of this period. In this example, the day is presumed to be an 8-hour day starting at 8:00 AM. If the case starts late (Example B) or finishes early (Example C), there is unutilized time. You can also have unutilized time between cases, as seen in Example D. Moreover, it must be emphasized that underutilized and overutilized time can occur in the same procedure room on the same day (Example E).

The NORA units appear to have higher rates of underutilization than traditional ORs. In an abstract presented at the 2016 American Society of Anesthesiologists (ASA), Tsai et al. compared 11,483 main OR suites with 3137 NORA locations at the University of Vermont. As illustrated in Figure 7.7, the underutilization as a percentage of inefficient time between the two locations was striking.

In a study from the University of Kentucky, Kimbrough et al. looked to improve OR efficiency by focusing on constraint management.[16] The principles and improvements in their study can be applied to NORA locations. Their method was 2-fold:

I. Identify system constraints
   - Missing documentation
   - Incomplete testing
   - Missing surgeon and/or resident
   - Noncurrent preference cards

II. Devise low-technology, practical solutions
   - Actively manage the schedule
   - Enforce quality initiatives
   - Use transparency of metrics
   - Provide a culture of efficiency and accountability

By doing this, they were able to increase first-time starts from 40% to over 80%. They were able to increase the number of cases performed between 7 AM and 5 PM with no increase in the number of cases performed between 5 and 11 PM. Plus, they increased utilization from about 73% to about 85%—which is realistically as high as might be desired.

In a study by Strum et al.,[17] the cost of overutilized time exceeds that of underutilized time. This is not only because of the cost of overtime, but also because of the alienation of staff members always being asked to stay late. Most health care workers anticipate emergencies. However, it is a poor staffing model to consistently rely on staff staying late to cover cases that routinely run late. This leads to high staff turnover and the associated recruitment costs.

Another factor to consider is that as utilization increases, access to the schedule decreases.[18] Anything above 80% utilization means that it will be difficult for additional interventionalists to add cases to the schedule (Figure 7.8). For units that perform mainly elective cases, this may actually be an advantage. However, in units that must have capacity for emergent add-ons, some capacity must remain for cases that are urgent.

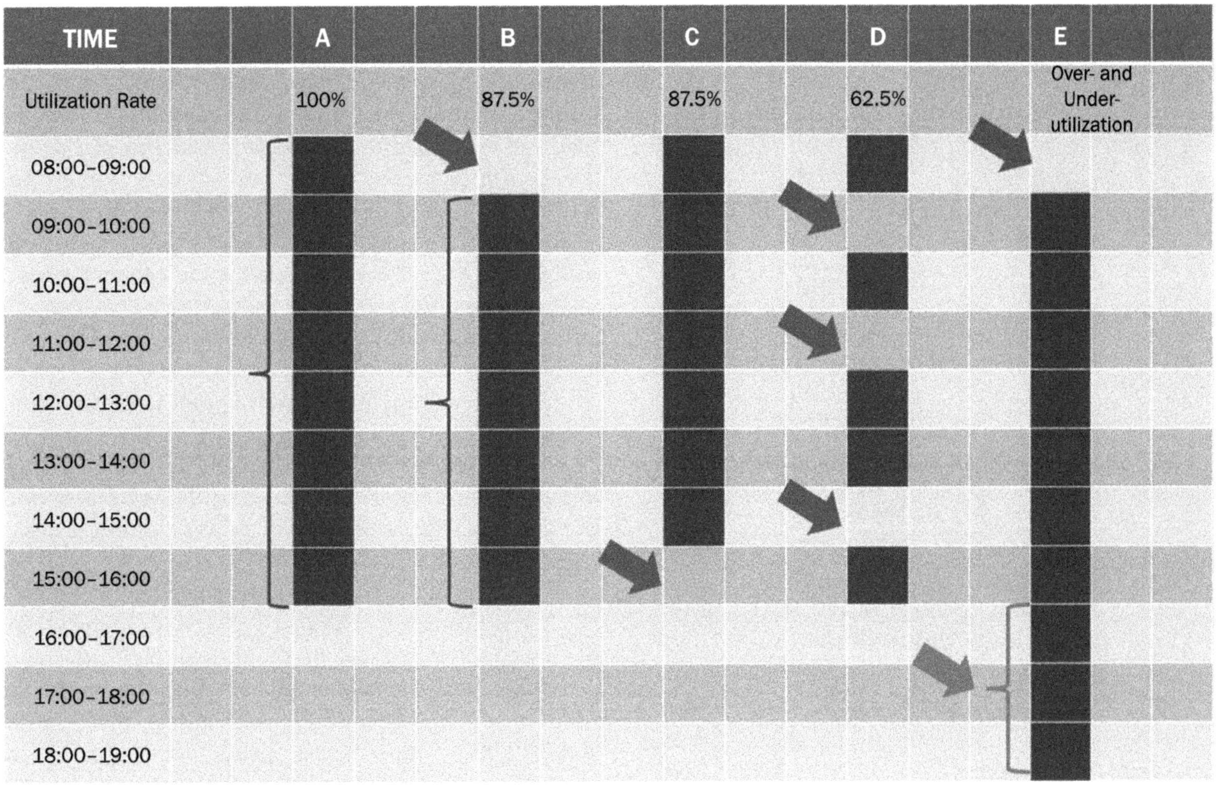

Figure 7.6. Examples of under- and overutilization.

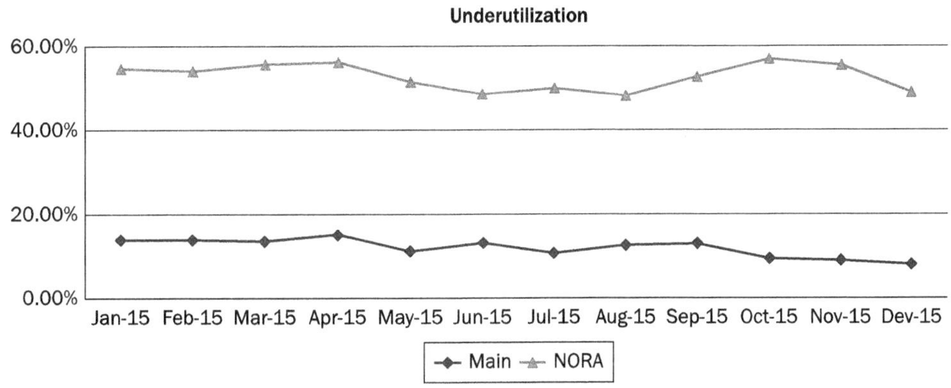

Figure 7.7. Underutilization as a percentage of inefficient time, main OR versus NORA locations.

Another factor to consider when running a unit is that when a manager uses the term *efficiency*, it is important to clarify what the manager means. A study from Sweden evaluated this concept.[19] Performing an intensive interview of 12 subjects, investigators found that anesthesiologists, surgeons, and experienced nurses defined efficiency as achieving desired results with the least resources and fast work with preserved quality. In contrast, nurse anesthetists and less-experienced nurses considered efficiency to be doing one's best, enjoying work, and adjusting energy to the situation. This underscores the importance of making sure that everyone knows exactly what goals are, including definitions, if process improvements are undertaken.

PROCEDURAL SCORECARD

Operating room literature documents well the importance of tracking certain metrics to improve OR financial performance.[20,21] Macario at Stanford has listed some of these, which include[22]

- Minimizing staffing costs
- Reducing start-time tardiness
- Reducing case cancellation rate
- Minimizing PACU admission delays

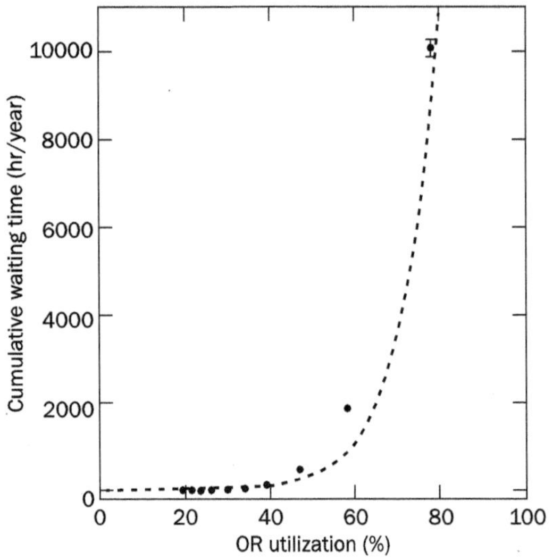

Figure 7.8. *Wait time as a function of OR utilization. (Originally printed by Antognini JMO, Antognini JF, Khatri V. How many operating rooms are needed to manage non-elective surgical cases? A Monte Carlo simulation study. BMC Health Serv Res. 2015;15:487. doi:10.1186/s12913-015-1148-x.)*

- Improving the contribution margin (mean) per hour
- Having rapid turnover times
- Improving prediction bias (estimation of case duration)
- Minimizing prolonged turnovers

For individual NORA locations (GI, electrophysiology, radiology, interventional radiology), these metrics are just now being measured. However, the direction in which each one of these metrics should be moving can be tracked in any given unit and optimized to enhance financial performance. Other scorecards have been proposed to address efficiency, quality, and outcome metrics.[21,23]

The Veterans Affairs uses a list of metrics to track reasons for cases being canceled, separating cancellation causes due to patient factors, facility factors, the patient's workup, anesthesia, and surgical reasons. As can be seen in Table 7.5, most of these factors can be applied to NORA locations.[24]

Gabriel and colleagues conjoined OR efficiency metrics with quality metrics.[21] These data would then be used to give feedback to anesthesiologists on a quarterly and annual basis. Physicians respond to feedback, and this method can be used to improve both operational and financial performance and to improve quality.[25]

TECHNOLOGY

Technological advancements have helped not only to increase the number of NORA procedures but also to ensure that appropriate scheduling of those procedures occurs. Variation in practice among institutions shows that some still utilize nontechnological means of NORA scheduling (i.e., phone calls or regular paper submissions to anesthesia schedulers).[13,26]

Dexter et al. set up a system wherein schedulers of various departments requiring NORA (radiology, GI, etc.) were given the ability to schedule cases themselves as needed through an electronic system. The schedule would then be reviewed by the anesthesia team and discrepancies addressed. Per their findings, there are several advantages to giving outside departments this ability. First, there are fewer phone calls or emails for the anesthesia scheduler to field on a given day; second, there is increased consistency in patient preoperative instructions; third, there is an increased ability to coordinate patient appointments (e.g., can receive a CT scan, then come for procedure afterward on the same day).[26]

There are several financial advantages to using technology for scheduling. By integrating the OR suites with the off-site locations receiving anesthesia, schedulers are better prepared to meet staffing needs, which in turn allows for better allocation of patient cases and resources and decreased over- and underutilization of OR time.[13,27]

For instance, if a certified registered nurse anesthetist (CRNA) scheduled for work for 10 hours is assigned to an off-site area, then it is in the best interest of both the anesthesia department and the off-site area to schedule enough cases to complete in a 10-hour block. Anticipating this "anesthesia" block, allows off-site physicians to improve their patient scheduling (higher throughput), which allows better preparation for case turnover and ancillary staffing. It also motivates an efficient work ethic by the proceduralist (knowing you have 10 cases to complete in 10 hours makes you waste less time).[13,28]

Improvements in utilization and staffing should occur on an ongoing, day-to-day basis. Use of computer systems can help analyze daily utilization patterns and help with future decision-making.[29] For instance, with NORA locations that consistently overuse their block time, based on historical data, the block time allocations should be extended for anesthesia services. This not only helps with anesthesia assignments but also helps nursing staff anticipate their workday requirements, thus decreasing overall overtime costs.

Information drawn from historical data can also be used to predict future case durations based on case type and proceduralist, another parameter to consider when scheduling cases.[13] Anesthesia groups that actively participate in data analysis, and assist in making corresponding management decisions, have the advantage of enhancing their position as OR stakeholders.[30]

However, it is important to keep in mind that data and data analysis alone cannot promote improvement and change. Staffing and employee skills must also be taken into account.[30] Therefore, when gathering and analyzing any information, one must be careful to place it within the correct context and use an appropriate, institution-specific, set of assumptions to avoid common statistical pitfalls.

ORGANIZATION

Organization is critical to the management of any NORA location. Because interventionists and ancillary staff in these areas are not as familiar with anesthesia requirements—and because anesthesia providers are, likewise, usually not fully aware of

TABLE 7.5. Veterans Affairs (VA) Categories for Surgical Case Cancellations

PATIENT	FACILITY	WORKUP	ANESTHESIA	SURGICAL
Patient refused or no consent	Equipment broken or not available	Surgeon workup needed	Anesthesia staff not available	Surgery staff not available
VA transportation	Implant(s) not available	Anesthesia workup needed		
Patient transportation	No ICU beds	Abnormal test		
Preoperative instructions not followed or patient not instructed adequately	No hospital beds	Change in medical status		
Patient substance abuse	Scheduling error	Change in treatment plan		
Patient cancels, had procedure performed elsewhere	Staff shortage, other than surgeons and anesthesia providers			
Patient cancels, but did not have the procedure performed elsewhere	No OR time			
Patient death	Emergency case			
Case aborted in OR	Blood products not available			
Patient is a no-show, no contact from patient	Facility environment			
	Weather/natural disaster			

ICU, intensive care unit; OR, operating room.

the requirements of the staff in these areas—organization is critical to improve unit performance.

Everyone involved in the case should be aware of what other team members are trying to accomplish. Effective teamwork in NORA locations, as in the OR, includes coordination, communication, cooperation, leadership, and monitoring.[31] This is especially critical when novel procedures are attempted. Team huddles at the beginning of the day or else before each case are a useful method to incorporate teamwork and team building not only into everyday work, but also into every case performed each day. Because of the constant changes that occur on the procedure list in many NORA locations, it is imperative that everyone be aware of alterations in the schedule. These factors will increase both safety and efficiency in these locations.

REFERENCES

1. Koenig L, Doherty J, Dreyfus J, Xanthopoulos J. An analysis of recent growth of ambulatory surgery centers [Report for ASC Coalition]. Available at: http://citeseerx.ist.psu.edu/viewdoc/download?doi=10.1.1.512.4498&rep=rep1&type=pdf. Published June 5, 2009. Accessed on April 7, 2018.
2. Bragg SM. *Budgeting: The Comprehensive Guide.* 3rd ed. Centennial, CO: Accounting Tools; 2013.
3. Teach E. No time for budgets: yesterday's budgets are too slow for today's volatile world. Here's how to pick up the planning pace. *CFO Magazine,* May 27, 2014. Available at: http://ww2.cfo.com/budgeting/2014/05/time-budgets/. Accessed on April 7, 2018.
4. Miller D, Fau AM, Fau SS, Hackman T. How rolling forecasting facilitates dynamic, agile planning. *Healthc Financ Manage.* 2013;67:80–82, 84.
5. Newberg A, Sutton J. Healthcare financial planning using rolling forecast. Crowe Horwath LLP. Available at: https://www.crowehorwath.com/insights/healthcare-connection/hc-rolling-forecast.aspx. Published February 23, 2016. Accessed on April 7, 2018.
6. Myers R. Budgets on a roll: recalculating a business' outlook several times a year. *J Accountancy.* 2001 Dec 1. Available at: https://www.journalofaccountancy.com/issues/2001/dec/budgetsonaroll.html. Accessed on April 7, 2018.
7. Johnson H. Rolling budgets catching on—more efficient and flexible forecasting tools. *Crain's New York Business,* July 31, 2011.
8. Cohen B, Ogorek D, Oifa S, Cattan A, Matot I. Smart marketing may improve public understanding of the anesthesia profession. *Isr J Health Policy Res.* 2015;4:16. doi:10.1186/s13584-015-0011-1. Available at: https://www.ncbi.nlm.nih.gov/pubmed/26078849. Accessed on April 7, 2018.
9. Liu R, Garcia PS, Fleisher LA. Interest in anesthesia as reflected by keyword searches using common search engines. *J Anesth Clin Res.* 2012;3:1000187. doi: 10.4172/2155-6148.1000187. Accessed on April 7, 2018.
10. Liu H, Waxman DA, Main R, Mattke S. Utilization of anesthesia services during outpatient endoscopies and colonoscopies and associated spending in 2003–2009. *JAMA.* 2012;307(11):1178–1184. doi:10.1001/jama.2012.270. Available at: https://www.ncbi.nlm.nih.gov/pubmed/22436958. Accessed on April 7, 2018.
11. National Institute for Clinical Excellence. Routine preoperative tests for elective surgery. Available at: https://www.nice.org.uk/guidance/ng45. Published April 5, 2016. Accessed on April 7, 2018.
12. Marjamaa R, Vakkuri A, Kirvela O. Operating room management: why, how and by whom? *Acta Anaesthesiol Scand.* 2008;52(5):596–600. doi:10.1111/j.1399-6576.2008.01618.x. Available at: https://www.ncbi.nlm.nih.gov/pubmed/18419711. Accessed on April 7, 2018.
13. Macario A. Proper scheduling of anesthesia services outside of the operating room suite. Available at: http://www.medscape.com/viewarticle/714107. Published December 29, 2009. Accessed on April 7, 2018.
14. Dexter F, Owens D. Staffing and case scheduling for anesthesia in geographically dispersed locations outside of operating rooms. In: Macario

A, ed., *Anaesthesia Outside of the Operating Room.* Philadelphia, PA: Lippincott & Williams; 2006:453–458.

15. Tsai M, Sanford JA, Genziano JL, O'Donnell SE, Urman RD.Information Management And Database Research. NORA Scheduling Error: A Game of Over and Under. A5017; 2016.
16. Kimbrough CW, McMasters KM, Canary J, et al. Improved operating room efficiency via constraint management: experience of a tertiary-care academic medical center. *J Am Coll Surg.* 2015;221(1):154–162. doi:10.1016/j.jamcollsurg.2015.02.032.
17. Strum DP, Vargas LG, May JH, Bashein G. Surgical suite utilization and capacity planning: a minimal cost analysis model. *J Med Syst.* 1997;21(5):309–322.
18. Antognini JMO, Antognini JF, Khatri V. How many operating rooms are needed to manage non-elective surgical cases? A Monte Carlo simulation study. *BMC Health Serv Res.* 2015;15(1):487. doi:10.1186/s12913-015-1148-x.
19. Arakelian E, Gunningberg L, Larsson J. How operating room efficiency is understood in a surgical team: a qualitative study. *Int J Qual Health Care.* 2011;23(1):100–106. doi:10.1093/intqhc/mzq063.
20. Fixler T, Wright JG. Identification and use of operating room efficiency indicators: the problem of definition. *Can J Surg.* 2013;56(4):224–226. doi:10.1503/cjs.020712. Available at: https://www.ncbi.nlm.nih.gov/pubmed/23883490. Accessed on April 7, 2018.
21. Gabriel RA, Gimlich R, Ehrenfeld JM, Urman RD. Operating room metrics score card-creating a prototype for individualized feedback. *J Med Syst.* 2014;38(11):144. doi:10.1007/s10916-014-0144-8. Available at: https://www.ncbi.nlm.nih.gov/pubmed/25315824. Accessed on April 7, 2018.
22. Macario A. Are your operating rooms being run efficiently? *Medscape Anesthesiology*, April 07, 2010. http://www.medscape.com/viewarticle/719542. Accessed on April 7, 2018.
23. Peccora CD, Gimlich R, Cornell RP, Vacanti CA, Ehrenfeld JM, Urman RD. Anesthesia report card—a customizable tool for performance improvement. *J Med Syst.* 2014;38:105. doi:10.1007/s10916-014-0105-2. Epub 2014 Jul 20.
24. Basson MD, Butler TW, Verma H. Predicting patient nonappearance for surgery as a scheduling strategy to optimize operating room utilization in a veterans' administration hospital [Abstract]. *Anesthesiology.* 2006;104:826–834.
25. Kaye AD, Okanlawon OJ, Urman RD. Clinical performance feedback and quality improvement opportunities for perioperative physicians. *Adv Med Educ Pract.* 2014;5:115–123. doi:10.2147/AMEP.S62165. Available at: https://www.ncbi.nlm.nih.gov/pubmed/24833948. Accessed on April 7, 2018.
26. Dexter F, Xiao Y, Dow AJ, Strader MM, Ho D, Wachtel RE. Coordination of appointments for anesthesia care outside of operating rooms using an enterprise-wide scheduling system. *Anesth Analg.* 2007;105(6):1701–1710. doi:10.1213/01.ane.0000287686.23187.3f.
27. Randa K, Heiser R, Gill R. Strategic investments in the operating room (OR): information technology (IT) to generate rapid ROI and long-term competitive advantage. Available at: http://dev.healthleadersmedia.com/content/242938.pdf. Published 2010. Accessed on August 15, 2015. Accessed on April 7, 2018.
28. md buyline, Research Library. Integrated operating rooms. Available at: http://www.mdbuyline.com/research-library/articles/integrated-operating-rooms/. Published 2017. Accessed on April 7, 2018.
29. Macario A, Vasanawala M. Technology and computing in the surgical suite: key features of an OR management information system and opportunities for the future. *Anesth Analg.* 2002;95(4):1120–1121. doi:10.1213/00000539-200210000-00067. Accessed on April 7, 2018.
30. Sanford JA, Macario A. Data, data, on the server: challenges in applying data analysis to operating room management. *Anesthesiology.* 2014;121(1):6–8. doi:10.1097/ALN.0000000000000288. Available at: https://www.ncbi.nlm.nih.gov/pubmed/24796683. Accessed on April 7, 2018.
31. Passauer-Baierl S, Baschnegger H, Bruns C, Weigl M. Interdisziplinare Teamarbeit im OP: Identifikation und Erfassung von Teamarbeit im Operationssaal. DEP—20130701 [Interdisciplinary teamwork in the OR: identification and measurement of teamwork in the operating room].. *Z Evid Fortbild Qual Gesundhwes.* 2014;108(5–6):293–298. doi:10.1016/j.zefq.2013.05.007. Available at: https://www.ncbi.nlm.nih.gov/pubmed/25066348. Accessed on April 7, 2018.

ADDITIONAL READINGS

Gabriel RA, Burton BN, Tsai MH, Ehrenfeld JM, Dutton RP, Urman RD. After-hour versus daytime shifts in non-operating room anesthesia environments: national distribution of case volume, patient characteristics, and procedures. *J Med Syst.* 2017;41(9):140.

Wu A, Sanford JA, Tsai MH, O'Donnell SE, Tran BK, Urman RD. Analysis to establish differences in efficiency metrics between operating room and non-operating room anesthesia cases. *J Med Syst.* 2017;41(8):120.

Tsai MH, Huynh TT, Breidenstein MW, O'Donnell SE, Ehrenfeld JM, Urman RD. A system-wide approach to physician efficiency and utilization rates for non-operating room anesthesia sites. *J Med Syst.* 2017;41(7):112.

8 | ANESTHESIA INFORMATION MANAGEMENT SYSTEMS (AIMS) FOR THE OOOR SETTING

KEITH J. RUSKIN, MD, ORI GOTTLIEB, MD

INTRODUCTION

Anesthesia information management systems (AIMSs) offer the same benefits to an anesthesiologist who practices beyond the operating room as they do to those managing inpatients undergoing complex surgical procedures. An electronic workflow allows the anesthesiologist to focus on patient care while facilitating tasks such as quality assurance, compliance, research, and billing. AIMSs have the potential to improve patient care because they deliver a customized, legible anesthesia record while storing the patient's physiologic data in an easily searchable database. This information can be used for quality assurance, to search for and track specific events and their outcomes, and to provide benchmarking for individual providers.

Anesthesiologists have been among the first to develop technology for keeping electronic health records (EHRs) and work with medical device manufacturers and standards organizations to create new devices that can communicate with AIMSs. In one study, 67% of all academic anesthesiology practices had adopted AIMSs. This same study predicted an 84% adoption rate between 2018 and 2020.[1] This ability to collect, store, and organize large amounts of data makes AIMSs ideal for quality assurance and clinical research. Although many office anesthesia practices still rely on paper records, these practitioners may soon begin to adopt EHRs.

BENEFITS

An EHR can facilitate preoperative screening and may ultimately decrease the incidence of outpatient procedures needing to be deferred, delayed, or canceled. A preoperative evaluation module makes the patient's history, physical examination, and pertinent laboratory data easily accessible to the anesthesiologist. A survey of anesthesiologists attending a large meeting revealed that missing information commonly caused cancellations on the day of surgery.[2] The ability to access a patient's medical information either on site or remotely, including the anesthesia record from prior surgeries, can help to prevent the cancellation of a procedure simply because the needed information was unavailable. This improves both patient and surgeon satisfaction while maximizing the use of valuable resources, making an EHR with a preoperative evaluation module a desirable component of an AIMS, whether it is used in the surgical or procedural setting.

In one example of how AIMSs can improve patient care, Nair et al. reported that including real-time alerts for prophylactic antibiotic administration increased the rate of timely administration by over 9%. The study concluded that a decision support system that includes real-time guidance and alerts could improve compliance with guidelines.[3] The Anesthesia Quality Institute (AQI), under the umbrella of the American Society of Anesthesiologists (ASA), is a nonprofit foundation that maintains the National Anesthesia Clinical Outcomes Registry (NACOR). Widespread use of information that NACOR produces helps anesthesiologists improve their practice. The AQI works with both AIMS vendors and practice groups to facilitate methods for transmitting anesthesia records to its database.

The development of widely used data transmission standards has made it possible to connect medical equipment together and to transmit medical information through existing networks to desktop computers, mobile devices, servers, or monitoring stations. Wireless networks (Wi-Fi) are inexpensive to set up and maintain and are highly versatile. The end result is that a core communication infrastructure is likely to be compatible with new devices and can be installed using commercially available equipment, even in an outpatient or office setting. These advantages, combined with the low cost and wide availability of Wi-Fi equipment, make this technology well suited for many health care applications. Most monitors are now capable of transmitting numbers and waveforms (e.g., an electrocardiogram or a blood pressure tracing) to a remote device, making this critical information immediately available to the clinician. A portable device capable of displaying this critical information allows a physician to be immediately available in the event of a sudden change in the patient's condition.[4,5] For example, an anesthesiologist can care for a patient in the operating room while being able to observe the vital signs of a patient who is in the recovery area.

CHOOSING A SYSTEM

When choosing an AIMS for an office-based practice, the questions that should be considered are fundamentally the same as those of a large, hospital-based practice. The practitioner should choose a system that allows him or her to provide high-quality perioperative care while keeping a comprehensive record that meets third-party payer and regulatory requirements. Several commercially available systems use wireless devices (e.g., an Apple iPad) to facilitate record-keeping in an office setting. Two systems (Anesthesiaos [Medical Information Records, Houston, TX] and PlexusTG [Plexus Technology Group, Birmingham, AL]) offer complete solutions that include compliance with PQRS (Physician Quality Reporting System) and QCDR requirements as well as electronic billing support. Evaluating a system on its return on investment (ROI) may not be productive because an AIMS may never pay for itself by increasing profits. Instead, the provider should do a cost-benefit analysis that includes such intangible benefits as reduced medication errors, improved resource utilization, and more rapid patient turnover.

Specific characteristics that should be evaluated before purchasing a system include compatibility issues, ability to access old records, safety and data security features, and usability. Whenever possible, it should be a system that is ideally integrated or, at the very least, compatible with existing EHR. This will allow the anesthesia record to be incorporated into the remainder of the patient record. This also improves patient flow because pertinent preoperative information may be available to the anesthesiologist. The system should also be able to display critical information, such as patient demographics and drug allergies.

The ability to extract information for quality assurance will help the provider to improve patient care as well as meet some state and third-party payer requirements. Such a system can be used to identify specific events that should be reviewed as part of a quality assurance process. It can also be used to create quality dashboards that can be used to identify areas for practice improvement.[6] A system that captures comorbidities and billing modifiers will help to improve revenue by charging for services that otherwise might have been missed by a billing service.

All patient information must be stored securely to prevent data breaches, and the system should maintain an audit trail that indicates who modified a record and what modifications were made. Most important, the system must be easy to use. A system that is not compatible with physiologic monitors, for example, and requires manual entry of vital signs will rapidly fall into disuse. Last, the vendor should have a solid record of successful installations in practices that are similar to the one in which it will be used. It is important to make several site visits to see the system in actual use, to speak with the anesthesia providers who are using it, and to see the reports that the system generates.

In many cases, the choice of an AIMS will be determined by its compatibility with existing information systems or be included as part of a larger purchase by a practice management group. In this case, it is critical for the anesthesiologists who will use the system to participate in the negotiations regarding the system, especially with respect to how it will be installed and integrated into existing workflow. The practice should also ensure that provisions have been made for training and troubleshooting.

BARRIERS TO IMPLEMENTATION

Despite the obvious advantages of EHRs, however, their complexity and costs have prevented many providers, particularly those working in small hospitals or in rural practices, from adopting this important technology. As many office-based anesthesiologists rely on the surgeon's medical records, an AIMS may not be available to them. As a result, few anesthesiologists who practice in an office setting will have the resources to adopt a comprehensive AIMS. Many of these systems can, however, provide an ROI by ensuring compliance with Physician Quality Reporting Initiative (PQRI) guidelines and Centers for Medicare and Medicaid Services (CMS) documentation requirements. AIMSs have also been shown to increase scheduling efficiency, decrease drug costs, and provide better charge capture and diagnosis and procedure coding.[7,8] However, at least the initial implementation period may be associated with decreased operating room efficiency.[9,10] The American Recovery and Reinvestment Act (ARRA) established programs to distribute approximately $19 billion to eligible health care professionals who participate in Medicare and adopt practices that make "meaningful use" (MU) of EHRs. Although most hospital-based anesthesiologists are specifically excluded from these incentives, office-based anesthesiologists or others who bill primarily under ambulatory service codes might be eligible for these payments. It is currently unknown, however, whether the CMS will consider offering incentives to office-based anesthesiologists who provide evidence of MU.

Although implementing an AIMS is initially time consuming and requires substantial resources, several studies have identified predictors of user satisfaction. At least one study has shown that physicians who have been using an EHR for at least 2 years are more likely to be satisfied or very satisfied with the system. This study, which focused on primary care physicians, also revealed that clinical notes, an easily accessible diagnosis, and off-site login capabilities were also important. Although anesthesiologists have different information needs, these predictors would seem to be important to any user of an AIMS.[11]

Perhaps the most significant difficulty in upgrading an AIMS occurs if it is necessary to migrate from one system to another that is provided by a different vendor. Although most systems store information in commercially available databases (e.g., Microsoft SQL Server), it may be difficult to move many patient records into a completely new system. It is therefore important to choose a system that can grow and adapt to a changing practice and that will be usable for the foreseeable future. It is also important to carefully explore problems related to data migration before migrating to a new system.

INFORMATION SECURITY

Electronic generation, transmission, and storage of health data have transformed patient care by making it easy to acquire, search, manipulate, and distribute large amounts of information. Information in the health record is also used for purposes not directly related to patient care, including insurance qualification, law enforcement, and litigation. Health information may also be used for clinical research, quality reporting, and outcome measurements and for other projects that improve public health. Unintentional release of information about disease processes, medication use, or visits to health care providers can result in stigmatization, difficulty in obtaining credit or employment, or disruption of friendships or family relationships. Most important, unintended release of information can result in a breach of trust between patient and physician. Patients and physicians are aware of how health information may be used and have legitimate concerns about how their information will be used and expect their health care providers to protect health information from unauthorized use.

Government regulations as well as ethical obligations require that patients' health information be protected. Most of the requirements for storage and transmission of medical records are covered under the Health Insurance Portability and Accountability Act of 1996 (HIPAA). These requirements extend beyond health professionals who collect information. Any provider of services to a health care organization that handles protected health information (PHI) is bound by HIPAA to defend the security of medical records. Any practice contemplating the implementation of an AIMS should develop a comprehensive information security plan that encompasses physical protection of hardware, access control, data storage, and encryption of sensitive information.[12]

Specific requirements for privacy and security of electronic medical records systems are included in HIPAA. The primary impact of the HIPAA Privacy Rule on the development of preanesthetic evaluation systems is to require user identification and authentication and to log every access to the EHR to allow the patient to have access to a list of all personnel who had accessed the record. Under HIPAA, health care organizations face a series of regulations that dictate how PHI must be stored, distributed, and used. These regulations apply not only to practitioners who collect the information but also to their business associates. If, for example, a physician in solo practice collects information that is then forwarded to a billing service, that billing service must comply with HIPAA privacy rules. Patients must give consent to the use of PHI, although HIPAA consents can be interpreted broadly. Compliance with HIPAA regulations will ultimately benefit health care providers by preventing or limiting disclosure or damage to PHI.[13] The Health Information Technology for Economic and Clinical Health (HITECH) Act was enacted as part of the ARRA of 2009 and is intended to promote the adoption and MU of health information technology. HITECH includes $20 billion in funding for health information and extends the privacy and data security regulations enacted as part of HIPAA. The act also includes provisions for the development of health information standards as well as even stronger privacy and security regulations. As interoperable EHRs become commonplace, however, the ability to share information between providers and institutions will require that the health care provider and the patient jointly determine who can access PHI and how it will be used.[12]

Attacks on personal computers in the form of viruses, keystroke loggers, ransomware, and "phishing" attacks are a growing threat and have the potential to interfere with patient care. Hundreds of viruses are released every day. Many health care applications rely on Intel-based computers running the Microsoft Windows operating system. As a result, they are vulnerable to the same kinds of viruses that affect home and office computers. In addition to rendering a computer unreliable, viruses and worms can compromise, steal, hide, or destroy health information. Ransomware encrypts PHI, rendering it unusable until the victim pays the attacker for a key to decrypt the data. Unfortunately, the latest trend is malware that allows the attacker to retain access to the data, permitting future attacks or allowing the data to be sold to other criminals. Because office based AIMSs may be readily accessible to a variety of staff, it is important to limit the number of programs installed on the computers that run patient care applications. Office staff should be educated regarding the critical nature of these computers and the impact on patient care should the computer become unusable because of a virus infection.

Fortunately, some simple precautions, combined with common sense, can minimize the risk of information theft or damage. Ideally, protection of computers on a network should involve a comprehensive approach that includes both hardware and software firewalls, antivirus software, and frequent security analyses. All access to sensitive information must be protected by a carefully chosen password, which should ideally consist of a series of letters, numerals, and punctuation marks. Remote access to hospital information systems from home computers and mobile devices, which may not have the latest security updates, should be allowed only when necessary, and these computers should be encrypted using security software installed by the hospital information technology department. Several security companies will, for a fee, attempt to break into the institution's computers to find and repair vulnerabilities. It is also possible to hire companies to send social engineering (phishing) messages to employees. These messages then redirect employees who fall for the ruse to educational sites that explain how to identify suspect email.

Firewalls determine if information traveling across a network should be allowed to continue. Software firewalls prevent unauthorized programs from using an Internet connection. Specific programs, such as a web client, are permitted to send information to a given address. If an unknown program attempts to establish a connection, a software firewall blocks the connection until the user grants access. By limiting the programs that can send information to external computers, software firewalls prevent information from being stolen by spyware or adware. A hardware firewall is a piece of equipment that is installed between a home or office network and potential threats from the Internet and helps to protect against attacks from outside computers. Hardware firewalls guard an entire network against an outside attack but usually permit any computer on the local network to establish an outbound connection. As a result, hardware firewalls do not protect against programs that harvest information. To maintain an adequate level of security, the firewall's firmware must be updated regularly, and the default user ID and password must be changed immediately on installation. One recent distributed denial of service attack used devices such as home routers and Internet-connected baby monitors that had been infected with malware.[14]

CONCLUSIONS

In conclusion, AIMSs offer a variety of benefits to any anesthesia provider, including those who practice beyond the operating room, such as in an office setting. The increasing requirement for anesthesia services in locations such as interventional radiology or endoscopy suites underscores the need for efficient, reliable AIMSs. Modern systems offer a sophisticated user interface, allowing multiple features to be accessed at the touch of a button. Online help systems can allow the clinician to find the particular feature that he or she was looking for, and newer systems are far more intuitive and easy to use. Clinical Decision Support (CDS) through an AIMS has matured to a point where it can offer significant help to the anesthesiologist. Furthermore, AIMS can improve operating room efficiency, decrease the number of canceled or deferred procedures, and provide important information that can be used for quality assurance and regulatory compliance. A variety of factors must be considered before purchasing an AIMS, including compatibility with existing EHRs and monitors, data security and integrity, and usability. If chosen carefully and implemented as part of a comprehensive information technology solution, an AIMS can be successfully adopted by the anesthesiologist practicing primarily beyond the operating room setting.

REFERENCES

1. Stol IS, Ehrenfeld JM, Epstein RH. Technology diffusion of anesthesia information management systems into academic anesthesia departments in the United States. *Anesth Analg.* 2014;118(3):644–650.
2. Holt NF, Silverman DG, Prasad R, Dziura J, Ruskin KJ. Preanesthesia clinics, information management, and operating room delays: results of a survey of practicing anesthesiologists. *Anesth Analg.* 2007;104(3):615–618.
3. Nair BG, Newman SF, Peterson GN, Wu WY, Schwid HA. Feedback mechanisms including real-time electronic alerts to achieve near 100% timely prophylactic antibiotic administration in surgical cases. *Anesth Analg.* 2010;111(5):1293–1300.
4. Cermak M. Monitoring and telemedicine support in remote environments and in human space flight. *Br J Anaesth.* 2006;97(1):107–114.
5. Kyriacou E, Pavlopoulos S, Berler A, et al. Multi-purpose healthcare telemedicine systems with mobile communication link support. *Biomed Eng Online.* 2003;2:7.
6. Doyle C. Health information technology: use for quality assurance and improvement. In: Ruskin KJ, Stiegler M, Rosenbaum S, eds. *Quality and Safety in Anesthesia and Perioperative Care.* New York, NY: Oxford University Press; 2016:80–98.
7. Sandberg WS, Sandberg EH, Seim AR, et al. Real-time checking of electronic anesthesia records for documentation errors and automatically text messaging clinicians improves quality of documentation. *Anesth Analg.* 2008;106(1):192–201.
8. Brovman EY, Preiss D, Urman RD, Gross WL. The challenges of implementing electronic health records for anesthesia use outside the operating room. *Curr Opin Anaesthesiol.* 2016;29:531–535. doi:10.1097/ACO.0000000000000349.
9. McDowell J, Wu A, Ehrenfeld JM, Urman RD. Effect of the implementation of a new electronic health record system on surgical case turnover time. *J Med Syst.* 2017;41:42. doi:10.1007/s10916-017-0690-y. Epub 2017 Jan 27.
10. Wu A, Kodali BS, Flanagan HL Jr, Urman RD. Introduction of a new electronic medical record system has mixed effects on first surgical case efficiency metrics. *J Clin Monit Comput.* 2016 Sep 13. [Epub ahead of print] PMID:27623949.
11. Menachemi N, Powers T, Au DW, Brooks RG. Predictors of physician satisfaction among electronic health record system users. *J Healthc Qual.* 2010;32(1):35–41.
12. Agrawal R, Johnson C. Securing electronic health records without impeding the flow of information. *Int J Med Inform.* 2007;76(5–6):471–479.
13. Gostin LO. National health information privacy: regulations under the Health Insurance Portability and Accountability Act. *JAMA.* 2001;285(23):3015–3021.
14. Perlroth N. Hackers used new weapons to disrupt major websites across U.S. *New York Times*, October 21, 2016.

9 | PROCEDURAL SEDATION BY NONANESTHESIA PROVIDERS

JULIA METZNER, MD, KAREN B. DOMINO, MD, MPH

INTRODUCTION

Although anesthesiologists and certified registered nurse anesthetists (CRNAs) are experts in sedation/analgesia outside of the operating room (OOOR), extensive demand in the face of limited resources has resulted in sedation being routinely performed by nonanesthesia health care providers. Sedation/analgesia is administered for minor office and hospital procedures in a variety of areas, including gastroenterology, radiology, cardiology, dentistry, and the emergency room. Given the extreme diversity of settings, it is understandable that procedural sedation and analgesia evolved to meet the unique needs of each of these specialties. However, to improve patient safety, the Joint Commission and the American Society of Anesthesiologists (ASA) issued standards that unify and standardize the various approaches across specialties and institutions.[1,2] This chapter briefly reviews the essential elements needed to develop a safe policy for sedation by nonanesthesia practitioners.

CONTINUUM OF SEDATION/GENERAL ANESTHESIA

An essential component of standardization is the definition of the "continuum" of sedation/anesthesia from minimal sedation to general anesthesia (Figure 9.1).[2] The continuum was developed to create nonequivocal terminology for the sedation levels. Previously, three levels of sedation (conscious sedation, deep sedation, and general anesthesia) were recognized. The notion of "conscious" sedation was frequently misinterpreted and abused, in reality meaning "deep" sedation or even "general" anesthesia. Therefore, it has been replaced with the clearer term of "moderate" sedation, a well-demarcated clinical state that is safe and optimal in everyday OOOR practice. Furthermore, the definitions crystallize what the different stages of sedation/analgesia represent clinically and the expected physiologic consequences in each state.

Minimal sedation involves anxiolysis during which the patient responds normally to verbal commands. The patient maintains normal airway reflexes and ventilation and normal cardiovascular responses. Types of sedative agents for this level include a single dose of sedative or analgesic administered orally for the purpose of alleviating anxiety or pain and nitrous oxide less than 50% with no other sedatives or analgesics.

Moderate sedation involves the depression of consciousness, but during which the patient still responds to verbal commands, either alone or accompanied by light tactile stimulations. Spontaneous respiration is usually adequate, and no interventions are required to maintain a patent airway. Cardiovascular function is usually maintained.

This type of sedation is the most common in OOOR procedures, and it is used for diagnostic and interventional procedures in gastroenterology, radiology, cardiac catheterization, and other OOOR locations. Intravenous drugs such as midazolam and fentanyl are popular and safe for moderate sedation.

Deep sedation/analgesia involves significant depression of consciousness during which patients cannot be easily aroused but may respond purposefully following repeated or painful stimulation. Patients may require assistance in maintaining a patent airway, and spontaneous ventilation may be inadequate. Cardiovascular function is usually adequate. Higher doses of midazolam or fentanyl, as well as sedative doses of propofol, are commonly used for deep sedation.

General anesthesia is a drug-induced loss of consciousness during which patients are not arousable, even by painful stimulation. Patients often require assistance in maintaining a patent airway, and positive-pressure ventilation may be required because of depressed spontaneous ventilation or drug-induced depression of neuromuscular function. Cardiovascular function may be impaired. Propofol may fairly easily and unexpectedly result in general anesthesia. If the patient loses consciousness and the ability to respond purposefully, the anesthesia care is a general anesthetic, irrespective of whether airway instrumentation is required.

It is crucial to understand that sedation represents a cascade of events with progressive alteration (a continuum) in level of responsiveness, airway patency, and respiratory and cardiac function as increased depths of sedation/anesthesia are achieved. The progression from minimal sedation to deep sedation/general anesthesia might represent a quick transition that lacks distinct separation between stages. In addition, the transition from one level of sedation to the next is often difficult to predict and varies from patient to patient, as well as with changing degrees of procedural stimulation and pain.

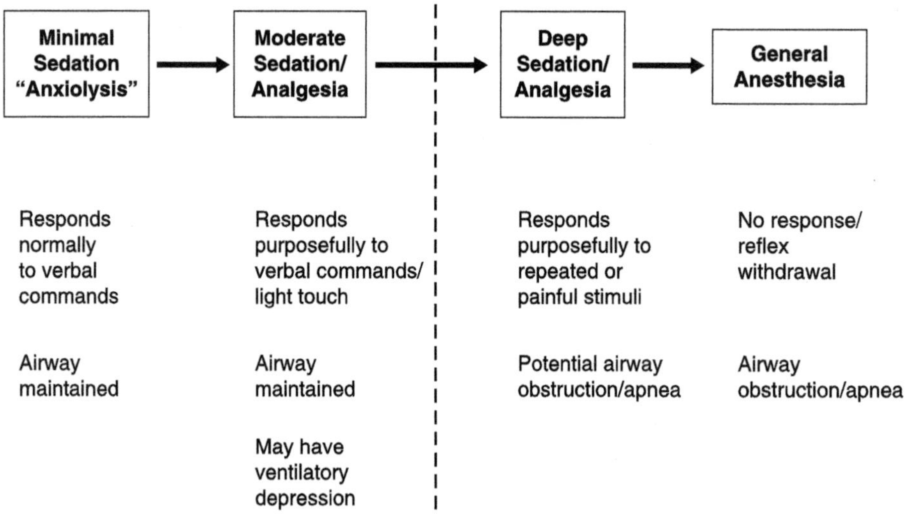

Figure 9.1. *Continuum of conscious sedation. (Adapted from American Society of Anesthesiologists. Practice guidelines for sedation and analgesia by non-anesthesiologists: an updated report by the American Society of Anesthesiologists Task Force on Sedation and Analgesia by Non-Anesthesiologists. Anesthesiology. 2002;96:1004–1017.)*

The sedation continuum is not drug specific, and levels from mild sedation to general anesthesia can be reached with virtually any commonly used sedative/analgesic agent. This is particularly true when drug combinations are used such as a sedative plus an opioid, when the dosing interval is too short and drug accumulation occurs (this may be hard to predict), and during changes in intensity of painful stimuli during the procedure. While patients may breathe during painful parts of procedures, spontaneous respiration may be severely depressed when the stimulation subsides.

The Centers for Medicare and Medicaid Services (CMS) state that only anesthesia professionals (anesthesiologist, nurse anesthetist, and anesthesiologist's assistant) or other qualified nonanesthesiologist physicians (as well as a dentist, oral surgeon, or podiatrist who is qualified to administer anesthesia under state law) are permitted to administer deep sedation and general anesthesia.[3] Registered nurses, advanced practice registered nurses, or physician assistants may not administer deep sedation per CMS. The 2010 ASA "Advisory on Granting Privileges for Deep Sedation to Non-Anesthesiologist Sedation Practitioners" was created to "assist health care facilities in developing a program" for the delineation of procedure-specific clinical privileges for nonanesthesiologist physicians to administer or supervise the administration of sedative and analgesic drugs to establish a level of deep sedation. The advisory outlines recommendations for education, training, licensure, performance evaluation, and performance improvement. In contrast, mild-to-moderate sedation usually can be administered safely by nonanesthesia practitioners who have had specialized training.[3] Knowledge of the pharmacologic profiles of sedation agents is necessary to maximize the likelihood that the intended level of sedation is targeted accurately. If cardiorespiratory compromise occurs, the nonanesthesia practitioners should possess the skills necessary to "rescue" a patient whose level of sedation is deeper than planned and return the patient to the intended level. Therefore, one person must be available whose only responsibility is to monitor the patient, identify cardiorespiratory compromise, and institute bag-mask ventilation and cardiopulmonary resuscitation if necessary. Backup emergency services, including protocols for summoning emergency medical services, must be established and maintained.

PERSONNEL AND TRAINING PROCEDURES FOR NONANESTHESIA PRACTITIONERS GIVING OR SUPERVISING MODERATE SEDATION

The Joint Commission requires that sedation providers have adequate training to administer the sedative drugs effectively and safely, the skills to monitor the patient's response to the medications given, and the expertise needed to manage all potential complications. This generally implies that sedation/analgesia at every location must be supervised by a competent physician who is appropriately trained and privileged. A qualified support person (nurse, respiratory therapist) should be present for the continuous monitoring of the patient. Such support persons must focus on the patient's status and not take part in the procedure. They should have "rescue capacity" to respond to a deeper level of sedation than intended, with expertise in airway management and advanced life support. They may assist with minor, interruptible tasks; however, they should have no other responsibilities that would interfere with the level of monitoring and documentation appropriate for the planned level of sedation. They should be free to monitor the patient from the start of the procedure through the completion of the recovery phase.

While The Joint Commission set forth standards for the procedural sedation care, the benchmarks of training required for privileges to perform procedural sedation actually depend on the individual institution or hospital. CMS recently issued revised interpretative guidelines for anesthesia services that require analgesia and sedation services in hospitals to be under the direction of one anesthesia service, under the direction of a qualified physician.[3] The anesthesia service is responsible for developing policies and procedures governing the provision of sedation/analgesia, including the minimal qualifications for each category of practitioner who may provide sedation, for all patients having all levels of sedation in all facility locations.

In 2006, the ASA issued guidelines for privileging nonanesthesiologists to provide moderate sedation; the guidelines are found in entirety on the ASA website.[4] This statement was created to give a foundation to any institution interested in developing sedation privileging policies. Included is specific training in administration of sedative/analgesic drugs, airway skills, resuscitation skills, patient presedation evaluation, monitoring and interpreting physiological variables, postprocedure transport and evaluation, and discharge criteria (Table 9.1).

PATIENT PREPARATION AND SELECTION

Table 9.2 illustrates patient preoperative factors that should prompt consultation of an anesthesiologist to evaluate the safety and provision of sedation. These factors include sicker patients (ASA status 4 and 5) as well as extremes of age, morbid obesity, sleep apnea, an anticipated difficult airway, chronic pain on opioid therapy, substance use disorder, history of difficult sedation, a prior adverse reaction to sedation/anesthesia, a long or complex procedure planned, and the prone position. Further details concerning preoperative patient selection and evaluation are described in Chapter 6.

FASTING GUIDELINES

A history of last oral intake is required before providing sedation/analgesia. Practitioners should follow the ASA fasting guidelines required for sedation/analgesia.[2] The concept behind these recommendations is that it is difficult to predict the exact depth of sedation that will result from a dose of a sedative in a given patient. Therefore, it should be assumed that airway reflexes may be lost and steps to minimize gastric aspiration risk should be taken.

TABLE 9.1. Training and Credentialing in Procedural Sedation and Analgesia for Nonanesthesia Providers

COMPETENCY CATEGORY	REQUIRED SKILLS AND KNOWLEDGE	COMMENTS
Administration of sedative/ analgesic drugs	Knows	Written test recommended for verification of knowledge
	1. Pharmacology: • Appropriate drug selection • Route of administration and dosage • Time of onset, duration of action, maximum dose, side effects 2. Treatment of oversedation: • Airway, breathing, circulation (ABC) • Reversal agents • Vasoactive drugs and antiarrhythmics	
Airway skills	1. Airway assessment: ability to examine airway and recognize potentially difficult airway Physical examination: • Habitus: significant obesity (BMI > 35); excessive facial hair; receding chin • Head and neck: short neck; limited neck extension; decreased hyoid-mental distance (<3 cm in adults); neck mass, cervical spine disease; dysmorphic facial features (e.g., Pierre-Robin, Down syndromes) • Mouth: small opening (<3 cm in adults); edentulous; protruding incisors; high arched palate; macroglossia, tonsillar hypertrophy; nonvisible uvula • Jaw: micrognathia, retrognathia, trismus, significant malocclusion 2. Recognize signs of airway obstruction • Stridor, noisy breathing, wheezing • Rocking motion of chest and abdomen 3. Ability to "rescue" a compromised airway • Neck, head repositioning • Perform jaw thrust, chin lift • Insert oral/nasal airway • Perform bag-mask ventilation	Airway skills training may include • Airway workshops • Airway simulator • Supervised practice on patients in operating room
Resuscitation skills	1. Basic life support (BLS) required 2. Moderate sedation: Advanced cardiac life support (ACLS) team available within 5 minutes 3. Deep sedation: Individual trained in ACLS present during the procedure (deep sedation should be performed only by anesthesia providers)	Institutions should conduct periodical "mock codes" to preserve and reinforce resuscitation skills and team response time.

(continued)

TABLE 9.1. *(Cont'd)*

COMPETENCY CATEGORY	REQUIRED SKILLS AND KNOWLEDGE	COMMENTS
Patient presedation evaluation	1. Obtaining consent • Explanation of risks/benefits and possible alternatives 2. Medical history • Abnormalities of major organ systems • Obesity with or without sleep apnea • History of previous adverse reactions to sedation/analgesia or regional or general anesthesia • Drug allergies • Current medications, including herbal products • Time of last oral intake • Tobacco, alcohol, or substance abuse	
	3. Physical examination • Body weight; BMI > 35 • Examination of the upper airway • Level of consciousness • Baseline vital signs, including blood pressure, heart rate, O_2 saturation via pulse oximetry • Heart/lung auscultation 4. Additional evaluation • Diagnostic and laboratory testing guided by comorbid conditions and possible interference with the course of sedation/analgesia • American Society of Anesthesiologists (ASA) physical status classification	Should be used for risk stratification and decision-making for anesthesiology consult (see Table 9.1).
Monitoring and interpreting physiologic variables	1. Vital signs that should be continuously monitored and recorded every 5 minutes: • Consciousness and level of responsiveness • Electrocardiogram (ECG) • Pulse rate • Blood pressure • Respiratory rate • Oxygen saturation via pulse oximetry • Capnography (end-tidal CO_2 monitoring optional)	For **moderate sedation**, there needs to be a designated person, other than the practitioner performing the procedure, who monitors the patient and, if necessary, may perform minor, interruptible tasks.
	2. Availability of resuscitative equipment and rescue drugs (see Table 9.4)	For **deep sedation**, the monitoring person should not perform any other tasks.
Postprocedure transport	1. A trained person capable of managing complications (airway, hemodynamic) should accompany the patient to recovery. 2. Oxygen via face mask administration 3. Emergency airway equipment and rescue drugs available 4. Pulse oximetry strongly recommended	
Postprocedure evaluation	1. Postsedation patients should be observed in an appropriately staffed and equipped area. 2. Consciousness and basic vital signs (oxygen saturation, blood pressure, respiratory rate, pulse rate) should be monitored until discharge criteria are reached. 3. Pain should be well controlled before discharge.	
Discharge criteria	Guidelines for discharge: 1. Patient alert and oriented 2. Vital signs stable and back to baseline 3. All patients who have received a reversal agent should be monitored for signs of resedation up to 60–90 minutes. 4. A responsible person should be available to accompany the patient home. 5. Written discharge instructions regarding diet, medications, and activities should be provided.	Every hospital should have its own discharge policy. See standardized recovery scoring systems similar to those used in their surgical postanesthesia recovery areas (see Table 9.7)

BMI, body mass index.

TABLE 9.2. Preoperative Factors That Prompt an Anesthesia Consult

ASA CLASS	MEDICAL DESCRIPTION	EXAMPLES	PRESENCE OF ANESTHESIOLOGIST
1	Healthy patient	Healthy without medications	Not needed unless special indications[a]
2	A patient with mild systemic disease—no functional limitation	• Mild asthma • Medically controlled hypertension • Well-controlled diabetes mellitus	Not needed unless special indications[a]
3	A patient with severe systemic disease—definite functional limitation	• Moderate-to-severe asthma • Poorly controlled hypertension • Poorly controlled diabetes mellitus with end-organ disease	Consider anesthesia consultation; special indications[a]
4	A patient with severe systemic disease that is a constant threat to life	• Morbidly obese with sleep apnea on oxygen therapy • End-stage renal failure requiring dialysis • Congestive heart failure	Often needed
5	A moribund patient who is not expected to survive without the operation	• Septic shock • Polytrauma	Needed

ASA, American Society of Anesthesiologists.

[a]Special indications for an anesthesia consult: extremes of age (under 5 years of age or over 80 years), morbid obesity, sleep apnea, a difficult airway, chronic pain on opioid therapy, substance use disorder, history of difficult sedation, prior adverse reaction to sedation/anesthesia, a long or complex procedure planned, and the prone position.

The ASA guidelines recommend at least 2 hours of fasting for clear liquids (fluids that light penetrates, not containing milk products), at least 4 hours for breast milk, at least 6 hours for a light meal, and 8 hours for a fatty meal (Table 9.3). These recommendations apply only to healthy patients undergoing elective procedures and do not guarantee that complete gastric emptying has occurred. They do not apply in many clinical situations, including for pregnant women beyond the first trimester of pregnancy; patients with severe pain on parenteral opioids; alcohol intoxication; patients with positional gastroesophageal reflux, nausea/vomiting, bowel obstruction, ascites, and other gastrointestinal disorders that reduce gastric emptying; morbid obesity; diabetes; and numerous other conditions. In adults, some institutions have found it practical and safest to add an additional conservative margin with nothing by mouth (nil per os, npo) status (such as at least 4 hours after clear liquids and 8 hours after a meal) due to frequent changes in schedules and the presence of patient medical conditions that may predispose to reductions in gastric emptying.

With the recommendations just outlined in mind, each practitioner will need to weigh the urgency of the procedure against the relative risk of pulmonary aspiration. Recognizing the lack of sufficient evidence pertaining to sedation/analgesia, the ASA, in its Task Force on Sedation/Analgesia by Non-Anesthesiologists, recommended that the potential for pulmonary aspiration of gastric contents should be considered in determining the target level of sedation, whether the procedure should be delayed, and whether the trachea should be protected by intubation.[2] Emergency room physicians routinely perform procedural sedations on patients noncompliant with the ASA fasting guidelines, and there is little indication that aspiration is a significant problem in this setting with mild/moderate sedation.[5,6] Caution with the use of drugs that may more easily result in oversedation and loss of airway reflexes, such as propofol or fospropofol, should be carefully considered. Although not supported in the literature, administration of metoclopramide or H_2 blockers may be considered with the goal of decreasing injury should aspiration occur.

EQUIPMENT AND SUPPLY

Because sedation and analgesia may result in untoward events, including oversedation, respiratory depression, or cardiopulmonary arrest, having the appropriate emergency equipment

TABLE 9.3. Fasting Recommendations to Reduce the Risk of Pulmonary Aspiration

INGESTED MATERIAL	MINIMUM FASTING PERIOD
Clear liquids[a]	2 hours
Breast milk	4 hours
Infant formula	6 hours
Nonhuman milk	6 hours
Light meal (toast and clear liquids)	6 hours
Fatty meal	8 hours

NOTE. These recommendations apply to healthy patients who are undergoing elective procedures. See text for other exceptions. Note that following the guidelines does not guarantee that complete gastric emptying has occurred, and patients with severe pain and those undergoing upper gastrointestinal procedures may have medical conditions that may place them at higher risk for aspiration of gastric contents.

[a]Examples of clear liquids include water, fruit juices without pulp, carbonated beverages, clear tea, and black coffee without milk.

in close vicinity to the sedation area is mandatory. Supportive equipment must include oxygen, suction, patient-monitoring devices, basic and advanced airway management equipment, a monitor/defibrillator/pacer, advanced life support medications, reversal or rescue agents, and vascular access equipment (Table 9.4).

MONITORING

RECOMMENDED MONITORS

Chapter 4 describes monitoring techniques in detail. Guidelines that follow the ASA recommendations for monitoring patients during sedation/analgesia have been developed by several professional societies, including gastroenterology, emergency medicine, and radiology. There is general agreement that the patient should be continuously monitored from the start of moderate sedation until the time discharge criteria are met. Baseline vital signs, including blood pressure measurement, oxygen saturation by pulse oximetry, heart rate and rhythm, and level of consciousness are the minimum assessment parameters to be monitored, recorded, and documented prior to, throughout, and after sedation (Table 9.4). The ASA also recommends continuous electrocardiographic (ECG) monitoring and use of supplemental oxygen during the administration of intravenous sedation.

TABLE 9.4. Equipment and Drugs for Procedural Sedation and Analgesia

IN THE PROCEDURAL ROOM	*READILY AVAILABLE*
1. High-flow oxygen source	Defibrillator/pacer
2. Suctioning apparatus	Emergency drugs
3. Airway management equipment • Face masks • Oral and nasal airways (different sizes) • Laryngeal mask airways (LMAs) • Laryngoscope handles (battery tested) • Laryngoscope blades (different sizes) • Endotracheal tubes cuffed and uncuffed for children • Stylet • Bag-valve-mask device (Ambu bag)	• Epinephrine • Ephedrine • Vasopressin • Atropine • Amiodarone • Lidocaine • Hydrocortisone • Glucose 50% • Diphenhydramine • Esmolol or metoprolol
4. Vascular access equipment • Gloves, tourniquets, alcohol wipes • Intravenous catheters (24;20;18 gauge) • Syringes and needles • Intravenous fluids and tubing	
5. Basic monitoring equipment (ECG, pulse oximeter, BP cuff, capnometer strongly encouraged)	
6. Supplemental O_2 during procedure	
7. Reversal agents • Naloxone • Flumanezil	

BP, blood pressure; ECG, electrocardiogram.

Pulse oximetry has become undeniably the standard monitor for the detection of desaturation and hypoxemia during sedation/analgesia. However, pulse oximetry is far from the ideal in detecting ventilatory compromise, including hypoventilation, airway obstruction, or apnea. Significant respiratory compromise can occur despite normal oxygen saturation, particularly when supplemental oxygen is administered.[7]

According to the ASA standards for monitoring during sedation, the adequacy of ventilation during moderate or deep sedation shall be evaluated by continual observation of qualitative clinical signs and monitoring for the presence of exhaled carbon dioxide unless precluded or invalidated by the nature of the patient, procedure, or equipment.[8] Capnography is more sensitive than clinical assessment of ventilation in detection of apnea. In a recent study in which the anesthesia provider was blinded to capnography, 10 of the 39 patients developed 20 seconds of apnea, missed by clinical signs and pulse oximetry but detected by capnography.[9] Adverse outcomes from oversedation that may be potentially avoided by capnography are described in Chapter 3.

Although capnography is not currently a standard requirement for all procedural sedation/analgesia in OOOR locations, its use in detecting adverse respiratory events associated with sedation has been the focus of multiple publications outside of the anesthesiology field.[10,11] A recent randomized controlled trial using the combination of an opioid and benzodiazepine (BDZ) for elective endoscopic retrograde cholangiopancreatography (ERCP) found significantly fewer episodes of hypoxemia in patients monitored with capnography.[12]

DEPTH-OF-SEDATION MONITORS

Depth of sedation may be monitored by processed electroencephalographic (EEG) activity; however, its usefulness is under debate. An example of this type of monitor is the bispectral index (BIS). The BIS is a continuously processed EEG parameter specifically developed to provide an estimate of the depth of consciousness. Sedation depth is scored on a unitless scale from 0 to 100. A BIS value of 100 is considered complete alertness, 0 is no cortical activity at all, and the range of 40 to 60 is believed to be consistent with general anesthesia.

Although this technology has been widely used to monitor depth of hypnosis in the operating room, its applicability for the purpose of sedation has yielded controversial data. It may be beneficial in preventing oversedation and reducing the time to discharge. Several investigations have suggested that its use may better guide the depth of sedation endpoint than traditional sedation scales, and it may have further benefit for sedation/analgesia in children as they frequently require deeper levels of sedation to prevent movement.[13,14] Other studies have found unacceptably wide ranges of BIS values compared with the clinical assessment and no improvement in clinical outcomes.[15,16] Although depth of sedation monitoring may have a beneficial role in the future for sedation/analgesia in the OOOR setting, the findings indicate that more data are required before its possible uses and benefits can be defined.

DRUGS USED FOR SEDATION/ANALGESIA

A variety of drugs can be chosen to provide sedation and analgesia for adults and children for OOOR procedures. In selecting agents, one should consider the requirements of the procedure (e.g., is the procedure painful or prolonged, or does the patient need to be motionless?) and the risks and benefits for the individual patient and situation. Every clinician will prefer a drug or combination of drugs that grant analgesia, anxiolysis, amnesia, and minimal hypnosis, that are easily titratable and reversible, and that lack respiratory and cardiovascular depression and other side effects. Unfortunately, such drugs have yet to be discovered.

From a practical standpoint, if the procedure is not painful (e.g., noninvasive radiologic procedures such as computed tomography scanning and magnetic resonance imaging), pure sedation may suffice, and BDZs may be used alone. Analgesic agents (opioids) should be added to any procedure that demands pain relief. Ketamine may be an excellent single-drug choice for painful or stimulating procedures in children and for restricted adult applications (e.g., fracture reduction). Most often, a combination of drugs consisting of hypnotics and analgesics is a reasonable choice. However, the practitioner should be aware that with combinations of hypnotics/analgesics, drug side effects are frequently synergistic and can potentiate untoward side effects.

The specific agents for procedural sedation, amnestic and analgesic properties, dosage recommendations for adult patients, and side effects are listed in Tables 9.5 and 9.6 and are described briefly in the next section. See Chapter 6 and other chapters in this volume for more detail and more specific applications of these drugs in different OOOR settings.

COMMON DRUGS FOR PROCEDURAL SEDATION/ANALGESIA

Benzodiazepines include *midazolam* (Versed®), *diazepam* (Valium®), and *lorazepam* (Ativan®). BDZs have antianxiety, anticonvulsant, sedative, muscle relaxant, and amnestic properties. However, they do not provide analgesia, and therefore, they are commonly coadministered with opioids, which potentiate their effects. Doses should be reduced in patients with hepatic or renal disease, as well as elderly, critically ill, and obese patients. In these patients, the clearance of midazolam is halved, leading to prolonged half-life and excessive sedation.[17] Adverse effects include pain on injection (diazepam and lorazepam), birth defects in first trimester of pregnancy, paradoxical reactions (agitation), and dose-related hypoventilation, hypoxemia, and hypotension (especially midazolam).

In contrast to all other sedative-hypnotics, there is a specific drug to reverse the sedative effects of BDZs, namely, *flumazenil* (Romazicon®). Its onset of action is rapid (1–2 minutes), its peak effects occur in 5–10 minutes, and it has a half-life of 45–90 minutes. Because the duration of flumazenil is shorter than most BDZs, the possibility of resedation exists, and continuous respiratory monitoring is advised. It should be titrated in doses of 0.1 to 0.2 mg IV every 1 to 2 minutes to the desired effect. A dose of 1 mg is generally sufficient. Flumanezil should be used with extreme caution in patients with BDZ dependence or a history of seizures as it may precipitate life-threatening status epilepticus. Seizures have been reported after the reversal of BDZs even in non-BDZ-dependent patients. For this reason, routine reversal with flumazenil is not recommended.

Opioids (*narcotics*) are administered for their analgesic properties. In the context of procedural sedation, they are used to supplement other agents (e.g., sedative-hypnotics) to provide optimal conditions for painful procedures. These drugs share the ability to interact with opiate receptors located throughout the central nervous system and inhibit nociception. Although they differ substantially in potency, the opioids are equally effective for most OOOR applications. The choice of one opioid instead of another is usually based on its onset and duration or adverse effects. The clinically available agents range from the naturally occurring alkaloid morphine to synthetic compounds like *fentanyl* and *meperidine* (Demerol®). The most commonly used opioids by nonanesthesia practitioners in OOOR procedures are fentanyl and meperidine.

Fentanyl is a synthetic opioid 100 times more potent than morphine. Owing to its rapid onset, short duration of action, lack of histamine release, and stable cardiovascular profile, it is the preferred analgesic for procedural sedation/analgesia. It is highly lipid soluble and rapidly crosses the blood-brain barrier, causing analgesia in less than 90 seconds for durations up to 30 to 40 minutes. Administered in incremental small doses (e.g., 25 to 50 μg), it is useful for short, painful procedures.

The drawback of fentanyl is respiratory depression that significantly overlaps its analgesic effects. The magnitude of respiratory depression can be greatly increased when fentanyl is used in combination with other sedatives, such as midazolam.[18] Supplemental oxygen and monitoring with pulse oximetry and capnography are strongly recommended with even small amounts of fentanyl. In small concentrations, fentanyl has limited effects on cardiovascular function, although significant decreases in blood pressure may occur with fentanyl/BDZ combinations[19] and in critically ill or hypovolemic patients.

As the first synthetic opioid, meperidine was often used to provide analgesia for procedures inside the operating room and OOOR. With the advent of short-acting fentanyl, its popularity faded. Presently (in combination with a BDZ), it has some limited residual use in endoscopic procedures. It may be given in doses of 25–75 mg IV every 5 minutes. Peak effects occur in 5 to 7 minutes; however, the elimination half-life is long, between 3–5 hours. Normeperidine, a toxic metabolite of meperidine, causes central nervous excitement and seizures. Meperidine has many drug interactions, but

TABLE 9.5. Drug Dosage and Administration of Commonly Used Drugs for Procedural Sedation by Nonanesthesiologists

DRUG	SEDATION/ AMNESIA	ANXIOLYSIS	ANALGESIA	ROUTE/DOSE	ONSET (MIN)	PEAK (MIN)	DURATION (MIN)	COMMENTS
Sedative/ hypnotics[a]								
Midazolam (Versed)	Yes	Yes	No	IV: 0.5–1 mg (titrate to effect up to 5-10 mg/h)	0.5–1	3–5	10–30	– Minimal cardiorespiratory depression
				IM: 0.08 mg/kg	10–15	20–45	60–120	– Reduce dose when used in combination with opioids
				PO: 0.5 mg/kg	15–30	35–45	60–90	– Midazolam is benzodiazepine of choice for short procedures – Antagonist: flumazenil
Diazepam (Valium)	Yes	Yes	No	IV: 2–3 mg (titrate to effect up to 15 mg)	1–2	8–15	15–45	
				PO: 5–10 mg	30–60	45–60	60–100	
Lorazepam (Ativan)	Yes	Yes	No	IV: 0.25 mg (titrate to effect up to 2 mg)	1–2	15–20	60–120	
				PO: 2–4 mg	60–120	120	>480	
Opioids[a]								
Fentanyl	No	No	Yes	IV: 25–50 µg intermittent boluses	1–2	5	30–40	– Respiratory depression; decreased response to hypercarbia and hypoxia
Meperidine (Demerol)	No	No	Yes	IV: 25–75 mg	3–5	5–7	60–180	– Synergistic sedative and respiratory depressant effects (reduce dose with sedatives) – Nausea, vomiting – Meperidine: histamine release – Antagonist: naloxone
Reversal agents (antagonists)								
Flumazenil (Anexate)	No	No	No	IV: 0.1–0.2 mg (titrate to effect to maximum of 5 mg)	1–2	5–10	45–90	– Short acting, repeat doses may be required – Avoid in patients receiving benzodiazepines for seizure control – Caution with chronic benzodiazepine therapy (withdrawal effect) or with tricyclic antidepressants
Naloxone (Narcan)	No	No	No	IV: 0.02–0.04 mg (titrate to effect)	1–2	2–3	30–60	– Short acting, repeat doses may be required – May cause hypertension and tachycardia – Pulmonary edema reported

[a]Alterations in dosing may be indicated based on the clinical situation and the practitioner's experience with these agents. Individual dosages may vary depending on age and coexistent diseases. Doses should be reduced for sicker patients and in the elderly. When using drug combinations, the potential for significant respiratory impairment and airway obstruction is increased. Drugs should be titrated to achieve optimal effect, and sufficient time for dose effect should be allowed before administering an additional dose or another medication.

TABLE 9.6. Drug Dosage and Administration of Anesthetic Drugs for Procedural Sedation

DRUG	SEDATION/ AMNESIA	ANXIOLYSIS	ANALGESIA	ROUTE/DOSE	ONSET (MIN)	PEAK (MIN)	DURATION (MIN)	COMMENTS
Sedative/hypnotics[a]								
Ketamine (Ketalar)	Yes	No	Yes	IV: 0.2–0.5 mg/kg (titrate to effect)	1	1–2	10–20	– Dissociative anesthetic – Emergence reactions blunted with midazolam
				IM: 2–5 mg/kg	5	15	15–30	– Minimal respiratory depression, bronchodilator – Hypersalivation, laryngospasm – Cardiac stimulant (increase in blood pressure and heart rate) – Increase in intracranial pressure and intraocular pressure
Propofol (Diprivan)	Yes	Yes	No	IV: 0.5 mg/kg (intermittent boluses) or infusion: 25–75 μg/kg/min	<1	1–2	5–8	– Cardiorespiratory depression – Pain on injection – Antiemetic properties
Dexmedeto-midine (Precedex)	Yes	Yes	Yes	IV loading dose: 0.5–1 μg/kg, slowly, over 10–20 min IV maintenance: 0.4–0.7 μg/kg per hour	5–10	60	Depends on infusion time: 4 min after 10 min infusion; 250 min after 8-h infusion	– Minimal respiratory depression – Decreases blood pressure and heart rate – Potentiates the central nervous system effects of sedatives – Safe in elderly

[a] Alterations in dosing may be indicated based on the clinical situation and the practitioner's experience with these agents. Individual dosages may vary depending on age and coexistent diseases. Doses should be reduced for sicker patients and in the elderly. When using drug combinations, the potential for significant respiratory impairment and airway obstruction is increased. Drugs should be titrated to achieve optimal effect, and sufficient time for dose effect should be allowed before administering an additional dose or another medication.

it is most notably contraindicated with monoamine oxidase inhibitors. Side effects include respiratory depression, hypotension, nausea, vomiting, and paradoxical agitation or anxiety.

Opioids can be reversed by *naloxone* (Narcan®). Naloxone antagonizes all of the central nervous system effects of the opioids, including respiratory depression, excessive sedation, and analgesia. Naloxone should be titrated slowly, in increments of 0.04 mg IV over 1–2 minutes, to the desired effect (e.g., responsiveness to stimulation and increase in respiratory rate over 8 breaths/minute). Absolute annihilation of analgesia may precipitate sympathetic discharge, manifested by hypertension, tachycardia, and at extremis, ventricular fibrillation and pulmonary edema. The effects are seen in 1–2 minutes; however, the duration of reversal is rather short, 30–60 minutes, and resedation may occur if long-acting narcotics have been used. Because of naloxone's side effects, it is safest to administer appropriate doses of opioids in the first place. If naloxone is required due to an accidental overdose of an opioid, close monitoring of the reversed patient for 60–120 minutes is essential due to the possibility of late respiratory depression.

DRUGS USED LESS FREQUENTLY BY NONANESTHESIA PRACTITIONERS

DISSOCIATIVE ANESTHETICS

Ketamine, a phencyclidine derivative, is unique because it possesses remarkable analgesic and amnestic properties, unlike other anesthetic-hypnotics. Ketamine causes disconnection between the thalamocortical and limbic systems, preventing the higher centers from perceiving sensory (auditory, visual) input or painful stimuli.[20] This leads to a cataleptic "dissociative" state, characterized by mental disconnection from the surroundings and deep analgesia. Although ketamine is usually administered by anesthesia personnel, ketamine in small doses (10–20 mg IV in an adult) has been used to enhance analgesia (Table 9.6), with minimal respiratory depression. Ventilatory drive is minimally depressed, and protective airway reflexes, including those of laryngeal muscles, are well preserved. Ketamine has sympathomimetic effects and is a potent bronchodilator. Ketamine can increase blood pressure, heart rate, and cardiac output, although these effects are blunted with concurrent administration of BZDs.

The major side effect of ketamine is emergence delirium. Hallucinations, nightmares, and agitation may occur at and after emergence in up to 15%–30% of adult patients who are administered ketamine without other sedative agents. It is rare among the pediatric population. Emergence reactions are blunted by concurrent administration of BZDs, such as midazolam.[21,22] Ketamine stimulates oral secretions and may induce laryngospasm, particularly during light planes of anesthesia. Children might benefit from pretreatment with glycopyrrolate, 0.01 mg/kg given 10 minutes before the ketamine. Ketamine increases intracranial and intraocular pressure, and its use is limited in head trauma or open globe injury.

OTHER ANESTHETIC AGENTS

Propofol has potent sedative and hypnotic properties with minimal analgesic effect.[23,24] Its high lipid solubility makes possible quick penetration into the central nervous system and rapid clearance from the blood, resulting in both rapid onset of action and quick recovery for doses used for procedural sedation. Propofol's duration of action is very short, between 2 and 8 minutes. The plasma concentration of propofol required for sedation depends on the targeted depth of sedation and is influenced by coadministration of other sedatives/analgesics. Usually, sedation will be achieved at a plasma concentration of 0.5–1.5 μg/mL, corresponding to a continuous infusion rate of approximately 25–75 μg/kg per minute.[17]

Awakening is fast, even after prolonged infusion of propofol, requiring a 50% decrease in the plasma concentration of the drug.[23] The pharmacokinetic parameters of propofol are altered by a variety of factors, including weight, sex, age, and concomitant disease; the presence of liver or renal failure does not significantly alter its pharmacokinetics. However, dose reduction is recommended in the elderly, as volume of distribution falls with age.[24]

Propofol is an appealing drug for procedural sedation/analgesia due to its rapid onset/offset effect, clear-head recovery, and antiemetic effects. Nevertheless, propofol has many undesirable side effects, including respiratory depression,[25] severe hypotension,[26] and pain on injection, especially when administered through small peripheral veins. The most concerning property of propofol is that the therapeutic window of propofol is very narrow. After even a single dose of propofol, the depth of sedation may move quickly on the sedation continuum scale and become deep sedation or general anesthesia. Furthermore, the Food and Drug Administration (FDA) restricts the use of propofol to practitioners trained in the administration of general anesthesia who are not involved in the conduct of the surgical/diagnostic procedure. Hence, in most OOOR settings in the United States, propofol administration is limited to anesthesia professionals.

There is a growing interest in the use of target-controlled infusion (TCI) devices and patient-controlled systems (PCSs) for moderate sedation for endoscopic procedures. Advances in the technology of intravenous delivery devices combined with sophisticated pharmacologic modeling made possible the invention of computer-controlled infusion pumps. On the basis of age and weight of the patient, the TCI infusion system calculates, by using a three-compartment pharmacokinetic model, the starting dose of propofol and the subsequent infusion rate required to achieve and maintain a desired target plasma concentration.[27] A recent prospective study found that a TCI of propofol in a range of 2 to 5 μg/mL provided adequate sedation for gastroenterology procedures of different degrees of difficulty without increasing the risk of drug-related side effects; the level of satisfaction with the sedation was high for patient, nurse, and endoscopist, and patients were discharged in about 30 minutes.[28]

In a PCS device, the medication is self-administered by the patient in response to pain; therefore, the patient has to be conscious enough to press the handheld button. Specialized pumps are used that deliver a preset dose of medication in response to a patient pressing a handheld button. A lockout time is programmed into the pump to prevent the delivery of additional doses until the previous dose has taken its full effect. Results from a randomized, crossover trial comparing propofol administered by intravenous boluses with PCS and patient-maintained sedation using TCI of propofol found that the mean time for titration to adequate sedation was longer with TCI than with PCS (9 vs. 6 minutes).[29] Although both techniques provided moderate sedation, two (9%) patients became oversedated during PCS.

SEDASYS (Ethicon Endo-Surgery, Inc., Cincinnati, OH) is a new propofol delivery system designed to provide moderate sedation in adult ASA 1 and 2 patients for colonoscopy and esophagogastroduodenoscopy. The device interfaces continuous monitoring of patient vital signs, including ECG, pulse oximetry, capnography, blood pressure, and patient responsiveness, with computer-controlled propofol delivery to facilitate precise control of sedation. With signs of oversedation, it automatically decreases or stops the propofol infusion rate, simultaneously increasing oxygen delivery through the nasal cannula attached to the patient. However, a practitioner can override the dose reduction and administer an additional propofol dose.

Studies conducted in the United States and Belgium demonstrated the feasibility of SEDASYS in administering minimal-to-moderate propofol sedation for endoscopic procedures by the gastroenterology team. The results were consistent with a low mean propofol dosage (65 mg) and a very rapid recovery time (29 seconds). Oxygen desaturation lasting less than 30 seconds occurred in 6% of patients, and 18 (38%) had at least one episode of apnea lasting more than 30 seconds. There was no need for airway support, and there were no device-related adverse events.[30] In May 2009, an advisory panel to the FDA recommended approval of the device with the following restrictions: use for colonoscopy and EGG procedures on adult patients under 70 years of age, develop a comprehensive training program, require a dedicated sedation delivery team, and require postapproval surveillance of adverse events. The device was eventually approved by the FDA in 2013. It was used in the United States by several endoscopy practices, until the company pulled it from the market in 2016.

Dexmedetomidine (Precedex®) is an α_2-receptor agonist drug. Dexmedetomidine interacts with both presynaptic and postsynaptic α_2-adrenergic receptors to decrease central sympathetic tone. It is rapidly distributed and extensively metabolized in the liver and eliminated in urine. Dexmedetomidine has many advantages over more commonly used hypnotics, especially in older patients. Although it produces sedative, analgesic, and anxiolytic effects, unlike other sedatives, it does not depress ventilation. When dexmedetomidine is administered as a continuous infusion, it is associated with a predictable and stable hemodynamic response. Less stability is seen with bolus dosing. However, care should be taken when administered to patients who are hypovolemic or have severe heart block because dexmedetomidine can cause hypotension and bradycardia.[31]

DISCHARGE CRITERIA

All patients receiving sedation/anesthesia should be monitored until they are no longer at risk for cardiorespiratory depression. To be discharged, they should be alert and oriented (or returned to age-appropriate baseline), and vital signs should be stable. Many hospitals have chosen to use standardized recovery scoring systems similar to those used in their surgical postanesthesia recovery areas (Table 9.7). Although there is no general agreement about the safe time to discharge, one large study performed in the emergency room found that in children with uneventful sedations using a variety of drugs, no serious adverse effects occurred more than 25 minutes after the final medication administration. The authors concluded that in most cases, prolonged observation beyond 60 minutes is rarely necessary.[32]

TABLE 9.7. Aldrete Scoring System

Respiration
Able to take deep breath and cough = 2
Dyspnea/shallow breathing = 1
Apnea = 0
Oxygen saturation
SaO_2 > 95% on room air = 2
SaO_2 > 90%–95% on room air = 1
SaO_2 < 90% even with supplemental O_2 = 0
Consciousness
Fully awake = 2
Arousable on calling = 1
Not responding = 0
Circulation
BP ± 20 mm Hg baseline = 2
BP ± 20–50 mm Hg baseline = 1
BP ± 50 mm Hg baseline = 0
Activity
Able to move 4 extremities = 2
Able to move 2 extremities = 1
Able to move 0 extremities = 0

NOTE: Monitoring may be discontinued and patient discharged to home or appropriate unit when Aldrete score is 9 or greater.

CONTINUOUS QUALITY IMPROVEMENT EFFORTS

Patient safety during procedural sedation should be monitored by the development of a vigorous continuous quality improvement program (see Chapter 3 for further details). At minimum, adverse events should be measured, such as O_2 desaturation below 85% for 20 seconds, apnea episodes, laryngospasm, need for positive-pressure ventilation, use of reversal agents, prolonged recovery stays, and serious adverse events such as aspiration of gastric contents, cardiac events, and unplanned admissions.[33,34,35,36]

SUMMARY

In summary, safe administration of procedural sedation/analgesia by nonanesthesia professionals requires an understanding of the continuum of sedation/general anesthesia; extensive training and credentialing of personnel performing these procedures; proper patient preparation and selection, with an anesthesia consult for higher-risk patients; adherence to fasting guidelines; standard equipment and monitoring procedures; and a thorough knowledge of the pharmacologic and physiologic properties of sedative and analgesic drugs. Due to the severity of adverse effects of sedative/opioid/anesthetic drugs and the potential for unexpected progression along the continuum to deep sedation or anesthesia, anesthesiologists should design the curriculum/training procedures and supervise credentialing of nonanesthesia health care practitioners who administer sedation/analgesia in the OOOR setting.

REFERENCES

1. Joint Commission. *Comprehensive Accreditation Manual for Hospitals: The Official Handbook CAMH, 2009.* Oakbrook, IL: Joint Commission Resources.
2. American Society of Anesthesiologists. Practice guidelines for sedation and analgesia by non-anesthesiologists: an updated report by the American Society of Anesthesiologists Task Force on Sedation and Analgesia by Non-Anesthesiologists. *Anesthesiology.* 2002;96:1004–1017.
3. Department of Health and Human Services, Centers for Medicare and Medicaid Services. Revised hospital anesthesia services interpretive guidelines–State Operations Manual (SOM) Appendix A. Advisory on granting privileges for deep sedation to non-anesthesiologist sedation practitioners. American Society of Anesthesiologists, 2010. Available at: https://www.cms.gov/. Accessed on March 3, 2018.

4. American Society of Anesthesiologists. Practice Guidelines for Moderate Procedural Sedation and Analgesia 2018: A Report by the American Society of Anesthesiologists Task Force on Moderate Procedural Sedation and Analgesia, the American Association of Oral and Maxillofacial Surgeons, American College of Radiology, American Dental Association, American Society of Dentist Anesthesiologists, and Society of Interventional Radiology. *Anesthesiology.* 2018;128(3):437–479.
5. Green SM, Roback MG, Miner JR, et al. Fasting and emergency department procedural sedation and analgesia: a consensus-based clinical practice advisory. *Ann Emerg Med.* 2007;49:454.
6. Green SM, Krauss B. Pulmonary aspiration risk during ED procedural sedation—an examination of the role of fasting and sedation depth. *Acad Emerg Med.* 2002;9:35.
7. Vargo JJ, Zuccaro G Jr, Dumot JA, et al. Automated graphic assessment of respiratory activity is superior to pulse oximetry and visual assessment for the detection of early respiratory depression during therapeutic upper endoscopy. *Gastrointest Endosc.* 2002;55:826–831.
8. American Society of Anesthesiologists. Standards for basic anesthetic monitoring, last affirmed on October, 2015. Available at: http://www.asahq.org/quality-and-practice-management/standards-guidelines-and-related-resources/standards-for-basic-anesthetic-monitoring. Accessed on March 1, 2018.
9. Soto RG, Fu ES, Vila H, Miguel RV. Capnography accurately detects apnea during monitored anesthesia care. *Anesth Analg.* 2004;99:379–382.
10. Krauss B, Hess DR. Capnography for procedural sedation and analgesia in the emergency department. *Ann Emerg Med.* 2007;50:172–181.
11. Anderson JL, Junkins E, Pribble C, Guenther E. Capnography and depth of sedation during propofol sedation in children. *Ann Emerg Med.* 2007;49:9–13.
12. Qadeer MA, Vargo JJ, Dumot JA, et al. Capnographic monitoring of respiratory activity improves safety of sedation for endoscopic cholangiopancreatography and ultrasonography. *Gastroenterology.* 2009;136(5):1568–1576.
13. Agrawal D, Feldman HA, Krauss B, Waltzman ML. Bispectral index monitoring quantifies depth of sedation during emergency department procedural sedation and analgesia in children. *Ann Emerg Med.* 2004;43:247–255.
14. Dominguez TE, Helfaer MA. Review of bispectral index monitoring in the emergency department and pediatric intensive care unit. *Pediatr Emerg Care.* 2006;22(12):815–821.
15. Drake LM, Chen SC, Rex DK. Efficacy of bispectral monitoring as an adjunct to nurse-administered propofol sedation for colonoscopy: a randomized controlled trial. *Am J Gastroenterol.* 2006;101(9):2003–2007.
16. Gill M, Green SM, Krauss B. A study of the Bispectral Index Monitor during procedural sedation and analgesia in the emergency department. *Ann Emerg Med.* 2003;41(2):234–241.
17. Gan TJ. Pharmacokinetic and pharmacodynamic characteristics of medications used for moderate sedation. *Clin Pharmacokinet.* 2006;45(9):855–869.
18. Bailey PL, Pace NL, Ashburn MA, et al. Frequent hypoxemia and apnea after sedation with midazolam and fentanyl. *Anesthesiology.* 1990;73:826–830.
19. Stanley TH, Webster LR. Anesthetic requirements and cardiovascular effects of fentanyl-oxygen and fentanyl-diazepam-oxygen anesthesia in man. *Anesth Analg.* 1978;57:411–416.
20. Vadivelu N, Schermer E, Kodumudi V, et al. Role of ketamine for analgesia in adults and children. *J Anaesthesiol Clin Pharmacol.* 2016;32(3):298–306.
21. Grace RF. The effect of variable-dose diazepam on dreaming and emergence phenomena in 400 cases of ketamine-fentanyl anaesthesia. *Anaesthesia.* 2003;58:904–910.
22. Chudnofsky CR, Weber JE, Stoyanoff PJ, et al. A combination of midazolam and ketamine for procedural sedation and analgesia in adult emergency department patients. *Acad Emerg Med.* 2000;7:228–235.
23. Smith I, White PF, Nathanson M, Gouldson R. Propofol. An update on its clinical use. *Anesthesiology.* 1994;81:1005–1043.
24. Bryson HM, Fulton BR, Faulds D. Propofol. An update of its use in anaesthesia and conscious sedation. *Drugs.* 1995;50(3):513–519.
25. Moerman AT, Struys MM, Vereecke HE, et al. Remifentanil used to supplement propofol does not improve quality of sedation during spontaneous respiration. *J Clin Anesth.* 2004;16:237–243.
26. Ebert TJ, Muzi M, Berens R, et al. Sympathetic response to induction of anesthesia in humans with propofol or etomidate. *Anesthesiology.* 1992;76:725–733.
27. Egan D. Target-controlled drug delivery: progress toward an intravenous "vaporizer" and automated anesthetic administration. *Anesthesiology.* 2003;99:1214–1219.
28. Fanti L, Agostoni M, Casati A, et al. Target-controlled propofol infusion during monitored anesthesia in patients undergoing ERCP. *Gastrointest Endosc.* 2004;60:361–366.
29. Rodrigo MR, Irwin MG, Tong CK, Yan SY. A randomised crossover comparison of patient-controlled sedation and patient-maintained sedation using propofol. *Anaesthesia.* 2003;58:333–338.
30. Pambianco DJ, Whitten CJ, Moerman A, et al. An assessment of computer-assisted personalized sedation: a sedation delivery system to administer propofol for gastrointestinal endoscopy. *Gastrointest Endosc.* 2008;68(3):542–547.
31. Carollo DS, Nossaman BD, Ramadhyani U. Dexmedetomidine: a review of clinical applications. *Curr Opin Anaesthesiol.* 2008;21(4):457–461.
32. Newman DH, Azer MM, Pitetti RD, Singh S. When is a patient safe for discharge after procedural sedation? The timing of adverse effect events in 1367 pediatric procedural sedations. *Ann Emerg Med.* 2003;42:627–635.
33. Woodward ZG, Urman RD, Domino KB. Safety of non-operating room anesthesia: a closed claims update. *Anesthesiol Clin.* 2017;35(4):569–581.
34. Chang B, Kaye AD, Diaz JH, et al. Complications of non-operating room procedures: outcomes from the national anesthesia clinical outcomes registry. *J Patient Saf.* 2015 Apr 7.
35. Karamnov S, Sarkisian N, Grammer R, et al. Analysis of adverse events associated with adult moderate procedural sedation outside the operating room. *J Patient Saf.* 2017;13(3):111–121.
36. Antonelli MT, Seaver D, Urman RD. Procedural sedation and implications for quality and risk management. *J Healthc Risk Manag.* 2013;33(2):3–10.

10 | OUTCOMES, REGULATION, AND QUALITY IMPROVEMENT

JULIA METZNER, MD, KAREN B. DOMINO, MD, MPH

INTRODUCTION

Providing anesthesia care in areas outside of the operating room (OOOR) has numerous challenges, including an unfamiliar environment; inadequate anesthesia support; deficient resources; cramped, dark, small rooms; and variability of monitoring modalities.[1,2] In addition, sicker patients are undergoing more complex procedures in areas that may be physically located far from the operating room (OR) environment. To improve the safety of patients undergoing procedures in remote locations, practitioners need to be familiar with the development of rigorous continuous quality improvement (CQI) systems, national and regulatory patient safety efforts, as well as complications related to anesthesia/sedation in OOOR settings. This chapter identifies severe outcomes and mechanisms of injury in these remote locations, national patient safety and regulatory efforts that may be adapted to the OOOR setting, and quality improvement efforts essential to track outcomes and improve patient safety.

SAFETY OF ANESTHESIA AND SEDATION IN OOOR LOCATIONS

Good multi-institutional outcome data concerning complications of anesthesia and sedation in OOOR locations are lacking. The best data have been obtained in the pediatric population, perhaps because of greater involvement of safety-oriented pediatric anesthesiologists in the sedation of children for radiologic and other procedures.

OUTCOME DATA IN PEDIATRIC SEDATION/ANESTHESIA FROM OUTSIDE THE OPERATING ROOM

There has been tremendous interest in outcomes of sedation and anesthesia in OOOR locations in the pediatric population. Cote et al.[3] used the Food and Drug Administration database to perform a critical incident analysis of sedation-related adverse events in children. Of the 95 cases investigated, 51 cases resulted in death and 9 in permanent brain injury. These severe injuries occurred more frequently in non–hospital-based facilities, such as dental offices (93% vs. 37%, Figure 10.1). Moreover, the majority of these deaths were judged to be preventable. Most were associated with failure to provide airway/ventilatory support in a timely fashion. Inadequate and inconsistent respiratory monitoring was another major factor contributing to poor outcome. Despite the lack of denominator data, this study was considered a breakthrough in the safety of pediatric procedural sedation.

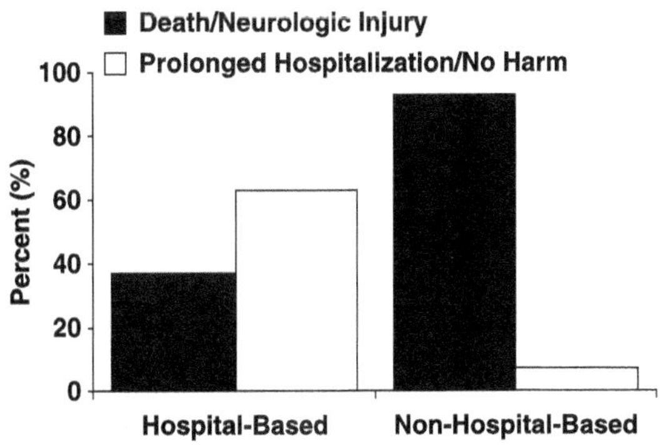

Figure 10.1. *Outcome of adverse sedation-related events in children sedated in hospital-based compared with non–hospital-based facilities ($p < .001$). (Reproduced with permission from Cote CJ, Notterman DA, Karl HW, et al. Adverse sedation events in pediatrics: a critical incident analysis of contributing factors. Pediatrics. 2000;105:805–814. Copyright 2000 by the AAP.)*

In 2003, with the collaboration of 37 institutions around the world, the Pediatric Sedation Research Consortium database was created with the goal to share information on the current pediatric sedation practice OOOR. In a prospective observational study, Cravero and colleagues[4] studied the incidence and nature of adverse events among the first 30,000 cases submitted to the registry. Data collection methods were standardized, and definitions were based on guidelines from professional societies. The most important findings were as follows: Overall rate of complications was 5.3%; there were no deaths; major complications included one cardiac arrest secondary to hypoxia and one aspiration pneumonia (Table 10.1). The majority of complications were related to adverse respiratory events, including desaturation below 90% and lasting more than 30 seconds; stridor, laryngospasm, wheezing, or apnea that could progress to a poor outcome if not managed adequately; and airway and ventilation interventions, including bag-mask ventilation, oral airway placement, or emergency intubation (Table 10.1). Eighty percent of patients were in the American Society of Anesthesiologists (ASA) class 1 or 2,

TABLE 10.1. Complications of Pediatric Sedation/Anesthesia in OOOR Locations

	INCIDENCE PER 10,000	*N*	*95% CI*
Adverse events			
Death	0.0	0	0.0–0.0
Cardiac arrest	0.3	1	0.0–1.9
Aspiration	0.3	1	0.0–1.9
Hypothermia	1.3	4	0.4–3.4
Seizure (unanticipated) during sedation	2.7	8	1.1–5.2
Stridor	4.3	11	1.8–6.6
Laryngospasm	4.3	13	2.3–7.4
Wheeze (new onset during sedation)	4.7	14	2.5–7.8
Allergic reaction (rash)	5.7	17	3.3–9.1
Intravenous-related problems/ complication	11.0	33	7.6–15.4
Prolonged sedation	13.6	41	9.8–18.5
Prolonged recovery	22.3	67	17.3–28.3
Apnea (unexpected)	24.3	73	19.1–30.5
Secretions (requiring suction)	41.6	125	34.7–49.6
Vomiting during procedure (nongastrointestinal)	47.2	142	39.8–55.7
Desaturation below 90%	156.5	470	142.7–171.2
Total adverse events	339.6 (1 per 29)	1020	308.1–371.5
Unplanned treatments			
Reversal agent required (unanticipated)	1.7	5	0.6–3.9
Emergency anesthesia consult for airway	2.0	6	0.7–4.3
Admission to hospital (unanticipated; sedation related)	7.0	21	4.3–10.7
Intubation required (unanticipated)	9.7	29	6.5–13.9
Airway (oral; unexpected requirement)	27.6	83	22.0–34.2
Bag-mask ventilation (unanticipated)	63.9	192	55.2–73.6
Total unplanned treatments	111.9 (1 per 89)	336	85.3–130.2
Conditions present during procedure			
Inadequate sedation, could not complete	88.9 (1 per 338)	267	78.6–100.2

OOOR, outside of the operating room.

SOURCE: Reprinted with permission from Cravero JP, Blike GT, Beach M, et al. Incidence and nature of adverse events during pediatric sedation/anesthesia for procedures outside the operating room: report from the Pediatric Sedation Research Consortium. *Pediatrics.* 2006;118:1087–1096. Copyright 2006 by the AAP.

and 76% were younger than 8 years; sedation/anesthesia was provided mostly by anesthesiologists, intensivists, and emergency physicians; and most procedures (62%) were radiologic. The most frequently used sedatives and analgesic agents were propofol (50%), midazolam (27%), ketamine (14%), and pentobarbital (13%). Although severe complications were infrequent, the data from Cravero et al.[4] suggest that continued attention to prevention of adverse respiratory events is necessary to improve patient safety in these low-risk procedures.

OUTCOMES OF ANESTHESIA AND PROCEDURAL SEDATION IN ADULTS

Pino[5] reviewed outcomes in over 63,000 patients undergoing diagnostic or therapeutic procedures under sedation or anesthesia in one hospital. Forty-one percent were sedated by nonanesthesia providers, with anesthesiologists providing monitored anesthesia care (MAC) in patients at extremes of age, ASA physical status 3–4, and in morbidly obese patients. There were 2 deaths and 17 cardiac arrests, but all were in the cardiac catheterization suite and were not related to sedation. It is important to note that respiratory events were likely to be underestimated because capnography, used to detect respiration and the presence of airway obstruction, was not used.

CLOSED MALPRACTICE CLAIMS IN OOOR LOCATIONS

Rare serious adverse outcomes have been studied by reviewing medicolegal records. Using the ASA Closed Claims database, we recently reviewed closed malpractice claims against anesthesiologists providing anesthesia care in remote locations.[6] The Closed Claims Project is a detailed structured evaluation of adverse anesthetic outcomes obtained from the closed malpractice claim files of 37 professional liability insurance companies throughout the United States. Claims for dental damage are excluded. Patterns of injury and liability associated with claims from anesthesia in remote locations arising since 1990 ($n = 87$) were compared with claims from OR procedures ($n = 3287$).

The facilities most commonly involved in the remote location claims were the gastrointestinal suite (32%) and cardiology catheterization/electrophysiology laboratory (25%), followed by the emergency room, interventional radiology, and lithotripsy suite. Patients in remote locations were older (20% more than 70 years, $p < .01$) and sicker (69% ASA physical status 3–5, $p < .005$) than patients in OR claims. There were also more children ($p < .01$) in remote locations. More than a third of remote location claims involved emergent procedures as compared with only 15% of OR claims ($p < .001$). These findings emphasize the high risk of many patients requiring care by anesthesia personnel as opposed to nonanesthesiologists for procedures OOOR.

Although the most frequently encountered anesthetic mishap in both remote and OR sites was of respiratory system origin, respiratory etiologies for remote location claims were double that of OR claims (44% vs. 20%, $p < .001$, Table 10.2). Inadequate oxygenation/ventilation was the most common single mechanism of injury in remote locations, occurring seven times more frequently than in OR claims (Table 10.2). Respiratory depression from oversedation was most common in the gastrointestinal suite during endoscopic retrograde cholangiopancreatography (ERCP) or upper gastrointestinal endoscopy. Propofol was most commonly used as the single agent or in combination with other drugs.

The severity of injuries for claims from remote locations was greater than those associated with the OR (Figure 10.2). The proportion of death was almost double in remote location claims (54% vs. 29%, $p < .001$). The anesthesia care was judged by closed claims reviewers as substandard in more than half of remote location claims. In addition, a third of the claims in remote locations were judged by the reviewers as being potentially preventable by better monitoring, including pulse oximetry, capnography, or both. A capnograph was employed in only a minority of claims associated with oversedation.[6]

The most recent ASA closed claims analysis demonstrated that OOOR claims had a higher proportion of claims for death than claims in the OR, and OOOR claims most frequently involved monitored anesthesia care.[7] About a third of OOOR claims were related to inadequate oxygenation/ventilation, and there was also a proportional increase of claims in cardiology and radiology.

The most common anesthetic technique was MAC in which the anesthesiologist administered sedation and monitored the patient, accounting for 50% of remote location claims. Respiratory depression due to an absolute or relative overdose of sedative-hypnotic-analgesic drugs and deficient monitoring were deemed responsible for the complication. MAC was the predominant technique in the gastroenterology suite, radiology, and cardiology catheterization laboratories.[6]

TABLE 10.2. Mechanisms of Injury in Remote Location Claims

	REMOTE LOCATION (N = 87) N (%)	OPERATING ROOM (N = 3287) N (%)
Respiratory event	38 (44%) [a]	671 (20%) [a]
Inadequate oxygenation/ ventilation	18 (21%) [a]	94 (3%) [a]
Cardiovascular event	9 (10%)	526 (16%)
Equipment failure/ malfunction	12 (14%)	438 (13%)
Event related to regional block	2 (2%) [a]	283 (9%) [a]
Medication-related event	5 (6%)	256 (8%)
Other events[b]	21 (24%)	1113 (34%)

[a] $p < .001$ remote location versus operating room claims by z test.

[b] Other events include surgical technique/patient condition, patient fell, wrong operation/location, positioning, failure to diagnose, other known damaging events, no damaging event, and unknown.

SOURCE: Reprinted with permission from Metzner J, Posner K, Domino K. The risk and safety of anesthesia at remote locations: the US closed claims analysis. *Curr Opin Anaesthesiol.* 2009;22:502–508.

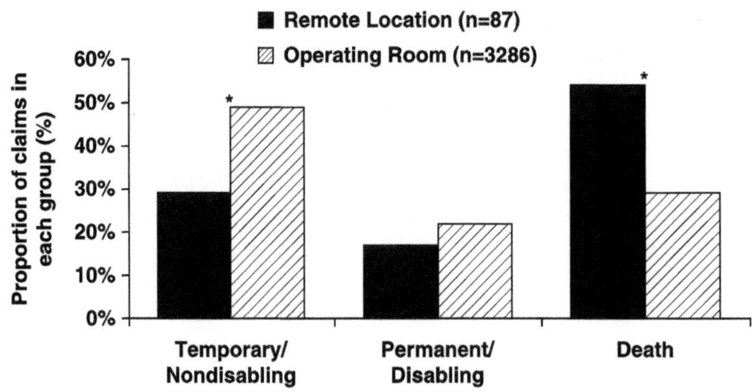

Figure 10.2. Severity of injury in remote location claims versus operating room claims. One claim with missing data excluded; $p < .001$ by Fisher exact test. (Reprinted with permission from Metzner J, Posner K, Domino K. The risk and safety of anesthesia at remote locations: the US closed claims analysis. Curr Opin Anaesthesiol. 2009;22:502–508.)

Bhananker et al.[8] used closed claims methodology to examine patterns of injury and liability during MAC in other settings. Death or permanent brain damage occurred in 41% of claims for MAC, comparable to the severity of injury during claims associated with general anesthesia. The findings were similar to those in remote location claims in that respiratory depression secondary to oversedation was the leading mechanism of injury, as most of these injuries could have been prevented by adequate monitoring of ventilation, especially end-tidal capnography. "Polypharmacy," including propofol in combination with other sedatives/opioids, was often involved in oversedation. These cases emphasize that pharmacokinetic features, changing levels of noxious stimulation, and variability in patient responses may contribute to accidental overdose.[9] The findings point out that sedation is a continuum, and that moderate sedation may fairly easily become deep sedation. In addition, the findings point out the roles of attitudes of anesthesia and surgical personnel and delayed recognition of respiratory depression so that cardiac arrest may be the initial signaling event.[9]

It is important to remember that closed claims are biased by severe, permanent injuries and lack denominator data (the total number of anesthetics/sedation performed), as well as nominator data (the total number of adverse outcomes). Hence, estimates of risk or safety cannot be made from this type of data. However, the data provide excellent clinical details of rare, severe complications.

The conclusions that can be drawn from the analysis of ASA Closed Claims Project data[6,8] are as follows:

- The most common etiology of death or permanent brain damage is inadequate oxygenation/ventilation.
- Respiratory depression from sedative agents is the leading cause of respiratory depression during sedation and MAC.
- Better monitoring of patient respiration, particularly end-tidal capnography, might prevent adverse respiratory events.
- General endotracheal anesthesia may be safer in some patients (e.g., those with morbid obesity with severe obstructive sleep apnea) and some procedures (e.g., ERCP and prone position procedures).

As a result of the Closed Claims findings, the ASA recently recommended use of end-tidal capnography to monitor adequacy of ventilation during propofol sedation, particularly because moderate sedation may quickly become deep sedation with this agent.[10] Better assessment of adequacy of ventilation should improve the safety of patients undergoing anesthesia and sedation in OOOR locations. Another recent study examining the National Anesthesia Clinical Outcomes Registry found that although non-OR cases appeared to have lower mortality rates compared to OR cases, there were increased complication rates in interventional cardiology and radiology locations.[2]

OTHER ADVERSE EVENTS IN REMOTE LOCATION CLAIMS

In addition to oversedation causing respiratory depression, the types of claims varied with the remote location.[6] Most of the claims from radiology involved anesthesia in the magnetic resonance imager (MRI) scanner, resulting in oversedation, burns from non–MRI-compatible electrodes, and a claim for brachioplexopathy in an obese patient whose arms were positioned above his head because he was too obese to allow arm positioning at his sides. Procedures in cardiology also had claims for difficult intubation with esophageal intubation during resuscitation and a variety of events related to invasive procedures in patients with cardiac disease. Claims from the emergency room also involved complications of emergency endotracheal intubation and resuscitation, including central line placement.[6]

REGULATORY EFFORTS AT IMPROVING QUALITY OF CARE

THE JOINT COMMISSION AND NATIONAL PATIENT SAFETY GOALS

In 2003, the Joint Commission, which accredits hospitals and health care organizations, began requiring health care organizations to comply with national patient safety goals (NPSGs) in an attempt to reduce medical errors and improve patient safety. The NPSGs are formulated based on the information provided by the Sentinel Event Advisory Group and should be viewed as a synthesis of the reported sentinel events (i.e., unexpected death or serious injury or potential for these injuries). The Joint Commission recommends program-specific (hospitals, ambulatory centers, offices) NPSGs for adoption, and if the surveys show improvement in a specific area, the goals will be implemented into the accreditation standards. Each year, the Joint Commission revises and updates the NPSGs and removes some goals while identifying new goals and requirements. The goals are found on the Joint Commission website (http://www.jointcommission.org/).

The NPSGs in 2009, relevant to anesthesia and sedation, focused on ways to improve the accuracy of patient identification, effectiveness of communication among caregivers and during transfer of care, medication safety, and reduction of iatrogenic infections and surgical fires (Box 10.1).[11]

Recently, The Joint Commission has focused attention on the application of the "Universal Protocol https://www.jointcommission.org/standards_information/up.aspx for Preventing Wrong Site, Wrong Procedure, and Wrong Person" to correctly identify the patient, the appropriate procedure, and the correct site of the procedure. Although distinct from the NPSGs, the Universal Protocol was inspired by the NPSGs and is particularly relevant to patient safety when anesthetized or sedated patients are undergoing procedures.

The protocol is based on three intertwined elements: conducting a preprocedure verification process, marking the procedure site (involve the patient directly if possible), and performing a time out before the procedure. The time out is standardized; is initiated by a designated member of the procedure team (e.g., either the anesthesiologist or the surgeon); involves the immediate members of the procedure team; has

BOX 10.1. 2009 NATIONAL PATIENT SAFETY GOALS RELEVANT TO ANESTHESIOLOGY

GOAL 1: IMPROVE THE ACCURACY OF PATIENT IDENTIFICATION

Use two patient identifiers, such as the individual's name, an assigned identification number, telephone number, or other person-specific identifier.

Prior to the procedures, mark the surgical site, and use time out to identify the patient and confirm the right procedure on the right side.

Eliminate transfusion errors related to patient misidentification.

Before initiating a blood or blood component transfusion, match the blood or blood component to the order, match the patient to the blood or blood component, and use a two-person verification process.

GOAL 2: IMPROVE THE EFFECTIVENESS OF COMMUNICATION AMONG CAREGIVERS

Report critical results of tests and diagnostic procedures on a timely basis.

"Read back" the critical lab/diagnostic results.

Use standardized abbreviations, acronyms, and symbols.

Use a "standardized" approach of handoff communication; allow clinicians to ask and answer questions pertinent to patient's care.

GOAL 3: IMPROVE THE SAFETY OF USING MEDICATIONS

Prevent errors with look-alike/sound-alike medications.

Label medications and solutions; discard unlabeled medications.

Reduce harm from anticoagulation therapy. Use approved protocols for the initiation and maintenance of anticoagulant therapy; use international normalized ratio for Coumadin therapy; use programmable infusion pumps for intravenous heparin therapy.

GOAL 4: REDUCE THE RISK OF HEALTH CARE–ASSOCIATED INFECTIONS

Improve compliance with hand hygiene guidelines.

Implement policies and practices aimed to reduce the risk of infections associated with a central line and surgical site infections.

GOAL 5: RECONCILE MEDICATIONS ACROSS THE CONTINUUM OF CARE

Complete a list of the patient's medications and communicate that information to the next provider of care.

GOAL 6: REDUCE THE RISK OF SURGICAL FIRES

Currently this goal is applicable only to the Joint Commission's ambulatory care and office-based surgery accreditation programs.

Educate staff members, including licensed independent practitioners and anesthesia care providers, in how to control heat sources, manage fuels, and provide enough time for patient preparation.

Provide guidelines to minimize oxygen concentration under drapes.

SOURCE: Based on the Joint Commission 2009 national patient safety goals (NPSGs).

team member agreement about the patient identity, correct site, and procedure to be performed; and has documentation of the time out. The surgical time out has recently been expanded to improve team communication concerning equipment readiness, patient conditions, and anticipated intraoperative or postoperative concerns (Figure 10.3). Implementation of a 19-item surgical safety checklist designed by the World Health Organization's (WHO's) Safe Surgery Saves Lives Program reduced death and complications after noncardiac surgery in a multi-institutional international study.[12] Adaptation of this checklist to procedure units in OOOR settings may be helpful to improve team communication and consistency of care.

In summary, as The Joint Commission continues to gather sentinel event statistics and correlate them with past and current NPSGs, new goals will emerge and new patient safety questions will be addressed. Although the purpose of most of the goals seems clear, there are some concerns about the challenges some goals might represent in their applicability in clinical care. The Joint Commission is reviewing current NPSGs, and, as a result, new NPSGs were developed for 2018.

NEVER EVENTS

In 2002, the National Quality Forum (NQF) published a report, *Serious Reportable Events in Healthcare*, that identified a list of 27 adverse events that should never happen in a safe hospital practice, defined as "never events."[13] In publishing this report, the NQF's goal was to provide the basis of systematic reporting of the most alarming health care errors and associated adverse events and ultimately to increase public accountability and stipulate a safer health care. To be included in NQF's list of never events, an event must be of concern to both the public and health care professionals; clearly identifiable and measurable; serious, resulting in death or significant disability; usually preventable; and important for public credibility or accountability.[14] Over time, the list has been revised and expanded, and it now includes 28 never events (Box 10.2).[15]

Events relevant to anesthesia practice include procedures performed on the wrong body part or wrong patient, the wrong procedure performed, patient death from medication error, administration of incompatible blood or blood products, and intraoperative or immediately postoperative death in an ASA class 1 patient. Over 25 states require hospitals to report all or several of the NQF-endorsed adverse events. Minnesota, the first state to implement an open adverse events reporting system and to perform root cause analysis (RCA; to be described further in this chapter), reported 154 adverse events that occurred between 2005 and 2006 (Figure 10.4).[16] The events that were reported most often (55%) were pressure ulcers and objects retained in a patient's body after an invasive procedure. Twenty-three percent of adverse events resulted in no harm to patients, while 20% led to either death or serious disability. Of the 24 deaths reported during this time period, 12 were due to falls, 3 were the result of suicide, 2 were related to the malfunction of a product or device, and 2 were related to medication errors. There were 23 cases of surgery on the wrong body part, 3 on the wrong patient, and 5 cases in which the wrong procedure was performed.

In an effort to improve patient safety, the Centers for Medicare and Medicaid Services and other major insurers moved to ban payments for certain adverse events that may be preventable with better care. Some of the selected events overlap with NQF's never events list and include surgery on the wrong body part, foreign body left in a patient after surgery, mismatched blood transfusion, major medication error, severe "pressure ulcer" acquired in the hospital, and preventable postoperative death. Other never events, like urinary tract infections and hospital-acquired pneumonia, are particular to the Medicare policy and contribute to the escalation of health care costs, as well as patient harm.

THE LEAPFROG GROUP

Hospitals also are facing increasing financial pressure from private stakeholders to do more to avoid never events. The Leapfrog Group was one of the leading organizations to adopt a never events policy and to ask hospitals to apologize to patients, report unexpected adverse outcomes to various safety agencies (such as the Joint Commission), perform RCAs, and waive all related costs when a preventable, serious adverse event occurs within their facility.[17]

Established in 2000 by a small number of health care purchasers, today the Leapfrog Group comprises more than 65 employers and agencies that purchase care for more than 30 million people. Since its inception, the group visionary was to exert its leverage toward improving health care quality, optimizing patient outcomes, and ultimately lowering health care costs nationwide. More information can be found on their website (http://www.leapfroggroup.org).

The goals of the Leapfrog Group are to reduce preventable medical mistakes and improve the quality and affordability of health care; encourage reporting of quality and outcomes so consumers can make informed health care choices; reward doctors and hospitals for improving the quality, safety, and affordability of health care; and help consumers reap the benefits of making smart health care decisions.

To achieve this goal, the Leapfrog Group proposed specific patient safety measures (leaps) to be implemented in hospitals across the United States. To evaluate the hospital's compliance with these safety measures, the group conducts periodic surveys and releases the data for the public on its website. Financial incentives and rewards are allocated to the well-performing sites.

The Leapfrog Group's "patient safety leaps" include intensive care specialist coverage in the intensive care unit, computerized physician order entry systems, referral to high-volume centers for high-risk procedures, and a good Safe Practices Score.[18] The Leapfrog Safe Practices Score is based on 13 safe practices audited by the group using voluntary hospital surveys. These safe practices include a safety culture, adequate nursing workforce, pharmacist involvement in medication use, patient readback of informed consent, documentation of end-of-life directives, prevention of mislabeled radiographs, anticoagulation and deep venous thrombosis prevention, prevention of central line sepsis, handwashing procedures, prevention of aspiration, and computerized medical record systems.[19] Based on the obtained data, hospitals are ranked by quartiles, and the information is displayed on the Leapfrog

** RETURN WITH PREFERENCE LIST TO MAIN OR PAVILION FRONT DESK**

PLEASE PLACE PATIENT STICKER HERE OR WRITE IN PATIENT NAME:	**SURGICAL SAFETY CHECKLIST** **WHO / SCOAP - SAFE SURGERY SAVES LIVES** **GLOBAL PATIENT SAFETY CHALLENGE** **Directions: Please place a check mark in the box for actions performed**

SIGN IN – PRIOR TO INDUCTION OF ANAESTHESIA, VERIFY:

□ PATIENT CONFIRMED IDENTITY, SITE, PROCEDURE AND CONSENT
□ SITE MARKED/NOT APPLICABLE

□ ANAESTHESIA SAFETY CHECK COMPLETED
□ PULSE OXIMETER ON PATIENT AND FUNCTIONING

DOES PATIENT HAVE A:
KNOWN ALLERGY
□ NO □ YES
DIFFICULT AIRWAY/ASPIRATION RISK
□ NO □ YES, AND NEEDED EQUIPMENT AND ASSISTANCE AVAILABLE

TIME OUT – PRIOR TO SKIN INCISION **(ATTENDING SURGEON BEGINS CHECKLIST HERE):**

□ CONFIRM ALL TEAM MEMBERS HAVE INTRODUCED THEMSELVES BY NAME AND ROLE

□ SURGEON, ANAESTHESIA PROFESSIONAL AND NURSE VERBALLY CONFIRM PATIENT, SITE, PROCEDURE, POSITION

ANTICIPATED CRITICAL EVENTS
□ SURGEON REVIEWS: WHAT ARE THE CRITICAL OR UNEXPECTED STEPS, OPERATIVE DURATION, ANTICIPATED BLOOD LOSS? RISK OF >500CC BLOOD LOSS (7CC/KG IN CHILDREN)? □ NO □ YES, AND ADEQUATE IV ACCESS AND FLUIDS PLANNED
□ ANAESTHESIA TEAM REVIEWS: WHAT ARE CRITICAL RESUSCITATION PLANS, PATIENT-SPECIFIC CONCERNS, IF ANY?
□ NURSING TEAM REVIEWS: WHAT ARE THE STERILITY INDICATOR RESULTS, EQUIPMENT ISSUES, OTHER PATIENT CONCERNS?

□ ANTIBIOTIC PROPHYLAXIS GIVEN IN LAST 60 MINUTES □ NOT APPLICABLE
□ ANTIBIOTIC REDOSING PLAN IN PLACE □ NOT APPLICABLE (CASE < 3 HOURS)

□ ESSENTIAL IMAGING DISPLAYED □ NOT APPLICABLE

□ ACTIVE WARMING IN PLACE □ NOT APPLICABLE (CASE < 1 HOUR)

□ GLUCOSE CHECKED FOR DIABETICS □ INSULIN STARTED FOR GLUCOSE > 125 □ NOT APPLICABLE

□ BETA BLOCKER PLANNED POSTOPERATIVELY □ NOT APPLICABLE (NOT ON PREOP BETA BLOCKER, NO INDICATIONS)

□ VTE PREVENTION PLAN IN PLACE □ NOT APPLICABLE

LAST YEAR THERE WERE 58 SHARPS INJURIES IN THIS OR-

□ THE OPERATING TEAM HAS AN AGREED PLAN TO PREVENT SHARPS INJURY? □ NOT APPLICABLE (NO SHARPS)

SIGN OUT – PRIOR TO WOUND CLOSURE:
□ SURGEON CONFIRMS INSTRUMENTS & SPONGES ARE OUT OF INCISION (SURGEON)

SIGN OUT – AT COMPLETION OF THE CASE & PRIOR TO THE PATIENT LEAVING THE OPERATING THEATRE:

NURSE VERBALLY CONFIRMS WITH THE TEAM:
□ INSTRUMENT, SPONGE AND NEEDLE COUNTS CORRECT

□ WHAT PROCEDURE WAS PERFORMED?

□ HOW IS THE SPECIMEN LABELLED (INCLUDING PATIENT NAME)?

□ ARE THERE ANY EQUIPMENT MALFUNCTIONS OR ISSUES TO BE ADDRESSED?

SURGEON, ANAESTHESIA PROFESSIONAL AND NURSE REVIEW:
□ WHAT ARE THE KEY CONCERNS FOR RECOVERY AND MANAGEMENT OF THIS PATIENT AND WHAT COULD HAVE BEEN DONE BETTER?

Return with PL
to
Main or Pavilion Front Desk.

______________________________ _______________
SIGNATURE (ON BEHALF OF ENTIRE TEAM) **DATE**

Figure 10.3. *World Health Organization's Safe Surgery Saves Lives checklist used at University of Washington Medical Center, Seattle, Washington, one of the participating hospitals in the Haynes et al. study.[12] VTE, venous thromboembolism*

BOX 10.2. NEVER EVENTS, 2006: SERIOUS REPORTABLE EVENTS IN HEALTH CARE

SURGICAL EVENTS

Surgery performed on the wrong body part

Surgery performed on the wrong patient

Wrong surgical procedure performed on a patient

Unintended retention of a foreign object in a patient after surgery or other procedure

Intraoperative or immediately postoperative death in an American Society of Anesthesiologists class 1 patient

Artificial insemination with the wrong sperm or donor egg

PRODUCT OR DEVICE EVENTS

Patient death or serious disability associated with the use of contaminated drugs, devices, or biologics provided by the health care facility

Patient death or serious disability associated with the use or function of a device in patient care, in which the device is used for functions other than as intended

Patient death or serious disability associated with intravascular air embolism that occurs while being cared for in a health care facility

PATIENT PROTECTION EVENTS

Infant discharged to the wrong person

Patient death or serious disability associated with patient elopement (disappearance)

Patient suicide, or attempted suicide resulting in serious disability, while being cared for in a health care facility

CARE MANAGEMENT EVENTS

Patient death or serious disability associated with a medication error (e.g., errors involving the wrong drug, wrong dose, wrong patient, wrong time, wrong rate, wrong preparation, or wrong route of administration)

Patient death or serious disability associated with a hemolytic reaction due to the administration of ABO/HLA-incompatible blood or blood products

Maternal death or serious disability associated with labor or delivery in a low-risk pregnancy while being cared for in a health care facility

Patient death or serious disability associated with hypoglycemia, the onset of which occurs while the patient is being cared for in a health care facility

Death or serious disability (kernicterus) associated with failure to identify and treat hyperbilirubinemia in neonates

Stage 3 or 4 pressure ulcers acquired after admission to a health care facility

Patient death or serious disability due to spinal manipulative therapy

ENVIRONMENTAL EVENTS

Patient death or serious disability associated with an electric shock or electrical cardioversion while being cared for in a health care facility

Any incident in which a line designated for oxygen or other gas to be delivered to a patient contains the wrong gas or is contaminated by toxic substances

Patient death or serious disability associated with a burn incurred from any source while being cared for in a health care facility

Patient death or serious disability associated with a fall while being cared for in a health care facility

Patient death or serious disability associated with the use of restraints or bedrails while being cared for in a health care facility

CRIMINAL EVENTS

Any instance of care ordered by or provided by someone impersonating a physician, nurse, pharmacist, or other licensed health care provider

Abduction of a patient of any age

Sexual assault on a patient within or on the grounds of the health care facility

Death or significant injury of a patient or staff member resulting from a physical assault (i.e., battery) that occurs within or on the grounds of the health care facility

SOURCE: Reproduced with permission from the National Quality Forum, © 2007.

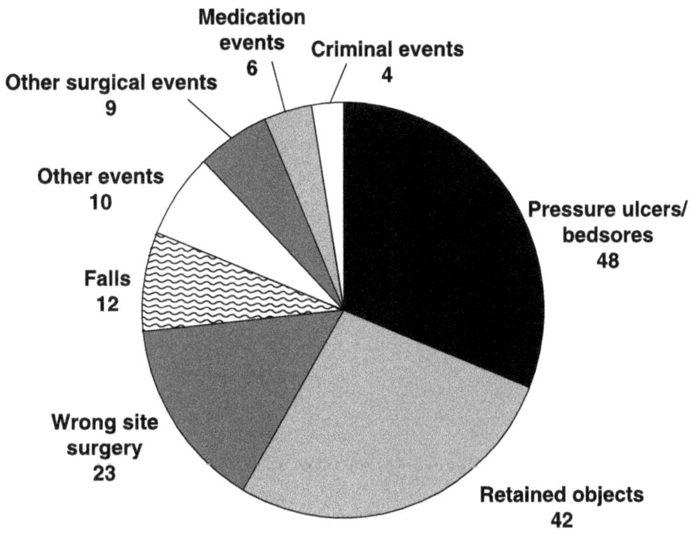

Figure 10.4. Reported adverse health events (154) by category in Minnesota, 2005–2006. (Reprinted with permission from "Adverse Health Events in Minnesota" 2007 public report, overview of reported events, page 5. Copyright Minnesota Department of Health 2007.)

Group website. To be rewarded for high-quality care, a hospital must score on the top quartile and show evidence of continuous improvement in the safety process.

To date, the impact of these initiatives on the quality and cost of health care have been discussed extensively in the literature, and whether they represent a real breakthrough is still under debate. A recent study analyzing the first initiatives collectively showed that hospitals performing according to the Leapfrog Group standards had lower mortality rates and better quality-of-care scores for acute myocardial infarction, pneumonia, and congestive heart failure.[20] Another study found that hospitals in California that met referral criteria for high-volume surgery for abdominal aortic aneurysm repair had a 51% reduction of in-hospital mortality compared with those who did not adhere to standards.[21] Moreover, a report published by the Leapfrog Group in 2008 indicated that implementing these leaps in nonrural hospitals could save more than 57,000 lives and save up to $12.0 billion each year.[18] Although a recent review did not show any significant improvement in risk-adjusted inpatient mortality rate in hospitals that completed the 2006 Safe Practice Score survey,[22] it is likely that the Safe Practice Score represents a major step for improving overall patient safety in hospitals.

CONTINUOUS QUALITY IMPROVEMENT IN THE OOOR SETTING

STRUCTURE, PROCESS, AND OUTCOME: THE BUILDING BLOCKS OF QUALITY

Quality improvement programs are generally guided by requirements of the Joint Commission. These programs are oriented toward improvements in the structure, process, and outcome of health care delivery.[23] *Structure* refers to the setting in which the process of care takes place and describes the organizational characteristics that facilitate delivery of care. Examples include organization and ownership of the facilities, ratio of practitioners to patients, qualifications of medical staff, and technological complexity. Structural characteristics are considered necessary but insufficient elements in the delivery of health services. They are considered indirect measures of quality in that their presence enables the provision of quality health services but does not ensure it, whereas the absence of these structural characteristics decreases the probability of quality outcomes.

Process encompasses includes not only all the medical activities performed for "good" patient care but also prevention, continuity of care, and physician-patient interaction. In the actual practice, process measures often imply compliance with standards of care, such as: Was the patient consented prior to procedure? Was the antibiotic timely administered? Was central venous access obtained under strict sterile technique? Although process characteristics are considered more proximal indicators of quality than the structural ones, they cannot guarantee a quality outcome; they can only increase its probability.

Outcome refers to the impact of treatments on patient status at the end of the care, including mortality, morbidity, length of hospital stay, and patient satisfaction. CQI programs focus on measuring and improving these basic components of care.

QUALITY IMPROVEMENT STRATEGIES

Episodic outcome assessment has a well-rooted tradition in medicine in the form of mortality and morbidity (M&M) conferences. Since the 1990s, CQI systems have taken a systems approach to identifying and improving quality of care, rather than the traditional medical approach of blaming the individual.

In the Joint Commission standards, routine tracking of outcomes requires analysis when trends exceed acceptable performance limits, performance or outcome varies excessively, and special adverse events occur, such as adverse drug reactions, adverse events related to anesthesia and sedation, and sentinel events. The goal is to identify

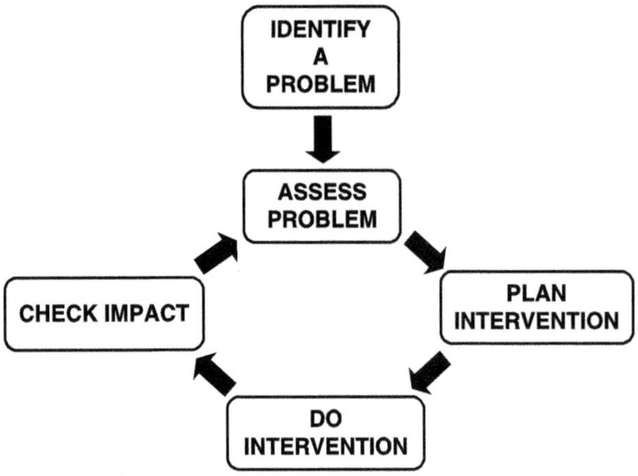

Figure 10.5. Continuous quality improvement (CQI) process. (Reprinted from Campion FX, Rosenblatt MS. Quality assurance and medical outcomes in the era of cost containment. Surg Clin North Am. 1996;76:139–159. Copyright 1996, with permission from Elsevier.)

and correct latent errors, effect change, and reassess to determine effect (Figure 10.5).[24]

SENTINEL EVENT MONITORING

Hospitals and health departments use the reporting of sentinel events to focus on interventions and structural engineering that can prevent subsequent patient injury and death. Sentinel events that mandate reporting, review, and a planned response mechanism include wrong site or wrong patient surgery, hemolytic transfusion reactions due to major blood group incompatibility, and awareness during general anesthesia if it results in significant psychological harm. Although reporting sentinel events to the Joint Commission is voluntary, RCA is mandatory within 45 days if the Joint Commission determines that an organization has had a reviewable sentinel event. Failure of the institution to conduct an RCA can result in the organization being placed on accreditation watch.

ROOT CAUSE ANALYSIS

Root cause analysis is a system-based approach to investigate the causal or contributing factors underlying adverse events or critical incidents. Initially developed to analyze aviation and industrial accidents, RCA is now widely implemented as an error analysis tool in health care. The goal is to determine what happened, why it happened, and what can be done to prevent it happening again. The fundamental theory of RCA is not to "name and blame" individuals for a mistake but rather identify the underlying problems and sequence of events in which the incident was rooted. A typical RCA process follows a structured approach, which begins with data collection and reconstruction of the event through record review and participant interviews. A multidisciplinary team analyzes the sequence of events with the goal to spot why and how the incident occurred. Although identification of "active" errors is important, the major goal of RCA is to uncover "latent" errors (i.e., system weaknesses) hidden in a faulty operating system.

The RCA method helps to determine the factors causing variation from the expected outcome. For example, a published RCA investigated the case of a patient who was mistakenly taken for another patient's invasive electrophysiology procedure.[25] A traditional analysis might have focused on assigning individual blame, perhaps to the nurse who sent the patient for the procedure despite the lack of a consent form. However, the subsequent RCA discovered at least 17 distinct errors, no single one of which could have caused this adverse event by itself. The case illustrates how these specific "active" errors interacted with a few underlying latent conditions to cause harm. The most remediable of these were absent or misused protocols for patient identification and informed consent, systematic faulty exchange of information among caregivers, and poorly functioning teams. This led the hospital to implement a series of systematic changes to reduce the likelihood of a similar error in the future.

The US Department of Veterans Affairs[26] and the Joint Commission pioneered RCA in the early 1990s; each developed its own programs, replacing older review methods with a more systematic approach. The Joint Commission now requires organizations to perform a RCA for every sentinel event.[27] In the Veterans Affairs system, facilities submit RCA reports for serious adverse events to the National Center for Patient Safety. Currently, 25 states require reporting of adverse events to the state health department. Although these institutions teach standard methods and have developed tools to help standardize reports, best practices have not been established for recommendations for action, follow-up, and analyzing results (Box 10.3).[28] Furthermore, there are no studies in peer-reviewed literature on the effectiveness of RCA in reducing risk or improving safety in medical care, and there are no evaluations of the cost or cost-effectiveness of the procedure compared with other tools to alleviate hazards.

CONTINUOUS QUALITY IMPROVEMENT SYSTEMS IN OOOR LOCATIONS

To improve patient safety by making system changes in anesthesia/sedation practices in OOOR procedure areas, a robust CQI system should be adopted. In addition to adherence to regulatory standards and measurement of "best practice" process indicators (e.g., performance of time out, antibiotic administration, etc.), outcomes must be measured and compared over time and to national standards. Outcome measurements for anesthesia and sedation practices need to include patient injuries, as well as escalation of care and identification of process problems (Table 10.3 provides outcome measurements).[29] Identification of management areas (Table 10.4) from which these adverse outcomes arose helps focus attention for improvement in various systems. For more severe quality indicators that result in unexpected temporary injuries, permanent injuries, or death, an RCA should be performed to determine system conditions that may have contributed to the adverse event and to make process changes

BOX 10.3. ROOT CAUSE ANALYSIS (RCA)

A root cause analysis has the following characteristics:

1. A process that is interdisciplinary, involving experts from the front-line services
2. A process that involves those who are the most familiar with the situation
3. A process that is continually digging deeper by asking why, why, why at each level of cause and effect
4. A process that identifies changes that need to be made to systems
5. A process that is as impartial as possible

To be thorough, a root cause analysis must include the following:

1. Determination of human and other factors
2. Determination of related processes and systems
3. Analysis of underlying cause-and-effect systems through a series of why questions
4. Identification of risks and their potential contributions
5. Determination of potential improvement in processes or systems

To be credible, a root cause analysis must do the following:

1. Include participation by the leadership of the organization and those most closely involved in the processes and systems
2. Be internally consistent
3. Include consideration of relevant literature

SOURCE: US Department of Veterans Affairs National Center of Patient Safety (NCPS).

TABLE 10.3. Continuous Quality Improvement (CQI) Anesthesia Outcomes

MAJOR INJURIES	ESCALATION OF CARE
Death	Prolonged intubation
Brain damage	Prolonged stay in postanesthesia care unit
Nerve damage	Prolonged hospital stay
Respiratory system injuries	Unscheduled admission of an outpatient
Airway trauma	Unscheduled intensive care unit admission
Adult respiratory distress syndrome/acute lung injury	Extra tests
Aspiration pneumonitis	Postoperative consult
Pneumothorax	Change in anesthetic plan
Prolonged ventilatory support	Naloxone
Pulmonary edema	Rule out myocardial infarction
Respiratory arrest	Reintubation
Other respiratory system injury	Extra drugs
Cardiovascular system injuries	Other escalation of care
Myocardial infarction	**Process problem**
Prolonged arrhythmia	Delay in procedure
Stroke	Time-out problem
Cardiac arrest	Cancellation of procedure
Localized vascular insufficiency	Patient arrived needing further tests, labs
Other cardiovascular system injury	Antibiotic administration
Other injuries	Equipment problem
Burn (thermal)	Other process problem
Skin inflammation	
Eye injury	***Quality assurance (QA) concern scores for outcomes:***
Dental injury	*0. No QA concern*
Seizure	*1. QA concern—no effect*
Awareness/recall	*2. QA concern—escalation of care*
Pain	*3. QA concern—temporary injury*
Other patient injury	*4. QA concern—permanent injury*
Other soft tissue	*5. QA concern—death*

TABLE 10.4. Continuous Quality Improvement (CQI) Management Areas

AIRWAY	INSTRUMENTATION
Airway obstruction	Central line
Aspiration of gastric contents	Equipment
Bronchospasm	Arterial line
Difficult intubation	Instrumentation (miscellaneous)
Endobronchial intubation	**IV infusion**
Esophageal intubation	Disconnect
Inability/difficult to ventilate	Infiltration
Accidental extubation	IV infusion (miscellaneous)
Inadequate ventilation/ oxygenation	**Metabolic**
Laryngospasm	Hypoglycemia
Premature extubation	Hyperglycemia

(Continued)

TABLE 10.4. *(Cont'd)*

AIRWAY	INSTRUMENTATION
Airway (miscellaneous)	**Peripheral nerve**
Circulatory	Peripheral nervous system
Air embolism	**Position**
Excessive blood loss	Hyperextension
Hypertension	Pressure
Hypotension	Position injury (miscellaneous)
Inadequate/ inappropriate fluid therapy	**Pulmonary**
Ischemia, cardiac	Pneumothorax
Circulatory management (miscellaneous)	Pulmonary management (miscellaneous)
Central nervous system	**Thermoregulation**
Central nervous system (miscellaneous)	Hypothermia
Medication	**Other**
Wrong dose	Preop evaluation
Wrong drug	Turnover
Allergic reaction	Miscommunication
Neuromuscular block management	Personnel delay
Drug action/interaction (miscellaneous)	Failure to diagnose/misdiagnosis
	Failure to treat/wrong treatment
	Inadequate monitoring
	Document issue
	Other

to prevent the event from occurring in the future. In addition to determination of rates of adverse events, current CQI systems also review production issues as well as patient satisfaction with care.

SUMMARY

Providing anesthesia and sedation in procedure areas OOOR is increasing in popularity, but it is associated with risks that may be greater than when provided to similar patients in the OR setting. Patient safety can be improved by adherence to respiratory monitoring (e.g., pulse oximetry and capnography), sedation standards/guidelines and national patient safety and regulatory efforts, and development of vigorous CQI systems to measure outcomes and effect system changes.

REFERENCES

1. Nagrebetsky A, Gabriel RA, Dutton RP, Urman RD. Growth of nonoperating room anesthesia care in the United States: a contemporary trends analysis. *Anesth Analg.* 2017;124(4):1261–1267.
2. Chang B, Kaye AD, Diaz JH, Westlake B, Dutton RP, Urman RD. Complications of non-operating room procedures: outcomes from the national anesthesia clinical outcomes registry. *J Patient Saf.* 2015. [Epub ahead of print].
3. Cote CJ, Notterman DA, Karl HW, et al. Adverse sedation events in pediatrics: a critical incident analysis of contributing factors. *Pediatrics.* 2000;105:803–814.
4. Cravero JP, Blike GT, Beach M, et al. Incidence and nature of adverse events during pediatric sedation/anesthesia for procedures outside the operating room: report from the Pediatric Sedation Research Consortium. *Pediatrics.* 2006;118:1087–1096.
5. Pino RM. The nature of anesthesia and procedural sedation outside of the operating room. *Curr Opin Anaesthesiol.* 2007;20:347–351.
6. Metzner J, Posner KL, Domino KB. The risk and safety of anesthesia at remote locations: the US closed claims analysis. *Curr Opin Anaesthesiol.* 2009;22:502–508.
7. Woodward ZG, Urman RD, Domino KB. Safety of Non-Operating Room Anesthesia: A Closed Claims Update. *Anesthesiol Clin.* 2017;35(4):569–581.
8. Bhananker SM, Posner KL, Cheney FW, et al. Injury and liability associated with monitored anesthesia care: a closed claims analysis. *Anesthesiology.* 2006;104:228–234.
9. Hug CC Jr. MAC should stand for maximum anesthesia caution, not minimal anesthesiology care. *Anesthesiology.* 2006;104:221–223.
10. American Society of Anesthesiologists. Statement on safe use of propofol, last amended 2014. Available at: http://www.asahq.org/quality-and-practice-management/standards-guidelines-and-related-resources/statement-on-safe-use-of-propofol. Accessed on March 4, 2018.
11. The Joint Commission. National patient safety goals. 2017. Available at: https://www.jointcommission.org/hap_2017_npsgs/. Accessed on March 4, 2018.
12. Haynes AB, Weiser TG, Berry WR, et al. A surgical safety checklist to reduce morbidity and mortality in a global population. *N Engl J Med.* 2009;360:491–499.
13. National Forum for Healthcare Quality Measurement and Reporting. *Serious Reportable Events in Healthcare: A Consensus Report.* Washington, DC: National Quality Forum; June 2002.
14. Henriksen K, Battles JB, Marks ES, Lewin DI, eds. *Advances in Patient Safety: From Research to Implementation. Vol. 4, Programs, Tools, and Products.* Rockville, MD: Agency for Healthcare Research and Quality; 2005. AHRQ Publication No. 05-0021-4.
15. National Quality Forum. *Serious Reportable Events in Healthcare 2006 Update: A Consensus Report.* Washington, DC: National Quality Forum; March 2007.
16. Minnesota Department of Health. Adverse health events in Minnesota. Available at: http://www.health.state.mn.us/patientsafety/ae/2016ahereport.pdf. Published February 2016. Accessed on March 9, 2017.
17. Milstein A, Galvin RS, Delbanco SF, et al. Improving the safety of health care: the Leapfrog initiative. *Eff Clin Pract.* 2000;3(6):313–316.
18. Lwin AK, Shepard DS. *Estimating Lives and Dollars Saved From Universal Adoption of the Leapfrog Safety and Quality Standards: 2008 Update.* Washington, DC: Leapfrog Group; 2008. Available at: http://citeseerx.ist.psu.edu/viewdoc/download?doi=10.1.1.537.1190&rep=rep1&type=pdf. Accessed on March 4, 2017.
19. Agency for Healthcare Research and Quality. Safe practices for better healthcare: summary. A consensus report. National Quality Forum. Available at: https://www.ahrq.gov/professionals/quality-patient-safety/index.html. Page last reviewed December 2016. Accessed on March 9, 2017.
20. Jha AK, Orav EJ, Ridgway AB, et al. Does the Leapfrog program help identify high-quality hospitals? *Jt Comm J Qual Patient Saf.* 2008;34(6):318–325.
21. Brooke BS, Perler BA, Dominici F, et al. Reduction of in-hospital mortality among California hospitals meeting Leapfrog evidence-based standards for abdominal aortic aneurysm repair. *J Vasc Surg.* 2008;47(6):1155–1156.
22. Kernisan LP, Lee SJ, Boscardin WJ, et al. Association between hospital-reported Leapfrog safe practices scores and inpatient mortality. *JAMA.* 2009;301(13):1341–1348.
23. Donabedian A. Evaluating the quality of medical care. *Milbank Mem Fund Q.* 1996;44(3)(suppl 1):166–206.

24. Campion FX, Rosenblatt MS. Quality assurance and medical outcomes in the era of cost containment. *Surg Clin North Am.* 1996;76:139–159.
25. Chassin MR, Becher EC. The wrong patient. *Ann Intern Med.* 2002;136(11):826–833.
26. Bagian JP, Gosbee J, Lee CZ, et al. The Veterans Affairs root cause analysis system in action. *Jt Comm J Qual Improv.* 2002;28(10):531–545.
27. The Joint Commission. Sentinel event. Available at: https://www.jointcommission.org/sentinel_event_policy_and_procedures/ Accessed on March 10, 2017.
28. US Department of Veterans Affairs. National Center for Patient Safety: root cause analysis (RCA). n.d. Available at: https://www.patientsafety.va.gov/professionals/onthejob/rca.asp. Accessed on March 10, 2017.
29. Posner KL, Kendall-Gallagher D, Wright IH, et al. Linking process and outcome of care in a continuous quality improvement program for anesthesia services. *Am J Med Qual.* 1994;9(3):129–137.

11 | CT- AND PET/CT-GUIDED INTERVENTIONAL RADIOLOGY PROCEDURES

SHARATH K. BHAGAVATULA, MD, DANIEL A. T. SOUZA, MD, MILANA FLUSBERG, MD, STUART G. SILVERMAN, MD, PAUL B. SHYN, MD

INTRODUCTION

Over the last several decades, computed tomography (CT) has become a valuable guidance modality for a large number of diagnostic and therapeutic percutaneous interventions.[1] Common diagnostic CT-guided interventions include tissue biopsies, fluid aspirations, and catheter drainages. Needle biopsies can be used to obtain tissue for cytologic or histologic assessment from almost any anatomical region of the body. In oncology, biopsy specimens provide both a fully detailed diagnosis and a genetic and molecular assessment that are vital in the care of virtually every type of cancer. Needle aspiration of fluid collections can be performed to obtain samples for microbiology, cytology, chemistry, and other tests. Some of the additional diagnostic interventions that can be accomplished under CT guidance include spinal diskography and fiducial marker placement to more accurately localize tumors prior to surgical resection or radiation.[1,2]

Catheter drainages are now the initial preferred approach to definitively manage many fluid collections, both infected and uninfected.[3] Types of fluid collections that can be drained include abscesses throughout the body (including thoracic empyemas), uninfected pleural and peritoneal collections, hematomas, seromas, and fluid collections due to fistulas such as bilomas, urinomas, lymphoceles, cerebrospinal fluid–omas, pancreatic collections, and collections due to bowel leaks. Some uninfected collections (e.g., lymphocele) and some symptomatic cysts, including those due to parasitic infection (e.g., echinococcus), can also be treated with sclerosing agents under CT guidance.[4] Catheter drainage of a viscus, such as percutaneous cholecystostomy, can also be used to temporize or palliate ill patients until their condition allows definitive surgical therapy. CT-guided gastrostomies and cystostomies can also be performed, particularly when there is concern for complex anatomy or intervening structures that precludes ultrasound (US) guidance.[1,5]

Percutaneous tumor ablation (e.g., radio-frequency [RF] ablation, cryoablation, and microwave ablation) is commonly performed under CT guidance; recent advances in these technologies and data regarding their efficacy have led to an increased number of tumors ablated for curative and palliative purposes. CT-guided neurolysis procedures, local anesthetic injections, vertebroplasties, and ablation procedures can be performed for pain management purposes.[1,6]

COMPUTED TOMOGRAPHY: HISTORICAL BACKGROUND AND RECENT ADVANCES

Computed tomography was introduced in the early 1970s. It was the first technology to incorporate computer reconstruction of images. The spatial and temporal resolution of CT scanners has improved substantially over the last few decades. With the introduction of spiral CT in the early 1990s, followed by multidetector CT (MDCT), rapid acquisition of volume data became possible, paving the way for the development of multiplanar re-formations (MPRs) and three-dimensional (3D) imaging (e.g., maximum intensity projection [MIP], surface-shaded display [SSD], and volume-rendering techniques [VRTs]), to play an important role in both diagnostic imaging and interventional CT guidance. More recently, improvements in computational power have promoted and facilitated developments in image processing and iterative reconstruction techniques for faster and higher-quality image acquisition and lower radiation exposure. The emergence of dual-energy CT has allowed improved characterization of tissue composition by assessing spectral tissue properties, and advances in cone beam technologies have allowed simultaneous imaging of tissue volumes during a single rotation.[7] These new features have led to the application of CT imaging to a wide spectrum of clinical indications, including CT myelography, angiography, urography, coronary calcium scoring, perfusion imaging, and virtual endoscopy.[8–10]

Computed tomographic fluoroscopy, also developed in the 1990s, represented a substantial technologic advance, combining the cross-sectional imaging capability of CT with real-time image display.[10–12] A foot pedal that initiates image acquisition, sterile drapes over the gantry table controls, and an image display monitor in the interventional CT suite permit the radiologist to stand alongside the patient during the procedure, affording more radiologist control, faster procedure times, and uninterrupted patient monitoring. This is especially useful for interventions in less-compliant and critically ill patients.[13–15] The development and commercialization of portable CT scanners now include fluoroscopy capabilities that expand further the use of CT to guide interventional procedures.[7]

THE INTERVENTIONAL CT SUITE: PLANNING AND SETUP

Any CT scanner can be used for CT-guided interventions; however, MDCT scanners are generally preferred because they allow faster coverage of important anatomy in three dimensions. This not only facilitates recognition of needle deviations in the craniocaudal direction but also is less susceptible to organ shift during the intervention.[11] Selection of a scanner with a large-bore gantry or a portable scanner with arms that rotate around the patient may also be helpful for certain procedures where longer instruments are used, as well as for large or claustrophobic patients (Figure 11.1). There should be sufficient space in the interventional CT suite for the radiologist, one or two assistants, one or two nurses, a sterile instrument table, and patient-monitoring devices. For selected procedures, more space is needed for additional equipment, such as a mechanical ventilator, anesthesia delivery systems, and ancillary interventional devices, such as ablation equipment. The location of wall gases and suction should be accessible from either side of the scanner. The scanner gantry and table control buttons are typically duplicated on both sides of the scanner. Anesthesia equipment and personnel are usually positioned on the side of the patient opposite from the interventional radiologist or at the head of the patient on the opposite side of the gantry.[12]

PREPROCEDURAL CONSIDERATIONS

RADIATION

A relative disadvantage of CT guidance is exposure of the patient, the interventionalist, and support personnel to ionizing radiation.[13–15] However, the x-ray beam in CT is well collimated, and there is a marked drop in radiation exposure beyond the gantry. Nevertheless, as with all medical imaging, the goal is to minimize the use of scanning during a CT-guided procedure to the extent necessary for safely and efficaciously accomplishing the procedure while minimizing radiation exposure under the ALARA (as low as reasonably achievable) principle. Because prior imaging studies are usually available at the time of the procedure, the planning and postprocedure scans should be limited to the organ or region of interest, including the planned approach and adjacent critical structures. The CT scanning technique parameters (kilovolts, milliamperes, and collimation), the number of sequential scans, and the total CT fluoroscopy time during a procedure should be optimized to reduce patient radiation yet allow identification of important structures and monitor for possible complications. CT dose index (CTDI) and dose-length product (DLP), measured in grays and gray-centimeters, respectively, are typically reported for all CT exams and allow quantification and monitoring of patient and staff dose during and after the procedure.[16]

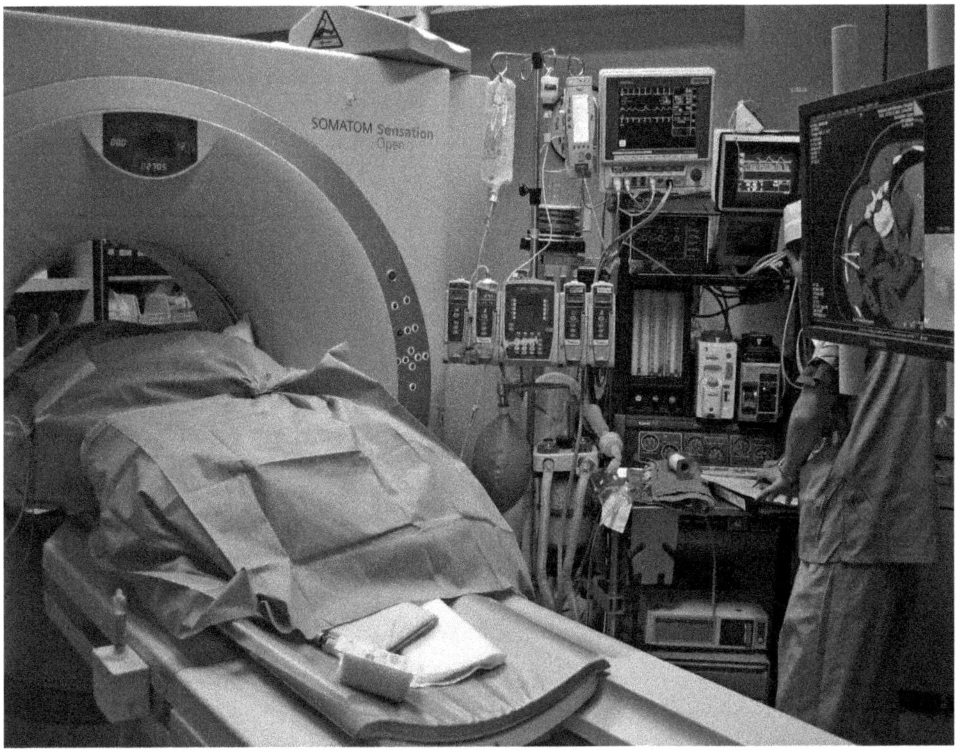

Figure 11.1. Computed tomography (CT)–guided percutaneous ablation: The wide-bore CT gantry depicted is a potential advantage in large patients because it allows comfortable scanning of the patient and the positioned percutaneous devices during the procedure.

Techniques to minimize radiation to the patient and staff include using lower radiation dose (milliamperes) than required for diagnostic purposes; intermittent rather than continuous CT fluoroscopy; covering areas of the patient outside the region of interest with lead drapes; and imaging the needle tip rather than the entire needle during the procedure.[13,16] It is particularly important to be aware of a potentially high patient skin dose from repeat scanning of the same area during the course of an intervention.[17]

When CT fluoroscopy is used, the interventionalist and other in-room personnel are also exposed to radiation. The interventional radiologist's hand should never extend into the primary x-ray beam. When continuous fluoroscopy is necessary, plastic needle holders are available that remove the hand from the primary beam.[17–19] Catheters and needles may also occasionally be prebent to allow manipulation from outside the scan plane. Scattered radiation from the patient's body is the dominant source of exposure to personnel in the procedure room, with smaller amounts of exposure resulting from source radiation leakage and direct radiation from the beam. Radiation scatter can be limited by placing a lead drape over the region of the patient's body closest to the interventionalist but not infringing on the scan coverage area.[19] Radiation protection measures for the interventional radiologist and other personnel within the CT suite are similar to those for other fluoroscopic interventions. A lead apron with 0.35-mm lead equivalent and thyroid shield must be worn. Protective lead goggles may reduce the risk of premature cataracts.[20,21] Personnel should maximize their distance from the patient during scan acquisitions to the extent possible because radiation levels decrease in proportion to the inverse square of the distance from the radiation source. This means that even small increases in distance from the patient result in large decreases in radiation exposure to personnel. When possible, stepping out of the CT suite or behind a lead glass radiation shield during scanning virtually eliminates radiation exposure to personnel.[18,19]

BLEEDING RISK

Bleeding is a potential complication of percutaneous interventions, and it is of particular concern in patients receiving anticoagulants or with bleeding disorders. Periprocedural management of these patients can be complex due to the wide range of procedural techniques, patient medications, and comorbidities.[22,23]

Guidelines for optimizing coagulation parameters prior to image-guided procedures exist, but they are not concrete and are often adapted to a particular patient's clinical history and risk factors.[22,24] Consideration is also given to the invasiveness and bleeding risk associated with the particular procedure, with many CT-guided biopsies, aspirations, and drainages considered of moderate or high bleeding risk. In general, the international normalized ratio (INR) should be below 1.5, the partial thromboplastin time (PTT) close to normal, and the platelet count above 50,000/mm^3 for most procedures. When possible, warfarin is discontinued 5–7 days prior to the procedure. Clopidogrel and aspirin are typically withheld for 5 days before the procedure, and fractionated heparin is held for 12 to 24 hours. Nonsteroidal anti-inflammatory drugs (NSAIDs) may be less critical but are preferentially withheld for 1–2 days. Heparin is typically stopped 4–6 hours before the procedure; PTT can be remeasured to confirm that the heparin effect is reduced sufficiently. Heparin can generally be resumed 12 to 24 hours after the procedure if necessary.[21] The use of closure devices, smaller-diameter catheters and biopsy devices, and adjunct hemostatic measures such as postbiopsy tract occlusion may also reduce the incidence of periprocedural bleeding complications.[25] Severe hypertension may increase the bleeding risk; however, this increased risk is likely minimal.[26]

LARGE PATIENTS

Several challenges can exist when planning a procedure in a large patient. Needles and catheters used in interventional radiology are designed with variable lengths, usually ranging up to 20 or 45 cm. In large patients, the skin-to-target distance may exceed the maximum length of available instruments. In this case, preprocedural planning becomes even more important; reviewing available imaging studies can help determine the optimal patient position and approach to achieve the shortest possible distance from the skin to the target lesion. Pillows, splints, foam pads, bolsters, and other devices may be used to position the patient optimally on the CT scanner table. Belts are commonly used to prevent patients from slipping from the table, and occasionally extremity restraints may be required for delirious or critically ill patients. These devices allow the patient to remain securely and comfortably positioned for the duration of the procedure.

Large patients have an increased incidence of diabetes and heart disease, and they are more prone to complications, including wound infections, pressure ulcers, myocardial ischemia, and respiratory compromise. Some large patients have obstructive sleep apnea or are at high risk for airway compromise. In such cases, the expertise and participation of the anesthesiologist is critical in managing these patients appropriately.[27]

ORAL CONTRAST MATERIAL

When precise bowel visualization is necessary, oral contrast can be administered prior to CT scanning. Oral contrast allows better differentiation of bowel loops from adjacent structures and can assist in planning a targeted approach to avoid bowel injury. We selectively utilize oral contrast prior to procedures in patients requiring intravenous sedation. Barium and iodine-based contrast are both used commonly; iodinated (water-soluble) oral contrast agents are increasingly being utilized and preferred when gastrointestinal perforation is suspected.[8] Low osmolar iodinated contrast are preferred in patients with potential for aspiration as they are less likely to induce pulmonary edema.[28] When monitored anesthesia care (MAC) or general anesthesia is planned, oral contrast may be withheld due to the potential risk of aspiration. However, when oral contrast is necessary, special intubation techniques may be helpful in reducing the risk of aspiration.[8]

INTRAVENOUS CONTRAST MATERIAL

Intravenous (IV) contrast administration is used in some cases to better delineate the target lesion or to better visualize surrounding anatomy, including arteries and veins. Intravenous contrast also can help characterize hypervascular tumors, vascular malformations, or nearby vascular structures that may represent relative or absolute contraindications for biopsy and other procedures.[29]

Intravenous contrast can be nephrotoxic, and it is therefore avoided in patients with an estimated glomerular filtration rate (eGFR) of less than 30 mL/min, unless they are on chronic dialysis. Careful consideration of risks and benefits is necessary in patients with acute renal failure, even if the eGFR is greater than 30, as contrast may exacerbate their condition. If intravenous contrast is absolutely necessary in these patients, aggressive hydration may decrease the risk of contrast-induced nephropathy.[30]

Adverse reactions to contrast can occur, and they can be of variable severity. Symptoms may be mild (e.g., sneezing, vomiting, mild rash) or severe (e.g., hypotension, hypertension, extensive urticaria, laryngeal edema, wheezing, shortness of breath, and anaphylaxis). In patients with a history of prior mild contrast reaction, premedication with corticosteroids is recommended prior to subsequent scans to reduce the risk of a contrast reaction.[31] Intravenous contrast is generally avoided following a severe reaction, particularly anaphylaxis.[28,30] Patients at risk for a reaction include those with active asthma or multiple allergies and those with previously documented reactions to contrast material.

Intravenous contrast may be injected by hand, but it is better delivered using a power injector that allows more precise injection volume, rate, and timing. A 20-gauge intravenous access is usually adequate. Many central lines, ports, and peripherally inserted central catheter (PICC) lines are not compatible with power injection; therefore, exact specifications of the access line should be reviewed prior to power injection. Although rare, power injection in a patient with a known patent foramen ovale may theoretically result in systemic air embolization and should be avoided when possible.[32] Finally, attention should be paid to compatibility of intravenous contrast with other drugs being administered through the same line.

ANESTHESIA CONSIDERATIONS

Most CT-guided interventions can be performed under intravenous conscious sedation (IVCS). In addition to relieving patient anxiety and discomfort, the reduction in respiratory rate and tidal volume with sedation can be helpful for thoracic and abdominal procedures, where target lesions move with respiratory motion. At the same time, however, reproducible breath holds may be necessary to allow accurate targeting of lesions, and oversedation can negatively affect patient cooperation.[33] Although IVCS can be administered or supervised by an appropriately certified radiologist, consultation with an anesthesiologist may be helpful in patients with significant comorbidities, a history of difficult intubation, chronic pain issues, sleep apnea, morbid obesity, or abnormal head and neck anatomy or movement. For more invasive procedures such as tumor ablations, deeper sedation or even general anesthesia may be required. For these patients, a full outpatient preprocedural assessment by an anesthesiologist is typically performed 1 week prior to the procedure.

INTERVENTIONAL CT PROCEDURES

CT-GUIDED BIOPSY

Percutaneous biopsies guided by CT provide a minimally invasive method of obtaining a definitive cytologic, histologic, or molecular diagnosis of lesions throughout the body. As with other image-guided procedures, CT-guided percutaneous biopsies are performed using sterile technique. Antibiotics are not routinely administered prior to the biopsy. Needle size can vary widely, although the majority of tissue samples are obtained using needles ranging from 16 to 25 gauge. Multiple samples are usually obtained. In some institutions, a cytotechnologist or cytopathologist is present in or nearby the interventional CT suite at the time of biopsy to evaluate for sample adequacy before the needles are removed; this immediate on-site feedback can potentially reduce the number of nondiagnostic procedures. Additional information regarding image-guided biopsy technique can be found in Chapter 12.

Patient positioning is usually determined by the shortest and safest route to the lesion. Liver mass biopsies are typically performed in the supine or slightly right anterior oblique position. Retroperitoneal mass, renal, and vertebral biopsies are most often performed with the patient in a prone, prone oblique, or lateral decubitus position. Pain can vary with the anatomic site and depth of needle penetration. Most biopsies are performed using a combination of local anesthesia and IVCS. The level of sedation required tends to be relatively constant throughout the procedure; however, the patient may experience increased pain or discomfort requiring additional intravenous and local anesthesia when the needle traverses sensitive structures such as the hepatic capsule or peritoneum. For lesions near the diaphragm, where respiratory motion can be significant, such as for liver and kidney lesions, it is preferable to begin sedation before the initial planning CT scan. Once sedated, visceral organs are in a more stable position for the duration of the procedure. This facilitates selection of an optimal skin entry site and trajectory. The majority of CT-guided biopsies can be completed in under 1 hour.

For some biopsies, a craniocaudal angled approach may be necessary, making the procedure technically more difficult. In these cases, reproducible breath holds or shallow respirations are even more important, as the most significant anatomic shifts with breathing will be in the craniocaudal direction. Multiplanar reformats may be helpful during the biopsy to assist needle guidance, but they can prolong procedure time.

Although most biopsies are straightforward, some patients require additional preprocedural planning. A transpleural path should generally be avoided to prevent pneumothorax or spread of infection or tumor from the abdomen into the thorax. Traversing the small bowel or colon can be done with fine needles (19 gauge or smaller) when necessary to biopsy a solid structure. We typically avoid traversing small bowel and colon with large needles (18 gauge or larger). The small bowel and colon are generally not transgressed with fine needles when targeting a fluid-containing structure so the patient is not infected or the sample contaminated.[25]

CATHETER DRAINAGES

Over the last several decades, image-guided abscess drainage has become common practice, replacing open surgical drainage in the vast majority of patients. Catheter drainage provides a rapid and simple means of therapy with a high success rate and few complications. CT is often the imaging modality of choice for guidance of abscess drainage procedures due to its excellent anatomic detail, including the ability to clearly differentiate bowel from surrounding structures. In general, deeper collections or those requiring crossing of large muscles tend to cause more pain and discomfort. Although the majority of abscesses are readily accessible and can be drained percutaneously, alternative access routes, such as transrectal or transvaginal approaches, may be necessary to facilitate the drainage of deep pelvic fluid collections.[34]

There are two general techniques used for drainage catheter placement. In the modified Seldinger technique, the catheter is placed into the collection over a guidewire after dilation of the tract. In the trocar technique, the catheter is placed into the collection in a single step. In either case, the dilation or catheter insertion steps may be painful. Additional information regarding techniques of catheter drainage can be found in Chapter 12.

THERMAL ABLATION

Percutaneous tumor ablation procedures are performed typically to manage malignant lesions, most commonly in the liver, kidney, adrenals, lung, or bone. A variety of technologies are currently being used, including RF ablation, microwave ablation, and cryoablation (discussed in further detail in Chapter 12) (Figure 11.2). Although some ablation procedures are completed in about 1 hour, other cases may require up to 3 or 4 hours.

Ablation procedures require the precise placement of one or more ablation applicators into the target organ or tissue. Some RF ablation devices allow placement of a single applicator with subsequent deployment of an expandable array of tines or electrodes into the target area; however, this is less commonly utilized.[35–37]

Radio-frequency ablation applies an alternating electric current to tissues from a needle applicator probe; the current causes high electrical power concentrated within the tissue surrounding the needle, which produces ionic agitation and frictional heating of this tissue.[38] Coagulative necrosis occurs when temperatures exceed 50°C. A 2- to 6-cm diameter thermal ablation zone can be produced with each RF ablation, although ablation of tumors greater than 3 cm is associated with higher local recurrence rates.[39,40] Reproducible levels of breath holding are often important in facilitating optimal and safe probe placement, and they can be accomplished either with a degree of intravenous sedation that allows patient cooperation or with general anesthesia and same-level interruption of ventilation. Analgesia is particularly important just prior to turning on the RF generator because the heating process may trigger significant pain, particularly for tumors located near sensitive structures such as the diaphragm and hepatic capsule. RF ablation tends to produce more pain than other ablation methods, such as cryoablation. Artificial ascites or pneumoperitoneum can be introduced prior to ablation to help insulate the ablation zone from adjacent critical structures[41]; this can also decrease pain when treating lesions close to the diaphragm.

Microwave ablation is a relatively new ablation modality with several advantages over RF ablation, including reduced

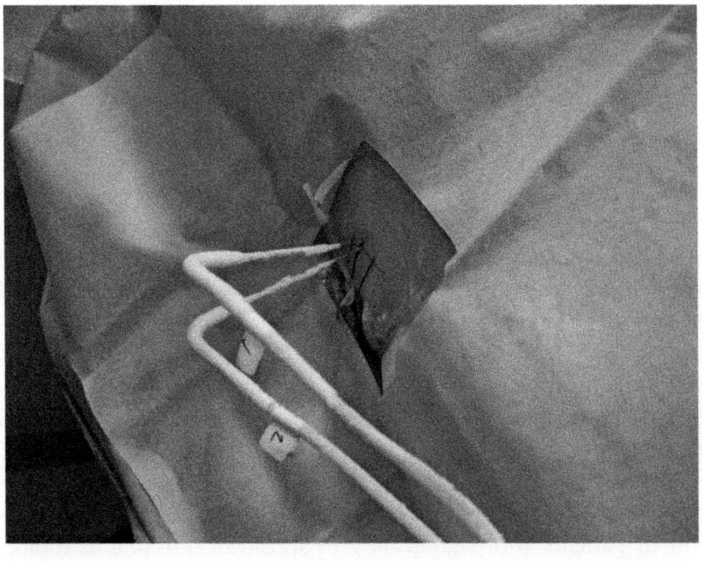

Figure 11.2. Manufacturers of radio-frequency and cryoablation applicators have designed flexible and right-angle handles in order to clear the gantry during scanning. Right-angle cryoapplicators are pictured here.

susceptibility to heat sink effect (which causes unwanted temperature heterogeneity within the ablation zone) and improved clinical efficacy for tumors greater than 5 cm.[42,43] A microwave antenna/probe is inserted into the tumor, and microwave energy emitted into the surrounding tissue results in rapid molecular realignment (dielectric hysteresis), which causes tissue heating.[43,44] Because microwaves pass readily through charred, necrotic tissues, there is typically more uniform tissue destruction relative to RF ablation. Again, analgesia prior to induction of heating is recommended, as the ablation process can be painful.

PAIN MANAGEMENT

Nerve blocks can be used for pain management and involve CT-guided placement of the needle adjacent to a nerve or nerve plexus that is responsible for pain.[45] Various neurolysis procedures that can be performed may target the pterygopalatine ganglion, trigeminal nerve, stellate ganglion, celiac plexus, pudendal nerve, and interiliac sympathetic plexus and ganglion. Although the ultimate goal is pain management, the procedure itself can be quite painful, and sedation is often required. Chemical ablation can be performed using the percutaneous injection of alcohol (95%) or phenol (6%) to induce neurolysis, and CT can be used to visualize the local extent of the neurolytic agent.[46] Injection of steroids for local pain management and anti-inflammatory effects may target various joints, such as the facet joints, sacroiliac joints, and others.

SPECIAL CONSIDERATIONS

PERCUTANEOUS BIOPSY OF CARCINOID TUMOR

In patients with carcinoid tumors, carcinoid crisis has been described in association with surgery and anesthesia, as well as other stresses. Stimulation of hormone (e.g., serotonin and histamine) release can result in hypertension or profound hypotension, flushing, bronchoconstriction, and tachycardia that can be life threatening and difficult to reverse. Although reports of complications from biopsy of carcinoid tumors are rare, severe and occasionally fatal cases of carcinoid crisis after percutaneous biopsy of carcinoid liver and lung metastases have been described in the literature.[47,48] Anesthesia consultation and premedication may be considered for interventional procedures involving carcinoid tumors. Somatostatin analogues such as octreotide and, more recently, methylene blue have been used to treat carcinoid crises and should be available in the procedure room prior to biopsy of a patient with suspected carcinoid tumor.[47]

BIOPSY AND ABLATION OF ADRENAL MASSES

Catecholamine-induced hypertensive crisis is a specific problem encountered with adrenal and extra-adrenal pheochromocytoma that can lead to labile blood pressures during biopsy. When pheochromocytoma is suspected, pharmacologic pretreatment strategies (e.g., α blockade) should be considered in conjunction with the anesthesiologist and endocrinologist, although pretreatment does not necessarily prevent such crises from occurring. Ablation of adrenal lesions can also trigger massive release of catecholamines, even if the lesion is not a pheochromocytoma but normal adrenal tissue is present; therefore, premedication is also performed prior to ablation.[49,50]

Both the radiologist and anesthesiologist should be prepared to treat a catecholamine-induced crisis when performing adrenal mass biopsies and ablations. Although historically there has been concern over intravenous contrast administration in patients with suspected pheochromocytoma, it is extremely rare for intravenous contrast alone to induce a crisis.[51,52]

ECHINOCOCCAL CYSTS

Percutaneous needle aspiration of hydatid cysts caused by echinococcal disease had historically been discouraged because of potential complications, such as anaphylactic shock and the spread of daughter cysts into the peritoneum (for hepatic cysts). However, recent data indicate that this is extremely rare, and percutaneous treatment of echinococcal cyst with puncture, aspiration, injection of antiparasitic agent, and reaspiration (PAIR) has been established as a safe alternative to surgical resection for certain cysts.[53] An antiparasitic agent (e.g., albendazole) is typically administered prior to and following aspiration, and an anesthesiologist should be readily available during the procedure given the potential for anaphylactic reaction.

POSTPROCEDURAL CONSIDERATIONS

After completion of a CT-guided percutaneous interventional radiology procedure, the skin entry site is sterilely bandaged. A CT scan of the target region is performed after the procedure if necessary to exclude immediate complications and to document the position of drainage catheters or other devices. Broader coverage may be required to detect post–lung biopsy pneumothorax. Outpatients are placed on bed rest for 1 to 6 hours, depending on the type of procedure. During that time, vital signs and pain levels are monitored. After thoracic interventions, a chest x-ray may be performed to exclude a pneumothorax. Following thermal ablations, patients are either discharged the same day or admitted overnight for observation, laboratory value assessment, and a follow-up CT or magnetic resonance imaging (MRI) to evaluate the ablation site.

Mild hemoptysis following lung biopsies can occur and should significantly decrease in volume over a period of a few hours. Massive hemoptysis (more than 200 mL in 1 hour) requires immediate intervention. After percutaneous interventions, signs or symptoms of hemorrhage generally warrant a CT scan. Large or active hemorrhage may necessitate bronchoscopy or angiographic embolization.[54,55]

Postprocedural pain control is sometimes a significant issue in patients after tumor ablation procedures performed adjacent to sensitive areas, such as peritoneal surfaces, liver capsule, and pleura. Ablations involving the diaphragm may lead to referred shoulder pain that can persist for days or even weeks after the procedure, but it tends to subside slowly over time. Postablation syndrome, characterized by flu-like symptoms, is common, particularly in larger tumors, but typically resolves within 1 to 2 weeks after the ablation and can be treated conservatively.[56]

POSITRON EMISSION TOMOGRAPHY/ COMPUTED TOMOGRAPHY

HISTORICAL BACKGROUND AND RECENT ADVANCES

Positron emission tomography (PET) is being increasingly used for the diagnosis, staging, and follow-up of various malignancies. By far the most common radiopharmaceutical employed in PET and PET/CT imaging is ^{18}F-fluorodeoxyglucose (FDG), a radiolabeled glucose analogue. Many other radiopharmaceuticals have been introduced, including three compounds recently approved by the Food and Drug Administration for prostate and somatostatin receptor–positive tumors and many other investigational agents currently undergoing preclinical evaluation.[57] Malignant cells often have increased glucose metabolism, reflecting increased cell membrane–facilitated transport and upregulation of intracellular hexokinase activity, among other factors. FDG is taken up by tumor cells but, unlike glucose, is not fully metabolized, thereby becoming trapped inside metabolically active cells.[58] FDG-PET has been used in the evaluation of solitary pulmonary nodules, non–small cell lung carcinoma, lymphoma, melanoma, breast cancer, colorectal cancer, and many other malignant and inflammatory conditions. FDG-PET can aid in the differentiation of malignant from benign lesions, assist in the staging of malignancies, and provide a means of monitoring response to therapy. PET can be especially useful in highly metabolic tumors and when there is a complicated appearance on CT or MRI due to postoperative changes or scar tissue. PET/CT incorporates the cross-sectional anatomic information provided by CT and the metabolic information provided by PET in a single scanner. PET/CT offers several advantages over PET alone, the most important of which is the ability to accurately localize increased metabolic activity to specific anatomic locations or structures.

PET/CT-GUIDED INTERVENTION

Increasingly, PET/CT is utilized in interventional radiology. PET/CT enables direct targeting of metabolically active portions of tumors, which are more likely to yield viable cells for diagnosis during biopsy (Figure 11.3). This is particularly useful with partially necrotic tumors, in which sampling of nonviable tissue can lead to nondiagnostic or false-negative biopsies. The emerging need to differentiate and sample clonal populations within heterogeneous tumors may also lead to a greater role for PET/CT guidance in the future.[57,59] Incorporation of metabolic targeting capabilities also improves the ability to target lesions that are not visible or poorly visible on CT, MRI, or US. PET/CT has also been used to guide tumor ablations, as it can be used to confirm that the ablation is complete. Particularly with microwave and RF ablation, the margin between ablated and unablated tissue is often not appreciated by US and CT; in these cases; PET/CT may provide more immediate evaluation of the ablation zone.[60] The CT component of the PET/CT is critical for determining a safe interventional approach during biopsy and ablation procedures.

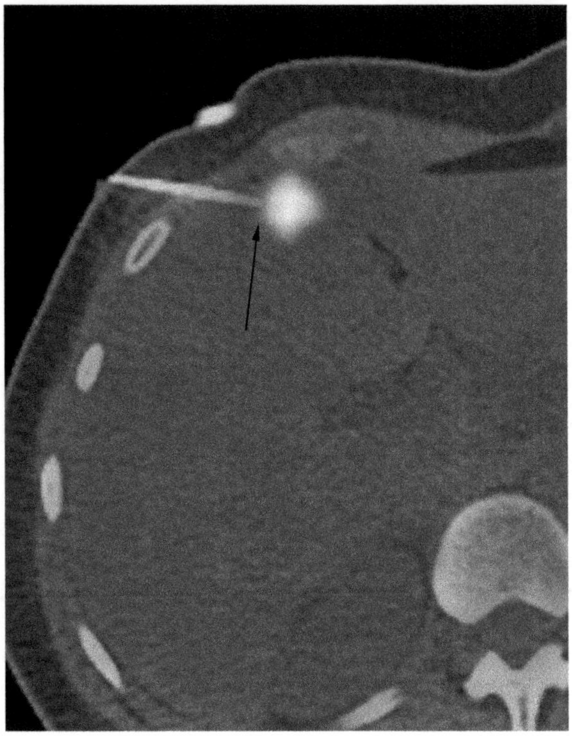

Figure 11.3. *Positron emission tomography (PET)/computed tomography (CT)–guided liver biopsy. The PET/CT image shown is the result of grayscale CT and color PET image fusion. The arrow indicates the tip of a biopsy needle entering the metabolically active liver metastasis in this patient with known breast cancer.*

Patients fast for approximately 4–6 hours prior to PET/CT to enhance FDG uptake by tumors as well as to minimize cardiac and muscle uptake. Before the injection of FDG, a blood glucose level of less than 150 mg/dL is preferred, as cellular FDG uptake is competitive with glucose. Pregnancy is a relative contraindication to FDG administration but can be administered following a risk-benefit assessment; there are no absolute contraindications. Imaging is initiated approximately 60 minutes following the injection of FDG. PET/CT scans are acquired as a series of sequential bed positions, with each bed position providing at least 15 cm of coverage along the patient's long axis. For interventional purposes, a single bed position may suffice in terms of anatomic coverage. A single bed position PET/CT scan can be completed in 2–6 minutes depending on equipment and imaging protocol.

Potential radiation exposure to operating personnel from positron-emitting radiopharmaceuticals should be considered, but it is not prohibitive.[41] Standard lead aprons are not useful in reducing exposure from the high-energy photons produced by PET radiopharmaceuticals; therefore, strategies of maintaining distance from the patient and minimizing close contact periods are most helpful.

A potential limitation of PET/CT-guided interventions is that of misregistration of the PET and CT image data sets. The PET and CT hardware is configured serially within a single long gantry, with metabolic and anatomic images obtained sequentially rather than simultaneously. As a result, there is potential for patient motion between the PET and CT scan acquisitions due to shifts in body position or, more commonly, due to differences in respiratory phase. For anatomic locations that do not move with respiration, such as much of the skeleton, neck, pelvis, and extremities, respiratory motion is rarely a significant problem. For structures close to the diaphragm, strategies are needed to minimize image misregistration, such as respiratory-triggered acquisitions and adequate sedation to reduce the rate and depth of inspiration. Several breath-hold techniques have also been demonstrated to reduce misregistration.[61]

The PET/CT scanners resemble MRI scanners, with a long gantry that can limit access to the patient by the medical team. As with procedures performed in a closed-bore MRI, tubing and monitoring leads must be long enough to allow free travel of the patient into the scanner gantry. A video camera system can be installed at the far end of the gantry to provide constant visual monitoring of the patient. Wall-mounted gas supplies, suction, and monitoring equipment should be considered when planning the layout of a PET/CT suite that may be used for interventional procedures.

In conclusion, CT is a well-established guidance modality for interventional procedures, and PET/CT is an emerging guidance modality for similar procedures. The anesthetic considerations are quite variable depending on the procedure, the patient, and the interventional radiologist. Close communication between the radiologist and the anesthesiologist will help ensure an uneventful procedure and an optimal outcome for the patient.

REFERENCES

1. Begemann P. CT-guided interventions—indications, technique, pitfalls. In: Mahnken A, Ricke J, eds. *CT- and MR-Guided Interventions in Radiology*. New York, NY: Springer New York; 2009:11–20.
2. Patel A, Khalsa B, Lord B, Sandrasegaran K, Lall C. Planting the seeds of success: CT-guided gold seed fiducial marker placement to guide robotic radiosurgery. *J Med Imaging Radiat Oncol.* 2013;57(2):207–211. doi:10.1111/j.1754-9485.2012.02445.x.
3. Haaga JR, Alfidi RJ, Havrilla TR, et al. CT detection and aspiration of abdominal abscesses. *Am J Roentgenol.* 1977;128(3):465–474. doi:10.2214/ajr.128.3.465.
4. Jang SY, Park SY, Tak WY, Kweon YO, Ryeom H. Long-term follow-up of large symptomatic hepatic cysts treated by percutaneous ethanol sclerotherapy. *Acta Radiol.* 2016;57(10):1205–1209. doi:10.1177/0284185115626476.
5. Tamura A, Kato K, Suzuki M, et al. CT-guided percutaneous radiologic gastrostomy for patients with head and neck cancer: a retrospective evaluation in 177 patients. *Cardiovasc Intervent Radiol.* 2016;39(2):271–278. doi:10.1007/s00270-015-1170-8.
6. Dodd GD, Soulen MC, Kane R a, et al. Minimally invasive treatment of malignant hepatic tumors: at the threshold of a major breakthrough. *Radiographics.* 2000;20(1):9–27. doi:10.1148/radiographics.20.1.g00ja019.
7. Ginat DT, Gupta R. Advances in computed tomography imaging technology. *Annu Rev Biomed Eng.* 2014;16:431–453. doi:10.1146/annurev-bioeng-121813-113601.
8. Rydberg J, Buckwalter KA, Caldemeyer KS, et al. Multisection CT: scanning techniques and clinical applications. *Radiographics.* 2000;20(6):1787–1806. doi:10.1148/radiographics.20.6.g00nv071787.
9. Flohr TG, Schaller S, Stierstorfer K, Bruder H, Ohnesorge BM, Schoepf UJ. Multi-detector row CT systems and image-reconstruction techniques. *Radiology.* 2005;235:756–773. doi:10.1148/radiol.2353040037.
10. Jolesz FA, Lorensen WE, Shinmoto H, et al. Interactive virtual endoscopy. *Am J Roentgenol.* 1997;169:1229–1235. Available at: https://www.spl.harvard.edu/archive/spl-pre2007/pages/papers/frank/virt_endoscopy/endoscopy.html. Accessed on November 13, 2017.
11. Haaga JR. Interventional CT: 30 years' experience. *Eur Radiol.* 2005;15(suppl 4):D116–D120.
12. Schenker MP, Martin R, Shyn PB, Baum RA. Interventional radiology and anesthesia. *Perioper Nurs Clin.* 2009;4(4):451–458. doi:10.1016/j.cpen.2009.09.010.
13. Kloeckner R, Dos Santos DP, Schneider J, Kara L, Dueber C, Pitton MB. Radiation exposure in CT-guided interventions. *Eur J Radiol.* 2013;82(12):2253–2257. doi:10.1016/j.ejrad.2013.08.035.
14. Brenner DJ, Hall EJ. Computed tomography—an increasing source of radiation exposure. *N Engl J Med.* 2007;357(22):2277–2284. doi:10.1056/NEJMra072149.
15. Fazel R, Krumholz HM, Wang Y, et al. Exposure to low-dose ionizing radiation from medical imaging procedures. *N Engl J Med.* 2009;361(9):849–857. doi:10.1056/NEJMoa0901249.
16. Sarti M, Brehmer WP, Gay SB. Low-dose techniques in CT-guided interventions. *RadioGraphics.* 2012;32(4):1109–1119. doi:10.1148/rg.324115072.
17. Jungnickel K. Radiation protection during CT-guided interventions. In: Mahnken AH, Ricke J, ed. *CT- and MR-Guided Interventions in Radiology.* New York, NY: Springer; 2009:35–38.
18. McCollough CH, Bruesewitz MR, Kofler JM. CT dose reduction and dose management tools: overview of available options. *Radiographics.* 2006;26(2):503–512. doi:10.1148/rg.262055138.
19. Nawfel RD, Judy PF, Silverman SG, Hooton S, Tuncali K, Adams DF. Patient and personnel exposure during CT fluoroscopy-guided interventional procedures. *Radiology.* 2000;216(1):180–184. doi:10.1148/radiology.216.1.r00jl39180.
20. Anastasian ZH, Strozyk D, Meyers PM, Wang S, Berman MF. Radiation exposure of the anesthesiologist in the neurointerventional suite. *Anesthesiology.* 2011;114(3):512–520. doi:10.1097/ALN.0b013e31820c2b81.
21. Rubin D. Anesthesia for ambulatory diagnostic and therapeutic radiology procedures. *Anesthesiol Clin.* 2014;32(2):371–380. doi:10.1016/j.anclin.2014.02.015.
22. Patel IJ, Davidson JC, Nikolic B, et al. Consensus guidelines for periprocedural management of coagulation status and hemostasis risk in percutaneous image-guided interventions. *J Vasc Interv Radiol.* 2012;23(6):727–736. doi:10.1016/j.jvir.2012.02.012.
23. Somerville P, Seifert PJ, Destounis S V, Murphy PF, Young W. Anticoagulation and bleeding risk after core needle biopsy. *AJR Am J Roentgenol.* 2008;191(4):1194–1197. doi:10.2214/AJR.07.3537.
24. Patel IJ, Davidson JC, Nikolic B, et al. Addendum of newer anticoagulants to the SIR consensus guideline. *J Vasc Interv Radiol.* 2013;24(5):641–645. doi:10.1016/j.jvir.2012.12.007.
25. Trumm C, Hoffmann R. Diagnostic interventions: biopsy. In: Mahnken A, Ricke J, eds. *CT- and MR-Guided Interventions in Radiology.* New York, NY: Springer; 2009:91–115.
26. Potretzke TA, Gunderson TM, Aamodt D, et al. Incidence of bleeding complications after percutaneous core needle biopsy in hypertensive patients and comparison to normotensive patients. *Abdom Radiol.* 2016;41(4):637–642. doi:10.1007/s00261-016-0653-7.
27. Uppot RN. Impact of obesity on radiology. *Radiol Clin North Am.* 2007;45(2):231–246. doi:10.1016/j.rcl.2007.03.001.
28. American College of Radiology. *ACR Manual on Contrast Media.* Version 10.2. Reston, VA: American College of Radiology; 2016.
29. Catanzano T. Radiation and contrast concerns. In: *How to Think like a Radiologist.* Cambridge, England: Cambridge University Press; 2009:1–7.
30. Bettmann MA. Frequently asked questions: iodinated contrast agents. *Radiographics.* 2004;24(suppl 1):S3–S10. doi:10.1148/rg.24si045519.
31. Kim S-H, Lee S-H, Lee S-M, et al. Outcomes of premedication for non-ionic radio-contrast media hypersensitivity reactions in Korea. *Eur J Radiol.* 2011;80(2):363–367. doi:10.1016/j.ejrad.2010.06.014.
32. Yeddula K, Ahmad I, Mohammed SHS, et al. Paradoxical air embolism following contrast material injection through power injectors in patients with a patent foramen ovale. *Int J Cardiovasc Imaging.* 2012;28(8):2085–2090. doi:10.1007/s10554-012-0017-5.

33. Mueller PR, Biswal S, Halpern EF, Kaufman JA, Lee MJ. Interventional radiologic procedures: patient anxiety, perception of pain, understanding of procedure, and satisfaction with medication—a prospective study. *Radiology.* 2000;215(3):684–688. doi:10.1148/radiology.215.3.r00jn33684.
34. Maher MM, Gervais DA, Kalra MK, et al. The inaccessible or undrainable abscess: how to drain it. *Radiographics.* 2004;24(3):717–735. doi:10.1148/rg.243035100.
35. Clasen S, Pereira PL, Lubienski A. Interventional radiology—radiofrequency ablation. In: Mahnken A, Ricke J, eds. *CT- and MR-Guided Interventions in Radiology.* New York, NY: Springer; 2009:159–248.
36. Gervais DA, McGovern FJ, Wood BJ, Goldberg SN, McDougal WS, Mueller PR. Radio-frequency ablation of renal cell carcinoma: early clinical experience. *Radiology.* 2000;217(3):665–672. doi:10.1148/radiology.217.3.r00dc39665.
37. Mayo-Smith WW, Dupuy DE. Adrenal neoplasms: CT-guided radiofrequency ablation—preliminary results. *Radiology.* 2004;231(28):225–230. doi:10.1148/radiol.2311031007.
38. Hong K, Georgiades C. Radiofrequency ablation: mechanism of action and devices. *J Vasc Interv Radiol.* 2010;21(suppl 8):S179–S186. doi:10.1016/j.jvir.2010.04.008.
39. Chen M-H, Yang W, Yan K, et al. Large liver tumors: protocol for radiofrequency ablation and its clinical application in 110 patients—mathematic model, overlapping mode, and electrode placement process. *Radiology.* 2004;232(1):260–271. doi:10.1148/radiol.2321030821.
40. Livraghi T, Goldberg SN, Lazzaroni S, et al. Hepatocellular carcinoma: radio-frequency ablation of medium and large lesions. *Radiology.* 2000;214(3):761–768. doi:10.1148/radiology.214.3.r00mr02761.
41. Bhagavatula SK, Chick JFB, Chauhan NR, Shyn PB. Artificial ascites and pneumoperitoneum to facilitate thermal ablation of liver tumors: a pictorial essay. *Abdom Radiol (NY).* 2017;42(2):620–630. doi:10.1007/s00261-016-0910-9.
42. Thamtorawat S, Hicks RM, Yu J, et al. Preliminary outcome of microwave ablation of hepatocellular carcinoma: breaking the 3-cm barrier? *J Vasc Interv Radiol.* 2016;27(5):623–630. doi:10.1016/j.jvir.2016.01.011.
43. Lubner MG, Brace CL, Hinshaw JL, Lee FT. Microwave tumor ablation: mechanism of action, clinical results, and devices. *J Vasc Interv Radiol.* 2010;21(suppl 8):S192–S203. doi:10.1016/j.jvir.2010.04.007.
44. Simon CJ, Dupuy DE, Mayo-Smith WW. Microwave ablation: principles and applications 1. *RadioGraphics.* 2005;25(suppl 1):S69–S83. doi:10.1148/rg.25si055501.
45. Koizuka S, Nakajima K, Mieda R. CT-guided nerve block: a review of the features of CT fluoroscopic guidance for nerve blocks. *J Anesth.* 2014;28(1):94–101. doi:10.1007/s00540-013-1675-8.
46. Baheti D, Bakshi S, Gupta S, Gehdoo R. *Interventional Pain Management: A Practical Approach.* New Delhi, India: Jaypee Brothers Medical; 2009.
47. Magabe PC, Bloom AL. Sudden death from carcinoid crisis during image-guided biopsy of a lung mass. *J Vasc Interv Radiol.* 2014;25(3):484–487. doi:10.1016/j.jvir.2013.10.054.
48. Bissonnette RT, Gibney RG, Berry BR, Buckley AR. Fatal carcinoid crisis after percutaneous fine-needle biopsy of hepatic metastasis: case report and literature review. *Radiology.* 1990;174:751–752. doi:10.1148/radiology.174.3.2406783.
49. Pua BB, Solomon SB. Ablative therapies in adrenal tumors: primary and metastatic. *J Surg Oncol.* 2012;106(5):626–631. doi:10.1002/jso.23191.
50. Ethier MD, Beland MD, Mayo-Smith W. Image-guided ablation of adrenal tumors. *Tech Vasc Interv Radiol.* 2013;16(4):262–268. doi:10.1053/j.tvir.2013.08.008.
51. Paulsen SD, Nghiem HV, Korobkin M, Caoili EM, Higgins EJ. Changing role of imaging-guided percutaneous biopsy of adrenal masses: evaluation of 50 adrenal biopsies. *Am J Roentgenol.* 2004;182(4):1033–1037.
52. Tsitouridis I, Michaelides M, Stratilati S, Sidiropoulos D, Bintoudi A, Rodokalakis G. CT guided percutaneous adrenal biopsy for lesions with equivocal findings in chemical shift MR imaging. *Hippokratia.* 2008;12(1):37–42.
53. Gupta N, Javed A, Puri S, Jain S, Singh S, Agarwal AK. Hepatic hydatid: PAIR, drain or resect? *J Gastrointest Surg.* 2011;15(10):1829–1836. doi:10.1007/s11605-011-1649-9.
54. Tai R, Dunne RM, Trotman-Dickenson B, et al. Frequency and severity of pulmonary hemorrhage in patients undergoing percutaneous CT-guided transthoracic lung biopsy: single-institution experience of 1175 cases. *Radiology.* 2016;279(1):287–296. doi:10.1148/radiol.2015150381.
55. Katoh M, Schneider G, Bucker A. Pre and postinterventional imaging. In: Mahnken A, Ricke J, eds. *CT and MR-Guided Interventions in Radiology.* New York, NY: Springer; 2009:3–9.
56. Dodd GD, Napier D, Schoolfield JD, Hubbard L. Percutaneous radiofrequency ablation of hepatic tumors: postablation syndrome. *Am J Roentgenol.* 2005;185(1):51–57. doi:10.2214/ajr.185.1.01850051.
57. Weissleder R, Schwaiger MC, Gambhir SS, Hricak H. Imaging approaches to optimize molecular therapies. 2016;8(355):1–8.
58. Kapoor V, McCook BM, Torok FS. An introduction to PET-CT imaging. *Radiographics.* 2004;24(2):523–543. doi:10.1148/rg.242025724.
59. Gerlinger M, Horswell S, Larkin J, et al. Genomic architecture and evolution of clear cell renal cell carcinomas defined by multiregion sequencing. *Nat Genet.* 2014;46(3):225–233. doi:10.1038/ng.2891.
60. Ryan ER, Sofocleous CT, Schöder H, et al. Split-dose technique for FDG PET/CT–guided percutaneous ablation: a method to facilitate lesion targeting and to provide immediate assessment of treatment effectiveness. *Radiology.* 2013;268(1):288–295. doi:10.1148/radiol.13121462.
61. Shyn PB, Tatli S, Sahni VA, et al. PET/CT-guided percutaneous liver mass biopsies and ablations: targeting accuracy of a single 20 s breath-hold PET acquisition. *Clin Radiol.* 2014;69(4):410–415. doi:10.1016/j.crad.2013.11.013.

12 | MAGNETIC RESONANCE IMAGING AND ULTRASOUND-GUIDED PERCUTANEOUS INTERVENTIONAL RADIOLOGY PROCEDURES

SHARATH K. BHAGAVATULA, MD, BIJAL PATEL, MD, KEMAL TUNCALI, MD, STUART G. SILVERMAN, MD, PAUL B. SHYN, MD

INTRODUCTION

The need for procedural sedation and anesthesia for minimally invasive procedures continues to grow as the number of procedures and interventional applications increases. This trend will continue as the population ages and the complexity and array of imaging-guided interventional procedures expand. Minimally invasive procedures performed with image guidance both supplement and in many situations replace surgeries.

Although image-guided procedures are less invasive than surgery, they still have potential complications and can result in patient anxiety, pain, and discomfort. Accordingly, there is an important role for monitored and general anesthesia for patient safety and comfort, as well as for facilitating the technical success of the procedure. Anesthesiologists are often present throughout the entire procedure or may be consulted if intravenous sedation is administered by the interventional radiologist. To select appropriate sedation and analgesia strategies, the anesthesiologist must assess the patient's current status, underlying medical conditions, and details of the procedure, including the type of the procedure, the expected duration and complexity of the procedure, patient's position, breath-holding concerns, the anticipated amount and type of pain, and potential complications. Frequent communication between the interventional radiologist and anesthesiologist before, during, and after the procedure is important for delivering sedation and analgesia in a safe, effective manner. This chapter focuses on the various types of interventional procedures performed with ultrasound (US) and magnetic resonance imaging (MRI) guidance.

MAGNETIC RESONANCE IMAGING

Magnetic resonance imaging is used principally as a diagnostic tool, and it has been used with increasing frequency to guide interventional radiology procedures. The principal advantages of MRI during intervention include high intrinsic soft tissue contrast resolution and its ability to provide images in any anatomic plane without the use of ionizing radiation. While the physics of MRI is beyond the scope of this chapter, MRI, in basic terms, utilizes magnetic fields and radio waves to generate images. The strength of the magnetic field is an important determinant of image contrast.[1] The magnetic field strength is measured in tesla (T). The field strength can range from low (0.1–0.5 T), medium (0.5–1.0 T), or high (1.5–3.0 T), to ultrahigh (>3.0 T).[2,3] The specific information depicted in MRI images can be manipulated or emphasized by altering the sequence parameters selected. For example, image sequences can be selected to help distinguish tissue types based on fat or water content, presence or absence of iron or hemosiderin, and degree of vascularity or perfusion. MRI may depict pathology and provide functional information that is not discernible with US or computed tomography (CT).

There are some limitations with MRI that affect diagnostic imaging and interventional radiology applications. For instance, evaluation of dense bone or heavy calcification is characterized by a signal void. Long image acquisition times can result in motion artifacts from respiratory motion, patient movement, bowel peristalsis, or cardiac and vascular pulsations. This motion artifact can degrade image quality, making both interpreting images and guiding interventional procedures difficult. Steady progress over the years has led to improvements in signal-to-noise ratio while decreasing the length of MRI sequences and maintaining anatomic coverage.[4] Nevertheless, MRI-guided procedures are usually more time consuming than those performed with CT or US.

ADVANTAGES OF MAGNETIC RESONANCE IMAGING–GUIDED PROCEDURES

Unlike CT scanning, MRI does not utilize ionizing radiation. Therefore, it is possible for the personnel to remain in the procedure room during scanning (however, because MRI scanning creates high decibel noise, it is advisable to limit exposure by providing earplugs and earmuffs for patients and personnel who will remain in the room). MRI provides direct multiplanar imaging. Acquiring images in any plane allows the entire needle path to be visualized regardless of needle angulation.[5] The excellent soft tissue contrast resolution of MRI is advantageous when a biopsy or ablation is required for lesions that cannot be discerned and targeted optimally with US or CT. Similarly, ablation zones, treatment responses, complications, thermal effects on adjacent structures, and tumor recurrences can often be imaged with superior tissue contrast resolution by MRI as compared to other imaging modalities.[6–8] The use of specially tailored sequences such as temperature-sensitive imaging during the procedure and subtraction contrast-enhanced imaging[9,10] after the procedure increases inherent contrast resolution. In addition, diffusion sequences can facilitate targeting of cellular tumor.[11]

CHOICE OF APPARATUS

Both open and closed MRI systems have been used for interventional procedures; however, development of closed-bore systems with higher field strengths and larger gantries have led to increased utility of the closed-bore system, particularly those with a wide bore.[12] Most diagnostic MRI examinations are now performed in closed-bore magnets of 1.5 to 3.0 T. These systems allow for greater signal-to-noise ratios and scan speeds that are sufficient for diagnostic imaging. However, closed-bore MRI systems can only be used to guide interventions intermittently because the patient must be repetitively moved in and out of the magnet for manipulation of the instruments. The confined space of the closed-bore MRI system limits access to the patient. Furthermore, the confined space limits the length of incrementally advanced biopsy needles or ablation applicators that can remain partially outside the patient's body during imaging. Newer wide-bore (70-cm or larger) and short -bore (125- to 150-cm) high-field systems have been developed that help increase access during interventional procedures and allow for instruments to be advanced incrementally between imaging acquisitions[12] (Figure 12.1).

Open MRI systems have been designed to image large or claustrophobic patients. Relative to closed systems, open MRI systems provide greater access to patients not only when manipulating the needle but also while acquiring images in near real time. However, open magnets are usually of lower field strength (0.2–1.0 T), which results in a lower signal-to-noise ratio and decreased spatial resolution. In addition, the image acquisition times may be longer, which results in patients having to hold their breath for extended periods of time. The available access to the patient, space limitations, and duration of image acquisition provided by the different systems will affect the anesthesiologist's management of the patient during the procedure.

PATIENT FACTORS

Magnetic resonance imaging–guided procedures can be contraindicated in patients with active implants (e.g., cardiac pacemakers, insulin pumps, cochlear implants, bone growth stimulators, implantable infusion pumps, and neurostimulators) and certain passive implants (e.g., aneurysm clips), particularly when in close proximity to critical structures.[13,14] Cardiac arrhythmias and burn injuries can be caused by radio-frequency–induced electrical currents or

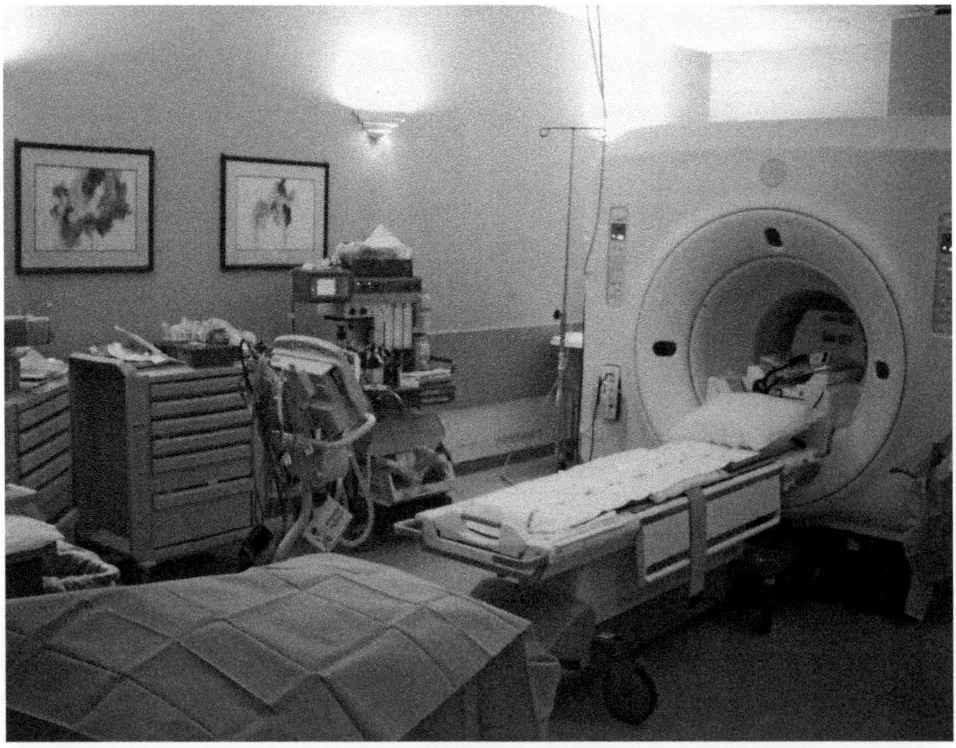

Figure 12.1. Closed-bore magnetic resonance imaging (MRI) interventional suite. All equipment in the MRI interventional room is MRI compatible. This particular system has a magnet bore diameter of 70 cm, which is comparable to that of many computed tomography (CT) scanners.

heating within intracardiac pacing wires and other indwelling metal-containing catheters or leads. Care should be taken when imaging patients with metallic objects (ferromagnetic or otherwise), which are susceptible to significant heating as compared with normal biologic tissues. Certain devices that are ferromagnetic, such as some cerebral aneurysm or vascular clips, can be dislodged. Similarly, metallic foreign bodies, such as bullets and other metallic fragments, can potentially move while being imaged.[15,16]

If MRI is to be performed in a patient with an implanted device, the documentation of the specific model implanted should be reviewed and assessed for safety.[14,17] An increasing number of implants and devices have been confirmed to be MRI compatible, including nonferromagnetic vascular clips, staples, and orthopedic implants or prostheses. In addition, many cardiac prosthetic valves and most recently certain cardiac pacemaker models can be scanned safely or conditionally (e.g., with certain magnetic field strengths). Patients who may have intraorbital metal, such as welders, or patients with a history of penetrating eye injury should be screened with radiographs of the orbits because metallic foreign bodies can dislodge and cause ocular injury and blindness.

DEVICE FACTORS

For most interventional procedures, continuous electrocardiogram (ECG) monitoring is required, especially when general anesthesia is used. Cardiac monitoring is affected by magnetic field–induced distortion of the electrocardiac signals.[18] Although MRI-compatible 3- and 4-lead ECG devices are available, these have lower sensitivity and may not detect silent cardiac ischemia; 12-lead magnetic resonance (MR) conditional ECG leads have recently been developed and may improve intraprocedural monitoring in the MRI environment.[19] However, patients with known active ischemic heart disease should not have their procedures performed in the MRI suite until these new technologies have been clinically validated.

All equipment in the interventional MRI room must be MRI compatible. This means that the equipment is MRI safe (will not cause harm to the patient), will not affect image quality,[20] and will not be damaged or have a loss of functionality in the MRI scanner. Access to the interventional MRI procedure room should be strictly controlled to prevent inappropriate objects and devices from entering. Many conventional interventional, surgical, and anesthesia instruments are ferromagnetic and are strongly attracted by the magnetic field. Regardless of size, these objects can become hazardous projectiles, accelerating within the magnetic field into the patient gantry.[5,14] In addition, contact burns may occur from MR-induced current induction within equipment placed on the patient (e.g., ECG leads, grounding pads, etc.).[20,21]

Equipment used during the procedure may adversely affect the image quality and scanner performance by interference with the magnetic field or radio-frequency signals. Patient monitoring equipment, such as pulse oximetry sensors, can produce radio-frequency interference that affects image quality.[20] A number of MRI-compatible interventional instruments, such as scissors, blades, needles, carts, and ablation equipment, have been developed, and MRI-compatible anesthesia equipment, such as patient monitors, infusion pumps, gas cylinders, and respirators, are also available.[12] Further information on MRI safety has been described.[13,14]

MAGNETIC RESONANCE IMAGING–GUIDED BIOPSY

Magnetic resonance imaging is not used as commonly as CT or US to guide percutaneous biopsies; however, MRI guidance may be advantageous if lesions are not visible or are poorly visualized with the other imaging modalities. Because of its multiplanar capability, MRI is useful also in guiding biopsies of lesions in the superior abdomen, where angulation of the needle is required to avoid diaphragmatic injury and pneumothrorax.[5] In these cases, the entire length of the needle path can be visualized. In addition, diffusion-weighted MRI has gained recent interest due to its potential to identify functionally diverse foci within a tumor.[11]

Magnetic resonance imaging is particularly helpful in guiding breast and prostate gland biopsies, as malignancies in these organs are often not well seen by other imaging modalities.[22,23] For example, MRI has been shown to detect breast cancer with higher cancer detection yield than mammography and US.[24] MRI-guided breast biopsies are performed with the patient in a prone position using a dedicated breast surface coil. Large-needle biopsy and wire localization are procedures usually performed in a closed MRI system.[23,25] MRI-guided biopsy (up to 9 gauge) with vacuum assistance has been accepted as a safe and accurate technique, allowing for sampling of lesions as small as 1 cm with a success rate of 95% to 100%.[23,26] During these procedures, gentle compression is applied to the breast. Local anesthesia and a small skin incision are usually sufficient, and intravenous sedation is not typically required.

Magnetic resonance imaging–guided prostate gland biopsy has rapidly gained widespread clinical use because MRI has been shown not only to depict cancers better than any other imaging modality but also to yield information that distinguishes aggressive cancers from indolent ones. As a result, data have emerged that demonstrate the utility of using MRI to target the cancers that are clinically significant and warrant treatment.[27] Technical improvements, such as robotic systems allowing in-bore transperineal and transrectal biopsies, have also been shown to be safe and effective.[28,29] Local anesthesia may be sufficient, although intravenous sedation is commonly preferable.[28]

TUMOR ABLATION

Percutaneous thermal ablation techniques (microwave, radio frequency, and cryoablation) are minimally invasive alternatives to surgery. While historically reserved for patients with significant comorbidities or unresectable disease, ablation is increasingly being utilized as first-line treatment in surgical candidates as well. Radio-frequency ablation with

MRI guidance is feasible but technically challenging due to difficulties in imaging changes in heated tissue and interaction between radio-frequency signals and MRI signals.[30] Recent technical advances have allowed successful MR guidance of microwave ablation, but CT and US guidance remains more common.[31] Microwave and radio-frequency ablation are discussed in more detail in Chapter 11.

Frozen tissue is well visualized by MRI; therefore, cryoablation is the most common ablation modality to be performed in the interventional MRI suite. In addition, there is no electromagnetic interference, and there is typically clear visualization of the ablation zone as a low-signal "ice ball." Cryoablation destroys the targeted tissues through a freezing-and-thawing process, resulting in cellular dehydration, intracellular disruption, cell membrane damage, local ischemia due to small-vessel injury, and other factors.[32] The distal end of the cryoablation applicators can reach temperatures as low as −185°C.[33] The critical temperature for complete tissue destruction ranges between −20°C and −50°C, depending on the tissue.[34]

Typically, one or more needle-like cryoablation applicators are placed into the targeted tissue, depending on the size of the tumor. During the cryoablation process, an ice ball is formed around the distal end of the cryoprobe as the heat is removed from the surrounding tissues. The ice ball can be visualized and monitored by MRI, CT, or US.[33] US is limited in that the entire ice ball cannot be visualized due to acoustic shadowing that obscures tissue deep to the ice ball. CT can be used to visualize the entire ice ball, but MRI provides better contrast between frozen and unfrozen tissues.[5] In addition, MRI can provide near real-time monitoring of the dynamic formation of ice and can visualize the irreversible effects in targeted tissues after the thawing process.[35] Optimal visualization of the ice ball allows for improved tumor coverage while reducing the risk of injury to adjacent organs (Figure 12.2). MRI-guided percutaneous cryoablation has been shown to be effective and safe for a variety of oncologic applications in the liver, kidney, breast, prostate, and musculoskeletal system.[36-39]In addition, cryoablation can be used to treat uterine fibroids.[40,41]

Cryoablation tends to cause less pain than the heating of radio-frequency ablation, a factor that affects sedation and anesthesia decisions.[42,43] Whether radio-frequency ablation or cryoablation is performed, reproducible levels of breath holding are often important for optimal and safe probe placement, particularly if the target organ is subject to respiratory motion. When general anesthesia is used, breath holding can be accomplished with same-level ventilation interruption. When intravenous sedation is used, it is often helpful to use smaller doses of sedatives and analgesics to control patient discomfort while allowing the patient to hold his or her breath on command. Once the ablation probes are in place, increased doses of medications may be appropriate during the actual heating or freezing periods of the procedure. Monitored anesthesia care, instead of intravenous sedation without anesthesia

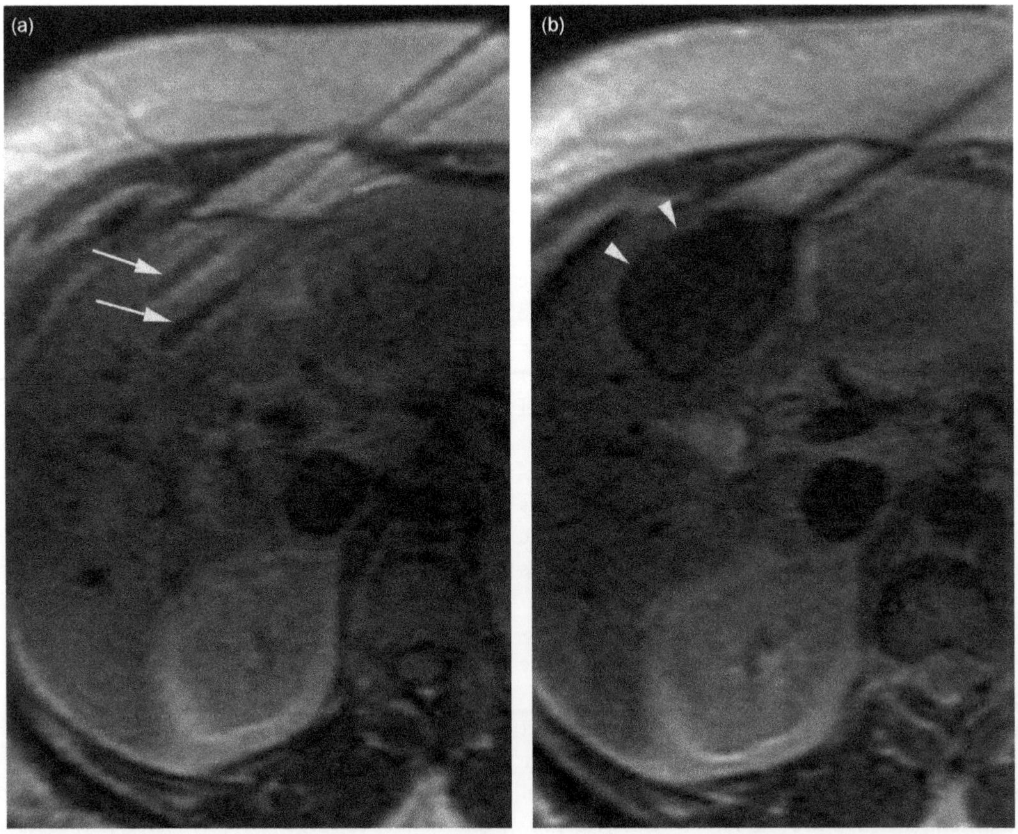

Figure 12.2. (a) Cryoablation. An axial magnetic resonance imaging (MRI) image (0.5 T; T2 weighted) demonstrates a hyperintense breast cancer metastasis in the liver with two percutaneous cryoprobes positioned in the lesion (arrows). (b) An axial MRI obtained during cryoablation demonstrates a hypointense ice ball (arrows) that completely surrounds the metastasis.

personnel, is often preferred for patients with comorbidities and those who cannot tolerate any discomfort or being in a restricted position for 2 to 4 hours.[6] At our institution, ablation procedures are most often performed with monitored anesthesia care.

When intravenous sedation is used, the patient can often be discharged the same day. If monitored anesthesia care or general anesthesia is used, patients are observed for a longer period of time or admitted overnight and observed for complications. Bleeding is the most common complication. Rarely, severe thrombocytopenia can occur after extensive liver cryoablations and may require platelet transfusions for management.[5] Extensive ablations also can induce myoglobinemia and myoglobinuria, which can lead to acute renal failure and require hydration or alkalinization of urine with sodium bicarbonate.[37,44] Cryoshock is another rare complication of cryoablation that can result in multiorgan failure, thought due to a systemic response to tissue necrosis.[44]

Cryoablation guided by MRI for adrenal tumors has been shown to be effective.[45] However, a specific problem that is encountered when performing cryoablation of the adrenal gland or structures near the adrenal gland is catecholamine-induced hypertension. This complication is more likely to occur when residual normal adrenal tissue is present and is less likely to occur when the adrenal gland is completely replaced with nonhormonally active tumor.[43] During cryoablation procedures, the hypertension occurs during or following thawing and not during freezing. This is in contrast to radiofrequency ablation procedures, which are more likely to induce hypertension during the application of heat.[43] Hypertension can also occur in the immediate postablation period.[45] Pretreatment medication with α blockade is recommended and has been shown to reduce the risk or severity of hypertensive crisis, although this is not entirely preventive.[45]

MAGNETIC RESONANCE IMAGING–GUIDED, HIGH-INTENSITY FOCUSED ULTRASOUND THERAPY

Magnetic resonance imaging–guided focused ultrasound (MRgFUS) is a noninvasive ablation modality that delivers US energy from an external probe to ablate tissue; MRI guidance is ideal because of its ability to detect temperature-sensitive tissue changes in near real time.[46] With this procedure, high-frequency US beams penetrate through the soft tissues and are focused to a specific target site; temperatures in the range of 55°C to 90°C can be generated in the targeted tissues. MRgFUS has been clinically approved for the treatment of uterine fibroids and painful osseous metastatic disease; clinical trials have demonstrated promise for indications in the prostate, brain, breast, and other locations.[47–51] For the treatment of uterine fibroids with focused US, patients are placed prone on a special MRI table that contains an embedded set of US transducers. During the procedure, intravenous sedation is used to ensure patient comfort and immobility while maintaining verbal communication throughout the procedure. It is important to search for scars on the anterior abdominal wall because these can absorb US energy, resulting in skin burns and discomfort. Hair removal may also be required to ensure optimal contact between the transducer and skin.[6] To avoid bladder filling during the procedure, a Foley catheter is placed. Once the target is localized and a safe pathway is established, therapeutic focal sonications are administered with continuous thermal feedback until predetermined appropriate temperature profiles have been reached.[52] After the procedure, intravenous gadolinium-enhanced images are performed to assess for adequate treatment response.

MAGNETIC RESONANCE IMAGING–GUIDED BRACHYTHERAPY

Brachytherapy involves the placement of radioactive seeds into a tumor to kill malignant cells. Brachytherapy has been effective for various malignancies, either as primary treatment or in combination with other treatment modalities.[53] For example, the combination of brachytherapy and external beam radiation has been shown to be more effective than external beam radiation alone,[54] and brachytherapy has also been recommended for definitive treatment of locally advanced cervical carcinoma.[55] As with other MRI-guided procedures, the superior contrast resolution of MRI often allows for more optimal visualization of the tumor, target organ, and surrounding structures. In addition, advances in MR robotic guidance tools continue to advance precise brachytherapy seed placement.[56] This allows for better targeting, which can maximize tissue destruction while reducing injury to adjacent normal structures.[57]

Various MRI approaches for seed delivery have been proposed that involve open- and closed-bore MRI configurations and patient positions. As with other MRI-guided procedures, open MRI scanners are less spatially restrictive but have lower resolution, while closed-bore scanners can be technically more challenging and have longer procedure times with higher precision.

In summary, MRI offers advantages in a variety of interventional applications and is likely to be used more often in the future for an increasing array of interventional procedures. MRI may make possible or facilitate minimally invasive procedures previously not possible or difficult to accomplish with CT or US guidance. Many issues, such as MRI-safe and MRI-compatible equipment, room safety, patient monitoring, and appropriate anesthesia levels, require special consideration in the MRI environment.

ULTRASOUND

Ultrasound has been a valuable method of imaging the body for decades and is currently one of the most widely used and versatile imaging modalities in radiology. US at current diagnostic energies poses no known risks to the patient and does not use ionizing radiation.[58] It does, however, have the potential to deposit enough energy into the tissues that local heating can occur; Doppler US in particular is capable of generating higher acoustic energies. Limitations on energy settings and time of scanning are therefore appropriate in certain settings, such as obstetrical US.[59,60] Another advantage of US is that it provides real-time assessment of moving structures such as the heart, blood vessels, and fetus. The ability to visualize respiratory motion of viscera during interventional procedures is extremely helpful. The multiplanar and real-time imaging capabilities of US allow for the rapid assessment of spatial relationships, a great advantage for interventional applications. When compared to other imaging modalities, such as CT or MRI, US has the added advantage of being portable and relatively inexpensive. Superficial structures and many deep structures can be readily assessed with satisfactory spatial resolution and tissue contrast. US offers various types of Doppler imaging that can be used to make qualitative and quantitative assessments of blood flow. Recently, contrast-enhanced US has also become feasible due to the availability and approval by the Food and Drug Administration (FDA) of microbubble contrast agents. US contrast agents are safe, and contrast reactions are extremely rare, with a reported life-threatening anaphylaxis reaction rate of 0.001%.[61]

There are some limitations with US imaging that affect diagnostic and interventional applications. Sound energy is nearly completely absorbed or reflected at interfaces between soft tissue and bone, such that structures deep to bone cannot be visualized. Air in bowel and in the lungs also strongly reflects the US beam, which limits visualization of deeper structures and in the chest, respectively. In these situations, repositioning the patient or scanning from different approaches may avoid these structures and allow visualization. Finally, large patients can present a challenge because sound waves must traverse greater depths to provide imaging of anatomical regions of interest.

Ultrasound-guided interventional procedures can range from quickly performed procedures requiring minimal patient cooperation and sedation to more prolonged, difficult cases requiring controlled breathing, patient cooperation, and adequate pain control. The most commonly performed US-guided interventional procedures include percutaneous biopsies of organs or masses and fluid aspirations or drainages, all of which can be performed in many body regions (Figure 12.3).

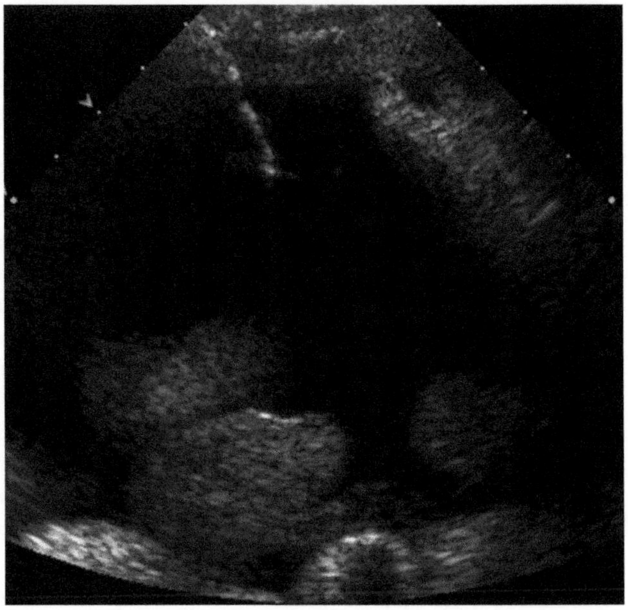

Figure 12.3. *Ultrasound-guided paracentesis. The percutaneously inserted needle is seen as a thin linear bright (echogenic) structure within the ascites. Loops of small bowel are seen in the inferior aspect of the image and are avoided.*

ULTRASOUND-GUIDED MASS BIOPSIES

Pain from US-guided needle biopsies varies with the anatomic site and depth of needle penetration. Unlike catheter placements, the level of sedation required tends to be relatively constant throughout the procedure.

Fine-needle aspiration biopsy (FNAB) is a minimally invasive and safe method for obtaining a tissue diagnosis. FNAB is usually performed with 19- to 25-gauge needles. The procedure can be performed with syringe aspiration or capillary action techniques. While these techniques usually obtain cellular material suitable for cytopathology or molecular analysis, these techniques can, on occasion, obtain tissue cores suitable for histopathology analysis as well. Large-needle (18-gauge and larger) biopsies, commonly using spring-loaded side-cutting needles, are also commonly employed and are more likely to yield an actual core of tissue for histopathology evaluation than FNAB techniques. Although spring-loaded core biopsy devices are available in sizes as small as 22 gauge, most such biopsies are performed with 18-gauge or larger systems. Although the diagnostic yield attained from core biopsies may be higher than FNAB,[62] the potential for bleeding complications may be increased, particularly with 14-gauge and larger needles.[62,63]

US-GUIDED LIVER PARENCHYMAL BIOPSY

Liver parenchymal biopsies are usually performed on an outpatient basis with large needle core biopsy devices. Parenchymal biopsies can be performed to evaluate for transplant rejection, treatment response, abnormal liver function tests, and unexplained jaundice. For hepatic parenchymal biopsies, an 18-gauge biopsy is usually obtained, and these are considered procedures with a higher bleeding risk. Relative contraindications to the procedure include uncorrectable coagulopathy, with international normalized ratio (INR) greater than 1.5 and platelets less than 50,000/μL.[64] Patients with chronic liver disease may have persistent abnormal coagulation parameters; these cases should be evaluated on a case-by-case basis. The presence of ascites is itself not a contraindication to liver biopsy. The procedure is usually performed with local anesthesia and intravenous sedation. If the right lobe is targeted, the patient can be scanned through an intercostal or subcostal approach in the right anterior oblique position. If the left lobe is targeted, an epigastric approach in the supine position can be used. With interventions performed near the diaphragm as in liver biopsy, intermittent breath holding is helpful for needle visualization and to prevent inadvertent injury to the target organ or surrounding structures. Even though it is important to maintain patient comfort during the procedure, oversedation can interfere with the patient's ability to follow breathing instructions. Potential complications include bleeding, infection, and bile duct injury. Rare complications may include gallbladder injury, pneumothorax, or bowel perforation.

US-GUIDED RENAL PROCEDURES

Both renal parenchymal and renal mass biopsies can be performed with US guidance. To decrease the risk of bleeding during parenchymal biopsies, a subcostal, posterolateral approach is preferred; typically, the lower pole cortex is targeted, and care is taken to avoid the renal hilum.[65,66] US can also be used to help guide percutaneous renal abscess drainages or facilitate percutaneous nephrostomy access. Accessing the renal collecting system allows for percutaneous nephrostomy, ureteral interventions, stone manipulations, or even fiber-optic endoscopy.

Renal interventions require local anesthesia administration and often intravenous sedation. Reproducible breath holding is important because the location of the kidney is dependent on the phase of respiration. Complications may include subcapsular or perinephric bleeding, hematuria, urinoma, infection, adjacent organ injury, and rarely tumor seeding.[67,68] Although infection risk is low, a nonurgent biopsy should be delayed if the patient has cystitis or pyelonephritis. With renal biopsies performed with large needles, there is a small risk of arteriovenous fistula formation. These patients can present with renin-mediated hypertension, hematuria, renal colic, or in severe cases, heart failure and hypotension. Preexisting hypertension is thought to be a risk factor for developing a fistula following a renal biopsy and could also increase bleeding risk.

TRANSRECTAL ULTRASOUND APPLICATIONS

Endocavitary transducers with biopsy guide attachments can be used for transrectal biopsies and drainages. One of the most common applications with this approach is prostate biopsy. The patient is placed in a left or right lateral decubitus position, which allows for easy probe insertion and manipulation. Pain encountered during the procedure can increase patient anxiety and result in pelvic muscle contraction, making the procedure more difficult. Administration of a local anesthetic in the periprostatic margins blocks the capsular nerve fibers.[69] Potential injury to the neurovascular bundles is reduced with real-time needle visualization. US-guided prostate biopsy has frequent minor and rare major complications. Immediate complications include hematuria (most common complication), rectal bleeding, and vasovagal episodes. Delayed complications, which may occur up to 7 days after the biopsy, include persistent hematuria, dysuria, vague pelvic discomfort, hematospermia, and hematochezia.

TRANSVAGINAL ULTRASOUND APPLICATIONS

Endovaginal US guidance is a useful alternative for needle biopsies of pelvic tumors if the transabdominal route is not feasible or safe.[70] A transvaginal route may be less painful and difficult than a posterior approach through the sacrosciatic notch, where multiple nerves and vessels are located. The transvaginal route is also an option for needle aspiration of pelvic fluid collections because they are often in close proximity to the vaginal fornices. Fluid collections, including sterile fluid collections (urinomas, seromas, lymphoceles, endometriomas, hemorrhagic cysts, loculated ascites, and peritoneal inclusion cysts), should generally be aspirated completely to minimize the risk of secondary infection.[71]

The lithotomy position is employed, and intravenous antibiotics may be given for prophylaxis. The procedure can be painful as the needle passes through the vaginal wall musculature, particularly if dilators and catheters are placed. For this reason, transvaginal catheter drainages are uncommonly performed. Intravenous sedation and analgesia are desirable. An 18-gauge needle of adequate length can be inserted through the attached needle guide, and local anesthetic can be applied before fully traversing the vaginal wall.[70] Complications can include bleeding and bowel injury.

US-GUIDED THORACENTESIS

Ultrasound is capable of detecting as little as 3 mL of fluid in the pleural space; however, even with US guidance, thoracentesis is usually indicated and more safely performed when larger amounts of fluid are present.[55] US guidance is particularly helpful in targeting small or loculated effusions or when previous attempts without imaging guidance have failed.

The ideal position for the patient is sitting upright and leaning slightly forward. A lateral decubitus or supine oblique position can be used in patients who cannot sit upright. Local anesthesia often suffices for these procedures and is applied from the skin to the parietal pleura. For anxious or uncooperative patients or when technical challenges are anticipated, intravenous sedation or even general anesthesia may uncommonly be required. Potential complications include pneumothorax, bleeding, lung or diaphragm injury, rarely reexpansion pulmonary edema, injury to upper abdominal viscera such as the liver or spleen, or infection. These risks are lower when using US guidance as compared to localization by physical examination.[72]

US-GUIDED PARACENTESIS

Ultrasound-guided paracentesis is a common procedure performed for both diagnostic and therapeutic indications. Complicated ascites may demonstrate echogenic debris or septations and may be difficult to completely drain. Relative contraindications include uncorrectable coagulopathy, an acute abdomen requiring immediate surgery, numerous intra-abdominal adhesions, abdominal wall cellulitis at the site of puncture, and pregnancy. Although large volumes of ascites, up to 10 L, may be safely drained in many patients, lower volumes are generally removed in patients with hypotension, hypoalbuminemia, or tenuous cardiovascular status. Albumin can be infused intravenously prior to paracentesis when appropriate and is recommended for large-volume paracentesis (>5 L) in cirrhotic patients.[73,74]

Desirable preprocedure coagulation parameters at many institutions are similar to those described previously for thoracentesis.[64] Local anesthesia applied from the skin to the peritoneal layer often suffices for these procedures, with only the exceptional patient requiring sedation or general anesthesia. The patient is typically placed in a supine position. Variations in positioning may facilitate the accumulation of a larger pocket of fluid in a safely accessible peritoneal location. Care is taken to avoid abdominal viscera and inferior epigastric vessels during needle/catheter placement. Real-time US visualization during needle placement is most helpful when targeting small or loculated collections and when critical structures are in close proximity to the fluid collection.

This is a relatively safe procedure with a low incidence of complications. Potential complications include persistent fluid leak from the puncture site, abdominal wall hematoma, and infection. Complications such as perforation of bowel and major blood vessel (e.g., inferior epigastric) laceration are reduced with real-time image guidance.[75]

ULTRASOUND-GUIDED NEEDLE ASPIRATION AND CATHETER DRAINAGE OF ABSCESSES

Percutaneous catheter drainages of abscesses yield high success rates with relatively low complication rates and are often preferred to open surgical drainage.[76] Percutaneous abscess drainage is often performed for definitive management but also is used as a temporizing measure in some cases prior to surgery.[76,77] Surgical drainage is still performed in patients where safe percutaneous access is not possible and in patients with fluid collections that are expected to be too viscous or multiloculated for effective percutaneous drainage. Similarly, when underlying conditions such as tumor, large-caliber bowel perforation, bowel necrosis, pancreatic necrosis, and other situations mandate surgical intervention, percutaneous drainage may not be appropriate.

Ultrasound is often an excellent method for detecting abscess collections in the neck, extremities, abdomen, and pelvis. Pulmonary abscesses may even be visible if they are contiguous with the chest wall such that no air-containing lung intervenes. Once the collection is located with US, a pathway is selected for approach. Usually, the shortest distance that avoids structures such as bowel or large vessels is chosen. Uninvolved solid organs are usually avoided but may be traversed if necessary and depending on the procedure. Traversing more than one body cavity is avoided when possible to avoid cross-contamination. If the collection is small or only a diagnostic sample is needed, US-guided needle aspiration may suffice. For larger collections and commonly for therapeutic purposes, percutaneous catheter drainage may be indicated.

Local anesthesia may suffice for superficial fine-needle aspiration procedures, just as with simple paracentesis or thoracentesis procedures. On the other hand, needle aspirations of deep collections and in particular catheter drainage procedures typically require intravenous sedation. Monitored anesthesia care and general anesthesia are rarely needed. For the interventional radiologist, having a relaxed and comfortable patient can mean the difference between a rapid, uncomplicated procedure and a prolonged, difficult procedure. For procedures near the diaphragm, such as liver abscess drainages, respiratory motion can also be a significant issue. Sedation may be helpful in decreasing the respiratory rate and tidal volume, resulting in less motion of the target organ or region. On the other hand, having the patient adequately sedated but not oversedated will provide the advantage of being able to have the patient suspend respirations when needed during critical points in the procedure. For procedures away from the diaphragm, such as pelvic or extremity drainages, respiratory motion is usually not a factor. Generally, the most painful portions of catheter drainage procedures are the serial dilation and catheter insertion steps. Certain access routes are more likely to cause significant pain for the patient, including approaches through the sacrosciatic notch for deep pelvic fluid collection drainages.

ULTRASOUND-GUIDED PERCUTANEOUS CHOLECYSTOSTOMY

Ultrasound-guided percutanous cholecystostomy is indicated in critically ill patients with acute cholecystitis who cannot undergo surgical cholecystectomy and in patients with severe acute cholecystitis, per Tokyo guidelines.[78] As the patient's condition improves, definitive treatment with cholecystectomy can be performed. In acalculous cholecystitis, percutaneous drainage may be adequate alone. A transhepatic approach is preferred for gallbladder drainages to reduce the risk of bile leakage into the peritoneum; a transperitoneal route is used when there is no transhepatic access or in patients with liver disease or coagulopathies. Complications of percutaneous cholecystostomy include bile peritonitis, hemobilia, gallbladder perforation, pneumothorax, and vagal effects due to catheter placement.[78] A mature fibrous tract should be allowed to form along the peritoneal catheter tract prior to catheter removal to decrease the risk of bile peritonitis. This may require leaving the catheter in place for 4–6 weeks, and potentially longer in patients with diabetes, malnutrition, steroid use, ascites, or other reason for delayed tract formation.[78] Percutaneous cholecystostomy may require an intercostal approach and will most commonly traverse the liver capsule in addition to entering the gallbladder. Small amounts of bile may leak into the peritoneum. When this occurs, bile is irritating to the peritoneum and can cause considerable pain. Adequate sedation and analgesia are therefore important; however, some of these patients may already be in the intensive care unit, medicated and intubated.

ULTRASOUND GUIDANCE IN REGIONAL ANESTHESIA

Ultrasound guidance can significantly improve the quality of nerve blocks in many types of regional anesthesia.[79] US may allow for direct visualization of the nerve, surrounding anatomic structures, and the local anesthetic solution during injection. It is important to ensure that the local anesthetic is administered around the nerve structures for successful regional anesthetic blocks.[79] Most nerve block procedures require high-frequency transducers, in the range of 10–14 MHz. The majority of peripheral nerves can be visualized over their entire course and are described to have a fascicular pattern with US.[79] Many potential complications can be avoided with US guidance as compared to traditional block techniques, which rely on anatomic landmarks. In particular, complications such as intraneuronal or intravascular injection are reduced with US guidance. A more complete description of specific nerve blocks is available.[79]

ULTRASOUND-GUIDED VASCULAR INTERVENTIONS

Vascular access can be challenging in volume-depleted or large patients. Intravenous drug users or patients with aberrant venous anatomy may also present difficulties in vascular access. This can be particularly problematic in the emergency setting or critical care setting. Traditional vascular access relies on anatomic landmarks, arterial palpation, or visible pulsations. These clinical clues, for example, during jugular vein access, can be limited or difficult to assess, resulting in multiple needle passes and complications such as pneumothorax or hemothorax. US guidance provides real-time visualization of the needle and vessel and can distinguish between arteries and veins, allowing for successful first-attempt access and shorter procedure times. Veins such as the basilic, cephalic, and subclavian veins may be difficult to see or access without US guidance.

Ultrasound can also be used for percutaneous embolization of pseudoaneurysms.[80] Traditionally, the management of pseudoaneurysms has been surgical resection. US embolization is relatively safe, simple, and quick to perform. Pseudoaneurysms can be occluded with transducer-applied direct pressure to interrupt blood flow through the pseudoaneurysm neck. This method, however, can take 30–60 minutes to complete. An alternative method is percutaneous US-guided thrombin injection into the pseudoaneurysm sac. Thrombosis is usually observed within seconds, and complications related to this technique are low.

Ultrasound can be used to guide many other types of interventions, which are beyond the scope of this chapter. FNAB of thyroid nodules and large-needle breast lesion biopsies are common procedures usually performed on an outpatient basis. US can be used to facilitate and assist in brachytherapy seed placements for pelvic neoplasms and to guide uterine dilation and curettage procedures.[81] In conclusion, US is a versatile and practical imaging modality for use in a wide range of image-guided interventional radiology procedures.

REFERENCES

1. Jacobs MA, Ibrahim TS, Ouwerkerk R. MR Imaging: brief overview and emerging applications. *RadioGraphics.* 2007;27(4):1213–1229. doi:10.1148/rg.274065115.
2. Bottomley PA, Foster TH, Argersinger RE, Pfeifer LM. A review of normal tissue hydrogen NMR relaxation times and relaxation mechanisms from 1–100 MHz: dependence on tissue type, NMR frequency, temperature, species, excision, and age. *Med Phys.* 1984;11:425–448. doi:10.1118/1.595535.
3. Edelstein W, Bottomley P, Hart H. Signal, noise, and contrast in nuclear magnetic resonance (NMR) imaging. *J Comput Assist Tomogr.* 1983. Available at: http://www.jcat.org/pt/re/jcat/abstract.00004728-198306000-00001.htm. Accessed on November 29, 2016.
4. Hoult DI, Lauterbur PC. The sensitivity of the zeugmatographic experiment involving human samples. *J Magn Reson.* 1979;34(2):425–433. doi:10.1016/0022-2364(79)90019-2.
5. Tatli S, Morrison PR, Tuncali K, Silverman SG. Interventional MRI for oncologic applications. *Tech Vasc Interv Radiol.* 2007;10(2):159–170. doi:10.1053/j.tvir.2007.09.008.
6. Silverman S, Jolesz F, Newman R, Morrison P. Design and implementation of an interventional MR imaging suite. *Am J Roentgenol.* June 1997. Available at: https://www.researchgate.net/profile/Ron_Kikinis/publication/14049429_Perspective_Design_and_implementation_of_an_interventional_MR_imaging_suite/links/54f38ca30cf2f9e34f07e5cd.pdf. Accessed on November 29, 2016.
7. Tuncali K, Morrison PR, Tatli S, Silverman SG. MRI-guided percutaneous cryoablation of renal tumors: Use of external manual displacement of adjacent bowel loops. *Eur J Radiol.* 2006;59(2):198–202. doi:10.1016/j.ejrad.2006.04.013.
8. Silverman SG, Collick BD, Figueira MR, et al. Interactive MR-guided biopsy in an open-configuration MR imaging system. *Radiology.* 1995;197(1):175–181. doi:10.1148/radiology.197.1.7568819.
9. Jolesz FA. From biopsy to intraoperative imaging: MRI-guided procedures. In: Jolesz FA, Young AR, eds. *Interventional MR, Techniques and Clinical Experience.* London, England: Dunitz; 1998:1–8.
10. Tempany CMC, Stewart EA, McDannold N, Quade BJ, Jolesz FA, Hynynen K. MR imaging-guided focused ultrasound surgery of uterine leiomyomas: a feasibility study. *Radiology.* 2003;226(3):897–905. doi:10.1148/radiol.2271020395.
11. Guimaraes MD, Gross JL, Chojniak R, Marchiori E. MRI-guided biopsy: a valuable procedure alternative to avoid the risks of ionizing radiation from diagnostic imaging methods. *Cardiovasc Intervent Radiol.* 2014;37(3):858–860. doi:10.1007/s00270-013-0677-0.
12. Kaye EA, Granlund KL, Morris EA, Maybody M, Solomon SB. Closed-bore interventional MRI: percutaneous biopsies and ablations. *Am J Roentgenol.* 2015;205(4):W400–W410. doi:10.2214/AJR.15.14732.
13. Kraff O, Ladd ME. MR safety update 2015 : where do the risks come from? *Curr Radiol Rep.* 2016;4(6):1–6. doi:10.1007/s40134-016-0163-y.
14. Kanal E, Barkovich AJ, Bell C, et al. ACR guidance document on MR safe practices: 2013. *J Magn Reson Imaging.* 2013;37(3):501–530. doi:10.1002/jmri.24011.
15. Shellock FG, Spinazzi A. MRI safety update 2008: Part 1, MRI contrast agents and nephrogenic systemic fibrosis. *Am J Roentgenol.* 2008;191(4):1129–1139. doi:10.2214/AJR.08.1038.1.
16. Shellock FG, Spinazzi A. MRI safety update 2008: Part 2, screening patients for MRI. *Am J Roentgenol.* 2008;191(4):1140–1149. doi:10.2214/AJR.08.1038.2.
17. Kanal E, Froelich JW, Barkovich AJ, et al. Standardized MR terminology and reporting of implants and devices as recommended by the American College of Radiology Subcommittee on MR Safety. *Radiology.* 2015;274(3):866. doi:10.1148/radiol.2015151108.
18. Shellock FG. *Reference Manual for MR Safety, Implants and Devices.* Los Angeles, CA: Biochemical Research Publishing Group; 2007.
19. Tse ZTH, Dumoulin CL, Clifford GD, et al. A 1.5T MRI-conditional 12-lead electrocardiogram for MRI and intra-MR intervention. *Magn Reson Med.* 2014;71(3):1336–1347. doi:10.1002/mrm.24744.
20. Keeler EK, Casey FX, Engels H, et al. Accessory equipment considerations with respect to MRI compatibility. *J Magn Reson Imaging.* 1998;8(1):12–18. doi:10.1002/jmri.1880080107.
21. Jolesz FA, Morrison PR, Koran SJ, et al. Compatible instrumentation for intraoperative MRI: expanding resources. *J Magn Reson Imaging.* 1998;8(1):8–11. doi:10.1002/jmri.1880080105.
22. Buchanan CL, Morris EA, Dorn PL, Borgen PI, Van Zee KJ. Utility of breast magnetic resonance imaging in patients with occult primary breast cancer. *Ann Surg Oncol.* 2005;12(12):1045–1053. doi:10.1245/ASO.2005.03.520.
23. Kuhl CK, Morakkabati N, Leutner CC, Schmiedel A, Wardelmann E, Schild HH. MR imaging–guided large-core (14-gauge) needle biopsy of small lesions visible at breast MR imaging alone. *Radiology.* 2001;220:31–39. doi:10.1148/radiology.220.1.r01jl0731.
24. Zhang Z, Zhang Z, Lehrer D, et al. Detection of breast cancer with addition of annual screening ultrasound or a single screening MRI

to mammography in women with elevated breast cancer risk. *JAMA*. 2012;307(13):1394. doi:10.1001/jama.2012.388.
25. Eby PR, Lehman C. MRI-guided breast interventions. *Semin Ultrasound, CT MRI*. 2006;27(4):339–350. doi:10.1053/j.sult.2006.05.008.
26. Imschweiler T, Haueisen H, Kampmann G, et al. MRI-guided vacuum-assisted breast biopsy: comparison with stereotactically guided and ultrasound-guided techniques. *Eur Radiol*. 2014;24(1):128–135. doi:10.1007/s00330-013-2989-5.
27. Moore CM, Robertson NL, Arsanious N, et al. Image-guided prostate biopsy using magnetic resonance imaging–derived targets: a systematic review. *Eur Urol*. 2013;63(1):125–140. doi:10.1016/j.eururo.2012.06.004.
28. Penzkofer T, Tuncali K, Fedorov A, et al. Transperineal in-bore 3-T MR imaging–guided prostate biopsy: a prospective clinical observational study. *Radiology*. 2015;274(1):170–180. doi:10.1148/radiol.14140221.
29. Meier-Schroers M, Homsi R, Kukuk G, et al. In-bore transrectal MRI-guided prostate biopsies: are there risk factors for complications? *Eur J Radiol*. 2016;85(12):2169–2173. doi:10.1016/j.ejrad.2016.09.029.
30. Zhang Q, Chung YC, Lewin JS, Duerk JL. A method for simultaneous RF ablation and MRI. *J Magn Reson Imaging*. 1998;8(1):110–114. doi:10.1002/jmri.1880080122.
31. Hoffmann R, Rempp H, Keßler D-E, et al. MR-guided microwave ablation in hepatic tumours: initial results in clinical routine. *Eur Radiol*. August 2016:1–10. doi:10.1007/s00330-016-4517-x.
32. Erinjeri JP, Clark TWI. Cryoablation: mechanism of action and devices. *J Vasc Interv Radiol*. 2010;21(8):S187–S191. doi:10.1016/j.jvir.2009.12.403.
33. Silverman SG, Tuncali K, Morrison PR. MR imaging-guided percutaneous tumor ablation. *Acad Radiol*. 2005;12:1100–1109. doi:10.1016/j.acra.2005.05.019.
34. Baust J, Gage AA, Ma H, Zhang CM. Minimally invasive cryosurgery—technological advances. *Cryobiology*. 1997;34:373–384. doi:10.1006/cryo.1997.2017.
35. Morrison PR, Silverman SG, Tuncali K, Tatli S. MRI-guided cryotherapy. *J Magn Reson Imaging*. 2008;27(2):410–420. doi:10.1002/jmri.21260.
36. Silverman SG, Tuncali K, VanSonnenberg E, et al. Renal tumors: MR imaging–guided percutaneous cryotherapy—initial experience in 23 patients 1. *Radiology*. 2005;236(2):716–724. doi:10.1148/radiol.2362041107.
37. Silverman SG, Tuncali K, Adams DF, et al. MR imaging-guided percutaneous cryotherapy of liver tumors: initial experience. *Radiology*. 2000;217(3):657–664. doi:10.1148/radiology.217.3.r00dc40657.
38. Han K, Cohen JK, Miller RJ, et al. Treatment of organ confined prostate cancer with third generation cryosurgery: preliminary multicenter experience. *J Urol*. 2003;170(4 Pt 1):1126–1130. doi:10.1097/01.ju.0000087860.52991.a8.
39. Tuncali K, Morrison PR, Winalski CS, et al. MRI-guided percutaneous cryotherapy for soft-tissue and bone metastases: Initial experience. *Am J Roentgenol*. 2007;189(1):232–239. doi:10.2214/AJR.06.0588.
40. Hesley GK, Gorny KR, Woodrum DA. MR-guided focused ultrasound for the treatment of uterine fibroids. *Cardiovasc Intervent Radiol*. 2013;36(1):5–13. doi:10.1007/s00270-012-0367-3.
41. Sakuhara Y, Shimizu T, Kodama Y, et al. Magnetic resonance-guided percutaneous cryoablation of uterine fibroids: early clinical experiences. *Cardiovasc Intervent Radiol*. 2006;29(4):552–558. doi:10.1007/s00270-004-6163-y.
42. Hinshaw JL, Lubner MG, Ziemlewicz TJ, Lee FT, Brace CL, Brace CL. Percutaneous tumor ablation tools: microwave, radiofrequency, or cryoablation—what should you use and why? *Radiographics*. 2014;34(5):1344–1362. doi:10.1148/rg.345140054.
43. Schenker MP, Martin R, Shyn PB, Baum RA. Interventional radiology and anesthesia. *Perioper Nurs Clin*. 2009;4(4):451–458. doi:10.1016/j.cpen.2009.09.010.
44. Foltz G. Image-guided percutaneous ablation of hepatic malignancies. *Semin Intervent Radiol*. 2014;31(2):180–186. doi:10.1055/s-0034-1373792.
45. Welch BT, Atwell TD, Nichols D a, et al. Percutaneous image-guided adrenal cryoablation: procedural considerations and technical success. *Radiology*. 2011;258(1):301–307. doi:10.1148/radiol.10100631.
46. Schlesinger D, Benedict S, Diederich C, Gedroyc W, Klibanov A, Larner J. MR-guided focused ultrasound surgery, present and future. *Med Phys*. 2013;40(8):080901. doi:10.1118/1.4811136.
47. Napoli A, Anzidei M, Ciolina F, et al. MR-guided high-intensity focused ultrasound: current status of an emerging technology. *Cardiovasc Intervent Radiol*. 2013;36(5):1190–1203. doi:10.1007/s00270-013-0592-4.
48. Medel R, Monteith SJ, Elias WJ, et al. Magnetic resonance-guided focused ultrasound surgery: Part 2: a review of current and future applications. *Neurosurgery*. 2012;71(4):755–763. doi:10.1227/NEU.0b013e3182672ac9.
49. Khan AT, Shehmar M, Gupta JK. Uterine fibroids: current perspectives. *Int J Womens Health*. 2014;6:95–114. doi:10.2147/IJWH.S51083.
50. Blana A, Walter B, Rogenhofer S, Wieland WF. High-intensity focused ultrasound for the treatment of localized prostate cancer: 5-year experience. *Urology*. 2004;63(2):297–300. doi:10.1016/j.urology.2003.09.020\rS0090429503010082 [pii].
51. Hynynen K, Pomeroy O, Smith DN, et al. MR imaging-guided focused ultrasound surgery of fibroadenomas in the breast: a feasibility study. *Radiology*. 2001;219(1):176–185. doi:10.1148/radiology.219.1.r01ap02176.
52. Voogt MJ, Trillaud H, Kim YS, et al. Volumetric feedback ablation of uterine fibroids using magnetic resonance-guided high intensity focused ultrasound therapy. *Eur Radiol*. 2012;22(2):411–417. doi:10.1007/s00330-011-2262-8.
53. Tanderup K, Viswanathan AN, Kirisits C, Frank SJ. Magnetic resonance image guided brachytherapy. *Semin Radiat Oncol*. 2014;24(3):181–191. doi:10.1016/j.semradonc.2014.02.007.
54. Spratt D, Soni P, McLaughlin P, Merrick G. The American Brachytherapy Society Task Group Report: combination of brachytherapy and external beam radiation for high-risk prostate cancer. *Brachytherapy*. 2017;16:1–12. Available at: http://www.sciencedirect.com/science/article/pii/S1538472116305505. Accessed on November 21, 2016.
55. Viswanathan AN, Thomadsen B, American Brachytherapy Society Cervical Cancer Recommendations Committee RM, et al. American Brachytherapy Society consensus guidelines for locally advanced carcinoma of the cervix. Part I: general principles. *Brachytherapy*. 1991;11(1):33–46. doi:10.1016/j.brachy.2011.07.003.
56. Podder TK, Beaulieu L, Caldwell B, et al. AAPM and GEC-ESTRO guidelines for image-guided robotic brachytherapy: report of Task Group 192. *Med Phys*. 2014;41(10):101501. doi:10.1118/1.4895013.
57. D'Amico A V., Cormack RA, Tempany CM. MRI-guided diagnosis and treatment of prostate cancer. *N Engl J Med*. 2001;344(10):776–777. doi:10.1056/NEJM200103083441017.
58. Hangiandreou NJ. AAPM/RSNA physics tutorial for residents. Topics in US: B-mode US: basic concepts and new technology. *Radiographics*. 2003;23(4):1019–1033. doi:10.1148/rg.234035034.
59. Abramowicz JS. Fetal Doppler: how to keep it safe? *Clin Obstet Gynecol*. 2010;53(4):842–850. doi:10.1097/GRF.0b013e3181fbae34.
60. Bly S, Van den Hof MC, Lewthwaite B, Gagnon R, Morin L, Salem S. Obstetric ultrasound biological effects and safety. *J Obstet Gynaecol Canada*. 2005;27(6):572–575. doi:10.1016/S1701-2163(16)30716-2.
61. Claudon M, Dietrich C, Choi B, et al. Guidelines and good clinical practice recommendations for contrast enhanced ultrasound (CEUS) in the liver—update 2012. *Ultraschall der Medizin—Eur J Ultrasound*. 2012;34(01):11–29. doi:10.1055/s-0032-1325499.
62. Kim MJ, Kim E-K. US-guided fine-needle aspiration of thyroid nodules: indications, techniques, results. *Radiographics*. 2008;28(7):1869–1889. doi:10.1148/rg.287085033.
63. Corapi KM, Chen JLT, Balk EM, Gordon CE. Bleeding complications of native kidney biopsy: a systematic review and meta-analysis. *Am J Kidney Dis*. 2012;60(1):62–73. doi:10.1053/j.ajkd.2012.02.330.
64. Patel IJ, Davidson JC, Nikolic B, et al. Consensus guidelines for periprocedural management of coagulation status and hemostasis risk in percutaneous image-guided interventions. *J Vasc Interv Radiol*. 2012;23(6):727–736. doi:10.1016/j.jvir.2012.02.012.
65. Bhagavatula S, Shyn PB. Image-guided renal interventions. *Radiol Clin North Am*. 2017;55(2):359–371.
66. Dyer RB, Regan JD, Kavanagh P V, Khatod EG, Chen MY, Zagoria RJ. Percutaneous nephrostomy with extensions of the technique: step by step 1. *Radiographics*. 2002;22(3):503–525. doi:10.1148/radiographics.22.3.g02ma19503.
67. Lane BR, Samplaski MK, Herts BR, Zhou M, Novick AC, Campbell SC. Renal mass biopsy—a renaissance? *J Urol*. 2008;179(1):20–27. doi:10.1016/j.juro.2007.08.124.
68. Sainani NI, Tatli S, Anthony SG, Shyn PB, Tuncali K, Silverman SG. Successful percutaneous radiologic management of renal cell carcinoma tumor seeding caused by percutaneous biopsy performed before ablation. *J Vasc Interv Radiol*. 2013;24:1404–1408. doi:10.1016/j.jvir.2013.04.034.
69. Nazir B. Pain during transrectal ultrasound-guided prostate biopsy and the role of periprostatic nerve block: what radiologists should know. *Korean J Radiol*. 2014;15(5):543–553. doi:10.3348/kjr.2014.15.5.543.
70. Park JJ, Kim CK, Park BK. Ultrasound-guided transvaginal core biopsy of pelvic masses: feasibility, safety, and short-term follow-up. *Am J Roentgenol*. 2016;206(4):877–882. doi:10.2214/AJR.15.15702.
71. O'Neill MJ, Rafferty EA, Lee SI, et al. Transvaginal interventional procedures: aspiration, biopsy, and catheter drainage. *Radiographics*. 2001;21(3):657–672. Available at: http://www.ncbi.nlm.nih.gov/pubmed/11353114. Accessed on November 29, 2016.

72. Jones PW, Moyers JP, Rogers JT, Rodriguez RM, Gary Lee YC, Light RW. Ultrasound-guided thoracentesis: is it a safer method? *Chest.* 2003;123(2):418–423. doi:10.1378/chest.123.2.418.
73. Runyon BA. Introduction to the revised American Association for the Study of Liver Diseases practice guideline management of adult patients with ascites due to cirrhosis 2012. *Hepatology.* 2013;57(4):1651–1653. doi:10.1002/hep.26359.
74. Umgelter A, Reindl W, Wagner KS, et al. Effects of plasma expansion with albumin and paracentesis on haemodynamics and kidney function in critically ill cirrhotic patients with tense ascites and hepatorenal syndrome: a prospective uncontrolled trial. *Crit Care.* 2008;12(1):R4. doi:10.1186/cc6765.
75. Bard C, Lafortune M, Breton G. Ascites: ultrasound guidance or blind paracentesis? *CMAJ.* 1986;135(3):209–210. Available at: http://www.ncbi.nlm.nih.gov/pubmed/3524781. Accessed on December 2, 2016.
76. vanSonnenberg E, Wittich GR, Goodacre BW, Casola G, D'Agostino HB. Percutaneous abscess drainage: update. *World J Surg.* 2001;25(3):362–369. doi:10.1007/s002680020386.
77. Bouali K, Magotteaux P, Jadot A, et al. Percutaneous catheter drainage of abdominal abscess after abdominal surgery. Results in 121 cases. *J Belge Radiol.* 1993;76(1):11–14. Available at: http://www.ncbi.nlm.nih.gov/pubmed/8320186. Accessed on November 29, 2016.
78. Venara A, Carretier V, Lebigot J, Lermite E. Technique and indications of percutaneous cholecystostomy in the management of cholecystitis in 2014. *J Visc Surg.* 2014;151(6):435–439. doi:10.1016/j.jviscsurg.2014.06.003.
79. Marhofer P, Chan VWS. Ultrasound-guided regional anesthesia: current concepts and future trends. *Anesth Analg.* 2007;104(5):1265–1269, tables of contents. doi:10.1213/01.ane.0000260614.32794.7b.
80. Ferrer J V, Soriano P, Zazpe C, Vicente F, Herrera J, Lera JM. Pseudoaneurysm of the inferior epigastric artery. Pathogenesis, diagnosis, and treatment. *Arch Surg.* 1996;131(1):102–103. Available at: http://www.ncbi.nlm.nih.gov/pubmed/8546568. Accessed on November 29, 2016.
81. Scanlan KA, Propeck PA, Lee FTJ. Invasive procedures in the female pelvis: value of transabdominal, endovaginal, and endorectal US guidance. *Radiographics.* 2001;21(2):491–506. doi:10.1148/radiographics.21.2.g01mr21491.

13 | INTERVENTIONAL NEURORADIOLOGY

RUTH THIEX, MD, PHD, KAI U. FRERICHS, MD

INTRODUCTION

Interventional neuroradiology—also known as endovascular neurosurgery—evolved as a new medical subspecialty in the 1980s and focuses on the treatment of cerebrovascular, head and neck, and spinal diseases by using endovascular or other percutaneous routes to reach the target. Rapid technical improvements in each successive generation of medical devices and materials (catheter technology, coils, and stents) brought interventional neuroradiology to the forefront in the management of aneurysms and various vascular malformations.

In 1927, Egas Moniz, professor of neurology in Lisbon, Portugal, pioneered the radiographic imaging of the intracranial vasculature in a living human subject.[1] The only approach at the time was Dandy's method of introducing air into the ventricular system to localize space-occupying lesions of the brain by the distortion of the ventricles.[2] Egas Moniz injected bromide into the surgically exposed carotid artery of a 48-year-old patient with postencephalitic Parkinson disease and took angiographic images.[1] However, the patient died 8 hours later from carotid thrombosis. The field of neuroangiography has since tremendously expanded as a result of improved imaging capabilities, technical equipment, and safer contrast media. In the era of noninvasive imaging such as computed tomographic (CT) angiography and magnetic resonance (MR) angiography, cerebral angiography still remains the gold standard for visualizing the cerebral vasculature given its unique high spatial resolution, high-speed real-time image acquisition, high-resolution road mapping, and indispensable information on hemodynamics. Cerebral angiography carries a very low risk when performed by experienced neurointerventional staff.[3–5] Besides the technical competences, a thorough understanding of pertinent anatomy and pathology is essential. The indications must be reviewed in light of all previous imaging studies, prior surgical procedures, and evolution of the anatomic pathology. Excellent diagnostic skills with noninvasive neuroimaging modalities are necessary to identify the presence of cerebrovascular diseases, identify potential candidates for neurointerventional procedures, provide routes of endovascular access, and define the scope of treatment options.

NEURORADIOLOGY TECHNIQUES

DIGITAL SUBTRACTION ANGIOGRAPHY AND ROAD-MAPPING TECHNIQUE

In angiography, images are acquired by exposing an area of interest with time-controlled x-rays while injecting contrast medium into the blood vessels. To remove the overlying structures besides the blood vessels in this area, first a mask image is acquired before contrast injection; this is then subtracted from subsequent images obtained during and after contrast injection. By doing so, contrast reduction from bone and soft tissues surrounding the vasculature is vastly reduced and vessel detail greatly enhanced (Figure 13.1). Digital subtraction angiography (DSA) requires that the patient ideally remains almost motionless during image acquisition. Road map fluoroscopic imaging has allowed interventional neuroradiologists to superimpose angiographic images of the vascular anatomy on the live fluoroscopic image by injecting a small amount of contrast medium during acquisition of a mask image to enable safe device navigation (Figure 13.2). Road map imaging in particular is easily degraded by patient movement.

ESSENTIALS OF RADIATION PROTECTION AND X-RAY IMAGE PRODUCTION

A basic understanding of radiation physics is essential to minimize the neuroanesthesia team's radiation exposure. Most nonpatient exposure is the result of scattered radiation produced as the primary x-ray beam passes from the tube through the patient and into the image intensifier. A common cause of exposure of anesthesiologists to the primary x-ray beam is reaching into the beam without alerting the operator. During fluoroscopy, the interventionalist is looking at the video monitors and will not see the anesthesiologist approaching the patient. Therefore, the anesthesiologist and interventionalist should coordinate any adjustments on the patient, his or her leads, and vascular accesses during nonfluoroscopy periods whenever possible. During DSA runs, both the anesthesiologist and the interventionalist should step out of the neuroangiographic suite whenever possible. The hand injection technique requires that the operator stays near the patient to inject the contrast in a manually controlled fashion in unfavorable vascular anatomies during DSA. The benefit of hand injections in lieu of using a power injector is the immediate feedback and ability to stop the injection in cases of catheter movement or malposition. The anesthesiologist, however, can step away from the table, therefore reducing his or her exposure to scattered radiation. This might not be justifiable in exceptional cases, such as unstable patients who require continuous attendance. Protective devices such as

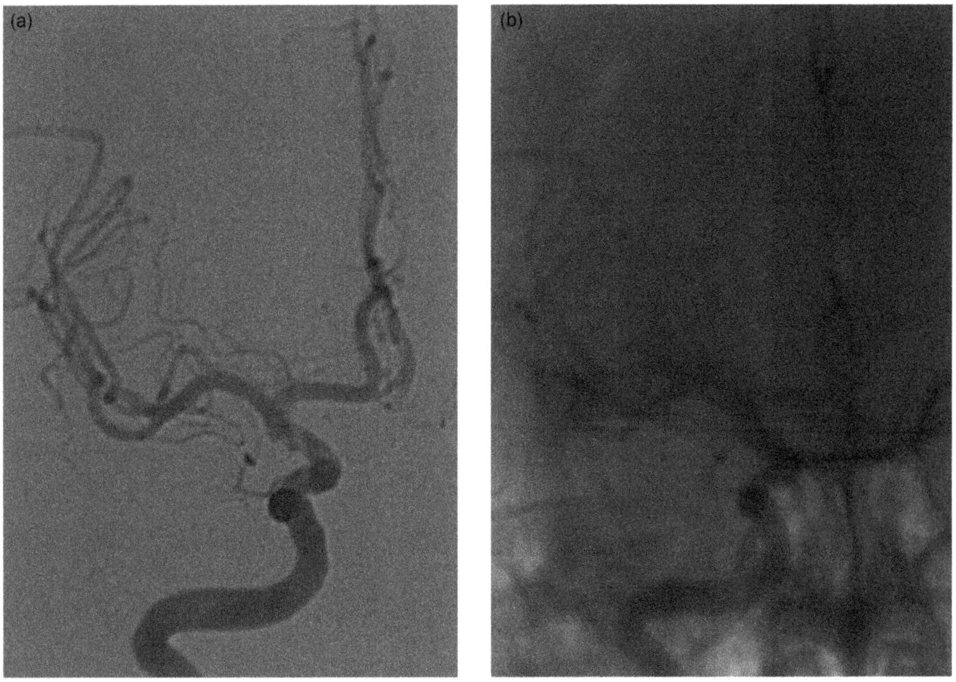

Figure 13.1. Right internal carotid artery injection (frontal plane) in a 38-year-old female patient with (a) and without (b) computer-generated subtraction. The vascular details become apparent during injection once the bony anatomy and soft tissue are digitally subtracted.

pull-in and ceiling-mounted lead acrylic window shields and lead aprons as well as increasing the distance from the primary beam should be used to protect from radiation exposure.[6–9]

CONTRAST MEDIUM AND SIDE EFFECTS

Acute adverse reactions occur in 5%–8% of patients in whom conventional, ionic, higher-osmolality contrast agents are administered intravascularly.[10] Nonionic contrast media (such as Omnipaque, Ultravist) are usually used in neuroangiography because of their lower osmolality and fewer side effects. Adverse reactions to intravascular contrast media are generally classified as either anaphylactoid (idiosyncratic) or nonidiosyncratic.[10] Anaphylactoid reactions occur independently of the dose or concentration of the agent. Their acuity and symptoms (vomiting, hot flushes, urticaria, pruritus, and diaphoresis) typically make them appear as allergic or hypersensitivity reactions; however, they do not result from an antigen-antibody interaction. Nausea/vomiting and scattered hives are usually minor, self-limited reactions. They should, however, be watched closely for other systemic symptoms because they might indicate early signs of a more severe reaction. Severe reactions are laryngeal edema, bronchospasm, pulmonary edema, hypotensive shock, respiratory arrest, or convulsions. For bronchospastic reactions without hypotension, oxygen (3 L/min), 0.1–0.2 mL (0.1–0.2 mg) of 1:1,000 solution of epinephrine subcutaneously or inhaled bronchodilators are recommended.[10] In severe anaphylactoid reactions, oxygen (3 L/min), intravenous (IV) fluids (normal saline or Ringer's solution), 0.1 mg epinephrine of 1:10,000 solution IV, 50 mg diphenhydramine IV, and 200 mg hydrocortisone IV are recommended. In patients with a history of previous radiocontrast media reaction, pretreating with prednisone and diphenhydramine reduces the risk to 9%.[11] Using low-osmolality radiocontrast media further reduces the risk to 0.5%.[11] In patients with a history of mild-to-moderate contrast reactions, the American College of Radiology recommends a regimen of prednisone 50 mg by mouth 13 hours, 7 hours, and 1 hour prior to contrast administration as an acceptable premedication regimen.[12]

Chemotoxic reactions are due to specific physiochemical effects of the injected agent on the organ or vessel it perfuses. They are directly dependent on the dose and concentration of the administered agent. Patients should be screened for the presence of clinically significant conditions (e.g., renal dysfunction, cardiovascular disease, seizures) that may place them at higher risk. In such patients, alternate diagnostic imaging modalities that do not require intravascular administration of a radiopaque contrast medium should be investigated first. If found inconclusive and administration of contrast medium is necessary, a lower-osmolality agent should be used. From et al. showed that contrast-induced nephropathy is associated with increased mortality. This risk is higher in patients in whom the contrast medium is administered intravenously as opposed to intra-arterially (IA).[13] For patients with renal insufficiency, prehydration with sodium bicarbonate (130 mEq/L IV solution at 3.5 mL/kg bolus over 1 hour, then 1.2 mL/kg per hour during the procedure and for 6 hours after the procedure) and administration of *N*-acetylcysteine (600 mg orally at 24 and 12 hours before and after the procedure) can prevent contrast-induced nephropathy.[14,15]

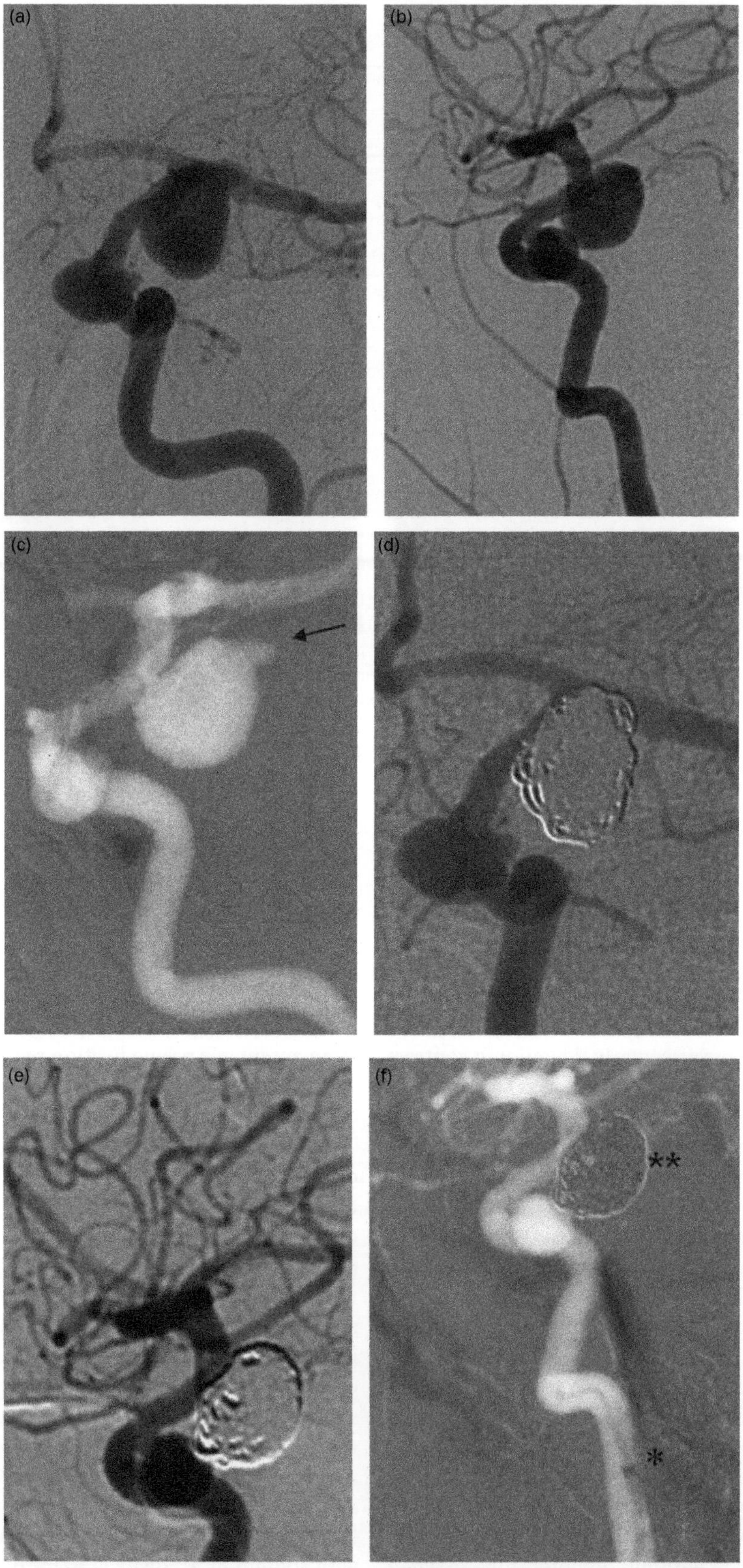

Figure 13.2. *Left internal carotid artery injection in frontal (a) and lateral (b) plane in an 83-year-old female patient who presented with a subarachnoid hemorrhage from a ruptured left-sided posterior communicating artery aneurysm measuring 11 by 8.9 mm with a daughter dome at its posterior and superior aspect representing the likely rupture site (c, arrow). The patient also had a medial variant clinoid aneurysm on the same side. Once the best trajectory was chosen, a road map (c) was used to guide the catheter to the proper location within the blood vessel so that coils could be deployed to treat a cerebral aneurysm. Complete obliteration of the aneurysm was confirmed on postembolization angiography (d, frontal; e, in lateral plane; f, road map with * indicating catheter tip and ** coils).*

NEURORADIOLOGY-NEUROANESTHESIA TEAM: GENERAL CONSIDERATIONS

Whereas diagnostic cerebral angiography is generally performed using conscious sedation or local anesthesia only, many of the interventional procedures require general anesthesia given their longer duration and the sensitivity of DSA and road map imaging to patient motion rather than significant pain associated with these procedures. However, certain procedures, such as the retrieval of an intracerebral intravascular clot using the MERCI (mechanical embolus retrieval in cerebral ischemia; Concentric Medical, Inc.) device can be painful and potentially result in sudden increases in heart rate and blood pressure. The operator should alert the neuroanesthesiologist prior to such maneuvers. Certain procedures, such as carotid stenting or tumor embolizations, benefit from the patient being kept awake and cooperative to evaluate neurological function throughout the procedure unless the risk of patient injury, such as arterial dissection, or inability to visualize the embolization process safely because of patient motion rises above a safe threshold. Many other procedures (e.g., kyphoplasty) can be performed safely using either method, and the choice of anesthesia relies highly on operator and patient preference and has to be decided on an individual basis.

To obtain a high-quality DSA cerebral angiogram, the patient must be able to refrain from moving, swallowing, or breathing for the duration of 10–15 seconds during each injection of contrast. Most patients can undergo diagnostic cerebral angiography without any sedation or with minimal-to-moderate sedation using fentanyl (25–200 μg) and midazolam (0.5–2 mg).

Uncooperative patients (i.e., any patient unable to refrain from moving, swallowing, or breathing on command because of impaired level of consciousness or neurological deficits such as global aphasia or neglect) may require general anesthesia and paralytics to adequately control movement and respiration. Particularly for the performance of urgently required cerebral angiography, such as for evaluation of subarachnoid hemorrhage (SAH), the threshold for use of general anesthesia will be low because diagnostic angiography in such cases is often followed by an intervention to treat the offending source of hemorrhage. In the absence of a neurological examination in the anesthetized patient, a bolt or external ventricular drainage (EVD) should be in place in patients with radiographic and clinical evidence of or potential for increased intracranial pressure (ICP). This can be easily performed in the angiography suite. This is particularly important in the angiography suite because the patient has to be positioned supine with no head elevation to stay in an isocenter position within the biplane radiographic environment. This may have a negative effect on the ICP and require additional pharmacological measures other than cerebrospinal fluid drainage to help with ICP control.

Neuropsychological monitoring allows for the assessment of the functional state of specific regions in the brain throughout a procedure, and it provides an indirect measure of regional ischemia while the patient is under general anesthesia. These techniques include electroencephalography (EEG), somatosensory or motor evoked potentials, as well as brainstem evoked potentials and are routinely performed in carotid endarterectomy, cerebrovascular surgery, and complex spinal surgery. Liu et al. described its use also in 35 patients undergoing 50 endovascular procedures (balloon test occlusion [*n* = 19], coil embolizations [*n* = 22], and permanent vessel occlusion [*n* = 9]).[16] They reported an alteration in management in 14% of the patients based on changes in EEG, somatosensory evoked potentials, or brainstem auditory evoked potentials. Neuropsychological monitoring is relatively insensitive in detecting ischemic changes in the cerebellum or posterior cerebral artery territories. Other limitations include confounding anesthesia-related effects that may mimic cerebral ischemia.[17] The implications for the neuroanesthesiologist are to use opioids intraprocedurally for analgesia and to avoid inhalational agents for their negative impact on EEG activity and evoked potentials.

As in the surgical operating room, to bring the case to a safe conclusion, both the neuroanesthesiologist and the neurointerventionalist need to have a good understanding of each other's procedural requirements within the neuroangiographic suite. Depending on the neuroangiographic suite layout, the neuroanesthesiologist will have to adapt the usual setup to this unique setting. The position of the anesthesiologist and anesthesia equipment relative to the patient is altered by the confines of the room and angiographic apparatus (Figure 13.3). Due to the size and proximity of the neuroangiography apparatus to the head, access to the patient is more limited than in the regular operating room.

Modern dedicated neuroangiography systems have simultaneous biplane (i.e., anteroposterior and lateral) imaging using paired x-ray tubes and image intensifiers that almost completely surround the patient's head and require large degrees of freedom of motion around the head to allow for projectional adjustments. In addition, the relatively fixed positions of the interventionalist and the video fluoroscopy monitors further limit access to the patient. Although unrestricted direct access to the patient's head and airway is generally desired by the neuroanesthesiologist, this is clearly not possible during most open or endovascular neurosurgical procedures. Whenever general endotracheal anesthesia is used, ventilator tubing and other support lines must be carefully positioned and extended so they are not accidentally caught during movements of the fluoroscopy equipment. Although adjustments can always be made and access to the airway obtained, this usually requires temporary withdrawal of the x-ray machines from the head. This may not matter during noncritical parts of a procedure, but it could cause serious interference during more critical parts of an intervention, when continuous visualization of the anatomy is required.

At our institution, the dedicated biplane neuroangiography suites allow best access to the patient when the neuroanesthesiologist and the ventilation machine are located to the patient's left side to minimize interference with the interventionalist and the imaging system (Figure 13.3). Anesthesia is induced before imaging equipment is brought into its working position, which allows unrestricted, direct access to the patient during induction. After the airway has

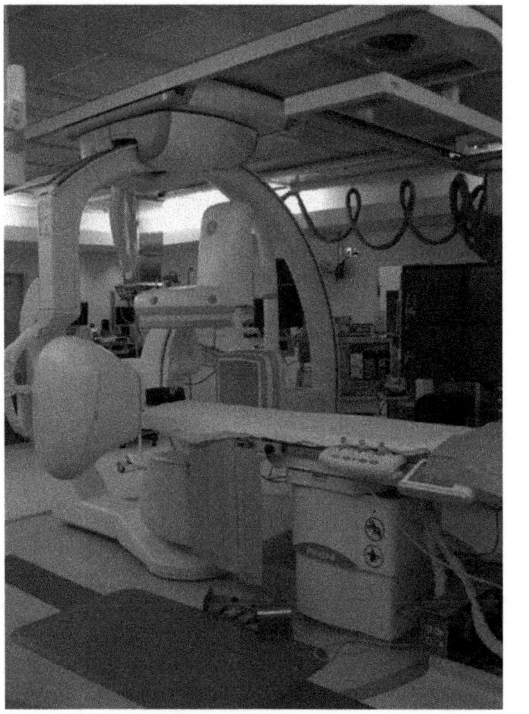

Figure 13.3. The GE Innova biplane angiography suite at the authors' facility provides images in two planes at the same time, thus allowing better visualization, fewer injections of contrast, and shorter procedure time. The technology features rotational angiography and 3D reconstruction; it is also capable of producing cross-sectional images like a computed tomographic (CT) scan. The neuroanesthesiologist and the ventilation machine are best located to the patient's left side given the confines of the angiography apparatus.

been secured and the patient stabilized, the imaging equipment is brought into its working position. The interventionalist on the patient's right side must assist the neuroanesthesia team to position equipment and arrange convenient airway and vascular access. While approaching the arch with the catheter, the operator can easily verify the correct position of the endotracheal tube and central venous lines and communicate this with the anesthesia team.

During monitored anesthesia care (MAC) or standby anesthesia care cases, rapid airway access is more critical than it is in cases performed under general endotracheal anesthesia because the patient's airway is not protected. In these cases, the neuroanesthesiologist's need for immediate airway access takes precedence and requires good communication with the interventionalist.

PATIENT MONITORING

Once the patient is brought to the neuroangiography suite and placed in the supine position, an 18- or 20-gauge intravenous line is started. Continuous monitoring of heart rate and rhythm, blood pressure, breathing rate and pattern, as well as peripheral oxygen saturation are mandatory for every procedure whether under local anesthesia, intravenous sedation, MAC, or general anesthesia. An arterial line is inserted for procedures requiring strict blood pressure monitoring and control, including patients with acute SAH or cardiovascular instability. In patients with an acute stroke, time is of the essence, and although desirable, insertion of a radial arterial line may cause an unnecessary delay for the revascularization attempt. Blood pressure control in both directions will frequently have to depend on the skillful administration of vasoactive medication based on frequently updated cuff pressures. Invasive blood pressure measurement including mean arterial pressure (MAP) and ICP monitoring via a bolt or EVD is mandatory in patients with raised ICP to monitor cerebral perfusion pressure (CPP). This is of paramount importance in patients with high-grade SAH during aneurysm embolization or vasospasm therapy. If the ICP rises, the level of the EVD and thereby the amount of drained cerebrospinal fluid has to be adjusted in close coordination with the operator. If ICP cannot be controlled to maintain adequate cerebral perfusion in the angiography suite setting, the procedure may have to be aborted to allow for optimized ICP management, including head elevation, a simple but highly effective maneuver.

VASCULAR ACCESS SITES

For a right-handed operator, the right common femoral artery is the preferred access point. However, both groin areas are prepped and draped in case the right common femoral artery cannot be accessed for anatomic reasons or if bilateral access is required. In case the anesthesiologist cannot put in an arterial line because of either limited time in acute stroke cases or for anatomic reasons, the operator can introduce a sheath that is 1 French larger in size than the intended one, which may allow transduction of the blood pressure via the femoral sheath. This increases the risk of injury to the femoral artery, particularly in stroke cases, in which the use of already very large access sheaths (8 French) is common. Complications of the transfemoral approach include groin hematoma, retroperitoneal hemorrhage, arteriovenous fistula and pseudoaneurysm formation, dissection, and femoral nerve injury.[18] The transbrachial approach obviates the need for prolonged bed rest and eliminates the risk of occult hematoma formation. This alternate approach is sometimes necessary when transfemoral access is impossible because of peripheral vascular disease or aortic occlusion (Figure 13.4). For diagnostic catheterization, a 4 or 5 French sheath is used, whereas 6 or 7 French sheaths are routinely used for embolizations. For revascularization procedures, 8 or 9 French sheaths are required. Once the sheath is in place, it is connected to continuous pressurized heparin saline flush (3000 IU of heparin in 1000 mL of normal saline).

Access site hemostasis following sheath removal can be achieved by simple or assisted manual (FemoStop II Plus Compression System, St. Jude Medical) compression or by the use of a collagen hemostatic puncture closure device (Angio-Seal, St. Jude Medical). Due to the increased risk of access site complications from the use of such devices,[19] our preferred method is manual compression whenever possible. The presence of peripheral pulses distal to the arterial puncture site should be ascertained before the patient leaves the neuroangiographic suite and monitored afterward.

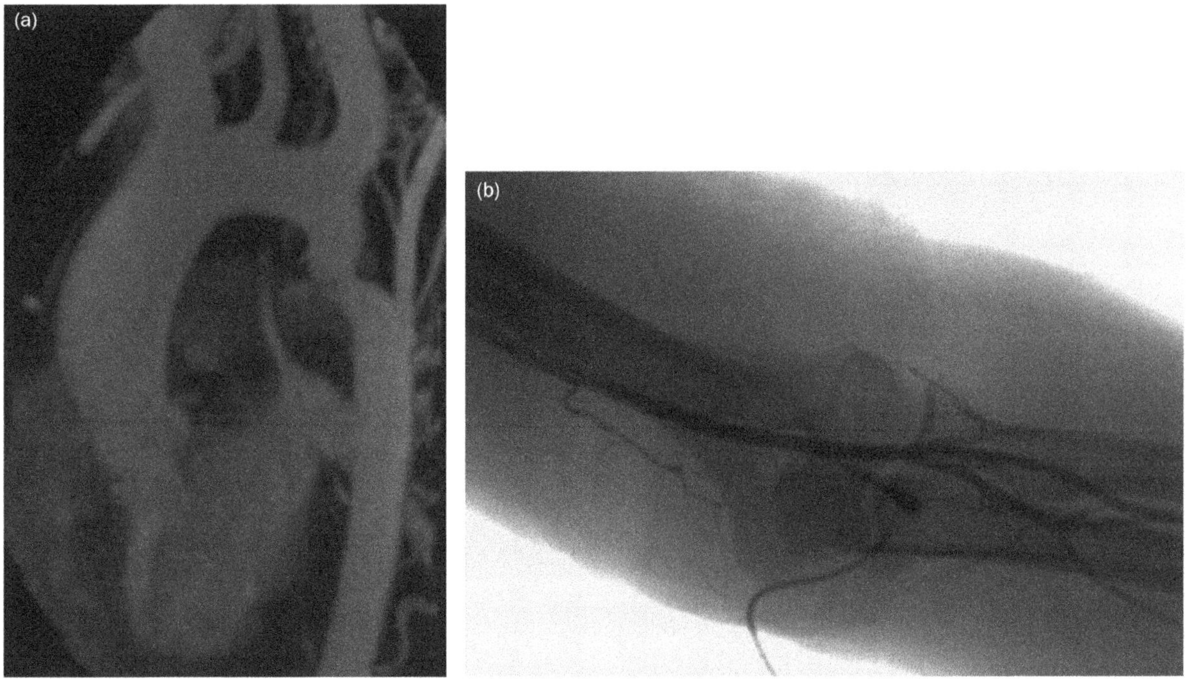

Figure 13.4. *Coronal maximum intensity projection (MIP) (a) of magnetic resonance angiography (MRA) in a 51-year-old male patient with episodic left arm tingling and numbness. Cerebral angiography was requested to evaluate the moya-moya-like pattern of his cerebral arteries and the configuration of the basilar tip aneurysm seen on MRA of the brain. Initial angiography was unsuccessful due to the inability to navigate from the descending aorta to the arch. An MRA of the chest revealed coarctation of the aorta. In a second attempt, the left brachial artery was catheterized (b), and cerebral angiography was performed.*

The timing and method of sheath removal needs to be discussed with the anesthesia team because this may affect the postextubation care of the patient, who must stay in a horizontal position for a prolonged period of time.

ANTICOAGULATION

To prevent embolic complications, interventions are performed under systemic heparinization and should be initiated after sheath placement. An 80-IU/kg loading dose is administered to target an activated clotting time (ACT) of two or three times baseline. The ACT is checked at intervals during the procedure, and additional heparin boluses are given to ensure targeted anticoagulation. At the end of the procedure, the patient's anticoagulation is allowed to correct spontaneously, and the access sheath is removed at a later time when coagulation parameters have reached a safe level.

COMMON INTERVENTIONAL NEURORADIOLOGY PROCEDURES AND NEUROANESTHESIA CONSIDERATIONS

ENDOVASCULAR MANAGEMENT OF CEREBRAL ANEURYSMS

The permanent obliteration of aneurysms and their exclusion from the circulation is the main goal of aneurysm therapy (Figure 13.2d, e). The choice of the appropriate endovascular technique depends on aneurysm size, location, and characteristics.

INTRA-ANEURYSMAL EMBOLIZATION

Direct *intra-aneurysmal embolization* of the aneurysm with preservation of the parent artery aims at complete exclusion of the aneurysm from the circulation analogous to surgical clip placement. In 1995, the Guglielmi Detachable Coil (GDC) (Target Therapeutics, Inc., South San Francisco, CA) achieved approval of the US Food and Drug Administration (FDA) for aneurysm *coiling*. This coil consists of soft platinum that is attached to a microguidewire by a thin stainless steel junction. If the coil conforms to the confines of the aneurysm in the desired fashion, it is released by passing a tiny positive current through the guidewire. After electrolysis of the junction, the guidewire is withdrawn while the coil is left within the aneurysm. Most aneurysms require placement of several progressively smaller coils to achieve complete obliteration (Figure 13.2). Since the original release of the GDC, numerous other coil designs from other manufacturers have entered the market, but the basic principle remains the same.

In a landmark study, endovascular treatment with coils was found to be associated with better patient outcomes compared to surgical clipping in patients who have had a SAH from the aneurysm.[20] The prerequisite for aneurysm coiling without assist techniques is a relatively small aneurysm neck that allows retention of coils without encroachment on the parent artery. Compaction of coils with time and regrowth of the aneurysm are potential limitations of the technique. Although controversial, cranial neuropathies due to aneurysm pressure may be less likely to improve after coiling than clipping.

The endovascular treatment of wide-neck aneurysms has been revolutionized by the introduction of highly flexible,

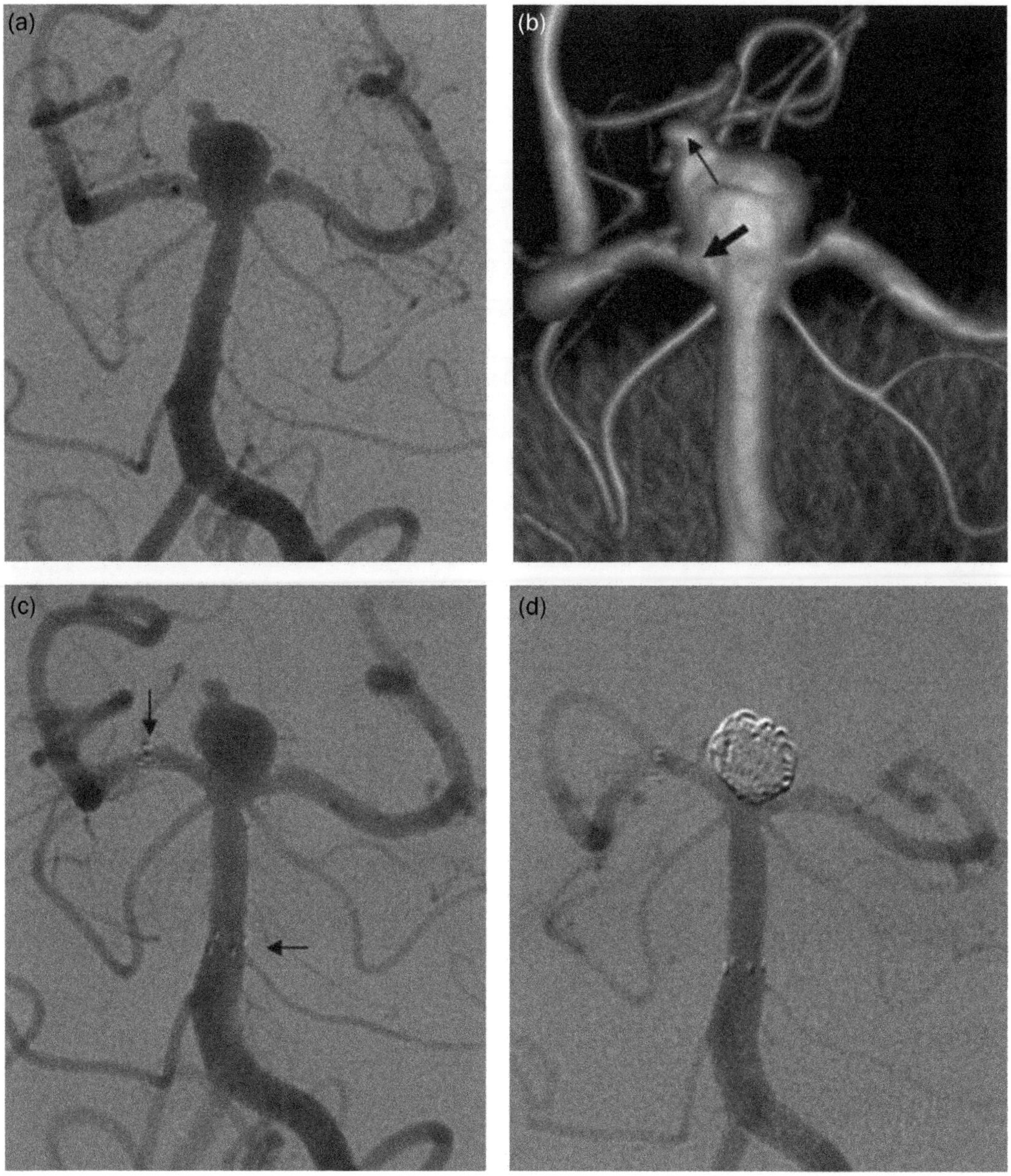

Figure 13.5. Left vertebral artery injection (frontal plane: a, before stent placement; b, after three-dimensional reconstruction; c, after stent placement; d, after coiling) in a 68-year-old female patient with a known basilar tip aneurysm that had been followed by magnetic resonance angiography (MRA) for 7 years with recently documented aneurysm growth. This broad-based, 7.4 by 7 mm basilar tip aneurysm (b) partially incorporated the right P1 segment (big arrow) and had a daughter dome (small arrow). A Neuroform III stent 3.5 by 20 mm was positioned in the right P1 and midbasilar segment bridging the aneurysm neck, thus preventing coil protrusion into the parent vessel during coil embolization 6 weeks later (arrows indicate proximal and distal stent markers).

self-expanding nitinol stents that can be navigated into the tortuous cerebral circulation. The stent implantation requires premedication with aspirin (325 mg/d) and clopidogrel (75 mg/d) for 5 days before treatment and at least 12 weeks thereafter. Coil embolization through the stent struts can follow stent placement immediately or in a second stage after endothelialization of the stent (Figure 13.5). As the required anticoagulation and antiplatelet therapy carry an excessively high risk for hemorrhagic complications, the stent-assisted technique is usually limited to unruptured aneurysms.

Complications during coil embolization include aneurysm rupture or thromboembolism. Aneurysm rupture during embolization is more common in recently ruptured and small aneurysms.[21] If a rupture is suspected, heparin should be immediately reversed using protamine sulfate (1 mg per 100 IU heparin) and an initial downward adjustment of the blood pressure by the anesthesiologist. The interventionalist will attempt to continue with obliteration of the aneurysm sac as quickly as possible. Usually, continued coiling results in cessation of the bleeding. If this fails, the outcome is likely to be catastrophic.

Thromboembolic complications are typically platelet-derived events and occur during aneurysm coiling in approximately 3% of cases, resulting in a permanent neurological disability in 1.7%–5% of the procedures.[22] Heparin is commonly used as an anticoagulant in the prevention and treatment of thromboembolism during the procedures. However, heparin has almost no effect on platelet aggregation and therefore may not always be able to prevent these complications.

Once a thromboembolic complication has occurred and been recognized, various pharmacological agents or mechanical techniques may be used to dissolve or remove the clot. This includes the use of additional heparin or IA administration of a thrombolytic or antiplatelet agent.[23] For example, abciximab (Rheopro) administered locally (2–10 mg) at the site of the thrombus has been successfully used to treat thromboembolic complications during coiling, even in cases with ruptured aneurysms.[24] Eptifibatide (Integrilin) is an alternative and binds to the platelet receptor glycoprotein (GP) IIb/IIIa of human platelets and inhibits platelet aggregation. The eptifibatide dosing regimen includes two systemic 180-μg/kg bolus doses given 10 minutes apart combined with a continuous infusion of 2.0 μg/kg per minute.[25,26]

PARENT VESSEL OCCLUSION AND PROVOCATIVE TESTING (BALLOON TEST OCCLUSION)

In some cases, direct aneurysm obliteration without parent artery sacrifice may not be possible. The majority of aneurysms treated by *parent vessel occlusion* are cavernous/petrous/extracranial internal carotid artery (ICA) aneurysms, extracranial vertebral artery aneurysms, dissecting aneurysms of the ICA or vertebral artery, and giant aneurysms in the subarachnoid space with ill-defined neck or inaccessible location. The prerequisite for parent vessel occlusion is adequate collateral circulation as proven by balloon test occlusion to prevent subsequent cerebral infarction. This information is also critical for the neurosurgeon if the aneurysm is treated surgically. A balloon is advanced to the target artery, either the internal or vertebral artery, at or near the site of proposed permanent vessel sacrifice, and a baseline neurological examination is obtained. After systemic anticoagulation to an ACT of 300–350 seconds, the balloon is inflated to occlude the artery, and continuous neurologic evaluation follows. Development of a new neurologic deficit indicates insufficient collateral blood supply.

In our institution, cerebral blood flow evaluation by technetium Tc 99m single-photon emission computed tomography (SPECT) is used to enhance the predictive value of the test. The radionucleotide Tc 99m hexamethyl-propylene-amine oxime (HMPAO) is injected once the patient tolerates test occlusion for 10 minutes during a hypotensive challenge. After successful 20-minute balloon test occlusion, the balloon is deflated, and the patient is transferred for nuclear imaging. If balloon test occlusion indicates adequate collateral circulation, permanent occlusion of the parent artery may be performed using microcoils. In patients with poor tolerance for parent artery occlusion, an extracranial-intracranial bypass has to be done surgically before parent artery occlusion.

TREATMENT OF VASOSPASM

The IA infusion of vasodilators has been proven beneficial for catheter-induced vasospasm and vasospasm following SAH.[27] Verapamil is a phenylalkylamine calcium channel blocker that inhibits voltage-gated calcium channels in the arterial wall smooth muscle cells and results in vasodilation (Figure 13.6).[27,28] Nimodipine and nicardipine, dihydropyridine agents, also improve the distal microcirculation and have a longer half-life than verapamil.[29,30] On selective catheterization of the targeted vessel, 5 mg verapamil diluted in 10 mL sterile water is slowly infused over 2 minutes while close attention is paid to cardiac side effects such as hypotension and bradycardia. The neuroanesthesiologist has to anticipate these effects because untoward elevation of ICP or reduction of systemic blood pressure by vasodilators can exacerbate the neurological injury. The infusion of the vasodilator can be done either via the proximal guide catheter, thus not requiring general anesthesia, or via superselective catheterization of the target vessel.

In case of severe flow limitation, urgent angioplasty may be necessary to avoid incipient infarction. Transluminal balloon angioplasty should be performed under general anesthesia using high-resolution digital road map imaging to avoid catastrophic vessel rupture or dissection. The pathophysiology underlying transluminal balloon angioplasty includes disruption of smooth muscle cells and extracellular matrix, thus causing smooth muscle and endothelial cell flattening.[31] Transluminal balloon angioplasty of the spastic segment is more durable for vasospasm therapy[32]; however, the IA administration of verapamil runs a significantly lower risk of vessel injury and allows treatment of distal and small-artery vasospasm not amenable to balloon angioplasty.

EMBOLIZATION OF CEREBRAL ARTERIOVENOUS MALFORMATIONS

In brain arteriovenous malformations (AVMs), arterial feeders are directly connected to the venous system without intervening capillaries, resulting in high-flow arteriovenous shunts (Figure 13.7). The risk of treating a brain AVM must be weighed against its natural history. Intracranial hemorrhage is the most common form of clinical presentation, with a quoted annual risk of 2%–4%.[33,34] The angiographic evaluation of patients with an AVM also includes superselective catheterization of the feeding arteries to rule out flow-related aneurysms or angiopathies. In patients with hemorrhage, it has to be determined which lesion, the AVM itself or an associated aneurysm, is responsible for the hemorrhage. The AVM should be addressed initially, when identified as the source of hemorrhage. Aneurysms associated with AVMs present an increased risk of hemorrhage and may regress spontaneously following AVM treatment.[35]

Current therapeutic options for brain AVMs include embolization, microsurgical resection, stereotactic radiosurgery, and various combinations. The goal of any combined therapy is to decrease the overall morbidity and mortality of AVM treatment. Preoperative AVM embolization is indicated to facilitate surgical excision of the AVM by reduction of the intraoperative bleeding. Embolization prior to radiosurgery aims at reducing the size of the nidus so that stereotactic

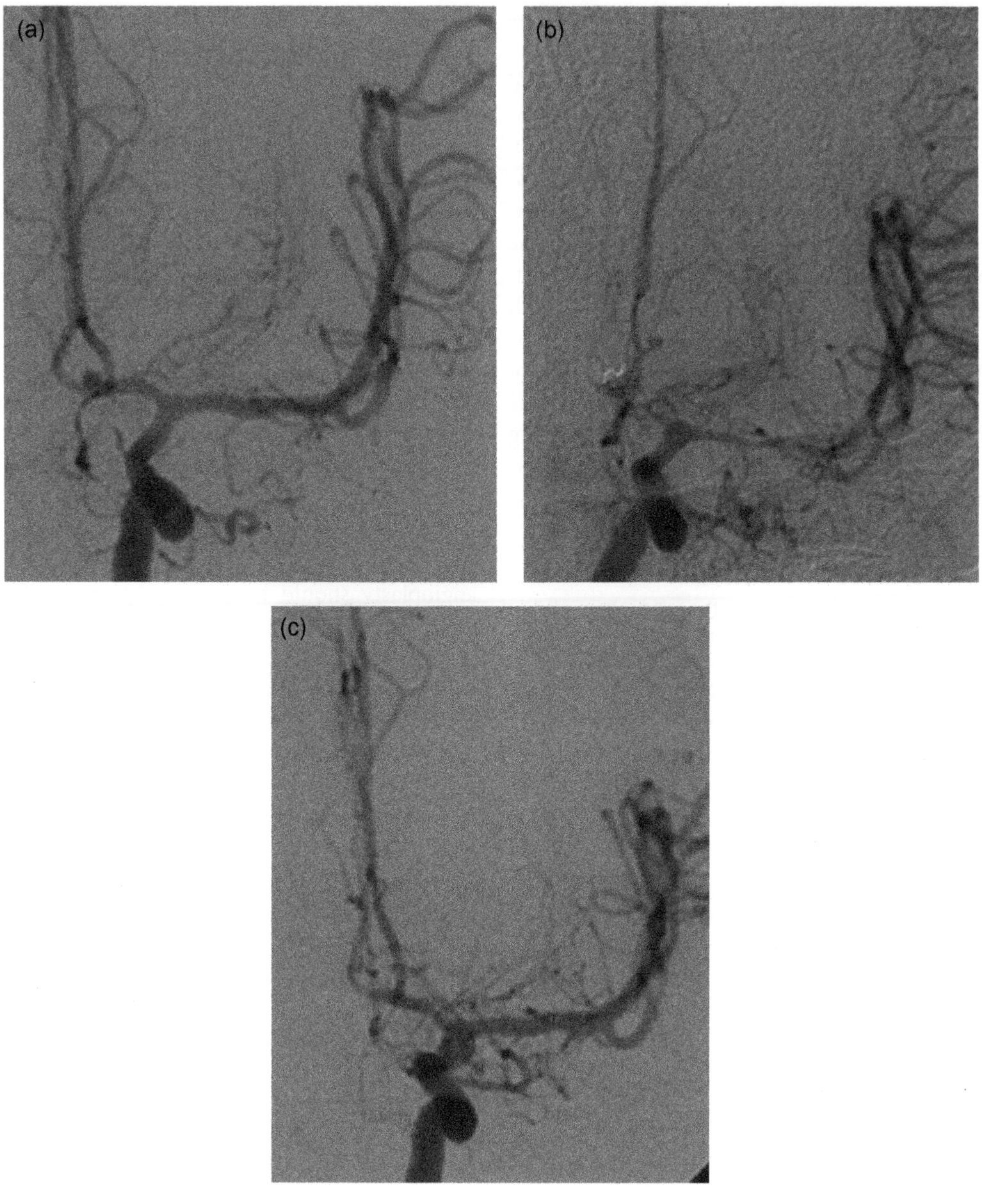

Figure 13.6. Left internal carotid artery injection in frontal plane on days 0 (a), 6 (b), and 9 (c) after subarachnoid hemorrhage. This 43-year-old patient presented with a subarachnoid hemorrhage from a ruptured anterior communicating artery aneurysm and underwent successful coil embolization of the aneurysm. On day 6 after coiling, he became somnolent and was found to have severe vasospasm in the left A1 and both A2 segments as well as in the left M1 segment. The vasospasm was treated with intra-arterial infusion of verapamil into the left internal carotid artery on four consecutive days. The patient was also subjected to "triple H therapy" (induced hypertension, hemodilution, and hypervolemia). The vessel diameter of the spastic segments gradually improved, and the mental status change subsided.

radiosurgery can target the remainder with a higher dose and a better chance of cure. In selected cases, small AVMs may be completely obliterated by embolization alone. Embolization of AVMs requires a special armamentarium, such as flow-directed microcatheters for safe and reliable navigation into the very distal aspects of an arterial feeder. Flow-directed navigation uses arterial blood flow to drag the very flexible distal microcatheter segment forward into the vessel with the highest flow, which is usually the desired feeder. In very high-flow AVMs, flow-guided microcatheters rapidly achieve very distal, often intranidal, positions at very low risk of vessel injury. Intravenous heparin is administered on an individual basis to prevent microemboli if there are small feeders or if there is slow flow.

For embolization, solid occlusive devices (coils, balloons), particulates (polyvinyl alcohol [PVA] particles), or liquid embolic agents such as Onyx or *N*-butyl cyanoacrylate (NBCA) are used. Complications associated with the liquid embolic agents include passage through the nidus before solidifying and lodging in veins draining the AVM, which can lead to AVM rupture if not yet completely embolized. Other complications include passage of embolic material into the pulmonary circulation. In case of microcatheter entrapment, cutting the catheter at the access site and leaving it in place, although not a desirable outcome, may be safer than continued or overly aggressive pulling on the device, which could lead to brain hemorrhage or catheter fracture.

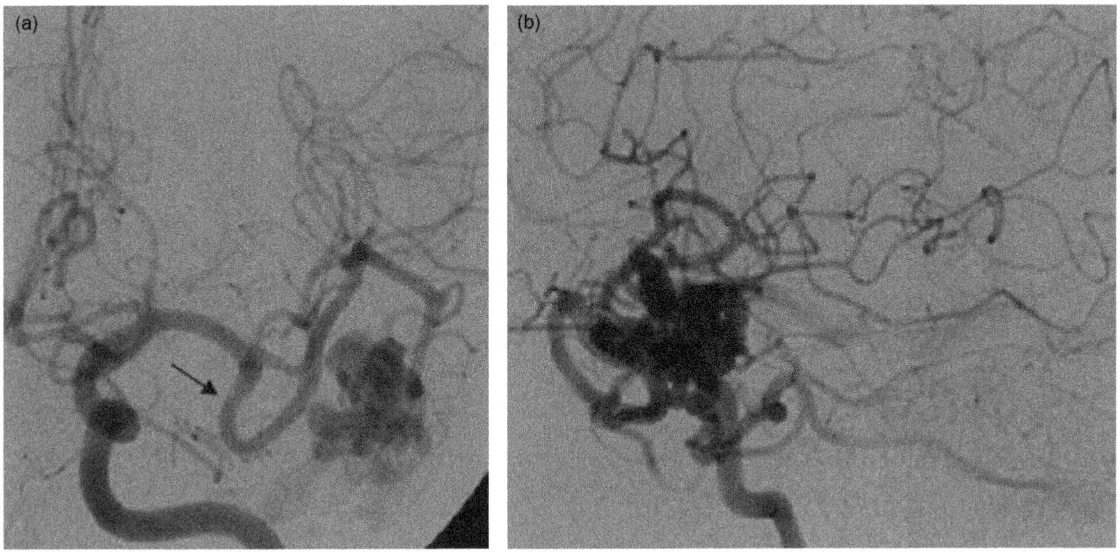

Figure 13.7. Left internal carotid artery injection (a, frontal; b, lateral plane) of a 67-year-old male patient who presented with seizures and was found to have a 1-cm left anterior temporal arteriovenous malformation (AVM) fed by the left anterior temporal artery (arrow) draining into the vein of Rosenthal and vein of Labbé.

Anesthetic considerations during cerebral AVM embolization primarily consist of tight control of arterial blood pressure. Once the microcatheter is in position, the patient's blood pressure is transiently lowered to slow flow through the AVM and allow more controlled embolization. Embolization can markedly reduce flow through the nidus, causing stagnation in the draining veins with subsequent thrombosis, hemorrhage, or venous ischemic infarct.[36] Another reason for hemorrhage may be normal perfusion pressure breakthrough. The chronically low perfusion pressure in the parenchyma adjacent to an AVM impairs cerebrovascular autoregulation. After removal of the shunt, parenchymal hyperperfusion can cause edema and hemorrhage.[37] Approximately 10% of brain AVM embolizations cause a permanent neurological deficit.[38] These deficits are often caused by embolization of branches arising from an AVM feeder that supply normal brain parenchyma.

ACUTE STROKE INTERVENTION

Intravenous administration of recombinant tissue plasminogen activator (r-tPA) within the first 3 hours of stroke onset was the first FDA-approved therapy for acute ischemic stroke based on two phase III National Institutes of Neurological Disorders and Stroke (NINDS) tissue plasminogen activator (tPA) trials completed in 1995.[39] In angiographic controlled pilot trials of intravenous r-tPA, the rate of recanalization of major arterial occlusions with intravenous r-tPA is low, with partial or complete recanalization of only 10% of occluded internal carotid arteries and 25% of occluded proximal middle cerebral arteries.[40] Patients with emergent large-vessel occlusion (ELVO) of a major intracerebral artery often have a large area of brain injury resulting in death or severe disability.[41]

With the publication of five randomized multicenter controlled clinical trials, the guideline recommendations for acute stroke treatment have changed tremendously.[42–46] These trials provide class 1, level A evidence that endovascular thrombectomy is the standard of care for patients with ELVO and first-line treatment for patients not eligible for r-tPA. In patients with acute occlusion of the intracranial ICA or M1 segment, endovascular thrombectomy results in significantly better clinical outcomes compared to best medical treatment. Besides the availability of a neurointerventionalist and his or her team, on-site expertise in vascular neurology and neurocritical care are of paramount importance to achieve good clinical outcomes.

At first, a detailed angiographic examination of the vascular anatomy, including the collateral circulation at the circle of Willis and the leptomeningeal levels, is performed. A microcatheter is then passed over the microguidewire to the level of occlusion. Contrast is injected into the microcatheter to locate the clot. The microcatheter is then advanced over the microguidewire through the clot, followed by a microinjection to assess the extent of the clot. Two milligrams of r-tPA are injected through the catheter starting beyond the thrombus; the microcatheter is then retracted into the thrombus.

Mechanical clot disruption or retrieval is performed by one of the following interventional techniques, alone or in combination:

- Clot extraction using a stent retriever (Solitaire FR, Medtronic or Trevo, Concentric Medical)
  - Clot fragmentation and aspiration using the Penumbra aspiration system (Penumbra, Inc., Alameda, CA)
  - Clot extraction device such as the MERCI retrieval system

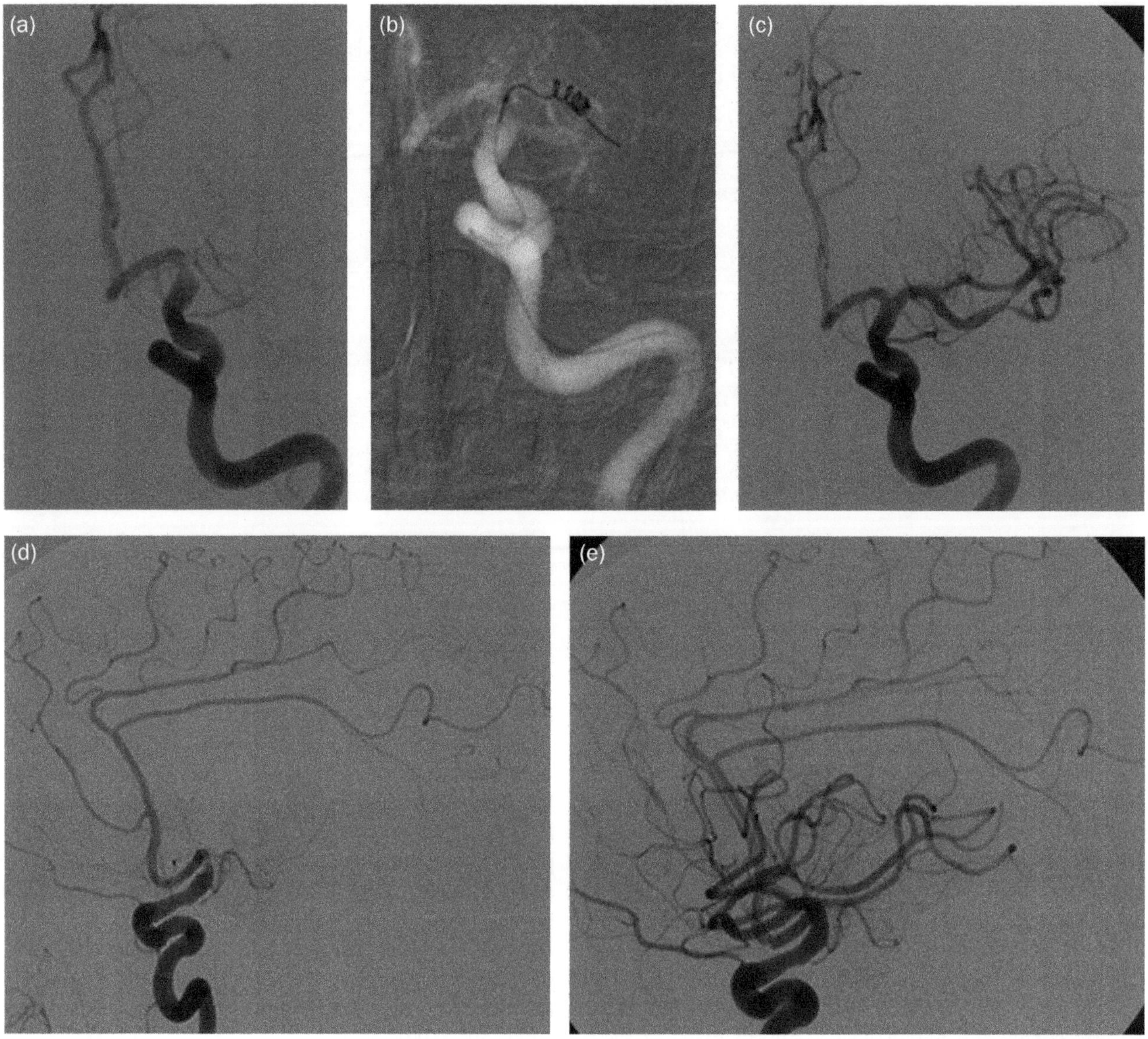

Figure 13.8. Left internal carotid artery injection (a and c, frontal plane; b, road map; d and e, lateral plane) in an 83-year-old male patient who presented with a 4- to 5-hour history of aphasia and right-side hemiplegia. The patient had received intravenous tissue plasminogen activator (tPA) in an outside hospital and was found to have a proximal M1 occlusion with clot partially extending into the A1 origin (a and d). After clot retrieval using the MERCI device (b), complete recanalization of the M1 segment and the superior and inferior division of the M2 segments was achieved (c and e).

The MERCI device is a flexible, helical-shaped, tapered tip made of nitinol wire with arcading filaments in its second and third generation (V series) to enhance friction between the device and the clot to increase the capture rate (Figure 13.8) This technique is used in conjunction with simultaneous flow reversal in the affected artery during retrieval. First-generation MERCI devices achieved recanalization rates of 48%, and, when coupled with IA thrombolytic drugs, recanalization rates of 60% have been reported.[47]

Multi MERCI was an international, multicenter, prospective, single-arm trial of thrombectomy in patients with large-vessel stroke treated *within 8 hours* of symptom onset.[48] Treatment with the L5 Retriever resulted in successful recanalization in 75 of 131 (57.3%) treatable vessels and in 91 of 131 (69.5%) after adjunctive therapy (IA tPA, mechanical). Favorable clinical outcomes (modified Rankin scale 0 to 2) occurred in 36%, and mortality was 34%; both outcomes were significantly related to vascular recanalization. Symptomatic intracerebral hemorrhage occurred in 16 patients (9.8%).

The Penumbra system (PS) is an embolectomy device that removes the thrombus in large-vessel thromboembolism via aspiration and extraction.[49] For aspiration, a reperfusion catheter is used in parallel with a microguidewire with a bulbous tip ("separator") and an aspiration source to break up the thrombus from proximal to distal and aspirate it from the occluded vessel. This is accomplished by slowly advancing the aspiration catheter into the clot while continuously moving the bulbous separator tip in and out of the distal end of the microcatheter.

Stent retrievers including the Solitaire FR and Trevo device are the newest iteration of mechanical approaches for revascularization. Once placed across the thrombus and deployed, they promote immediate reperfusion in 80%–90%

of cases by displacing the thrombus outside the stent between the stent tines and the vessel wall. Flow restoration may rapidly reestablish oxygen supply to the ischemic brain region. Once deployed for 5–10 minutes, the deployed stent is pulled back into the guide catheter under proximal aspiration through the guide catheter. If unsuccessful, they can be resheathed and used repeatedly. Compared to permanent self-expanding stents, there is no need for precase loading of dual antiplatelet agents. Safety and astonishing recanalization results were reported for both devices in the Solitaire FR With the Intention for Thrombectomy (SWIFT)[50] and Thrombectomy Revascularization of large Vessel Occlusions (TREVO 2)[51] randomized trials.

Anesthesia considerations in the management of patients with acute stroke include a rapid response by the anesthesia provider to decrease the time from onset of symptoms to the onset of treatment given the limited therapeutic window for IA thrombolysis (6 hours after patient was last seen normal) or aggressive mechanical clot disruption (8 hours after patient was last seen normal). In addition, there is evidence that earlier recanalization improves the chance for a good outcome. Therefore, it is critical to proceed expeditiously, even though a complete medical history or other circumstances may not be fully known or retrievable at the time of induction. For example, not infrequently, the patient may have arrived at our institution by airlift, while family has not arrived yet or other caregivers cannot be reached to obtain more detailed information.

General anesthesia is advocated in patients with a significantly altered level of consciousness and the inability to communicate and cooperate because of aphasia or neglect, whereas the majority of acute stroke interventions are done under conscious sedation. Communication between the interventionalist and neuroanesthesiologist regarding the optimal blood pressure management in each individual case is essential to enforce good perfusion of the collaterals but to avoid hemorrhage into the reperfused brain tissue.

OTHER NEUROINTERVENTIONAL PROCEDURES

Other neurointerventional procedures that may involve specialized anesthesia care include preoperative embolizations of head, neck, and spinal tumors; embolization of dural fistulas of the brain and spine; elective intracranial and extracranial stent/angioplasty; sclerotherapy of vascular malformations of the head and neck; and others. A detailed discussion covering all of these procedures is beyond the scope of this chapter. Similar principles of neuroanesthetic considerations as outlined previously, however, apply to a great extent to these procedures as well.

CONCLUSION

As the scope of endovascular neurosurgery continues to expand, so does the need for anesthesia support outside the normal operating room environment. A close cooperation and familiarity with the endovascular procedure by the neuroanesthesiologist is required for optimal results.

REFERENCES

1. Moniz EL. *L' Angiographie Cérébrale*. Paris, France: Masson & Cie; 1934:142–214.
2. Dandy WE. Ventriculography following the injection of air into the cerebral ventricles. *Ann Surg*. 1918;68:5–11.
3. Johnston DC, Chapman KM, Goldstein LB. Low rate of complications of cerebral angiography in routine clinical practice. *Neurology*. 2001;57:2012–2014.
4. Krings T, Willmes K, Becker R, et al. Silent microemboli related to diagnostic cerebral angiography: a matter of operator's experience and patient's disease. *Neuroradiology*. 2006;48:387–393.
5. Thiex R, Norbash AM, Frerichs KU. The safety of dedicated-team catheter-based diagnostic cerebral angiography in the era of advanced noninvasive imaging. *Am J Neuroradiol*. 2010;31:230–234
6. Chopp M, Portnoy HD, Schurig R, Croissant P. Clinical dosimetry during cerebral angiography. *Neuroradiology*. 1980;20:79–81.
7. Kemerink GJ, Frantzen MJ, Oei K, et al. Patient and occupational dose in neurointerventional procedures. *Neuroradiology*. 2002;44:522–528.
8. Kuon E, Schmitt M, Dahm JB. Significant reduction of radiation exposure to operator and staff during cardiac interventions by analysis of radiation leakage and improved lead shielding. *Am J Cardiol*. 2002;89:44–49.
9. Layton KF, Kallmes DF, Cloft HJ, Schueler BA, Sturchio GM. Radiation exposure to the primary operator during endovascular surgical neuroradiology procedures. *Am J Neuroradiol*. 2006;27:742–743.
10. Bush WH, Swanson DP. Acute reactions to intravascular contrast media: types, risk factors, recognition, and specific treatment. *Am J Radiol*. 1991;157:1153–1161.
11. Greenberger PA, Patterson R. The prevention of immediate generalized reactions to radiocontrast media in high-risk patients. *J Allergy Clin Immunol*. 1991;87:867–872.
12. American College of Radiology. *Manual on Contrast Media*. 4th ed. Reston, VA: ACR; 1998.
13. From AM, Bartholmai BJ, Williams AW, Cha SS, McDonald FS. Mortality associated with nephropathy after radiographic contrast exposure. *Mayo Clin Proc*. 2008;83:1095–1100.
14. Tepel M, Van DerGiet M, Schwarzfeld C, et al. Prevention of radiographic-contrast-agent-induced reductions in renal function by acetylcysteine. *N Engl J Med*. 2000;343:180–184.
15. Merten GJ, Burgess WP, Gray LV, et al. Prevention of contrast-induced nephropathy with sodium bicarbonate: a randomized controlled trial. *JAMA*. 2004;291:2328–2334.
16. Liu AY, Lopez JR, Do HM, et al. Neurophysiological monitoring in the endovascular therapy of aneurysms. *Am J Neuroradiol*. 2003;24:1520–1527.
17. Lopez JR. Intraoperative neuropsychological monitoring. *Int Anesthesiol Clin*. 1996;34:33–54.
18. Dion JE, Gates PC, Fox AJ, et al. Clinical events following neuroangiography: a prospective study. *Stroke*. 1987;18:997–1004.
19. Carey D, Martins JR, Moore CA, et al. Complications of femoral artery closure devices. *Cathet Cardiovasc Interv*. 2001;52:3–7.
20. Molyneux A, Kerr R, Stratton I, et al. International Subarachnoid Aneurysm Trial (ISAT) of neurosurgical clipping versus endovascular coiling in 2143 patients with ruptured intracranial aneurysms: a randomised trial. *Lancet*. 2002;26:1267–1274.
21. Brisman JL, Niimi Y, Song JK, Berenstein A. Aneurysmal rupture during coiling: low incidence and good outcomes at a single large volume center. *Neurosurgery*. 2008;62(6)(suppl 3):1538–1551.
22. Workman MJ, Cloft HJ, Tong FC, et al. Thrombus formation at the neck of cerebral aneurysms during treatment with Guglielmi detachable coils. *Am J Neuroradiol*. 2002;23(9):1568–1576.
23. Gralla J, Rennie AT, Corkill RA, et al. Abciximab for thrombolysis during intracranial aneurysm coiling. *Neuroradiology*. 2008;50:1041–1047.
24. Jones RG, Davagnanam I, Colley S, West RJ, Yates DA. Abciximab for treatment of thromboembolic complications during endovascular coiling of intracranial aneurysms. *Am J Neuroradiol*. 2008;29:1925–1929.
25. Katsaridis V, Papagiannaki C, Skoulios N, Achoulias I, Peios D. Local intra-arterial eptifibatide for intraoperative vessel thrombosis during aneurysm coiling. *Am J Neuroradiol*. 2008;29:1414–1417.

26. Yi HJ, Gupta R, Jovin TG, et al. Initial experience with the use of intravenous eptifibatide bolus during endovascular treatment of intracranial aneurysms. *Am J Neuroradiol.* 2006;27:1856–1860.
27. Feng L, Fitzsimmons BF, Young WL, et al. Intraarterially administered verapamil as adjunct therapy for cerebral vasospasm: safety and 2-year experience. *Am J Neuroradiol.* 2002;23:1284–1290.
28. Keuskamp J, Murali R, Chao KH: High-dose intraarterial verapamil in the treatment of cerebral vasospasm after aneurismal subarachnoid hemorrhage. *J Neurosurg.* 2008;108:458–463.
29. Badjatia N, Topcuoglu MA, Pryor JC, et al. Preliminary experience with intra-arterial nicardipine as a treatment for cerebral vasospasm. *Am J Neuroradiol.* 2004;25:819–826.
30. Biondi A, Ricciardi GK, Puybasset L, et al. Intra-arterial nimodipine for the treatment of symptomatic cerebral vasospasm after aneurysmal subarachnoid hemorrhage: preliminary results. *Am J Neuroradiol.* 2004;25:1067–1076.
31. Megyesi JF, Findlay JM, Vollrath B, et al. In vivo angioplasty prevents the development of vasospasm in canine carotid arteries. Pharmacological and morphological analyses. *Stroke.* 1997;28:1216–1224.
32. Muizelaar JP, Zwienenberg M, Rudisill NA, et al. The prophylactic use of transluminal balloon angioplasty in patients with Fisher grade 3 subarachnoid hemorrhage: a pilot study. *J Neurosurg.* 1999;91:51–58.
33. Crawford PM, West CR, Chadwick DW, et al. Arteriovenous malformations of the brain: natural history in unoperated patients. *J Neurol Neurosurg Psychiatry.* 1986;49:1–10.
34. Ondra SL, Troupp H, George ED, et al. The natural history of symptomatic arteriovenous malformations of the brain: a 24-year follow-up assessment. *J Neurosurg.* 1990;73:387–391.
35. Meisel HJ, Mansmann U, Alvarez H, et al. Cerebral arteriovenous malformations and associated aneurysms: analysis of 305 cases from a series of 662 patients. *Neurosurgery.* 2000;46:793–800.
36. Haw CS, terBrugge K, Willinsky R, et al. Complications of embolization of arteriovenous malformations of the brain. *J Neurosurg.* 2006;104:226–232.
37. Spetzler RF, Wilson CB, Weinstein P, et al. Normal perfusion pressure breakthrough theory. *Clin Neurosurg.* 1978;25:651–672.
38. Arteriovenous Malformation Study Group. Arteriovenous malformations of the brain in adults. *N Engl J Med.* 1999;18:1812–1818.
39. National Institute of Neurological Disorders and Stroke rt-PA Stroke Study Group. Tissue plasminogen activator for acute ischemic stroke. *N Engl J Med.* 1995;333:1581–1587.
40. Wolpert S, Bruckmann H, Greenlee R, et al. Neuroradiologic evaluation of patients with acute stroke treated with recombinant tissue plasminogen activator. *Am J Neuroradiol.* 1993;14:3–13.
41. Lima FO, Furie KL, Silva GS, et al. Prognosis of untreated strokes due to anterior circulation proximal intracranial arterial occlusions detected by use of computed tomography angiography. *JAMA Neurol.* 2014;71:151–157.
42. Berkhemer OA, Fransen PS, Beumer D, et al. A randomized trial of intraarterial treatment for acute ischemic stroke. *N Engl J Med.* 2015;372:11–20.
43. Goyal M, Demchuk AM, Menon BK, et al. Ranomized assessment of rapid endovascular treatment of ischemic stroke. *N Engl J Med.* 2015;372:1019–1030.
44. Jovin TG, Chamorr A, Cobo E, et al. Thrombectomy within 8 hours after symptom onset in ischemic stroke. *N Engl J Med.* 2015;372:2296–306.
45. Saver JL, Goyal M, Bonafe A, et al. SWIFT PRIME Investigators. Stent-retriever thrombectomy after intravenous t-PA vs. t-PA alone in stroke. *N Engl J Med.* 2015;372:2285–2295.
46. Campbell BC, Mitchell PJ, Kleinig TJ, et al. Endovascular therapy for ischemic stroke with perfusion-imaging selection. *N Engl J Med.* 2015;372:1009–1018.
47. Smith WS, Sung G, Starkman S, et al. Safety and efficacy of mechanical embolectomy in acute ischemic stroke: results of the MERCI trial. *Stroke.* 2005;36:1432–1438.
48. Smith WS, Sung G, Saver J, et al. Mechanical thrombectomy for acute ischemic stroke: final results of the Multi MERCI trial. *Stroke.* 2008;39:1205–1212.
49. Bose A, Henkes H, et al. for the Penumbra Phase 1 Stroke Trial Investigators. The Penumbra System: a mechanical device for the treatment of acute stroke due to thromboembolism. *Am J Neuroradiol.* 2008;29:1409–1414.
50. Saver JL, Jahan R, Levy EI, et al. Solitaire flow restoration device versus Merci retriever in patients with acute ischaemic stroke (SWIFT): a randomised, parallel group, non-inferiority trial. *Lancet.* 2012;380:1241–1249.
51. Nogueira RG, Lutsep HL, Gupta R, et al. Trevo versus MERCI retrievers for thrombectomy revascularization of large vessel occlusions in acute ischaemic stroke (TREVO 2): a randomised trial. *Lancet.* 2012;380:1231–1240.

14 | INTERVENTIONAL RADIOLOGY PROCEDURES

LESLIE B. SCORZA, MD, FSIR

INTRODUCTION

The specialty of interventional radiology (IR) is called on often to help solve many different clinical problems. Despite its recognized value, IR has always suffered somewhat from a recognition problem. The specialty has been known under many different names and acronyms; most of these persist today. Examples include the following:

1. Interventional radiology
2. IR
3. Cardiovascular and interventional radiology
4. CVI (cardiovascular imaging)
5. CVIR (cardiovascular and interventional radiology)
6. Angio
7. Special procedures
8. CVI/R (Cardiovascular Imaging/Radiology)
9. Vascular radiology

Even the specialty's major society, the Society of Interventional Radiology (SIR; sometimes pronounced as in Yes, Sir) has gone through name changes. Formerly, it was known as the Society of Cardiovascular and Interventional Radiology (SCVIR; pronounced "skiver," rhymes with "shiver"). Before that, the society began in 1973 as the Society of Cardiovascular Radiology or SCVR.[1]

To this day, when asked, "What do you do?" many practitioners of IR will simply reply, "I am a physician." If the questioner persists, the next question will often be, "What type of practice?" When the words "interventional radiology" are given in response, too many of us are confronted with a relatively blank stare, all due to the recognition problem of IR.

This chapter is an effort to correct some of that recognition problem and to offer a summary, albeit incomplete, of the scope of practice of interventional radiologists. Clarification of the spectrum of IR cases is appropriate before further discussions in subsequent chapters of the anesthetic needs for such cases. Please note that lists of indications and contraindications are not intended to be exhaustive. Discussions of complications center on those acute complications that will be of particular interest to providers administering off-site anesthesia for these cases. Specific anesthetic considerations for radiologic procedures are discussed in Chapter 15.

Before describing the practice of IR physicians, some details about these practitioners themselves might be helpful. A survey of radiologists in 2003 with a special focus on interventional radiologists was performed by the American College of Radiology and was published in 2005.[2] Some interesting findings from that study included the following:

- About 10% of radiologists called themselves *interventional radiologists.*
- Less than one-half of those who called themselves interventional radiologists actually did IR cases more than 70% of the time.
- Interventional radiologists worked more hours than their non-IR counterparts.
- Fewer than 6% of IRs were female.
- The average age for interventional radiologists was the mid- to late 40s.

Another important point is that the percentage of practitioners who perform IR procedures *and who are radiologists* continues to decrease. Cardiologists, vascular surgeons, general surgeons, neurosurgeons, as well as some nephrologists, urologists, and even neurologists today perform some cases previously performed almost exclusively by interventional radiologists. That fact may have ramifications for those providing anesthesia for some of these cases because the operators' expectations of those providing anesthesia may vary based on their backgrounds.

To return to the initial focus of this chapter, the question must be asked: What kinds of procedures are in fact performed in IR? To sum it up simply, in IR we perform a vast array of diagnostic and interventional procedures, mostly through *very small holes.*

Examples discussed in the subsequent sections of this chapter include

- Abscess drainage
- Arterial procedures and interventions

- Biliary procedures and interventions
- Gastrointestinal (GI) procedures and interventions
- Genitourinary (GU) procedures and interventions
- Intraoperative cases (e.g., thoracic and abdominal aortic stent grafts)
- Noninvasive vascular imaging
- Percutaneous oncologic interventions
- Percutaneous biopsies
- Venous procedures and interventions
- Venous access

ABSCESS DRAINAGE

An abscess is a collection of pus that has formed in a confined space in the body in response to an infection. The confined space can be an organ or simply body tissue, and abscesses can arise in almost any location in the body. The contents of abscesses can include varying amounts of fluid, bacteria (usually), dead and dying tissue, live and dying neutrophils, and other debris. Abscesses can be related to disease processes (e.g., appendicitis and diverticulitis) or trauma, or they may be postoperative.

Postoperative abscesses are more common with contaminated surgical procedures, but even "clean" procedures can occasionally result in abscess formation. Treatment includes antibiotics (which do not readily penetrate the abscess cavity but do treat the surrounding inflammation and infection) and drainage.

Some abscesses need no image guidance (Figure 14.1) to allow effective drainage. Surgical incision and drainage is in many cases the preferred method, and when open drainage is performed, it is usually done by providers other than interventional radiologists.

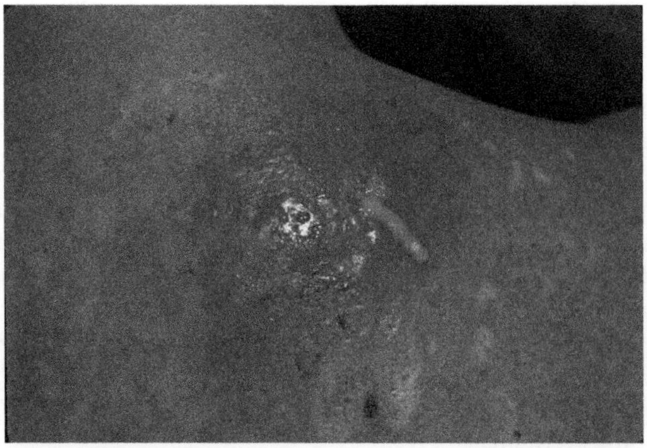

Figure 14.1. Superficial cutaneous abscess for which no imaging is needed for incision and drainage (I&D).

Suitable anesthesia (this can be local, regional, general, or some combination) is needed regardless of the method of drainage. From an IR standpoint, abscesses can be drained using several modalities, including

- Computed tomography (CT) (Figure 14.2)
- Ultrasound
- Fluoroscopy (Figure 14.3)
- Magnetic resonance (MR)
- Some combination

In all cases, the target area needs to be localized and identified. Also, important nontarget structures (e.g., large vessels, bowel, lung, and other viscera) must be identified and avoided in the planned path of access. Imaging aids greatly in both identifying the target and avoiding undesired structures.

The use of a disposable metallic grid in a CT scan can help identify positioning. In ultrasound and fluoroscopy, structures are visualized in real time during access. Magnetic resonance is used less frequently because special (translation: *expensive*) nonferromagnetic equipment must be employed. In some cases, a procedure may be begun with one modality (e.g., CT or ultrasound), and once access is established, the procedure may be completed with fluoroscopic guidance.

Acute complications from abscess drainage include

1. Acute infection/sepsis from disrupted abscess
2. Injury to undesired target, which can lead to bleeding, bowel injury, peritonitis, or pneumothorax

ARTERIAL PROCEDURES AND INTERVENTIONS

Arterial procedures can be performed purely for diagnostic purposes or they may be therapeutic in nature. Most purely diagnostic procedures do not require more than sedation and analgesia (moderate sedation). Some of the more complex procedures may indeed require a more intensive level of anesthesia support. Currently, many purely diagnostic arterial evaluations are performed through the use of CT angiography which avoids arterial puncture completely.

Arteriography represents the purely diagnostic arterial procedures. In these procedures, the patient is generally placed supine on the angiography table. The planned site of entry is prepped and draped using sterile technique. After the administration of local anesthesia, access into the arterial system is gained with a needle and a wire. Most commonly, access is gained via the common femoral artery, but other access sites can be used as well. The most common alternate site is the brachial artery, left preferable to right (fewer great vessel origins are crossed from the left). Radial artery access is used in coronary angiography, but the small vessel size and distance to

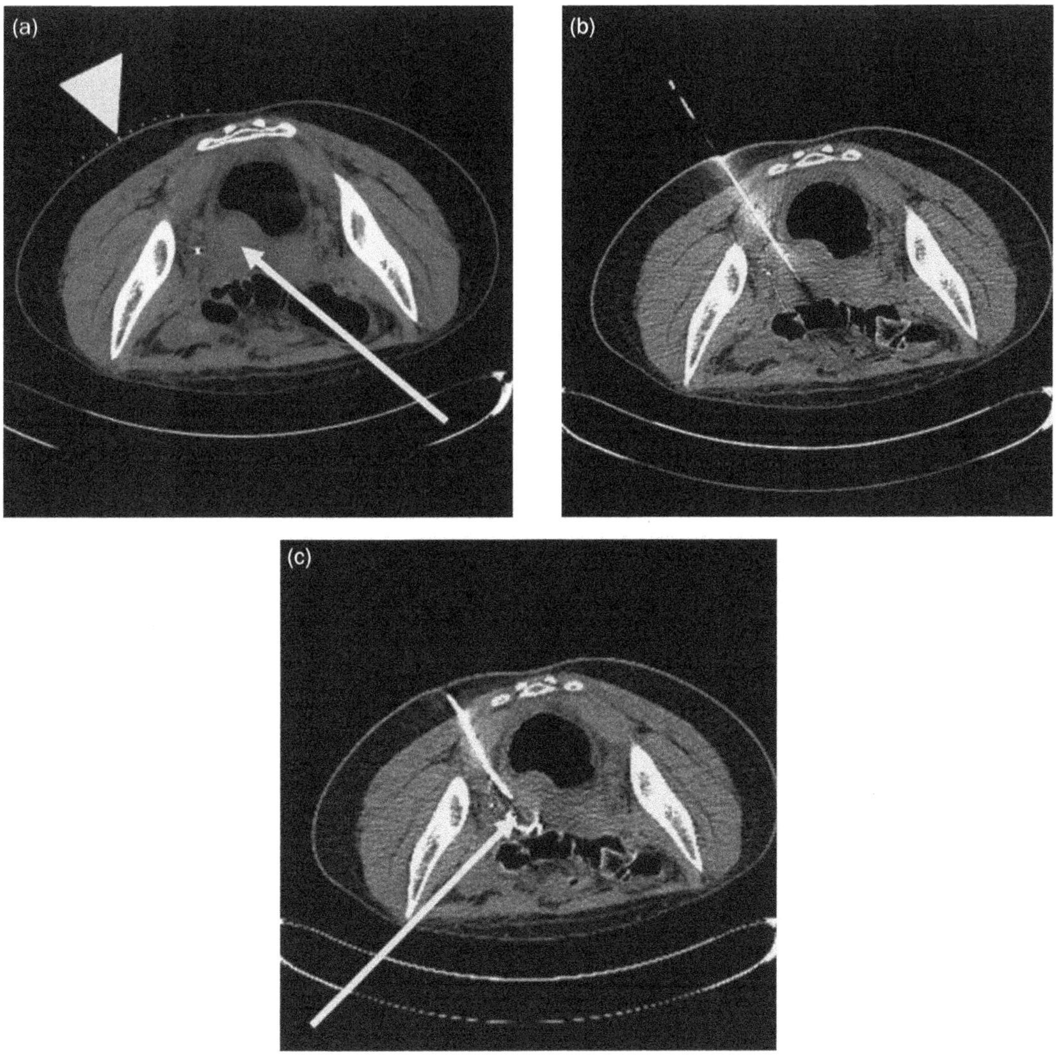

Figure 14.2. *Computed tomography (CT)–guided abscess drainage. (a) Prone CT scan with metallic grid (arrowhead) in place; the abscess is identified (arrow). (b) Prone CT scan with narrow-gauge finder needle in place. (c) Prone CT scan demonstrating drain within abscess collection; the Cope loop (arrow) of the drainage catheter has been formed.*

common arterial targets might preclude its use in peripheral arterial procedures, although some IRs currently do employ radial access.

A sheath with a hemostatic valve may be inserted at the operator's discretion. Reasons to use a sheath are listed next. Catheters of varying shapes, sizes, materials, and hole configurations (some have only a single end hole, while others have many additional side holes) are inserted and navigated to the desired locations. Contrast is injected, either by hand or using a power injector, while imaging is acquired. In many institutions, much diagnostic arteriography has been replaced with CT angiography (CTA), which is discussed further in this chapter.

Some reasons to use a vascular sheath (Figure 14.4) include

1. Planned frequent catheter exchanges
2. Planned intervention (reduces injury to the vessel or damage to devices)
3. Scarred access site (when in the common femoral artery, it is known as the "hostile groin")
4. When the sheath is needed for arterial pressure monitoring during the case
5. When the operator is working alone
6. A deep groin in an obese patient
7. Heavily calcified vessels (minimizes trauma with catheter exchanges)
8. Planned repeat intervention in the near future (e.g., thrombolysis)

Cut-film imaging has been nearly completely supplanted by digital subtraction angiography (DSA). When acquiring images during DSA, one or more images are acquired before the introduction of contrast material to serve as a "mask." Then, the contrast is injected while the patient remains

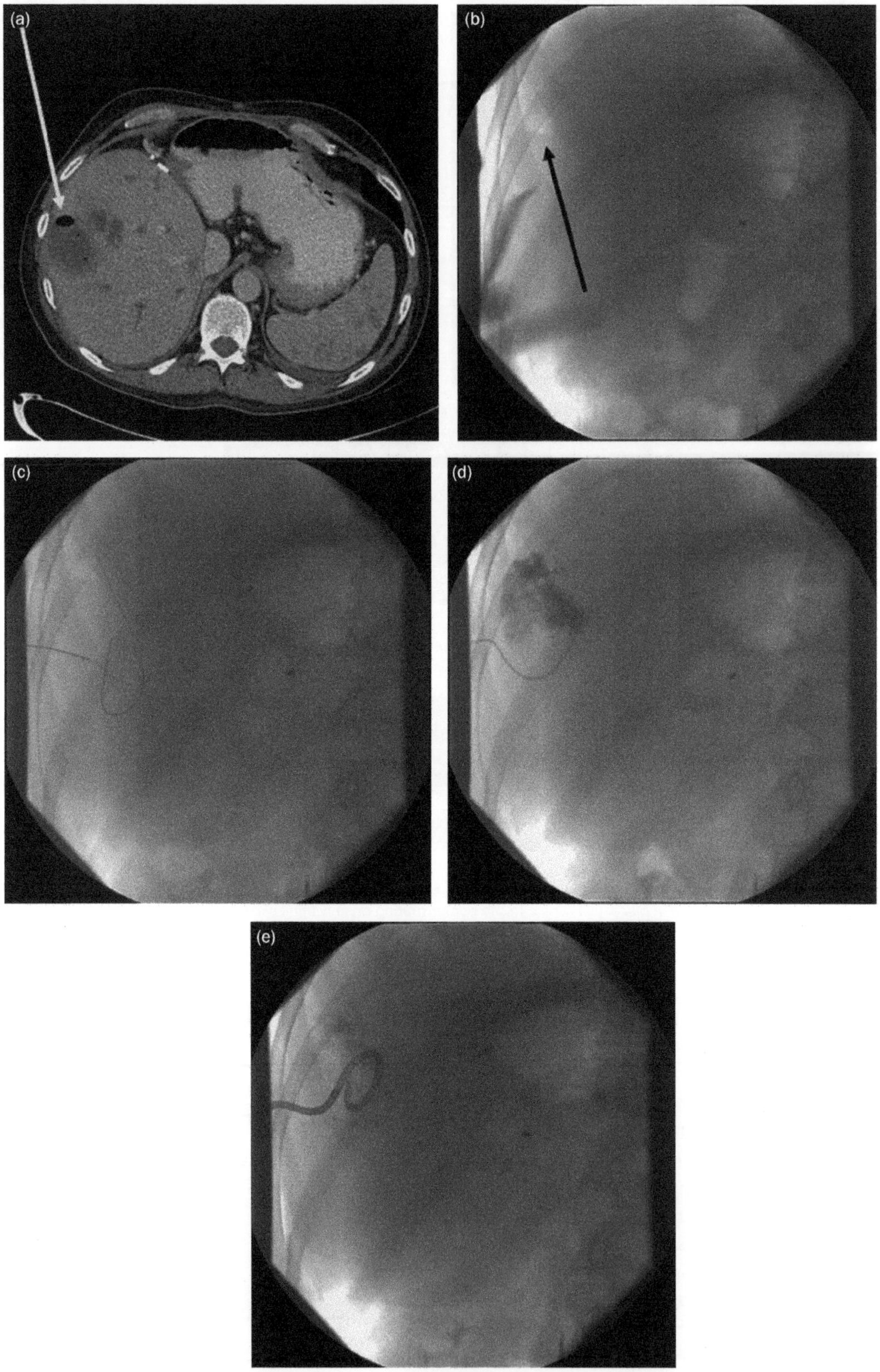

Figure 14.3. *Fluoroscopy-guided abscess drainage. (a) Supine computed tomography (CT) scan identifying intrahepatic abscess with air (arrow). (b) Supine fluoroscopic image demonstrating same air pocket (arrow). (c) Fluoroscopic image demonstrating needle into fluid collection below air with wire (through a needle) coiled in collection. (d) Contrast injected through micropuncture catheter confirming positioning within abscess. (e) Drainage catheter (with Cope loop coiled) within abscess.*

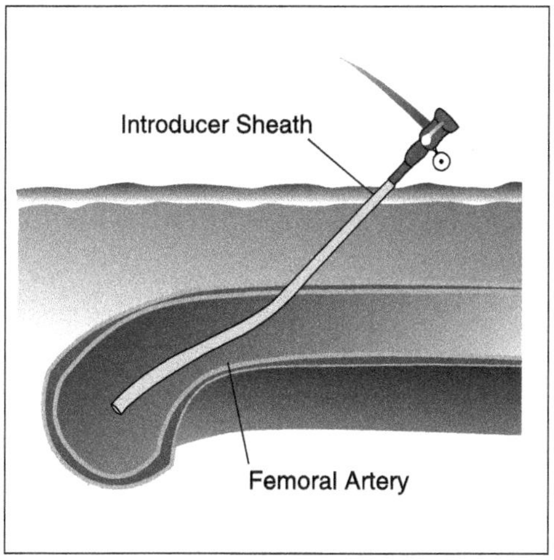

Figure 14.4. *Vascular sheath. (Used with permission from Vascular Solutions, Inc.)*

motionless. Using a noncontrast image as a mask, its findings are digitally subtracted from the findings on the postcontrast imaging. The difference in the before and after images results in a depiction of the newly contrast-filled arteries. This technique can be quite accurate with excellent resolution; however, it is negatively affected by patient motion.

There are many indications for diagnostic arteriography, including

1. Evaluation of the extent of atherosclerotic disease
2. Evaluation of ischemia
3. Evaluation of the arterial supply to a neoplasm, vascular anomaly, or planned flap
4. Evaluation for presence and extent of arterial trauma

In some instances, the diagnostic information obtained will serve as a preoperative guide for the surgeon. In other cases, the intervention will be performed percutaneously, either at the same time or at a separate sitting.

Contraindications to diagnostic arteriography include gross hemodynamic instability, uncorrectable bleeding diathesis, prior severe reaction to iodinated contrast material, and significant renal insufficiency (unless dialysis is planned). A patient who cannot control his or her breathing or remain still may be imaged, but anesthesia support may be required.

Arterial interventions can include

- Percutaneous transluminal angioplasty (PTA)
- Arterial stenting
- Thrombolytic therapy
- Embolic therapy

Percutaneous transluminal angioplasty (Figure 14.5) and arterial stenting are mechanisms to dilate arteries that have become stenotic or even occluded. In these techniques, the precise location of the significant stenosis to be treated is identified angiographically, and its significance may be confirmed with hemodynamic (pressure) measurements. Intravenous heparin is usually administered prior to crossing the stenosis. Next, a catheter and wire are passed through and beyond the stenosis. In the case of an occlusion, the occluded segment may actually be recanalized (this can be through the occlusion itself or in a subintimal plane) with a small catheter and wire.

The catheter is removed, leaving the wire in position. Over this wire, an angioplasty balloon (generally about 20% larger than the native vessel) or a stent (equal to or up to about 10% larger than the native vessel) of appropriate size is positioned. The balloon is inflated and held in position, usually for 1 to 2 minutes. In the case of a stent, it is deployed at the correct site. If it is a "self-expanding" stent, it is allowed to open and then angioplastied with a balloon as needed; if it is a "balloon-mounted" stent, then inflation of the included balloon deploys and expands the stent to the desired size. In all cases, follow-up arteriography is mandatory to evaluate the result.

Thrombolytic therapy (Figure 14.6) is utilized to dissolve or lyse a thrombus in blood vessels, and these vessels can be arteries, veins, or artificial conduits. A thrombus is most readily and successfully treated early during its course. Many thrombolytic agents available today are enzymes that work by converting plasminogen to the natural fibrinolytic plasmin. Plasmin lyses a clot by breaking down fibrin and other compounds contained in the clot. Various agents are currently utilized, among them alteplase (recombinant tissue plasminogen activator or r-tPA), urokinase, tenecteplase, and reteplase. Streptokinase is not used much in the United States.

With thrombolytic therapy, higher success rates are achieved when a wire can be passed through the clotted segment, a technique known as the *wire traversal test.* Once the wire is confirmed to be intravascular and beyond the thrombosed segment, a special catheter designed for thrombolysis is positioned just into the clot, with its infusion segment spanning as much of the clot as possible. Thrombolytic agent is infused at specified rates and for specified durations, after which additional angiography is performed. These subsequent results guide whether catheter repositioning, continuation of thrombolysis, cessation of thrombolysis, or additional treatment (e.g., angioplasty, stenting, or surgical intervention) is warranted.

Indications for thrombolytic therapy include

1. Thrombosis of native vessel (arterial or venous)
2. Thrombosis of conduit vessel, including venous bypass graft, prosthetic bypass graft, or dialysis graft
3. Embolization of thrombus occurring during percutaneous thrombolysis or open surgical procedure

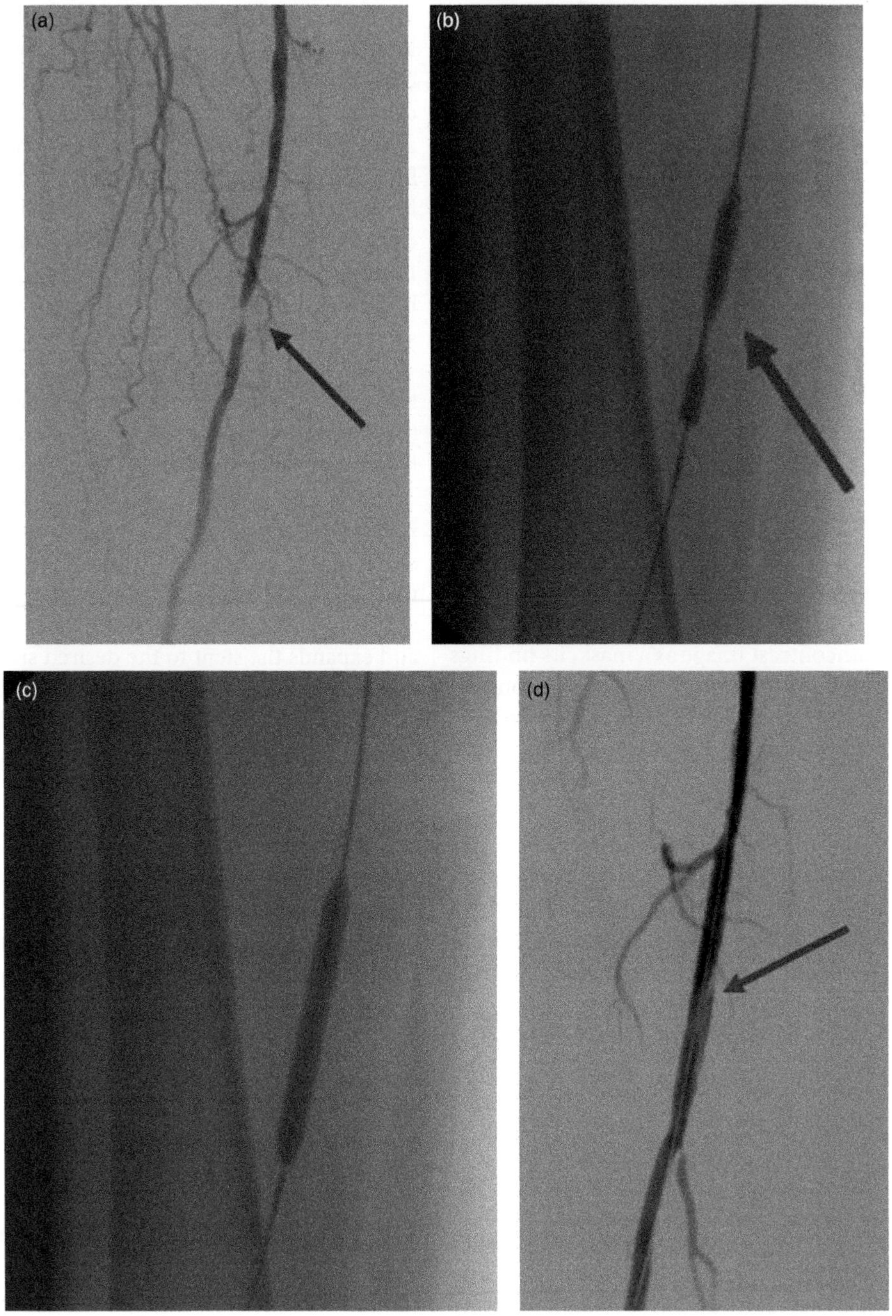

Figure 14.5. (a) Digital subtraction angiography (DSA) image of the distal right superficial femoral artery (SFA) with high-grade stenosis (arrow). (b) Angioplasty balloon partially inflated demonstrating stenosis at the "waist" (arrow). (c) Angioplasty balloon fully inflated demonstrating no residual stenosis. (d) Follow-up postangioplasty image showing resolution of stenosis; a small dissection flap (arrow) was not flow limiting.

Contraindications to thrombolytic therapy include

1. Active bleeding (e.g., GI bleeding, bleeding ulcer) or uncorrected bleeding diathesis
2. Recent bleeding (e.g., recent surgery or trauma, recent hemorrhagic stroke)
3. Pregnancy
4. Previous allergic reaction to thrombolytic agent
5. Known intracranial neoplasm or vascular malformation
6. Suspected aortic dissection
7. A nonviable extremity

With embolization therapy (Figure 14.7), various agents can be used to effect either permanent or temporary occlusion of blood vessels, more commonly of arteries but also of veins. Among the agents that have been used are the following:

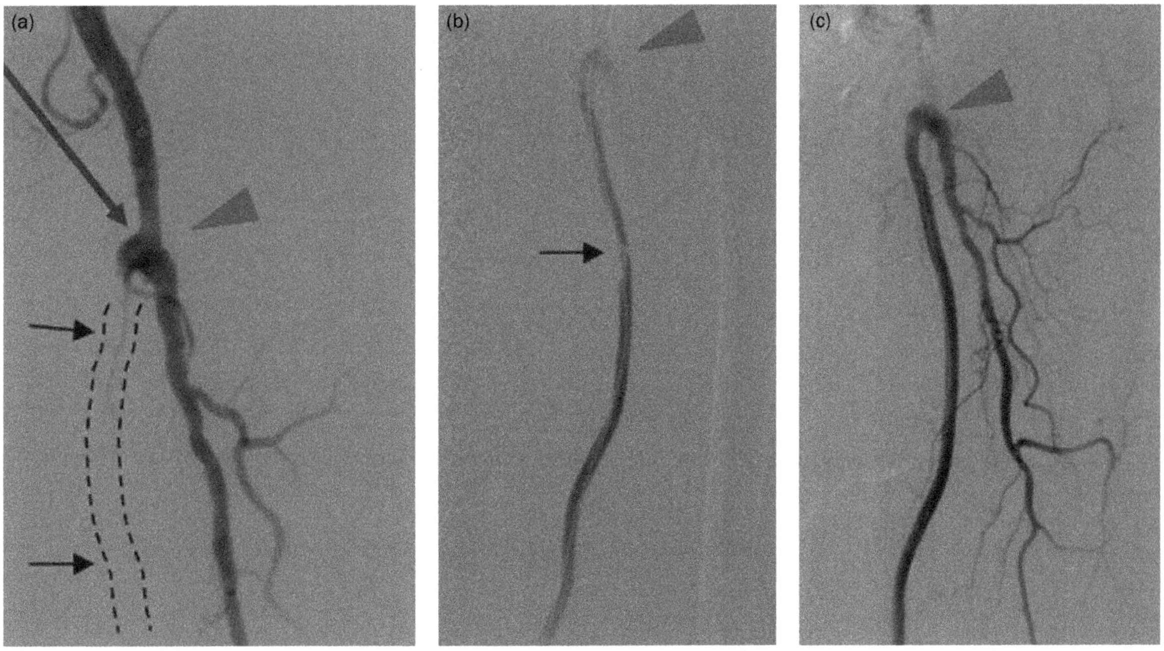

Figure 14.6. *(a) Occluded femoral-to-distal graft (short arrows and dashed lines show path of the occluded graft); stump of occluded graft (long arrow) guides placement of the thrombolysis catheter. (b) Partial thrombolysis noted after 7 hours; some clot still present (short arrow). (c) After 24 hours, graft is now completely eradicated of clot; a distal lesion (not shown) was treated with angioplasty. Note that the arrowhead points to the same anatomic location in each image.*

- Permanent agents
- Polyvinyl alcohol (PVA)—particles or spheres
- Absolute alcohol
- Sodium tetradecyl sulfate (Sotradecol®; Bioniche Pharma, USA, Inc., Bogart, GA)
- Coils (platinum or steel)
- Balloons
- Glue (*N*-butyl cyanoacrylate or NBCA, known as TRUFILL®; Cordis Neurovascular, Miami Lakes, FL)
- Onyx® liquid embolic system (ev3, Inc., Plymouth, MN)
- 50% glucose
- Boiling contrast
- Silk thread
- Temporary agents
- Gelfoam (as a slurry or as "torpedoes") (Pharmacia and Upjohn Company, Kalamazoo, MI)
- Autologous blood

Sites/reasons for embolization therapy may include

- Trauma
- GI hemorrhage
- Hemoptysis
- Spontaneous bleeding (e.g., rectus sheath hematoma)
- Postoperative or postpartum bleeding
- Vascular anomalies
- Varicoceles/pelvic congestion
- Uterine arteries for fibroids
- Aneurysms
- Chemoembolization or radioembolization (^{90}Y) for cancer treatment.

Arterial embolization techniques involve arteriography to identify the artery or arteries to be treated. A catheter is positioned as close to the desired site as is feasible. The embolic agent is carefully administered, taking care to avoid reflux into uninvolved vessels or embolization of undesired vessels ("nontarget embolization"). As with other arterial interventions, follow-up arteriography is mandatory to evaluate efficacy. Venous embolization is carried out similarly, although often a tourniquet is applied to control outflow if the treatment site is an extremity.

Acute complications for diagnostic arterial procedures are relatively infrequent, but they can include

1. Bleeding from the entry site or other vessel
2. Thrombosis at the entry site or other vessel
3. Embolus from thrombus
4. Dissection (which may be flow limiting)
5. Contrast reaction

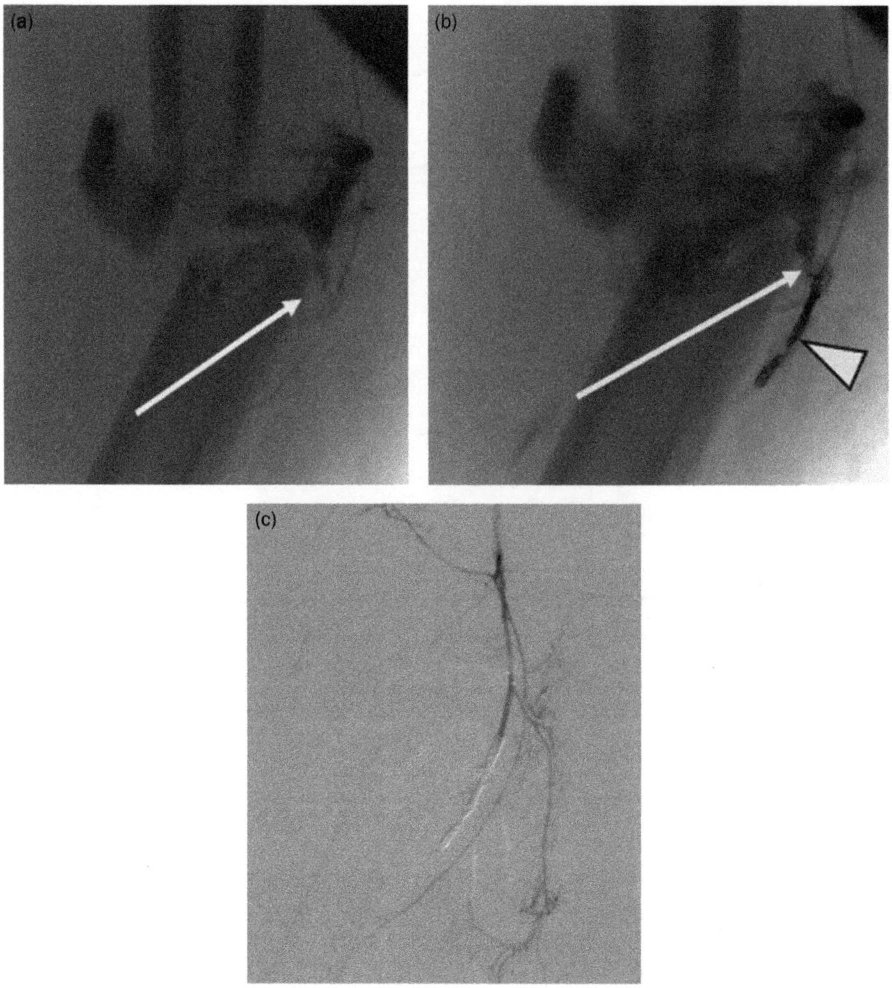

Figure 14.7. *(a) Extravasation (arrow) from injured artery near site of femur fracture; image is unsubtracted. (b) After deposition of some coils (arrowhead), there is still extravasation (arrow) from injured artery near site of femur fracture; image is unsubtracted. (c) After completion of coil embolization, no further extravasation is seen on this digital subtraction angiography (DSA) image.*

With the addition of interventions to the diagnostic arterial procedure, the complications include those just listed, as well as the following:

1. With thrombolysis, unrelated bleeding may ensue (e.g., intracranial, GI).
2. With embolization procedures, nontarget embolization may occur.
3. Angioplasty or stenting can result in vessel disruption.

BILIARY PROCEDURES AND INTERVENTIONS

The biliary system may be accessed via direct puncture through the liver, or diagnostic information related to the biliary system may be obtained by a transvenous route. Biliary procedures performed by direct puncture include percutaneous transhepatic cholangiography and percutaneous transhepatic biliary drainage.

Indications for diagnostic percutaneous biliary procedures include

1. Evaluation for source of obstructive jaundice (including stone, mass, or stricture)
2. Evaluation of medically treatable jaundice
3. Determination of the etiology of cholangitis
4. Determination of the location of a bile duct leak (if endoscopic retrograde cholangiopancreatography [ERCP] cannot do so)
5. Evaluation for presence and extent of biliary ductal system abnormalities (e.g., choledochal cysts or atresias)

Contraindications to percutaneous biliary procedures include

1. Uncorrectable bleeding diathesis
2. Previous severe reaction to iodinated contrast
3. Hydatid disease, documented or suspected

4. Large vascular hepatic lesions (tumors or vascular malformations)
5. Extensive undrained ascites
6. Severe contrast reaction that has not been pretreated

The technique of biliary drainage (Figure 14.8) involves placing the patient supine on the angiography table. The right arm should be placed above the head. Intravenous sedation (or general anesthesia, if indicated) is administered. A suitable lateral location in the midaxillary line at or below the 10th intercostal space (to minimize pleural transgression) is identified using fluoroscopy. Local anesthesia is instilled. A long 22-gauge Chiba needle is inserted obliquely into the hepatic parenchyma. With magnified fluoroscopic visualization, contrast is gently instilled as the needle is slowly withdrawn.

The goal is to opacify a bile duct and then the entire biliary ductal system. Structures other than bile ducts that may be opacified include hepatic parenchyma, portal vein branches, hepatic vein branches, hepatic arterial branches (not particularly common), the gallbladder, lymphatics, and even extrahepatic structures (inferior vena cava [IVC], aorta, peritoneal cavity, and right kidney). If the first attempt is unsuccessful, additional attempts with slightly altered angulations are performed until a bile duct is opacified.

Once a bile duct is opacified, additional contrast is instilled while multiple images are acquired. If intervention is warranted, a suitable duct (assuming the duct entered for the initial cholangiogram was not suitable) for definitive access is identified. Using complex angulation, that duct can be entered with a separate needle-stick. A guidewire is carefully advanced into the ductal system. The needle is exchanged for a transitional dilator set or a directional catheter, as indicated. Conversion to a drainage catheter can follow.

Another percutaneous biliary procedure is cholecystostomy tube placement. In patients with acute cholecystitis who are unsuitable for operative intervention, gallbladder drainage can be performed with temporary amelioration of symptoms. The patient is placed in a position similar to the position for biliary drainage. The gallbladder is identified with imaging (ultrasound is commonly used, but CT or fluoroscopy alone can be used). The gallbladder is accessed with a needle (which should traverse some hepatic parenchyma to allow closure of the tract when the tube is removed) and then a guidewire. Over the wire, an appropriate drainage catheter is placed and secured.

Transvenous (usually transjugular, but the transfemoral route can sometimes be used as well) hepatic and biliary procedures include hepatic venography, hepatic hemodynamic pressure measurement, liver biopsy (these three are often performed at one sitting, referred to by some as a "hepatic triple package"), and transjugular intrahepatic portosystemic shunt (TIPS) creation.

Indications for hepatic venography and hemodynamic evaluation include suspicion for hepatic venous pathology (e.g., Budd-Chiari syndrome) and determination of the presence and severity of portal hypertension. Random liver biopsies can be obtained at the same time.

For most cases, sedation and analgesia (moderate sedation) are sufficient. With the patient supine and head slightly to the left, ultrasound is used to identify and subsequently access the right internal jugular (IJ) vein. Through the access needle, a wire is inserted with fluoroscopic guidance. Ultimately, a long vascular sheath is inserted. Through this sheath, access through the right atrium into the IVC is gained. An angled catheter is used to engage a right or middle hepatic vein (the left can be chosen as well). Contrast hepatic venography is performed. Simultaneous

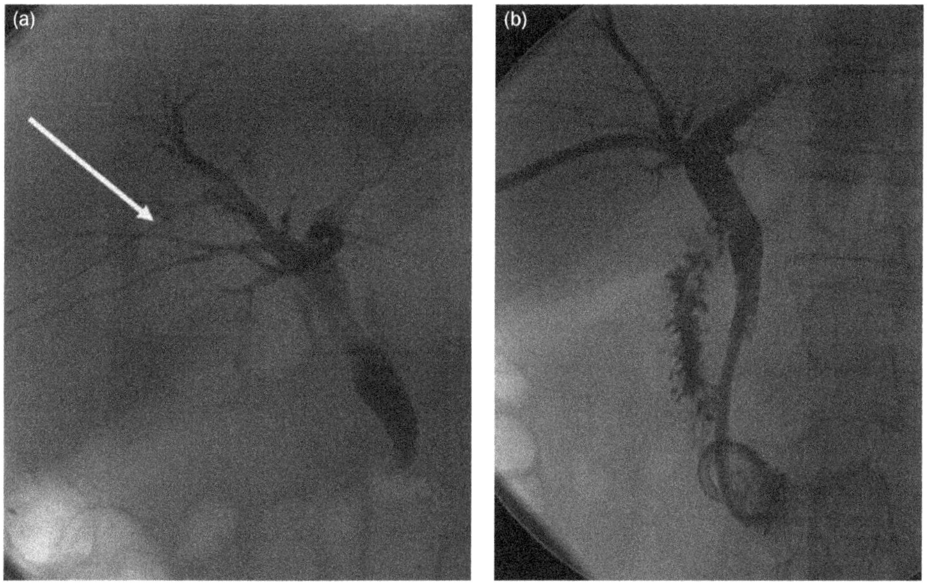

Figure 14.8. *(a) Chiba needle (arrow) has been used to access and opacify the biliary ducts; the point of entry is in a right anterior duct. (b) After separate access into a right posterior duct, this access was converted to a drainage catheter (its Cope loop is coiled in the duodenum).*

right atrial (via the sheath) and free (i.e., not yet wedged) hepatic venous (via the catheter) pressures are measured.

Next, the catheter is advanced over a wire to a wedged position in the periphery of the hepatic vein. The wedged position allows an indirect estimate of the portal venous pressure in a manner similar to the way pulmonary capillary wedge pressure approximates left atrial pressure. The sheath can either remain positioned in the right atrium or be advanced into the free hepatic vein position. Additional hemodynamic measurements are made. The corrected sinusoidal pressure (CSP), which is the difference between wedged and free pressures, determines the presence and severity of portal hypertension.

Creation of a portosystemic shunt can be performed percutaneously via the transjugular route. Indications and contraindications are listed next.

Indications for TIPS creation can include (Figure 14.9)

1. Repeated episodes of esophageal variceal bleeding
2. Upper GI bleeding due to esophageal varices that have failed endoscopic treatments
3. As a "bridge" to liver transplantation to prevent variceal bleeding
4. Intractable ascites or hepatic hydrothorax

Contraindications to TIPS creation include

1. Preexisting hepatic encephalopathy
2. Failure of cessation of alcohol use (precluding subsequent liver transplantation)
3. Younger patients who may require years of portal decompression (although many of these are now managed with transplantation)
4. Significant heart failure, valvular disease, or pulmonary hypertension

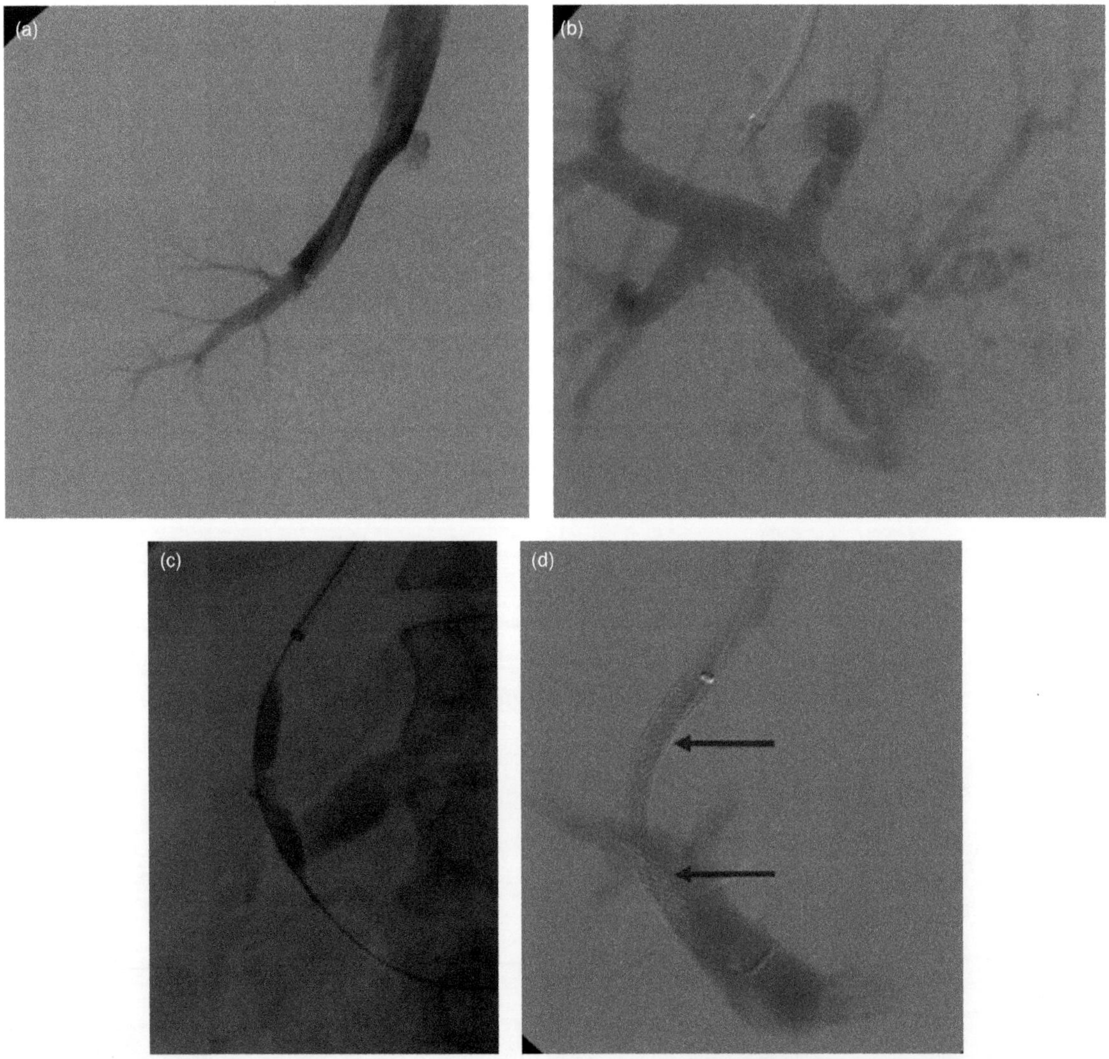

Figure 14.9. (a) A right-sided hepatic vein (later proven to be the middle hepatic vein) is injected with digital subtraction angiography (DSA) imaging. (b) After probing with the needle from the hepatic vein, a portal vein branch is identified; the portal system is opacified by a catheter passed into the main portal vein. (c) The hepatic parenchymal tract is dilated with an 8-mm × 4-cm angioplasty balloon. (d) The metallic stent (arrows) has been inserted spanning from the portal vein inferiorly, through the parenchymal tract, and into the hepatic vein more superiorly.

Technically, the procedure begins similarly to the hepatic venography described previously. However, these cases are generally longer and more painful. In our institution, we use general endotracheal anesthesia. Once access to the right hepatic vein (preferred) is obtained, the position of the right portal vein is estimated. Experience and cross-sectional imaging are helpful here; alternatively, injection of CO_2 or contrast from a wedged hepatic vein position may yield images of the portal vein. A newer adaptation is simultaneous transsplenic access to the portal venous system.

A special needle for this purpose is thrust anteriorly out of the right hepatic vein, through the hepatic parenchyma, and it is hoped into the portal vein (a maneuver sometimes jokingly referred to as the "poke and hope"). Aspiration is performed, and, if venous blood is returned, contrast is instilled to confirm successful entry into the portal venous system. If not, the technique is repeated using slightly different angulations (requiring more pokes and more hope) until entry into the portal venous system is obtained. Transsplenic access can be used to place a snare in the desired portal vein, thereby providing a target.

Once the portal venous system has been engaged, a guidewire and catheter are advanced into the portal vein. Hemodynamic measurements are made before creation of the portosystemic communication. The parenchymal tract is predilated with an angioplasty balloon. Ultimately, a metallic stent or, more commonly, a combined covered/uncovered stent (VIATORR®, W. L. Gore & Associates, Newark, DE) is inserted spanning from the portal venous end, through the parenchymal tract, and to the hepatic venous end near the IVC. Hemodynamic measurements are again made to determine reduction of the portosystemic gradient. Final contrast images should be obtained.

Another newer biliary procedure is portal vein embolization (PVE). PVE is performed in patients who are scheduled to undergo hepatic resection, but in whom insufficient liver volume would be left behind after resection. In these cases, the portal vein branches to the segments that contain the tumor are embolized. With the decrease in blood flow to those segments, the remaining segments that were not embolized are thereby stimulated to hypertrophy. In a matter of weeks, sufficient hypertrophy can occur so that the resection can proceed as planned, now leaving adequate hepatic parenchyma for sufficient postoperative liver function and patient survival.

Technically, PVE is initially prepared like a percutaneous biliary drainage. With adequate sedation and local anesthesia, passes through the liver are made with a long needle. Contrast is gently injected until portal vein branches, rather than bile ducts, are opacified. Once a portal vein branch is entered, a wire is advanced. Catheters and wires as appropriate are used to engage the desired portal vein branches. Transsplenic access can be used in PVE as well. Embolization is then performed with PVA and coils.

Acute complications from biliary interventions include

1. Bleeding into the tube tract from portal venous injury (more commonly than from hepatic arterial injury)
2. Bile leak
3. Bleeding from the liver capsule or skin
4. Pleural transgression (can result in hemothorax, pneumothorax, or bile in the thorax)
5. Contrast reaction

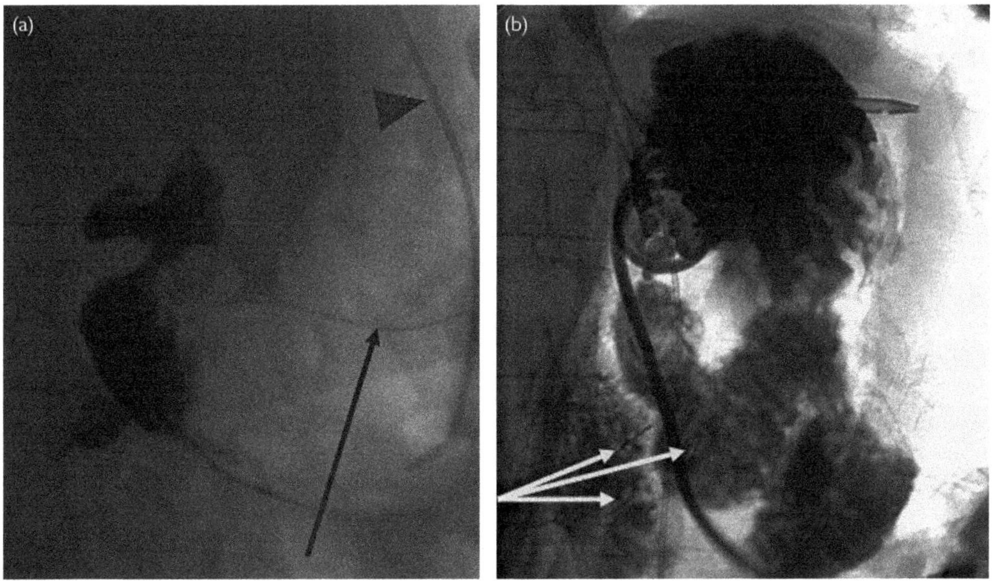

Figure 14.10. (a) The stomach has been distended with air delivered via a nasally placed 5-French catheter (arrowhead); a wire (arrow) has been inserted through a needle (not seen). (b) Three metallic gastropexy anchors (arrows) have been placed, as has a gastrostomy tube; there is contrast in the stomach, and peristalsis has brought contrast into small bowel loops as well.

GASTROINTESTINAL PROCEDURES AND INTERVENTIONS

Gastrointestinal interventions by interventional radiologists mostly consist of access procedures. The most common of these is percutaneous gastrostomy, although percutaneous gastrojejunostomy, percutaneous cecostomy, and direct percutaneous jejunostomy are performed as well.

Gastrostomy placement (Figure 14.10) usually requires distention of the stomach with air (by an existing or a temporarily placed nasogastric tube). Once the stomach is distended, fluoroscopy and possibly ultrasound are used to identify a path that will avoid important adjacent structures (particularly colon, liver, and lung).

Some practitioners perform gastropexy with specially designed gastropexy anchors, while others choose not to do so. Next, the stomach is entered with a needle, then a wire. Over the wire, the tract can be dilated, and then an appropriate tube (either a gastrostomy tube or a gastrojejunal tube) is placed.

Cecostomy and direct jejunostomy are performed similarly, but without the nasogastric tube. These can be a bit more challenging than gastric access. Another variation of GI procedures includes CT-guided gastrostomy into the distal gastric remnant after a gastric bypass procedure because the remnant is often already distended with air or fluid.

Acute complications from GI procedures include

1. Bleeding (from access site or from the entered viscus, usually stomach)
2. Peritonitis (from leak of gastric or other contents)
3. Transgression of undesired structures (e.g., colon, pleura, liver, spleen)

GENITOURINARY PROCEDURES AND INTERVENTIONS

Genitourinary interventions can be safely performed in the IR suite, usually with sedation and analgesia. Most commonly, direct access into the renal collecting system is requested. Access down the ureter into the bladder can be performed as well, leaving behind either an internal/external nephroureteral tube or abandoning external access and leaving only an internal double-J nephroureteral tube. Direct access into the bladder, via suprapubic cystostomy, is another GU procedure performed by IR practitioners. Balloon ureteroplasty can be performed for strictures, although subsequent prolonged stenting of ureters treated this way is required. Last, reverse nephroureteral tube placement or exchange via an ileal conduit (following cystectomy) can be performed.

With the exception of cystostomy and reverse nephroureteral tube procedures, most GU procedures performed in the IR suite require that the patient be prone. This positioning presents its own anesthetic and airway management issues.

The most frequent indication for nephrostomy tube placement is to divert urine in the face of obstruction, most commonly related to nephrolithiasis. Other less-common indications for nephrostomy tube placement include

- Access for other procedures, such as nephrolithotomy
- Diversion of urine and stenting of the ureter to allow healing after ureteral injury
- Treatment of complications related to renal transplantation
- Access for medication infusion, including chemotherapy and antimicrobial agents
- Treatment of urinary tract obstruction related to pregnancy

From a technical standpoint, percutaneous nephrostomy tube placement requires the patient to be prone except in very unusual circumstances. The three major steps can be reduced to *opacify/identify*, *access*, and *drain*.

To *opacify* the collecting system, contrast must be given. This can be done by administering intravenous contrast and waiting for the pyelographic phase of the intravenous urogram (usually 3 to 5 minutes) to identify the renal pelvis. Alternatively, direct puncture over the suspected region of the renal pelvis can be performed with a 22-gauge Chiba needle, using fluoroscopic guidance and bony (or calcified) landmarks. Ultrasound may help. Once the renal pelvis is entered, aspiration on the needle will result in the return of urine.

At this point, a small amount of contrast and air is injected. The contrast outlines the collecting system and, because the patient is prone and the air will rise (which in this case is posteriorly), a suitable posterior calyx can be *identified* for definitive access.

To *access* the posterior calyx, oblique lateral angulation is preferred. This technique allows passage of the second needle through the relatively avascular plane of Brödel (Figure 14.11).

Once the needle is deemed to be in line with the desired calyx, fluoroscopic imaging is performed at a 90° angle so the appropriate depth to the desired calyx can be

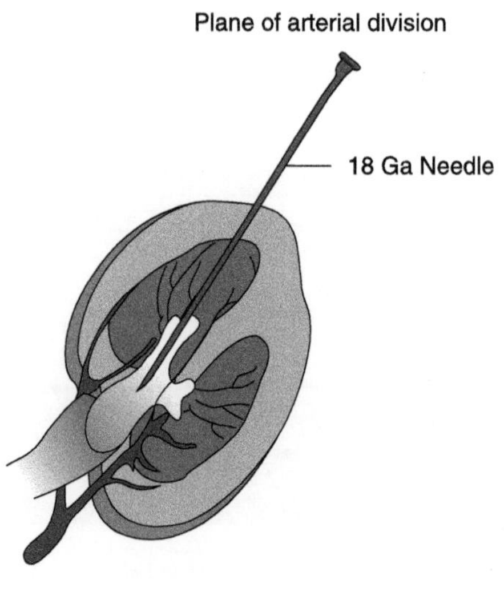

Figure 14.11. Needle through the avascular plane of Brödel.

ascertained. Once the needle enters the calyx, probing with a guidewire is performed to confirm positioning within the calyceal system. From this point, conversion to a catheter (for navigating down the ureter if needed) is carried out, and ultimately, placement of the *drainage* tube of choice is performed (Figure 14.12). Tubes can be secured using a number of securement devices; in our institution, we prefer 2-0 nylon suture.

Acute complications from GU procedures include

1. Bleeding (can cause hematuria or retroperitoneal bleeding)
2. Pneumothorax (risk is lowest when access is below the 12th rib)
3. Contrast reaction

INTRAOPERATIVE CASES

In many facilities, intraoperative cases (e.g., thoracic and abdominal aortic stent grafts) (Figure 14.13) are no longer performed by the interventional radiologists. In other facilities, these cases are performed as a combined effort with vascular or cardiothoracic surgeons working jointly with IR physicians. Inasmuch as these cases are performed either in the operating room or in a hybrid endovascular suite (quite analogous to an operating room), they often do not constitute an "off-site" location. They are mentioned here only to be included among the varied scope of procedures in which IR physicians may be involved.

Acute complications of intraoperative cases include

1. Access site complications
2. Stent malposition or migration
3. Vessel injury with bleeding
4. Contrast reaction

NONINVASIVE VASCULAR IMAGING

Noninvasive vascular imaging has greatly expanded in the last decade or two. Formerly consisting only of duplex ultrasound, noninvasive imaging now also includes peripheral CTA, cardiac CT with coronary CTA, MR angiography (MRA), and cardiac MR imaging (MRI).

Again, interventional radiologists are involved in these modalities in varying degrees, depending on institutional practices. For most of these procedures, anesthesia support is not needed, with the occasional exception of some of the MR studies in patients who cannot adequately control motion, respirations, or both. Diagnostic and interventional procedures in CT, MR, and ultrasound are covered in more detail elsewhere in this text.

The most significant complications from noninvasive studies are related to contrast reaction (much more common with iodinated contrast for CT than with gadolinium-based contrast for MR) and intravenous site problems.

PERCUTANEOUS ONCOLOGIC INTERVENTIONS

The field of percutaneous oncologic interventions has experienced rather rapid expansion in the last several years, with

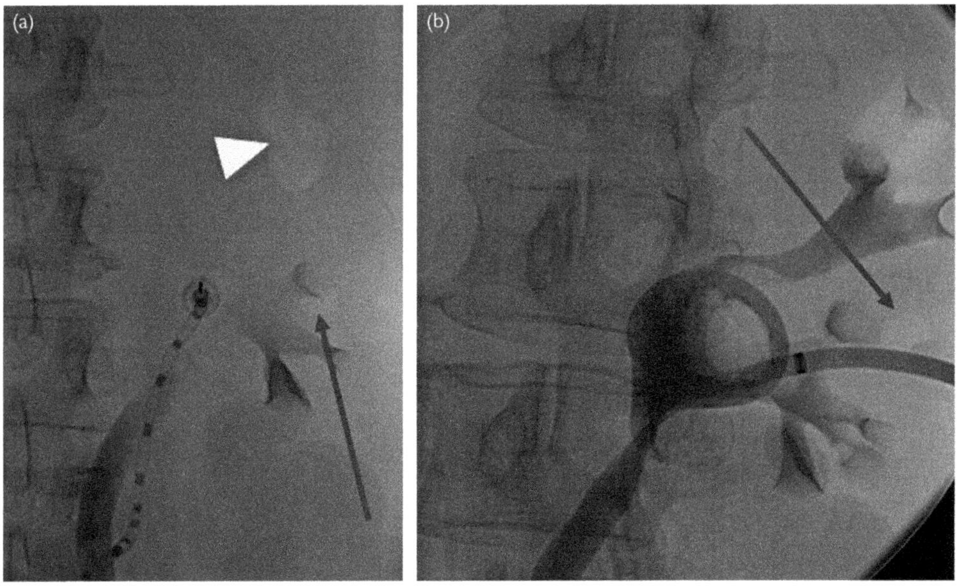

Figure 14.12. *(a) The collecting system has been entered with a needle, and both contrast and air have been instilled; a posterior upper pole calyx (arrowhead) overlies the 12th rib, so a smaller posterior midpole calyx (arrow) was chosen for final access. (b) The posterior midpole access (the arrow points to the air in the calyx) was converted to the nephrostomy tube; the Cope loop of the tube is coiled in the renal pelvis.*

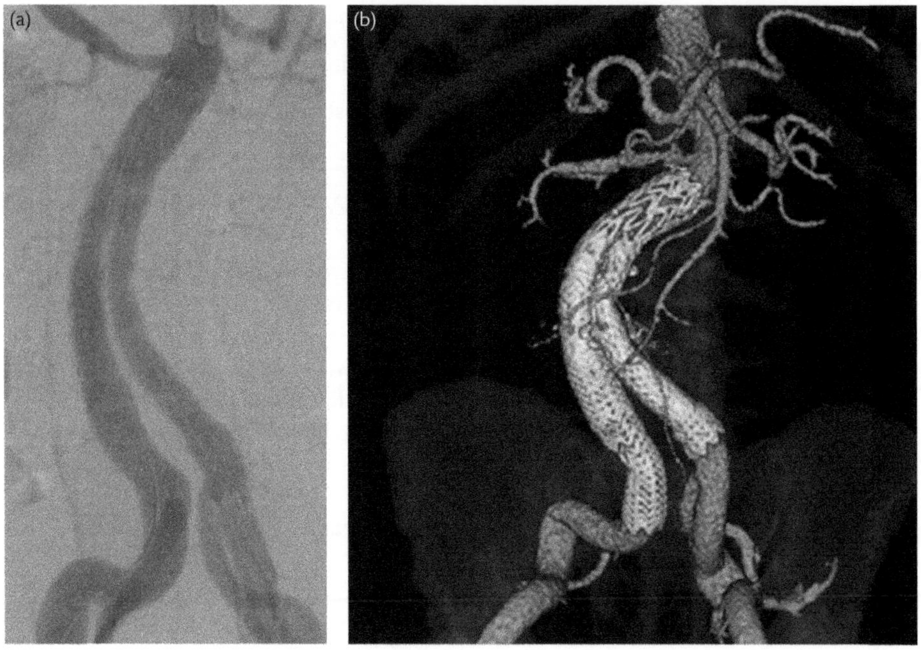

Figure 14.13. *(a) Intraoperative digital subtraction angiography (DSA) imaging of abdominal aortic aneurysm (AAA) endograft repair. (b) Postoperative computed tomographic angiography (CTA) of the same patient demonstrating stable position of the endograft at almost 6 months postoperative.*

many significant advances having been made. Examples of these interventions include

1. Percutaneous transarterial chemoembolization (TACE)
2. Percutaneous ablation most commonly using radiofrequency waves or cryoablation, but microwaves, laser, alcohol instillation, and acetic acid instillation have been used as well. (Figure 14.14)
3. Image-guided insertion of radioactive agents, such as hepatic arterial insertion of ^{90}yttrium spheres

Some of these procedures can be done with sedation and analgesia, but in selected patients, general anesthesia may be warranted (claustrophobic patients, those who cannot remain still for extended periods, and those with questionable airways).

Percutaneous ablation treatments may be discussed in more detail elsewhere. Briefly, image guidance (usually CT or ultrasound, but fluoroscopy can be used as well) is used to safely gain access into the lesion(s). Lesions to be treated are most commonly in the liver (hepatocellular carcinoma or metastases), but treatment of lesions in kidney, lung, bone, and adrenal have been performed. Once the location is ensured, treatment begins by either using specialized devices to deliver ablation energy (radio frequency, laser, microwave, or cryoablation) or less commonly by instilling a measured amount of liquid ablation agent (alcohol or acetic acid).

Transarterial chemoembolization and ^{90}yttrium spheres are delivered after arteriography identifies the vessel or vessels supplying the lesion(s). Once access as peripheral as desired is obtained, either chemotherapeutic agent combined with embolic agent or the radioactive spheres are delivered via the catheter through the selected hepatic arterial branches. Postprocedure care is according to established protocols.

Acute complications from oncologic interventions are dependent on the type of access:

1. If percutaneous access is used, then the acute complications are similar to other percutaneous procedures, including bleeding, injury to nontarget structures, and transgressing pleura. Also, injury (from heat or cold) to nontarget structures may occur.
2. If transarterial access is used, acute complications are similar to other transarterial embolization cases.

PERCUTANEOUS BIOPSIES

Interventional radiologists perform percutaneous biopsies at some facilities, whereas at other institutions, body imagers and others perform these procedures. Suffice it to say that the maxim from Samuel Shem's 1978 book, *The House of God*, which states that "there is no body cavity that cannot be reached with a #14 needle and a good strong arm" is not far from true.[3] One alteration is that it is wiser to use a smaller needle (e.g., 22 gauge) in case undesired targets are encountered. Some representative images are shown in Figure 14.15.

Acute complications from biopsies are generally site specific and can include

1. Bleeding
2. Acute injury to nontarget structures (including pneumothorax and pancreatitis)
3. Inadequate specimen

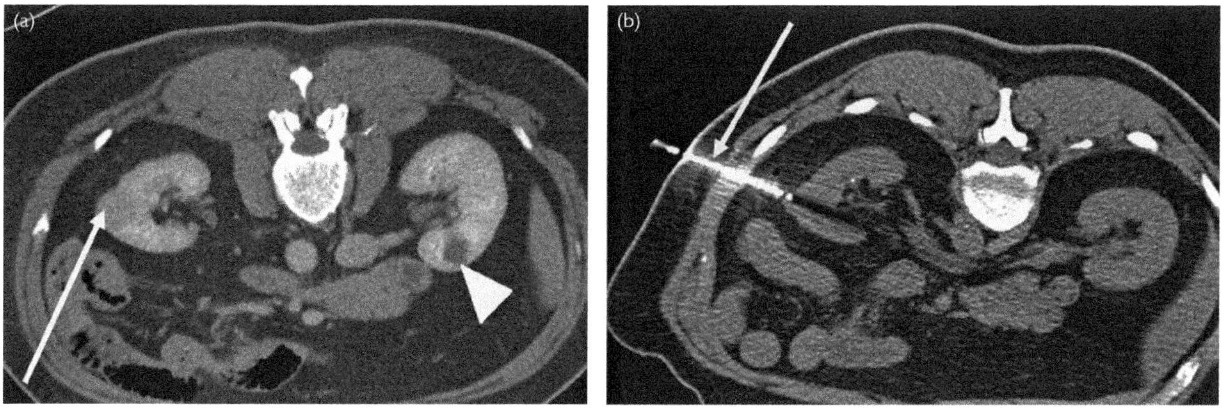

Figure 14.14. (a) Prone contrast computed tomography (CT) shows a hyperdense lesion (arrow) representing a left renal cell cancer; the hypodense right kidney lesion (arrowhead) represents a cyst. (b) The cryotherapy ablation probe (arrow) has been positioned into the left renal mass on this noncontrast prone CT scan.

VENOUS PROCEDURES AND INTERVENTIONS

Apart from venous access, venous procedures are less common than arterial procedures. However, the breadth of venous procedures is greater than that of arterial procedures. Some venous procedures have were discussed in the section Biliary Procedures and Interventions, including hepatic venography with hemodynamic evaluation, transjugular liver biopsy, and TIPS.

Other venous procedures include

1. Venography
2. Angioplasty (Figure 14.16)
3. Stent placement (Figure 14.17)
4. IVC filter placement and retrieval
5. Minimally invasive treatment of varicose veins
6. Selective venous sampling (SVS; e.g., adrenal veins, renal veins, petrosal veins, and parathyroid)
7. Pulmonary arteriography (accessed via the venous system)
8. Embolization of pulmonary arteriovenous malformations (PAVMs)
9. Foreign body retrieval
10. Venous thrombolysis

Venography is angiography (the general term for imaging of the vessels) of the veins. The technical aspects are similar in many ways to arteriography. More often than with arteriography, ultrasound is used during access because the precise location of a vein is not as evident as the palpable pulse of an artery. Otherwise, sheaths, catheters, and wires are used to navigate to various areas for evaluation or treatment. Contrast is administered with DSA imaging to obtain venograms. For extremity venography, often a temporary tourniquet is applied to allow filling of deeper veins.

Angioplasty can be performed in the venous system similarly to the arterial system. The need for central venous angioplasty is often related to indwelling venous devices (e.g., ports, central lines, and pacer/defibrillator wires). Not infrequently, venous angioplasty needs to be repeated.

Stents can be placed in the venous system for stenoses refractory to angioplasty. Some promising short-term results are reported, but the restenosis and occlusion rates for venous stents appear to be higher than for arterial stenting. In some cases, the stent can allow for antegrade flow long enough for sufficient collateral venous channels to develop before the stent occludes.

Placement of an IVC filter is used to reduce the risk of emboli originating from lower extremity or pelvic deep vein thrombosis (DVT) reaching the lung (pulmonary embolus, or PE). While most DVTs can be managed with anticoagulation, in certain instances, patients who cannot receive anticoagulation are treated with IVC filter placement.

Indications for IVC filter placement include

1. Failure of anticoagulation (i.e., DVT or PE while adequately anticoagulated)
2. Allergy to anticoagulants (includes heparin-induced thrombocytopenia)
3. Contraindication to anticoagulation (recent surgery, active bleeding, recent trauma, known intracranial lesion, noncompliance, and others)
4. Patient at high risk for PE

Currently, retrievable (also known as removable, temporary, or optional), convertible (from a filter to a stent), and permanent filters are available. Most can be placed via either the transfemoral or transjugular route. The technique involves access into the vein, performance of IVC venography, selection of an appropriate location (usually below the lowest renal vein and above the iliac confluence), deployment of the filter, and follow-up venography. On occasion, a suprarenal IVC filter can be placed; even

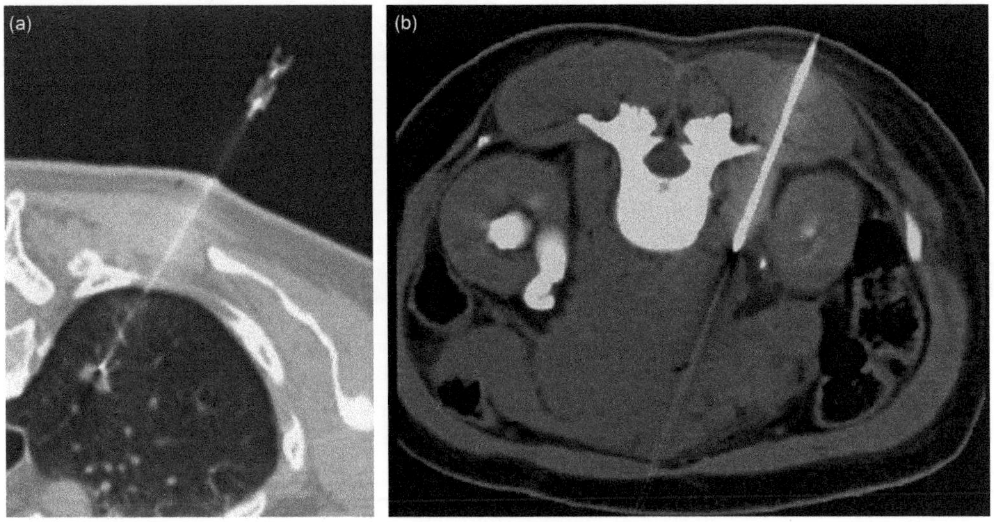

Figure 14.15. *(a) A fine needle has been advanced into a lung lesion with computed tomographic (CT) guidance. (b) A fine needle was passed through enlarged paravertebral lymph nodes by CT; the needle will have to be withdrawn slightly before sampling.*

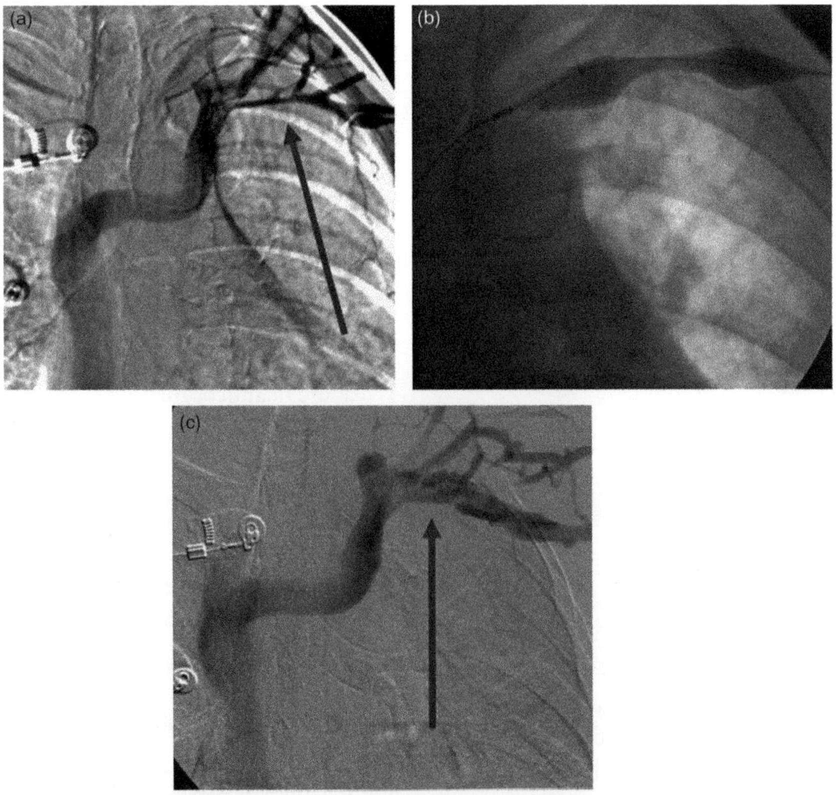

Figure 14.16. *(a) Severe stenosis of the left subclavian vein (arrow). (b) Angioplasty balloon is partially inflated revealing the "waist" at the stenosis. (c) Angiographic improvement noted at the site of previous stenosis (arrow) after angioplasty.*

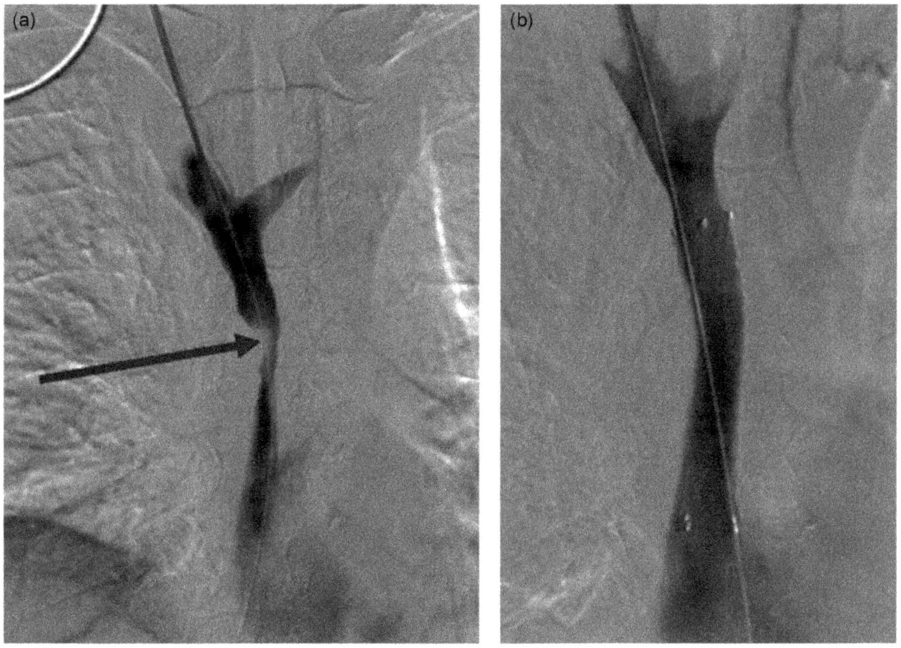

Figure 14.17. *(a) High-grade stenosis in the mid–superior vena cava (SVC) (arrow). (b) Successful resolution of stenosis in the mid-SVC following stent placement; a stent was used because the compression of the SVC was caused by a large paratracheal neoplasm in a terminally ill patient.*

less common is superior vena cava (SVC) filter placement, performed to prevent an upper extremity DVT from embolizing centrally.

The procedures can be performed with little or no sedation. Before orthopedic surgery, I personally had a retrievable IVC filter placed (Figure 14.18) via the transjugular route (without sedation, so I could resume performing cases immediately afterward); it was removed 2 months later (also without sedation) without incident.

Minimally invasive varicose vein procedures (Figure 14.19) include endovenous ablation (by radio frequency or laser) of incompetent superficial lower extremity veins (most commonly the greater and lesser saphenous veins), phlebectomy, and injection sclerotherapy. These procedures can all be accomplished without sedation in many patients; in others, sedation and analgesia can be used. Imaging requirements usually consist only of ultrasound for access. A detailed description of the techniques is beyond the scope of this chapter.

Selective venous sampling can be used to identify veins draining various organs. In some cases, establishing laterality of the abnormality is desired, such as adrenal vein sampling for aldosterone and cortisol or renal vein sampling for renin. In other cases, SVS helps establish or refute a diagnosis. For example, bilateral simultaneous venous sampling for ACTH (corticotropin) levels from the inferior petrosal sinuses after peripheral injection of CRH (corticotropin-releasing hormone) can confirm or refute a central (pituitary) source of ACTH. The diagnosis of Cushing disease is supported by detecting a significant gradient between the central (pituitary) and peripheral values of plasma ACTH. In parathyroid sampling, multiple veins that could potentially drain parathyroid tissue are accessed and sampled. An elevated parathyroid hormone level from one sample suggests the site of a parathyroid adenoma.

Pulmonary arteriography (Figure 14.20) is used less frequently than in the past given the speed, availability, and excellent results of pulmonary CTA. Nonetheless, it remains a procedure that interventional radiologists are at times requested to perform. In some cases, it is used to evaluate for PEs in the presence of a high clinical suspicion but a negative or equivocal noninvasive test (pulmonary CTA or nuclear medicine test). Other indications include evaluation for chronic PE, evaluation and treatment of PAVMs or pseudoaneurysms, or evaluation of pulmonary hypertension. Percutaneous treatment of PEs (by thrombolysis or thrombectomy) is returning to favor at some sites.

Technically, either the jugular or femoral venous approach can be employed. Once access is gained to the right atrium, one of several catheters can be used to navigate through the tricuspid valve, through the right ventricle, and into the pulmonary outflow tract. The left and right pulmonary arteries are selected and power injected as needed. Control of the patient's respirations is mandatory here. DSA imaging is acquired in the anteroposterior (AP) projection and at least one obliquity.

If pulmonary AVMs are identified, they can be embolized with coils or metallic occlusion devices, taking care to avoid passage of the embolization device through the fistula and to

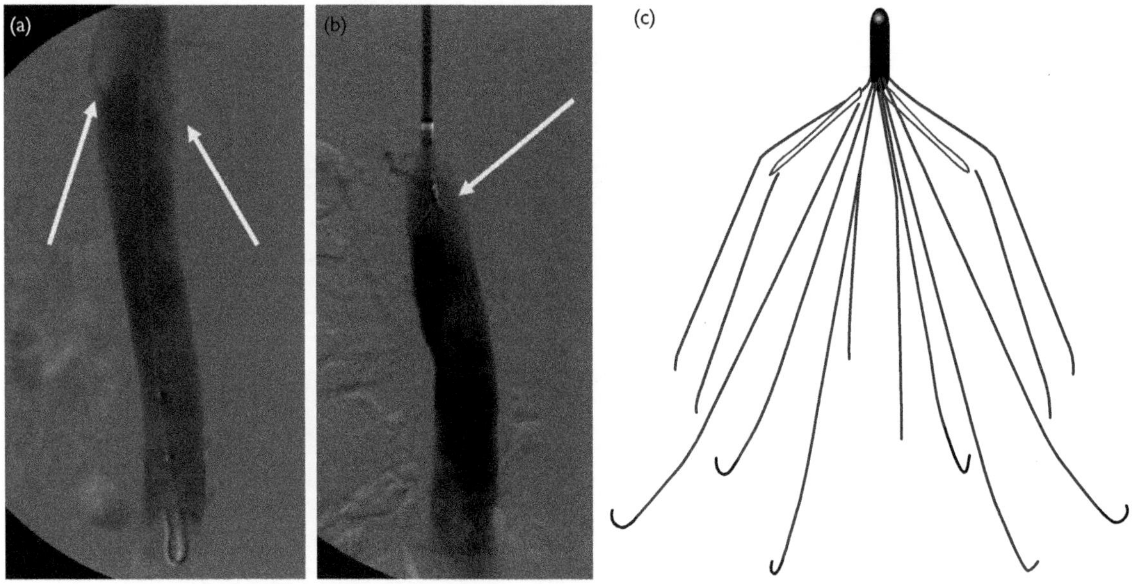

Figure 14.18. (a) Inferior vena cava (IVC) gram (my own) showing normal caliber; note inflow defects from unopacified blood from renal veins bilaterally (arrows). (b) The IVC filter has been successfully deployed. (c) Photo of an IVC filter.

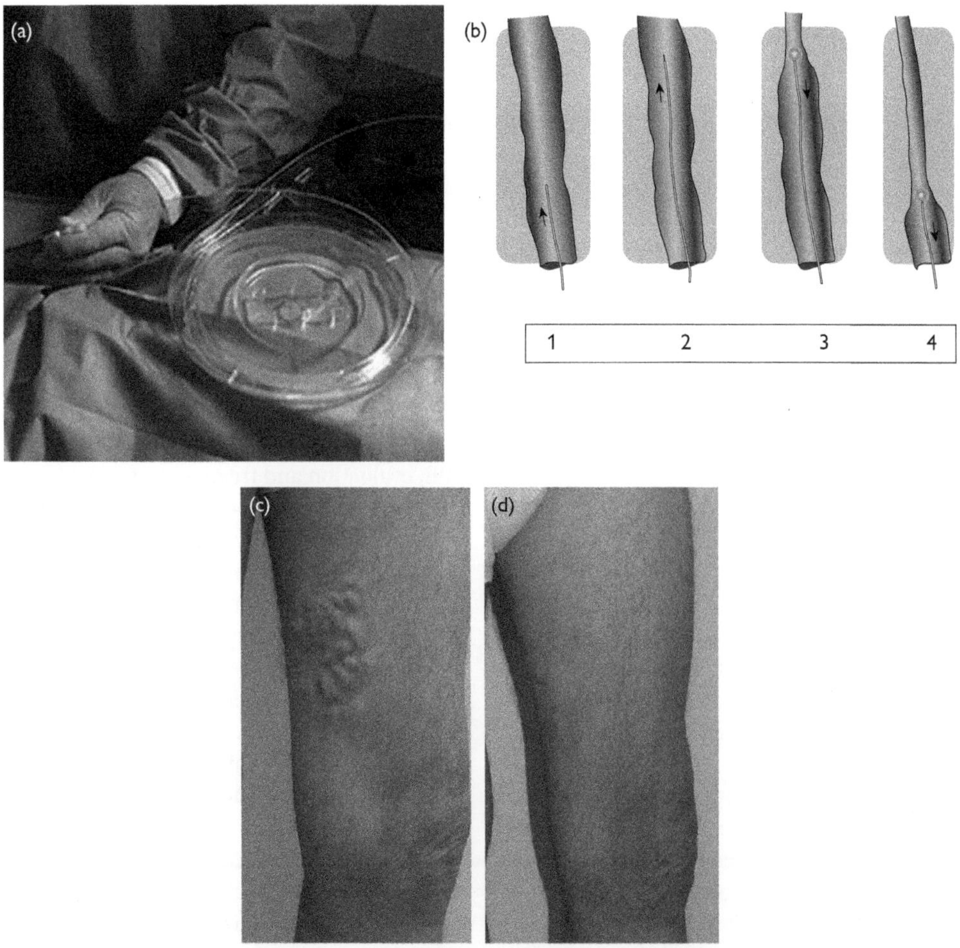

Figure 14.19. (a) A photo of an endovenous laser being used during a procedure. (b) The laser fiber is inserted and positioned (frames 1 and 2), then activated and withdrawn (frames 3 and 4), causing thermal damage to the lining of the treated vein, ultimately resulting in its occlusion (frame 4). (c) A "before" photo showing large medial thigh varicose veins. (d) An "after" photo showing resolution of the large medial thigh varicose veins following ablation of the incompetent source vein, in this case the left greater saphenous vein. (All images used with permission from Vascular Solutions, Inc.)

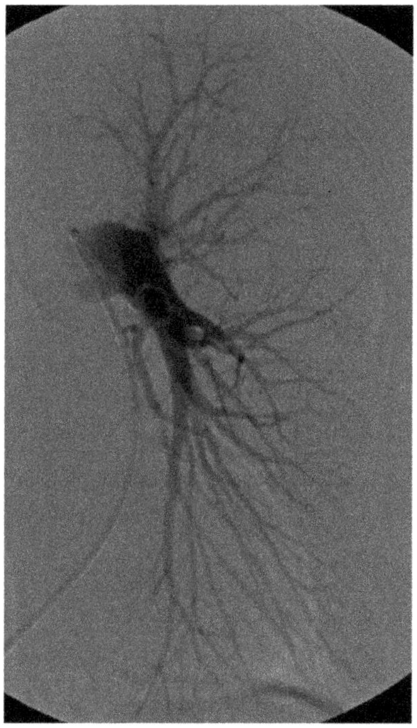

Figure 14.20. Normal left pulmonary arteriogram obtained with digital subtraction angiography (DSA) imaging.

the left atrium, left ventricle, and ultimately, the systemic arterial circulation.

Foreign body retrieval (Figure 14.21) most commonly consists of retrieving a broken venous catheter fragment. These fragments often reside in the heart or pulmonary arterial tree. Many are asymptomatic, identified on an unrelated chest radiograph. Retrieval via the transfemoral route is most commonly attempted using one or more of a variety of snare products to grab the fragment and pull it out through a sheath in the access vein.

Venous thrombolysis is less commonly employed than arterial thrombolysis, but the principles are similar. For lower extremity DVT thrombolysis, sometimes the patient must remain prone while access via the popliteal vein is gained and maintained during infusion of thrombolytic.

Acute complications from venous procedures include

1. Access issues (bleeding, thrombosis, pneumothorax)
2. Contrast reaction
3. Vessel injury with bleeding
4. Thrombosis
5. Embolism (of thrombus or of the foreign body to be retrieved)
6. Device malposition (e.g., IVC filter)
7. Cardiac irritation with dysrhythmia

VENOUS ACCESS (INCLUDING HEMODIALYSIS ACCESS)

Central venous access (Figure 14.22) encompasses a large portion of many IR practices. Access into the central circulation can be performed for infusion of medications (antibiotics, chemotherapeutic agents, blood products) or for withdrawal of blood for treatment (pheresis therapy or hemodialysis). Catheters can be partially tunneled under the skin (providing more comfortable access and a low infection rate), implanted completely (subcutaneous ports), or inserted directly into the vein (nontunneled). Catheters range greatly in size, from 3 or 4 French to 16 French and potentially even more, based on patient size, vein size, and planned usage.

Ultrasound is frequently used to access the desired vein, both to identify a nonpalpable structure (the soft vein) and to avoid adjacent nontarget structures (including arteries and lung). Fluoroscopy is used to follow the course of the wire once needle access into the vein is gained. Also, contrast can be given via the needle, and DSA imaging can be performed if the wire path is unusual in some respect.

Many different veins can be selected for access. In our institution, the IJ is the route of choice, largely to reduce potential subclavian stenosis.[4] For nontunneled catheters, there is evidence that the infection rate for subclavian access may be lower than for IJ puncture.[5]

Other less-common and less-preferable sites include

1. Common femoral veins
2. Saphenous veins
3. Arm veins (basilic, cephalic, or brachial)
4. External jugular veins
5. Translumbar access into the IVC
6. Transhepatic access into the hepatic veins and then to the IVC

Along with catheter insertion, catheter exchange and removal are part of the array of central venous procedures performed by IR physicians. Additionally, management of noncatheter hemodialysis access (arteriovenous [AV] fistula and AV grafts) is frequently performed. These techniques include diagnostic contrast studies as well as angioplasty and sometimes stent placement. Peritoneal dialysis catheter

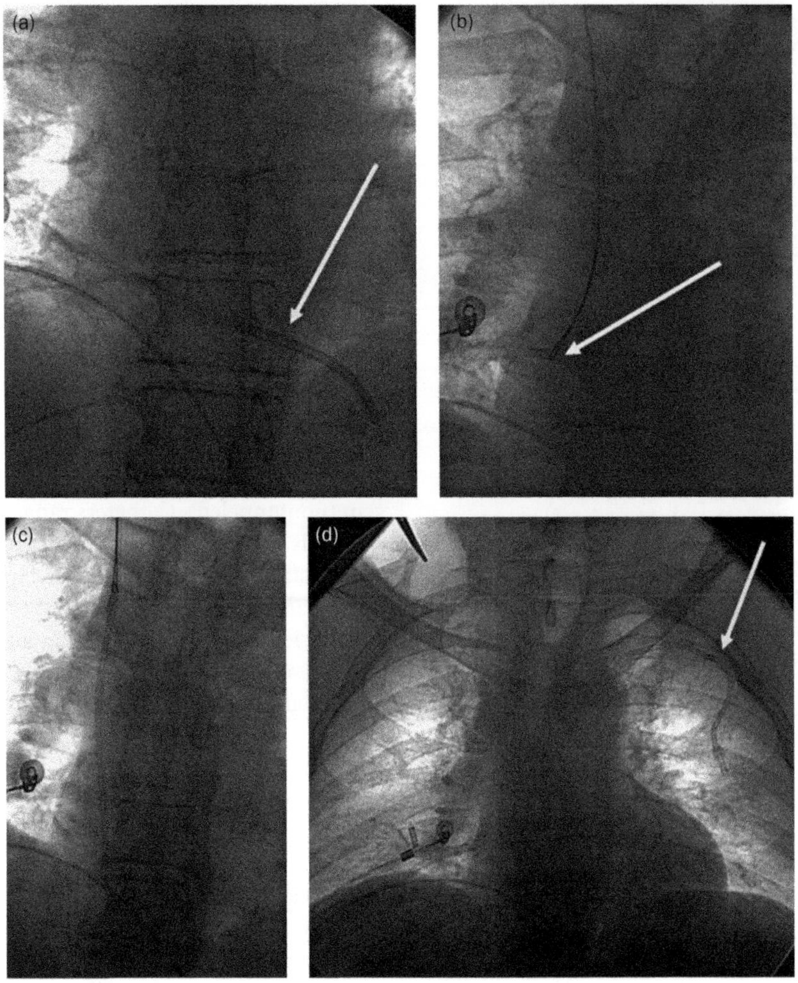

Figure 14.21. *(a) Fragment of catheter (arrow) seen over lower chest, spanning right atrium and right ventricle. (b) One end of catheter fragment has been grasped with a snare (arrow). (c) Ensnared fragment is being removed via a right internal jugular (IJ) sheath. (d) The fragment has been completely removed; only the subcutaneous portion remains (arrow), and it can be easily removed externally.*

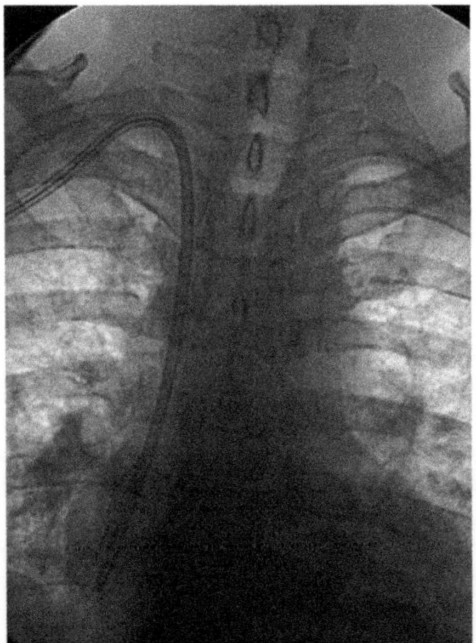

Figure 14.22. *A right internal jugular (IJ) tunneled hemodialysis catheter has been inserted and is ready for use.*

(obviously not venous, but included here for discussion) positions can be manipulated percutaneously as well, although the success rate is not exceedingly high.

Acute complications from venous access procedures can be similar to any of those listed previously for other venous procedures.

SUMMARY

The scope of procedures that are performed regularly by interventional radiologists has been outlined here to give a summary of its breadth. Clearly, that list of procedures encompasses many different indications, organ systems and body areas, techniques, and outcomes. As summed earlier, we who work in IR do indeed perform a vast array of diagnostic and interventional procedures, mostly through *very small holes*.

Individual practices vary based on need and practice history of the particular institution and region. In many instances, the addition of sedation and analgesia (moderate sedation) is needed for comfortable performance of these procedures. In other cases, deep sedation or general anesthesia may be required to permit the successful performance of the procedures. The details of anesthesia involvement in IR procedures are discussed in Chapter 15.

REFERENCES

1. Baum S, Athanasoulis CA. The beginnings of the Society of Interventional Radiology (SIR, née SCVIR, SCVR). *J Vasc Interv Radiol.* 2003;14:837–840.
2. Sunshine JH, Lewis RS, Bhargavan M. A portrait of interventional radiologists in the United States. *Am J Radiol.* 2005;185:1103–1112.
3. Shem, S. *The House of God. Berkley Books*, Reissue Edition, New York, 2010.
4. Barrett N, Spencer S, McIvor J, Brown EA. Subclavian stenosis: a major complication of subclavian dialysis catheters. *Nephrol Dial Transplant.* 1988;3(4):423–425.
5. Mermel LA. Prevention of intravascular catheter-related infections. *Ann Intern Med.* 2000;132:391–402.

15 | ANESTHESIA FOR DIAGNOSTIC AND THERAPEUTIC RADIOLOGIC PROCEDURES

ANNIE AMIN, MD, THOMAS W. CUTTER, MD, MAED

INTRODUCTION

Radiology procedures can be diagnostic, therapeutic, or both. Diagnostic procedures are anatomic or functional, minimally invasive or noninvasive, cause little pain or discomfort, and seldom require anesthesia support. When anesthesia assistance is requested, it is typically because of the patient's physiological or psychological needs. Therapeutic techniques are often more invasive and more likely to require the services of an anesthesiologist because of the complexity of the procedure and the comorbidities and discomfort of the patient. All therapeutic procedures are to some degree interventional, but many diagnostic procedures are not, although an *interventional radiologist* may perform them.

Patient safety is paramount during any radiological procedure. For many patients, comfort can be achieved with as little as reassurance or local anesthesia. Patients having more complex or invasive procedures may benefit from the administration of sedative or analgesic medications (sedo-analgesia) titrated to effect or require a regional or general anesthetic. Safety ensues from the judicious administration by a trained and vigilant practitioner of sedo-analgesia to a patient in optimal medical condition. The American Society of Anesthesiologists (ASA) has defined the sedation continuum that derives from titrating medication and its concomitant impact on level of responsiveness and physiologic function (Table 15.1).[1]

Noninvasive and many minimally invasive procedures (e.g., chest x-ray and breast needle localization, respectively) can be managed without medication, although some patients receive nominal sedation, anxiolysis, or analgesia. If the patient requests or requires moderate sedation (i.e., sedo-analgesia that might result in the loss of protective mechanisms such as the gag reflex, airway tone, and ventilatory drive), additional precautions are warranted to detect and mitigate its consequences. Among these are the evaluation and preparation of the patient, monitoring during the procedure, and postanesthesia care. Guidance can be found in the ASA "Practice Guidelines for Sedation and Analgesia by Non-anesthesiologists."[1] If more than moderate sedation is planned (i.e., deep sedation or regional or general anesthesia) or for patients with significant comorbidities, a trained and dedicated provider should care for the patient.

Conducting anesthetics in the radiology department can be challenging because of the patient's comorbidities, the procedure, the anesthetic, the radiology equipment, and the environment. The ASA "Practice Advisory for Preanesthesia Evaluation"[2] should be followed, and anesthetics should be administered by qualified and credentialed anesthesia personnel. After the anesthetic, the patient's recovery should be guided by the ASA "Practice Guidelines for Postanesthetic Care."[3] Remote locations often preclude immediate assistance, so thorough preparation, including access to a crash cart and defibrillator, is essential, and a system to provide reinforcements should be in place. Preparations must also be made for monitoring and support if the patient will be transported to another site for postanesthesia recovery. Patient safety is best ensured through following the "Guidelines for Nonoperating Room Anesthetizing Locations" as promulgated by the ASA.[4]

Care delivered by anesthesia professionals can be one of three types: monitored anesthesia care (MAC), regional anesthesia, or general anesthesia. Selection depends on the procedure and the relative risks and benefits to the patient. MAC, the least-invasive anesthetic, is indicated when a procedure requires deep sedation or increased monitoring.[1] The anesthesiologist administers intravenous sedation and analgesia while the proceduralist may give an additional local anesthetic at the site. MAC is a physician service that is distinct from moderate sedation because the anesthesia provider must be able to apply resources to support life and ensure patient comfort and safety during diagnosis or therapy.[5] For regional anesthesia, the anesthesiologist performs a nerve block. Blocks may be central (neuraxial) blocks (e.g., spinal, lumbar epidural) or peripheral (e.g., brachial plexus, paravertebral). General anesthesia is used when the patient or procedure requires it. For all anesthetics, patient safety through selection and monitoring are critical components of an anesthesiologist's care.

DIAGNOSTIC RADIOLOGY

CONTRAST MEDIA

Iodinated contrast media are frequently employed in both diagnostic and interventional radiology procedures and may result in adverse (anaphylactoid) reactions or renal dysfunction. Adverse reactions involve direct cellular effects, including enzyme induction and activation of the complement, fibrinolytic, kinin, and other systems.[6] Manifestations range

TABLE 15.1. Continuum of Depth of Sedation: Definition of General Anesthesia and Levels of Sedation/Analgesia

	MINIMAL SEDATION (ANXIOLYSIS)	MODERATE SEDATION/ ANALGESIA (CONSCIOUS SEDATION)	DEEP SEDATION/ANALGESIA	GENERAL ANESTHESIA
Responsiveness	Normal response to verbal stimulation	Purposeful[a] response to verbal or tactile stimulation	Purposeful[a] response after repeated or painful stimulation	Unarousable, even with painful stimulus
Airway	Unaffected	No intervention required	Intervention may be required	Intervention often
Spontaneous ventilation	Unaffected	Adequate	May be inadequate	Frequently inadequate
Cardiovascular function	Unaffected	Usually maintained	Usually maintained	May be impaired

NOTE: Minimal sedation (anxiolysis) is a drug-induced state during which patients respond normally to verbal commands. Although cognitive function and coordination may be impaired, ventilatory and cardiovascular functions are unaffected. Moderate sedation/analgesia (conscious sedation) is a drug-induced depression of consciousness during which patients respond purposefully to verbal commands, either alone or accompanied by light tactile stimulation. No interventions are required to maintain a patent airway, and spontaneous ventilation is adequate. Cardiovascular function is usually maintained. Deep sedation/analgesia is a drug-induced depression of consciousness during which patients cannot be easily aroused but respond purposefully following repeated or painful stimulation. The ability to independently maintain ventilatory function may be impaired. Patients may require assistance in maintaining a patent airway, and spontaneous ventilation may be inadequate. Cardiovascular function is usually maintained. General analgesia is a drug-induced loss of consciousness during which patients are not arousable, even by painful stimulation. The ability to independently maintain ventilatory function is often impaired. Patients often require assistance in maintaining a patent airway, and positive pressure ventilation may be required because of depressed spontaneous ventilation or drug-induced depression of neuromuscular function. Cardiovascular function may be impaired. Because sedation is a continuum, it is not always possible to predict how an individual patient will respond. Hence, practitioners intending to produce a given level of sedation should be able to rescue patients whose level of sedation becomes deeper than initially intended. Individuals administering moderate sedation/analgesia (conscious sedation) should be able to rescue patients who enter a state of deep sedation/analgesia, while those administering deep sedation/analgesia should be able to rescue patients who enter a state of general anesthesia.

[a]Reflex withdrawal from a painful stimulus is not considered a purposeful response.

SOURCE: Reprinted with permission from American Society of Anesthesiologists Task Force on Sedation and Analgesia by Non-Anesthesiologists. Practice guidelines for sedation and analgesia by non-anesthesiologists. *Anesthesiology*. 2002;96(4):1005.

from relatively benign itching to life-threatening cardiovascular or ventilatory collapse. Prophylaxis and treatment for the former include antihistamines and steroids. Anaphylaxis is quite rare and is probably not a result of the iodine in the contrast material.[7]

Patient risk factors for renal complications include chronic renal disease, diabetes mellitus, heart failure, older age, anemia, and left ventricular systolic dysfunction. Contrast risk factors are high osmolarity, viscosity, volume, and ionic media. For patients with renal disease, diabetes, proteinuria, hypertension, gout, or congestive heart failure, serum creatinine levels should guide the radiologist's administration of the contrast material. Adequate hydration, the use of bicarbonate, and low volumes of iso- or low-osmolar contrast are necessary in patients at risk. *N*-Acetylcysteine or ascorbic acid may be of value in very high-risk patients.[8] Diabetic patients with preexisting renal dysfunction who also take metformin have developed severe lactic acidosis after an iodinated contrast study. Thus, metformin should be discontinued at the time of or before the procedure, withheld for 48 hours subsequent to the procedure, and reinstituted only after renal function has been reevaluated and found to be normal.[9]

Intravenous gadolinium may be employed for magnetic resonance imaging (MRI) contrast studies and is not problematic during the anesthetic. Gadolinium-based contrast agents (GDBAs) have been associated with nephrogenic systemic fibrosis in patients with a glomerular filtration rate below 30 $mL/min/1.73\ m^2$. Nephrogenic systemic fibrosis is a rare but serious disease characterized by fibrosis of the skin and other tissues. The incidence of cases has decreased drastically since the implementation of restrictive guidelines in 2006. The US Food and Drug Administration (FDA) is currently evaluating the clinical implications of the discovery of residual gadolinium deposits in the brain from patients who have had multiple imaging studies with GDBAs over their lifetime. To date, there have been no adverse sequelae reported.[10]

Although barium is an oral and not an intravenous contrast agent, it should be mentioned because it may pose an aspiration risk after ingestion if deep sedation or general anesthesia is necessary.

Ultrasound contrast is achieved through the intravenous administration of microbubbles, which are echogenic during an ultrasound examination. They carry an FDA warning that patients with pulmonary hypertension or unstable cardiopulmonary conditions should be closely monitored during and for at least 30 minutes after administration.

ANATOMIC IMAGING

MAGNETIC RESONANCE IMAGING

The MRI suite is typically divided into four zones (Figure 15.1).[12] The ASA has issued a specific practice advisory[13] suggesting a location or position for optimal patient observation and vigilance during delivery of care in zones III and IV. The ASA also suggests procedures for entering zones III and IV, with special emphasis on hazards in these environments, effects on monitoring capabilities, potential health hazards (e.g., high decibel levels and high-intensity magnetic fields), and the need for precautions to ensure the safety of MRI scanners. The American College of Radiologists and the Joint Commission also have established standards, guidelines, and recommendations for the MRI suite.[14–17]

Patient monitoring and the administration of an anesthetic in the MRI suite can be difficult because the anesthesia provider

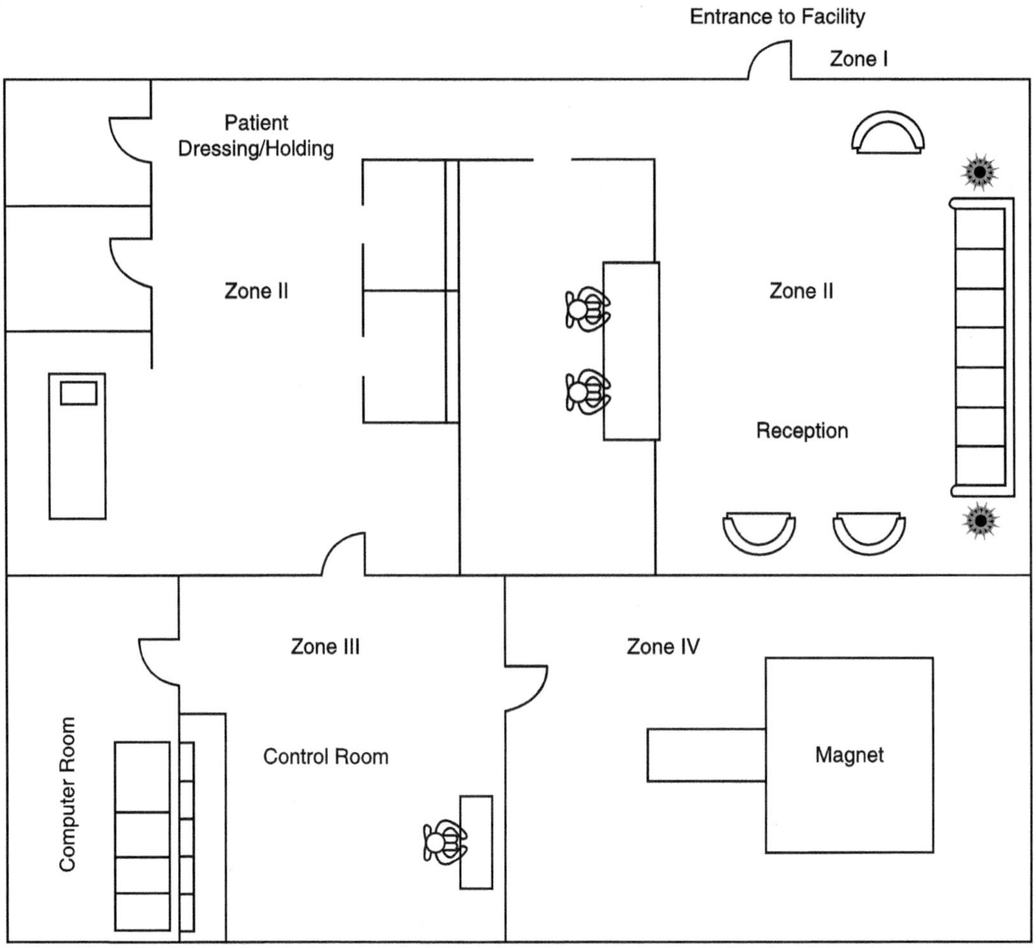

Figure 15.1. Layout of a typical magnetic resonance imaging (MRI) suite.

is often physically separated from the patient during the study. The patient must be observed continually, either through a window into the scanner room or with a camera trained on the patient and a video monitor in the control booth. Vital signs must be monitored through a window or via a camera trained on a monitor in the scanner room or a slave monitor in the control room. Airway management must be scrupulous because of the distance and barriers between the anesthesiologist and the patient. As with monitors, anesthesia devices, including airway equipment, must conform to the criteria of the American Society for Testing and Materials and the FDA. It may be best to secure the airway outside the scanner room and then transport the patient into the room.

Anesthesia providers should be familiar with the revised terminology for labeling of MRI implants and devices, specifically as it pertains to commonly used anesthesia equipment.[18] *MRI safe* refers to items that pose no known hazards in all MR (magnetic resonance) imaging environments. The items are nonconducting, nonmetallic, and nonmagnetic.[18] *MR conditional* poses no known hazards in a specified MRI environment with specified conditions of use. *MR unsafe* poses hazards in all MRI environments.[18] Some anesthesia devices that are frequently used are found to have a degree of magnetic attraction that, depending on severity, increases the risk of device movement or dislodgement. However, even devices with low movement forces can produce artifact depending on their metallic components. Comparison of imaging artifact during MRI with six different supraglottic devices concluded that artifact was most prominent with the LMA Proseal™ and nonexistent with the Ambu® disposable laryngeal mask and the i-gel® supraglottic airway.[19] If the region of imaging is near the airway, devices with little or no metal should be used. Consultation with a radiologist is always warranted if there are any concerns.

Monitor placement and the length and routing of leads, wires, and tubing should be considered to avoid entanglement or traction as the MRI table moves. Monitor wires (e.g., pulse oximeter, electrocardiogram) should not be coiled because coiling has resulted in patient burns.[20] Patient temperature should be monitored because it may increase from the heat of radio-frequency radiation within the magnetic field,[21] or it may decrease by radiation, conduction, convection, and evaporation. Monitoring temperature intermittently instead of continuously may prevent burns from the thermistor during long sessions or in critically ill patients.[22]

Medical emergencies must be anticipated, and a plan must be in place to treat them. Although advanced cardiac life support may be instituted for a patient still in the scanner, prompt relocation outside the scanner room gives better access to the patient and is safer for the staff. If the magnet is shut down too quickly, called "quenching,"[23] the liquid cryogen boils off rapidly and releases enormous amounts of helium vapor that may displace air, so an evacuation plan must be in place. The scanner is noisy, and there have been reports of hearing loss following MRI scan, so some form of ear protection is advisable, even for unconscious patients.[24] Positioning of patients can be difficult and care must be taken to avoid injury to obese patients or patients with preexisting neurologic disease.[25] The patient's entrance into and exit from the scanner warrants vigilance as well.

Most MRI studies are associated with minimal patient discomfort. After ensuring a patient's safety, the primary goal is to keep the patient still. Frequently, patient cooperation is all that is required and little or no sedative or analgesic medication is needed. If medications are used, they should be titrated to effect. Doses that are too large may lead to confusion and disinhibition, resulting in an agitated and uncooperative patient. An anesthesiologist should be consulted if the patient requires more than moderate sedation and is at risk for the loss of consciousness or protective reflexes. When a patient's medical condition is painful or if the procedure induces pain, regional[26] or general anesthesia may be chosen.

For pediatric patients, options for completing imaging studies include a patient who is awake, sedated, or under general anesthesia. If the patient is expected to be uncooperative during the procedure because of young age or claustrophobia, then general anesthesia is indicated. Table 15.2 lists the guidelines for selecting sedo-analgesia in pediatric patients based on age, developmental status, position, study duration, coexisting disease, and type of imaging study.[27] A selective list of sedative, analgesic, and general anesthetic agents used in imaging studies is found in Table 15.3.[27] Sedation with ketamine, midazolam, and propofol is adequate, safe, and comparable to that used for general anesthesia with endotracheal intubation (Table 15.4).[28] Infants who are at increased risk for adverse effects (Table 15.5) may require an experienced and skilled practitioner.[28] When intravenous propofol, oral chloral hydrate, and intravenous pentobarbital were compared for anesthesia in infants, propofol produced the fastest induction and recovery (Table 15.6) and lowest failure rate (Table 15.7), although the incidence of respiratory events was high.[29] Dexmetomidine can be used as a sole sedative for pediatric imaging studies. Mason et al. showed that by increasing the bolus to 3 μg/kg/min from 2 μg/kg/min over 10 minutes and the infusion rate to 2 μg/kg/min from 1.5 μg/kg/min, the rate of successful sedation was increased from 91.8% to 97.8%, and the need for pentobarbital rescue was reduced. There was a 16% incidence of bradycardia, but mean arterial blood pressure remained within 20% of "awake" values and was not associated with adverse sequelae.[30]

X-RAY, FLUOROSCOPY, AND COMPUTED TOMOGRAPHY

Electromagnetic waves (x-rays) have been incorporated into a number of different imaging modalities. The traditional x-ray refers to two-dimensional still images, although the same frequency of electromagnetic radiation is used for two-dimensional moving images (fluoroscopy) and "three-dimensional" computed tomography (CT). Concerns in these environments include the anesthesia provider's radiation exposure and distance from the patient. The former is addressed by distance, lead shielding, and radiation monitoring (personal dosimeter) and the latter by following protocols for monitoring similar to those in the MRI suite. The US Occupational Safety and Health Administration has established limits for the exposure of individuals to radiation in restricted areas,[31] and institutional guidelines should adhere to these standards. The presence of radiographic equipment (e.g., C-arm or CT aperture) can make airway management and access to the patient difficult, while the anesthesia machine and cart often compete for space with radiology equipment and supplies. The configuration of the table and other equipment means that patient positioning, especially lateral or prone, can be problematic. If the anesthesia provider remains in the procedure room, the anesthetic is performed with the encumbrance of a lead apron.

For diagnostic fluoroscopy procedures (Table 15.8), contrast material may be ingested (e.g., barium swallow), administered per rectum (e.g., barium enema), or injected intravenously (e.g., intravenous pyelogram) or intra-arterially (e.g., aortogram). Many procedures can be performed without anesthesia support unless a patient's comfort, comorbidities, or cooperation requires it. For example, diagnostic angiography is often performed with no or only light-to-moderate sedo-analgesia by cardiologists; percutaneous transhepatic cholangiography may be performed by a radiologist using the same regimen. Unstable or claustrophobic patients may require anesthesia assistance.

Computed tomography is a benign procedure for most patients and is relatively safe for personnel because the x-ray beam is tightly focused. Although studies are performed in a few seconds or minutes, they require a still patient, so cooperation must be ensured through either patient education or pharmacologic intervention. A variant is CT angiography, in which thin-section CT and contrast material produce vascular maps that equal or exceed those provided by classic angiography.[32]

ULTRASOUND

Like diagnostic x-rays, diagnostic ultrasound imaging is noninvasive and easily tolerated. For noninvasive techniques, anesthesia support is not warranted; if it is indicated, no encompassing techniques or precautions are necessary.

FUNCTIONAL BRAIN IMAGING

Functional brain imaging reveals blood flow, metabolism, or electrical activity. Electrical activity is demonstrated by the electroencephalogram (EEG), which directly measures the electrical potential between two scalp electrodes. Many anesthesiologists are familiar with this technology from its use in electroconvulsive shock therapy or intraoperative monitoring during carotid endarterectomy. Variants of the EEG used intraoperatively are the BIS®, Narcotrend®, PSI®, Entropy®, SNAPII®, and Cerebral State Monitor®. The EEG is spatially limited by the number of electrodes, a limitation that has been improved by high-density arrays of over 120 electrodes.[33] Magnetoencephalography is a more sensitive technology that

TABLE 15.2. Guidelines for Scheduling Imaging Studies as Awake, Sedated, or Under Anesthesia

TECHNIQUE	IMAGING FACTORS			PATIENT FACTORS		
	STUDY	DURATION (MIN)	POSITION	AGE (YR)	DEVELOPMENTAL STATUS	COEXISTING DISEASE
Awake	CT, NM	<30	Constant	< 0.3, >3	Normal	Minimal or none
	MRI	<60	Constant	> 7	Normal	Minimal or none
Sedate	CT, NM	>30	Changing	< 0.3	Normal	Minimal or none
	MRI	<60	Changing	< 4.5	Normal	Minimal or none
Anesthesia	CT, NM	Any	Any	Any	Severe delay	Any
	MRI	>60–90	Any	Any	Any	Any

CT, computed tomography; MRI, magnetic resonance imaging; NM, nuclear medicine.

Coexisting diseases include severe sleep apnea, refractory seizure disorders, preliver transplantation, patients unable to lie flat for extended periods of time, and American Society of Anesthesiologists physical status 3 or 4. In addition to changes, position may be an indication for sedation or anesthesia if it will be extremely uncomfortable for an extended period of time.

SOURCE: Reprinted with permission from Taghon TA, Bryan YF, Kurth CD. Pediatric radiology sedation and anesthesia. *Int Anesthesiol Clin.* 2006;44(1):65–79.

TABLE 15.3. Medications Commonly Used in Radiology Sedation and Anesthesia

DRUG	DOSAGE RANGE	RADIOLOGY-SPECIFIC SEDATION COMMENTS	CLASS
Propofol anesthetic	150–200 µg/kg per minute 2 mg/kg per IV bolus	Potential for apnea and airway obstruction	General
Sevoflurane anesthetic	2%–3% inhaled	Potential for airway obstruction and larnygospasm	General
Choral hydrate	25–100 mg/kg orally	Potential for prolonged duration of action and toxicity with impaired liver function	Hypnotic
Pentobarbital	3–8 mg/kg IV or orally	Potential for paradoxical reaction: can use orally in infants and small children or intravenously	Barbiturate sedative
Midazolam	0.3–1 mg/kg orally	Adjunct; may be sufficient as single agent in severe neurologic disease	Benzodiazepine anxiolytic
Fentanyl	1–2 µg/kg	Painful condition exacerbated by position in scanner	Opioid
Morphine	0.1 mg/kg IV	Adjunct with pentobarbital or midazolam	Opioid
Meperidine	2 mg/kg IV or orally	Adjunct with pentobarbital may be particularly useful with adolescents	Opioid
Dexmedetomidine	2–5 µg/kg per hour, 1 µg/kg per loading dose	Centrally acting alpha-1 agonist, with minimal respiratory depression	Hypnotic

SOURCE: Reprinted with permission from Taghon TA, Bryan YF, Kurth CD. Pediatric radiology sedation and anesthesia. *Int Anesthesiol Clin.* 2006;44(1):65–79.

records local magnetic fields produced by neuronal electrical activity in the brain via extremely sensitive instruments, such as superconducting quantum interference devices. It may be useful in multiple sclerosis, Alzheimer disease, schizophrenia, Sjögren syndrome, chronic alcoholism, and facial pain and has demonstrated efficacy in epilepsy.[34,35]

Other functional brain imaging techniques rely on the remarkably consistent relationship between regional changes in the cellular activity of the brain and changes in the blood flow and metabolism of the region.[36] Blood flow is revealed by functional MRI (fMRI), positron emission tomography (PET), and single-photon emission computed tomography (SPECT). Functional MRI can use blood as a contrast medium because oxygenated hemoglobin is diamagnetic (negative magnetic susceptibility) and deoxygenated hemoglobin is paramagnetic (positive magnetic susceptibility), resulting in distinct magnetic resonance signals. A less-common technique uses arterial spin labeling to magnetically alter the protons in the water molecules of the arterial blood in the neck and then identify them as they perfuse the brain. Functional MRI has been useful in determining the functional relationship between tumors and surrounding tissues.[37]

TABLE 15.4. Study Durations, Case Turnover, and Incidence of Side Effects in Children Subjected to Magnetic Resonance Imaging (MRI) Under Either General Anesthesia (GET Group) or Intravenous Anesthesia (MKP Group)

MKP	GROUP GET (N = 313)	GROUP MKP (N = 342)
Time to start scan (min)	9.6 (1.5)	4.2 (1.1)*
Duration of scan (min)	27.3 (7.9)	29.3 (11.4)
Emergence (min)	8.7 (5.5)	6.7 (4.1)
Time to discharge (min)	32.7 (10.9)	29.7 (9.7)
Case turnover	4–5 cases/5 h	5–6 cases/5 h
Side effects		
Discontinued	0 (0)	2 (0.6)
Repeat the scan	1 (0.3)	8 (2.3)*
Desaturation	10 (3.2)	16 (4.7)
Laryngospasm	8 (2.6)	0 (0)
Shivering	4 (1.3)	0 (0)
Total	23 (7.0)	26 (7.7)

NOTE: Data are mean (SD) or *n* (%).

*$p < .05$.

SOURCE: Reprinted with permission from Shorrab AA, Demian AD, Atallah MM. Multidrug intravenous anesthesia for children undergoing MRI: a comparison with general anesthesia. *Paediatr Anaesth.* 2007;17(12):1187–1193.

TABLE 15.5. Side Effects in Patients Subjected to Magnetic Resonance Imaging (MRI) Under Either General Anesthesia (Group GET) or Intravenous Anesthesia (Group MKP)

	GROUP GET (N = 313)			GROUP MKP (N = 342)		
	<1 YEAR	1–4 YEARS	>4 YEARS	<1 YEARS	1–4 YEARS	>4 YEARS
Number	93	134	86	98	138	106
Discontinued	0 (0)	0 (0)	0 (0)	2 (2)	0 (0)	0 (0)
Repeat the scan	1 (1.1)	0 (0)	0 (0)	4 (4.1)	3 (2.1)	1 (0.9)
Desaturation	5 (5.3)	3 (2.2)	2 (2.3)	8 (8.1)	5 (3.6)	3 (2.8)
Total	6 (6.4)[a]	3 (2.2)	2 (2.3)	14 (14.2)[b]	8 (5.8)	4 (3.7)

NOTE: Data are *n* (%).

[a] Significant ($p < .05$) compared with the older age strata within GET group.

[b] Significant ($p < .05$) compared with the older age strata within MKP group and compared with the same age stratum of GET group.

SOURCE: Reprinted with permission from Shorrab AA, Demian AD, Atallah MM. Multidrug intravenous anesthesia for children undergoing MRI: a comparison with general anesthesia. *Paediatr Anaesth.* 2007;17(12):1191.

During a PET scan, after injection of a positron-emitting radionuclide molecule, gamma rays can be detected by a scanner. When the positrons emitted by the tracer annihilate with electrons up to a few millimeters away, two gamma photons are emitted; the amount of imaged tracer reflects blood flow and concomitant brain activity. A PET scan also shows regional metabolic activity if the radionuclide molecule contains [^{18}F]-2-fluoro-deoxy-d-glucose (FDG), which concentrates in the more active areas. PET has been used in stroke patients to assess the magnitude of injury and the viability of areas at risk,[38,39] in seizure patients to map brain areas to predict surgical morbidity and outcome, in Parkinsonian syndromes as an adjunct to clinical diagnosis, in dementia for early diagnosis and differentiation, and in the prognosis and efficacy of treatment for brain tumors. PET is often combined with CT or MRI to provide an anatomic correlate for the functional image. Like PET, SPECT detects gamma rays, but the tracer material itself emits gamma radiation as it decays. More material indicates greater blood flow.

TABLE 15.6. Mean (± SD) Values of Time in Minutes After Three Different Anesthetics

TIMES	CHLORAL HYDRATE[a]	PENTOBARBITAL	PROPOFOL
	(*n* = 101[b])	(*n* = 66[b])	(*n* = 68)
Sedation ready	23.5 (13.4)	12.7 (8)	9.1* (6.7)
Procedure duration	48.11 (20.8)	49.3 (15.7)	58.5* (19.5)
Time to discharge	61.2 (31.9)	80.3 (39.2)†	53.9 (30.1)

n, number of cases.

[a]Values in parentheses indicate ± SD values.

[b]One patient each in the chloral hydrate and the pentobarbital group was excluded due to sedation failure requiring transfer back to the induction room and assumption of care and further sedation with propofol by an anesthesiologist.

*$p < .05$, propofol versus chloral hydrate and propofol versus pentobarbital.

† $p < .05$, pentobarbital versus propofol and pentobarbital versus chloral hydrate.

SOURCE: Reprinted with permission from Dalal PG, Murray D, Cox T, et al. Sedation and anesthesia protocols used for magnetic resonance imaging studies in infants: provider and pharmacologic consideration. *Anesth Analg.* 2006;103(4):863–868.

TABLE 15.7. Adverse Events After Administration of the Primary Sedative Drugs in Three Groups

ADVERSE EVENT	CHLORAL HYDRATE (N = 102)	PENTOBARBITAL (N = 67)	PROPOFOL (N = 68)
Cardiorespiratory events	3* (2.9%)	9 (13.4%)	9[a] (13.6%)
Gastrointestinal events	Emesis (2)	Hiccups (1)	0
Movement in scanner	23 (22.5%)†	8 (12.2%)	1 (1.4%)
Scan aborted completely	4 (3.9%)*	1 (1.4%)	0
Scan completed with additional/rescue sedation/ Pedialyte	12 (11.7%)*	7 (10.4%)	1 (1.4%)
Scan completed with repositioning, bundling, etc.	7 (5.9%)	0	0

n, number of cases.

[a] Significant respiratory event in two cases; referred to anesthesiologist.

*$p < .05$.

† $p < .001$.

SOURCE: Reprinted with permission from Dalal PG, Murray D, Cox T, et al. Sedation and anesthesia protocols used for magnetic resonance imaging studies in infants: provider and pharmacologic consideration. *Anesth Analgesia.* 2006;103(4):863–868.

Metabolic activity can be directly revealed through magnetic resonance spectroscopy, which detects signals from hydrogen or phosphorous to determine the concentration of brain metabolites such as *N*-acetyl aspartate, choline, creatine, and lactate in tissue. Greater levels indicate greater metabolic activity. It is used in the diagnosis and treatment of certain neuropsychiatric disorders, such as schizophrenia, affective diseases, or autism; in the pathogenetic interpretation of some Parkinsonian neurodegenerative disorders[40]; in tumor diagnosis, prognosis, and therapeutic outcome; in dementia diagnosis and prognosis; and in multiple sclerosis, infections, trauma, stroke, and perinatal ischemia.[41] These procedures are often performed on awake individuals, although occasionally a patient's psychological or physical condition may require the use of sedation or general anesthesia.

Administering anesthetic psychotropes may result in artifacts that disrupt the remarkably consistent relationship between regional changes in the cellular activity of the brain and changes in its circulation and metabolism. For example, unresponsiveness induced with isoflurane was associated with a relatively uniform reduction in brain glucose metabolism during PET with FDG.[42] Halothane resulted in a similar reduction. Propofol was associated with larger absolute metabolic reductions, a greater suppression of cortical metabolism than either inhalational agent, and significantly less suppression of basal ganglia and midbrain metabolism.[43] Propofol preferentially decreased cerebral blood flow (CBF) in brain regions previously implicated in the regulation of arousal, performance of associative functions, and autonomic control and was more regionally than globally active.[44] With fMRI, morphine had a regional effect, decreasing the signal in cortical areas, as did propofol or midazolam. Activation was observed in endogenous analgesic regions, such as the periaqueductal gray, the anterior cingulate gyrus (decreased signal), and hypothalamus

TABLE 15.8. Diagnostic Fluoroscopy Procedures

UPPER GASTROINTESTINAL SERIES
Air contrast colon
Intravenous pyelogram (IVP)
Small bowel enteroclysis
Fluoroscopic-guided biopsy
Arthography
Myelography
Modified barium swallow
Hystersalpingogram
Venogram
Arterogram
Barium enema
Percutaneous transhepatic cholangiography

(increased signal).[45] Midazolam affects fMRI by significantly altering the signal in the brain's auditory and visual cortices.[46] Nonpharmacologic interventions can also influence imaging outcomes, such as increased mean airway pressure (e.g., continuous positive airway pressure) reducing the fMRI signal in the primary visual cortex.[47]

There are no strong recommendations for anesthetic technique for these diagnostic procedures. Indeed, functional brain imaging techniques such as PET and fMRI have been used to *study* the effects of general anesthesia on the brain, and a systematic baseline response to anesthetics has not yet been developed.[48–50] If an anesthetic is required, the anesthesiologist should consider the anesthetic's impact on CBF, metabolism, and electrical activity and choose agents with minimal effect, combine agents to minimize their effects, and maintain steady-state anesthetic conditions.

THERAPEUTIC RADIOLOGY

Therapeutic radiology has grown from percutaneous procedures for aspiration/drainage to the more complex placement of arterial stents or embolization of arteriovenous malformations (AVMs). Table 15.9 lists some common interventional therapeutic radiologic procedures and imaging methods. Biliary tube placement or exchange, tunneled catheter placement, vascular interventions, and other catheter insertions have been performed using moderate sedation for the patient, during which nurses, trained in critical care, monitor the patient and administer low-dose midazolam and fentanyl.[51] Adverse events are few (Table 15.10) and minor without clinical impact.[51] Tables 15.11 and 15.12 list various procedures and compare the utilization of different methods of anesthesia in Europe and the United States.[52] Less rather than more sedation is the rule in Europe, although general anesthesia is more common in Europe. In one East Coast academic center, MAC or general anesthesia was used for only 10% of cases for interventional radiology.[53]

As interventional radiology cases increase in volume and complexity, it is more often being performed in an emergency setting and includes high-risk patients who cannot tolerate a more invasive method, making an anesthesiologist necessary.[54] The conditions for performing an anesthetic for therapeutic radiology procedures include monitoring from afar, avoiding radiation exposure, working around radiology equipment (Figure 15.2), and prohibiting ferrous materials in the MRI suites. The choice of anesthetic technique for interventional radiology is procedure specific with wide variations, depending on the patient and the skill sets of the interventionalist and associated personnel. The anesthetic presents more challenges because the procedure is invasive and the patient may have several comorbidities. The requirement of a completely still patient, both for the success of the procedure and the safety of the patient, can be fulfilled by sedo-analgesia administered by either the proceduralist or an anesthesia professional. If a predictable ventilatory pattern in the patient is desired, it can be achieved by the judicious administration of sedo-analgesia to a cooperative patient or by general anesthesia with controlled ventilation. Some particularly painful procedures (e.g., radiofrequency ablation [RFA] of osteoid osteomas) require a subarachnoid block or general endotracheal intubation by an anesthesiologist.[55] Other procedures associated with extreme fluid shifts (e.g., drainage of ascites fluid or blood loss during a uterine artery embolization) benefit from the presence of someone who is well versed in securing intravenous access and who knows how to use it. Some procedures may require anticoagulation and the means to measure its effects (e.g., activated coagulation time). Because interventional neuroradiology has virtually become a subspecialty unto itself, it is discussed in a separate section of this chapter.

FLUOROSCOPY

ENDOVASCULAR STENTS

Fluoroscopy is the common imaging technique for stent placement. Anesthesiologists are requested for these procedures because of the potential for complications and because the patient population comprises patients who were previously considered "too sick for open surgery."[56] Among the anesthetic techniques used for endovascular aortic repair are general, epidural, combined epidural/spinal, spinal, continuous spinal paravertebral block, and local anesthesia with intravenous sedation.[57] Analysis of a large database of endovascular aortic repairs in Europe (EUROSTAR) showed a benefit of regional and local anesthesia over general anesthesia in morbidity, mortality, and length of intensive care unit (ICU) and hospital stays in high-risk groups and encouraged use of minimally invasive anesthesia techniques when possible.[58] When performed under MAC, one must be prepared for significant blood loss and invasive monitoring.[59] Mild hypotension, using nitroglycerin,[60] nitroprusside, nicardipine, or esmolol,[61] and an immobile patient are important when deploying the stent. Spinal cord injury may be decreased by

TABLE 15.9. Therapeutic Radiology Procedures and Imaging Techniques

PROCEDURE IMAGING	ARTERIAL/VENOUS INTERVENTIONS	CANCER TREATMENT	ABLATION RADIO FREQUENCY, ETHANOL, MICROWAVE, CRYO-LASER	VASCULAR ACCESS	VERTEBROPLASTY KYPHOPLASTY	EMBOLIZATION	PERCUTANEOUS PROCEDURES
Fluoroscopy	Stenting, balloon angioplasty, catheter-directed thrombolysis, inferior vena cava filter, transjugular intrahepatic portosystemic shunt	Chemoembolization: Hepatic cancer		Artery, vein	Vertebral compression fractures	Brain aneurysm, uterine fibroids, arteriovenous malformation, varicocele, esophageal varices	Biliary drainage, nephrolithotomy, nephrolithotripsy
Computed tomography (CT)		Cryotherapy: Prostate cancer, liver cancer, cervical cancer, retinoblastoma	Kidney, liver, lung		Vertebral compression fractures		
Ultrasound	Magnetic resonance imaging (MRI)		Cryotherapy: Prostate cancer, liver cancer, cervical cancer, retinoblastoma	Kidney, liver, lung			

TABLE 15.10. Frequency of Adverse Events Occurring in Five Common Interventional Radiology Procedures

PROCEDURE CATEGORY (N = 539)	RESPIRATORY EVENTS (%)	SEDATION EVENTS (%)	MAJOR EVENTS (%)
Biliary procedures (n = 183)	8.7[a] (p = .044)	6.0 (p > .05)	2.2 (p > .05)
Tunneled catheters (n = 135)	3.0 (p > .05)	3.7 (p > .05)	1.5 (p > .05)
Diagnostic arteriogram (n = 125)	4.0 (p > .05)	4.0 (p > .05)	2.4 (p > .05)
Vascular interventions (n = 51)	2.0 (p > .05)	2.0 (p > .05)	2.0 (p > .05)
Other procedures (n = 45)	0.0 (p > .05)	2.2 (p > .05)	2.2 (p > .05)

[a] Statistically significant for respiratory events (p = .044) and any adverse event (p = .015) during biliary procedures.

SOURCE: Reprinted with permission from Arepally A, Oechsle D, Kirkwood S, et al. Safety of conscious sedation in interventional radiology. *Cardiovasc Intervent Radiol.* 2001;24(3):188.

TABLE 15.11. Preferred Levels of Sedation for All Procedures

PROCEDURE	AWAKE/ALERT	DROWSY/AROUSABLE	ASLEEP/AROUSABLE	DEEP SEDATION	GENERAL ANESTHESIA
Vascular					
Angiography	74% (163)	24% (53)	1% (2)	1% (2)	0.5% (1)
Pulmonary angiography	74% (136)	24% (45)	0.5% (1)	0.5% (1)	1% (2)
Angioplasty	62% (130)	33% (69)	3% (7)	2% (4)	0.5% (1)
Caval filter placement	67% (120)	29% (53)	3% (5)	1% (1)	0.5% (1)
Embolization	36% (71)	46% (91)	9% (18)	5% (10)	4% (8)
TIPSs	9% (11)	26% (32)	21% (26)	14% (17)	30% (37)
Thrombolysis	59% (118)	35% (70)	5% (9)	0.5% (1)	0.5% (1)
Atherectomy	58% (60)	36% (37)	5% (5)	0% (0)	1% (1)
Venous access	53% (78)	38% (56)	7% (10)	1% (1)	1% (2)
Genitourinary					
Nephrostomy	17% (26)	56% (85)	23% (35)	2% (3)	1% (2)
Nephrolithotomy	7% (5)	16% (11)	11% (8)	11% (8)	54% (38)
Stricture dilation	11% (11)	33% (32)	39% (38)	7% (7)	9% (9)
Abscess drainage	33% (50)	52% (80)	12% (19)	2% (3)	1% (1)
Abdominal/pelvic					
Abscess drainage	36% (69)	49% (93)	13% (24)	2% (3)	1% (2)
Biliary drainage	12% (22)	38% (68)	32% (57)	11% (19)	8% (14)
Cholecystostomy	14% (15)	49% (53)	25% (27)	7% (8)	4% (4)
Thora-/paracentesis	50% (54)	34% (37)	12% (13)	4% (4)	1% (1)
Tube procedure	47% (47)	37% (37)	13% (13)	3% (3)	1% (1)

(continued)

TABLE 15.11. *(Cont'd)*

PROCEDURE	AWAKE/ALERT	DROWSY/AROUSABLE	ASLEEP/AROUSABLE	DEEP SEDATION	GENERAL ANESTHESIA
Biopsy	62% (110)	32% (57)	5% (9)	1% (2)	0.5% (1)
Biliary dilation	7% (10)	34% (49)	35% (50)	14% (20)	11% (16)
Gastro-/jejunostomy	17% (16)	55% (53)	18% (17)	8% (8)	2% (2)
Stent placement	17% (31)	46% (83)	22% (39)	7% (12)	8% (15)
Chest					
Biopsy	67% (104)	29% (46)	3% (4)	0% (0)	1% (2)
Fluid drainage	61% (83)	31% (46)	6% (8)	0% (0)	2% (2)
Chest tube placement	45% (40)	42% (37)	11% (10)	1% (1)	1% (1)

TIPSs, transjungular intrahepatic portosystemic shunts.

NOTE: Figures in parentheses are the number of responders.

SOURCE: Reprinted with permission from Haslam PJ, Yap B, Mueller PR, et al. Anesthesia practice and clinical trends in interventional radiology: a European survey. *Cardiovasc Intervent Radiol.* 2000;23(4):256–261.

TABLE 15.12. Preferred Level of Sedation for Selected Procedures and Comparison With US Data

	ALERT/ AWAKE		DROWSY/ AROUSABLE		ASLEEP/ AROUSABLE		DEEP SEDATION		GENERAL ANESTHESIA	
PROCEDURE	EUROPEAN	US	EUROPEAN	US	EUROPEAN	US	EUROPEAN	US	EUROPEAN	US
Diagnostic vascular										
Vascular angiography	74	20	24	73	1	7	1	0	0.5	0
Pulmonary angiography	74	24	2	67	0.5	3	0.5	0	1	0
Therapeutic vascular										
Angioplasty	62	14	33	72	3	13	2	0	0.5	1
Caval filter placement	66	23	30	71	3	35	1	0	1	0
Embolization	35	7	47	60	9	29	5	2	4	2
Thrombolysis	59	15	36	68	5	17	0.5	1	0.5	0
Venous access	53	27	38	62	7	10	1	1	1	0
Diagnostic visceral										
Abdominal/pelvic biopsy	62	35–50	32	50–60	5	3–5	1	1	1	0
Chest biopsy	67	48	29	48	3	17	0	1	1	0
Therapeutic visceral										
Biliary drainage	12	0	38	25	31	48	10	22	8	5
Abdominal/pelvic										
Abscess drainage	36	5–8	49	65	12	25	2	3	1	0
Nephrostomy	17	0–1	57	20–45	23	45	2	12	1	1–2
Biliary stent placement	17	3	47	50	21	37	7	42	8	1
Tube manipulation/change	47	30	37	57	13	12	3	1	1	0

NOTE: Data are presented as percentages. Each percentage is an approximation for that procedure at the level of sedation.

SOURCE: Reprinted with permission from Haslam PJ, Yap B, Mueller PR, et al. Anesthesia practice and clinical trends in interventional radiology: a European survey. *Cardiovasc Intervent Radiol.* 2000;23(4):256–261.

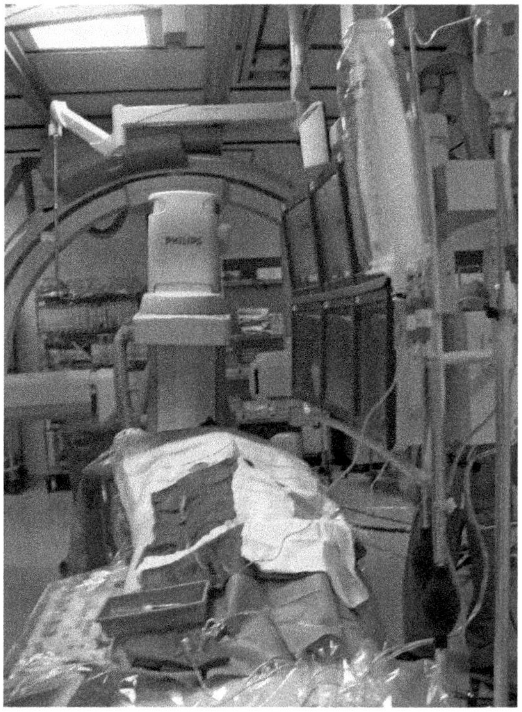

Figure 15.2. Picture of an interventional radiology suite.

limiting hypotension, monitoring evoked potentials and cerebrospinal fluid (CSF) pressure, and measuring CSF proteins (S100 β) during thoracic aneurysm repair.[62] An intrathecal drain may be beneficial for thoracic aneurysm repairs,[63] but it may also lead to catheter-related complications.[64]

Carotid artery stenting is an alternative to carotid artery endarterectomy in high-risk surgical patients, although numerous randomized, controlled studies have not demonstrated a difference in long term (>3 years) benefits in regard to stroke, myocardial infarction, and death.[65] The American College of Cardiology and American Heart Association (AHA) guideline states that carotid stenting is recommended as an alternative to endarterectomy in *symptomatic* patients with an average surgical risk when the anticipated risk of periprocedural stroke or mortality is less than 6% and also is preferred when carotid lesions are anatomically unfavorable (i.e., in cases of restenosis, high cervical or intrathoracic lesions, or following radiation therapy). Carotid artery stenting may be considered in highly selected *asymptomatic* patients with 60% or greater angiographic stenosis.[66] Aspirin and clopidrogel are often administered before the procedure, and heparin is given intraoperatively while activated clotting time is monitored. Stenting may be performed in a patient under MAC, with close attention paid to central nervous system (CNS) changes and bradycardia, or under general anesthesia. General anesthesia depressed barorecepter reflex sensitivity and induced hemodynamic stability, potentially decreasing complications.[67] Hypertension should be treated postoperatively to avoid neurological complications.

Stenting to improve blood flow through iliac, popliteal, subclavian, or renal arteries does not mandate the presence of an anesthesiologist[68] unless the patient's condition warrants it. Stenting of venous outflow has been used for chronic nonmalignant or malignant obstruction of the femoroiliocaval vein,[69] and patients with neoplastic superior vena cava syndrome have received palliative stents without sedation.[70]

A transjugular intrahepatic portosystemic shunt treats complications of portal hypertension (e.g., esophageal varices) with an expandable metallic stent to create an artificial parenchymal channel between portal and hepatic vein branches. It may be performed under MAC or general anesthesia.[71] The patient's mental status, ability to tolerate the procedure without moving, overall hemodynamic status, and ease of airway management dictate the type of anesthesia. Significant comorbidities can include pathological shunting in vascular beds, leading to increased cardiac output and heart failure. Ascites, pleural effusions, intrapulmonary shunting, pulmonary hypertension, hepatorenal syndrome, encephalopathy, and coagulopathies are common in these patients. Because of hepatic insufficiency, the anesthetic agents selected should not depend on the liver for clearance.[72] A cirrhotic cardiomyopathy may be associated with a prolonged Q-Tc interval, which may deteriorate into a torsades de pointes arrhythmia.

CATHETER-DIRECTED THROMBOLYSIS

Thrombolysis is accomplished by the local infusion of tissue plasminogen activators that create plasmin for fibrinolysis. Common agents include streptokinase, urokinase, and recombinant formulations. Thrombolysis is used in patients with myocardial infarction, ischemic stroke, pulmonary embolism, thrombosed dialysis access, portal vein thrombosis, and acute limb ischemia. Anesthesia is seldom required, but if it is, the anesthetic depends on the patient's comorbidities and preventing trauma during airway maneuvers. Neuraxial regional anesthesia is contraindicated.[73]

INFERIOR VENA CAVA FILTER

Inferior vena cava filters are placed in patients who have a history of, or who are at risk for, deep vein thromboses in the legs that may then embolize to the right heart and lungs. Access is obtained through the right internal jugular vein or a femoral vein. The procedure may be performed without sedation, although sedo-analgesia may be administered by the interventional radiologist. General anesthesia or MAC is occasionally necessary after evaluation of the patient's comorbidities.

BALLOON ANGIOPLASTY

In balloon angioplasty, a narrowed or obstructed blood vessel is widened with a balloon-tipped catheter. Carotid angioplasty has been performed with deep cervical plexus blockade,[74] MAC, or general anesthesia. The same concerns apply to carotid stenting, which is commonly preceded by balloon angioplasty. Relatively minor procedures, such as percutaneous transluminal angioplasty of the infrarenal aorta, can be safely performed with local anesthesia by the interventionalist.[75]

CHEMOEMBOLIZATION

Chemoembolization is currently limited to hepatic tumors, either primary or metastatic. A catheter is inserted into the femoral artery and guided under fluoroscopy into the hepatic artery; contrast material is then injected to identify the arterial supply to the tumor. A chemotherapeutic agent such as doxorubicin is injected, followed by an embolic agent such as iodized poppy seed oil, which both limits the tumor's blood supply and traps the agent in close proximity to the tumor. Combination therapy with cisplatin, doxorubicin, and mitomycin C often enhances the tumor-specific toxicity.[76] The procedure is typically performed without an anesthesiologist. If anesthesia is requested, the primary anesthetic concerns are patient comorbidities, coagulopathies, and hepatic insufficiency.

VASCULAR ACCESS

Vascular access refers to the placement of catheters in large veins for the infusion of medications (e.g., chemotherapy, parenteral feedings, antibiotics), dialysis, or blood sampling. Adults seldom require anesthesia care for catheter placement, but if anesthesia is needed, special attention is given to the patient's coexisting diseases and to the risk of air emboli through an open, large-bore catheter during spontaneous ventilation.

VASCULAR OCCLUSION PROCEDURES

Uterine fibroids, varicoceles, esophageal varices, and AVMs can be embolized under fluoroscopy. A catheter is inserted through a large artery or vein with the tip positioned near the structure to be embolized. Particles (e.g., gelfoam or particulate agents such as gelatin-impregnated acrylic polymer spheres), sclerosing agents (e.g., alcohols), metal coils, or liquid glue is used. The procedure is typically performed without an anesthesiologist. The primary concerns are patient comorbidities.

For the placement of balloon occlusion catheters in parturients at risk for hemorrhage, both general[77] and epidural[78] anesthesia have been utilized. An epidural catheter is placed before the balloon catheter is inserted to prevent displacement of the balloon when the patient is positioned and to provide analgesia should the patient undergo a cesarean section. Preparations should be in place for adequate intravenous access and invasive monitoring.

PERCUTANEOUS PROCEDURES

In percutaneous nephrolithotomy, medium-size or larger renal calculi are extracted from the urinary tract with a nephroscope. The patient is placed prone, and a track is created through a small incision above the kidney, through which dilators and finally the nephroscope are inserted. If the stones are small, they may be removed directly. For larger stones, percutaneous nephrolithotripsy breaks up the calculi into manageable pieces; the procedure requires a neuraxial block or general anesthesia.[79] Attention is paid to fluid absorption, dilutional anemia, hypothermia, the potential for significant blood loss,[80] renal insufficiency, and the effects of placing the patient in the prone position. Potential complications include pneumothorax or hydrothorax, pneumonia/atelectasis, paralytic ileus, nephrostomy tube dislodgement, urine drainage from the flank lasting more than 1 week, infection, urinoma formation, renal pelvic laceration, ureteral avulsion, ureteropelvic or ureteral stricture, bowel injury, or escape of stone fragments into the retroperitoneum.[81]

Percutaneous biliary drainage may be performed with local anesthesia at the site of the drain tube and with supplemental intravenous sedo-analgesia. When pain is anticipated from large drainage catheters or dilation of the transhepatic tracts, epidural or general anesthesia is recommended.[82] Hepatic insufficiency and the potential for blood loss should be considered in the anesthetic plan.

COMPUTED TOMOGRAPHY, MAGNETIC RESONANCE IMAGING, AND ULTRASOUND IMAGING

ABLATION PROCEDURES

Ablative therapies require cross-sectional images for accurate needle, probe, or catheter placement with the aid of CT, MRI, or ultrasound imaging. The same general imaging-specific caveats apply as for other therapeutic and diagnostic procedures. Thus, radiation exposure in the CT suite is monitored, and precautions against ferrous materials are taken in the MRI suite. The preanesthesia evaluation focuses on patient comorbidities.

Hyperthermic ablation includes RFA, microwave or laser ablation. In RFA, the most common procedure, electrical currents in the radio-frequency range heat an electrode that has been percutaneously or directly placed within a tumor. Because healthy tissue is better able to withstand heat, radio-frequency energy preferentially destroys the tumor and only a small edge of normal tissue around its perimeter. The heat also "cauterizes" small blood vessels and reduces the risk of bleeding. Kidney, lung, breast, bone, and liver tumors are common targets. Moderate sedation is often adequate for a percutaneous approach.[83] Radio-frequency techniques may be effective for hepatocellular carcinoma because ablation energy can be applied without pain.[84] General and epidural anesthesia are often used for RFA of renal cell tumors.[85] Because the process involves heat, precautions must be taken when the electrode is adjacent to critical structures. For example, during RFA for a mediastinal lymph node, a temperature probe was applied to the endotracheal tube cuff to monitor the tracheal temperature. When the temperature rose, chilled saline was substituted for air in the cuff to avoid tracheal trauma.[86]

Cryoablation is used for tumors in the lung, liver, breast, kidney, or prostate. Liquid nitrogen or gaseous argon destroys tissue by direct freezing, denaturation of cellular proteins, cell rupture, cell dehydration, and ischemia. Patient comfort and safety have been provided with local or general anesthesia.[87] In lung cryoablation, inflammation may result from the thawing phase of the ablated tissue. Cracking of a cryoablated liver may cause hemorrhage.[76]

INTERVENTIONAL NEURORADIOLOGY

Interventional neuroradiologists use imaging techniques combined with catheters and other devices to treat vascular lesions in the CNS and surrounding tissues by either occluding blood flow through abnormal vessels or by increasing blood flow in occluded vessels.[88] Cross-sectional imaging techniques assist in diagnosis, and the procedures are performed under fluoroscopy. Box 15.1 lists some procedures offered at a teaching hospital in the Midwest.

BOX 15.1 INTERVENTIONAL NEURORADIOLOGY PROCEDURES

1. Transarterial embolization of cerebral and spinal arteriovenous malformations and arteriovenous fistulas
2. Transarterial and transvenous embolization of cranial and spinal dural arteriovenous fistulas
3. Endosaccular embolization of intracranial aneurysms
4. Temporary and permanent balloon occlusion of intracranial and brachiocephalic vessels
5. Endovascular trapping of intracranial and extracranial aneurysms
6. Intracranial percutaneous transluminal angioplasty and stenting (e.g., internal carotid, middle cerebral, vertebrobasilar arteries)
7. Extracranial brachiocephalic percutaneous transluminal angioplasty and stenting (e.g., innominate, common and internal carotid, subclavian, and vertebral arteries)
8. Management of acute thromboembolic stroke with superselective intra-arterial chemical thrombolysis and percutaneous transluminal angioplasty
9. Chemical and mechanical angioplasty of intracranial vasospasm
10. Tumor embolization via transarterial and direct puncture
11. Embolization of congenital and acquired arteriovenous malformations and arteriovenous fistulas via transarterial, transvenous, and direct puncture
12. Direct puncture sclerotherapy of low-flow vascular malformations (e.g., venous, lymphatic, mixed)
13. Percutaneous vertebroplasty of benign and malignant vertebral compression fractures
14. Combined computed tomography and fluoroscopic-guided percutaneous biopsies, drainage procedures, and therapeutic embolization of spinal pathologies

Anesthesiologists are often needed because of the complexity of the procedure, the medical status of the patient, or the need for immobility. The preanesthesia assessment focuses on the patient's neurologic status and comorbidities. An anesthetic plan must consider the potential for disease progression or iatrogenic complications. Consultation with a neuroradiologist determines whether the patient must be responsive for continuous CNS evaluation or whether rapid emergence from general anesthesia is preferred. Anesthetic medications for a responsive patient include propofol, dexmedetomidine, and fentanyl; for general anesthesia, they include propofol, sevoflurane, and desflurane.[90] Nitrous oxide is not used because of the potential for enlarging emboli. Laryngeal mask airways may be considered for airway management.

Among the intraprocedural concerns are elevated intracranial pressure, hemorrhage, blood pressure issues, and cerebrovascular occlusion. Control of carbon dioxide may be necessary for selected procedures. Hypercapnia has been used to vasodilate cerebral vessels for catheter entry, to enhance catheter propagation during superselective cerebral catheterization, and to increase cerebral venous outflow, thereby favoring movement of an embolizing agent away from intracranial drainage pathways.[91] Hypocapnia may decrease CBF and lower intracranial pressure. Patient considerations include temperature, either warm for comfort or cool for cerebral protection[92]; padding; positioning; and bladder distention, the last because intravascular volume/renal perfusion must be maintained in the presence of a dye load. Table 15.13 lists some anesthetic considerations for various interventional neuroradiologic procedures.[93]

In addition to routine monitors, an arterial line may be needed if the procedure requires hypertension or hypotension. An arterial line enables the anesthesiologist to maintain the delicate balance between intracranial pressure and cerebral perfusion pressure or intravascular pressure if there is a potential for hemorrhage. If arterial monitoring will be needed after the procedure, a peripheral site (e.g., radial artery) may be preferred to the side port of the introducer sheath. Intravenous access should always be adequate and blood products should be available as needed.

Before certain obliterative procedures, awake patients may undergo Wada testing, in which a barbiturate is selectively injected into each cerebral hemisphere via the internal carotid artery to determine the dominant side for speech and memory. The superselective anesthesia functional examination (SAFE) is a variant of Wada testing that improves the specificity of the test by positioning the tip of the catheter closer to the targeted region.

PROCEDURES

Vertebroplasty and kyphoplasty are typically used to treat vertebral compression fractures in osteoporotic elderly patients with significant comorbidities, such as diminished pulmonary function associated with the vertebral fracture. These procedures may be performed with general anesthesia or sedation with local anesthesia. In either procedure, after the patient is placed prone, trocars are inserted on each side of the vertebral body under fluoroscopic or CT guidance. Polymethylmethacrylate (PMMA) is injected via a trocar into the medulla of the vertebral body under direct visualization. In kyphoplasty, a balloon is inserted through the trocar to restore

TABLE 15.13. Interventional Neuroradiologic Procedures and Primary Anesthetic Considerations

PROCEDURE	POSSIBLE ANESTHETIC CONSIDERATIONS
Therapeutic embolization of vascular malformation	
Intracranial AVMs	Deliberate hypotension, postprocedure NPPB
Dural AVM	Existence of venous hypertension, deliberate hypercapnia
Extracranial AVMs	Deliberate hypercapnia
Carotid cavernous fistula	Deliberate hypercapnia, postprocedure NPPB
Cerebral aneurysms	Aneurysmal rupture, blood pressure control[a]
Ethanol sclerotherapy of AVMs or venous malformations	Brain swelling, airway swelling, hypoxemia, hypoglycemia, intoxication from ethanol, cardiorespiratory arrest
Balloon A&S of occlusive cerebrovascular disease	Cerebral ischemia, deliberate hypertension, concomitant coronary artery disease
Balloon angioplasty of cerebral vasospasm secondary to aneurismal SAH	Cerebral ischemia, blood pressure control[a]
Therapeutic carotid occlusion for giant aneurysms and skull base tumors	Cerebral ischemia, blood pressure control[a]
Thrombolysis of acute thromboembolic stroke	Postprocedure ICH (NPPB), concomitant coronary artery disease, blood pressure control[a]
Intra-arterial chemotherapy of head and tumors	Airway swelling, intracranial hypertension
Embolization for epistaxis	Airway control

A&S, angioplasty and stenting; AVM, arteriovenous malformation; ICH, intracranial hemorrhage; NPPB, normal perfusion pressure breakthrough; SAH, subarachnoid hemorrhage.

[a] Blood pressure control refers to deliberate hypo- or hypertension.

SOURCE: From Young WL. Anesthesia for endovascular neurosurgery and interventional neuroradiology. *Anesthesiol Clin.* 2007;25(3):391–412. Copyright Elsevier 2007.

the intervertebral distance before PMMA is injected.[94] Risks of extravasations are increased by the presence of osteoporotic and osteolytic lesions. If PMMA leaks into perivertebral veins, it can cause radiculopathy, embolization, or interference with pulse oximetry readings. The most severe complication of PMMA leakage is spinal cord compression that requires immediate surgical decompression. Other complications associated with PMMA leaks are hypotension, hypoxemia, cardiac arrhythmias, and pulmonary embolism.[95]

Anesthesia for the endovascular coiling of cerebral aneurysms ranges from none to general anesthesia. Many radiologists prefer general anesthesia to obtain optimal conditions for imaging and patient comfort and safety, even though general anesthesia may mask the clinical signs that guide the progress of the procedure.[96] Patients with subarachnoid hemorrhage caused by a leaking or ruptured aneurysm are at greater risk for increased intracranial pressure, cerebral ischemia, and hydrocephalus. Patients with a ventricular drain are at risk for transmural pressure changes and rebleeding with elevated arterial pressure.[90]

Patients with an AVM often have a redistribution of blood flow from a steal phenomenon that may lead to the loss of autoregulation in the surrounding brain tissue as the chronic vasodilation compensates for the steal from the AVM. They may suffer spontaneous hemorrhage and have seizures or other neurological symptoms because of the ischemia resulting from this steal phenomenon or from venous hypertension.[97]

General anesthesia is often preferred for embolization of an AVM because it facilitates visualization of structures and avoids patient movement. Blood pressure is controlled by reducing the anesthetic or administering vasoactive agents that may help "float" a flow-directed catheter into the desired vessels. The most common AVM embolic agents are the fast-polymerizing liquid adhesive *N*-butyl cyanoacrylate (NBCA) and Onyx, which has a theoretical advantage of slow solidification, which allows for a more controlled injection. As newer agents become available and microcatheter technology improves, endovascular treatment of AVMs may expand.[98] During injection, Valsalva maneuvers and controlled hypotension may reduce the gradient across the AVM and diminish the amount of distal adhesive embolization.[99] When the AVM is embolized and the steal phenomenon ceases, the surrounding brain may suffer hyperperfusion injury unless the CBF is aggressively controlled with nitroprusside or other agents.

Pial and dural arteriovenous fistulas (AVFs) are direct shunts between an artery and a vein and may be associated with extremely high blood flow. Clinical characteristics include bruit, neurologic symptoms, or intracranial hemorrhage. Children may have concomitant high-output cardiac failure.[100] Transarterial embolization for high-flow, single-hole fistulas is performed with balloons, coils, stents, or NBCA.[90]

Cerebral thrombolytic procedures are most often performed on awake individuals, but their tenuous medical status may mandate an anesthesiologist's presence. Anesthesia concerns include altered mental status, airway protection, control of patient movement, and management of intracranial pressure.

Cerebral tumor embolization may be indicated for hemangioblastomas, intracranial metastases, meningiomas, hemangiopericytomas, neurogenic tumors (e.g., schwannomas), paragangliomas, juvenile nasopharyngeal angiofibromas, hemangiomas, esthesio-neuroblastomas, benign bone tumors, malignant bone tumors, and extracranial metastases.[101] As with an AVM, a steal phenomenon can result because of the hypervascular nature of these tumors. Hypotension should be prevented before embolization, and hypertension should be prevented after it. Other concerns include greater intracranial pressure from brain edema, which may be treated with steroids.

Neurophysiologic monitoring helps gauge the progress of an intervention. In a patient under general anesthesia, it signals impairment so that the cause of the insult can be reversed promptly. The EEG, somatosensory evoked potentials (SSEPs), and brainstem auditory evoked potentials are valuable adjuncts to endovascular treatment of cerebral aneurysms under general anesthesia.[102] Muscle motor evoked potentials can indicate spinal cord perfusion in the anterior spinal artery during endovascular procedures and complement SSEPs.[103] Transcranial Doppler ultrasonography directly measures regional cerebral blood flow (rCBF) in AVMs, aneurysms, and arterial stenoses.[104] Other direct measures of rCBF include radionuclide CBF (e.g., technetium) studies and xenon CT.[102] Because anesthetics often have an effect on measurements, the anesthesiologist must be in close communication with monitoring personnel to distinguish between anesthetic artifact and a new neurologic deficit.

Two serious complications of interventional neuroradiology procedures are intracranial hemorrhage and thromboembolic stroke.[105] The incidence of these two complications during coiling of cerebral aneurysms is 2.4% and 3.5%, respectively; during embolization of AVM, it is 1%–8%.[106] Arterial pressure increases suddenly with acute intracranial hemorrhage and should be controlled immediately. Heparin reversal may be necessary along with decreasing arterial pressure. Hyperventilation and mannitol should be considered to reduce intracranial pressure. Hemorrhage from a perforation can often be treated with coiling, although emergency craniotomy and clipping may be required if coiling fails.

Occlusive events can be thrombotic, embolic, or vasospastic. For all, the arterial pressure should be raised to increase collateral blood flow while normocarbia is maintained. Thrombi may be treated by mechanical lysis with a guidewire, normal saline, or thrombolytics. Misplaced coils may be retrieved endovascularly or via craniotomy. Vasospasm may be treated by increasing arterial pressure and volume while decreasing blood viscosity through hemodilution[107]; papaverine or nicardipine[108] or cerebral angioplasty[109] is also used. Maintaining hypotension with antihypertensive agents such as labetolol or esmolol may be beneficial after AVM embolization to avoid cerebral edema and hemorrhage. Using phenylephrine or norepinephrine can elevate mean arterial pressure 20%–30% above normal and maintain cerebral perfusion in patients with occlusion or vasospasm.[90]

Revascularization after an acute stroke is an emergency procedure that must be performed in a timely manner. Patients who have presented outside of the window for, or have contraindications to, systemic thrombolytics should be considered for endovascular treatment of acute ischemic stroke. Anesthesiologists are often involved due to the acute nature of the procedure. Preoperative assessment may be difficult if the patient's mental status is altered, but it is important to proceed promptly as even a 30-minute delay has been associated with worse outcomes at 3 months.[110] There are conflicting data to guide practitioners on anesthetic choice: Some data indicated worse outcomes with general anesthesia in retrospective studies in which the choice of general anesthesia was guided by institutional preference or severity of symptoms at presentation.[110] Thus, choice of general anesthesia with endotracheal intubation or local anesthesia with MAC should be based on patient condition and made in close communication with the neurointerventionalist. Placement of an arterial line is warranted to maintain strict hemodynamic goals of a systolic blood pressure between 140 and 180 mm Hg and a diastolic blood pressure less than 105 mm Hg, but placement should not delay the procedure.[110] After revascularization, blood pressure goals should be communicated with the neurointerventionalist to prevent the risk of hyperperfusion leading to hemorrhagic conversion. Euvolemia, normothermia, and normoglycemia should be maintained. Glucose should be monitored every hour and maintained between 140 and 70 mg/dL. Glucose-containing solutions should be started only if the blood sugar is below 50 mg/dL.[110]

RECOVERY

Recovery of the patient is governed by the ASA standards for postoperative care.[3] Nursing care should conform to the standards of the American Society of Perianesthesia Nurses. The facilities and equipment for recovery should be commensurate with the complexity of the patient's medical condition. Medically stable patients who have undergone innocuous procedures (MRI, inferior vena cava filter) under MAC can often recover en suite, provided that the nurses are trained and an anesthesiologist is available. Patients who have received regional or general anesthesia who are at risk for pain (e.g., RFA for hepatocellular carcinoma) or procedural complications (e.g., aortic stent graft) recover in a dedicated poastanesthesia care unit or an intensive care unit. Resuscitation equipment, oxygen, and monitors should be available for transport from the radiology suite.

SUMMARY

As minimally invasive techniques in radiology suites become more common, the need for anesthesia support will increase. Recognizing and addressing a patient's comorbidities and other concerns are similar to care given in the surgical setting. The additional requirements and constraints of the imaging environment and the procedure are unique and call for specific solutions. Just as in the operating room, there is frequently no single best anesthetic technique for a given procedure. The anesthetic should be aligned with the demands of the procedure and the skill sets of the providers. Patient safety always takes precedence, and the location should never be permitted to compromise care.

The radiologist serves a critical function, for it is the radiologist who decides whether to consult the anesthesiologist or perform a procedure alone. If the decision is to proceed with moderate sedation (administered by a nonanesthesia professional), the importance of vigilant clinical monitoring cannot be understated. In all cases, the patient deserves care that is consistent with the parameters, guidelines, and standards established by the various accrediting agencies and professional societies. There should be no exceptions.

REFERENCES

1. American Society of Anesthesiologists Task Force on Sedation and Analgesia by Non-Anesthesiologists. Practice guidelines for sedation and analgesia by non-anesthesiologists. *Anesthesiology.* 2002;96:1004–1017.
2. American Society of Anesthesiologists Task Force on Preanesthesia Evaluation. Practice advisory for preanesthesia evaluation: a report by the American Society of Anesthesiologists Task Force on Preanesthesia Evaluation. *Anesthesiology.* 2012;116:522–538.
3. American Society of Anesthesiologists Task Force on Postanesthetic Care. Practice guidelines for postanesthetic care: a report by the American Society of Anesthesiologists Task Force on Postanesthetic Care. *Anesthesiology.* 2013;118:291–307.
4. American Society of Anesthesiologists. Guidelines for nonoperating room anesthetizing locations, last amended 2013. Available at: http://www.asahq.org/quality-and-practice-management/standards-guidelines-and-related-resources/statement-on-nonoperating-room-anesthetizing-locations. Last accessed March 1, 2018.
5. American Society of Anesthesiologists. Distinguishing monitored anesthesia care (MAC) from moderate sedation/analgesia (conscious sedation). Last amended 2013. Available at: http://www.asahq.org/quality-and-practice-management/standards-guidelines-and-related-resources/distinguishing-monitored-anesthesia-care-from-moderate-sedation-analgesia. Last accessed March 1, 2018.
6. Bush WH, Swanson DP. Acute reactions to intravascular contrast media: types, risk factors, recognition, and specific treatment. *Am J Roentgenol.* 1991;157:1153–1161.
7. Almen T. The etiology of contrast medium reactions. *Invest Radiol.* 1994;29(suppl 1):S37–S45.
8. Paunnu N, Wiebe N, Tonelli M. Albert Kidney Disease Network. Prophylaxis strategies for contrast-induced nephropathy. *JAMA.* 2006;295:2765–2779.
9. Bush WH, Bettmann MA. Update on metformin (Glucophage®) therapy and the risk of lactic acidosis: change in FDA-approved package insert. *ACR Bulletin.* 1998;54(3):15.
10. American College of Cardiology. *ACR Manual on Contrast Media.* V10.2; 2016. Available at: https://www.acr.org/Clinical-Resources/Contrast-Manual. Last accesed March 1, 2018.
11. Kanal E, Borgstede JP, Barkovich AJ, et al. American College of Radiology white paper on MR safety: 2004 update and revisions. *Am J Roentgenol.* 2004;182:1111–1114.
12. American Society of Anesthesiologists. Practice advisory on anesthetic care for magnetic resonance imaging: a report by the American Society of Anesthesiologists Task Force on Anesthetic Care for Magnetic Resonance Imaging. *Anesthesiology.* 2009;110:459–479.
13. American College of Radiology. ACR/SIR practice parameter for sedation/analgesia, revised 2015. Available at: https://www.acr.org/-/media/ACR/Files/Practice-Parameters/sed-analgesia.pdf. Accessed on March 1, 2018.
14. American College of Radiology. ACR practice guideline for pediatric sedation/analgesia, revised 2005. Available at: http://www.spitjudms.ro/_files/protocoale_terapeutice/radiologie/12262.pdf. Accessed March 1, 2018.
15. Joint Commission on Accreditation of Healthcare Organizations. *Standard and Intents for Sedation and Anesthesia Care: Comprehensive Accreditation Manual for Hospitals.* Chicago, IL: JCAHO; 2001. Report TX. 2-2.4.1.
16. Kanal E, Barkovich AJ, Bell C, et al. ACR guidance document for safe MR Practices: (2007). *Am J Roentgenol.* 2007;188:1–27.
17. Shellock FG, Woods TO, Crues JV. MR labeling information for implants and devices: explanation of terminology. *Radiology.* 2009;253:26–30.
18. Zaballos M, Bastida E, del Castillo T, de Villoria JG, Jiménez C. In vitro study of magnetic resonance imaging artifacts of six supraglottic airway devices. *Anaesthesia.* 2010;65:569–572.
19. Dempsey MF, Condon B. Thermal injuries associated with MRI. *Clin Radiol.* 2001;56(6):457–465.
20. Bryan YF, Templeton TW, Nick TG, et al. Brain magnetic resonance imaging increases core body temperature in sedated children. *Anesth Analg.* 2006;102:1674–1679.
21. Hall SC, Stevenson GW, Suresh S. Burns associated with temperature monitoring during magnetic resonance imaging [letter]. *Anesthesiology.* 1992;76:152.
22. Bucsko JK. MRI facility safety: understanding the risks of powerful attraction. *Radiol Today.* 2005;6:22.
23. Peden CJ, Menon DK, Hall AS, et al. Magnetic resonance for the anaesthetist. Part II Anaesthesia and monitoring in the MR units. *Anaesthesia.* 1992;47:508–517.
24. Wegliniski MR, Berge KH, Davis DH. New-onset neurologic deficits after general anesthesia for MRI. *Mayo Clin Proc.* 2002;77(1):101–103.
25. Gozal D, Gozal Y. Spinal anesthesia for magnetic resonance imaging examination. *Anesthesiology.* 2003;99:764.
26. Taghon TA, Bryan YF, Kurth CD. Pediatric radiology sedation and anesthesia. *Int Anesthesiol Clin.* 2006;44(1):65–79.
27. Shorrab AA, Demian AD, Atallah MM. Multidrug intravenous anesthesia for children undergoing MRI: a comparison with general anesthesia. *Paediatr Anaesth.* 2007;17:1187–1193.
28. Dalal PG, Murray D, Cox T, et al. Sedation and anesthesia protocols used for magnetic resonance imaging studies in infants: provider and pharmacologic considerations. *Anesth Analg.* 2006;103:863–868.
29. Mason KP, Zurakowski D, Zgleszewski SE, et al. High dose dexmedetomidine as the sole sedative for pediatric MRI. *Paediatr Anaesth.* 2008;18:403–411
30. Occupational Safety & Health Administration Standards: Ionizing radiation. Available https://www.osha.gov/pls/oshaweb/owadisp.show_document?p_table=STANDARDS&p_id=10098. Accessed March 1, 2018.
31. Fishman EK. From the RSNA refresher courses CT angiography: clinical applications in the abdomen. *RadioGraphics.* 2001;21:S3–S16.
32. Lantz G, Grave de Peralta R, Spinelli L, Seeck M, Michel CM. Epileptic source localization with high density EEG: how many electrodes are needed? *Clin Neurophysiol.* 2003;114(1):63–69.
33. Georgopoulos AP, Karageorgiou E, Leuthold AC, et al. Synchronous neural interactions assessed by magnetoencephalography: a functional biomarker for brain disorders. *J Neural Eng.* 2007;4(4):349–355.
34. Ossenblok P, de Munck JC, Colon A, Drolsbach W, Boon P. Magnetoencephalography is more successful for screening and localizing frontal lobe epilepsy than electroencephalography. *Epilepsia.* 2007;48(11):2139–2249.
35. Raichle ME. Functional brain imaging and human brain function. *J Neurosci.* 2003;23(10):3959–3962.
36. Jack CR Jr, Thompson RM, Butts RK, et al. Sensory motor cortex: correlation of presurgical mapping with functional MR imaging and invasive cortical mapping. *Radiology.* 1994;190:85–92.
37. Yasaka M, Read SJ, O'Keefe GJ, et al. Positron emission tomography in ischaemic stroke: cerebral perfusion and metabolism after stroke onset. *J Clin Neurosci.* 1998;5:413–416.
38. Powers WJ, Zazulia AR. The use of positron emission tomography in cerebrovascular disease. *Neuroimaging Clin North Am.* 2003;13(4):741–758.
39. Federico F, Simone IL, Lucivero V, et al. Proton magnetic resonance spectroscopy in Parkinson's disease and progressive supranuclear palsy. *J Neurol Neurosurg Psychiatry.* 1997;62:239–242.
40. Lin AP, Tran TT, Ross BD. Impact of evidence-based medicine on magnetic resonance spectroscopy. *NMR Biomed.* 2006;19(4):476–483.
41. Alkire MT, Haier RJ, Shah NK, Anderson CT. Positron emission tomography study of regional cerebral metabolism in humans during isoflurane anesthesia. *Anesthesiology.* 1997;86:549–557.
42. Alkire MT, Pomfrett C. Functional brain imaging during anesthesia in humans: effects of halothane on global and regional cerebral glucose metabolism. *Anesthesiology.* 1999;90:701–709.
43. Fiset P, Paus T, Daloze T, et al. Brain mechanisms of propofolinduced loss of consciousness in humans: a positron emission tomographic study. *J Neurosci.* 1999;19(13):5506–5513.
44. Becerra L, Harter K, Gonzalez RG, Borsook D. Functional magnetic resonance imaging measures of the effects of morphine on central nervous system circuitry in opioidnaive healthy volunteers. *Anesth Analg.* 2006;103:208–216.
45. Kiviniemi VJ, Haanpää H, Kantola JH, et al. Midazolam sedation increases fluctuation and synchrony of the resting brain BOLD signal. *Magn Reson Imaging.* 2005;23(4):531–537.
46. Lorenz IH, Kolbitsch C, Hörmann C, et al. Increasing mean airway pressure reduces functional MRI (fMRI) signal in the primary visual cortex. *Magn Reson Imaging.* 2001;19(1):7–11.
47. Purdon PL, Pierce ET, Bonmassar G, et al. Simultaneous electroencephalography and functional magnetic resonance imaging of general anesthesia. *Ann NY Acad Sci.* 2009;1157(1):61–70.
48. Ramani R, Wardhan R. Understanding anesthesia through functional imaging. *Curr Opin Anaesthesiol.* 2008;21(5):530–536.
49. Rogers R, Wise R, Painter D, et al. Noninvasive brain imaging: an investigation to dissociate the analgesic and anesthetic properties of ketamine using functional magnetic resonance imaging. *J Pain.* 2004;5(suppl 1):S2.
50. Arepally A, Oechsle D, Kirkwood S, et al. Safety of conscious sedation in interventional radiology. *Cardiovasc Intervent Radiol.* 2001;24(3):185–190.

51. Haslam PJ, Yap B, Mueller PR, et al. Anesthesia practice and clinical trends in interventional radiology: a European survey. *Cardiovasc Intervent Radiol.* 2000;23(4):256–261.
52. Schenker MP, Martin R, Shyn PB, et al. Interventional radiology and anesthesia. *Anesthesiol Clin.* 2009;27:87–94.
53. Watkinson AF, Francis IS, Torrie P, et al. Commentary: the role of anaesthesia in interventional radiology. *Br J Radiol.* 2002;75:105–106.
54. Callstrom MR, Charboneau W, Goetz MP, et al. Painful metastases involving bone: feasibility of percutaneous CT- and US- guided radiofrequency ablation I. *Radiology.* 2002;224:87–97.
55. Ellis JE, Pai SS. Pro. Vascular stents in the radiology suite—an anesthesiologist is needed. *J Cardiothorac Vasc Anesth.* 2005;19:801–804.
56. Flaherty, J, Horn, J, Derby R. Regional anesthesia for vascular surgery. *Anesthesiology Clin.* 2014;32:639–659.
57. Ruppert V, Leurs LJ, Rieger J, et al; EUROSTAR Collaborators. Risk-adapted outcome after endovascular aortic aneurysm repair: analysis of anesthesia types based on EUROSTAR Data. *J Endovasc Ther.* 2007;14:12–22.
58. Henretta JP, Hodgson KJ, Mattos MA, et al. Feasibility of endovascular repair of abdominal aortic aneurysms with local anesthesia with intravenous sedation. *J Vasc Surg.* 1999;29:793–799.
59. Bernard EO, Schmid ER, Lachat ML, et al. Nitroglycerin to control blood pressure during endovascular stentgrafting of descending thoracic aortic aneurysms. *J Vasc Surg.* 2000;31:790–793.
60. Strachan AN, Edwards ND. Anaesthesia for stent graft repair of thoracic aneurysm and coarctation of the aorta. *Eur J Anaesthesiol.* 2001;18:759–762.
61. Winnerkvist A, Anderson RE, Hansson Lo, et al. Multilevel somatosensory evoked potentials and cerebrospinal proteins: indicators of spinal cord injury in thoracoabdominal aortic aneurysm surgery. *Eur J Cardiothorac Surg.* 2007;31:637–642.
62. Tiesenhausen K, Amann W, Koch G, et al. Cerebrospinal fluid drainage to reverse paraplegia after endovascular thoracic aortic aneurysm repair. *J Endovasc Ther.* 2000;7:132–135.
63. Cheung AT, Pochettino A, McGarvey ML, et al. Strategies to manage paraplegia risk after endovascular stent repair of descending thoracic aortic aneurysms. *Ann Thorac Surg.* 2005;80:1280–1288.
64. White CJ. Carotid artery stenting vs endarterectomy expert analysis. Available at: http://www.acc.org/latest-in-cardiology/articles/2016/04/27/09/38/carotid-stenting-vs-endarterectomy. Published April 27, 2016. Last accessed March 1, 2018.
65. Brott TG, Halperin JL, Abbara S, et al. 2011 ASA/ACCF/AHA/AANN/AANS/ACR/ASNR/CNS/SAIP/SCAI/SIR/SNIS/SVM/SVS guideline on the management of patients with extracranial carotid and vertebral artery disease: executive summary: a report of the American College of Cardiology Foundation/American Heart Association Task Force on Practice Guidelines, and the American Stroke Association, American Association of Neuroscience Nurses, American Association of Neurological Surgeons, American College of Radiology, American Society of Neuroradiology, Congress of Neurological Surgeons, Society of Atherosclerosis Imaging and Prevention, Society for Cardiovascular Angiography and Interventions, Society of Interventional Radiology, Society of NeuroInterventional Surgery, Society for Vascular Medicine, and Society for Vascular Surgery. *J Am Coll Cardiol.* 2011;57:1002–1044.
66. Nagata S, Kazekawa K, Aikawa H, et al. Hemodynamic stability under general anesthesia in carotid artery stenting. *Radiat Med.* 2005;23(6):427–431.
67. Steib A, Collange O. Anesthesia for other endovascular stenting. *Curr Opin Anesthesiol.* 2008;21:519–522.
68. Neglen P, Holis KC, Olivier J, et al. Stenting of the venous outflow in chronic venous disease: long-term stent-related outcome, clinical, and hemodynamic result. *J Vasc Surg.* 2007;46:979–990.
69. Bierdrager E, Lampmann LE, Lohle PN, et al. Endovascular stenting in neoplastic superior vena cava syndrome prior to chemotherapy or radiotherapy. *Neth J Med.* 2005;63:20–23.
70. Pivalizza EG, Gottschalk LI, Cohen A, et al. Anesthesia for transjugular intrahepatic portosystemic shunt placement. *Anesthesiology.* 1996;85:946–947.
71. Scher C. Anesthesia for transjugular intraheptaic portosystemic shunt. *Int Anesthesiol Clin.* 2009;47(2):21–28.
72. Slaughter TF. Ambulatory regional anesthesia and anticoagulation. In: Steel SM, Nielsen KC, Klein SM, eds. *The Ambulatory Anesthesia and Perioperative Analgesia Manual.* New York, NY: McGraw-Hill; 2004:445–451.
73. Alessandri C, Bergeron P. Local anesthesia in carotid angioplasty. *J Endovasc Surg.* 1996;3(1):31–34.
74. De Vries JP, van Den Heuvel DA, Vos JA, et al. Freedom from secondary interventions to treat stenotic disease after percutaneous transluminal angioplasty of infrarenal aorta: long-term results. *J Vasc Surg.* 2004;39:427–431.
75. Leyendecker JR, Dodd GD III. Minimally invasive techniques for the treatment of liver tumors. *Semin Liver Dis.* 2001;21(2):283–291.
76. Sundaram R, Brown AG, Koteeswaran SK, et al. Anaesthetic implications of uterine artery embolisation in management of massive obstetric haemorrhage. *Anaesthesia.* 2006;61:248–252.
77. Harnett MJ, Carabuena JM, Tsen LC, Kodali BS. Anesthesia for interventional radiology in parturients at risk of major hemorrhage at cesarean secion delivery. *Anesth Analg.* 2006;103:1329–1330.
78. Kuzgunbay B, Turunc T, Akin S, Ergenoglu P, Aribogan A, Ozkardes H. Percutaneous nephrolithotomy under general versus combined spinal-epidural anesthesia. *J Endourol.* 2009;23:1835–1838.
79. Rozentsveig V, Neulander AZ, Roussabrov E, et al. Anesthetic considerations during percutaneous nephrolithotomy. *J Clin Anesth.* 2007;19:351–355.
80. Lee WJ, Smith AD, Cubelli V, et al. Complications of percutaneous nephrolithotomy. *Am J Roentgenol.* 1987;148:177–180.
81. Barth KH. Percutaneous biliary drainage for high obstruction. *Radiol Clin North Am.* 1990;28(6):1223–1235.
82. McGhana JP, Dodd GD III. Radiofrequency ablation of the liver: current status. *Am J Roentgenol.* 2001;176:3–16.
83. Kurokohchi K, Watanabe S, Yoneyama H, et al. A combination therapy of ethanol injection and radiofrequency ablation under general anesthesia for the treatment of hepatocellular carcinoma. *World J Gastroenterol.* 2008;14(13):2037–2243.
84. Ukimura O, Kawauchi A, Fujito A, et al. Radio-frequency ablation of renal cell carcinoma in patients who were at significant risk. *Int J Urol.* 2004;11:1051–1057.
85. Hanazaki M, Taga N, Nakatsuka H, et al. Anesthetic management of radiofrequency ablation of mediastinal metastatic lymph nodes adjacent to the trachea. *Anesth Analg.* 2006;103:1041–1042.
86. Shingleton WB, Sewell PE Jr. Percutaneous renal tumor cryoblation with magnetic resonance imaging guidance. *J Urol.* 2001;165:773–776.
87. Taylor W, Rodesch G. Recent advances: interventional neuroradiology. *BMJ.* 1995;311:789–792.
88. Varma MK, Price K, Jayakrishnan V, et al. Anaesthetic considerations for interventional neuroradiology. *Br J Anaesth.* 2007;99(1):75–85.
89. Lai YC, Bulusu R, Manninen PH. Anesthesia for interventional neuroradiology: general considerations. *Semin Anesthesia Perioperative Med Pain.* 2000;19(4):248–253.
90. Busto R, Dietrich WD, Globus MY, et al. Small differences in intraischemic brain temperature critically determine the extent of ischemic neuronal injury. *J Cereb Blood Flow Metab.* 1987;7:729–738.
91. Biebuyck JF, Young WL, Pile-Spellman J. Anesthetic considerations for interventional neuroradiology. *Anesthesiology.* 1994;80:427–456.
92. Wiles MD, Nowicki RW, Hancock SM, et al. Anaesthesia for vertebroplasty and kyphoplasty. *Curr Anaesth Crit Care.* 2009;20:38–41.
93. Frost EA, Johnson DM. Anesthetic considerations during vertebroplasty, kyphoplasty, and intradiscal electrothermal therapy. *Int Anesthesiol Clin.* 2009;4(2):45–55.
94. Jones M, Leslie K, Mitchell P. Anaesthesia for endovascular treatment of cerebral aneurysms. *Clin Neurosci.* 2004;11:468–470.
95. Crawford PM, West CR, Chadwick DW, Shaw MD. Areteriovenous malformations of the brain: natural history in unoperated patients. *J Neurol Neurosurg Psychiatry.* 1986;49:1–10.
96. Bruno CA, Meyers PM. Endovascular management of arteriovenous malformations of the brain. *Interv Neurol.* 2013;1(3–4):109–123.
97. Cockroft KM, Hwang SK, Rosenwasser RH. Endovascular treatment of cerebral arteriovenous malformations: indications, techniques, outcome, and complications. *Neurosurg Clin N Am.* 2005;16:367–380.
98. Söderman M, Pavic L, Edner G, et al. Natural history of dural arteriovenous shunts. *Stroke.* 2008;39:1735–1739.
99. American Society of Interventional and Therapeutic Neuroradiology. Head, neck, and brain tumor embolization. *Am J Neuroradiol.* 2001;22(suppl 8):S14–S15.
100. Liu AY, Lopez JR, Do HM, et al. Neurophysiological monitoring in the endovascular therapy of aneurysms. *Am J Neuroradiol.* 2003;24:1520–1527.
101. Sala F, Niimi Y, Berenstein A, Deletis V. Neuroprotective role of neurophysiological monitoring during endovascular procedures in the spinal cord. *Ann NY Acad Sci.* 2001;939:126–136.
102. Lai YC, Manninen PH. Neurophysiologic monitoring and future monitoring modalities during interventional neuroradiology. *Sem Anesth Perioperative Med Pain.* 2000;19(4):309–314.

103. Young WL. Anesthesia for endovascular neurosurgery and interventional neuroradiology. *Anesthesiol Clin.* 2007;25(3):391–412.
104. Martin NA, Khanna R, Doberstein C, Bentson J. Therapeutic embolization of arteriovenous malformations: the case for and against. *Clin Neurosurg.* 2000;46:295–318.
105. Treggiari MM, Walder B, Suter PM, et al. Systematic review of the prevention of delayed ischemic neurological deficits with hypertension, hypervolemia, and hemodilution therapy following subarachnoid haemorrhage. *J Neurosurg.* 2003;98:978–984.
106. Badjatia N, Topcuoglua MA, Pryor JC, et al. Preliminary experience with intra-arterial nicardipine as a treatment for cerebral vasospasm. *Am J Neuroradiol.* 2004;25:819–826.
107. Brothers MF, Holgate RC. Intracranial angioplasty for treatment of vasospasm after subarachnoid hemorrhage: technique and modifications to improve branch access. *Am J Neuroradiol.* 1990;11(2):239–247.
108. Talke PO, Sharma D, Heyer EJ, et al. Society for Neuroscience in Anesthesiology and Critical Care expert consensus statement: anesthetic management of endovascular treatment for acute ischemic stroke: endorsed by the Society of Neuro Interventional Surgery and the Neurocritical Care Society. *J Neurosurg Anesthesiol.* 2014;26:95–108.

16 | ANESTHESIA IN THE RADIATION ONCOLOGY SUITE

ERIC A. HARRIS, MD, MBA, KEITH CANDIOTTI, MD

INTRODUCTION

Cancer continues to be a leading cause of death in the developed world, with physicians and scientists constantly devising new weapons to combat it. Among the pediatric population (age 0–14 years), it is estimated that 15,780 cases are diagnosed annually,[1] making it the second leading cause of death within this age group (accidents remain the primary culprit). Leukemia (especially acute lymphocytic leukemia) is the most common malignancy in this age group, followed by brain and central nervous system (CNS) tumors, soft tissue sarcomas, Wilms tumors, and non-Hodgkin's lymphoma.[2] Chemotherapy, surgery, nutrition, and holistic medicine all have a place in the multimodal approach that can prolong longevity and ameliorate quality of life. As part of this armamentarium, radiation therapy (XRT) has proven to be a safe and effective technique for the management of various malignant (and occasionally nonmalignant) lesions. XRT can be used for both curative and palliative purposes; in the latter case, patients benefit from decreased pain, preserved organ function, and the maintenance of lumen patency in hollow organs.[3] The medical team, led by a radiation oncologist, often includes a physicist, a dosimetrist, several radiation therapists (technologists), and the patient's primary care physician.[4] Anesthesiologists are increasingly being asked to join this team, as our services are recognized as a vital component for patient safety and comfort.

SELECTION CRITERIA

Because XRT is a painless procedure, the vast majority of patients can complete their treatment without the use of anesthesia or sedation. Many others can be managed with small amounts of a benzodiazepine administered by a nurse certified in patient sedation. A small fraction of patients, however, will require the expertise of an anesthesia team. In general, the following populations may require anesthesia services:

1. *Children:* Surprisingly, many children are able to handle XRT without any medication. Parental reassurance and possibly the promise of a small reward afterward provide enough motivation for many children to remain still. Clearly, babies and younger toddlers are not receptive to such enticement, and these are the patients who make up the vast majority of XRT anesthesia cases. Older children may be distressed by the absence of a parent next to them, but they often respond well to pictures attached to the ceiling within their field of view or the presence of music in the room. Indicators that suggest the need for anesthesia include young age, anxiety, treatment complexity (e.g., prone position), emotional immaturity for age, and a history of noncompliance.[5] Children up to age 3 almost always require some degree of sedation or anesthesia, with the incidence decreasing in an age-dependent fashion after that point (50% at age 7–8, 10% at age 12 or greater). There is no apparent correlation between gender and the need for anesthesia.[6]
2. *Patients with mental disabilities:* These patients may present as anxious, uncooperative, and combative. The application of physical restraints may only worsen the situation, and anesthetic intervention is often the only way to proceed. These patients may remain uncooperative throughout the entire course of treatment and are therefore some of the most challenging cases faced in the XRT suite.
3. *Patients with movement disorders:* Conditions such as tardive dyskinesia, choreiform disorders, and Parkinson disease make it difficult or impossible for these patients to remain still. Because effective treatment relies on precise anatomical targeting, such movements may be detrimental to the patient's course of therapy. These patients may therefore require general anesthesia with skeletal muscle paralysis.
4. *Claustrophobic patients:* In general, these patients do not find XRT as disturbing as magnetic resonance imaging (MRI) or computed tomographic (CT) scanning. However, if the head or neck is being treated, a plastic shield must be secured over the face. Many claustrophobic patients will not tolerate this unless they are deeply sedated.
5. *Procedures that are sufficiently painful:* Examples include treatment planning for prostate and cervical cancer (due to the exquisite neural innervation of these areas), where monitored anesthesia care (MAC) or general anesthesia may be required.

ANESTHESIOLOGY IN REMOTE LOCATIONS

The provision of anesthesia for patients undergoing radiotherapy procedures may present a deceptively simple challenge to the anesthesiologist. These cases are often very short in duration, sometimes lasting no more than 10 minutes. Furthermore, they can usually be accomplished without the use of general anesthesia. The patients themselves are typically young, and from a cardiopulmonary standpoint they are often healthy. There is no blood loss or fluid shift present. How then can we explain the discomfort that anesthesia providers experience when faced with performing cases in the XRT suite?

In general, many clinicians experience a palpable sense of angst when asked to do cases anywhere outside of the "comfort zone" of the operating room. The personnel employed in the XRT suite are well trained in their field of expertise; unfortunately for us, that field has little to do with anesthesiology. Assistance with lines, difficult airways, or anesthetic emergencies may be delayed or completely unavailable. Anesthesia staff and the anesthesia technicians might not be familiar with the location of the XRT suite, making it difficult and time consuming to acquire personnel support, extra drugs, or equipment. However, the greatest source of concern seems to be the physical distance that must be maintained from the patients. While many remote anesthetizing locations force the anesthesiologist to be a considerable distance from the patient, perhaps even in a different room (CT scanner, MRI suite), the XRT area is unique in that there is no means of directly viewing the patient or the monitors. Instead, once the procedure has begun, we must rely solely on the use of closed-circuit television monitoring. While "tele-anesthesia" has long been postulated as a possible future direction of the field (see Chapter 36), few practitioners are excited about being the mavericks forced to incorporate this technology into their current practice.

FUNDAMENTALS OF XRT

Before anesthesiologists can feel more comfortable providing anesthesia in the XRT suite, they must first have a basic understanding of what is accomplished there. When the actual treatment room is first entered, the most obvious piece of equipment is the linear accelerator (Figure 16.1). Inside of this machine, atomic particles are accelerated to very high energy states within a vacuum. The particles are then forced to collide with a material such as tungsten, which releases energy in the form of x-rays.[7] This energy is then focused at specific sites within the patient in an effort to degrade the genetic material within the tumor cells. The energy absorbed by the tissues is measured in terms of gray (Gy), which has replaced the more antiquated unit of rad, with 1 Gy equal to the deposition of 1 J/kg and equivalent to 100 rad units.[8] While most patients receive this type of x-ray therapy, other types of lesions respond better to bombardment with electron, proton, or neutron beam therapy. In any event, the anesthetic considerations are essentially identical despite the type of subatomic particle that is utilized.

SIMULATION

When a patient is accepted as a candidate for XRT, he or she must first undergo a treatment-planning session, referred to as a simulation. The physical setup of the simulation suite is similar to the XRT therapy room (Figure 16.2). However, the simulation machine is incapable of delivering therapeutic doses of radiation. Instead, it is used to provide radiographs and CT images of each treatment field, which will aid the XRT team in planning radiation doses and points of entry. Simulation serves several functions at the outset of therapy:

1. Simulation allows the radiation oncologist to prescribe the proper treatment by reproducing the exact conditions that will be encountered during the weeks of therapy. The number and location of anatomic fields that will need treatment will be decided; the XRT team may typically treat anywhere from one to six fields, depending on the type and size of the lesion. Ideal patient positioning will also be determined. Most patients can be treated in the supine position; however, craniospinal axis radiotherapy will necessitate the patient remaining in the prone position throughout therapy while two lateral whole-brain fields are supplemented with a posterior field of the spine.[9] This adds another layer of challenge to the anesthetic management.
2. Once these sites are determined, the therapist will mark the skin with ink to denote targets for future treatment. These markings will remain on the patient for the duration of the therapy and may be reapplied by the therapist as necessary. The markings increase accuracy and greatly enhance the speed of the future therapy sessions.
3. Plaster immobilization casts of the head (Aquaplast RT, Q-Fix, Avondale, PA; Figure 16.3) or body (Alpha Cradle, Smithers Medical Products Inc., North Canton, OH; Figure 16.4) are made, depending on the sites that are to be treated. These casts are designed to hold the patient in a fixed, uniform position during the treatment sessions, ensuring that the radiation is directed at its target and not at normal surrounding tissue. Inadequate immobilization can result in treatment failure[10,11] as well as damage to normal tissue.[12]
4. The radiation oncologist will determine whether blocks will be necessary during the treatment period. Blocks are radiopaque shields that are attached to the linear accelerator (Figure 16.5) to shield radiosensitive organs (e.g., kidneys, eyes) from the ionizing radiation.
5. If the team is still questioning the need for anesthesia, the simulation offers an ideal trial, without the risk of radiation, to see whether the patient will be cooperative and can remain immobile during the session.

The simulation session takes anywhere from 20 to 90 minutes, depending on the level of cooperation of the patient

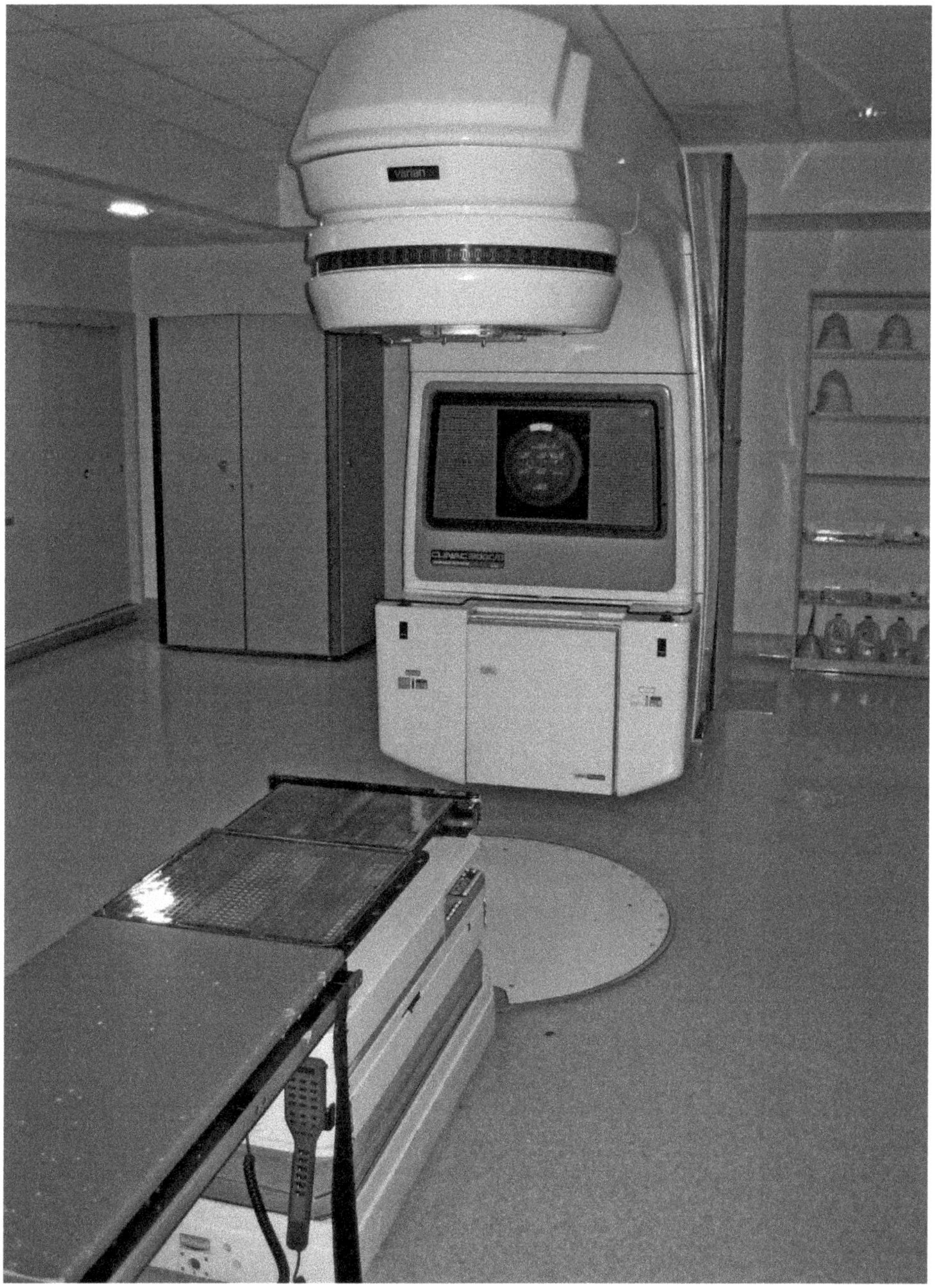

Figure 16.1. The linear accelerator.

and the number and location of the fields that need to be marked. Most patients who will require anesthesia for XRT do well during the simulation with MAC. Because therapeutic radiation is not used, the anesthesia team can remain with the patient during the majority of the simulation. When conventional radiographs are taken, the anesthesia and radiation oncology teams can remain in the room while wearing lead shielding or can safely observe the patient through a panel of leaded glass from an adjacent room. Medications can be given freely throughout the procedure as dictated by patient anxiety and motion. If general anesthesia is required, the anesthesia machine must be placed in a location that will not interfere with the lateral x-ray fields. Circuit hose extensions may be needed to place the machine at an appropriate distance from the patient. At the conclusion of the simulation, patients may be recovered in the XRT suite, provided there is adequate nursing supervision. Alternatively, the patient can recover in the main postanesthesia care unit.

The simulation phase may immediately be followed by the first treatment, but it is more common for the patient to return within the next day or two to begin the actual XRT. This gives the team adequate time to map the coordinates of the sites that will be irradiated and to decide on dose and duration parameters. Total dose varies between 25 and 80 Gy, with a median value of 60 Gy. Lower doses are used for hematological cancers (leukemia, lymphoma) and seminomas; higher doses are reserved for solid tumors such as sarcomas and gliomas. The total dose of radiation is typically divided

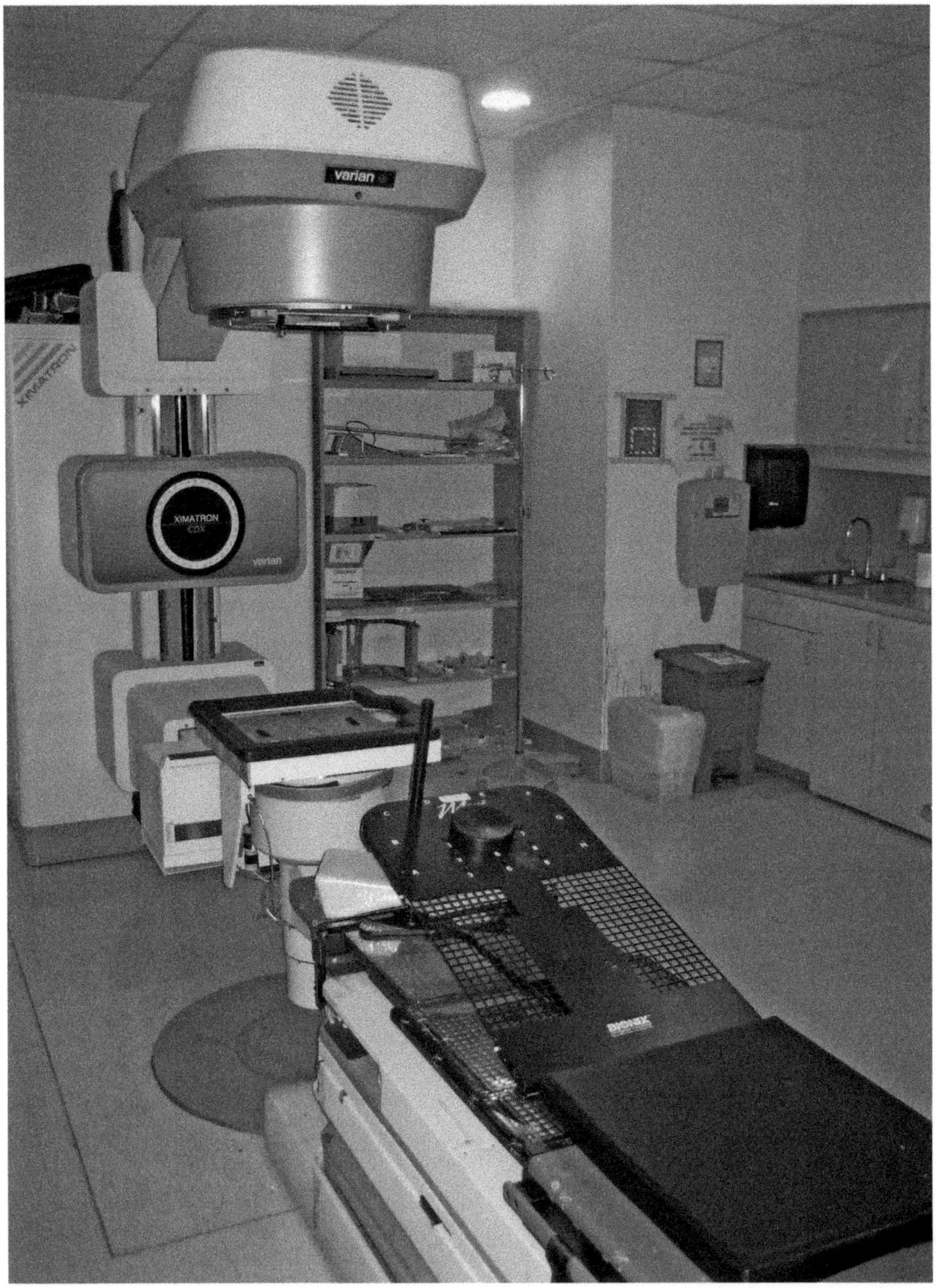

Figure 16.2. The simulation machine.

into 30 equal portions and administered once daily, 5 days per week, over a 6-week period. Certain patients may benefit from hyperfractionated irradiation or the administration of XRT more than once daily.[13] Each field requires up to 90 seconds of irradiation; after this is completed, the radiation therapists must adjust the couch, reset the coordinates of the linear accelerator, and change the blocks so that the next field can be treated. Depending on the number of fields (typically no more than six), the entire process can be completed in anywhere from 5 to 20 minutes. At specified time intervals (usually once per week), the therapists will repeat the radiographs to ensure that the anatomic targeting of the radiation beam is still accurate. This should add no more than another 5 minutes to the procedure.

ANESTHETIC MANAGEMENT OF XRT TREATMENT

The majority of patients who require anesthetic intervention can tolerate the daily therapeutic regimen with only MAC. Even patients who may have required general anesthesia for the simulation typically do well with heavy sedation during the therapy phase due to the brief time required for treatment. One significant exception is the patient being treated for retinoblastoma; in this case, the globe must be kept completely immobile. MAC sedation, especially if ketamine is used (with a resultant lateral nystagmus), cannot accomplish this.[14] The room will be evacuated during the treatment period; however, it is safe to reenter in between doses; therefore, it is unusual to

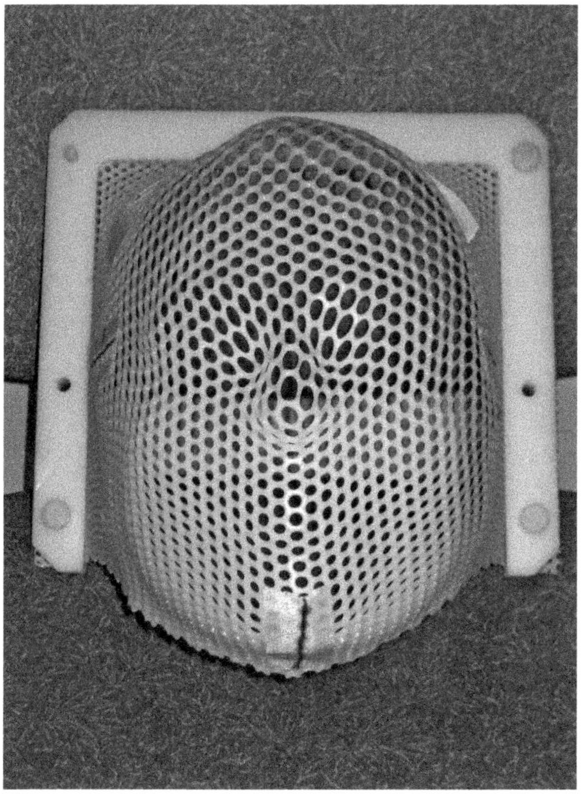

Figure 16.3. A premolded Aquaplast.

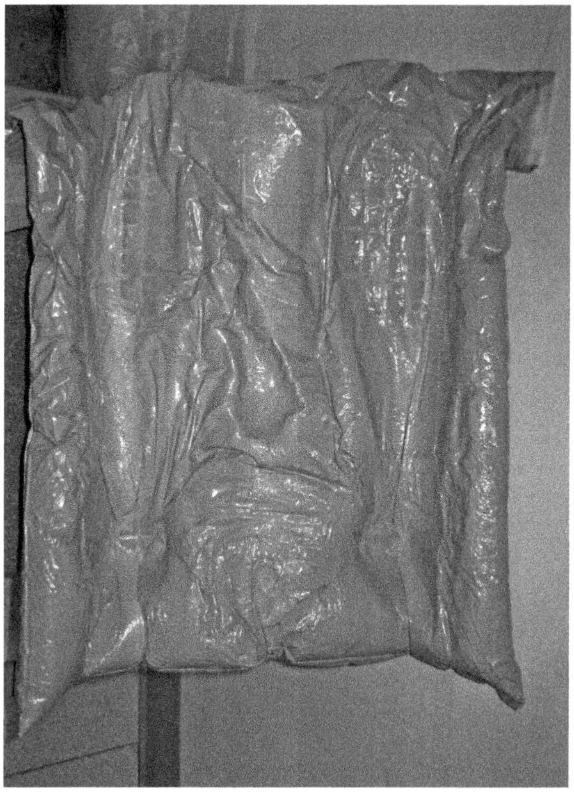

Figure 16.4. A premolded Alpha Cradle.

be away from the patient for more than 3 minutes. Of course, any reasonable request to reenter the room at any time should be honored by the radiation therapist; the treatment can be aborted before it is completed to allow safe entry into the room.

Patients are advised to follow fasting guidelines typical for all ambulatory patients. If the tumor or medical condition is impairing gastric emptying, stricter guidelines may need to be enforced. Parents are encouraged to allow infants and children to ingest solid food up to 4 hours before the procedure, and clear liquids and breast milk are generally permitted up to 2 hours beforehand.[15,16]

The intravenous route is the preferred method of administering medication to these patients. While intramuscular drugs such as ketamine are effective, the repeated trauma of a painful injection daily for 6 weeks is often worse than the prospect of the XRT therapy. A large majority of these patients have either recently completed a course of chemotherapy or are receiving it concomitant with the XRT and will therefore have an intravascular port present. Typically, the port can be accessed with a Huber needle (Figure 16.6) on the morning prior to the first treatment, and the access can be left in place throughout the week and removed after the week's final treatment on Friday. The port remains dormant over the weekend, and the cycle repeats the following week. Caregivers can apply EMLA cream (AstraZeneca, London, England) to the site 1 hour before arriving Monday morning to make the access less traumatic. Alternatively, if the patient does not have a port, intravenous access via a peripheral vein can be obtained Monday morning, left in throughout the week, and removed on Friday, thereby following the same schedule.[17] Again, EMLA can greatly facilitate the process. In either case, the port or catheter should be flushed with a heparin flush solution (typically 300 units of heparin in 3 mL of normal saline) at the conclusion of each treatment to ensure continued patency throughout the week.

Aseptic technique is imperative when accessing a port or placing an intravenous catheter. These patients are typically neutropenic from the XRT or chemotherapy, as well as their disease state, and cannot tolerate the threat of bacterial infection. Large case series estimated the risk of sepsis between 7%[5] and 15%.[18] The use of propofol, which can act as a potent culture medium for bacteria, may enhance the risk.[19]

Even with strict aseptic technique, it is unfortunately common for these children to develop concomitant medical conditions that increase the risk of anesthesia administration. Upper respiratory infection (often secondary to neutropenia) and serum electrolyte disturbances (usually as a result of prolonged emesis) are the most common.[20] The natural instinct to delay such a case until the abnormality is corrected must be weighed against the risk of delaying the XRT. Consultation with the radiation oncologist is therefore of paramount importance.

Fortunately, the advent of short-acting sedative agents has replaced much of the use of such pediatric favorites as rectal methohexital,[21] chloral hydrate, and the DPT (meperidine, promethazine, and chlorpromazine) cocktail.[22] Intravenous midazolam has been the cornerstone of pediatric sedation since its introduction into clinical practice. The anxiolytic and amnestic profile is so good that many patients can complete their entire series of treatments with

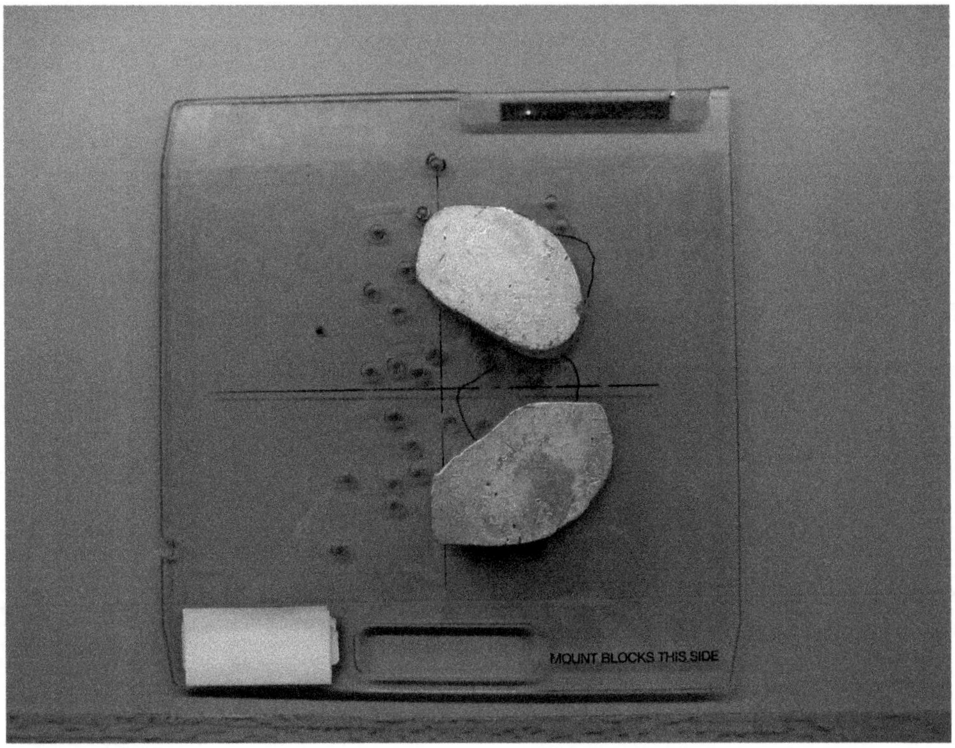

Figure 16.5. Blocks used to shield radiosensitive organs.

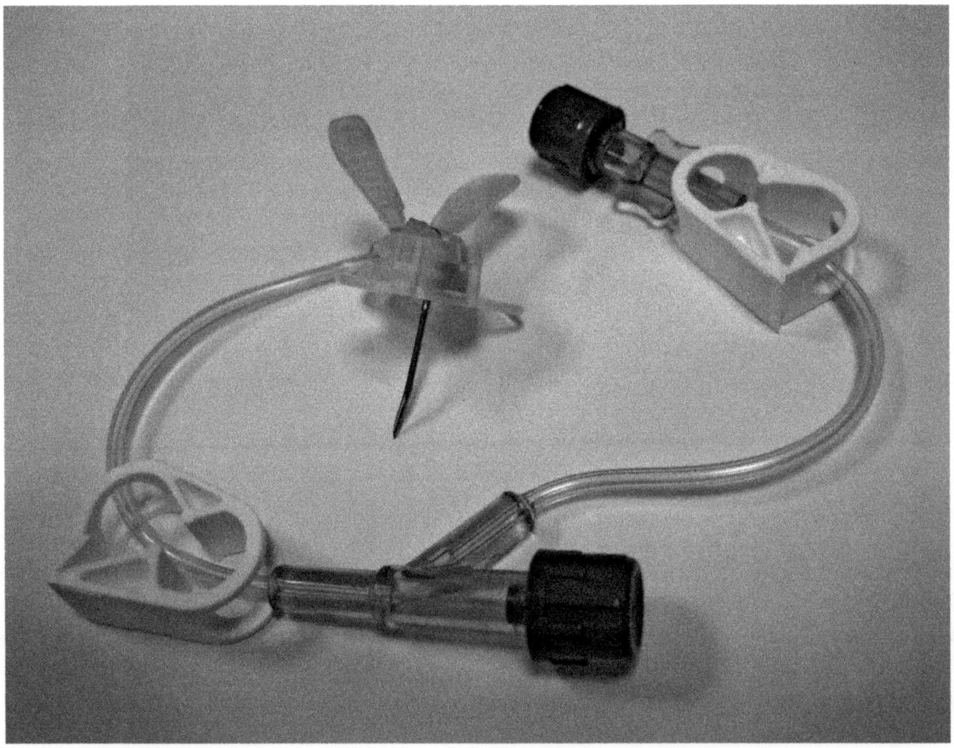

Figure 16.6. A Huber needle used to access an intravascular port.

the aid of only this drug. If this is the case, participation of an anesthesiologist is rarely warranted.[23] The safety record of intravenous midazolam used in the absence of other sedative drugs is extensive. Because XRT is a painless procedure, it is unnecessary to supplement the benzodiazepine with narcotics. Therefore, with adequate monitoring of vital signs, the sedation can typically be managed by a registered nurse.

Patients who require more extensive therapy often still benefit from the concomitant use of midazolam. An initial dose of 0.05 mg/kg IV often provides enough sedation to allow for the placement of monitors. If ketamine is to be used, midazolam may decrease the incidence of postprocedure delirium.[24] After this initial dose of midazolam, the patient should be dosed with a more potent agent to allow for transfer to the treatment couch and placement of therapeutic restraining devices. If necessary, midazolam can be readministered; cumulative doses greater than 0.2 mg/kg are rarely necessary.

When benzodiazepine therapy is insufficient, propofol has become the agent of preference for many anesthesiologists, especially when dealing with children.[25] (One large study of 1033 procedures noted successful sedation in 68% of the patients who received meperidine, chloral hydrate, or midazolam, versus 97% successful sedation in patients who received more potent drugs, such as propofol.[5]) After benzodiazepine pretreatment as previously described, an initial propofol bolus in the range of 0.5–0.8 mg/kg has been shown to provide adequate sedation for positioning and manipulation on the XRT couch while allowing for spontaneous respiration and airway control.[26] This is followed by a continuous propofol infusion in the range of 7.4–10 mg/kg per hour throughout the treatment phase.[27,28] Spontaneous eye opening was noted within 4 minutes of discontinuing the infusion.[26] Initial concerns about tachyphylaxis to propofol[29] have been disproven by more recent studies,[30–32] one of which even suggested a decreasing propofol requirement as therapy progresses.[33] Thus, propofol, combined with midazolam, provides excellent therapeutic conditions throughout the entire course of treatment.[34] The safety profile of propofol has been confirmed by the publication of the largest study to date of these patients: Owusu-Agyemang et al. reported a series of 9328 pediatric proton beam therapy procedures in which propofol was used (97.9% as the sole anesthetic, 2.1% supplemented with dexmedetomidine) and reported a complication rate of only 0.05%.[35]

The infusion of the α_2-agonist dexmedetomidine in the XRT suite has been described,[36] although it has not been widely adopted. Likely reasons for its infrequent use include the prolonged time needed to administer the initial bolus (which can be as long as the entire case itself) and the fact that analgesia is not necessary in these painless cases.

Ketamine is another drug that is also used successfully, following midazolam pretreatment,[37] to manage patients in the XRT suite.[38,39] Ketamine can be given as a continuous infusion (25 mg/kg per hour),[40] but the α-phase serum half-life of 11 minutes[41] and the short duration of these cases often makes this unnecessary. An initial dose of 0.5–0.75 mg/kg given at the start of therapy is often all that is required to accomplish the procedure. If the patient becomes agitated during the treatment, a supplemental dose of 0.25 mg/kg can be given to extend the period of cooperation. At some institutions, the use of ketamine has become so standardized that it is used in the XRT suite in the absence of an anesthesiologist.[42]

Several case series have reported a complication rate of between 23%[43] and 24%[44] associated with the use of ketamine. However, these complications are minor (the most commonly reported were sialorrhea, delayed recovery, and emergence delirium) and commonly associated with this drug. The prior administration of midazolam and an antisialogogue are useful adjuncts to decrease the incidence of these unwanted side effects.

Unlike propofol, it is not uncommon to witness tachyphylaxis develop to the effects of ketamine. By the fifth or sixth week of therapy, the patient may require twice the dosage to obtain the same effect as seen during the first or second week. Clinical experience has shown that recovery time is not prolonged in the later phases of treatment, suggesting that the metabolism of the drug is also enhanced.

When general anesthesia is required, the brevity of the procedure must be kept in mind when choosing an induction agent. A muscle relaxant may not be necessary (the exception, as stated previously, is XRT for retinoblastoma, which requires paralysis of the extraocular muscles). The subglottic swelling that may develop with repeated daily intubations can be obviated by the use of a supraglottic airway, such as the LMA (LMA North America Inc., San Diego, CA).[45,46]

Antiemetic therapy is suggested at the conclusion of each day's treatment. The emetic effects of XRT can exacerbate the nausea from chemotherapy and stress and result in vomiting in the recovery area. Ondansetron 0.1 mg/kg is perhaps the agent of choice for most practitioners, but others report the use of steroids or phenothiazines with good results. Haloperidol, while showing some promise for the relief of postoperative nausea and vomiting, has been shown to be of little value in the XRT suite.[47]

Some practitioners use psychosocial methods either in lieu of or as a supplement to pharmacologic sedation. These interventions work best among the pediatric population and may begin before the child enters the XRT suite. One center constructed an imitation linear accelerator in the children's playroom, complete with a large doll who received mock treatments. The children were allowed to act as the physicians and via transference were able to quell some of their apprehensions.[5] Other reports described the use of music and videos,[48] gradually immersing the patient by slowly introducing him or her to what is expected and rewarding each successful step,[49] and using an interactive Barney character[50] in an attempt to keep patients calm and motionless. While the last study showed a statistically significant decrease in patients' heart rates, there was no difference in the incidence of observed behavioral distress or the need for sedation. A large series consisting of 2- to 5-year-old patients conducted in the United Kingdom showed a need for pharmacologic sedation in only 10.8% of cases (exclusively among the 2- and 3-year-old patients) after the implementation of a behavioral desensitization program that included interactive rehearsal, emotive imagery, modeling, and positive incentive.[51] Unfortunately, a busy XRT service might not be able to devote the necessary time and patience to foster the atmosphere necessary for such methods.

MONITORING DURING XRT

Remote monitoring of the patient receiving XRT therapy has progressed to the point where it is on par with technology found in the operating room. The days of rigging together makeshift monitoring devices[52] have been supplanted by the use of crystal-clear, closed-circuit monitoring. The typical configuration (Figure 16.7) uses two cameras to provide visual monitoring. Each camera is controlled by switches next to the television screens, allowing individual control of zoom and focus.[53] One camera is directed at the patient to observe for consistent breathing and the absence of other movements. The other camera is focused on the monitors, which typically include (at minimum) the American Society of Anesthesiologists (ASA) standards for electrocardiography (ECG), noninvasive blood pressure (NIBP), pulse oximetry, and qualitative end-tidal CO_2. If the patient is receiving general anesthesia, the field of vision can be widened to include the ventilator and anesthesia machine as well. A microphone is also present to transmit the pulse oximeter tone. Remote audio monitoring of an esophageal stethoscope has been reported[54] but is not widely practiced.

ANESTHETIC COMPLICATIONS DURING XRT

Complications during XRT therapy that are attributable to the anesthetic regimen are extremely rare, ranging from a low incidence of 0.0074%[55] to a significantly higher, but still relatively low, rate of 1.3%.[33] The variability in the reported rate is mainly a factor of how the authors choose to define complications, with those reporting a lower rate limiting the definition to more significant occurrences (aspiration, falls). Rates above 1% typically include a very broad scope of events under the umbrella of "complications," including brief desaturation below 90% or airway obstruction requiring chin lift. Anghelescu et al. used univariate analysis to discover four factors that were positively correlated with a higher complication rate: a larger amount of propofol given, the need for adjunct drugs in addition to propofol, longer procedure times, and simulation (vs. treatment). The presence of retinoblastoma was also positively correlated to complication frequency. Position, age, and weight were discovered to have no relationship to the frequency of complications. On further multivariate analysis, the procedure duration and the total propofol dose were the only factors predictive of anesthetic risk after adjustment for age, weight, type of anesthetic, and type of therapy.[33]

XRT IN REMOTE SITES

The provision of XRT is not limited solely to the XRT suite; indeed, it has begun to make inroads into the operating room. Brachytherapy, or the intracavity implantation of radiotherapeutic material (e.g., radioactive prostate seeds, intrauterine isotopes) has been used successfully for years. Patient fears about "becoming radioactive" are largely exaggerated; because the radioactive material is sealed, only a small area around the site will be radioactive. The body as a whole will not emit radioactivity, and it is generally safe for the patient to resume contact with others. In contrast, a patient receiving external beam XRT will emit no radioactivity whatsoever. Patients who receive intravenous radioactive isotopes, however, will continue

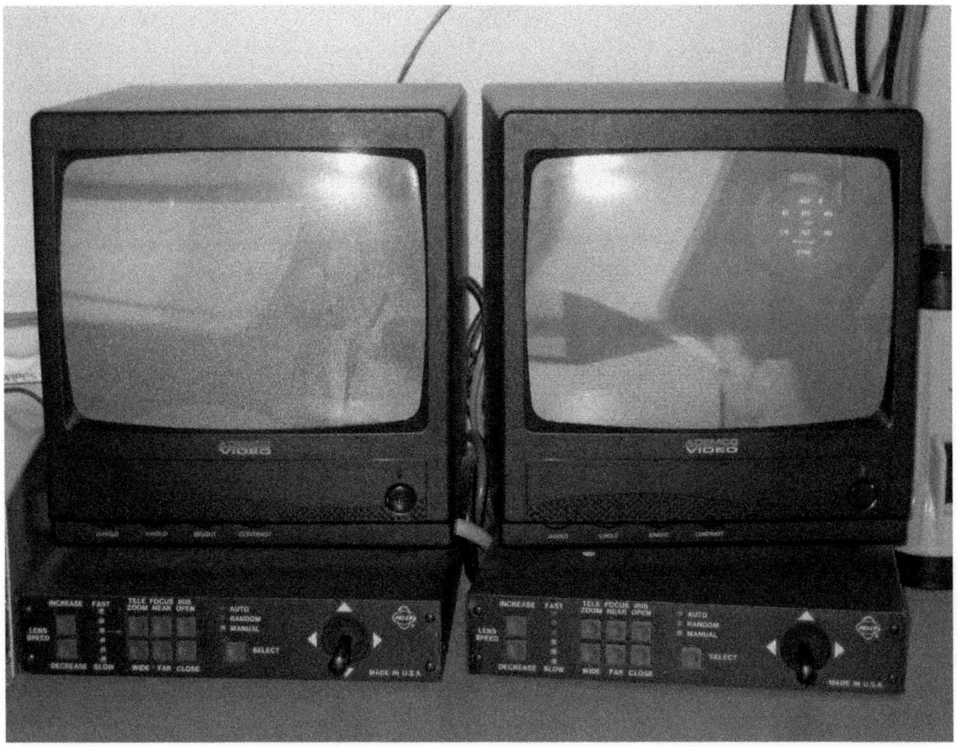

Figure 16.7. A remote monitor bank.

to discharge radioactive material in their saliva, sweat, and urine. The duration of this is dependent on the half-life of the agent used.[56]

Surgeons, radiation oncologists, and anesthesiologists can also work as a team to provide intraoperative radiation therapy (IORT).[57] This is especially useful for tumors that cannot be fully resected or have a high probability of local recurrence. In these cases, the treatment begins in the operating room, where surgical exposure and debulking of the tumor occurs. The wound is then covered, and the patient is then transported to the XRT suite to receive high-dose external beam radiation directly to the exposed tissue. The patient is then returned to the operating room for closure of the surgical site. These cases, typically performed under general anesthesia, require a great degree of coordination between all parties involved. Transport of the patient with an open surgical site requires careful attention to maintaining a sterile field, as well as continued provision of anesthesia and analgesia. The patient should be stable from a cardiovascular standpoint prior to leaving the operating room; full monitoring, airway, and advanced cardiac life support (ACLS) supplies should accompany the patient during the transit phase.[58]

Stereotactic radiosurgery is another XRT venue where anesthesiology services may be necessary. This procedure is used to treat conditions as diverse as malignancies, arteriovenous malformations, acoustic neuromas, and trigeminal neuralgia. The most widely used device, the Gamma Knife® (Elekta Instruments Inc., Stockholm, Sweden) focuses 201 beams of gamma radiation (derived from cobalt-60) on the lesion[59] (Figure 16.8). In contrast to XRT derived from a linear accelerator, only a single session of radiotherapy is needed to treat the disease. (However, the patient may require several doses administered consecutively, each targeted to a different surface of the lesion.)

Anesthetic management is much like what has been described for traditional XRT. MAC usually provides sufficient anesthesia, although general anesthesia may be required for very young patients and in other special circumstances. The patient must first have the stereotactic frame placed, which involves having four anchoring screws placed into the soft tissue of the head. The neurosurgeon or oncologist applying the frame will use local anesthesia to numb the areas; however, a small dose of ketamine or propofol immediately beforehand will make the procedure less traumatic. The patient will then proceed to the MRI suite, where scans will be taken of the patient's brain with the external frame in place. It is imperative that all practitioners are aware of the hospital's protocols for MRI safety. The patient will likely be transferred to an MRI-compatible stretcher, and all monitoring devices will be replaced with appropriate alternatives. Oxygen cylinders must be removed from the vicinity of the magnet. The patient must be interrogated about the presence of any metallic implants, and the medical staff must remove any objects that may become a projectile hazard. Because the frame will limit access to the patient's airway, it is imperative that the patient is transported with the appropriate tools to quickly remove the frame in case airway access is necessary. If a vascular lesion is present, the patient may also be taken to the neuroangiography suite for a diagnostic cerebral angiogram to further elucidate the anatomy. Afterward, the patient is permitted to rest while the physicians and physicists perform a three-dimensional reconstruction of the MRI, plotting the coordinates that will most effectively target the intracranial pathology. The patient is then placed into the Gamma Knife unit, where several doses of radiation are administered (each lasting from 4 to 10 minutes). On completion, the stereotactic frame is removed, antibiotic ointment is applied to the puncture sites left by the screws, and the patient is transported to the recovery area.

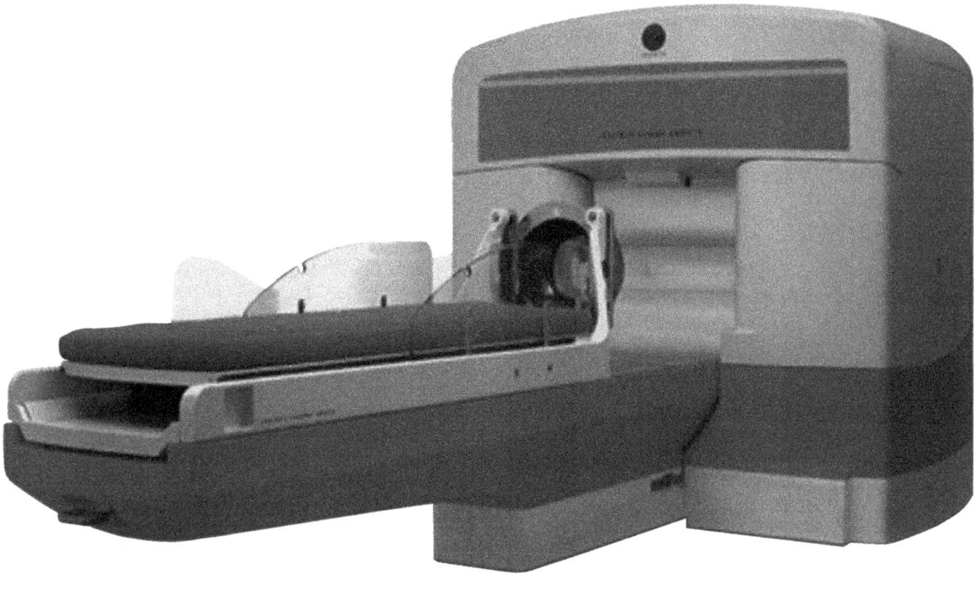

Figure 16.8. The Gamma Knife machine. (Courtesy of Elekta Instruments, Inc.)

CAREGIVER CONCERNS

One of the many concerns voiced by caregivers is the possible effect of repeated anesthetic exposure on these patients at an early age of neurodevelopment. It is difficult for the anesthesia provider to give a definitive assessment of the risk, as studies are currently ongoing to evaluate the immediate and long-term effects. While single exposure in an otherwise healthy child seems to be safe, neither of those conditions apply to this population. Animal studies have shown that agents as diverse as barbiturates, propofol, ketamine, chloral hydrate, benzodiazepines, and inhalational volatile anesthetics[60] can result in apoptotic neurodegeneration if given during vulnerable neurodevelopmental periods.[61] These periods of rapid synaptogenesis are believed to extend in humans through the age of 3 years.[62,63] Dexmedetomidine is perhaps the single agent that has been shown not to result in neural apoptosis.[60]

Current evidence seems to support the hypothesis that repeated exposure to anesthetic agents during this period results in anesthetic-mediated neurotoxicity.[64] Among this specific population, however, there are so many other confounding variables that may also affect neurodevelopment (the effects of chemotherapy, hospitalization, surgeries, etc.[65]) that it is impossible to distill out the unique effects of the anesthetic agents. In addition, if the XRT involves craniospinal fields, that irradiation itself has been shown to independently decrease the intelligence quotient.[66] Of course, XRT is given either as a life-sustaining effort (in which case the risk of neurodevelopmental delay is justified) or as a palliative measure in a terminal patient (in which case it is inconsequential). Depriving the child of sedation or anesthesia during the therapy may in itself result in poor neurocognitive outcome, as early emotional stress and trauma can result in impairment of the nocioceptive system, long-term adverse behavioral patterns, and learning difficulties.[60] Thus, while no blanket reassurances can be given to the concerned caregivers of these patients, they can be assured that the provision of anesthesia will make the process much more tolerable for the child while adding only one more element to the already crowded pool of potential risk factors.

CONCLUSION

Remote site anesthesiology has become more routine over the last decade as hospitals realize they can reduce costs and increase efficiency by "outsourcing" some types of cases out of the operating room. While some clinicians still feel uncomfortable emerging from the "protection" of the operating room, others have embraced the chance to expand their practice beyond its traditional borders. XRT offers the anesthesiologist both a physical layout and a patient population that can be challenging initially, but ultimately extremely rewarding. The fact that these patients return daily, for up to 6 weeks, allows the anesthesia providers to develop a rapport with them more typical of a primary care practice. For the patient, the doctor with the scary needles gradually morphs into the trusted friend who has made the XRT possible; for the anesthesiologist, the room with the scary monitors and machines has become another conquered boundary.

REFERENCES

1. Ward E, DeSantis C, Robbins A, et al. Childhood and adolescent cancer statistics, 2014. *CA Cancer J Clin.* 2014;64:83–103.
2. Jemal A, Seigel R, Ward E, et al. Cancer statistics, 2009. *CA Cancer J Clin.* 2009;59:225–249.
3. Singapuri K, Russell GB. Anesthesia and radiotherapy. In: Russell GB, ed. *Alternate-Site Anesthesia: Clinical Practice Outside the Operating Room.* Boston, MA: Butterworth-Heinemann; 1997:365–380.
4. Rubin S. *Clinical Oncology: A Multidisciplinary Approach for Physicians and Students.* 7th ed. Philadelphia, PA: Saunders; 1993.
5. Seiler G, DeVol E, Khafaga Y, et al. Evaluation of the safety and efficacy of repeated sedations for the radiotherapy of young children with cancer: a prospective study of 1033 consecutive sedations. *Int J Rad Oncol Biol Phys.* 2001;49(3):771–783.
6. McMullen KP, Hanson T, Bratton J, Johnstone PAS. Parameters of anesthesia/sedation in children receiving radiotherapy. *Radiat Oncol.* 2015;10:65.
7. DeVita V, Hellman S, Rosenberg S. *Principles and Practice of Anesthesiology.* 4th ed. Philadelphia, PA: Lippincott; 1993.
8. Johns HE, Cunningham JR. *The Physics of Radiology.* Springfield, IL: Thomas; 1983.
9. Glauber DT, Audenaert SM. Anesthesia for children undergoing craniospinal radiotherapy. *Anesthesiology.* 1987;67(5):801–803.
10. Jereb B, Krishnawami S, Reid A, Allen JC. Radiation of medulloblastoma adjusted to prevent recurrence to the cribriform plate region. *Cancer.* 1984;54(3):602–604.
11. Carrie C, Hoffstetter S, Gomaz F, et al. Impact of targeting deviation on outcome in medulloblastoma: study of the French Society of Pediatric Oncology (SFOP). *Int J Rad Oncol Biol Phys.* 1999;45(2):435–439.
12. McCormick B, Ellsworth R, Abramson D, et al. Radiation therapy for retinoblastoma: comparison of results with lens-sparing v. lateral beam techniques. *Int J Rad Oncol Biol Phys.* 1988;15(3):567–574.
13. Menache L, Eifel PJ, Kennamer DLL, Belli JA. Twice-daily anesthesia in infants receiving hyperfractionated irradiation. *Int J Rad Oncol Biol Phys.* 1990;18(3):625–629.
14. Pradhan DG, Sandridge AL, Mullaney P, et al. Radiation therapy for retinoblastoma: a retrospective review of 120 patients. *Int J Rad Oncol Biol Phys.* 1997;39(1):3–13.
15. Schreiner MS, Triebwasser A, Keon TP. Ingestion of liquids compared with preoperative fasting in pediatric outpatients. *Anesthesiology.* 1990;72(4):593–597.
16. Nicholson SC, Schreiner MS. Feed the babies. *Breastfeeding Abstracts.* 1995;15(1):3–4.
17. Rodarte, A. Heparin-lock for repeated anesthesia in pediatric radiation therapy. *Anesthesiology.* 1982;56(4):316–317.
18. Fortney J, Halperin E, Hertz C, Schulman S. Anesthesia for pediatric external beam radiation therapy. *Int J Rad Oncol Biol Phys.* 1999;44(3):587–591.
19. Bow EJ, Kilpatrick MG, Clinch JJ. Totally implantable venous access ports systems for patients receiving chemotherapy for solid tissue malignancies: a randomized controlled clinical trial examining the safety, efficacy, costs, and impact on quality of life. *J Clin Oncol.* 1999;17(4):1267–1273.
20. 19 McFadyen JG, Pelly N, Orr R. Sedation and anesthesia for the pediatric patient undergoing radiation therapy. *Curr Opin Anesthesiol.* 2011;24:433–438.
21. Varner PD, Ebert JP, McKay RD, et al. Methohexital sedation of children undergoing CT scan. *Anesth Analg.* 1985;64(6):643–645.
22. Snodgrass WR, Dodge WF. Lytic/"DTP" cocktail: time for rational and safe alternatives. *Pediat Clin North Am.* 1989;36(5):1285–1291.
23. Sievers TD, Yee JD, Foley ME, et al. Midazolam for conscious sedation during pediatric oncology procedures: safety and recovery parameters. *Pediatrics.* 1991;88(6):1172–1179.
24. Cartwright PD, Pingel SM. Midazolam and diazepam in ketamine anaesthesia. *Anaesthesia.* 1984;39(5):439–442.
25. Cravero JP, Havidich JE. Pediatric sedation—evolution and revolution. *Paediatr Anaesth.* 2011;21:800–809.
26. Weiss M, Frei M, Buehrer S, et al. Deep propofol sedation for vacuum-assisted bite-block immobilization in children undergoing proton radiation therapy of cranial tumors. *Paediatr Anaesth.* 2007;17(9):867–873.

27. Scheiber G, Ribeiro FC, Karpienski H, Strehl K. Deep sedation with propofol in preschool children undergoing radiation therapy. *Paediatr Anaesth.* 1996;6(3):209–213.
28. Buehrer S, Immoos S, Frei M, et al. Evaluation of propofol for repeated prolonged deep sedation in children undergoing proton radiation therapy. *Br J Anaesth.* 2007;99(4):556–560.
29. Deer TR, Rich GF. Propofol tolerance in pediatric patients. *Anesthesiology.* 1992;77(4):828–829.
30. Martin LD, Pasternak LR, Pudimat MA. Total intravenous anesthesia with propofol in pediatric patients outside the operating room. *Anesth Analg.* 1992;74(4):609–612.
31. Fassoulaki A, Farinotti R, Mantz J, Desmonts JM. Does tolerance develop to the anaesthetic effects of propofol in rats? *Br J Anaesth.* 1994;72(1):127–128.
32. Keidan I, Perel A, Shabtai EL, Pfeffer RM. Children undergoing repeated exposures for radiation therapy do not develop tolerance to propofol: clinical and bispectral index data. *Anesthesiology.* 2004;100(2):251–254.
33. Anghelescu DL, Burgoyne LL, Liu W, et al. Safe anesthesia for radiotherapy in pediatric oncology: St. Jude Children's Research Hospital experience, 2004–2006. *Int J Radiat Oncol Biol Phys.* 2008;71(2):491–497.
34. Setlock MA, Palmisano BW, Berens RJ, et al. Tolerance to propofol generally does not develop in pediatric patients undergoing radiation therapy. *Anesthesiology.* 1996;85(1):207–209.
35. Owusu-Agyemang P, Grosshans D, Arunkumar R, et al. Non-invasive anesthesia for children undergoing proton radiation therapy. *Radiother Oncol.* 2014;111:30–34.
36. Shukry M, Ramadhyani U. Dexmedetomidine as the primary sedative agent for brain radiation therapy in a 21-month old child. *Pediatric Anesth.* 2005;15(3):241–242.
37. Sherwin TS, Green SM, Khan Am Chapman DS, et al. Does adjunctive midazolam reduce recovery agitation after ketamine sedation for pediatric procedures? A randomized double-blind placebo-controlled trial. *Ann Emerg Med.* 2000;35(3):229–238.
38. Bennett JA, Bullimore JA. The use of ketamine hydrochloride anaesthesia for radiotherapy in young children. *Br J Anaesth.* 1973;45(2):197–201.
39. Worrell JB, McCune WJ. A case report: the use of ketamine and midazolam intravenous sedation for a child undergoing radiotherapy. *AANA J.* 1993;61(1):99–102.
40. Kozek-Langenecker SA, Marhoffer P, Sator-Katxenschlager SM, Dieckmann K. S(+)-Ketamine for long-term sedation in a child with retinoblastoma undergoing interstitial brachytherapy. *Pediatr Anesth.* 2005;15(3):248–250.
41. Weiber J, Gugler R, Hengstmann JH, Dengler HJ. Pharmacokinetics of ketamine in man. *Anaesthesist.* 1975;24(6):260–263.
42. Mason KP, Michna E, DiNardo JA, et al. Evolution of a protocol for ketamine-induced sedation as an alternative to general anesthesia for interventional radiologic procedures in pediatric patients. *Radiology.* 2002;225(2):457–465.
43. Lo J, Buckley JJ, Kim TH, et al. Anesthesia for high-dose total body irradiation in children. *Anesthesiology* 1984;61:101–103.
44. Casey WF, Price V, Smith HS. Anaesthesia and monitoring for pediatric radiotherapy. *J R Soc Med.* 1986;79:454–456.
45. Waite K, Filshie J. The use of laryngeal mask airway for CT radiotherapy planning and daily radiotherapy [letter]. *Anaesthesia.* 1990;45(10):894.
46. Grebenik CR, Ferguson C, White A. The laryngeal mask airway in pediatric radiotherapy. *Anesthesiology.* 1990;72(3):474–477.
47. Büttner M, Walder B, von Elm E, Tramèr MR. Is low-dose haloperidol a useful antiemetic? A meta-analysis of published and unpublished randomized trials. *Anesthesiology.* 2004;101(6):1454–1463.
48. Slifer KJ, Bucholtz JD, Cataldo MD. Behavioral training of motion control in young children undergoing radiation treatment without sedation. *J Pediatr Oncol Nurs.* 1994;11(2):55–63.
49. Slifer KJ. A video system to help children cooperate with motion control for radiation treatment without sedation. *J Pediatr Oncol Nurs.* 1996;13(2):91–97.
50. Klosky JL, Tyc VL, Srivastava DK, et al. Brief report: evaluation of an interactive intervention designed to reduce pediatric distress during radiation therapy procedures. *J Pediatr Psychol.* 2004;29(8):621–626.
51. Scott L, Langton F, O'Donoghue J. Minimising the use of sedation/anaesthesia in young children receiving radiotherapy through an effective play preparation programme. *Eur J Oncol Nurs.* 2002;6(1):15–22.
52. Bashein G, Russell AH, Momii ST. Anesthesia and remote monitoring for intraoperative radiation therapy. *Anesthesiology.* 1986;64(6):804–807.
53. Davies DJ. Anesthesia and monitoring for pediatric radiation therapy. *Anesthesiology.* 1986;64(3):406–407.
54. Pandya JB, Martin JT. Improved remote cardiorespiratory monitoring during radiation therapy. *Anesth Analg.* 1986;65(5):529–530.
55. Buchsbaum JC, McMullen KP, Douglas JG, et al. Repetitive pediatric anesthesia in a non-hospital setting. *Int J Radiat Oncol Biol Phys.* 2013;85(5):1296–1300.
56. National Cancer Institute. Radiation therapy for cancer. Available at: http://www.cancer.gov/CANCERTOPICS/FACTSHEET/THERAPY/RADIATION. Last reviewed June 30, 2010. Accessed on July 18, 2010.
57. Tepper JE, Wood WC, Cohen AM, et al. Intraoperative radiation therapy. In: De Vita VT, Hellman S, Rosenberg SA, eds. *Important Advances in Oncology.* Philadelphia, PA: Lippincott; 1985:97–113.
58. DeCosmo G, Gualtiere E, Bonomo V, et al. Intraoperative radiotherapy: anesthesiologic problems during transport of patients. *Minerva Anestesiol.* 1991;57(6):373–377.
59. International RadioSurgery Association. Gamma Knife® surgery. n.d. Available at: http://www.irsa.org/gamma_knife.html. Accessed on July 18, 2010.
60. Cote J, Lerman J, Anderson B. Surgery, anesthesia, and the immature brain. In: *A Practice of Anesthesia for Infants and Children.* 5th ed. Philadelphia, PA: Elsevier Saunders; 2013:475–491.
61. Cravero JP, Blike GT, Beach M, et al. Incidence and nature of adverse events during pediatric sedation/anesthesia for procedures outside the operating room. Report from the Pediatric Sedation Research Consortium. *Pediatrics.* 2006;118:1087–1096.
62. Loepke A. Developmental neurotoxicity of sedatives and anesthetics: a concern for neonatal and pediatric critical care medicine? *Pediatr Crit Care Med.* 2010;11:217–226.
63. Sun L. Early childhood general anesthesia exposure and neurocognitive development. *Br J Anesth.* 2010;105:61–68.
64. Wang X, Zheng X, Chang-Hong M. Current clinical evidence on the effect of general anesthesia on neurodevelopment in children: an updated systematic review with meta-regression. *PLoS One.* 2014;9:1–7.
65. Verma V, Beethe AB, LeRiger M, et al. Anesthesia complications of pediatric radiation therapy. *Pract Rad Oncol.* 2016;6:143–154.
66. Mulhern RK, Merchant TE, Gajjar A, et al. Late neurocognitive sequelae in survivors of brain tumors in childhood. *Lancet Oncol.* 2004;5:399–408.

17 | RADIATION SAFETY

ERIN M. MADDY, MD, KEVIN ABNET, MD, GEOFFREY SCRIVER, MRINAL SHUKLA

INTRODUCTION

Modern anesthesia practice requires anesthetists to perform cases with exposure to ionizing radiation in ever-increasing numbers. Radiation exposure to anesthetists has grown due to the combined increase in both number of procedures facilitated and the expanding role of imaging in surgical practice. Globally, medical radiation is the leading cause of ionizing radiation exposure, with an average annual number of radiologic diagnostic procedures of over one per capita in countries with advanced medical systems.[1]

Anesthetists are increasingly called to care for patients in non–operating room anesthesia (NORA) locations, such as cardiac catheterization labs, gastroenterology suites, and interventional radiology, which utilize ionizing radiation. A retrospective study of the National Anesthesia Clinical Outcomes Registry found that between the years 2010 and 2014, the number of anesthetics given in NORA radiology nearly tripled.[2]

The anesthetist's exposure to radiation can often exceed that of the interventionalist.[3,4] This is attributed both to NORA locations being optimized for the interventionalist's safety and a workflow that requires anesthetists be in close proximity to the patient. In the neurointerventional suite, exposure to the anesthesiologist's eyes was 3-fold higher than that of the interventional radiologist,[3] and during thoracoabdominal aortic aneurysm repairs the dose received by the anesthesia machine was double that of the vascular surgeon.[4] The mere presence of a catheterization lab doubled the radiation dose for an entire group of 30 anesthetists.[5] Despite known exposure to radiation, knowledge of both radiation safety practices and the dangers of radiation is often lacking among anesthetists. Studies of British and Turkish anesthetists found that the majority were routinely exposed to radiation; however, only 30% of Turkish anesthesiologists wore lead aprons, and only 17% of British anesthetists knew of the hazards of radiation to the eye.[6,7] Professional societies for cardiology, interventional radiology, and vascular surgery have released consensus statements, guidelines, and curriculums regarding safe practices surrounding radiation; to date, anesthesiology has not.[8–10]

The International Commission on Radiological Protection (ICRP) recommends that physicians who assist with radiation procedures be educated on the basics of radiation, including units, effects of radiation exposure, and radiation protection for both providers and patients.[11] The format of this chapter mirrors the recommendations of the ICRP and includes an introduction to radiation production, terminology, units, effects on the human body, dose limits, best practices for radiation protection, and safety infrastructure.

BACKGROUND

X-rays were first discovered by Roentgen a few days before Christmas in 1895. By February 1896, x-rays were being used to diagnose kidney stones, followed shortly in 1897 by reports of radiation injuries, such as hair loss and skin burns. The early pioneers of radiation medicine were unwitting martyrs to their field, suffering burns, vision loss, disfiguring injuries (most commonly loss of fingers), tumors, and death.[12,13] Current practitioners, armed with knowledge of the past, do not need to martyr themselves to deliver safe and effective care.

Radiation is transmission of energy in the form of either a wave or a particle. Radiation can be classified as either ionizing or nonionizing. Ionizing radiation carries enough energy to cause ionization of atoms in the matter through which it travels. Examples of ionizing radiation are alpha particles, beta particles, neutrons, x-rays, gamma rays, and high-energy protons. Nonionizing radiation is radiation with insufficient energy to cause ionization, such as ultrasound.[14]

X-rays used for medical imaging are produced using an x-ray tube and a tungsten target. A voltage, expressed in units of peak kilovoltage [kV(p)], is applied to the tube that accelerates electrons, creating a current, expressed in units of milliamps (mA). The electrons flow from the cathode filament to strike the tungsten anode, creating x-rays and heat.[10,14] Both the current and the voltage can be adjusted to change the resulting image. Increasing the amperage increases the amount of x-rays being produced. Increasing the voltage produces more penetrating x-rays and decreases image contrast.[10,15] Fluoroscopy, defined as continuous x-ray imaging, is often done in an automatic brightness control (ABC) mode, which automatically optimizes the image brightness and contrast.[15]

Different units are used to discuss the amount of radiation being produced and the dose received by the human body. The units that the fluoroscopy machine uses to track exposure to the patient will vary based on model. The amount of radiation generated is expressed in a total amount roentgen (amount of energy required to ionize air under standard conditions) or as an amount per unit time (roentgens/minute). More modern fluoroscopy machines may also calculate better indicators of patient dose, such as cumulative air kerma (CAK, the amount of energy per unit mass of air) expressed in grays (Gy); air kerma area product (KAP, cumulative air kerma over beam area; expressed in Gy/cm^2); and peak skin dose (PSD, highest amount of energy per unit mass of skin area; expressed in Gy).[16]

When the ionizing radiation contacts matter, in this case the human body, energy is absorbed most often in the form of heat. The terminology and units used to discuss this energy vary by quality and weighting factors. Absorbed dose, most commonly used to discuss doses of therapeutic radiation, is the total amount of energy absorbed by matter and is measured in grays (1 Gy = 1 J/kg = 100 rad). Equivalent dose, measured in sieverts (Sv), more accurately describes the effect of radiation because it uses a quality factor (Q) that accounts for how much energy the type of radiation has (i.e., an x-ray has a quality factor of 1, while an alpha particle has a quality factor of 20). In addition to factoring in the type of radiation, the effective dose (measured in Sv) uses a tissue weighting factor that accounts for the susceptibility of the exposed tissue and is used mainly for regulatory purposes.[17]

RADIATION EXPOSURE TO ANESTHETISTS

The radiation doses received by anesthetists vary by location and by procedure type. Not surprisingly, the highest doses for anesthetists are found in environments with frequent use of fluoroscopy: endovascular procedures, 15–268 μSv/case[4,18]; neurointerventional radiology, 4–6.5 μSv/case[3,18]; and the cardiac catheterization labs, 1.03 mSv/month.[19] These doses can be compared to common medical procedures, such as chest x-ray (posteroanterior and lateral), 0.06 mSv; computed tomography (CT) of the head, 2 mSv; and coronary angiogram, 5–15 mSv.[14]

The highest recorded doses received by anesthesiologists are during endovascular procedures. Arii et al.[18] and Mohapatra and coworkers[4] investigated exposure to anesthesiologists during endovascular aortic aneurysm repairs (EVARs). Arii et al. measured exposure of 15 μSv/case, which correlated to the number of interventions, mainly interruptions in mechanical ventilation, made by the anesthesiologist. Mohapatra and coworkers placed badges on the unshielded anesthesia equipment and found that the exposure was 268 μSv/case and was double that of the vascular surgeon. The anesthesiologists in Arii's study followed best practices, while the anesthesia machine was left unshielded and did not maintain distance from the patient. Arii et al. concluded that an anesthesiologist at their institution would need to deliver anesthesia for about 1300 EVAR before exceeding dose limits. Applying the same dose limits, if an anesthesiologist did not follow best practices (like the machine in Mohapatra and coworkers' study), the anesthesiologist should perform no more than 75 EVAR/year.[4,18]

The neurointerventional suite utilizes lateral beam imaging more frequently than body endovascular procedures. The lateral beam has the detector on the side of the interventionalist and the x-ray source on the side of the anesthetist. This minimizes the exposure to scatter radiation to the interventionalist and increases exposure to scatter radiation to the unshielded anesthetist. There are no studies with unshielded anesthetists (or machines) in neurointerventional radiology. Two studies by Arii et al. and Anastasian both stated that the anesthesiologists involved used structural shielding.[3,18] Arii studied 32 neurointerventional cases and found an average exposure of 4 μSv/case.[18] Anastasian studied 22 interventional cases with an average exposure of 6.5 μSv/case, which was three times higher than that for the interventional radiologist. Exposure during nine noninterventional neuroradiology cases was 1.0 μSv/case. Anastasian correlated the increased exposure to an increased number of pharmacologic interventions. Of note, one anesthesiologist was removed from Anastasian's study due to having a radiation dose over 10 times higher than colleagues.[3]

Exposure to the anesthesiologist in the catheterization lab was studied by Henderson et al. in 1994. Sixteen anesthesia fellows working in a children's hospital were rotated through a cardiac catheterization lab for 2-month rotations. During the rotation, the fellows wore dosimetry badges on their foreheads. The average monthly dose was 103 ± 66 mrem/month (1.03 mSv/month).[19] Katz looked at the exposure to an entire group of anesthesiologists and certified registered nurse anesthetists (CRNAs) before and after addition of an electrophysiology (EP) laboratory. After addition of the EP lab, the group's cumulative dose doubled without changes in other caseloads.[5] The role of the interventional cardiologist is expanding with ever more complex procedures, such as transaortic valve replacements, that have potential for additional radiation exposure to NORA personnel.

EFFECTS OF RADIATION ON THE HUMAN BODY

Ionizing radiation damages cells by depositing energy as it passes through the cell. Any molecule within a cell is a potential target for ionization. The consequence of the ionization is determined by which molecules were damaged, how important those molecules are to the cell, how many copies of the molecules are present in the cell, and how the cell responds to loss of working copies. As an example, a cell only has one copy of DNA, and the loss of the one working copy of DNA will lead to cell death.[20] Effects of radiation can be described as either stochastic or deterministic.

Stochastic effects are defined as those effects for which there is no minimum dose required; an increasing dose leads to increasing probability of developing the effect, and the latency period may be long. Stochastic effects develop when DNA is damaged, leading to mutation in an all-or-none phenomenon. Stochastic effects are responsible for induction of cancer and heritable effects.[8,14,17,21]

Deterministic effects are dose-dependent cell death and resultant tissue injury when a threshold dose of radiation has been exceeded. Higher doses of radiation lead to greater injury. The time course for deterministic effects is shorter and more predictable than that for stochastic effects. When enough cells within a tissue are damaged, symptoms will occur, and this is determined as the minimal threshold dose.[8,14,15,17] In medicine, the most commonly seen deterministic effect is skin damage, such as erythema, desquamation, hair loss, or, in severe cases, dermal necrosis. The time course for skin effects is 1–4 weeks.[14]

DOSE LIMITS

Dose limit recommendations are determined by the ICRP and the National Council on Radiation Protection (NCRP). Dose limits are for radiation workers, which is any occupationally exposed individual anticipated to exceed 1 mSv of exposure in one calendar year. The ICRP recommends maximum allowable whole-body exposure of 20 mSv/year averaged over 5 years, with no 1 year to exceed 50 mSv. The NCRP recommends whole-body exposure of less than 50 mSv/year, with lifetime exposure not to exceed 10 times the worker's age in years. Both the NCRP and ICRP recommend no more than 500 mSv/year for extremities and skin. In the United States, legislation varies state to state but is guided by NCRP recommendations.[17,21,22]

Of special note is the evolving understanding of the sensitivity of the lens of the eye and the debate whether the observed changes are due to stochastic or deterministic effects. Both the ICRP and NCRP recently decreased their dose limits from 150 mSv/year to 20 mSv/year and 50 mGy/year, respectively.[22–24]

Exposure to radiation during pregnancy is a special situation for both medical providers and patients. In the United States, a pregnant radiation worker is recommended, but not required, to disclose her pregnancy to the radiation safety officer (RSO).[17] Once a pregnancy is declared, an additional dosimetry badge is issued to be worn under personal shielding at the level of the waist. The ICRP recommends less than 1 mSv of effective dose to the fetus after disclosure of the pregnancy, and the NCRP recommends 5 mSv for the duration of the pregnancy, with no 1 month to exceed 0.5 mSv.[17,21]

LONG-TERM HEALTH CONSEQUENCES OF RADIATION EXPOSURE

The long-term health risks from radiation exposure have been determined from epidemiologic data from populations known to be exposed to radiation, such as atomic bomb survivors and more recently occupationally exposed workers. These epidemiologic studies have found increased rates of leukemias; solid tumors (thyroid, melanoma); and cataracts; however, there are numerous confounding variables in epidemiologic studies, especially when the inciting event is years, if not decades, from the studied effect.[25–27] The lifetime attributable risk of developing malignancy from radiation less than 100 mSv total-body radiation is small in comparison to non–radiation-associated malignancies. The rate of malignancy in the nonexposed population is 42 of 100 people. For populations with exposure to 100 mSv of radiation, the rate of malignancy is 43 of 100 people, with the additional malignancy being attributed to exposure to ionizing radiation.[28]

The nominal dose threshold, the dose where 1% of exposed individuals will develop an effect, for cataracts is 0.5 Gy (500 mGy).[22] There are still significant gaps in knowledge regarding the mechanism of cataractogenesis. Cataractogenesis could be from oxidative damage, DNA damage, or alterations in intracellular communication. Posterior subcapsular cataracts were seen in 25% of Chernobyl cleanup workers, have an increased incidence in medical workers even with a dose less than 0.5 Gy, and were found to have a relative risk of occurrence of 11 in interventional and cardiology nursing staff versus nonexposed nursing staff.[27] As mentioned, the study of cataract formation has multiple confounding variables, and follow-up of personnel at the currently recommended guidelines will take decades.

The psychological effects of radiation exposures have been studied in community-wide disasters, such as in Goiania, Brazil, and in Three Mile Island, Pennsylvania. Within these communities, both individuals exposed and those not exposed to radiation demonstrated a stress response with fear, depression, psychosomatic symptoms, decreased cognitive function, increased neuroendocrine stress hormones, and cardiovascular effects.[29,30] Klein et al. commented that radiation exposure is the "cost of doing business" to an interventionalist, and that some interventionalists have developed coping mechanisms to deal with the stress, such as ignoring the danger and deferring dosimeter badges.[9] The psychologic effect of a constant hazard and its associated coping mechanisms and effect on team dynamics in the medical setting has not been adequately studied.

BEST PRACTICES FOR RADIATION PROTECTION

The sources of radiation exposure during fluoroscopy are the primary beam, x-ray tube leakage current, and scatter from persons or objects within the primary beam. The primary source of radiation exposure to all personnel is scatter from the patient. Radiation from the primary beam is collimated by the interventionalist and does not contribute significantly to exposure unless a provider is present in the image being generated. Leakage from the x-ray tube is monitored and cannot exceed 100 mR/hour at 1 meter at maximal settings. The amount of scatter depends on the patient dose (exposure rate, area being exposed, fluoroscopy time) and beam energy. The scatter is the most intense on the beam side of the patient (Figure 17.1a). Anesthetists can have greater exposure to ionizing radiation than interventionalists due to scatter and proximity; however, well-informed anesthetists can minimize radiation to themselves and their patients.

The best way to avoid medical ionizing radiation exposure is not to use radiation. Imaging that uses radiation such as x-rays, CT scans, and fluoroscopy should be justified and the risks discussed with the patient, especially in special circumstances such as those involving pediatric and pregnant patients. When radiation is deemed necessary, its use should be optimized and exposure to providers minimized by using time, distance, and shielding.[1,11]

The idea of radiation being as low as reasonably achievable (ALARA) reminds providers to use the least amount of radiation to achieve the intended result because there is no lower limit to safe exposure. Any exposure to radiation has

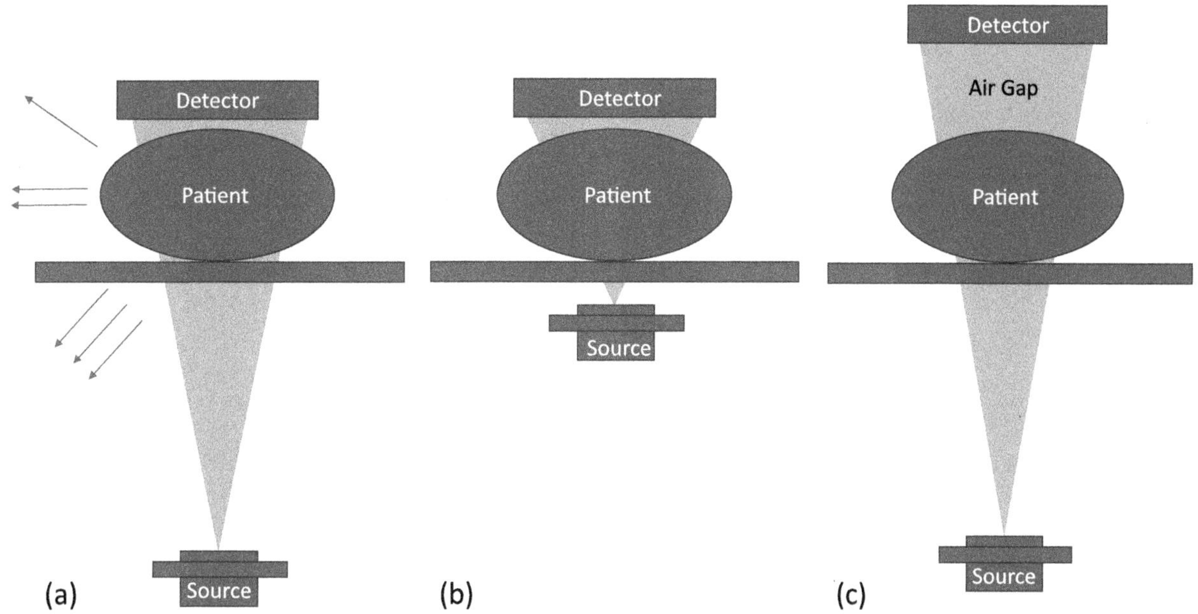

Figure 17.1 Demonstration of scatter. (a). Scatter is greatest on the side of the source. (b). Too small source-to-patient distance which can result in high patient skin dose and poor image quality. (c). Too large patient-to-detector distance will require higher dose to reach the detector and increase scatter to personnel. (34, 35)

the potential to cause stochastic effects. When able, providers should use nonionizing imaging modalities such as magnetic resonance imaging (MRI) and ultrasound. The dose of radiation given during procedures in NORA locations is rarely under the control of the anesthetist; however, there are guides for the interventionalist to minimize risk of radiation injury to the patient during the procedure.[8,10] Some recommendations for interventionalists are as follows:

- Minimize fluoroscopy time—only use fluoroscopy while looking at the screen
- Position the patient and collimate the beam without using fluoroscopy
- Minimize frame rates
- Use pulse fluoroscopy whenever possible
- Minimize use of "high dose," cine, and magnification
- Minimize number of acquisitioning runs
- Keep current low and tube potential as high as possible
- Use collimation
- Use filters on the x-ray tube output to reduce unnecessary x-ray photons
- Maximize source-to-skin distance (Figure 17.1b)
- Minimize patient-to-detector distance, reduce the "air gap" (Figure 17.1c)
- Minimize the angulation of the beam to reduce the x-ray beam path in the patient
- Do not work in one view exclusively to vary skin exposed to radiation[8]

Minimizing time that x-ray imaging is used will limit the amount of overall radiation exposure. This is under control of the interventionalist. More applicable to the anesthetist is rotation of personnel through radiation environments. As shown by Henderson et al.,[19] fellows on a cardiac catheterization lab rotation had significantly higher doses than peers on general operating room rotations. Rotating anesthetists through these environments will minimize any one individual's exposure by spreading the dose so no one provider receives an unsafe dose.

Distance is the hardest tenet of radiation safety for the anesthetist to accomplish. Proximity and immediate access are inherent needs for anesthetists to provide safe and effective care. During the procedure, the source of radiation exposure for the anesthetist is primarily scatter from the patient. The American Society of Anesthesiologists (ASA) guidelines for anesthetic monitoring allow for remote monitoring when a known hazard such as radiation is present.[31] The ability to remotely monitor is based on the available equipment, stability of the patient, and the anesthetist's discretion. The inverse square law states that the power of scattered radiation is inversely proportional to the square of the distance (Exposure = $1/d^2$).[14] If the anesthetist is unable to leave the room, increasing the distance from the patient will decrease the amount of ionizing radiation exposure.

In addition to maintaining distance, shielding should be used. Shielding can be structural or personal. Structural shielding includes mobile acrylic shields, leaded under-table drapes, and leaded walls. Structural shielding should be placed to minimize scatter. Personal shielding includes lead-equivalent aprons, thyroid collars, caps, and glasses. When lead aprons are worn, the front of the gown should face the source of scatter and be worn according to manufacturer recommendations with the appropriate amount of overlap. Lead equivalent of 0.25 mm will attenuate 96% of the dose and 0.5 mm will attenuate 99%. Standard prescription glasses offer poor protection from ionizing radiation, and leaded glasses should be worn with a minimum 0.75 mm equivalent, with side shields covering the temples to attenuate 98% of exposure.[1,14,21,32]

To date, interventional suites have been designed to minimize exposure to the interventionalist. An anesthetist can similarly optimize his or her surroundings prior to the start of the case. The greatest source of scatter radiation is the patient at the site where the x-ray beam first contacts the patient. Therefore, if possible, stay on the opposite side of the patient (the same side as the image detector) during the procedure. Place an acrylic shield between the patient and the anesthesia work area, then position intravenous equipment and the anesthesia machine so that providing interventions does not require radiation exposure (this will likely require circuit and intravenous extensions).[3,33]

There are several other measures that can be taken to minimize scatter radiation. Minimize scatter by minimizing the distance between the patient and the image intensifier, often referred to as the "air gap" (Figure 17.1).[8] An anesthetist can see the image detector and the air gap and encourage adherence to best practices. Conversely, maximizing the distance between the patient and the source minimizes the risk of radiation injury to the patient. Techniques with lower overall radiation exposure, such as low current and high voltage, will also lower scatter generation.

Anesthetists frequently exposed to radiation are eligible for dosimetry monitoring. Monitoring is important to identify unsafe working conditions and individuals whose dose is higher than expected. Individuals whose dose is higher than expected need a review of their habits and education regarding radiation protection.[8] The preferred method for monitoring is with two badges, one placed on the outside of personal shielding at the level of the thyroid and one placed on the inside of personal shielding between the waist and the shoulders. If only one badge is worn, it should be worn on the outside of personal shielding at the level of the thyroid. If a worker is pregnant, a third badge should be worn under personal shielding at the level of the waist.[17]

The ICRP recommends that physicians who assist with radiation procedures receive 8–12 hours of training in radiation protection. Topics to be included in this training are radiation hazards, radiation quantities and units, principles of radiation protection, radiation legislation, and factors affecting patient and staff doses. Training should be done by someone familiar with both radiation protection and the environment where the radiation exposure will occur; in most institutions, this training will be provided by the RSO.[11]

During the procedure, all personnel involved should be aware of the dose being administered to the patient and how the dose is being tracked. Fluoroscopy units provide estimates of fluoroscopy time, CAK, or PSD. When a high dose of radiation is used, a threshold dose will prompt a pause in the procedure (Table 17.1). During this pause, the operator considers the dose already delivered to the patient and weighs the risks and potential benefits of continuing the procedure versus the risk of continued radiation exposure. It may be possible to do a staged procedure and defer a portion of the procedure for a later date. If the procedure is going to continue, pause to assess for best practices that may have lapsed during the procedure to further minimize risk to patient and personnel.[36]

If the patient has received a high dose of radiation or has been identified as having increased risk for radiation injury, the patient will need follow-up. Follow-up should occur 10–14 days following the procedure to allow time for skin changes to manifest. Follow-up should focus on evaluation for skin erythema, and if present, this should be reported to the RSO, and the patient should be further evaluated to determine the severity of radiation injury (Table 17.1).[36]

SAFETY INFRASTRUCTURE

The responsibility for regulating radiation is shared between many federal and state agencies. Jurisdiction between these agencies frequently overlaps, with no single agency having primary responsibility. The Occupational Safety and Health Administration (OSHA) is responsible for occupational safety, including of health care workers. In radiology, however, OSHA does not typically perform inspections, measure compliance, or enforce standards. This is under the jurisdiction of the Center for Devices and Radiological Health (CDRH), a part of the Food and Drug Administration, which is responsible for setting standards for radiological equipment. However, the CDRH does not set exposure limits for workers who have occupational exposure to radiation; this in turn is regulated by the Nuclear Regulatory Commission (NRC). Any radioactive material produced by a nuclear reactor (except for enriched plutonium or uranium) is considered "byproduct material" by the NRC. This includes the radioisotopes used commonly in nuclear medicine examinations. The NRC closely regulates the

TABLE 17.1. Dose Notification Alerts and Recommended Thresholds Doses for Follow-Up

DOSE NOTIFICATION ALERTS

PARAMETER	FIRST NOTIFICATION	SUBSEQUENT NOTIFICATIONS	THRESHOLD FOR FOLLOW-UP
Peak skin dose	2000 mGy	500 mGy	3000 mGy
Kerma area product	300 Gy/cm^2	100 Gy/cm^2	500 Gy/cm^2
Fluoroscopy time	30 min	15 min	60 min

SOURCE: Reference 36.

production, transport, use, and disposal of these radioisotopes. The NRC exposure limits to radiation workers have been applied to all radiology personnel even if they do not work with nuclear byproduct materials.[34,35]

While these federal agencies share responsibility, it is state organizations that assume the role of regulating radiation safety for both patients and those with occupational exposure to radiation. This includes all sources of radiation, including fluoroscopy. It is impossible to list the requirements of each state; however, the Conference of Radiation Control Program Directors (CRCPD) has created a list of suggested state regulations, which can provide more specific information. At the local level, some individual institutions may elect to create policies stricter than either federal or state regulations.[34,35]

There is a robust safety infrastructure in place at most institutions regarding fluoroscopy and its use. Each medical facility must be authorized by a medical authority to use ionizing radiation. The NRC requires that each institution "develop, document, and implement a Radiation Protection Program" (RPP). In addition to byproduct materials, the RPP will address all ionizing radiation producing equipment at the institution. The implementation, maintenance, and enforcement of the RPP is the responsibility of the radiation safety committee headed by the RSO.[34,35] In addition to the RPP, the responsibilities of the RSO include radiation safety (including fluoroscopic safety); developing an ALARA program; facility design, including shielding; instruction of workers; machine registration and evaluation; personnel monitoring; patient protection; and managing fetal exposures of pregnant workers.[35]

While there are numerous radiation safety requirements in every fluoroscopic unit, all personnel should be made specifically aware of two. The first is a timer, which signals an audible alarm to alert the operator after every 5 minutes of fluoroscopy and will continue to sound until manually reset. The second requirement is that if the fluoroscopic unit has a "high-level" option a continuous signal will sound to indicate that a high radiation dose is being administered.[34,35]

SUMMARY AND RECOMMENDATIONS

With the rising use of medical ionizing radiation, anesthetists will encounter radiation more frequently, especially in NORA locations. Minimizing occupational exposure to ionizing radiation requires a systematic approach that includes the tenets of radiation safety: ALARA, time, distance, and shielding. Before the start of a procedure, discuss how the patient's dose can be minimized with techniques such as ultrasound and how the patient's dose will be monitored. In addition to safe practices to reduce radiation exposure, a rotation of personnel through areas with high exposure to radiation to minimize the amount of time any single provider is exposed.

In addition to structural and personal shielding (lead equivalent caps, aprons, thyroid shields, and glasses). Optimizing distances, specifically by minimizing the air gap and maximizing the distance between the patient and the radiation source, protects the patient and reduces scatter

Anesthetists benefit by maintaining distance from sources of radiation. Utilize remote monitoring when able and, whenever possible, set up the anesthesia machine and workstation as far as possible from the source of radiation, ideally over 6 feet away. Adding intravenous or circuit extensions allows interventions to be made from a safer distance.

The best radiation safety practices require clear and open communication. Prior to ionizing radiation use, we suggest that the entire team verify that all personnel are adequately shielded and the principles of ALARA have been fully applied.

REFERENCES

1. ICRP Publication 105. Radiological protection in medicine. *Ann ICRP.* 2007;37(6):1–63.
2. Nagrebetsky A, Gabriel RA, Dutton RP, Urman RD. Growth of nonoperating room anesthesia care in the United States: a contemporary trends analysis. *Anesth Analg.* 2017;124(4):1261–1267.
3. Anastasian ZH, Strozyk D, Meyers PM, Wang S, Berman MF. Radiation exposure of the anesthesiologist in the neurointerventional suite. *Anesthesiology.* 2011;114(3):512–520.
4. Mohapatra A, Greenberg RK, Mastracci TM, Eagleton MJ, Thornsberry B. Radiation exposure to operating room personnel and patients during endovascular procedures. *J Vasc Surg.* 2013;58(3):702–709.
5. Katz JD. Radiation exposure to anesthesia personnel: The impact of an electrophysiology laboratory. *Anesth Analg.* 2005;101:1725–1726.
6. Tüfek A, Tokgöz O, Aycan IÖ, Çelik F, Gümüş A. Current attitudes of Turkish anesthesiologists to radiation exposure. *J Anesth.* 2013;27:874–878.
7. Aizad M, Yusof M, Alrifai Z, Czernicki M. Radiation safety awareness for anaesthetists. Paper presented at: Anesthesiology Annual Meeting, American Society of Anesthesiologists; October 2016; Chicago, IL.
8. Bashore TM, Balter S, Barac A, et al. 2012 American College of Cardiology Foundation/Society for Cardiovascular Angiography and Interventions expert consensus document on cardiac catheterization laboratory standards update: a report of the American College of Cardiology Foundation Task Force. *J Am Coll Cardiol.* 2012;59(24):2221–2305.
9. Klein LW, Miller DL, Balter S, et al. Occupational health hazards in time for a safer environment. *Radiology.* 2009;250(2):538–5344.
10. Mitchell EL, Furey P. Prevention of radiation injury from medical imaging. *J Vasc Surg.* 2011;53:22S–27S.
11. Vañó E, Rosenstein M, Liniecki J, Rehani MM, Martin CJ, Vetter RJ. ICRP Publication 113. Education and training in radiological protection for diagnostic and interventional procedures. *Ann ICRP.* 2009;39(5):7–68.
12. Assmus A. Early history of X rays. *Beam Line.* 1995;25(2):10–24.
13. Sansare K, Khanna V, Karjodkar F. Early victims of X-rays: a tribute and current perception. *Dentomaxillofacial Radiol.* 2011;40(2):123–125.
14. Cheng SWK. Radiation safety. In: Cronenwett J, Johnston KW, eds. *Rutherford's Vascular Surgery.* Philadelphia, PA: Elsevier/Saunders; 2014:325–333.
15. Rathmell JP. Radiation safety and use of radiographic contrast agents in pain medicine. In: Benzon HT, Rathmell JP, Wu CL, Turk DC, Argoff CE, Hurley RW, eds. *Practical Management of Pain.* Philadelphia, PA: Elsevier/Mosby; 2014:981–993.
16. Panuccio G, Greenberg RK, Wunderle K, Mastracci TM, Eagleton MG, Davros W. Comparison of indirect radiation dose estimates with directly measured radiation dose for patients and operators during complex endovascular procedures. *J Vasc Surg.* 2011;53(4):885–894.
17. The 2007 recommendations of the International Commission on Radiological Protection. ICRP Publication 103. *Ann ICRP.* 2007;37(2–4):1–332.
18. Arii T, Uchino S, Kubo Y, Kiyama S, Uezono S. Radiation exposure to anaesthetists during endovascular procedures. *Anaesthesia.* 2015;70(1):47–50.
19. Henderson KH, Lu JK, Strauss KJ, Treves ST, Rockoff MA. Radiation exposure of anesthesiologists. *J Clin Anesth.* 1994;6:37–41.
20. Zeman EM, Schreiber EC, Tepper JE. Basics of radiation therapy. In: Niederhuber JE, Armitage JO, Doroshow JH, Kastan MB, Tepper JE, eds. *Abeloff's Clinical Oncology.* 5th ed. Philadelphia, PA: Elsevier/Saunders; 2013:393–422.
21. Dagal A. Radiation safety for anesthesiologists. *Curr Opin Anesthesiol.* 2011;24(4):445–450.
22. Dauer LT, Ainsbury EA, Dynlacht J, et al. Status of NCRP Scientific Committee 1-23 commentary on guidance on radiation dose limits for the lens of the eye. *Health Phys.* 2016;110(2):182–184.

23. Boal TJ, Pinak M. Dose limits to the lens of the eye: International Basic Safety Standards and related guidance. *Ann ICRP*. 2015;44(1)(suppl):112–117.
24. Boice J, Blakely E, Passmore C, Boice J. Lens of Eye Guidance—Next Steps [Conference brochure]. New York, NY; August 29, 2016.
25. Yoshinaga S, Mabuchi K, Sigurdson AJ, Doody MM, Ron E. Cancer risks among radiologists and radiologic technologists: review of epidemiologic studies 1. *Radiology*. 2004;233(2):313–321.
26. Sont WN, Zielinski JM, Ashmore JP, et al. First analysis of cancer incidence and occupational radiation exposure based on the National Dose Registry of Canada. *Am J Epidemiol*. 2001;153(4):309–318.
27. Ainsbury EA, Barnard S, Bright S, et al. Ionizing radiation induced cataracts: recent biological and mechanistic developments and perspectives for future research. Mutat Res Rev Mutat Res. 2016;770:238–2361.
28. Council, NR, *Health Risks from Exposure to Low Levels of Ionizing Radiation: BEIR VII Phase 2*. 2006, Washington, DC: The National Academies Press. 65–79.
29. Collins DL, Baum A, Singer JE. Coping with chronic stress at Three Mile Island: psychological and biochemical evidence. *Health Psychol*. 1983;2(2):149–166.
30. Landauer M, Young R, Hawley A. Physiological and psychological impact of low-level radiation: an overview. *Mil Med*. 2002;167(2)(suppl):141–142.
31. Committee on Standards and Practice Parameters (2015). *Standards for Basic Anesthetic Monitoring - American Society of Anesthesiologists (ASA)*. [online] Asahq.org. Available at: http://www.asahq.org/quality-and-practice-management/standards-guidelines-and-related-resources/standards-for-basic-anesthetic-monitoring.
32. Reeves RR, Ang L, Bahadorani et al. Invasive cardiologists are exposed to greater left sided cranial radiation: the BRAIN study (Brain Radiation Exposure and Attenuation During Invasive Cardiology Procedures). *JACC Cardiovasc Interv*. 2015;8(9):1197–206.
33. Miller DL, Vañó E, Bartal G, et al. Occupational radiation protection in interventional radiology: a joint guideline of the Cardiovascular and Interventional Radiology Society of Europe and the Society of Interventional Radiology. *Cardiovasc Interv Radiol*. 2010;33(2):230–239.
34. Brateman L. The AAPM/RSNA physics tutorial for residents: radiation safety considerations for diagnostic radiology personnel 1. *Radiographics*. 1999;19(4):1037–1055.
35. Committee on Education of the Commission on Medical Physics, American College of Radiology and Professional Council, American Association of Physicists in Medicine. ACR-AAPM Radiation Safety Officer Resources. American College of Radiology. Reston, VA. 2017.
36. Stecker MS, Balter S, Towbin RB, Miller DL, Vañó E, Bartal G, Angle JF, Chao CP, Cohen AM, Dixon RG, Gross K. Guidelines for patient radiation dose management. *Journal of Vascular and Interventional Radiology*. 2009;20(7):S263–273.

18 | GASTROINTESTINAL ENDOSCOPY PROCEDURES

MARK A. GROMSKI, MD, KAI MATTHES, MD, PHD

INTRODUCTION

A wide array of gastrointestinal (GI) endoscopy procedures are carried out in the GI endoscopy suite and operating room. Although the colonoscopy is the most widely performed procedure (approximately 15 million procedures completed per year in the United States alone) due to national guidelines for screening/surveillance colonoscopies for colorectal cancer detection and prevention, other procedures are routinely utilized to diagnose and treat various GI pathologies.[1,2] Procedures range from minimally invasive, such as a routine screening colonoscopy, to much more invasive and complicated, such as endoscopic submucosal dissection (ESD) and per oral endoscopic myotomy (POEM). Sedation and anesthesia are integral parts of each GI endoscopy procedure. Adequate sedation and anesthesia optimize patient comfort and create a favorable environment for the physician to safely and efficiently carry out the necessary procedure. Understandably, levels of sedation and anesthesia vary with the invasiveness of the GI endoscopic procedure and the individual patient. Thus, cogent plans for sedation and anesthesia should be devised for each patient expecting a GI endoscopic procedure. Anesthetic considerations are discussed in detail in Chapter 16.

Gastrointestinal endoscopy is a large field, and there are many advanced and developmental therapeutic techniques that are not covered in this chapter, as this chapter is meant to serve as an overview of the most common aspects of GI endoscopy. The aims of this chapter are to (a) briefly describe the most common endoscopic procedures and delineate events that are most stimulating during each procedure and (b) introduce the wide array of advanced GI endoscopic procedures that may be encountered by the anesthesia provider in the endoscopy suite.

COMMON PROCEDURES IN GASTROINTESTINAL ENDOSCOPY

A brief description of the most common GI endoscopy procedures is provided, along with stimulating events within each procedure. The procedures covered herein are as follows:

1. Esophagogastroduodenoscopy (EGD)
2. Sigmoidoscopy/colonoscopy
3. Endoscopic retrograde cholangiopancreatography (ERCP)

ESOPHAGOGASTRODUODENOSCOPY

Esophagogastroduodenoscopy is the diagnostic or therapeutic examination of the upper GI tract using a flexible endoscope (Box 18.1). This procedure provides the possibility to obtain tissue specimens by performing a mucosal biopsy or staining of GI layers. Diagnostic EGD can be performed with topical oropharyngeal sedation alone (as is often performed outside of the United States) or minimal or moderate sedation. The anticipation of advanced procedures such as esophageal dilation, treatment of Barrett's esophagus, treatment of esophageal varices, endoscopic mucosal resection (EMR), or ESD may require increased levels of anesthesia. Additionally, if there is a suspicion for brisk upper GI bleeding, gastric outlet obstruction, or retained gastric contents, it may be prudent to secure the airway with endotracheal intubation to decrease the risk of significant aspiration of gastric contents.

SIGMOIDOSCOPY/COLONOSCOPY

Sigmoidoscopy is the examination of the sigmoid colon and rectum using either rigid or (more likely) flexible endoscopes. The colonoscopy is the examination of the entire lower GI tract from anus to cecum (and occasionally including the terminal ileum) using a flexible endoscope. Endoscopy of the lower GI tract is considered less stimulating than the upper GI tract because there is no gag reflex involved (Box 18.2). There are aspects of the lower GI tract examination, however, that are stimulating enough to require adequate sedation, including gas distention

BOX 18.1. STIMULATING EVENTS DURING ESOPHAGOGASTRODUODENOSCOPY (EGD)

1. Intubation of the esophagus with endoscope (passing endoscope beyond pyriform sinus and traversing the upper esophageal sphincter)
2. Passing the endoscope through the pylorus
3. Overinsufflation of stomach or duodenum
4. Endoscopic interventions:
    a. Endoscopic hemostasis (argon plasma coagulation, clips, injection, heater probe, etc.)
    b. Esophageal/gastric/duodenal biopsy
    c. Esophageal stenting
    d. Dilation of esophageal or duodenal strictures
    e. Endoscopic mucosal resection (EMR)
    f. Endoscopic submucosal dissection (ESD)

BOX 18.2. STIMULATING EVENTS DURING SIGMOIDOSCOPY/COLONOSCOPY

1. Introduction of the endoscope
2. Gas (air or carbon dioxide) insufflation of the colon, causing distention of bowel
3. Advancement of the endoscope through sigmoid colon, splenic flexure, and hepatic flexure
4. Looping of the colonoscope on insertion
5. Endoscopic interventions:
   a. Mucosal biopsy
   b. Polypectomy
   c. Endoscopic hemostasis (argon plasma coagulator, clips, injection, heater probe, etc.)
   d. Endoscopic mucosal resection (EMR)
   e. Endoscopic submucosal dissection (ESD)
   f. Dilation and stenting of malignant strictures

BOX 18.3. STIMULATING EVENTS DURING ENDOSCOPIC RETROGRADE CHOLANGIOPANCREATOGRAPHY (ERCP)

1. Intubation of the esophagus with endoscope (passing endoscope beyond pyriform sinus and traversing the upper esophageal sphincter)
2. Shortening the endoscope in the duodenum (to create critical view of the duodenal papillae)
3. Insufflation of duodenum
4. Endoscopic interventions:
   a. Sphincterotomy (biliary or pancreatic) or sphincteroplasty
   b. Balloon or basket extraction of biliary stones
   c. Direct pancreaticobiliary visualization (e.g., SpyGlass)
   d. Laser lithotripsy
   e. Dilation of biliary or pancreatic duct strictures

of the colon, approach to right colon/cecum, and retroflexion in the rectum. Generally, insertion of the endoscope is more stimulating than the withdrawal or examination phase. Also, interventions such as the appropriation of biopsies, removal of polyps, or other treatments may require adequate sedation to minimize movement of the patient.

ENDOSCOPIC RETROGRADE CHOLANGIOPANCREATOGRAPHY

Endoscopic retrograde cholangiopancreatography is the radiographic examination of the biliary or pancreatic ducts via endoscopically injected contrast through the major or minor duodenal papilla (Box 18.3). Two-dimensional black-and-white fluoroscopic images are produced using this technique, along with the possibility of a variety of interventional endoscopic techniques, guided by the fluoroscopic information. Through the passage of catheters and guidewires, the biliary ductal system and pancreatic ductal system may be accessed, and a variety of interventions can be accomplished, including biliary and pancreatic sphincterotomy, stricture dilation, stone removal, stent placement, and sampling of tissue. ERCP requires a skillful delivery of sedation and analgesia. If the patients are too lightly sedated, they may gag, move, or become agitated, which would be potentially dangerous considering the precise interventions required during ERCP. If patients are too deeply sedated, they may develop airway obstruction, hypoventilation, hemodynamic instability, and delayed emergence and recovery. Due to these considerations, general anesthesia is often considered in an anesthetic/sedation plan for patients undergoing ERCP.

ADVANCED THERAPEUTIC AND DIAGNOSTIC TECHNIQUES

The following techniques are discussed:

1. Endoscopic hemostasis
2. Double-balloon enteroscopy
3. Direct pancreaticobiliary visualization
4. Endoscopic mucosal resection (EMR)
5. Endoscopic submucosal dissection (ESD)
6. Endoscopic ultrasound (EUS)
7. Per oral endoscopic myotomy (POEM)
8. Natural orifice translumenal endoscopic surgery (NOTES)

ENDOSCOPIC HEMOSTASIS

Acute and subacute GI bleeding may be treated with medical, endoscopic, or surgical approaches. For acute GI bleeding, endoscopy is a mainstay of therapy. There are a number of techniques and devices available for the endoscopic treatment of acute and subacute GI bleeding (bleeding peptic ulcer disease, arteriovenous malformations, diverticular bleeding, postpolypectomy bleeding, variceal hemorrhage, etc.).[3] Current modalities fall into four broad categories, including injection therapies (e.g., epinephrine), mechanical devices (e.g., endoclip, variceal banding), contact thermal therapy (e.g., bipolar coagulation probe), and noncontact thermal therapy (e.g., argon plasma coagulation), all of which are operable through the working channels of the endoscope.

Key components of the endoscopic procedure include care for airway protection if brisk upper GI bleeding is suspected. For instance, in active peptic ulcer bleeding or variceal hemorrhage, the patient may have a stomach entirely full of blood and blood clot, raising risk of significant aspiration intraprocedurally or periprocedurally. In the patient with active blood loss, the situation is complicated by a need for providing adequate sedation, especially given the endoscopic treatment modalities for hemostasis can be stimulating. Thus, it is essential for patients to be adequately resuscitated from a hemodynamic standpoint prior to endoscopy. Endoscopic therapy may include more than one modality.[4] For instance, endoscopists will often use both a mechanical device or a contact coagulation therapy in conjunction with an injection therapy for hemostasis purposes.

INJECTION THERAPY

Injection/sclerosis needles allow the injection of hemostatic agents into the area of interest through a syringe attached at the handle of the endoscope. Hemostasis is achieved by the cytochemical mechanisms of the injected solution (e.g., epinephrine) and by mechanical tamponade.[5] Furthermore, injection of glue materials such as 2-octyl-cyanoacrylate using either a standard upper endoscope or an EUS endoscope is utilized for management of significant varices, particularly gastric varices.[6] These variceal injections with glue materials have rare complications, including systemic embolization and laceration of the varix with the needle causing worsening of bleeding.

MECHANICAL DEVICES

Endoscopic clips create hemostasis via mechanical forces on the target lesion. Standard endoscopic clips are made by many manufacturers and are composed of a delivery catheter deployed through the endoscopic working channel with a handle to deploy the clip and a preloaded pronged metal clip.[5] These devices are closed on bleeding areas and provide mechanical tamponade on the area. Newer over-the-scope clips (OTSC, Tubingen, Germany) have also been used in severe or refractory bleeding.[7,8] These devices fit on the tip of the endoscope and are deployed in a similar fashion to band ligation systems. This device creates a slightly more difficult intubation of the esophagus with the scope given the larger diameter of the endoscopic attachment; thus, it can be stimulating to the patient during reintroduction of the scope.

Band ligation systems, often used for the banding of varices, house rubber or latex stretched bands in a catheter. Similar to the OTSC clip, this is a distal attachment that fits on the end of the scope, and it can cause increased stimulation during introduction of the scope and device. During treatment, the lesion is captured within the endoscopic cap, and the band is deployed around the base to create tight compression that leads to hemostasis and subsequent necrosis and sloughing of the lesion.[9]

DIRECT CONTACT THERMAL THERAPY

The heater probe (HP) is a device that is composed of an inner heating coil surrounded by a Teflon-coated metal cylinder, which transfers direct heat to the specimen for tissue coagulation. A thermocoupling device at the tip of the probe maintains a constant and precise temperature.[5] This probe is applied to a bleeding source and both desiccates the tissue and coapts together the walls of the vessel.

The hemostatic grasper is similar to a rotatable biopsy forceps. Monopolar electrocautery desiccates tissue that is grasped with the tool.[5]

The bipolar electrocautery probe (gold probe) delivers thermal energy to tissue by creating a local electrical circuit composed of two electrodes on the probe and the viable tissue in between.[5] With the bipolar probe, electrical conductivity decreases as tissue desiccates, which limits maximum tissue injury potential and maximum temperature production.[5]

NONCONTACT THERMAL THERAPY

The argon plasma coagulator (APC) utilizes argon plasma as a conduit to deliver high-frequency monopolar coagulation to desired tissues, creating noncontact coagulation. When initiated, the argon plasma becomes electrically active, creating desiccation of tissues at the tissue-argon interface. When the tissue becomes desiccated, it loses its electrical conductivity and is unable to transmit excessive energy. The plasma stream migrates to adjacent tissue that is electrically conductive.[5]

Additionally, the gas is only ignited when the catheter is near target tissue. These features limit the scope and depth of destruction of tissue.[5] In addition to hemostasis, the APC has been explored in other arenas, such as for the endoscopic ablation of Barrett's esophagus and residual adenomatous-appearing tissue after polypectomy/EMR.[10]

BALLOON-ASSISTED AND SPIRAL ENTEROSCOPY

Balloon-assisted enteroscopy is a diagnostic modality for the traditionally hard-to-reach regions of the small bowel. Here, special endoscopic units have overtubes with either one or two balloons to help progress the long enteroscope through small bowel. Unlike video capsule endoscopy, balloon-assisted enteroscopy allows for biopsy and therapeutic manipulation of small bowel pathology. Furthermore, balloon-assisted enteroscopy can be used to reach target tissue in postsurgical anatomy (such as after roux-en-Y gastric bypass) for evaluation or intervention.

In double-balloon enteroscopy, there are two balloons in the system in association with a specialized overtube. By repeated and sequential inflation and deflation of the balloons, the loops of bowel may be examined and then reduced on the overtube in a pleated fashion, creating little stretch on the small bowel.[11–14] The balloons serve as anchors on the bowel, allowing the bowel to be withdrawn back onto the overtube and maintained in that pleated position.[11–14] The technique may be used in either an antegrade approach (initiating the sequence in the jejunum) or a retrograde approach (initiating the sequence in the terminal ileum). Indications for double-balloon enteroscopy include abnormalities identified on capsule endoscopy, obscure GI bleeding, and polyposis syndromes.[15,16]

A novel, yet similar, approach is spiral enteroscopy. This approach is similar to balloon-assisted enteroscopy, with the exception of small bowel being advanced by reducing excess small bowel in an accordion style onto a special overtube system that has a series of spirals. Due to the length of small bowel that must frequently be examined in enteroscopies, the procedure times are often prolonged. Due to prolonged procedure times (often > 90 minutes), some physicians prefer general anesthesia for these procedures.[16]

DIRECT CHOLANGIOPANCREATOSCOPY

Direct pancreaticobiliary visualization (cholangiopancreatoscopy) is performed when a small-caliber cholangioscope is inserted into the biliary tree (or pancreatic duct if adequately dilated) after sphincterotomy and cannulation of the bile duct in a conventional ERCP procedure. As opposed to a purely fluoroscopic image in conventional ERCP, direct cholangioscopy allows for real-time direct video imaging of the biliary tract while also providing the capability for directed diagnostic and therapeutic maneuvers. Direct cholangioscopy has become more accessible as a single-operator procedure due to recent technological innovations, such as the newer generation SpyGlass™ direct visualization system, which is a mother-daughter scope system that utilizes a flexible daughter scope with independent controls that fit through the device channel of a therapeutic duodenoscope (Boston Scientific, Natick, MA, USA).[17] In this system, directed biopsies may be performed with proprietary biopsy forceps (SpyBite™; Boston Scientific) for suspicious biliary strictures. Furthermore, large biliary or pancreatic duct stones may be treated with directed electrohydraulic lithotripsy probes.[17] Complications are primarily related to the initial ERCP, but they may include a slightly higher incidence of postprocedural bacteremia, although there are few data on the newest imaging systems.[18] Also, lithotripsy slightly increases the possibility of the rare complication of perforation of the bile duct.[19] The antecedent ERCP procedure is already a significantly stimulating procedure that requires deep sedation. The direct pancreaticobiliary visualization, especially with interventions, further heightens the stimulation of the procedure.

ENDOSCOPIC MUCOSAL RESECTION

Both EMR and ESD were developed primarily in Asia as a treatment for cancerous lesions in the upper GI tract due to the overwhelming incidence of gastroesophageal cancers in Asia[17,20] In addition to resection of early gastric cancer and treatment of Barrett's esophagus, EMR is now widely utilized in the United States, predominantly for removal of large colonic polyps, including flat and sessile polyps.[21,22] In EMR, the mucosal lesion is resected and removed, predominantly with either a diathermic snare or band ligator, at the mucosal/submucosal plane.[20,21] There are a variety of EMR techniques, including the "inject, lift, and cut" method, EMR-cap technique, strip-off biopsy, and EMR with band ligation method.[20,21] For colonic EMR, usually a fluid such as normal saline or hetastarch tinted with a colorant such as methylene blue (to identify the submucosal fibers) is injected into the submucosal layer to facilitate resection and to serve to expand a protective submucosal barrier to decrease the risk of perforation. One limitation of EMR is that, for large lesions, it often results in piecemeal resection, which can limit defining an R0 resection if there is cancer present within the pathology specimen. Both EMR and ESD can be stimulating procedures. Complications of EMR include bleeding and perforation.

ENDOSCOPIC SUBMUCOSAL DISSECTION

Endoscopic submucosal dissection allows for en bloc resections of mucosal-based lesions, compared to the piecemeal resections of large mucosal lesions in EMR. In ESD, a circumferential area around the lesion is first demarcated by electrocautery markings. A viscous solution such as hyaluronic acid or methylcellulose is then injected into the submucosal layer to separate the muscularis from the mucosa and to maintain a "safety cushion" to prevent unintentional perforation. An electrocautery knife is then used to perform an en bloc dissection of the previously demarcated lesion within the plane of the submucosal space. The indications for ESD include mucosal-based dysplastic or malignant lesions in the esophagus or stomach or large lateral spreading tumors in the colon.[21,23,24] Bleeding, pain, perforation, and stricture are the major complications for both EMR and ESD, with significant bleeding and perforation more common in ESD.[21,23,24]

Of note, ESD is a meticulous procedure that requires the patient to be cooperative and still. The procedure can also be prolonged, with alternating dissection and hemostasis phases of the procedure. Due to this, many endoscopists will prefer deep or general anesthesia for these procedures. As with most advanced endoscopic procedures, the complication and efficacy rates do vary with the experience of the endoscopist. Currently, ESD in the United States is predominantly limited to very highly specialized academic centers.

ENDOSCOPIC ULTRASOUND

Endoscopic ultrasound has increased the diagnostic capability of endoscopy and has taken a prominent role in the staging of cancers in and around the GI tract[16] (Figure 18.1). Echoendoscopes use a combination of both video endoscopy and ultrasound systems integrated into the distal tip of the scope that provide an ultrasound image of surrounding tissue. Currently, there are two broad categories of echoendoscopes: radial and linear. Radial scanning echoendoscopes have an ultrasound transducer that rotates, creating an image of all tissue perpendicular to the long axis of the endoscope at the tip. Most radial echoendoscopes, however, do not have the capability to perform a directed biopsy or fine-needle aspiration (FNA). Linear array echoendoscopes provide

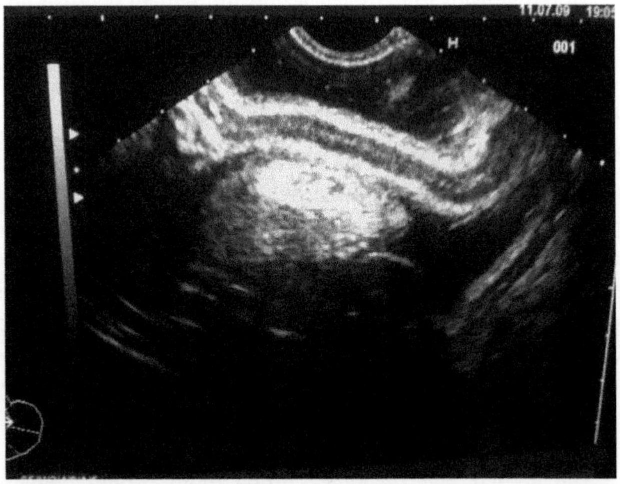

Figure 18.1. *An endoscopic ultrasound (EUS) image of a mass adjacent to the stomach wall. (Photo courtesy of Mark Gromski, MD.)*

images in an 80° to 105° arc along the long axis of the endoscope, which allows imaging of a needle as it is advanced into the ultrasonic field (and target lesion). This allows for ultrasound-guided needle access of tissues, which is essential for FNA, needle core biopsies, and fine-needle injection (FNI).

From a diagnostic and prognostic point of view, EUS has emerged as a valuable tool in the staging of esophageal,[25] gastric,[26,27] rectal,[28,29] and pancreatic cancers.[30,31] From a therapeutic perspective, EUS-guided pseudocyst drainage,[32] celiac plexus neurolysis and block,[33] and EUS-guided FNI for directed anticancer treatment[34–36] have emerged, in addition to a number of other advanced dual procedures and experimental approaches (e.g., rendezvous EUS-ERCP for directed access of the pancreatobiliary system, EUS-guided gallbladder drainage/stenting).

PER ORAL ENDOSCOPIC MYOTOMY

Per oral endoscopic myotomy is a recently developed endoscopic treatment. It has quickly become a option for treatment of achalasia, to be added in a menu of other therapeutic modalities, including pneumatic balloon dilation and Heller myotomy. POEM is an interventional endoscopic procedure performed by creating a submucosal tunnel in the esophagus, which extends from midesophagus through the gastroesophageal junction. The muscular layers (circumferential with or without longitudinal muscles) are then cut, and the endoscopic tunnel is closed using standard endoscopic clips.[37–39] The endoscopic release of the muscular layers through POEM has been highly effective for patients with achalasia. Risks of the procedure include perforation, pneumothorax, pneumomediastinum, and bleeding. Given the precise endoscopic maneuvers required in this procedure and the monitoring of respiratory status due to the proximity of the endoscopic tunnel to the mediastinum, anesthesia support and general anesthesia are often requested for these procedures.

NATURAL ORIFICE TRANSLUMENAL ENDOSCOPIC SURGERY

Natural orifice translumenal endoscopic surgery is an experimental scarless approach to abdominopelvic pathology that combines expertise of endoscopy and minimally invasive surgery. This approach, currently being extensively explored in animal studies and in a few hybrid laparoscopic-NOTES human protocols, will likely drive further industry and academic research and development into minimally invasive approaches to GI pathologies. The NOTES approach is discussed in more detail in Chapter 21.

COMPLICATIONS AND SPECIAL POPULATIONS

Complications during GI endoscopy result primarily from interventional procedures. Hemorrhage following polypectomy, EMR, or ESD is encountered with relative frequency but is nearly always able to be managed endoscopically—in only very rare circumstances does an intraprocedure or postprocedure bleeding complication require surgical intervention. Perforation from a variety of interventional procedures may lead to pneumomediastinum, pneumoperitoneum, or pneumothorax, depending on the location of the defect. This may result in venous compromise and hemodynamic responses due to decreased preload. Endoscopic management of perforations has improved with development of endoscopic suturing devices and new endoscopic clips (e.g., OTSC clip). Occasionally, significant clinical compromise may require prompt needle decompression of the body cavity involved or emergent surgical intervention. Variceal bleeding may lead to significant blood loss, which may lead to circulatory compromise and death. Complication profiles for more experimental techniques, such as NOTES, are not well characterized at this point in humans.

The complications of each endoscopic procedure must be known, and there needs to be a backup plan should the complication occur. Depending on the invasiveness of the procedure, the complication profile of the procedure, and the level of sedation desired for the patient, health care personnel skilled in airway management and emergency resuscitative techniques should be present or immediately available during the procedure.

When determining endoscopic management, including sedation, the gastroenterologist and anesthesiologist must also take into account special populations, such as the elderly, obese, pregnant, and patients with comorbid conditions. For example, obesity is an independent risk factor for complications in ambulatory endoscopic procedures. A study by Qadeer and colleagues found increased body mass index (BMI) to be a risk factor for hypoxemia in subjects undergoing a variety of ambulatory endoscopic procedures.[40] In another study, BMI greater than 28 was an independent risk factor for hypoxemia in subjects undergoing upper endoscopy.[41] Should endotracheal intubation become necessary during an endoscopic procedure, it is important to be aware that numerous studies correlated the difficulty of endotracheal intubation with obesity.[42–44]

REFERENCES

1. Seeff LC, Richards TB, Shapiro JA, et al. How many endoscopies are performed for colorectal cancer screening? Results from CDC's survey of endoscopic capacity. *Gastroenterology*. 2004;127:1670–1677.
2. Joseph DA, Meester RG, Zauber AG, et al. Colorectal cancer screening: estimated future colonoscopy need and current volume and capacity. *Cancer*. 2016;122:2479–2486.
3. Liu JJ, Saltzman JR. Endoscopic hemostasis treatment: how should you perform it? *Can J Gastroenterol*. 2009;23:481–483.
4. Marmo R, Rotondano G, Piscopo R, Bianco MA, D'Angella R, Cipolletta L. Dual therapy versus monotherapy in the endoscopic treatment of high-risk bleeding ulcers: a meta-analysis of controlled trials. *Am J Gastroenterol*. 2007;102:279–289; quiz 469.
5. Conway JD, Adler DG, Diehl DL, et al. Endoscopic hemostatic devices. *Gastrointest Endosc*. 2009;69:987–996.
6. Kahloon A, Chalasani N, DeWitt J, et al. Endoscopic therapy with 2-octyl-cyanoacrylate for the treatment of gastric varices. *Digest Dis Sci*. 2014;59:2178–2183.
7. Wedi E, von Renteln D, Jung C, et al. Treatment of acute colonic diverticular bleeding in high risk patients, using an over-the-scope clip: a case series. *Endoscopy*. 2016;48:E383–E385.
8. Wedi E, Gonzalez S, Menke D, Kruse E, Matthes K, Hochberger J. One hundred and one over-the-scope-clip applications for severe gastrointestinal bleeding, leaks and fistulas. *World J Gastroenterol*. 2016;22:1844–1853.

9. Liu J, Petersen BT, Tierney WM, et al. Endoscopic banding devices. *Gastrointest Endosc.* 2008;68:217–221.
10. Kelty CJ, Ackroyd R, Brown NJ, Stephenson TJ, Stoddard CJ, Reed MW. Endoscopic ablation of Barrett's oesophagus: a randomized-controlled trial of photodynamic therapy vs. argon plasma coagulation. *Aliment Pharmacol Ther.* 2004;20:1289–1296.
11. Matsumoto T, Moriyama T, Esaki M, Nakamura S, Iida M. Performance of antegrade double-balloon enteroscopy: comparison with push enteroscopy. *Gastrointest Endosc.* 2005;62:392–398.
12. May A, Nachbar L, Schneider M, Ell C. Prospective comparison of push enteroscopy and push-and-pull enteroscopy in patients with suspected small-bowel bleeding. *Am J Gastroenterol.* 2006;101:2016–2024.
13. Yamamoto H, Sekine Y, Sato Y, et al. Total enteroscopy with a nonsurgical steerable double-balloon method. *Gastrointest Endosc.* 2001;53:216–220.
14. Yamamoto H, Yano T, Kita H, Sunada K, Ido K, Sugano K. New system of double-balloon enteroscopy for diagnosis and treatment of small intestinal disorders. *Gastroenterology.* 2003;125:1556; author reply 1557.
15. Gerson LB. Double-balloon enteroscopy: the new gold standard for small-bowel imaging? *Gastrointest Endosc.* 2005;62:71–75.
16. Greenberger NJ, ed. *Current Diagnosis and Treatment: Gastroenterology, Hepatology, and Endoscopy*. 3rd ed. New York, NY: McGraw-Hill; 2009.
17. de Villiers WJ. Anesthesiology and gastroenterology. *Anesthesiol Clin.* 2009;27:57–70.
18. Chen MF, Jan YY. Bacteremia following postoperative choledochofiberscopy—a prospective study. *Hepatogastroenterology.* 1996;43:586–589.
19. Binmoeller KF, Bruckner M, Thonke F, Soehendra N. Treatment of difficult bile duct stones using mechanical, electrohydraulic and extracorporeal shock wave lithotripsy. *Endoscopy.* 1993;25:201–216.
20. Shim CS. Endoscopic mucosal resection. *J Korean Med Sci.* 1996;11:457–466.
21. Ahmadi A, Draganov P. Endoscopic mucosal resection in the upper gastrointestinal tract. *World J Gastroenterol.* 2008;14:1984–1989.
22. Puli SR, Kakugawa Y, Gotoda T, Antillon D, Saito Y, Antillon MR. Meta-analysis and systematic review of colorectal endoscopic mucosal resection. *World J Gastroenterol.* 2009;15:4273–4277.
23. Fujishiro M. Perspective on the practical indications of endoscopic submucosal dissection of gastrointestinal neoplasms. *World J Gastroenterol.* 2008;14:4289–4295.
24. Kakushima N, Fujishiro M. Endoscopic submucosal dissection for gastrointestinal neoplasms. *World J Gastroenterol.* 2008;14:2962–2967.
25. Kelly S, Harris KM, Berry E, et al. A systematic review of the staging performance of endoscopic ultrasound in gastro-oesophageal carcinoma. *Gut.* 2001;49:534–539.
26. Matthes K, Bounds BC, Collier K, Gutierrez A, Brugge WR. EUS staging of upper GI malignancies: results of a prospective randomized trial. *Gastrointest Endosc.* 2006;64:496–502.
27. Yasuda K. EUS in the detection of early gastric cancer. *Gastrointest Endosc.* 2002;56:S68–S75.
28. Bianchi P, Ceriani C, Palmisano A, et al. A prospective comparison of endorectal ultrasound and pelvic magnetic resonance in the preoperative staging of rectal cancer. *Ann Ital Chir.* 2006;77:41–46.
29. Savides TJ, Master SS. EUS in rectal cancer. *Gastrointest Endosc.* 2002;56:S12–S18.
30. Horwhat JD, Paulson EK, McGrath K, et al. A randomized comparison of EUS-guided FNA versus CT or US-guided FNA for the evaluation of pancreatic mass lesions. *Gastrointest Endosc.* 2006;63:966–975.
31. Turner BG, Cizginer S, Agarwal D, Yang J, Pitman MB, Brugge WR. Diagnosis of pancreatic neoplasia with EUS and FNA: a report of accuracy. *Gastrointest Endosc.* 2010;71:91–98.
32. Fockens P. EUS in drainage of pancreatic pseudocysts. *Gastrointest Endosc.* 2002;56:S93–S97.
33. Hoffman BJ. EUS-guided celiac plexus block/neurolysis. *Gastrointest Endosc.* 2002;56:S26–S28.
34. Chang KJ. EUS-guided fine needle injection (FNI) and anti-tumor therapy. *Endoscopy.* 2006;38(suppl 1):S88–S93.
35. Matthes K, Mino-Kenudson M, Sahani DV, Holalkere N, Brugge WR. Concentration-dependent ablation of pancreatic tissue by EUS-guided ethanol injection. *Gastrointest Endosc.* 2007;65:272–277.
36. Matthes K, Mino-Kenudson M, Sahani DV, et al. EUS-guided injection of paclitaxel (OncoGel) provides therapeutic drug concentrations in the porcine pancreas (with video). *Gastrointest Endosc.* 2007;65:448–453.
37. Pannala R, Abu Dayyeh BK, Aslanian HR, et al. Per-oral endoscopic myotomy (with video). *Gastrointest Endosc.* 2016;83:1051–1060.
38. Stavropoulos SN, Modayil R, Friedel D. Per oral endoscopic myotomy for the treatment of achalasia. *Curr Opin Gastroenterol.* 2015;31:430–440.
39. Stavropoulos SN, Harris MD, Hida S, Brathwaite C, Demetriou C, Grendell J. Endoscopic submucosal myotomy for the treatment of achalasia (with video). *Gastrointest endosc.* 2010;72:1309–1311.
40. Qadeer MA, Rocio Lopez A, Dumot JA, Vargo JJ. Risk factors for hypoxemia during ambulatory gastrointestinal endoscopy in ASA I-II patients. *Digest Dis Sci.* 2009;54:1035–1040.
41. Dhariwal A, Plevris JN, Lo NT, Finlayson ND, Heading RC, Hayes PC. Age, anemia, and obesity-associated oxygen desaturation during upper gastrointestinal endoscopy. *Gastrointest Endosc.* 1992;38:684–688.
42. Lavi R, Segal D, Ziser A. Predicting difficult airways using the intubation difficulty scale: a study comparing obese and non-obese patients. *J Clin Anesth.* 2009;21:264–267.
43. Lundstrom LH, Moller AM, Rosenstock C, Astrup G, Wetterslev J. High body mass index is a weak predictor for difficult and failed tracheal intubation: a cohort study of 91,332 consecutive patients scheduled for direct laryngoscopy registered in the Danish Anesthesia Database. *Anesthesiology.* 2009;110:266–274.
44. Shiga T, Wajima Z, Inoue T, Sakamoto A. Predicting difficult intubation in apparently normal patients: a meta-analysis of bedside screening test performance. *Anesthesiology.* 2005;103:429–437.

19 | ANESTHESIA FOR GASTROINTESTINAL ENDOSCOPIC PROCEDURES

LORI KRAL BARTON, MD, REGINA Y. FRAGNETO, MD

INTRODUCTION

For years, the number of endoscopic procedures performed by gastroenterologists in the United States has grown, and this trend continues. The escalating demand for endoscopic services can be attributed to an aging patient population, increased public awareness of cancer-screening benefits, and Medicare reimbursement for surveillance colonoscopies.[1] In addition, the complexity and invasiveness of procedures that can be accomplished via endoscopy has increased, with these procedures often requiring a more complex anesthetic than the conscious sedation commonly associated with the endoscopy suite. This may include general anesthesia with endotracheal intubation. Confounding this surge in complex procedures, there has also been an increase in the severity and number of patient comorbidities as American Society of Anesthesiologists physical class 3 (ASA 3) and ASA 4 patients now account for a greater proportion of patients being cared for in the endoscopy suite. Just as the procedures and the patients have evolved, so has the delivery of anesthesia. Not only has there been an increase in the use of general anesthetics, but also there has been continued investigation of both non–anesthesiologist-administered propofol (NAAP) as well as patient-administered sedation and target-controlled infusions (TCIs) as an attempt to balance the increased need for sedation services with the shortage of available anesthesiologists.[2]

Sedation for endoscopy facilitates the procedure, improves patient tolerance and satisfaction, and increases the likelihood that the patient will agree to further interventions.[3] Historically, sedation regimens for endoscopy have consisted of a benzodiazepine combined with an opioid administered by nursing personnel under direction of the endoscopist. In the United States, the most common combination is midazolam with fentanyl.[1] For screening colonoscopies in low-risk patients, this model usually proves successful. However, many modern endoscopic procedures are prolonged and complex, necessitating the need for deep sedation or general anesthesia. Along with an increasing volume of pediatric patients, these factors are altering sedation practices in the endoscopy suite. Although options for non–anesthesiologist-administered sedation are common for many endoscopic procedures, in situations such as these, the use of an anesthesiologist is increasing.

The administration of anesthesia or sedation for endoscopy is associated with unique challenges that often differ from those encountered when providing anesthesia care in the operating room (OR). The location where procedures are performed (Figure 19.1), inconsistencies in preoperative preparation, postanesthesia recovery issues, and the management of complications are all areas requiring distinctive management strategies in the non–operating room anesthesia (NORA) environment.

LOCATIONS

A 2006 survey of randomly selected members of the American College of Gastroenterology attempted to determine the locations where endoscopy procedures are commonly performed in the United States as well as the types of sedation utilized for these procedures. The survey revealed that the majority (55.2%) of gastrointestinal (GI) endoscopies are still being performed in the hospital setting, although a significant number are being performed in ambulatory surgery centers.[1] Procedures performed in an office-based setting remain uncommon. Of note, there were significant regional differences in facility preference as well as sedation methods and percentage of cases in which an anesthesia professional administered the sedation.[1] While there have been several publications within the gastroenterology literature documenting and supporting the administration of propofol by nurses supervised by the gastroenterologist,[4–6] this practice does not yet seem to have achieved widespread acceptance. A variety of factors likely explain this, including the restriction in the product labeling of propofol (which is discussed further in the chapter) as well as state-specific nursing regulations. Several state nursing boards do not allow registered nurses to administer propofol for procedural sedation.

SEDATION VERSUS GENERAL ANESTHESIA

Sedation for every procedure in the endoscopy suite is not ubiquitous; indeed, a small number of patients will tolerate simple GI endoscopic procedures without any sedation. While over 98% of colonoscopies and esophagogastroduodenoscopies (EGDs) are performed with sedation in the United States,[1] unsedated examinations are more common in other countries. European studies have

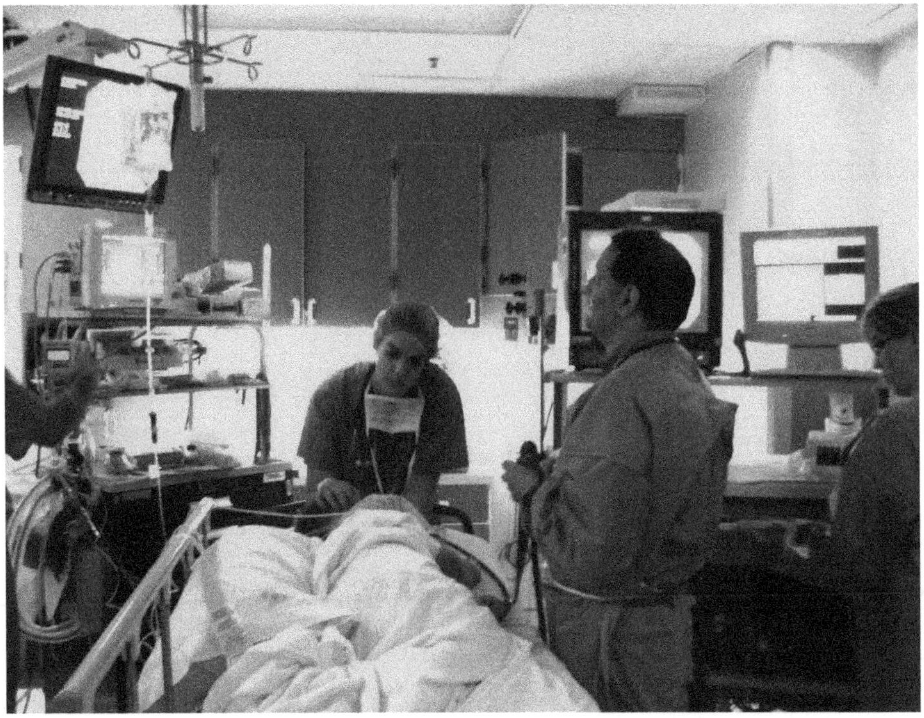

Figure 19.1. *Typical procedure room in gastrointestinal (GI) endoscopy suite.*

sought to elucidate patient factors that might predict poor tolerance of endoscopy without sedation.[7] Apprehension about the procedure and elevated levels of anxiety were both associated with poor patient tolerance. Recent studies have also been performed to determine factors that influence increased sedation needs. These characteristics include female gender, younger age, difficult endoscopy, current use of opioids or benzodiazepines, and involvement of a trainee during the procedure.[8,9]

Healthy patients undergoing simple procedures such as screening colonoscopies or EGDs will generally tolerate these procedures well with light-to-moderate sedation. While some centers will utilize anesthesia care providers for these cases, a majority of gastroenterologists will direct nurse-administered sedation for these routine procedures. Most GI endoscopy centers will consult anesthesiologists for specific patient groups (Box 19.1), such as pediatric patients, patients with a history of being difficult to sedate, mentally challenged patients, and patients with life-threatening medical conditions. In these more challenging situations, it is likely that deep sedation or general anesthesia will be required to achieve patient comfort and cooperation.

To choose the appropriate level of sedation for an endoscopic procedure, the anesthesia provider must consider several variables. The patient's medical status is paramount in this decision, including whether the patient is at risk for aspiration, thus requiring endotracheal intubation. The logistics of the procedure also come into play when formulating an anesthetic plan, namely, the complexity and length of the planned procedure, positioning requirements, and proximity of the anesthesiologist to the patient's airway during the case.

BOX 19.1. PATIENTS LIKELY TO REQUIRE SEDATION FOR GASTROINTESTINAL ENDOSCOPY

Pediatric patients
Patients with a history of being difficult to sedate or history of difficult intubation
Substance abusers
Mentally challenged patients
Patients undergoing complex/long procedures
Patients with serious or life-threatening medical conditions

SCHEDULING AND THE PREPROCEDURE EVALUATION

The same principles of preanesthetic evaluation for surgical cases should apply to GI endoscopic procedures.[10] This may require significant coordination between the anesthesia provider and the endoscopist, especially when dealing with medically complex patients. While many patients are evaluated by the gastroenterologist in an office visit prior to the procedure, the open-access model has become increasingly popular.[11] In this model, patients are referred by a primary care provider and scheduled for procedures without first being seen by the endoscopist. Most centers that employ an open-access scheduling system have a patient-screening process in place. For example, the endoscopy scheduler will conduct a telephone interview and review the patient's medical history. Affirmative answers to specific questions (i.e., history of heart failure, anticoagulant therapy) trigger a preprocedure office visit with the physician who will be performing the endoscopy.

It is critical that the gastroenterologist and anesthesiologist communicate, and the expectations regarding preanesthetic evaluations are understood. A well-defined process of evaluating each patient preendoscopy for anesthetic risks helps to avoid the frustrating scenario in which the anesthesiologist is faced with an inadequately evaluated patient moments before the procedure is scheduled to begin.

An excellent example of a situation that requires preprocedure planning is that of managing antiplatelet medications and anticoagulants in preparation for endoscopic procedures where bleeding is expected, such as esophageal varices banding or endoscopic retrograde cholangiopancreatography (ERCP) with sphincterotomy. As the indications for long-term anticoagulant/antiplatelet therapy expand, the number of patients presenting to the endoscopy suite who are taking these medications also is increasing. This issue is of particular importance in patients who have drug-eluting coronary stents. As with surgical patients, the decision whether to withhold these medications during the periprocedure period is complex and must be made in collaboration with the gastroenterologist, cardiologist, and anesthesiologist. An approach that has been studied and shown to be cost effective is to perform a primary diagnostic endoscopy while the patient remains on the usual anticoagulation regimen. An informed decision can then be made on how to manage the anticoagulants if a therapeutic procedure is deemed necessary.[12] It is somewhat reassuring that a retrospective case-control study concluded that antiplatelet agents were not significantly associated with bleeding after endoscopic sphincterotomy.[13] However, a recent survey indicated that as many as 26% of 239 US endoscopists felt that they would advise discontinuation of all antiplatelet agents before performing any endoscopic procedure, including low-risk procedures, despite the recommendations of previous American Society of Gastrointestinal Endoscopy (ASGE) guidelines.[14] This information further justifies the need for a multidisciplinary approach to decision-making about withholding these medications for each patient.

An important aspect of the preanesthetic evaluation is determining whether the endoscopy suite is the most appropriate location for performing the procedure. Unlike other nonsurgical procedures requiring anesthesia services, the equipment necessary to perform many GI procedures is relatively portable. From the anesthesiologist's perspective, the OR may be the safest environment for performing endoscopy in the most medically challenging patients. Specialized monitoring and airway equipment as well as additional anesthesiology personnel are more readily available if anesthesia complications arise.

REIMBURSEMENT

Payers do not typically provide separate reimbursement for sedation when a gastroenterologist both performs the procedure and oversees the sedation; the sedation component is included. As an increasing number of endoscopists have turned to anesthesiologists to provide sedation, charges to Medicare for anesthesia for colonoscopy have increased markedly. Between 2001 and 2003, the number of colonoscopies in which anesthesiologists provided sedation more than doubled, and charges to Medicare increased 86%.[15] This rapid growth attracted increased scrutiny from commercial payers and Medicare contractors. Many carriers distinguish between anesthesia for low-risk and high-risk patients, allowing reimbursement for the latter only. Carriers set guidelines to define a high-risk patient or procedure, and case-specific reasons that necessitate the participation of an anesthesia care provider must be documented accordingly.

In addition, significant regional differences exist that highlight disparities in reimbursement policies across the country, and this explains why anesthesia for endoscopy tends to be handled differently depending on the location. For instance, a 2004 survey showed that in the northeastern states, where carriers are generally unfavorable toward anesthesiologist involvement, only 7% of gastroenterologists used propofol sedation. In the mid-Atlantic states where more favorable policies exist, 43% of gastroenterologists utilized anesthesiologists to administer propofol.[1]

Despite these regional variations, 2016 brought with it a significant decrease in colonoscopy reimbursement across all regions, which has further complicated the participation of anesthesia providers. Prior to the reduction in reimbursement, studies had indicated that the actual procedure times were significantly less than the times on which the relative values for endoscopy had been based. This led the Centers for Medicare and Medicaid Services (CMS) to enact lower reimbursement for GI endoscopy beginning in 2016. They upheld their standard that colonoscopy coding still includes moderate sedation, thus preventing an endoscopist from adding additional coding for supervision of moderate sedation. However, they did stipulate that a second physician, other than the one performing the procedure, may report the codes for moderate sedation or anesthesia if he or she provides this service, thus acknowledging the importance of a dedicated anesthesia provider in some circumstances.[16]

Finally, in the interest of making preventive care more widely available, a provision of the Affordable Care Act waived "colorectal cancer screening test" copayments and deductibles for Medicare and other beneficiaries. Included in this ruling on physician fee schedules is the inclusion of anesthesia services furnished in conjunction with a screening colonoscopy, thus preventing a separate bill to the patient for a copay or deductible.[17] By including anesthesia services within the necessity of preventive medicine, the CMS further validated the role of the anesthesia provider even for screening procedures.

MEDICATIONS FOR SEDATION AND ANALGESIA

The sedation regimen for the majority of GI endoscopic procedures consists of a benzodiazepine combined with an opioid titrated to mild-to-moderate sedation.[18] As procedure numbers climb and techniques become more sophisticated, some limitations of this traditional sedation practice are discovered. There are patients who simply cannot be adequately sedated with a benzodiazepine/opioid combination, leading to failed procedural attempts or a poor experience for the patient. Onset of sedation can be prolonged with these two classes of drugs, and significant side effects are not uncommon in the recovery period, including nausea, vomiting, prolonged sedation, and respiratory depression. For these reasons, alternative drugs have been sought that offer improved pharmacodynamic profiles coupled with fewer side effects.[19]

PROPOFOL

While the issue of propofol administration by nonanesthesia personnel is controversial, there is little doubt that propofol is perhaps the most desired agent for endoscopic sedation.[20] High patient satisfaction, quick onset, rapid recovery, and improved operational efficiency are all factors that have led to increased demand for propofol use in the endoscopy suite. Depending on the type and duration of procedure, it can be administered as either intermittent boluses or a continuous infusion. One of the drug's disadvantages, though, is its very narrow therapeutic window. Due to significant variation among patients, it is not uncommon for a dose that typically produces moderate sedation to lead to a level of deep sedation or even general anesthesia in some patients. Unlike use of opioids and benzodiazapines, propofol currently does not have a reversal agent in case of oversedation. As a result, the US Food and Drug Administration (FDA) includes on propofol's product label a statement that it "should only be administered by persons trained in the administration of general anesthesia."[21] In addition, the American Society of Anesthesiologists "Practice Guidelines for Sedation and Analgesia by Non-anesthesiologists"[22] and The Joint Commission state that practitioners providing sedation should be able to manage patients who reach a deeper level of sedation than was planned. In the case of propofol administration, therefore, the practitioner should be competent in managing airway obstruction and respiratory depression, which could include the need for endotracheal intubation, as well as cardiovascular side effects such as hypotension. It is these positions by regulatory and accrediting agencies, which are supported by the American Society of Anesthesiologists, that have made the administration of propofol by nonanesthesia professionals, including registered nurses under the supervision of an endoscopist, a controversial topic.

In an article published in 2009, the argument for endoscopist-directed propofol (EDP) administration was made citing over 646,000 patients who received propofol for either upper endoscopy or colonoscopy in which there were just 4 deaths and 11 endotracheal intubations. Not all studies that were included in this analysis included data on the use of positive pressure ventilation, airway assist devices such as oral airways, or periods of apnea.[23] This retrospective study is limited based on reliance of self-reporting by each institution, including reporting based on memory rather than formal records and no uniform method of sedation with both single-agent propofol and balanced anesthesia with inclusion of opioids and benzodiazepines along with propofol, used by facilities providing data for the analysis.

The incidence of complications such as oxygen desaturation and airway obstruction associated with Nurse Administered Propofol Sedation (NAPS) is not well defined. Some gastroenterologists are now reporting the use of NAPS for more complex endoscopic procedures, such as endoscopic ultrasound (EUS).[24,25] In a retrospective study of more than 800 patients, 0.5% of patients required positive pressure ventilation during the procedure, and oxygen saturation decreased below 90% in 0.7% of patients.[24] This led one proponent of NAPS for simple endoscopic procedures to caution about adopting this technique for more advanced procedures.[26]

A meta-analysis that looked at the pooled results of sedation comparing NAPS with an anesthesia provider (anesthesiologist or certified registered nurse anesthetist [CRNA]) sedation for complex procedures including ERCP, EUS, and small intestine deep enteroscopy had interesting results. The NAPS sedations tended to use less propofol and require less airway intervention; however, patient and endoscopist satisfaction were significantly higher in the anesthesia professional group. Both groups had similar rates of desaturation.[27]

In 2015, the European Society of GI Endoscopy and the European Society of Gastroenterology and Endoscopy Nurses issued updated guidelines with recommendations limiting the scope of NAPS based on the patient's physical status, airway classification, body mass index (BMI), and anticipated long or complex procedures. Also included in these guidelines was the recommendation that propofol be used only as a single agent rather than as part of a balanced anesthetic. They further recommended use of propofol as patient-controlled sedation (PCS) or a TCI.[28]

Patient-controlled sedation is a delivery model that has been investigated for use in endoscopic procedures as a way to provide adequate sedation while minimizing the problem of oversedation that can occur due to propofol's narrow therapeutic window.[29,30] Although PCS with propofol and other medications has been investigated for endoscopy and has been shown to be safe and effective, PCS has not gained widespread acceptance for these procedures within the United States. Multiple studies have shown that when comparing PCS to both anesthesia provider- and nurse-administered sedation, medication doses tended to be lower, sedation levels lighter, and recovery times faster for PCS.[31–37] However, varying results have been found with PCS in regard to patient and endoscopist satisfaction.[33,35,37]

A prospective randomized study from France compared PCS with propofol administration by an anesthesiologist for patients undergoing colonoscopy. Patients in the patient-controlled group self-administered 20-mg boluses of propofol as needed with a 1-minute lockout time. Patients in the anesthesiologist-controlled group received a continuous infusion of propofol that was titrated to effect. Procedural success, which was defined as reaching the cecum with the colonoscope, and technical ease of the procedure as rated by the gastroenterologist did not differ between the groups. Patient satisfaction was similar between the groups as well. Patients in the patient-controlled propofol group experienced a lighter depth of sedation and used significantly less propofol than patients in the anesthesiologist-controlled group. In addition, fewer episodes of desaturation occurred in the patient-controlled group, and the time to discharge was also shorter in this group.[38]

Target controlled infusion systems also continue to be investigated and are used in about 90 countries; however, they are not FDA approved in the United States. A TCI of propofol uses a pharmacokinetic model to achieve and maintain a selected target blood propofol concentration, thereby avoiding the peaks and troughs associated with bolus dosing. A 2014 study comparing patients undergoing colonoscopy and EGD procedures with fentanyl/midazolam sedation versus NAPS with a TCI of propofol found that both patient and endoscopist satisfaction were significantly higher for the TCI group.[39] Research has been done comparing a manually controlled infusion of propofol with a TCI infusion, with both administered by nonanesthesia personnel. Although the TCI infusion offered some promising results, there were adverse events in both groups (including prolonged hypoxemia) that required advanced airway management.[40]

In 2013, the FDA approved the propofol-based sedation product SEDASYS, a computer-assisted personalized anesthesia system.[41] By integrating real-time patient data into a computer program, the system managed the delivery of propofol for both colonoscopies and EGD procedures. The ASA had recommended that the system be limited to patients over the age of 18 and only in locations where anesthesia professionals were immediately available. Concerns with the system included its use in patients who could develop airway complications, such as the morbidly obese population, patients with obstructive sleep apnea, and patients with respiratory complications. However, by March 2016 Johnson and Johnson had discontinued the device due to poor sales.[42]

While it may not be clear which practitioners and delivery methods will be used most commonly in the future, it is certain that propofol will continue to be a popular drug administered for sedation and anesthesia during endoscopic procedures.

DEXMEDETOMIDINE

Approved by the FDA in 1999 for sedation for intubated patients in the intensive care unit, dexmedetomidine is a highly selective α_2-adrenergic receptor agonist with sedative and analgesic effects.[43] Agonism at presynaptic receptors in peripheral sympathetic nerves inhibits the release of norepinephrine, while stimulation at central postsynaptic receptors serves to inhibit sympathetic activity. As the drug's mechanism of action is unrelated to the γ-aminobutyric acid (GABA) system, the quality of sedation is purportedly different.[44] Patients tend to appear quite sedated yet are more easily arousable than patients sedated by a GABA-potentiating agent such as midazolam or propofol. A relatively new agent in the anesthesiologist's armamentarium, dexmedetomidine's role in sedation for GI endoscopy has not been entirely established.

Few studies have been performed evaluating the use of dexmedetomidine specifically for endoscopic procedures. A Turkish study published in 2007 compared dexmedetomidine and midazolam in a cohort of 60 ASA 1 and 2 adult patients undergoing EGD.[45] Endoscopist satisfaction with sedation quality was higher and total side effects were lower in the dexmedetomidine group. Recovery time and hemodynamic parameters were comparable between the two groups. A 2014 study evaluated upper endoscopy with midazolam sedation versus dexmedetomidine sedation. This small study (n = 60) concluded that patients sedated with dexmedetomidine had higher oxygen saturations and improved satisfaction as compared to the group sedated with midazolam.[46]

A study from Poland evaluating dexmedetomidine for sedation during colonoscopy found it to be less than ideal, and indeed, the study was terminated due to adverse events in the dexmedetomidine group.[47] Compared with patients receiving meperidine and midazolam or fentanyl as a single agent, patients receiving dexmedetomidine had the longest recovery time as well as significant bradycardia and hypotension not seen in the other groups. When evaluating dexmedetomidine sedation with propofol sedation, researchers found minimal differences in oxygen saturation and respiratory rate variability, yet patients in the propofol group had lower mean arterial pressures (MAPs), while those in the dexmedetomidine group experienced more bradycardia. Patients reported greater satisfaction with dexmedetomidine, and endoscopist satisfaction was comparable between the dexmedetomidine and propofol groups.[48]

KETAMINE

A synthetic phencyclidine derivative, ketamine is a rapidly acting anesthetic agent that produces rapid sedation, amnesia, and analgesia.[49] Functioning as an *N*-methyl-D-aspartate (NMDA) receptor antagonist, ketamine acts to dissociate the limbic and cortical systems, producing a cataleptic state that does not resemble normal sleep patterns.[50]

Airway reflexes are generally maintained, and cardiovascular and respiratory side effects are minimal.

Ketamine has been examined both as a sole agent for sedation and in combination with other sedatives in both adults and children. Most literature references address its use in the pediatric population. Gigler et al. performed a retrospective analysis of 402 pediatric patients receiving various combinations of midazolam, meperidine, and ketamine for simple endoscopy procedures.[51] They concluded that the group that received midazolam and ketamine in combination had the lowest rate of complications as well as an equal rate of adequate sedation when compared with other sedation regimens. A study from Hong Kong sought to evaluate the effectiveness of intramuscular ketamine as a sole sedative agent in 60 children undergoing basic GI endoscopic procedures as well as bronchoscopy.[52] It was determined that a single intramuscular dose of ketamine (2–3 mg/kg) was safe and effective for children aged 7 years and older. A high failure rate was noted in children younger than 7 years, with the highest failure rates among infants. Kirberg et al. described their successful use of ketamine, primarily as an adjunct to other sedatives, in over 900 pediatric endoscopic procedures.[53] Ketamine use in difficult-to-sedate adult patients undergoing ERCP and EUS has been explored.[54] In patients who were inadequately sedated with meperidine and diazepam, it was found that ketamine administration offered a better depth of sedation and shorter recovery time than additional dosing of meperidine and diazepam.

BENZODIAZEPINES

Long an integral part of sedation for endoscopy, early benzodiazepines, such as diazepam, were not water soluble, leading to problems with administration. Once water-soluble midazolam became available in the late 1980s, it quickly gained favor.[55]

The majority of intravenous sedation for endoscopy today involves administration of midazolam in combination with an opioid, usually by a nonanesthesia professional.[1] Serious side effects from midazolam are uncommon, although dose-dependent respiratory depression does occur. This respiratory depression is more likely in patients who have underlying respiratory disease and in those receiving concomitant opioids for sedation.[18] A large prospective study of 2635 pediatric endoscopies at the Children's Hospital of Philadelphia found only two serious adverse events (apnea) and concluded that administration of midazolam and fentanyl is safe for pediatric endoscopy.[56]

OPIOIDS

The second component of the conventional sedation combination for endoscopy is an opioid. Twenty-five years ago, meperidine was the primary choice.[55] Today, meperidine has been supplanted by fentanyl as the predominant opioid used. Alternative opioids have been investigated for use in procedural sedation, such as the ultrashort-acting remifentanil. One study examined the use of remifentanil combined with a benzodiazepine in the sedation of 40 patients undergoing various procedures, including endoscopy.[57] While discharge times were short and analgesia was profound in the remifentanil group, the dose to achieve adequate sedation frequently led to apneic episodes requiring intervention. It was concluded that remifentanil use for sedation during brief procedures is not useful.

REMIMAZOLAM

Remimazolam is a benzodiazepine derivative now in phase 2 trials. Midazolam is the parent drug of remimazolam, which has been modified to include the pharmacokinetics of remifentanil.[58] GABA is the primary inhibitory neurotransmitter in the central nervous system, and like other anesthetics, remimazolam acts at GABA receptors (GABA-α) to elicit its sedative effects. Because the drug undergoes ester hydrolysis, which is dose independent, accumulation of the drug is not seen in clinical doses. In the phase 2 trials performed thus far, the time to recovery from sedation was shorter and more consistent with remimazolam when compared to midazolam. However, respiratory depressant effects have been reported in numerous studies.[59,60]

SEDATION/ANESTHESIA FOR SPECIFIC PROCEDURES

Gastrointestinal endoscopy procedures vary significantly in their complexity, duration, and degree of patient stimulation. Therefore, the anesthesiologist must tailor the sedation regimen to focus on not only individual patient requirements but also the unique variables associated with the procedure being performed.

ESOPHAGOGASTRODUODENOSCOPY

While many EGDs are performed successfully with a combination of a benzodiazepine and opioid, the majority of EGD sedations performed by anesthesiologists utilize propofol. A nationwide survey of gastroenterologists reported higher satisfaction rates with propofol compared to conventional benzodiazepine/opioid sedation.[1] The median satisfaction score for propofol was 10 on a scale where 10 was defined as best, while benzodiazepine and opioid in combination yielded a score of 8. Also, a majority of these physicians selected propofol as the agent they would choose to receive for their own endoscopy. Reasons given for favoring propofol included better sedation and analgesia, fast return to normal activity, and improved quality of the endoscopic examination.

While successful EGD exams can generally be performed under moderate sedation in most patients, individuals with a history of being difficult to sedate or a history of substance abuse will generally require deep sedation or general anesthesia. However, even when moderate sedation is the intended endpoint, studies have shown that deep sedation is often achieved. In one study, 60% of patients undergoing EGD reached a level of deep sedation despite a preprocedure plan for moderate sedation.[61]

A patient's need for endotracheal intubation is another factor to consider when choosing between sedation and general anesthesia for EGD. Many of the indications for EGD, such as persistent vomiting or severe gastroesophageal reflux disease, may dictate protection of the airway with an endotracheal tube. Other patients who may not tolerate the level of sedation needed for EGD include patients with obstructive sleep apnea or morbid obesity. Significant airway obstruction should be expected in these patients, and endotracheal intubation should be strongly considered.

One unique technique that has been employed for EGD under general anesthesia in pediatric patients is use of the ProSeal™ laryngeal mask airway (LMA).[62] The ProSeal LMA features a modified cuff and a drain tube that provides gastric access. The drain tube is of a sufficient size to accept pediatric-size gastroscopes. When compared with oxygen delivery via nasal cannula, the ProSeal group had overall higher SpO_2 values and fewer episodes of hypoxemia with no discernible difference between groups in ease of endoscopy.

An adjunct to sedation for EGD that is often overlooked is topical pharyngeal anesthesia. While there are studies that have reported no additional benefit from topical anesthesia in sedated patients,[63] other studies[64] as well as a meta-analysis[65] have reported an improvement in the ease of endoscopy in patients receiving topical pharyngeal anesthesia. It should be noted that commercially available local anesthetic sprays such as HurriCaine® and Cetacaine® sprays contain benzocaine, which has been associated with the development of methemoglobinemia.[66] Another novel method for topical anesthesia that has been described is use of a lidocaine lollipop.[67] In a study of

50 patients undergoing EGD, approximately one-third of those receiving the lidocaine lollipop did not require any further sedation throughout the procedure.

COLONOSCOPY

Like EGD, the majority of patients can be adequately sedated for colonoscopy with a combination of midazolam and opioid. One study found that when moderate sedation was planned, fewer patients progressed to deep sedation during colonoscopy than during EGD, ERCP, or EUS.[61] This might be explained by the less-stimulating nature of the colonoscopy exam when compared to the other procedures. However, most anesthesia providers who sedate patients for colonoscopy typically use propofol and aim for deep sedation or even general anesthesia. It seems likely that even in situations where the endoscopist is directing sedation, they and their patients prefer a deeper level of sedation. In a study of nurse-administered propofol sedation performed under the direction of a gastroenterologist, the mean bispectral index (BIS) score was found to be 59, indicating a state of general anesthesia.[68]

Several sedation techniques for colonoscopy have been studied. Moerman et al. compared intravenous remifentanil to intravenous propofol in 40 adult patients scheduled for complete colonoscopies. They found that measures of early recovery, such as spontaneous eye opening and following commands, occurred sooner in patients who received remifentanil than in patients who received propofol. In addition, recovery of cognitive function was quicker in the remifentanil group. However, patient satisfaction was lower in the remifentanil group, and respiratory depression was more common in this group as well.[69] Another study evaluating the use of remifentanil for sedation during colonoscopy found postprocedure nausea and vomiting to be a significant problem.[70] General anesthesia using an inhalational technique of sevoflurane/nitrous oxide also has been compared with total intravenous anesthesia (TIVA) using propofol/fentanyl/midazolam for colonoscopy.[71] While emergence was quicker in the TIVA group, patients who received an inhalational anesthetic were less sedated 20 minutes after completion of the procedure. The TIVA group also experienced psychomotor impairment lasting 30–90 minutes longer than the inhalational group.

Propofol as a sole agent for sedation during colonoscopy has been compared to a combination of lower-dose propofol in combination with fentanyl or midazolam titrated to moderate sedation. Patients in the propofol-only group reached a deeper level of sedation than any of the combination groups. No differences in vital signs, adverse respiratory events, or patient satisfaction were found among the groups, although patients in the propofol-only group remembered less procedural pain. Patients who received a combination of propofol with midazolam or fentanyl were discharged more quickly, however.[72]

In a small study comparing propofol sedation versus midazolam and meperidine, the authors examined the cardiovascular effects between the two dosing regimens. The rates of hypotension, hypoxemia, and bradycardia were statistically insignificant between the two groups, yet the length of recovery for the propofol group was significantly longer.[73] Of note, this study looked primarily at ASA 1 and 2 patients. Only a small percentage of patients in each sedation group were ASA 3 patients, which might explain why there were no significant differences in cardiovascular effects between the sedation regimens. Further investigation including a patient population with significant comorbidities might find some subtle differences between sedation drugs that could not be identified when studying relatively healthy patients.

ENDOSCOPIC RETROGRADE CHOLANGIOPANCREATOGRAPHY

Endoscopic retrograde cholangiopancreatography combines endoscopy and fluoroscopy (Figure 19.2) in a technique used to diagnose and treat diseases of the biliary and pancreatic ductal systems. Patients who present for ERCP are typically more severely ill than patients undergoing EGD or colonoscopy. Common presenting diagnoses include pancreatitis, bile duct or pancreatic cancer, sphincter of Oddi dysfunction, and cholangitis. The systemic illnesses in this patient population may partly account for the high risk of cardiopulmonary complications associated with ERCP. An Australian study that looked at ERCP complications related to patient age found that approximately 25% of patients 65 years or older developed new electrocardiographic changes (ischemia, arrhythmias) during or after ERCP. Elevated cardiac troponin I levels were documented in 11% of patients in this age group.[74] In comparison with colonoscopy or EGD, complex therapeutic procedures of significant duration are often undertaken during ERCP. Interventional techniques commonly employed include placement of biliary stents, biliary sphincterotomy, removal of bile duct stones, and stricture dilation. Patient immobility is paramount for successful performance of these often time-consuming and challenging procedures. Adding to the challenge for the anesthesia provider is the prone position that most gastroenterologists prefer for performing ERCP.

Given the multiple comorbidities that often accompany patients undergoing ERCP, it is not surprising that multiple studies have found higher incidences of cardiovascular and respiratory adverse events such as hypotension and hypoxemia during ERCP compared with other GI procedures, even when sedation is administered by anesthesiology personnel.[75,76] When comparing a sedation regimen of dexmedetomidine/ketamine versus propofol/fentanyl during ERCP, one study found fewer episodes of hypotension, desaturation, and bradycardia in the dexmedetomidine/ketamine group, yet this group also exhibited a significantly longer recovery time when compared to the propofol/fentanyl group.[77]

While many anesthesiologists prefer general anesthesia for ERCP, some do successfully provide moderate or deep sedation for this procedure. The preferred sedative drug is invariably propofol. Midazolam versus propofol sedation has been studied in the setting of ERCP.[78] Successful procedure completion was more likely in patients receiving propofol (97.5% vs. 80%), and recovery time was significantly shorter in the propofol group. TCI techniques have also been studied for use in ERCP sedation. Although cost effectiveness of the

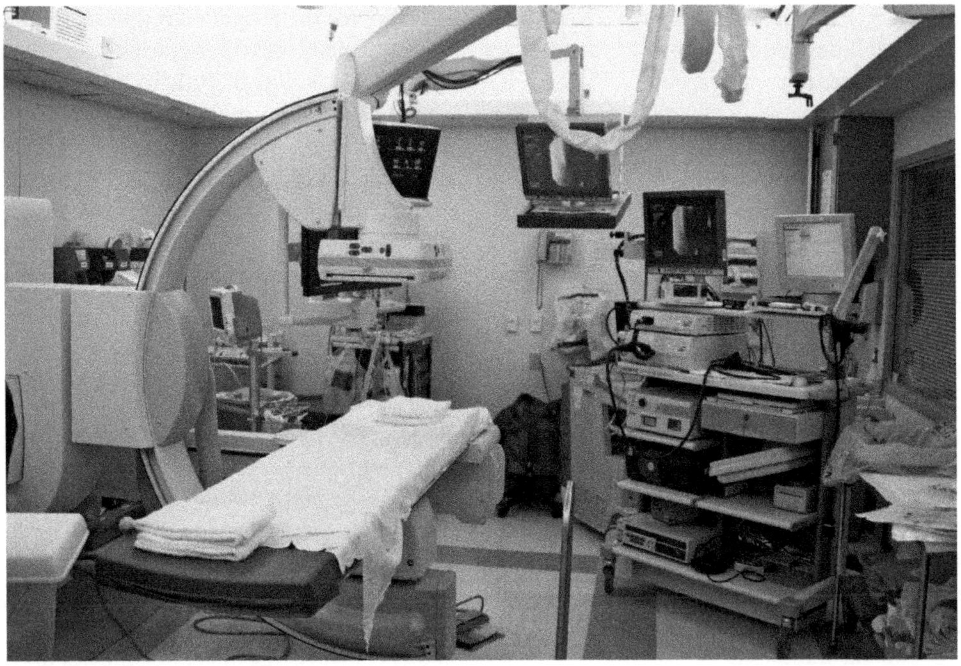

Figure 19.2. Endoscopic retrograde cholangiopancreatography (ERCP) procedure room.

system requires further investigation, successful sedation for ERCP has been reported by titrating propofol to a target concentration of 2–5 μg/mL.[79] Mazanikov and colleagues from Helsinki, Finland, have done extensive research into PCS and have investigated numerous sedation methods for ERCP. In one study, they compared propofol delivery via TCI and PCS during ERCP. In the PCS group, propofol consumption was less, while patients were at comparable levels of sedation in the recovery room when compared to TCI.[31] Mazanikov and colleagues also investigated PCS with propofol and remifentanil versus propofol and alfentanil. They concluded that PCS sedation with propofol and remifentanil was more likely to be associated with respiratory depression and postprocedural nausea than PCS sedation with propofol and alfentanil.[35]

The challenges associated with sedation for ERCP have led many anesthesiologists to prefer general anesthesia for the procedure. Data exist that support this clinical approach. A retrospective study of over 1000 ERCP procedures found the procedure failure rate with sedation to be double the failure rate with general anesthesia, usually due to inadequate sedation.[80] Complication rates may also be lower in patients receiving general anesthesia for therapeutic ERCP. The lower complication rate with general anesthesia is hypothesized to result from less patient movement and aperistalsis of the duodenum.[81]

Due to the prone position, inaccessibility of the airway to the anesthesiologist, and the presence of aspiration risk factors in many patients, endotracheal intubation is often performed when general anesthesia is chosen for ERCP. However, the use of the LMA for ERCP has been described by investigators, even in the prone position. In a group of 20 patients, no airway complications were encountered, and there were no technical difficulties with endoscope placement or ERCP performance.[82] In a study comparing TIVA without versus with endotracheal intubation in patients undergoing ERCP, they cited a 4.8% conversion rate to general endotracheal anesthesia. Reasons for having to place an endotracheal tube included retained food in the stomach or esophagus, patient movement, length of procedure, ventilation problems, and aspiration. In this study, the patients who were managed without intubation had shorter nonprocedural anesthesia times when compared to those who were intubated.[83]

ENDOSCOPIC ULTRASONOGRAPHY

Endoscopic ultrasonography is used for diagnosing and staging GI and pancreatic tumors and, like ERCP, is a more complex and stimulating procedure than EGD or colonoscopy. Frequently, needle aspiration biopsies are taken that must be examined by a pathologist before completion of the procedure. The long duration of the procedure coupled with the larger size of the ultrasound-containing endoscope results in an elevated level of patient discomfort when compared with simple EGD. As a result, adequate sedation for EUS typically requires deep sedation or general anesthesia.

Because achieving an appropriate level of sedation while avoiding hypoxemia and airway obstruction may be more challenging during EUS, many patients will not tolerate the procedure with the conventional benzodiazepine and opioid combination. Alternative strategies for sedation have been investigated. In one study, moderate doses of benzodiazepine and opioid were given before the EUS procedure began. This baseline sedation was then supplemented during the procedure with either ketamine or additional benzodiazepine and opioid. The degree of patient comfort, technical ease of the study, and recovery times were all improved in the patients who received ketamine supplementation. In addition, approximately one-third of the patients randomized to receive additional benzodiazepine/opioid had to cross over to the ketamine group to obtain a sedation level adequate to complete the EUS.[54]

A propofol infusion controlled by an anesthesiologist is, of course, another popular option for EUS sedation. Other unique techniques have been explored, including propofol TCI and PCS. One group of investigators studied the effect of midazolam dosing on the amount of propofol required to successfully complete the EUS procedure. They found that preprocedure administration of midazolam did not significantly affect the dose of propofol used, but it also did not delay the time to discharge.[84] PCS using boluses of 3.75 μg fentanyl and 4.25 mg propofol without a lockout interval has also proved successful for sedation during EUS.[85] A retrospective cohort study found improved diagnostic yield during EUS with fine-needle aspiration of pancreatic masses when general anesthesia was provided for the procedure by an anesthesiologist compared to conscious sedation provided by a registered nurse.[86]

NATURAL ORIFICE TRANSLUMENAL ENDOSCOPIC SURGERY

Natural orifice translumenal endoscopic surgery (NOTES) is an emerging technique within the field of minimally invasive surgery. The aim of NOTES is to perform intra-abdominal procedures with peritoneal access via natural orifices in lieu of conventional abdominal incisions. Proposed advantages include fewer skin flora–based infections, elimination of incisional hernias, a reduction in postoperative pain, and a lower incidence of postoperative adhesions.[87]

Multiple experiments have been carried out in animal models evaluating the feasibility of NOTES for various operations, including cholecystectomy,[88] gastrojejunostomy,[89] tubal ligation,[90] and splenectomy.[91] The use of NOTES in humans is just beginning, although several groups have published case reports of successful transvaginal cholecystectomy.[92–94] Auyang et al. have described a transgastric approach to cholecystectomy in humans utilizing a hybrid of endoscopic and laparoscopic techniques.[95] The most common procedures by orifice that have been performed are transvaginal cholecystectomy, followed in descending order by transgastric peritoneoscopy, transgastric cholecystectomy, and transvaginal appendectomy. The majority of these procedures have been performed outside of the United States, accounting for 86% of the reported cases, versus just 14% performed within the United States.[96]

Most cases of NOTES in humans have been performed with the patient under general anesthesia, with a few exceptions.[97] Some have suggested a potential advantage of NOTES might be the ability to avoid general anesthesia because there is no skin incision.[98] While avoidance of an abdominal incision would certainly lessen analgesia requirements, most published descriptions of the technique have involved creation of a pneumoperitoneum in patients who are under general anesthesia. Peritoneal insufflation is generally poorly tolerated in the lightly sedated patient and can lead to cardiopulmonary embarrassment. While laparoscopic surgery has been performed under spinal anesthesia, its success hinges on specialized techniques to ensure patient comfort. Successful laparoscopic cholecystectomy under spinal anesthesia has been described in a small number of patients using nitrous oxide to create the pneumoperitoneum, utilizing low insufflation pressures, minimizing surgical traction, and inserting trochars below the umbilicus.[99] Whether spinal anesthesia is a useful technique for NOTES is a subject for future study.

In the future, with technological and surgical advancements, it is quite possible that natural orifice surgery will be performed in locations outside the OR. Like conventional endoscopy, the necessary equipment is portable and the approach is minimally invasive. If techniques are developed in which pneumoperitoneum can be avoided or its side effects minimized, it may be possible to perform NOTES under sedation or regional anesthesia. For now, it seems this unique blend of endoscopy and general surgery is best performed in the OR under general anesthesia.

ENDOSCOPY FOR PEDIATRIC PATIENTS

The majority of pediatric patients will not tolerate GI endoscopy without deep sedation or general anesthesia. Anesthesiologists are therefore more likely to participate in pediatric procedures than adult procedures and, in some centers, are responsible for all or most pediatric sedations and anesthetics. While many of the techniques and drugs used are consistent across patient age groups, the pediatric population presents unique challenges. Typically, pediatric patients require larger doses of sedative medications on a per weight basis than adults. A group of investigators evaluating the median effective concentration of propofol required for EGD found that children aged 3–10 years required substantially higher plasma levels than adult patient groups undergoing the same procedure.[100]

One of the greatest challenges faced by the anesthesiologist in the endoscopy suite is obtaining intravenous access in children. In contrast with the OR where intravenous lines are generally started after inhalational induction of general anesthesia, it is often not practical to have an anesthesia machine available in this practice setting. Techniques to aid in placement of the intravenous line as well as separation from the parent are invaluable. In one study, preprocedural administration of oral midazolam (0.5 mg/kg) was found to improve the ease of intravenous line placement, facilitate parental separation, improve patient comfort, and result in lower overall propofol use for upper endoscopy.[101] Recovery time was substantially longer in the children who had received midazolam, but it still averaged just 26 minutes.

The ideal sedation combination is still being investigated in children who undergo upper endoscopy without intubation. In a recent study that looked at upper endoscopy in children over the age of 4, it was found that a combination of ketamine and midazolam offered better tolerance of the procedure when compared to propofol and fentanyl. Neither group developed major complications, including aspiration, cardiac arrest, laryngospasm, or apnea; however, the ketamine/midazolam group did develop significantly more recovery side effects, including emergence reactions, delirium, dizziness, and nausea and vomiting. Those in this group also had a statistically significant longer recovery period when compared to the group sedated with propofol and fentanyl.[102]

MANAGING COMPLICATIONS

A large prospective cohort study has been performed examining the incidence of cardiopulmonary complications during propofol sedation for upper endoscopy and colonoscopy. Nearly 12,000 colonoscopies and 6000 EGDs in which patients received propofol sedation were examined. The overall rate of complications was 0.86% for colonoscopy and 1.01% for EGD. Serious adverse events, defined as death, perforation, or bleeding, occurred in just 18 patients receiving colonoscopy and 17 patients undergoing EGD. Of note, the complication rate was lower for both procedures when sedation was provided by anesthesia providers rather than the gastroenterologist.[103] A large, retrospective, nonrandomized, observational cohort study examined 1.38 million procedures including upper endoscopy and colonoscopy. The authors of this study concluded that the use of anesthesiology professionals in ASA 1 or ASA 2 patients undergoing colonoscopy was associated with a lower incidence of serious adverse events (0.20%) as compared to sedation provided by endoscopists (0.28%). Interestingly, they found that the incidence of serious adverse events with upper endoscopy was lower with endoscopist-led sedation as compared to sedation provided by anesthesia professionals. However, the study authors admitted limitations given the retrospective nature of the study. All serious adverse events might not have been documented, and decisions about the use of anesthesia professionals might have been affected by complexity of the procedure or patient.[104]

Despite the low incidence of adverse events, the anesthesiologist should anticipate that complications will occasionally occur when administering sedation for GI endoscopy.[105,106] The general principles for management of these complications is the same as for cases performed in the OR; however, the resources available to aid the provider can be limited in the endoscopy suite. While the support personnel in the OR may be comfortable assisting the anesthesiologist during episodes of patient decompensation, nursing staff in the endoscopy center may not be able to provide the same level of assistance. In addition, equipment that is readily accessible in the OR, such as that needed for advanced airway management, may not be immediately available in the endoscopy area. These limitations put special importance on adequate preparation for each case. Any special equipment that might be required should be brought to the anesthetizing location and made ready for use before the case begins. Additionally, a plan to obtain additional assistance should be in place should a serious adverse event occur. If a patient is of sufficiently high risk, it may be advisable to perform the procedure in the OR, where serious complications can be dealt with in a more efficient manner.

POSTANESTHESIA RECOVERY

The anesthesiologist must fully appreciate the capabilities of the nursing staff responsible for monitoring patients after endoscopy. GI endoscopy units are often staffed to provide nursing care at the level necessary to recover patients who have received moderate sedation. However, it is essential that patients who have received deep sedation or general anesthesia in the endoscopy suite receive the same level of recovery care they would receive in the postanesthesia care unit of the OR. Accrediting organizations such as The Joint Commission require that equivalent postanesthesia care be delivered in all locations within the health care center. Determining whether an equivalent level of postprocedure patient care can be provided in the endoscopy center depends on whether nursing staff in the endoscopy recovery unit have received similar training as the nurses in the surgical postanesthesia care unit and also whether the appropriate nurse-patient ratio can be maintained. If the anesthesia provider is not comfortable with the level of postprocedure care offered for a particular patient, the patient should be transferred to the surgical recovery unit.

Discharge criteria should be the same as those used for patients who have been anesthetized in the OR. Recovery nurses must understand these criteria and also must know how to reach anesthesia personnel should issues arise during the recovery period. Postanesthesia management of patients with obstructive sleep apnea may be especially challenging as they may require an extended period of monitoring before satisfying criteria for discharge, which include maintaining an acceptable oxygen saturation while breathing room air. If staffing issues in the endoscopy recovery area do not allow such extended monitoring, arrangements should be made for recovery in a more suitable location.

REFERENCES

1. Cohen LB, Wecsler JS, Gaetano JN, et al. Endoscopic sedation in the United States: results from a nationwide survey. *Am J Gastroenterol.* 2006;101:967–974.
2. Clergue F. The challenges of anaesthesia for the next decade: the Sir Robert Macintosh Lecture 2014. *Eur J Anaesthesiol.* 2015;32:223–229.
3. McCloy R, Nagengast F, Fried M, et al. Conscious sedation for endoscopy. *Eur J Gastroenterol Hepatol.* 1996;8:1233–1240.
4. Heuss LT, Schnieper P, Drewe J, et al. Risk stratification and safe administration of propofol by registered nurses supervised by the gastroenterologist: a prospective observational study of more than 2000 cases. *Gastrointest Endosc.* 2003;57:664–671.
5. Rex DK, Heuss LT, Walker JA, et al. Trained registered nurses/endoscopy teams can administer propofol safely for endoscopy. *Gastroenterology.* 2005;129:2080–2083.
6. Rex KD, Overley CA, Walker J. Registered nurse-administered propofol sedation for upper endoscopy and colonoscopy: why? when? how? *Rev Gastroenterol Dis.* 2003;3:70–80.
7. Campo R, Brullet E, Montserrat A, et al. Identification of factors that influence tolerance of upper gastrointestinal endoscopy. *Eur J Gastroenterol Hepatol.* 1999;11:201–204.
8. Shingina A, Ou G, Takach O, et al. Identification of factors associated with sedation tolerance in 5000 patients undergoing outpatient colonoscopy: Canadian tertiary center experience. *World J Gastrointest Endosc.* 2016;8:770–776.
9. Braunstein ED, Rosenberg R, Gress F, et al. Development and validation of a clinical prediction score (the SCOPE score) to predict sedation outcomes

in patients undergoing endoscopic procedures. *Aliment Pharmacol Ther.* 2014;40:72–82.
10. Chang B, Urman RD. Non-operating room anesthesia: the principles of patient assessment and preparation. *Anesthesiol Clin.* 2016;34(1):223–240.
11. Pike IM: Open-access endoscopy. *Gastrointest Endosc Clin N Am.* 2006;16:709–717.
12. Mathew A, Riley TR 3rd, Young M, et al. Cost-saving approach to patients on long-term anticoagulation who need endoscopy: a decision analysis. *Am J Gastroenterol.* 2003;98:1766–1776.
13. Hussain N, Alsulaiman R, Burtin P, et al. The safety of endoscopic sphincterotomy in patients receiving antiplatelet agents—a case-control study. *Aliment Pharmacol Ther.* 2007;25:579–584.
14. Kanakadandi V, Parasa S, Sihn P, et al. Patterns of antiplatelet agent use in the US. *Endosc Int Open.* 2015;3:E173–E178.
15. Aisenberg J, Brill JV, Ladabaum U, et al. Sedation for gastrointestinal endoscopy: new practices, new economics. *Am J Gastroenterol.* 2005;100:996–1000.
16. Savarise MT. Coding and reimbursement for colonoscopy. *Bull Am Coll Surg.* 2016;101:40–43.
17. Centers for Medicare and Medicaid Services, HHS. Medicare program; revisions to payment policies under the Physician Fee Schedule, Clinical Laboratory Fee Schedule, access to identifiable data for the Center for Medicare and Medicaid innovation models and other revisions to Part B for CY 2015. *Fed Regist.* 2014, November 13; 79(219):67547–68010.
18. Cohen LB, Delegge MH, Aisenberg J, et al. AGA Institute review of endoscopic sedation. *Gastroenterology.* 2007;133:675–701.
19. Vargo JJ, Bramley T, Meyer K, et al. Practice efficiency and economics: the case for rapid recovery sedation agents for colonos-copy in a screening population. *J Clin Gastroenterol.* 2007;41:591–598.
20. Trummel J. Sedation for gastrointestinal endoscopy: the changing landscape. *Curr Opin Anaesthesiol.* 2007;20:359–364.
21. United States Food and Drug Administration. Propofol product label. Available at: https://www.accessdata.fda.gov/drugsatfda_docs/label/2014/019627s062lbl.pdf. Accessed on March 9, 2018.
22. American Society of Anesthesiologists Task Force on Sedation and Analgesia by Non-Anesthesiologists. Practice guidelines for sedation and analgesia by non-anesthesiologists. *Anesthesiology.* 2002;96:1004–1017.
23. Rex DK, Deenadayalu VP, Eid E, et al. Endoscopist-directed administration of propofol: a worldwide safety experience. *Gastroenterology.* 2009;137:1229–1237.
24. Fatima H, DeWitt J, LeBlanc J, et al. Nurse-administered propofol sedation for upper endoscopic ultrasonography. *Am J Gastroenterol.* 2008;103:1649–1656.
25. Dewitt J, McGreevy K, Sherman S, et al. Nurse-administered propofol sedation compared with midazolam and meperidine for EUS: a prospective, randomized trial. *Gastrointest Endosc.* 2008;68:499–509.
26. Cohen LB. Nurse-administered propofol sedation for upper endoscopic ultrasonography: not yet ready for prime time. *Nat Clin Pract Gastroenterol Hepatol.* 2009;6:76–77.
27. Goudra BG, Singh PM, Gouda G, et al. Safety of non-anesthesia provider-administered propofol (NAAP) sedation in advanced gastrointestinal endoscopic procedures: comparative meta-analysis of pooled results. *Dig Dis Sci.* 2015;60:2612–2627.
28. Dumonceau J, Riphaus A, Schreiber F, et al. Non-anesthesiologist administration of propofol for gastrointestinal endoscopy: European Society of Gastrointestinal Endoscopy, European Society of Gastroenterology and Endoscopy Nurses and Associates Guideline–updated June 2015. *Endoscopy.* 2015;47:1175–1189.
29. Crepeau T, Poincloux L, Bonny C, et al. Significance of patient-controlled sedation during colonoscopy. Results from a prospective randomized controlled study. *Gastroenterol Clin Biol.* 2005;29:1090–1096.
30. Mandel JE, Tanner JW, Lichtenstein GR, et al. A randomized, controlled, double-blind trial of patient-controlled sedation with propofol/remifentianil versus midazolam/fentanyl for colonoscopy. *Anesth Analg.* 2008;106:434–439.
31. Manzanikov M, Udd M, Kylanpaa L, et al. A randomized comparison of target-controlled propofol infusion and patient-controlled sedation during ERCP. *Endoscopy.* 2013;45:915–919.
32. Manzanikov M, Udd M, Kylanpaa L, et al. Dexmeditomidine impairs success of patient-controlled sedation in alcoholics during ERCP: a randomized, double-blind, placebo-controlled study. *Surg Endosc.* 2013;27:2163–2168.
33. Maurice-Szamburski A, Loundou A, Auquier P, et al. Effecto of patient-controlled sedation with propofol on patient satisfaction: a randomized study. *Ann Fr Anesth Reanim.* 2013;32:171–175.
34. Nguyen NQ, Toscano L, Lawrence M, et al. Patient-controlled analgesia with inhaled methoxyflurane versus conventional endoscopist-provided sedation for colonoscopy: a randomized multicenter trial. *Gastrointest Endosc.* 2013;78:892–901.
35. Manzanikov M, Udd M, Kylanpaa L, et al. Patient-controlled sedation with propofol and remifentanil for ERCP: a randomized, controlled study. *Gastrointest Endsoc.* 2011;73:260–266.
36. Kulling D, Fantin AC, Biro P, et al. Safer colonoscopy with patient-controlled analgesia and sedation with propofol and alfentanil. *Gastrointest Endosc.* 2001;54:1–7.
37. Ng JM, Kong CF, Ny MD. Patient-controlled sedation with propofol for colonoscopy. *Gastrointest Endosc.* 2001;54:8–13.
38. Crepeau T, Poincloux L, Bonny C, et al. Significance of patient-controlled sedation during colonoscopy. Results from a prospective randomized controlled study. *Gastroenterol Clin Biol.* 2005;29:1090–1096.
39. Fanti L, Rossi G, Gemma M, et al. Target controlled infusion for non-anaesthesiologist propofol sedation during gastrointestinal endoscopy: the first double blind randomized controlled trial. *Gastrointest Endosc.* 2015;47(7):566–571.
40. Seo SI, Ryu JY, Kang SS. Safety of target-controlled propofol infusion by gastroenterologists in patients undergoing endoscopic resection. *Dig Dis Sci.* 2016;61:3199–3206.
41. Urman RD, Maurer WG. Computer-assisted personalized sedation: friend or foe? *Anesth Analg.* 2014;119(1):207–211.
42. Periello B. Johnson & Johnson bails on Sedasys anesthesia device. *Mass Device.* March 15, 2016. Available at: http://www.massdevice.com/johnson-johnson-bails-sedasys-automated-anesthesia-device/. Accessed on January 7, 2017.
43. Aantaa R, Scheinin M. Alpha 2-adrenergic agents in anaesthesia. *Acta Anaesthesiol Scand.* 1993;37:433–448.
44. Shelly MP. Dexmedetomidine: a real innovation or more of the same? *Br J Anaesth.* 2001;87:677–678.
45. Demiraran Y, Korkut E, Tamer A, et al. The comparison of dexmedetomidine and midazolam used for sedation of patients during upper endoscopy: a prospective, randomized study. *Can J Gastroenterol.* 2007;21:25–29.
46. Wu W, Chen Q, Zhang LC, Chen WH. Dexmedetomidine versus midazolam for sedation in upper gastrointestinal endoscopy. *J Int Med Res.* 2014;42:516–522.
47. Jalowiecki P, Rudner R, Gonciarz M, et al. Sole use of dexmedetomidine has limited utility for conscious sedation during outpatient colonoscopy. *Anesthesiology.* 2005;103:269–273.
48. Wu Y, Zhang Y, Hu X, et al. A comparison of propofol vs. dexmedetomidine for sedation, haemodynamic control and satisfaction, during esophagogastroduodenoscopy under conscious sedation. *J Clin Pharm Ther.* 2015;40:419–425.
49. Vadivelu N, Schermer E, Kodumudi V, Belani K, Urman RD, Kaye AD. Role of ketamine for analgesia in adults and children. *J Anaesthesiol Clin Pharmacol.* 2016;32(3):298–306.
50. White PF, Way WL, Trevor AJ. Ketamine-its pharmacology and therapeutic uses. *Anesthesiology.* 1982;56:119–136.
51. Gilger MA, Spearman RS, Dietrich CL, et al. Safety and effectiveness of ketamine as a sedative agent for pediatric GI endoscopy. *Gastrointest Endosc.* 2004;59:659–663.
52. Law AK, Ng DK, Chan KK. Use of intramuscular ketamine for endoscopy sedation in children. *Pediatr Int.* 2003;45:180–185.
53. Kirberg A, Sagredo R, Montalva G, et al. Ketamine for pediatric endoscopic procedures and as a sedation complement for adult patients. *Gastrointest Endosc.* 2005;61:501–502.
54. Varadarajulu S, Eloubeidi MA, Tamhane A, et al. Prospective randomized trial evaluating ketamine for advanced endoscopic procedures in difficult to sedate patients. *Aliment Pharmacol Ther.* 2007;25:987–997.
55. Keeffe EB, O'Connor KW. 1989 A/S/G/E survey of endoscopic sedation and monitoring practices. *Gastrointest Endosc.* 1990;36:S13.
56. Mamula P, Markowitz J, Neiswender K, et al. Safety of intravenous midazolam and fentanyl for pediatric endoscopy: prospective study of 1578 endoscopies. *Gastrointest Endosc.* 2007;65:203–210.
57. Litman RS. Conscious sedation with remifentanil during painful medical procedures. *J Pain Symptom Manage.* 2000;19:468–471.
58. Wesolowski AM, Zaccagnino MP, Malapero RJ, Kaye AD, Urman RD. Remimazolam: pharmacologic considerations and clinical role in anesthesiology. *Pharmacotherapy.* 2016;36(9):1021–1027.
59. Rogers WK, McDowell TS. Remimazolam, a short-acting GABA(A) receptor agonist for intravenous sedation and/or anesthesia in day-case surgical and non-surgical procedures. *IDrugs.* 2010;13:929–937.
60. Pambiano DJ, Cash BD. New horizons for sedation: The ultrashort acting benzodiazepine remimazolam. *Tech Gastrointest Endosc.* 2016;18:22–28.

61. Patel S, Vargo JJ, Khandwala F, et al. Deep sedation occurs frequently during elective endoscopy with meperidine and midazolam. *Am J Gastroenterol.* 2005;100:2689–2695.
62. Lopez-Gil M, Brimacombe J, Diaz-Reganon G. Anesthesia for pediatric gastroscopy: a study comparing the ProSeal laryngeal mask airway with nasal cannulae. *Paediatric Anaesthia.* 2006;16:1032–1035.
63. Davis DE, Jones MP, Kubik CM. Topical pharyngeal anesthesia does not improve upper gastrointestinal endoscopy in conscious sedated patients. *Am J Gastroenterol.* 1999;94:1853–1856.
64. Ristikankare M, Hartikainen J, Heikkinen M, et al. Is routine sedation or topical pharyngeal anesthesia beneficial during upper endoscopy? *Gastrointest Endosc.* 2004;60:686–694.
65. Evans LT, Saberi S, Kim HM, et al. Pharyngeal anesthesia during sedated EGDs: is "the spray" beneficial? A meta-analysis and systematic review. *Gastrointest Endosc.* 2006;63:761–766.
66. Byrne MF, Mitchell RM, Gerke H, et al. The need for caution with topical anesthesia during endoscopic procedures, as liberal use may result in methemoglobinemia. *J Clin Gastroenterol.* 2004;38:225–229.
67. Ayoub C, Skoury A, Abdul-Baki H, et al. Lidocaine lollipop as single-agent anesthesia in upper GI endoscopy. *Gastrointest Endosc.* 2007;66:786–793.
68. Chen SC, Rex DK. An initial investigation of bispectral monitoring as an adjunct to nurse-administered propofol sedation for colonoscopy. *Am J Gastroenterol.* 2004;99:1081–1086.
69. Moerman AT, Foubert LA, Herregods LL, et al. Propofol versus remifentanil for monitored anaesthesia care during colonoscopy. *Eur J Anaesthesiol.* 2003;20:461–466.
70. Akcaboy ZN, Akcaboy EY, Albayrak D, et al. Can remifentanil be a better choice than propofol for colonoscopy during monitored anesthesia care? *Acta Anaesthesiol Scand.* 2006;50:736–741.
71. Theodorou T, Hales P, Gillespie P, et al. Total intravenous versus inhalational anaesthesia for colonoscopy: a prospective study of clinical recovery and psychomotor function. *Anaesth Intensive Care.* 2001;29:124–136.
72. VanNatta ME, Rex DK. Propofol alone titrated to deep sedation versus propofol in combination with opioids and/or benzodiazepines and titrated to moderate sedation for colonoscopy. *Am J Gastroenterol.* 2006;101:2209–2217.
73. Gurbulak B, Uzman S, Kabul Gurbulak E, et al. Cardiopulmonary safety of propofol versus midazolam/meperidine sedation for colonoscopy: a prospective, randomized, double-blinded study. *Iran Red Crescent Med J.* 2014;16:e19329.
74. Fisher L, Fisher A, Thomson A. Cardiopulmonary complications of ERCP in older patients. *Gastrointest Endosc.* 2006;63:948–955.
75. Coté GA, Hovis RM, Ansstas MA, et al. Incidence of sedation-related complications with propofol use during advanced endoscopic procedures. *Clin Gastroenterol Hepatol.* 2010;8:137–142.
76. Lordan JT, Woods J, Keeling P, Paterson IM. A retrospective analysis of benzodiazepine sedation vs. propofol anaesthesia in 252 patients undergoing endoscopic retrograde cholangiopancreatography. *HPB (Oxford).* 2011;13:174–177.
77. Goyal R, Hasnain S, Mittal S, Shreevastava S. A randomized, controlled trial to compare the efficacy and safety profile of a dexmedetomidine-ketamine combination with a propofol-fentanyl combination for ERCP. *Gastrointest Endosc.* 2016;83:928–933.
78. Jung M, Hofmann C, Kiesslich R, et al. Improved sedation in diagnostic and therapeutic ERCP: propofol is an alternative to midazolam. *Endoscopy.* 2000;32:233–238.
79. Fanti L, Agostoni M, Casati A, et al. Target-controlled propofol infusion during monitored anesthesia in patients undergoing ERCP. *Gastrointest Endosc.* 2004;60:361–366.
80. Raymondos K, Panning B, Bachem I, et al. Evaluation of endoscopic retrograde cholangiopancreatography under conscious sedation and general anesthesia. *Endoscopy.* 2002;34:721–726.
81. Martindale SJ. Anaesthetic considerations during endoscopic retrograde cholangiopancreatography. *Anaesth Intensive Care.* 2006;34:475–480.
82. Osborn IP, Cohen J, Soper RJ, et al. Laryngeal mask airway—a novel method of airway protection during ERCP: comparison with endotracheal intubation. *Gastrointest Endosc.* 2002;56:122–128.
83. Hagan K, Ruiz J, Thirumurthi S, et al. Total intravenous anesthesia without an endotracheal tube for endoscopic retrograde cholangiopancreatography and the incidence of conversion to endotracheal intubation: a retrospective review. *Gastrointest Endosc.* 2015;81:AB308.
84. Fanti L, Agostoni M, Arcidiacono PG, et al. Target-controlled infusion during monitored anesthesia care in patients undergoing EUS: propofol alone versus midazolam plus propofol. A prospective double-blind randomised controlled trial. *Dig Liver Dis.* 2007;39:81–86.
85. Agostoni M, Fanti L, Arcidiacono PG, et al. Midazolam and pethidine versus propofol and fentanyl patient controlled sedation/analgesia for upper gastrointestinal tract ultrasound endoscopy: a prospective randomized controlled trial. *Dig Liver Dis.* 2007;39:1024–1029.
86. Ootaki C, Stevens T, Vargo J, et al. Does general anesthesia increase the diagnostic yield of endoscopic ultrasound-guided fine needle aspiration of pancreatic masses: *Anesthesiology.* 2012;117:1044–1050.
87. Ko CW, Kalloo AN. Per-oral transgastric abdominal surgery. *Chinese J Digest Dis.* 2006;7:67–70.
88. Pai RD, Fong DG, Bundga ME, et al. Transcolonic endoscopic cholecystectomy; a NOTES survival study in a porcine model. *Gastrointest Endosc.* 2006;64:428–434.
89. Kantsevoy SV, Jagannath SB, Niiyama H, et al. Endoscopic gastrojejunostomy with survival in a porcine model. *Gastrointest Endosc.* 2005;62:287–292.
90. Jagannath SB, Kantsevoy SV, Vaughn CA, et al. Peroral transgas-tric endoscopic ligation of fallopian tubes with long-term survival in a porcine model. *Gastrointest Endosc.* 2005;61:449–453.
91. Kantsevoy SV, Hu B, Jagannath SB, et al. Transgastric endoscopic splenectomy: is it possible? *Surg Endosc.* 2006;20:522–525.
92. Marescaux J, Dallemagne B, Peretta S, et al. Surgery without scars: report of translumenal cholecystectomy in a human being. *Arch Surg.* 2007;142:823–826.
93. Zorron R, Maggioni LC, Pombo L, et al. NOTES transvaginal cholecystectomy: preliminary clinical application. *Surg Endosc.* 2008;22:542–547.
94. Ramos AC, Murakami A, Galvao Neto M, et al. NOTES transvaginal video-assisted cholecystectomy: first series. *Endoscopy.* 2008;40:572–575.
95. Auyang ED, Hungness ES, Vaziri K, et al. Human NOTES cholecystectomy: transgastric hybrid technique. *J Gastrointest Surg.* 2009;13:1149–1150.
96. Clark MP, Qayed ES, Kooby DA, et al. Natural orifice transluminal endoscopic surgery in humans: a review. *Minim Invasive Surg.* 2012;2012:189296.
97. Marks JM, Ponsky JL, Pearl JP, McGee MF. PEG "rescue": a practical NOTES technique. *Surg Endosc.* 2007;21:816–819.
98. Pearl JP, Ponsky JL. Natural orifice translumenal endoscopic surgery: a critical review. *J Gastrointest Surg.* 2008;12:1293–1300.
99. Hamad MA, El-Khattary OA Ibrahim, et al. Laparoscopic cholecystectomy under spinal anesthesia with nitrous oxide peritoneum: a feasibility study. *Surg Endosc.* 2003;17:1426–1428.
100. Hammer GB, Litalien C, Wellis V, et al. Determination of the median effective concentration (EC50) of propofol during oesophagogastroduodenoscopy in children. *Paediatr Anaesth.* 2001;11:549–553.
101. Paspatis GA, Charoniti I, Manolaraki M, et al. Synergistic sedation with oral midazolam as a premedication and intravenous propofol versus intravenous propofol alone in upper gastrointestinal endoscopies in children: a prospective, randomized study. *J Pediatr Gastroenterol Nutr.* 2006;43:195–199.
102. Akbulut UE, Saylan S, Sengu B, et al. A comparison of sedation with midazolam-ketamine versus propofol-fentanyl during endoscopy in children: a randomized trial. *Eur J Gastroenterol Hepatol.* 2017;29:112–118.
103. Vargo JJ, Holub JL, Faigel DO, et al. Risk factors for cardiopulmonary events during propofol-mediated upper endoscopy and colonoscopy. *Aliment Pharmacol Ther.* 2006;24:955–963.
104. Vargo JJ, Niklewski PJ, Williams JL, et al. Patient safety during sedation by anesthesia professionals during routine upper endoscopy and colonoscopy: an analysis of 1.38 million procedures. *Gastrointest Endosc.* 2017;85:101–108.
105. Chang B, Kaye AD, Diaz JH, Westlake B, Dutton RP, Urman RD. Complications of non-operating room procedures: outcomes from the national anesthesia clinical outcomes registry. *J Patient Saf.* 2015. [Epub ahead of print].
106. Woodward ZG, Urman RD, Domino KB. Safety of non-operating room anesthesia: a closed claims update. *Anesthesiol Clin.* 2017;35(4):569–581.

20 | ANESTHESIA FOR INTERVENTIONAL PULMONOLOGY

BASEM ABDELMALAK, MD

INTRODUCTION

As a part of the overall growth of OOOR anesthesia,[1] there is an increasing demand for providing anesthesia services for interventional pulmonology (bronchoscopic) procedures. This is a direct result of the proliferation of these procedures and the expansion of indications for performing them. Many of the traditional maximally invasive thoracic procedures, such as mediastinal staging, are now done as minimally invasive outpatient procedures.[2] Moreover, more of the new interventional pulmonology procedures are performed through the flexible bronchoscope in bronchoscopy suites outside of the operating room (OOOR). Even though the more invasive procedures such as those utilizing the rigid bronchoscope continue to be performed in the operating rooms, increased demand has led to the establishment of specialized OOOR interventional pulmonology centers that can accommodate these procedures. Many health care facilities aim to develop centers of excellence for such highly specialized care, utilizing standardized yet individualized protocols to improve safety and clinical outcomes in these so-called non–operating room anesthesia (NORA) service locations.

The majority of patients presenting for interventional pulmonology procedures are high-risk patients. This represents a challenge for the anesthesiologist, who must simultaneously consider the severity of the patient's lung pathology and other comorbidities. Other complicating factors may stem from the nature of the procedure when anesthesiologists share managing the airway with pulmonologists and the dynamic nature of the procedure given the continuously changing airway, fraction of inspired oxygen (FiO_2), and ventilation mode to accommodate the procedure being performed. In addition, sometimes more than one procedure may be performed in the same setting on the same patient. As a result, the anesthesiologist needs to be familiar with all of the planned procedures and needs to develop an anesthetic and airway management plan for these high-risk patients.

BRONCHOSCOPIC SURGICAL PROCEDURES

COMMON TRADITIONAL PROCEDURES

ENDOTRACHEOBRONCHIAL STENTING

Bronchoscopic surgical procedures are summarized in Table 20.1. In the last two decades, considerable progress has been made in the endoscopic management of central airway obstruction resulting from causes such as benign airway stenosis or neoplasia. In particular, the use of self-expanding metallic stents (SEMSs) placed bronchoscopically has provided important clinical options.[3] In addition, Metallic and silicone stents (Figure 20.1) are frequently used to support and maintain the tracheal lumen, restore integrity of a disrupted trachea, and support a collapsing tracheal wall (using a silicone stent) from a compressing mediastinal mass.

ENDOTRACHEOBRONCHIAL BIOPSY AND ENDOTRACHEOBRONCHIAL LASER

Biopsy of an endotracheal or bronchial lesion is done through either the flexible or the rigid bronchoscope. Nd:YAG (neodymium-doped yttrium aluminum garnet) and argon lasers are generally used to debulk an endotracheal or bronchial granuloma or a mass to maintain an open airway and treat airway stenosis.

ENDOBRONCHIAL ELECTROCAUTERY

Endobronchial electrocautery is equally effective but less expensive than Nd:YAG laser therapy for intraluminal airway obstruction.[4,5] It also leads to less airway scarring and subepithelial fibrosis compared to the Nd:YAG laser.[6]

BRONCHOSCOPIC BALLOON DILATION

The bronchoscopic balloon dilation procedure is customary in the treatment of stenosis of various etiologies, such as idiopathic subglottic stenosis commonly seen in female patients in their 40s. Bronchoscopic balloon dilation is also used to manage stenosis resulting from granulomatous diseases such as Granulomatosis with polyangiitis (formerly known as Wegner's Granulomatosis).

BRONCHOSCOPIC CRYOTHERAPY

Bronchoscopic cryotherapy entails the therapeutic application of extreme cold for local destruction of tissue. Nitrous oxide is used as a cryogen applied through a flexible fiber-optic bronchoscope. Frozen tissue is destroyed by coagulation necrosis. In short, cryotherapy is an alternative to laser treatment. Advantages of cryotherapy include ease of use, lower cost compared to laser therapies, reusability of the cryoprobe, and no risk of fire. Complications include airway perforation and bleeding.

TABLE 20.1. Bronchoscopic Surgery Procedures

COMMON TRADITIONAL PROCEDURES	NEW PROCEDURES	PROCEDURES UNDER INVESTIGATION
• Endotracheobronchial stenting	• Endobronchial ultrasound-guided transbronchial needle aspiration (EBUS-TBNA)	• Bronchoscopic lung volume reduction (BLVR)
• Endobronchial biopsy • Endotracheobronchial laser • Bronchoscopic balloon dilation • Bronchoscopic cryotherapy	• Complete mediastinal staging using EBUS-TBNA • Electromagnetic navigational bronchoscopy (ENB) • ENB + 3D cone computed tomographic biopsy	• Bronchial thermoplasty for treatment of poorly controlled asthma (started to make its way into a viable option to treat severe bronchial asthma)
• Endotracheobronchial electrocautery	• Fiducial marker implantation	

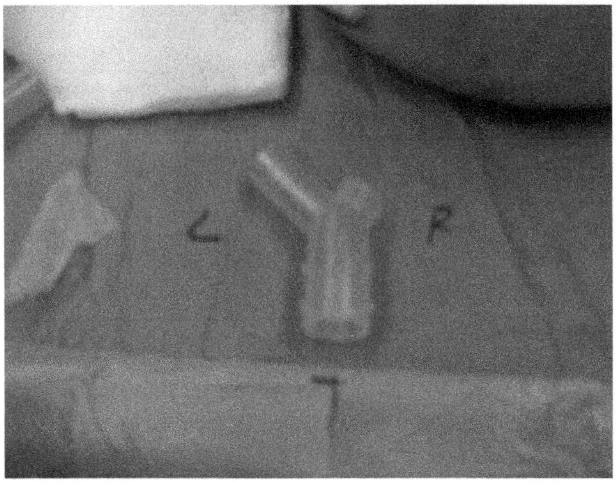

Figure 20.1. Y-shaped silicone stent. L, left (bronchus); R, right (bronchus); T, trachea. (Reprinted with permission, Cleveland Clinic Center for Medical Art & Photography © 2018. All rights reserved.)

NEW PROCEDURES

ENDOBRONCHIAL ULTRASOUND-GUIDED TRANSBRONCHIAL NEEDLE ASPIRATION AND ITS USE IN COMPLETE MEDIASTINAL STAGING

Through endobronchial ultrasound (EBUS), the tracheobronchial wall and adjacent structures can be well visualized. It is an accurate, safe, and cost-effective technique that allows biopsy of mediastinal lymph nodes and peribronchial lesions.[7,8] EBUS transbronchial needle aspiration (TBNA) has proved valuable for mediastinal lymph node staging of lung cancer.[9]

ELECTROMAGNETIC NAVIGATIONAL BRONCHOSCOPY

Electromagnetic navigational bronchoscopy (ENB) is designed to enable the pulmonologist to biopsy lesions within the periphery of the bronchial tree. The system components include the following[10]:

1. A sensor probe able to navigate the bronchial tree
2. An electromagnetic location board
3. A bronchoscope with an extended working channel
4. Computer software that converts computed tomographic (CT) scans of the lung into multiplanar images with three-dimensional (3D) virtual lung reconstruction. This setup allows navigational guidance within the lungs to bronchoscopically invisible targets and subsequent biopsy, almost in the same fashion as stereotactic brain biopsy.

FIDUCIAL MARKER IMPLANTATION

Stereotactic radiosurgery (CyberKnife; Accuray Inc., Sunnyvale, CA) is a treatment option for a lung tumor. For precise tumor ablation, fiducial markers are placed in or near the target tumor. For bronchoscopically invisible peripheral lung lesions, ENB may offer an attractive alternative to CT-guided placement of these fiducials.[11]

PROCEDURES UNDER INVESTIGATION

Two procedures are worth mentioning. *Bronchoscopic lung volume reduction* (BLVR) is being investigated for treatment of emphysema to replace open lung volume reduction surgery, given the very invasive nature and associated morbidity and mortality of the latter. Available technologies include one-way endobronchial valves, BioGlue®, and coils. In the *bronchial thermoplasty* procedure, controlled heat is applied endobronchially to reduce the mass of the airway smooth muscle as a treatment for poorly controlled asthma.[12] Bronchial Thermoplasty is gaining more acceptance and being used more frequently now.

ANESTHETIC CARE

PREOPERATIVE EVALUATION

The extent of preoperative evaluation depends on several important considerations. Important questions to ask are the following: Is the procedure elective or emergent? How stable or critical is the airway? In elective cases, preoperative assessment is usually conducted in the customary fashion with special attention to the following:

- Airway evaluation, symptoms of compromise: dysphagia, hoarseness, orthopnea, stridor, the use of accessory muscles of respiration

- Review of the pulmonologist's notes regarding the size and location of the lesion or tumor and the intended procedure(s)
- Review of CT scan of the neck and chest to rule out airway abnormalities and mediastinal masses
- Prior chemotherapy and any effects on vital organs (especially the heart and lungs)
- Commonly associated conditions, such as heavy tobacco smoking and alcohol use
- Common comorbidities: coronary artery disease and chronic obstructive/restrictive pulmonary disease, chronic alcoholism, malnutrition, and aspiration pneumonitis

PREMEDICATION

Premedication with sedatives and anxiolytics should be considered only for a very anxious patient because the respiratory status of patients has already been compromised, and many of the typically used medications are known to have respiratory depressant effects. Nevertheless, when it is considered necessary to use them, small titrated doses should be given. Once medicated, patients should not be left alone without appropriate monitoring. As an added safety precaution, supplemental oxygen should be provided before sedation.

MONITORED ANESTHESIA CARE

The commonly used technique of monitored anesthesia care (MAC), especially in OOOR/NORA settings, can be used for selected patients undergoing minimally invasive procedures. The majority of uncomplicated and routine diagnostic flexible bronchoscopic procedures can be performed under light sedation. However, ventilation support may be necessary if the lung is compromised or when a patient becomes unable to tolerate the respiratory depressant effects of many of the commonly used sedatives. On the whole, because of their understanding of the lung pathology in question and their knowledge of the patient's respiratory status, pulmonologists can make accurate judgments regarding the type of sedation for the patient. Options might include mild or moderate sedation provided by the sedation nurse and supervised by the proceduralist or MAC/general anesthesia provided by an anesthesiologist. Midazolam, fentanyl, morphine, remifentanil, alfentanil, ketamine, and propofol are among the medications successfully used as part of sedation and total intravenous anesthesia (TIVA) techniques. More recently, dexmedetomidine and fospropofol have been added to the list of acceptable choices.[13-15]

GENERAL ANESTHESIA

A TIVA technique is preferred over an inhalational anesthetic technique for the following reasons:

- It ensures continuous delivery of the anesthetic compared to an inhalation anesthetic-based technique when ventilation leaks occur around the rigid bronchoscope[16] or while the flexible bronchoscope is being inserted into and removed from the airway. TIVA is more practical when instruments such as balloons and techniques such as intermittent apnea or jet ventilation are used.
- It prevents pollution of the operating room by inhalational anesthetic agents.
- It avoids the risk of sedating operating room personnel, including the anesthesia team, pulmonology team, and the operating room nursing and support staff (advantages of TIVA are summarized in Box 20.1.).

Total intravenous anesthesia can be initiated as a pure propofol infusion (administered at 50–200 μg/kg per minute) Finally, it should be noted that while administering TIVA, the practitioner may consider using an EEG brain function monitor (bispectral index or Sedline) to prevent intraoperative recall and to titrate intravenous anesthetic agent to the appropriate anesthetic depth.[17]

THE USE OF MUSCLE RELAXATION

First, muscle relaxation facilitates supraglottic airway (SGA)/endotracheal tube (ETT) insertion. In addition, relaxing the jaw muscles makes insertion of the rigid laryngoscope (for suspension laryngoscopy) and rigid bronchoscope much easier and safer. It also improves overall lung compliance by eliminating the chest wall component, which would be very helpful during jet ventilation. Regardless of the airway choice—SGA versus ETT—muscle paralysis can be advantageous because unexpected patient movement during the procedure can result in unintended airway injury. For example, during laser therapy, a motionless patient dramatically decreases the risk of unwanted misdirection of the laser beam; sudden movement by the patient could result in damage to healthy tissues and possible major vessel or esophageal injury. If a SGA is used, the use of muscle relaxation also helps minimize trauma to the vocal cords caused by the frequent insertion and removal of the bronchoscope against contracted cords (the advantages of muscle relaxants are listed in Box 20.2).

BOX 20.1 ADVANTAGES OF TOTAL INTRAVENOUS ANESTHETIC TECHNIQUE (TIVA) IN BRONCHOSCOPIC SURGERY

- Ensures continuous delivery of the anesthetic
- Prevents pollution of the operating room by inhalational agents
- Avoids risk of sedating operating room personnel
- Enables certain techniques, such as intermittent apnea and jet ventilation

BOX 20.2 ADVANTAGES OF MUSCLE RELAXANTS IN BRONCHOSCOPIC SURGERY

- Facilitates SGA/ETT and rigid bronchoscope insertion
- Improves overall lung compliance
- Provides a motionless patient
- Helps minimize trauma to the vocal cords

ETT, endotracheal tube; SGA, supraglottic airway.

FLUID MANAGEMENT IN BRONCHOSCOPIC SURGERY

It is wise to restrict all administered fluids to the minimum needed because many of the patients present with a limited lung reserve. Pulmonary congestion may aggravate their lung condition. This is especially true if they have concomitant cardiac disease, such as left-sided or right-sided heart failure, which may be a complication of their long-standing lung pathophysiology (e.g., cor pulmonale).

THE USE OF STEROIDS IN BRONCHOSCOPIC SURGERY

Many anesthesiologists and surgeons use corticosteroids, in particular dexamethasone, as a prophylactic measure to decrease airway edema after airway surgery. Common scenarios when steroids may help reduce postoperative vocal cord swelling include cases where the flexible fiber-optic bronchoscope (alone or through an SGA and in the absence of an ETT) has been inserted into and removed from the airway several times, if the bronchoscope continually rubs against the vocal cords, or if a rigid bronchoscope has been used for a prolonged duration. Steroids also are used if extensive tracheobronchial tissue trauma is caused by a prolonged procedure.

However, the use of steroids is defended on the basis only of their putative clinical advantage because evidence of their real advantage is controversial at best. Evidence supporting the use of steroids includes their beneficial effects prior to certain maxillofacial procedures due to their proven benefit in reducing postoperative edema and inflammation.[18–20] However, Hughes et al. have shown that steroids are ineffective in reducing airway edema following carotid endarterectomy.[21] Additionally, steroids are beneficial as a preventive measure for postoperative nausea and vomiting.[22] Finally, many bronchoscopic surgery patients with underlying lung conditions (e.g., granulomatosis with polyangiitis, formerly known as Wegener granulomatosis) that require chronic steroid therapy are treated by many clinicians with 100 mg of hydrocortisone (the so-called stress dose steroids) to avoid adrenocortical insufficiency in the setting of a chronically suppressed suprarenal gland by the exogenous steroid. However, the effectiveness of this "stress dose" treatment has not been demonstrated conclusively.[23]

ANTINAUSEA AND ASPIRATION PROPHYLAXIS

Pulmonary aspiration can be detrimental to patients with limited pulmonary reserve. Additionally, because ETT is used only in a limited number of cases, the majority of the procedures are done with techniques that might not protect against pulmonary aspiration—the risk is higher when a rigid bronchoscope, SGA, or no airway is used. The use of maximum antinausea prophylaxis, especially in patients with risk factors for pulmonary complications, is therefore justified. In such cases, the use of propofol as part of the TIVA technique is helpful because propofol has antiemetic properties. The avoidance of inhalation anesthetics and of nitrous oxide also may be justified. Effective postoperative nausea and vomiting prophylaxis drugs include steroids (e.g., 4–8 mg of dexamethasone), dopamine receptor antagonists (e.g., 10–20 mg of metochlopramide), and 5-HT3 receptor antagonists (2–4 mg of ondansetron).[21]

MANAGEMENT OF THE F_{IO_2}

Administrating 100% FiO_2 in such procedures is common. However, during thermal treatment with Nd:YAG lasers, EBES (endobronchial electric surgery), or thermoplasty, it is usually necessary to maintain it at the lowest tolerable level, that is, below 40%. Periods of extended apnea and complete airway obstruction can be expected during more challenging cases. Complete airway occlusion frequently occurs during the critical phase of removing the stent or stent fragments or the inflated balloon dilators used for tracheobronchial dilation. Therefore, it is always advisable to return to ventilation with 100% oxygen before extraction of the stent, prior to exchange of airways, and prior to extubation.

Finally, during thermal treatment, if the patient cannot tolerate lower oxygen levels, it may become necessary to defer treatment temporarily and ventilate with higher oxygen concentrations.

AIRWAY CHOICE

WITHOUT ARTIFICIAL AIRWAYS

Treatment without artificial airways is a popular technique, especially when relatively short procedures are performed in a remote bronchosopy suite where an anesthesia machine is unavailable. An intravenous sedation technique is more appealing for these procedures, with the goal of maintaining spontaneous ventilation. Great emphasis should be placed on airway topicalization to tolerate the bronchoscope without the need for deeper planes of sedation and their associated risks.

ENDOTRACHEAL TUBE

Intubation with a large-diameter (e.g., size ≥ 8.0) ETT facilitates ventilation around the relatively large-diameter flexible bronchoscope. Many pulmonologists prefer to have the ETT cut short following intubation and securing the tube with tape. This is because a shorter tube can facilitate navigation of the flexible fiber-optic bronchoscope (Figure 20.2). Intubation of patients with a tracheal stent, whether a SEMS or a silastic type stent, requires caution because it can dislodge the stent distally or cause other complications. A shortened large-bore ETT could be used via an existing tracheotomy inserted with the use of a flexible bronchoscope.

RIGID BRONCHOSCOPE

A rigid bronchoscope (Figure 20.3) is preferred for procedures such as insertion and removal of silicone stents due to their size and noncompressible nature, removal of large broncholiths and granulation tissue, coring out of a large tumor invading the tracheobronchial tree, and supporting airway patency if a large mediastinal mass is compressing the airway. When the rigid bronchoscope is used, ventilation can be accomplished either by attaching the breathing circuit to the bronchoscope side port or through jet ventilation, where the jetting device is attached through a special adaptor to the bronchoscope side port. Leaks around the rigid bronchoscope are common when positive pressure ventilation is used, but they can be easily remedied by maximizing the fresh gas flow and packing the mouth with saline-soaked gauze to facilitate positive pressure ventilation. Special attention should be given to removing all the gauze to avoid subsequent airway obstruction from retained gauze pieces when the bronchoscope is removed.

SUPRAGLOTTIC AIRWAY

In cases where the tracheal lesion is high up in the trachea, a SGA device (e.g., laryngeal mask airway [LMA]) can be effective[24,25] because the device does not enter the glottis. The SGA provides a conduit for the flexible bronchoscope to access the subglottic lesion and at the same time allows ventilation of the patient. However, because it is a less-"definitive" airway compared to the ETT, the SGA device does not guarantee reliable protection against aspiration. Use of a fiber-optic swivel connector adaptor will allow continuous ventilation. The techniques just described require clear communication between the anesthesiologist and the pulmonologist.

THE USE OF AIRWAY EXCHANGE CATHETERS IN BRONCHOSCOPIC SURGERY

Exchange of the airway is often needed during bronchoscopic surgery because of the dynamic nature of the procedures and because of situations in which the airway is judged to be difficult to intubate. Accordingly, it is advisable to start with awake intubation and with a relatively small-size ETT, such as 7.5-mm inside diameter (ID) Parker Flex-Tip® tracheal tube. Compared to the standard tube, the use of the Parker tube has reduced the need to reposition the tube during insertion into the trachea from 89% to 29% ($p < .0001$).[26] After the Parker tube is in place, an airway exchange catheter can be used to replace it with a larger tube to facilitate the flexible bronchoscopic procedure. If a rigid bronchoscope is required, the exchange catheter can be used for access to the airway until the laryngeal inlet is visualized through the rigid bronchoscope and the scope is secured in position. The same principle can be applied again at the end of the procedure after finishing with the rigid bronchoscope: The exchange catheter can be introduced through it and used to insert an ETT after removing the rigid bronchoscope. The exchange catheter is also effective for intubation through an LMA.[27]

POSTOPERATIVE CARE

Most of the procedures described previously are performed as same-day outpatient procedures. However, patients with significant comorbidities or advanced disease undergoing a complicated resection or lasering of endotracheobronchial lesions may benefit from overnight admission. Still, this compares favorably with invasive thoracic surgery, which often requires postoperative intensive care unit admission and a prolonged hospital stay.

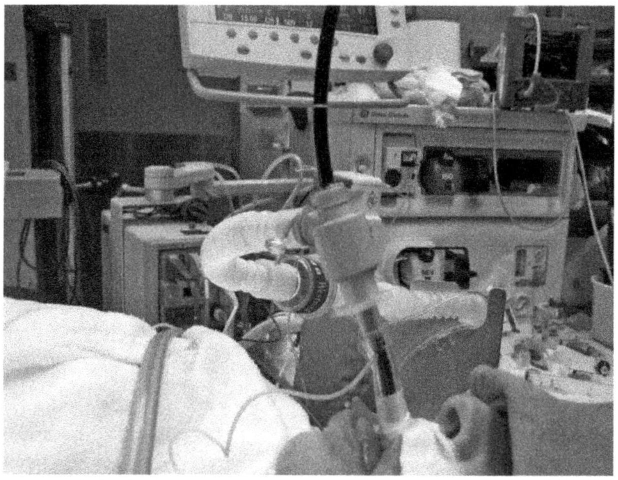

Figure 20.2. A large, 8.5-mm inside diameter (ID) endotracheal tube cut short with the bronchoscope through it. Ventilation around the bronchoscope is made possible by attaching the circuit to a swivel adapter (Reprinted with permission, Cleveland Clinic Center for Medical Art & Photography © 2018. All rights reserved.)

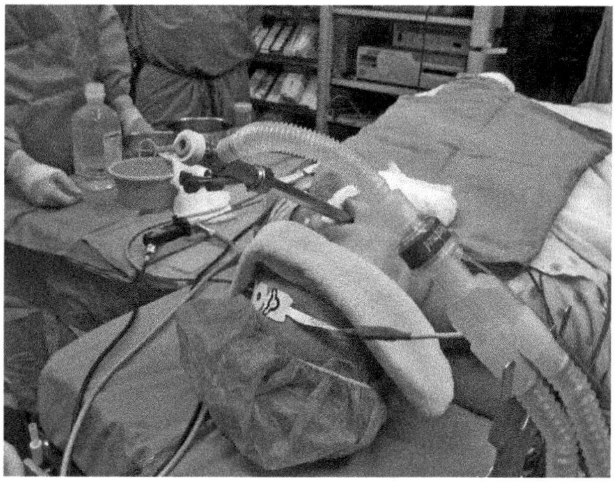

Figure 20.3. Positive pressure ventilation through connecting the breathing circuit to the side port of a rigid bronchoscope. Note the wet gauze packing around the rigid bronchoscope barrel to minimize leakage around the scope. (Reprinted with permission, Cleveland Clinic Center for Medical Art & Photography © 2018. All rights reserved.)

MANAGEMENT OF SPECIAL AIRWAY CASES

MANAGEMENT OF AN ANTERIOR MEDIASTINAL MASS

The presence of an anterior mediastinal mass (AMM) can predispose patients to severe respiratory and cardiovascular complications during anesthesia. These may include airway narrowing or obstruction, compression of the cardiac chambers, and compression of the pulmonary artery.[28–34] Extreme caution is required in managing these patients.

Airway obstruction is a serious complication of general anesthesia in patients with an AMM. Spontaneous ventilation has been highly recommended in the anesthetic management of AMM patients because it eliminates the use of muscle relaxants and maintains negative intrapleural pressure.[35]

Several conservative anesthetic plans have been proposed for managing AMM.[36] Under one plan, the patient should be intubated awake after being topicalized and mildly sedated while in the least symptomatic position (possibly through use of the flexible fiber-optic scope). An inhalational agent-based technique that maintains spontaneous respiration is another effective course of action.

Another option is to use dexmedetomidine, a selective α_2 agonist with sedative, analgesic, amnestic,[37] and antisialagogue properties.[38] Dexmedetomidine helps maintain spontaneous respiration with minimal respiratory depression. Its maintenance of spontaneous ventilation in the management of AMM has been described.[39] Patients under dexmedetomidine sedation are generally easy to arouse,[40] making it a useful drug for awake fiber-optic–assisted intubation.[13] However, these advantages may not hold with higher doses (off label).

Cases that include the management of patients with larger AMM (causing > 50% reduction in airway diameter as seen on a CT scan) should be considered for management in the main operating room Vs. OOOR location. Some authorities recommend that cardiopulmonary bypass be available on standby and that femoral vessel cannulation should be achieved prior to induction.[29,36]

COMPLICATIONS

POTENTIAL COMPLICATIONS OF BRONCHOSCOPIC PROCEDURES

Potential complications of bronchoscopic procedures are numerous and range from hypercarbia and minor levels of hypoxemia to major bleeding, tracheal rupture, and loss of airway integrity.

Stent removal provides an example of a potentially risky interventional procedure. Possible complications include retention of stent pieces, mucosal tears with bleeding, reobstruction, the need for postoperative mechanical ventilation, pneumothorax, and damage to the pulmonary artery.[41] When the stent is fractured during removal, unwanted fragments may remain permanently embedded in the tissue. In one report, critical airway obstruction occurred during removal of a tracheal stent using a rigid bronchoscope under general anesthesia, and cardiopulmonary bypass had to be instituted urgently. The stent was eventually removed by directly opening the trachea.[42]

The jet ventilation technique can lead to barotrauma and may result in a pneumothorax, necessitating chest tube insertion. Laser airway fire, although rare, is also a potential complication.

Suggested steps to take in case of an airway fire are as follows:

1. Discontinue lasering and turn off O_2 (and N_2O if it was mistakenly used).
2. Remove the burning ETT and drop it in a bucket of water.
3. Flush area with water or normal saline.
4. Reintubate immediately and resume ventilation with 100% O_2.
5. When the patient's condition has stabilized, assess damage to the airway with a ventilating rigid bronchoscope. Remove any debris or foreign bodies.
6. Consider the use of intravenous steroids (however, their efficacy has not been proven).
7. Consider administering antibiotics.
8. Implement supportive therapy, including ventilation, and extubate when clinically indicated.
9. Consider tracheotomy, if necessary.

TRACHEAL RUPTURE

Tracheal rupture or loss of tracheal integrity can complicate any of the aforementioned interventional pulmonology procedures. However, these complications occur more frequently with balloon dilation or complicated stent removal. Reported risk factors for tracheal rupture include advanced age; chronic obstructive pulmonary disease; weakened tracheal walls, usually secondary to chronic airway inflammation; previous procedures; infection; and prior steroid therapy.[43–46]

The signs and symptoms of tracheal rupture are nonspecific, but a combination of the associated symptoms or signs in the clinical setting should lead to a high degree of suspicion. Dyspnea and a dry cough are sometimes the only signs evident in an awake patient. Cyanosis and tachycardia may also be evident. Other signs include hemoptysis, persistent air leak, subcutaneous emphysema, pneumomediastinum, and pneumothorax.[47–49]

Bronchoscopy is the gold standard for the diagnosis of tracheal rupture. It is also critical in differentiating between small tears (<1 cm), which may be treated conservatively, and more severe injuries requiring surgical management. Routine chest radiographs and bronchoscopy are usually sufficient for diagnosis in 90% of cases.

The management of a tracheal tear can be observational (conservative) or surgical, depending on the extent of the injury, the presenting signs and symptoms, and the general condition of the patient. In general, small, shallow tears that do not lead to severe compromise in ventilation and oxygenation can be treated conservatively.[50,51] If the patient is dependent on positive pressure–assisted ventilation, however, surgical treatment is mandatory. Regardless of the choice of management, the status of the trachea should be monitored with tracheoscopy.

Ventilatory management consists of adequate oxygenation and ventilation of the patient and prevention of worsening subcutaneous emphysema, pneumomediastinum, or pneumothorax. This is best accomplished by positioning the ETT so that the cuff is distal to the level of the injury and also by keeping the airway pressures as low as possible. A higher FiO_2 and respiratory rate may be required. Selective or bilateral bronchial intubation can be performed in tears located above or near the carina. It is important to note that standard direct intubation can be potentially hazardous because a false passage can be easily created. Fiber optic guided intubation may be safer.

Other possible options in management include high-frequency oscillating ventilation and hyperbaric oxygen therapy in patients who are difficult to oxygenate or ventilate.[52,53] In rare situations, cardiopulmonary bypass or percutaneous cardiopulmonary support systems have been used.[54,55] Other management goals include treating pneumothoraces with chest tubes, controlling pain, and supporting the patient's hemodynamic status.

SUMMARY

Interventional pulmonology is a fast-growing field. These procedures are at times very complex, and the patient population often has many comorbidities. Many of the interventional pulmonology procedures are performed OOOR. Anesthesiologists need to stay abreast of the advances in this field and be prepared to deal with the anesthetic challenges that may arise. The key to favorable outcomes lies in understanding the underlying lung pathology, open two-way communication between the anesthesiologist and pulmonologist, understanding the nature of the procedure, and above all, extreme vigilance and preparedness.

REFERENCES

1. Nagrebetsky A, Gabriel RA, Dutton RP, Urman RD. Growth of nonoperating room anesthesia care in the United States: a contemporary trends analysis. *Anesth Analg.* 2017;124(4):1261–1267.
2. Eckardt J, Petersen HO, Hakami-Kermani A, Olsen KE, Jorgensen OD, Licht PB. Endobronchial ultrasound-guided transbronchial needle aspiration of undiagnosed intrathoracic lesions. *Interact Cardiovasc Thorac Surg.* 2009;9(2):232–235.
3. Ernst A, Feller-Kopman D, Becker HD, Mehta AC. Central airway obstruction. *Am J Respir Crit Care Med.* 2004;169(12):1278–1297.
4. Petrou M, Kaplan D, Goldstraw P. Bronchoscopic diathermy resection and stent insertion: a cost effective treatment for tracheobronchial obstruction. *Thorax.* 1993;48(11):1156–1159.
5. Boxem T, Muller M, Venmans B, Postmus P, Sutedja T. Nd-YAG laser versus bronchoscopic electrocautery for palliation of symptomatic airway obstruction: a cost-effectiveness study. *Chest.* 1999;116(4):1108–1112.
6. van Boxem AJ, Westerga J, Venmans BJ, Postmus PE, Sutedja G. Photodynamic therapy, Nd-YAG laser and electrocautery for treating early-stage intraluminal cancer: which to choose? *Lung Cancer.* 2001;31(1):31–36.
7. Cameron SE, Andrade RS, Pambuccian SE. Endobronchial ultrasound-guided transbronchial needle aspiration cytology: a state of the art review. *Cytopathology.* 2010;21(1):6–26.
8. Eberhardt R, Becker HD, Herth FJ. Endobronchial ultrasound for diagnosis of the mediastinum [in German]. *Chirurg.* 2008;79(1):50–55.
9. Yasufuku K, Nakajima T, Fujiwara T, et al. Role of endobronchial ultrasound-guided transbronchial needle aspiration in the management of lung cancer. *Gen Thorac Cardiovasc Surg.* 2008;56(6):268–276.
10. Eberhardt R, Anantham D, Herth F, Feller-Kopman D, Ernst A. Electromagnetic navigation diagnostic bronchoscopy in peripheral lung lesions. *Chest.* 2007;131(6):1800–1805.
11. Anantham D, Feller-Kopman D, Shanmugham LN, et al. Electromagnetic navigation bronchoscopy-guided fiducial placement for robotic stereotactic radiosurgery of lung tumors: a feasibility study. *Chest.* 2007;132(3):930–935.
12. Cox G, Miller JD, McWilliams A, Fitzgerald JM, Lam S. Bronchial thermoplasty for asthma. *Am J Respir Crit Care Med.* 2006;173(9):965–969.
13. Abdelmalak B, Makary L, Hoban J, Doyle DJ. Dexmedetomidine as sole sedative for awake intubation in management of the critical airway. *J Clin Anesth.* 2007;19(5):370–373.
14. Silvestri GA, Vincent BD, Wahidi MM, Robinette E, Hansbrough JR, Downie GH. A phase 3, randomized, double-blind study to assess the efficacy and safety of fospropofol disodium injection for moderate sedation in patients undergoing flexible bronchoscopy. *Chest.* 2009;135(1):41–47.
15. Abdelmalak B, Gutenberg L, Lorenz RR, Smith M, Farag E, Doyle DJ. Dexmedetomidine supplemented with local anesthesia for awake laryngoplasty. *J Clin Anesth.* 2009;21(6):442–443.
16. Abernathy JH 3rd, Reeves ST. Airway catastrophes. *Curr Opin Anaesthesiol.* 2010;23(1):41–46.
17. Avidan MS, Zhang L, Burnside BA, et al. Anesthesia awareness and the bispectral index. *N Engl J Med.* 2008;358(11):1097–1108.
18. Weber CR, Griffin JM. Evaluation of dexamethasone for reducing postoperative edema and inflammatory response after orthog-nathic surgery. *J Oral Maxillofac Surg.* 1994;52(1):35–39.
19. Montgomery MT, Hogg JP, Roberts DL, Redding SW. The use of glucocorticosteroids to lessen the inflammatory sequelae following third molar surgery. *J Oral Maxillofac Surg.* 1990;48(2):179–187.
20. Gersema L, Baker K. Use of corticosteroids in oral surgery. *J Oral Maxillofac Surg.* 1992;50(3):270–277.
21. Apfel CC, Korttila K, Abdalla M, et al. A factorial trial of six interventions for the prevention of postoperative nausea and vomiting. *N Engl J Med.* 2004;350(24):2441–2451.
22. Hughes R, McGuire G, Montanera W, Wong D, Carmichael FJ. Upper airway edema after carotid endarterectomy: the effect of steroid administration. *Anesth Analg.* 1997;84(3):475–478.
23. Goichot B, Vinzio S, Luca F, Schlienger JL. Do we still have glu-cocorticoid-induced adrenal insufficiency? *Presse Med.* 2007;36(7–8):1065–1071.
24. Abdelmalak B, Ryckman JV, AlHaddad S, Sprung J. Respiratory arrest after successful neodymium:yttrium-aluminum-garnet laser treatment of subglottic tracheal stenosis. *Anesth Analg.* 2002;95(2):485–486.
25. Hung WT, Liao SM, Su JM. Laryngeal mask airway in patients with tracheal stents who are undergoing non-airway related interventions: report of three cases. *J Clin Anesth.* 2004;16(3):214–216.
26. Kristensen MS. The Parker Flex-Tip tube versus a standard tube for fiberoptic orotracheal intubation: a randomized double-blind study. *Anesthesiology.* 2003;98(2):354–358.
27. Zura A, Doyle DJ, Avitsian R, DeUngria M. More on intubation using the Aintree catheter. *Anesth Analg.* 2006;103(3):785.
28. Bittar D. Respiratory obstruction associated with induction of general anesthesia in a patient with mediastinal Hodgkin's disease. *Anesth Analg.* 1975;54(3):399–403.
29. Azizkhan RG, Dudgeon DL, Buck JR, et al. Life-threatening airway obstruction as a complication to the management of mediastinal masses in children. *J Pediatr Surg.* 1985;20(6):816–822.
30. King DR, Patrick LE, Ginn-Pease ME, McCoy KS, Klopfenstein K. Pulmonary function is compromised in children with mediastinal lymphoma. *J Pediatr Surg.* 1997;32(2):294–300.
31. Piro AJ, Weiss DR, Hellman S. Mediastinal Hodgkin's disease: a possible danger for intubation anesthesia. Intubation danger in Hodgkin's disease. *Int J Radiat Oncol, Biol Phys.* 1976;1(5–6):415–419.
32. Ferrari LR, Bedford RF. General anesthesia prior to treatment of anterior mediastinal masses in pediatric cancer patients [published erratum appears in *Anesthesiology.* 1990;73(2):372]. *Anesthesiology.* 1990;72(6):991–995.
33. Turoff RD, Gomez GA, Berjian R, et al. Postoperative respiratory complications in patients with Hodgkin's disease: relationship to the size of the mediastinal tumor. *Eur J Cancer Clinl Oncol.* 1985;21(9):1043–1046.

34. Bechard P, Letourneau L, Lacasse Y, Cote D, Bussieres JS. Perioperative cardiorespiratory complications in adults with mediastinal mass: incidence and risk factors. *Anesthesiology.* 2004;100(4):826–834; discussion 825A.
35. Slinger P, Karsli C. Management of the patient with a large anterior mediastinal mass: recurring myths. *Curr Opin Anaesthesiol.* 2007;20(1):1–3.
36. Goh MH, Liu XY, Goh YS. Anterior mediastinal masses: an anaesthetic challenge. *Anaesthesia.* 1999;54(7):670–674.
37. Ebert TJ, Hall JE, Barney JA, Uhrich TD, Colinco MD. The effects of increasing plasma concentrations of dexmedetomidine in humans. *Anesthesiology.* 2000;93(2):382–394.
38. Scher CS, Gitlin MC. Dexmedetomidine and low-dose ketamine provide adequate sedation for awake fibreoptic intubation. *Can J Anaesth.* 2003;50(6):607–610.
39. Abdelmalak B, Marcanthony N, Abdelmalak J, Machuzak M, Gildea T, Doyle DJ. Dexmedetomidine for anesthetic management of anterior mediastinal mass. *Anesthesia.* 2010;25:607–610.
40. Shukry M, Miller JA. Update on dexmedetomidine: use in nonin-tubated patients requiring sedation for surgical procedures. *Ther Clin Risk Manag.* 2010;6:111–121.
41. Doyle DJ, Abdelmalak B, Machuzak M, Gildea TR. Anesthesia and airway management for removing pulmonary self-expanding metallic stents. *J Clin Anesth.* 2009;21(7):529–532.
42. Kao SC, Chang WK, Pong MW, Cheng KW, Chan KH, Tsai SK. Welded tracheal stent removal in a child under cardiopulmonary bypass. *Br J Anaesth.* 2003;91(2):294–296.
43. Luna CM, Legarreta G, Esteva H, Laffaire E, Jolly EC. Effect of tracheal dilatation and rupture on mechanical ventilation using a low-pressure cuff tube. *Chest.* 1993;104(2):639–640.
44. Putnam TD, Wu Y. Tracheal rupture following cervical manipulation: late complication posttracheostomy. *Arch Phys Med Rehabil.* 1986;67(1):48–50.
45. Harris R, Joseph A. Acute tracheal rupture related to endotracheal intubation: case report. *J Emerg Med.* 2000;18(1):35–39.
46. Irefin SA, Farid IS, Senagore AJ. Urgent colectomy in a patient with membranous tracheal disruption after severe vomiting. *Anesth Analg.* 2000;91(5):1300–1302.
47. Tcherveniakov A, Tchalakov P, Tcherveniakov P. Traumatic and iatrogenic lesions of the trachea and bronchi. *Eur J Cardiothorac Surg.* 2001;19(1):19–24.
48. Massard G, Rouge C, Dabbagh A, et al. Tracheobronchial lacerations after intubation and tracheostomy. *Ann Thorac Surg.* 1996;61(5):1483–1487.
49. Olson RO, Johnson JT. Diagnosis and management of intrathoracic tracheal rupture. *J Trauma.* 1971;11(9):789–792.
50. Zettl R, Waydhas C, Biberthaler P, et al. Nonsurgical treatment of a severe tracheal rupture after endotracheal intubation. *Crit Care Med.* 1999;27(3):661–663.
51. Marquette CH, Bocquillon N, Roumilhac D, Neviere R, Mathieu D, Ramon P. Conservative treatment of tracheal rupture. *J Thorac Cardiovasc Surg.* 1999;117(2):399–401.
52. Lin JC, Maley RH Jr, Landreneau RJ. Extensive posterior-lateral tracheal laceration complicating percutaneous dilational tracheostomy. *Ann Thorac Surg.* 2000;70(4):1194–1196.
53. Ratzenhofer-Komenda B, Offner A, Kaltenbock F, et al. Differential lung ventilation and emergency hyperbaric oxygenation for repair of a tracheal tear. *Can J Anaesth.* 2000;47(2):169–175.
54. Yamazaki M, Sasaki R, Masuda A, Ito Y. Anesthetic management of complete tracheal disruption using percutaneous cardiopulmonary support system. *Anesth Analg.* 1998;86(5):998–1000.
55. Hirsh J, Gollin G, Seashore J, Kopf G, Barash PG. Mediastinal "tamponade" of a tracheal rupture in which partial cardiopulmonary bypass was required for surgical repair. *J Cardiothorac Vasc Anesth.* 1994;8(6):682–684.

21 | ANESTHETIC IMPLICATIONS OF NATURAL ORIFICE TRANSLUMENAL ENDOSCOPIC SURGERY (NOTES) AND SINGLE-INCISION LAPAROSCOPIC SURGERY (SILS)

MARK A. GROMSKI, MD, KAI MATTHES, MD, PHD

NATURAL ORIFICE TRANSLUMENAL ENDOSCOPIC SURGERY

Natural orifice translumenal endoscopic surgery (NOTES) describes a minimally invasive approach to surgical diseases in which instruments are passed transluminally (predominantly transvaginal or transgastric, although other sites, such as transcolonic, have also been investigated) to achieve access to the desired location within the body. This approach obviates the need for standard abdominal incisions required in open or laparoscopic surgery.

There are actually a variety of procedures characterized as "NOTES" in the media and the medical literature. "Pure NOTES" implies the performance of a surgical procedure through a natural orifice without making any abdominal incisions (e.g., transvaginal cholecystectomy or transgastric appendectomy). At this developmental stage, many studies remain investigational animal research projects. Human studies and case series are dominated by "Hybrid NOTES" procedures, with additional laparoscopic port(s) for visualization, retraction, and technical assistance (e.g., if hemostasis or ligation is required). Some NOTES procedures involve the use of rigid laparoscopic instruments, and others involve flexible endoscopic instruments. The modern-day concept of NOTES procedures was initially conceptualized by Kalloo and colleagues at Johns Hopkins.[1]

Even though NOTES claims to be a novel approach, rudimentary techniques existed in culdoscopy many decades ago. Culdoscopy is the endoscopic examination of the female pelvic viscera by an endoscope (usually rigid) introduced into the pelvic cavity through the posterior vaginal fornix.[2] Before the introduction of modern-day NOTES, these transvaginal operations were performed safely and were shown to decrease postoperative pain, improve recovery, and cause fewer complications than conventional open or laparoscopic procedures.[3] Other early reports of transvaginal organ resection include procedures for gastric tumors, gallbladder, and rectal tumors during laparoscopic surgery.[4–6]

The American Society for Gastrointestinal Endoscopy (ASGE) and the Society of American Gastrointestinal and Endoscopic Surgeons (SAGES) founded the Natural Orifice Consortium for Assessment and Research (NOSCAR). This consortium has served as a think tank, funding source, and research engine for this novel approach. At the outset of the surge of enthusiasm for NOTES, a white paper outlined many of the limitations and potential benefits of NOTES.[7]

Natural orifice translumenal endoscopic surgery is attractive due to (a) avoidance of surgical scars (improved cosmesis); (b) avoidance of complications of transabdominal incisions, including herniation and infection; and (c) potentially improved postprocedure pain as no incisions cross abdominal wall musculature.[7] The less-invasive character of the approach may lead to a faster recovery with less perioperative pain. Due to the less-invasive character of the procedure, there likely is a decreased requirement for intraoperative and postoperative opioids, which may decrease or even avoid the risk of postoperative ileus, although this has not been investigated rigorously in a comparative fashion at this point. Furthermore, the development of NOTES as a surgical concept has advanced the research and development of more advanced endoscopic equipment.

ANESTHETIC CONSIDERATIONS OF NOTES

Preliminary data suggest that, in the porcine model, NOTES peritoneoscopy with air insufflation is associated with higher peak inspiratory pressures and marked increase in median intra-abdominal pressure, with wide variation compared to laparoscopic peritoneoscopy.[8] This increase in intra-abdominal pressure leads to a decrease in cardiac output based on decreased cardiac return, or preload. One study found that on-demand carbon dioxide endoscopic insufflation in NOTES procedures with the aid of a transabdominal Veress needle minimized risks of hemodynamic or respiratory compromise and had lower intra-abdominal pressures when compared to laparoscopic controls.[9] Today, any pure NOTES procedures undertaken in humans (generally in research and academic settings) are carried out with carbon dioxide as the insufflation medium and with peritoneal pressure measurements. A comparative porcine study of NOTES versus laparoscopic peritoneoscopy demonstrated no clinically significant differences in multiple hemodynamic parameters.[10] Nonetheless, more data about hemodynamic changes during NOTES still need to be generated.

In a recent systematic analysis of the most common classic NOTES procedure, the transvaginal hybrid cholecystectomy, it was found that there was less postoperative pain after NOTES compared to laparoscopic cholecystectomy patients on the day of surgery and postoperative day 1.[11] Furthermore, the NOTES cholecystectomy patients had a better quality-of-life score on postoperative day 10 compared to the laparoscopic cholecystectomy patients.[11] Also, the study concluded that the complication rates were similar, and on long-term follow-up, there were no significantly increased adverse effects on sexual health in the transvaginal NOTES group.[11] The current standard for NOTES procedures performed in humans is to use general endotracheal anesthesia. However, a few cases of NOTES have been performed under moderate sedation.[12]

COMPLICATIONS OF NOTES

One of the challenges of providing anesthesia for NOTES procedures is the limited knowledge or experience with unexpected complications. In the setting of vascular injury during a pure NOTES procedure, the ability to achieve hemostasis is limited by lack of access and functionality of flexible endoscopic devices—particularly if a large vessel is involved. This may result in unexpected blood loss and a potential conversion to laparoscopy or laparotomy if hemostasis cannot be achieved endoscopically. Limited visualization of the abdominal cavity with flexible endoscopes could lead to minor bleeding that may remain unrecognized. The translumenal access involves potential injuries of adjacent organs, particularly in a nonhybrid procedure with lack of visualization of the access procedure.

Another point of potential complication is the closure of the transluminal access point that is chosen. The closure of a transvaginal access port may be less critical because the bacterial flora of the vagina is rather benign and may unlikely lead to a significant infection of the abdomen. Also, these transvaginal port sites can often be closed with existing approaches well known to gynecologists. However, with transgastric or transcolonic access, the efficacy of closure is of utmost importance due to the increased potential of an intra-abdominal infection in the setting of closure insufficiency. When providing perioperative care for patients undergoing NOTES procedures, significant abdominal discomfort, tenderness, or clinical signs of infection may point toward peritonitis as a complication related to the translumenal closure.

If flexible endoscopy is chosen for a NOTES approach, the increased length of the endoscopic instruments is associated with an increased risk of infection because the instruments may touch unsterile areas of the operating room table or even the floor. This may be unrecognized, especially because this is a new technique and the operating team may be too focused on the procedure. Here, the anesthesiologist needs to be aware of these potential sources of infection and inform the surgeons accordingly. Finally, NOTES is best performed in a team-driven format with immediate availability of therapeutic endoscopists and surgeons. Potential significant adverse events may occur if a gasteroenterologist performs NOTES and encounters a significant complication that requires conversion to laparoscopy or laparotomy. If timely availability of a surgeon is not readily available, there may be serious consequences.

SINGLE-INCISION LAPAROSCOPIC SURGERY OR SINGLE-PORT ACCESS SURGERY

Single-incision laparoscopic surgery (SILS) is a minimally invasive approach carried out as an extension of traditional laparoscopic surgery. In SILS, a single cutaneous incision is created, within which a single-port access (SPA) device with multiple ports or several single ports adjacent to each other may be placed to laparoscopically approach the abdominal cavity. Commonly, the periumbilical location is the choice for the operating surgeon. One major potential benefit of SILS is improved cosmesis. Improved pain, however, has not been a consistently realized benefit, likely due to extensive surgical manipulation of the fascial wall beneath the skin incision. Due to the slightly increased size of the incision in comparison to multiple ports at various locations with standard laparoscopy, the risk of abdominal wall infection or hernia is also most likely not reduced. A recent meta-analysis of SILS versus standard multiport laparoscopic splenectomy demonstrated no differences in pain scores, operative time, or complications.[13] In SILS, standard laparoscopic instruments or slightly modified instruments with angled handles or a curved shape can be used to avoid interference of the surgeon's hands while manipulating the instruments. Some endoscopic cameras (EndoEye, Olympus America, Inc., Center Valley, PA) provide a flexible tip that allows visualization of structures around bends. Retraction of large organs, such as the liver for cholecystectomy, may provide a challenge if attempted through a single port. Some surgeons use additional needle ports to supplement retraction capabilities independent from the trajectory of the multiport in the umbilicus. In general, SILS is generally considered to be technically more challenging due to the ergonomic constraints and some difficulties with triangulation.[14] Many believe these constraints have limited widespread adoption of the technique.

ANESTHETIC CONSIDERATIONS OF SILS

The combination of SILS with a bilateral transverse abdominal plane block with ultrasound guidance provides the advantage of reduced use of perioperative opioids or even no use. There are reports of single-site surgeries for placement of an adjustable gastric band and gynecological oncology applications that required no opioids postoperatively.[15,16] We have also described performing SILS cholecystectomy combined with a bilateral transversus abdominis plane (TAP) block that allowed the avoidance of any perioperative opioids.[17] The TAP block is a useful adjunct regional anesthetic technique that may result in significantly decreased postoperative pain and thus decreased amounts of postoperative opioid use, as shown in prospective, randomized trials involving cesarean delivery, gynecological surgery, and colorectal surgery.[18,19] The TAP block has also reduced postoperative pain in observational studies in open retropubic prostatectomy and laparoscopic colorectal surgery.[20,21]

Anatomically, the abdominal wall consists of three lateral muscle layers, from internal to external: transversus abdominis, internal oblique, and external oblique. The anterior abdominal wall consists of the three previous layers, in addition to the more superficial rectus abdominis and fascial sheaths. The afferent nerves that communicate pain from the anterior abdominal wall are located in the potential space deep to the internal oblique muscles and superficial of the transversus abdominis muscles. This space is referred to as the *transversus abdominis plane*. The nerves supplying the anterior abdominal wall that course through this space may be blocked with local anesthetics. The addition of the TAP block, which blocks the afferent nerves affected by the anterior body wall manipulation in a SILS cholecystectomy, is a logical choice for adjunct pain relief.

In addition, anesthesiologists can consider combining ketamine with preoperative ketorolac for analgesia. In our experience, the response to the intubation was blunted using a combination of propofol, ketamine, and lidocaine. Ketorolac was given for visceral pain associated with the procedure. The reduction or avoidance of perioperative opioids provides advantages in patients sensitive to consumption of opioid medications, including the morbidly obese, those with pulmonary compromise, or those with previous poor tolerance for opioids.

"NEW NOTES": PER ORAL ENDOSCOPIC MYOTOMY AND ENDOSCOPIC FULL-THICKNESS RESECTION

The classic NOTES procedures have been relegated currently predominantly to the domain of the academic surgeon. There has been flourishing interest in novel endoscopic therapies, including per oral endoscopic myotomy (POEM) and endoscopic full-thickness resection (EFTR). These are procedures performed predominantly, but not exclusively, by therapeutic endoscopists and traverse the gastrointestinal (GI) lumen, thus qualifying as NOTES procedures.

Performed with a flexible endoscope, POEM is used for the treatment of achalasia and other esophageal motility disorders. In this procedure, the endoscopist creates a submucosal tunnel in the esophagus to tunnel to the gastroesophageal junction, where the circular or full-thickness myotomy is performed.[22] The early results of POEM have been promising, with multiple nonrandomized studies that have compared POEM to laparoscopic Heller myotomy. In general, these have demonstrated equivalent efficacy and reflux rates with shorter hospital stay and postprocedure pain in the POEM groups.[23–26] With the encouraging preliminary data, there are multiple randomized clinical trials ongoing.

The anesthesiologist needs to be aware of potential complications of the POEM procedure. Despite the procedure being carried out in close relation to critical mediastinal structures (e.g., aorta), there have been very few mortalities reported in the literature. Adverse events of the procedure that have been reported include pneumonia, bleeding, capnomediastinum, capnoperitoneum, capnothorax, and subcutaneous emphysema.[22] Carbon dioxide is used nearly universally in POEM, and the presence of gas on radiographs nearly always resolves in a short time without clinical consequence. Occasionally, capnoperitoneum has required needle decompression. Low-flow carbon dioxide insufflators have been used in response to this adverse event.

Other important considerations for anesthesia include retained esophageal contents prior to induction, as the most common indication for the procedure is achalasia, and these patients often retain fluid and food within the esophagus. In some cases, a general upper GI endoscopy is recommended prior to induction and intubation to ensure no residual debris is in esophagus in an effort to decrease the incidence of aspiration.[27,28] Generally, positive pressure ventilation under general anesthesia is recommended to minimize effects of pneumomediastinum.[27–29] Peak airway pressures should be monitored closely. One recent study demonstrated the ability to perform routine POEM procedures in the endoscopy unit.[30,31]

Endoscopic full-thickness resection is a minimally invasive approach to the resection of GI subepithelial masses. The procedure has some similarities to endoscopic submucosal dissection (ESD) and is basically an outgrowth of that technology, using tools dedicated to ESD. In this procedure, the submucosal layer of the GI wall is injected, followed by a circumferential incision around the subepithelial lesion. Finally, dissection of the tumor is performed, usually resulting in a full-thickness defect in the GI lumen.[32] Closure of the luminal defect is performed in a variety of different ways, including standard through-the-scope endoclips, Endoloops® (Ethicon, West Somerville, NJ), endoscopic suturing device, or over-the-scope (OTSC) "bear-claw" clips.[32] Finally, in most cases needle decompression of pneumoperitoneum is required.[32] There is far less clinical experience in North America with EFTR compared to POEM. Potential complications to be aware of include pneumoperitoneum, localized peritonitis, failure of luminal closure, or bleeding.

THE NEXT FRONTIER

The next frontier of minimally invasive endoscopic surgery is vast, with innumerable projects ongoing in the animal laboratory. One procedure that is gaining attention is the per oral pyloromyotomy (POP), also known as the G-POEM. This procedure is similar in technique to the POEM procedure, but the myotomy is created at the pylorus and is a treatment of refractory gastroparesis. Clinical experience is starting, yet further study is needed to determine long-term efficacy and safety.[33–36] Another emerging field is the drainage of intra-abdominal collections through endoscopic stenting and necrosectomy. One newly developed technique describes gallbladder drainage in cases of cholecystitis in patients deemed poor surgical candidates; this technique places, guided by endoscopic ultrasound (EUS), a transluminal lumen-apposing metallic stent.[37–39] Furthermore, management of walled-off pancreatic necrosis is developing with the transluminal lumen-apposing metallic stent placement, which involves the placement of a metallic stent, usually transgastric, into an area of walled-off necrosis.[40] The lumen of the stent is large enough to allow subsequent endoscopic necrosectomy through the stent directly into the necrotic collection.

REFERENCES

1. Kalloo AN, Singh VK, Jagannath SB, et al. Flexible transgastric peritoneoscopy: a novel approach to diagnostic and therapeutic interventions in the peritoneal cavity. *Gastrointest Endosc.* 2004;60:114–117.
2. Diamond E. Diagnostic culdoscopy in infertility: a study of 4,000 outpatient procedures. *J Reprod Med.* 1978;21:23–30.
3. Brosens I, Gordts S, Campo R, Rombauts L. Transvaginal access heralds the end of standard diagnostic laparoscopy in infertility. *Hum Reprod.* 1998;13:1762–1763.
4. Delvaux G, Devroey P, De Waele B, Willems G. Transvaginal removal of gallbladders with large stones after laparoscopic cholecystectomy. *Surg Laparosc Endosc.* 1993;3:307–309.
5. Kim J, Shim M, Kwun K. Laparoscopic-assisted transvaginal resection of the rectum. *Dis Colon Rectum.* 1996;39:582–583.
6. Taniguchi E, Ohashi S, Takiguchi S, et al. Laparoscopic surgery assisted by a transvaginal approach. *Surg Laparosc Endosc.* 1999;9:53–56.
7. Rattner D. Introduction to NOTES white paper. *Surg Endosc.* 2006;20:185.
8. von Delius S, Huber W, Feussner H, et al. Effect of pneumoperitoneum on hemodynamics and inspiratory pressures during natural orifice transluminal endoscopic surgery (NOTES): an experimental, controlled study in an acute porcine model. *Endoscopy.* 2007;39:854–861.
9. Navarro-Ripoll R, Martinez-Palli G, Guarner-Argente C, et al. On-demand endoscopic CO_2 insufflation with feedback pressure regulation during natural orifice transluminal endoscopic surgery (NOTES) peritoneoscopy induces minimal hemodynamic and respiratory changes. *Gastrointest Endosc.* 2012;76:388–395.
10. Bingener J, Michalek J, Winston J, et al. Randomized blinded trial comparing the cardiopulmonary effects of NOTES with standard laparoscopy in a porcine survival model. *Surg Endosc.* 2008;22:1430–1434.
11. Bulian DR, Knuth J, Lehmann KS, Sauerwald A, Heiss MM. Systematic analysis of the safety and benefits of transvaginal hybrid-NOTES cholecystectomy. *World J Gastroenterol.* 2015;21:10915–10925.
12. Lee CK, Lee SH, Chung IK, et al. Human diagnostic transgastric peritoneoscopy with the submucosal tunnel technique performed with the patient under conscious sedation (with video). *Gastrointest Endosc.* 2010;72:889–891.
13. Wu S, Lai H, Zhao J, et al. Systematic review and meta-analysis of single-incision versus conventional multiport laparoscopic splenectomy. *J Minim Access Surg.* 2016 December 21. doi:10.4103/0972-9941.195573. [Epub ahead of print]
14. Santos BF, Enter D, Soper NJ, Hungness ES. Single-incision laparoscopic surgery (SILS) versus standard laparoscopic surgery: a comparison of performance using a surgical simulator. *Surg Endosc.* 2011;25:483–490.
15. Fader AN, Escobar PF. Laparoendoscopic single-site surgery (LESS) in gynecologic oncology: technique and initial report. *Gynecol Oncol.* 2009;114:157–161.
16. Teixeira J, McGill K, Binenbaum S, Forrester G. Laparoscopic single-site surgery for placement of an adjustable gastric band: initial experience. *Surg Endosc.* 2009;23:1409–1414.
17. Matthes K, Gromski MA, Schneider BE, Spiegel JE. Opioid-free single-incision laparoscopic (SIL) cholecystectomy using bilateral TAP blocks. *J Clin Anesth.* 2012;24:65–67.
18. Yoshida T, Furutani K, Watanabe Y, Ohashi N, Baba H. Analgesic efficacy of bilateral continuous transversus abdominis plane blocks using an oblique subcostal approach in patients undergoing laparotomy for gynaecological cancer: a prospective, randomized, triple-blind, placebo-controlled study. Br J Anaesth. 2016;117:812–820.
19. Tikuisis R, Miliauskas P, Lukoseviciene V, et al. Transversus abdominis plane block for postoperative pain relief after hand-assisted laparoscopic colon surgery: a randomized, placebo-controlled clinical trial. *Tech Coloproctol.* 2016;20:835–844.
20. McDonnell JG, O'Donnell B, Curley G, Heffernan A, Power C, Laffey JG. The analgesic efficacy of transversus abdominis plane block after abdominal surgery: a prospective randomized controlled trial. *Anesth Analg.* 2007;104:193–197.
21. O'Donnell BD, McDonnell JG, McShane AJ. The transversus abdominis plane (TAP) block in open retropubic prostatectomy. *Reg Anesth Pain Med.* 2006;31:91.
22. Bechara R, Inoue H. POEM, the prototypical "new NOTES" procedure and first successful NOTES procedure. *Gastrointest Endosc Clin N Am.* 2016;26:237–255.
23. Bhayani NH, Kurian AA, Dunst CM, Sharata AM, Rieder E, Swanstrom LL. A comparative study on comprehensive, objective outcomes of laparoscopic Heller myotomy with per-oral endoscopic myotomy (POEM) for achalasia. *Ann Surg.* 2014;259:1098–1103.
24. Kumbhari V, Tieu AH, Onimaru M, et al. Peroral endoscopic myotomy (POEM) versus laparoscopic Heller myotomy (LHM) for the treatment of type III achalasia in 75 patients: a multicenter comparative study. *Endosc Int Open.* 2015;3:E195–E201.
25. Hungness ES, Teitelbaum EN, Santos BF, et al. Comparison of perioperative outcomes between peroral esophageal myotomy (POEM) and laparoscopic Heller myotomy. *J Gastrointest Surg.* 2013;17:228–235.
26. Chan SM, Wu JC, Teoh AY, et al. Comparison of early outcomes and quality of life after laparoscopic Heller's cardiomyotomy to peroral endoscopic myotomy for treatment of achalasia. *Dig Endosc.* 2016;28:27–32.
27. Tanaka E, Murata H, Minami H, Sumikawa K. Anesthetic management of peroral endoscopic myotomy for esophageal achalasia: a retrospective case series. *J Anesth.* 2014;28:456–459.
28. Inoue H, Tianle KM, Ikeda H, et al. Peroral endoscopic myotomy for esophageal achalasia: technique, indication, and outcomes. *Thorac Surg Clin.* 2011;21:519–525.
29. Inoue H, Minami H, Kobayashi Y, et al. Peroral endoscopic myotomy (POEM) for esophageal achalasia. *Endoscopy.* 2010;42:265–271.
30. Pannu D, White JD, Draganov PV. Peroral endoscopic myotomy in the endoscopy unit: location, location, location. *Gastrointest Endosc.* 2016;83:126–128.
31. Yang D, Pannu D, Zhang Q, White JD, Draganov PV. Evaluation of anesthesia management, feasibility and efficacy of peroral endoscopic myotomy (POEM) for achalasia performed in the endoscopy unit. *Endosc Int Open.* 2015;3:E289–E295.
32. Cai M, Zhou P, Lourenco LC, Zhang D. Endoscopic full-thickness resection (EFTR) for gastrointestinal subepithelial tumors. *Gastrointest Endosc Clin N Am.* 2016;26:283–295.
33. Gonzalez JM, Lestelle V, Benezech A, et al. Gastric per-oral endoscopic myotomy with antropyloromyotomy in the treatment of refractory gastroparesis: clinical experience with follow-up and scintigraphic evaluation (with video). *Gastrointest Endosc.* 2017;85:132–139.
34. Gonzalez JM, Vanbiervliet G, Vitton V, et al. First European human gastric peroral endoscopic myotomy, for treatment of refractory gastroparesis. Endoscopy. 2015;47(suppl 1) UCTN:E135–E136.
35. Lebaras C, Swanstrom LL. Per-oral pyloromyotomy (POP): an emerging application of submucosal tunneling for the treatment of refractory gastroparesis. *Gastrointest Endosc Clin N Am.* 2016;26:257–270.
36. Shlomovitz E, Pescarus R, Cassera MA, et al. Early human experience with per-oral endoscopic pyloromyotomy (POP). *Surg Endosc.* 2015;29:543–551.
37. Anderloni A, Buda A, Vieceli F, Khashab MA, Hassan C, Repici A. Endoscopic ultrasound-guided transmural stenting for gallbladder drainage in high-risk patients with acute cholecystitis: a systematic review and pooled analysis. *Surg Endosc.* 2016;30:5200–5208.
38. Barbera C, Grande G, Alberghina N, Manno M, Conigliaro RL. Single-step endoscopic ultrasound-guided fluoroless gallbladder drainage using the Axios lumen-apposing metal stent. *Endoscopy.* 2016;48(suppl 1):E254.
39. Kumta NA, Lordello Passos M, Rodela Silva GL, Novikov A, Kahaleh M. Endoscopic ultrasound-guided transmural gallbladder drainage with a lumen-apposing metal stent using an electrocautery enhanced delivery system. *Endoscopy.* 2016;48:E327.
40. Sharaiha RZ, Tyberg A, Khashab MA, et al. Endoscopic therapy with lumen-apposing metal stents is safe and effective for patients with pancreatic walled-off necrosis. *Clin Gastroenterol Hepatol.* 2016;14:1797–1803.

22 | NEW CHALLENGES FOR ANESTHESIOLOGISTS OUTSIDE OF THE OPERATING ROOM: THE CARDIAC CATHETERIZATION AND ELECTROPHYSIOLOGY LABORATORIES

WENDY L. GROSS, MD, MHCM, LEBRON COOPER, MD, ROBERT T. FAILLACE, MD, SCM, DOUGLAS C. SHOOK, MD, SUANNE M. DAVES, MD, ROBERT M. SAVAGE, MD, FACC

INTRODUCTION

The character of invasive cardiology procedures has changed dramatically over the past 5–10 years. With technological advancement, diagnostic and therapeutic procedures have become broader in scope and complexity; patient acuity has dramatically escalated as well. In parallel, the involvement of anesthesiologists has grown. In this chapter, we present an overview of the laboratory environment(s), the evolution and future pathways of current practice(s), cases performed in each venue, and current anesthetic approaches.

Invasive cardiology procedures performed in the cardiac catheterization laboratory (CCL), the electrophysiology laboratory (EPL), and the transesophageal echocardiography (TEE) laboratory have become the purview of anesthesiologists. Common CCL procedures include the following: diagnostic cardiac catheterizations, percutaneous coronary interventions (PCIs), peripheral vascular diagnostic and therapeutic procedures, implantation of percutaneous left ventricular assist devices (p-LVADs), placement of septal defect or atrial appendage occlusion devices, and percutaneous valve repair or replacement procedures. Common EPL procedures consist of electrophysiology studies (EPSs), atrial and ventricular radio-frequency (RF) ablation procedures, implantation and removal of pacing and cardioverter/defibrillator devices, and electrical cardioversion. TEE procedures include diagnostic TEE and combined TEE/direct current cardioversions (DCCVs). All of these procedures may require the involvement of anesthesiologists if the patient has significant comorbidities or if the procedure requires that the patient be absolutely still or asleep.

Even without the added concern of patient comorbidities, modern procedures are often lengthy, requiring technical precision and focus on the part of the proceduralist. In such situations, preservation of hemodynamic stability and maintenance of a sedated or asleep state is often best left to anesthesiologists. In this new and changing arena, collaboration and planning between cardiologists and anesthesiologists maximize patient safety and increase the probability of procedural success. A thorough understanding of the procedure to be performed is required in order for anesthesiologists to define and delineate the extent of their involvement and is a clear prerequisite for the formulation of a safe and effective anesthetic plan. A common knowledge base and mutual respect for each contributing discipline form the basis for integration of cardiology and anesthesia services in pursuit of optimized patient care.

THE LABORATORY ENVIRONMENT: MAKING ROOM FOR ANESTHESIOLOGISTS

The laboratory environment differs significantly from that of the operating room. It is imperative that anesthesiologists become familiar with this new venue by understanding the objectives and flow of procedures as well as the structure and function of equipment and the responsibilities of personnel. Innovative flexibility on the part of the anesthesiologist is frequently necessary with respect to equipment availability/positioning and the tempo of anesthesiology-cardiology interaction.

All labs include a separate control station and procedure room. The control station, shielded from radiation, is the vantage point from which a technician usually records the progress of the procedure. The technician communicates with the cardiologist from outside of the procedure room and controls recording of data, patient monitoring, video recording and editing, and digital record-keeping. Robotic equipment is usually stationed outside of the procedure room as well, and catheter manipulations are sometimes made by the proceduralist from outside of the procedure room if a robotic device is used.

Within the procedure room itself, cardiologists, anesthesiologists, nurses, and other (radiology and cardiovascular) technicians care for the patient during the procedure. The procedure room includes fluoroscopy equipment, the procedure table, screens for viewing the procedure, sterile tables for the cardiologist, closets or portable storage units for various catheters and wires for the procedures, and blood analysis machines. The anesthesiologist should become familiar with the contents of each procedure room, which varies from institution to institution. Gas outlets and suction, monitors for vital signs, cardioverter/defibrillator, emergency medications, and airway equipment are critical and may not be optimally or even obviously placed. The anesthesiologist may have to become familiar with equipment not typically found in the operating room. Consistent locations for a ventilator, anesthesia machine, anesthesia cart, and fiber-optic cart should also be identified. Other frequently utilized equipment includes ventricular assist devices, intra-aortic balloon pumps, device programmers, cardiopulmonary bypass pumps, and echocardiography machines.

Catheterization labs and EP labs are designed for cardiologists, not for anesthesiologists. Space becomes an issue in complex cases, particularly when additional equipment is utilized. The fluoroscopy table and fluoroscopy equipment may be controlled by radiology technicians under the direction of cardiologists or by the cardiologists/electrophysiologists themselves. These move during the procedure to facilitate imaging. Extensions for intravenous lines, extra oxygen tubing, and long breathing circuits are often needed to allow for movement of the table and to accommodate fluoroscopy equipment.

Basic monitoring equipment for sedation, regional, or general anesthesia may not be present in the CCL and EPL. Capnography monitoring in all procedure rooms is as important for safe patient care outside of the operating room as it is in the operating room, perhaps even more so. Assisting with a sedation problem during a procedure can be more difficult if end-tidal CO_2 monitoring is not available. Similarly, the local availability of extra airway equipment and an emergency airway cart becomes essential when the anesthesia workroom is not nearby. An anesthesia cart stocked with intravenous equipment, medications, airway equipment, malignant hyperthermia cart, and medication essentials is important in the CCL and EPL. All personnel in the laboratory should know the location and names of emergency equipment because the anesthesiologist will be occupied with the patient if called emergently to a procedure area. Collaboration and preprocedure planning are truly essential.

ANESTHESIA CONSULTATION: WHEN SHOULD ANESTHESIOLOGISTS BE INVOLVED

Each institution has established guidelines for anesthesia consultation in the CCL and EPL, but criteria vary widely. Emergencies can be minimized by preprocedure planning and review of patient sedation needs. When patients present with significant comorbidities or when the procedure promises to be complicated or unusual, the covering anesthesiologist should be involved. Sometimes it is necessary to decide between sedation and general anesthesia, and often the determination must be made by both the cardiologist and the anesthesiologist together. Consultation based on patient presentation or procedure complexity is often initiated by nurses or physician assistants (PAs) involved in the case. Continuous communication is important so that all team members are aware of pertinent issues. Case management decisions and planning should include all team members to the extent possible.

Patient airway characteristics that should trigger an anesthesia consultation include morbid obesity, obstructive sleep apnea, inability to lie flat, and known or suspected difficult airways (Mallampati class III or IV). Nonanesthesiology personnel should be taught how to perform basic airway histories and exams in order to establish the need for consultation. Other pertinent patient comorbidities include chronic obstructive pulmonary disease, low oxygen saturation, current congestive heart failure, hemodynamic instability, psychiatric disorders, chronic pain syndromes, neurological disorders, inability to handle oral secretions, and the presence of acute ongoing syndromes. In addition, patients taking medications that could complicate the administration or alter the effectiveness of sedative agents should be seen by an anesthesiologist.

Sometimes the nature of the procedure itself prompts a provider to seek an anesthesia consultation. If the potential need for immediate surgical backup is increased, such as with unprotected left main coronary artery stenting or percutaneous valve procedures, the anesthesiologist may be asked to see the patient, either to provide support during the case or to be available in case of emergency. If the nature of the case is likely to precipitate instability (i.e., valvuloplasties in very elderly and frail patients), a consultation is also warranted. Such procedures are typically long and technically sophisticated. The undivided attention of the cardiologist is required, and there is benefit in having an anesthesiologist in the room whose attention is focused solely on airway and hemodynamic control. Complex arrhythmia ablation procedures, complicated lead extractions requiring laser equipment, and biventricular pacemaker procedures should also invite the attention of anesthesiologists because the procedures are potentially long and complex and the patients are typically challenging. Of course, any procedure performed under general anesthesia requires a preprocedure anesthesia workup.

Criteria for anesthesia consultation will lead to more efficient and safer patient care, but the criteria will fluctuate as drugs, personnel, and technology change. Better preprocedure planning, including interdisciplinary discussion to establish route of catheterization (radial vs. femoral), planned modification of patient positioning to accommodate body habitus, and avoidance of sedation-induced airway obstruction are critical so that intraprocedural complications are avoided. In this way, nonanesthesia personnel administering sedative medication can increase their vigilance about important details, cardiologists are free to focus on the fine points of the procedure at hand, and anesthesiologists are alerted to the potential complications they may be called on to manage during the case.

PATIENT ASSESSMENT FOR CARDIAC PROCEDURES OUTSIDE OF THE OPERATING ROOM

For some patients, a comprehensive preprocedure evaluation by an anesthesiologist is essential. A complete history not only includes a standard preanesthetic assessment but also must encompass a comprehensive review of all previous cardiac interventions: diagnostic catheterizations; stent placement (type, location, and age); known left- and right-sided cardiac pressures; surgical interventions; arrhythmia interventions and ablations; echocardiograms (ventricular function and dimensions, valve disease); chest x-rays, and a comprehensive medication list, along with recent changes to the medication regimen, particularly with respect to anticoagulation.

Many patients present for procedures after failed interventions, during or immediately after myocardial infarctions, during acute exacerbations of heart failure, or with uncontrolled arrhythmias. These patients represent a population not normally cared for electively in the operating room because current American College of Cardiology (ACC)/American Heart Association (AHA) guidelines for preoperative assessment[1] recommend cancellation of elective surgery under these conditions. In cardiac procedure rooms, as in the operating room, anesthesiologists must be keenly aware of the overall current medical condition of their patients. In some cases, due to the urgency of the case, the anesthesiologists may be the only care providers aware of recent changes in health status. The focus of the cardiologist may be on the cardiac and technical aspects of the intervention at hand. Frequently, the patient is referred from an outside source.

Establishing the true urgency of the procedure is important both for optimal outcome and in order to identify potential intra- and postprocedural complications and management considerations. Communication among nurses, radiology/cardiology technicians, anesthesiologists, interventionalists, and electrophysiologists is critical. Different perspectives and lack of common understanding may generate conflict. What may seem essential to an anesthesiologist may seem of secondary importance to a cardiologist and vice versa. Maintenance of patient flow can assume undue importance if the urgency of a case is not articulated. Patient optimization prior to procedures is important if it is possible to achieve. Diuresis, adjustment of medication, resolution of acute infection, and improvement of respiratory function may permit the patient to lie flat during the procedure, thereby increasing the probability of a successful result. Radial rather than femoral artery catheterization may be a better option in some patients because this permits the patient to sit up to some extent during the procedure. When patients present emergently, however, options are limited, and direct involvement of an anesthesiologist for sedation or general anesthesia becomes necessary. Under these circumstances, clear and direct communication between anesthesiology and cardiology attending physicians is critical.

Emergent airway management in an already-sedated patient can be challenging, particularly in the CCL and EPL environment. The fluoroscopy table is more limiting for anesthesiologists than an operating room table. The head of the bed cannot be elevated, and the cardiologist has the table controls, usually at the foot of the bed. Fluoroscopy equipment, particularly in rooms with biplane imaging capability, usually surrounds the patient's head. In addition, the patient may be hemodynamically unstable, further complicating airway management. Finally, personnel in the CCL and EPL do not have training in advanced airway management and are often not helpful or may even be unintentionally obstructive in an emergency.

Preprocedure and ongoing airway assessment is therefore critical in this environment. Not only should ease of endotracheal intubation be assessed, but also the ability to mask ventilate should be evaluated. Mask ventilation often bridges a moment of oversedation during a procedure. Langeron et al. identified five independent criteria associated with difficult mask ventilation (age > 55, body mass index [BMI] > 26, beard, lack of teeth, and history of snoring); the presence of two of these indicates possible difficult mask ventilation.[2] A history of difficult intubation or possible difficult intubation does not preclude sedation, but it should be a warning that rescue from oversedation might be problematic. Under such circumstances, all personnel involved in the procedure should be alerted. Training in mask ventilation should be ubiquitous so that the patient is covered if the anesthesiologist must come from another location to attend to the patient. The location of airway supplies should be standardized and known to all personnel. Early communication of and prompt response to sedation problems during the procedure are imperative. Remember that undersedation can be as dangerous as oversedation because it can lead to tachycardia, hypertension, and excessive patient movement.

THE SEDATION CONTINUUM: WHERE DO ANESTHESIOLOGISTS BELONG?

Many procedures in the CCL and EPL are performed under mild-to-moderate sedation administered by trained nonanesthesiologists, usually nurses who are supervised by nonanesthesiologist physicians. Local anesthetic infiltration at the site of catheter placement by the cardiologist alleviates pain while the proceduralist gains access. Nonanesthesia personnel administering mild-to-moderate sedation should be trained in the pharmacology of commonly used agents and in the use of monitoring equipment. Early recognition and management of abnormal respiratory patterns and hemodynamic problems that evolve during mild, moderate, and deep sedation[3] are also important. Personnel administering sedative agents should be able to safely manage the next deeper level of sedation. Caregivers must understand the potentially synergistic drug interactions of benzodiazepines, opioids, and other commonly administered sedatives, such as diphenhydramine (given to patients who have intravenous contrast reactions), especially in patients with complicated airways or diminished respiratory capacity. Anesthesiologists should take an active role in developing and maintaining sedation standards for nonanesthesia personnel throughout the hospital.[3]

Patients in the CCL and EPL are often sedated with fentanyl and midazolam. Minimal sedation with liberal use of local anesthetic is usually recommended for patients with complicated airways, obstructive symptoms, or respiratory or hemodynamic compromise. For these patients, anxiety and fear can be treated with verbal comfort, reassurance, and a small amount of midazolam. Avoidance of fentanyl eliminates the synergistic respiratory depressant effect and is usually well tolerated because most pain is alleviated once local anesthesia has been administered. Ondansetron, dexamethasone, and haloperidol can be used as antiemetics.

Anesthesiologists have a broad spectrum of medications available to them. Many are more conducive to rapid deepening of sedation than midazolam and fentanyl, and they have shorter redistribution times. Management of sedation needs must be based on a firm understanding of the procedure and a thorough grasp of the patient's comorbidities. It is critical to know when the patient is likely to be stimulated so that deeper sedation can be administered. Tachypnea and tachycardia resulting from inadequate sedation can be just as dangerous as airway obstruction or snoring from oversedation. Both situations can make interventions more difficult for the cardiologist and less safe for patients. In circumstances where brief unconsciousness is necessary during a procedure, the assistance of an anesthesiologist should be sought (i.e., implanted cardioverter/defibrillator [ICD] testing after implantation, deployment of percutaneous valves, and cardioversion during ablation).

In some cases, dexmedetomidine (α_2-agonist) may be ideal for sedation because there is less respiratory depression associated with its administration.[4] In EPL patients, dexmedetomidine should be carefully considered because it may cause sympatholysis, which can be counterproductive when trying to induce arrhythmias for either diagnosis or treatment (ablation).

If the complexity of the procedure or comorbidities of the patient indicate that nurse-administered sedation is not appropriate, then an anesthesiologist should be involved in the care so that deep sedation or general anesthesia can be administered. Persistent oversedation with repeated reversal using naloxone and flumazenil is not recommended and is considered a reportable event in some jurisdictions. In most instances, it is safer to start a procedure with general anesthesia than to convert during the procedure. However, recent studies suggested that there may be an advantage to anesthesiologist-administered sedation, versus general anesthesia, in percutaneous aortic valve procedures.[5]

MONITORING

Patient monitoring in the CCL and EPL is often designed with the cardiologist in mind. The fluoroscopy screen and patient vital signs are easy for the cardiologist to see, but they may be 90° from the anesthesiologist if he or she is at the head of the bed. Establishing the best location from which to view the necessary monitors may involve changing the current room setup. Being able to see the fluoroscopy screen is helpful in monitoring the progress of the procedure and is helpful in anticipating changes in hemodynamics or comfort level. The anesthesiologist may have to ask the cardiologist frequently for progress reports if the fluoroscopy screen is not visible from the head of the bed.

Because some monitoring functions, such as cycling of blood pressure cuffs and adjustment of pulse oximetry volume, are typically controlled by cardiovascular technicians outside of the actual procedure room, the anesthesiologist may find that utilizing his or her equipment is preferable. During prolonged cases or with compromised patients (or both), invasive arterial monitoring with a display visible to the anesthesiologist may be preferable. It is worth remembering that blood pressure cuffs may not function during fast or erratic heart rhythms. It may be difficult for the anesthesiologist to see pressure waveforms if they are displayed only on the cardiologists screen. Therefore, it may be worth the effort to attach a Y-adapter at the transducer in order to display the arterial waveform at the anesthesia machine or other equipment close to the anesthesiologist. Some CCLs and EPLs may not have end-tidal CO_2 monitoring readily available. End-tidal CO_2 monitoring is recommended, especially for patients who might unintentionally become deeply sedated or whose respiratory status is difficult to ascertain.[3] The American Society of Anesthesiologists (ASA) has established monitoring guidelines for sedation by anesthesia and nonanesthesia personnel in non–operating room locations.[3,6]

Many centers rely on TEE to guide procedures and monitor the patient during various CCL and EPL procedures. Cardiac anesthesiology presence is therefore preferred, although some institutions utilize cardiology TEE staff for this purpose. A complete TEE exam encompassing standard views and assessment of cardiac function allows the anesthesiologist to assist the cardiologist in evaluating the progress of the case, the hemodynamic status of the patient, and any potential complications. If hemodynamic instability occurs, TEE provides instant assessment of contractility, volume status, and valve function. In some labs, the TEE image is incorporated into the screen visible to the cardiologist; if this is not the case, it is helpful to position the TEE screen so that it is visible to the cardiologist performing the procedure as well as the anesthesiologist performing the TEE. Often, fluoroscopy and TEE together are critical to guide the progress of an intervention.

MEDICATIONS

In addition to the standard medications used for sedation and general anesthesia, the anesthesiologist must be aware of medications used in the CCL and EPL, including their pharmacokinetics and pharmacodynamics. Medications include heparin, glycoprotein IIb/IIIa platelet receptor inhibitors, clopidogrel, direct thrombin inhibitors such as bivalirudin, and vasoactive and inotropic medications. In addition, many patients in the EPL are treated with a variety of antiarrhythmic agent classes. Common medications include sodium channel blockers (class 1: quinidine, lidocaine, flecainide); β-blockers (class 2: metoprolol, sotalol); potassium channel blockers (class 3: amiodarone, sotalol, ibutilide, dofetilide); and calcium channel blockers (class 4: verapamil, diltiazem).

Prior to the procedure, it must be made clear how medications will be delivered to the patient and who will administer them. The cardiologist usually directs the nurse in the room to administer drugs such as heparin and vasoactive and inotropic medications. In addition, the cardiologist may directly bolus medications such as nitroglycerine or calcium channel blockers into cardiac catheters, which can have a profound effect on the patient's hemodynamics. Communication must be clear so that cardiologists and anesthesiologists are both aware of when drugs are administered and so that subsequent hemodynamic effects can be anticipated and double dosing can be avoided.

A clear understanding of the procedure to be performed is important in order to be able to anticipate the anesthetic needs of the patient. Many of the procedures performed in the CCL and EPL are individually tailored for patients, so it is frequently necessary for the anesthesiologist to ask the cardiologist what is going on. Unlike in the operating room, it is often difficult to ascertain the progress of an intervention. It is important not only that each practitioner communicates his or her thoughts and actions but also that each ascertains that the other is aware of any intervention. The following section describes the history and process of common interventions, along with some of the relevant anesthetic considerations. Considerable attention must be given to room setup, availability and choice of anesthesia equipment, and preprocedure patient evaluation, as previously indicated.

PERCUTANEOUS CORONARY INTERVENTIONS

In recent years, PCI procedures for patients with both stable coronary artery disease and acute coronary syndromes have proliferated.[7] In 2007, a total of 525,654 PCI stent (79,769 non–drug-eluting and 445,885 drug-eluting stents) procedures were performed in the United States.[7] Presently, the spectrum of PCIs include coronary angioplasty mostly performed immediately prior to coronary stenting, with use of both bare metal stents and drug-eluting stents; atherectomy procedures with use of a diamond-tipped burr catheter applied at high rotational speeds to "pulverize" atherosclerotic plaque; and intracoronary thrombectomy procedures for removal of intracoronary thrombus in patients with acute ischemic syndromes (unstable angina, non-ST elevation myocardial infarction, or more commonly with ST elevation myocardial infarction).[8] In the stable coronary artery disease setting, PCI procedures are commonly performed on patients with 70% or greater intracoronary luminal atherosclerotic obstruction and demonstrated myocardial ischemia. Although PCI has not been shown to decrease the risk of myocardial infarction or prolong life in stable nonacute ischemic syndrome, its major benefit is to reduce or relieve symptoms of ischemic heart disease and increase aerobic capacity.[9] The COURAGE Trial demonstrated that no significant difference in total mortality, nonfatal myocardial infarction, or other major cardiovascular events existed between randomized patients treated with aggressive medical therapy or aggressive medical therapy along with PCI angioplasty with bare metal stenting.[10] However, in patients presenting with acute coronary syndromes, PCI has been shown to decrease mortality and decrease recurrent myocardial infarction when compared to medical treatment without invasive intervention.[11–13]

Recent studies demonstrated a similar benefit of PCI for left main coronary artery disease in selected patients.[14–16] The SYNTAX trial demonstrated that there was no significant difference at 1 year in the composite endpoint of death, myocardial infarction, stroke, or repeat revascularization between the subgroup with left main coronary artery disease who underwent coronary artery bypass surgery versus those who underwent PCI with stenting.[17]

The most recent 2009 guideline update for PCI has now made left main coronary artery stenting a class IIB indication (usefulness/efficacy less well established by evidence/opinion) as an alternative to coronary bypass graft therapy in patients who may be at increased surgical risk and who have anatomic left main coronary obstruction that is associated with low risk of a PCI complication.[8] An analysis of the American college of Cardiology-National Cardiovascular Data Registry (ACC-NCDR) demonstrated an increase in the use of stenting for unprotected (>50% stenosis without prior coronary artery bypass graft [CABG] surgery) left main coronary artery disease in both elective and urgent/emergent clinical settings along with a concomitant decrease of CABG.[18] A recent meta-analysis of 16 observational studies involving 1278 patients undergoing drug-eluting stent PCI for left main coronary artery disease demonstrated a 2.3% in-hospital mortality rate and a 5.5% mortality rate at a median of 10 months following the procedure.[19]

Although target-vessel revascularization was significantly higher in those patients who received stents (hazard ratio, 4.76; 95% confidence interval, 0.75 to 1.62), the Korean-based MAIN-COMPARE study demonstrated no difference in either death or a composite outcome of death, Q-wave myocardial infarction, or stroke for those patients who underwent either PCI (with bare metal or drug-eluting stents) or CABG surgery in matched cohorts of patients with unprotected left main coronary artery disease followed on average for 3 years.[14,20] However, this study showed that patients who received drug-eluting stents had a better outcome, with a trend toward lower rates of death and the composite endpoint of death, Q-wave myocardial infarction, or stroke compared to those patients who underwent CABG.

Percutaneous coronary interventions are commonly performed using mild-to-moderate sedation under the direction of the cardiologist. Anesthesiologists are usually involved when patients present with respiratory insufficiency or hemodynamic compromise.

When sedation-related complications or acute patient decompensation occur, anesthesiologists are called emergently. Close communication with the cardiologist is imperative because management decisions usually need to be made expeditiously. Information such as recent medications given, intravenous access, invasive monitoring, and stage of the procedure must be obtained. Access to the patient's head can be difficult, as mentioned previously. If an airway needs to be established, priority must be given to the anesthesiologist to temporarily move the table and fluoroscopy equipment. Placement of an endotracheal tube is preferred to a laryngeal mask airway (LMA). In general, LMAs are not recommended in the CCL and EPL because the constant movement of the fluoroscopy equipment and table can dislodge the LMA. In addition, patients can become acutely unstable, and having an endotracheal tube eliminates the need to further manage an airway in a crisis.

PERCUTANEOUS VENTRICULAR ASSIST DEVICES

Percutaneous left ventricular assist devices are placed in the CCL to support the failing heart in various clinical settings, that is, cardiogenic shock associated with myocardial infarction or hemodynamic compromise with severe left ventricular dysfunction from other etiologies. These p-LVADs have the capability to support patients in cardiogenic shock until either a recovery occurs or more definitive therapy is administered in the acute setting.[21] These devices are also utilized to support patients who are undergoing high-risk PCI procedures.[21] The TandemHeart (Cardiac Assist, Inc., Pittsburg, PA) and the Impella Recover LP 2.5 and 5.0 (Abiomed, Inc., Danvers, MA) are two commercially available percutaneous ventricular assist devices.[21–26]

The TandemHeart comprises a transeptal cannula, an arterial cannula, and an externally located centrifugal blood pump. This device is percutaneously inserted via the femoral vein and transeptally placed in the left atrium to create a left atrial to (contralateral) left femoral artery bypass system. The pump can deliver flow rates of up to 4.0 L/min at a maximum speed of 7500 rpm.[21] Use of the TandemHeart device has been reported to be associated with a 30-day survival rate of 61% in 18 patients (11 in cardiogenic shock and 7 undergoing high-risk PCI) in one center. The device helped patients in cardiogenic shock improve their cardiac index from 1.57 ± 0.31 L/min/m^2 to 2.60 ± 0.34 L/min/m^2.[21] The mean duration of p-LVAD support was 88 ± 74.3 hours (range, 4–264 hours).[21]

Similar p-LVADs are the Impella Recover LP 2.5 and 5.0 pump devices.[22] The Impella Recover LP 2.5 and 5.0 pump systems both utilize a cannula inserted in a retrograde fashion, via the femoral artery, across the aortic valve and into the left ventricle.[23] Their ease of implantation, avoidance of the need for a transeptal puncture, and smaller catheter size (13 French vs. 17 French) are advantages over the TandemHeart. In addition, there is no extracorporeal blood because the microaxial pump is integrated directly into the catheter system. Circulatory support of either 2.5 L/min or 5.0 L/min can be achieved with the Impella devices. Patient selection must be carefully considered.[23]

Percutaneous ventricular assist devices (TandemHeart and Impella Recover LP 2.5 or 5.0) are placed in patients who are having high-risk PCI (unprotected left main) or high-risk ablation procedures or who are or may become hemodynamically compromised (cardiogenic shock) during any procedure.[21,24,25] The anesthesiologist is most often consulted for these procedures because the patient is usually already unstable or the procedure can have both airway and hemodynamic complications. Depending on the procedure and state of the patient, either sedation or general anesthesia can be used to care for the patient. Communication between anesthesiologist and cardiologist should determine the type of anesthetic most appropriate for the case.

The TandemHeart and Impella LP 5.0 produce cardiac outputs that can completely replace left ventricular function. During this time, pulse oximetry and noninvasive blood pressure cuffs may not work properly because blood flow may not be pulsatile. The Impella LP 2.5 uses a smaller cannula that achieves a maximum cardiac output of 2.5 L/min. The patient must have some intrinsic cardiac function to maintain hemodynamic stability.

Invasive monitoring is available because arterial cannulation is used during the procedure. Large-bore intravenous access is desirable because significant blood loss is possible during the procedure.[26] Blood loss is more likely with the TandemHeart or Impella LP 5.0 because the cannulas used are larger. Surgical backup may be necessary during these procedures. The anesthesiologist should be in touch with the operating room and confirm that backup is available.

PERCUTANEOUS CLOSURE OF SEPTAL DEFECTS

The placement of intracardiac atrial septal occluder devices requires an anesthesiologist if TEE is used to guide placement of the device; the alternative is for the cardiologist to use intracardiac or intravascular echo. In 2001, the US Food and Drug Administration (FDA) approved the AMPLATZER™ Septal Occluder (AGA Medical Corp., Golden Valley, MN) as a treatment for a secundum atrial septal defect (ASD) and for patients who have undergone a fenestrated Fontan procedure requiring closure of the fenestration.[27] In 2005, the FDA approved the Gore Helex septal occluder (W. L. Gore and Associates, Flagstaff, AZ) for the percutaneous, transcatheter closure of ostium secundum ASDs. The Helex implant (W. L. Gore and Associates); the Premere PFO Closure System (St. Jude Medical, Inc., Maple Grove, MN); the Solysafe Septal Occluder (Swissimplant AG, Soluthurn, Switzerland); the IntraSept Occluder (CARDIA, Inc., Burnsville, MN); the Occlutech Device (Occlutech, Jena, Germany); the SeptR Occluder (Secant Medical, Perkasie, PA); the BioSTAR Septal Occluder, the first partially bioabsorbable septal repair implant (NMT Medical, Boston, MA); the SuperStich Device (Sutura, Inc., Fountain Valley, CA); and the PFx System (Cierra, Inc., Redwood City, CA) are other devices that are currently available.[28] A unique occluder device, the PFx System uses vacuum suction to hold the septum primum and secundum in place and RF energy to directly close the patent foramen ovale (PFO).[28] Despite widespread use, there presently has not been any prospective randomized controlled trial of percutaneous closure of PFOs in patients who have suffered from a cryptogenic stroke. Therefore, the FDA has not approved the use of percutaneous occluder devices for the prevention of recurrent cryptogenic stroke.[29] Nonetheless, we describe the AMPLATZER and the CardioSEAL™ (Nitinol Medical Technologies, Inc., Boston, MA) devices because they are routinely utilized in clinical practice.

The AMPLATZER Septal Occluder provides a permanently implanted, percutaneous-based delivery system comprising a two-sided "clamshell"-appearing occluder.[30] This clamshell comprises two flat disks with a middle or "waist." Nitinol wire mesh, a wire made from an alloy of nickel and titanium, along with polyester fabric inserts are the materials that comprise the disks. These fabric inserts provide a foundation for growth of tissue over the occluder after placement on either side of a PFO or an ASD.[29] Advantages of the AMPLATZER Septal Occluder include the following:

1. Smaller overall size with the delivery through smaller catheters
2. Round retention disks that extend radially beyond the defect, allowing firmer contact and enhancing endothelialization, therefore reducing the risk of residual shunting
3. Easy repositioning with a self-centering mechanism[31]

The CardioSEAL device is composed of two self-expanding Dacron patch–covered umbrellas that attach to either side of the intra-atrial septum. The umbrellas are formed by four central radiating metal arms attached to each other in the center. In order to minimize arm fractures and protrusion of the arm through the ASD, the device was reengineered with a self-centering mechanism consisting of nitinol springs. These springs connect the two umbrellas and a flexible core wire with a pin-pivoting connection. The name of the device is the STARflex, and it has significantly reduced the rate of arm fractures.[32,33]

Patients with recurrent cryptogenic stroke due to presumed paradoxical embolism through a PFO and who have failed conventional drug therapy have undergone atrial septal occlusion, although these devices have not yet been approved for this indication.[34] Muscular and perimembranous ventricular septal defects (VSDs; either congenital or acquired) have also been successively closed 96% of the time with a 2% major complication rate with these devices.[35] Success rates for closure of PFOs and ASDs have ranged from 79% to 100% after several years.[26]

Complications of percutaneous closure devices include, but are not limited to, the following: intraprocedure air embolism; device embolization; device malpositioning; device thrombosis and embolization (cerebral embolization may occur from air, a piece of the device itself, or a thrombus) during or following the procedure; device-related arrhythmias (usually atrial but include sudden death); and cardiac perforation with or without cardiac tamponade.[26,36–40] These complications must be immediately recognized, evaluated, and treated to either prevent permanent sequelae or minimize their impact.[38] TEE or intracardiac echocardiography (ICE) help guide the placement of these devices at the time of implantation. Because the procedure requires that the patient remain still and quiet, the use of TEE requires endotracheal intubation and general anesthesia. Although intracardiac ultrasound does not require endotracheal intubation or general anesthesia, implantation of septal occluder devices still demands the presence of a cardiac anesthesiologist. This team approach allows the operator to focus his or her attention on proper device placement and to remain vigilant for any complication that may arise while patients receive optimal anesthetic care.

Procedures such as these are used to close PFOs, ASDs, and VSDs. Patient history is important to determine the reason to close the defect. Closure of PFOs tends to be simpler than closure of ASDs. In patients with ASDs, it is important to determine whether right ventricular function and pulmonary arterial pressures are normal because the right side of the heart has been volume overloaded due to the typical left-to-right shunt through the ASD. In patients with VSDs, the anesthesiologist needs to determine whether the VSD is congenital or acquired (postmyocardial infraction) and the direction of flow through the defect. Typically, VSDs have left-to-right flow. Patients with postmyocardial infarction VSDs can be hemodynamically unstable and may be more likely to have complications (hypotension, arrhythmias) during closure of the defect.[41,42] Complications with any device placement in the CCL include air embolism, device embolization, malposition, thrombosis and embolization (pulmonary or systemic), arrhythmias (atrioventricular [AV] nodal block), hypotension, valve dysfunction, and cardiac perforation.[26,40,43]

Echocardiography is used during the procedure to help guide placement and confirm a successful result. If TEE is used, then general anesthesia will be necessary for the procedure. ICE can also be used to guide the procedure. If ICE is used, the procedure can be performed under sedation.[44] The determination of sedation versus general anesthesia should be based on the complexity of the closure and patient medical history.

If arterial monitoring is needed and the cardiologist is not planning femoral arterial access, a radial arterial line should be placed by the anesthesiologist. Two intravenous lines should be available so that one can be used for boluses and the other for infusions. The cardiologist can place a femoral venous line for infusions if necessary.

PERIPHERAL ARTERIAL DISEASE

The prevalence of peripheral arterial disease (PAD) increases with age and occurs more commonly in African Americans.[45] At the present time, it is estimated that PAD afflicts approximately 8 million Americans.[45] Atherosclerotic occlusion of the peripheral arteries is the main etiologic factor.[46] Men have a slightly higher prevalence than women.[47] Intermittent claudication and rest pain are the principal symptoms. *Claudicare* is the Latin derivative of "claudication" and means "to limp."[48] Claudication symptoms are due to insufficient arterial blood flow and leg ischemia. Patients suffering from intermittent claudication have symptoms of pain, aching, and a sense of fatigue or other discomfort that is experienced in the affected muscle group during exercise, especially walking, and relieved at rest.[48] Symptoms are most often experienced in the muscle bed supplied by the most proximal stenosis.[48] Buttock, hip, or thigh claudication is related to obstruction of the aorta or iliac flow. Calf claudication commonly is a result of either femoral or popliteal arterial stenosis, and either tibial or peroneal disease causes ankle or pedal claudication.[48]

According to ACC/AHA guidelines, percutaneous revascularization in patients with intermittent claudication should be considered when any one of the following circumstances is encountered:

1. Claudication symptoms significantly disable the patient, resulting in an inability to perform normal work or other activities that are important.
2. The patient is able to benefit from an improvement in claudication (i.e., exercise is not limited by another cause, such as angina, heart failure, chronic obstructive pulmonary disease, or orthopedic problems).
3. Exercise rehabilitation and pharmacologic therapy have not been successful in providing the patient with an adequate response.
4. A very favorable risk-benefit ratio to performing the procedure exists with a high likelihood of initial and long-term success.
5. The characteristics of the lesion permit appropriate intervention at low risk with a high likelihood of initial and long-term success; and/or the patient has limb-threatening ischemia, as manifested by rest pain, ischemic ulcers, or gangrene.[47–50]

Epidural anesthesia may attenuate stress responses and reduce the production of acute-phase reactants, leading to reduction in hypercoagulation-related complications in lower extremity stent procedures.[51] Equipment for general anesthesia must be available if regional anesthesia is to be administered. As most of these patients are on antithrombotic medications (e.g., clopidogrel, aspirin, warfarin, or heparin) given during the procedure, a major concern is the risk for an epidural or a spinal hematoma.[52,53] However, the anesthesiologist may be critical to the interventional cardiologist/vascular surgeon during a peripheral vascular intervention because many of these patients are unable to lie still during the procedure because of resting claudication symptoms. In addition, painful transient ischemia may occur as a result of the procedure itself. The resulting patient movement may further increase the risk of complication.

PERCUTANEOUS VALVE REPAIR AND REPLACEMENT

Newer percutaneous techniques for the treatment of mitral regurgitation and percutaneous aortic valve replacement have recently been developed and are presently under investigation and in clinical trials.[54–56]

Percutaneous Mitral Valve Repair

At the present time, cardiac surgical mitral valve repair is the procedure of choice for the treatment of symptomatic mitral regurgitation or mitral regurgitation with "impaired" left ventricular ejection fraction (<60%). However, current techniques under investigation for percutaneous mitral valve repair include coronary sinus annuloplasty, direct annuplasty, leaflet repair, and chamber plus annular remodeling.[57]

The annular circumference of the mitral annulus can be decreased with placement of a device in the coronary sinus because the sinus overlies the annulus.[57] One device utilizes a connecting spring to bridge anchors or stents percutaneously placed in the coronary sinus ostium and the distal coronary sinus (Monarc device, Edwards Lifesciences, Inc., Orange, CA). As the spring shortens, tension develops and the coronary sinus is pulled, diminishing the annular diameter. Another percutaneous coronary device system, the Carillon Mitral Contour System (Cardiac Dimensions, Kirkland, WA), uses a Nitinol wire-shaping ribbon between the proximal and distal anchors.[58–60] These devices are presently in clinical trials. In about half of patients, however, the coronary sinus crosses over branches of the circumflex coronary artery, and in many patients the coronary sinus does not directly parallel the mitral annulus.[61] Therefore, circumflex coronary artery compression can occur at the time of implantation, and cinching the coronary sinus may not change annular diameter. In the case of the Monarc device, circumflex coronary artery compression may occur later as the biodegradable material in the spring spaces absorbs and the spring element shortens over a period of weeks to months.[57] Coronary sinus erosion and thrombosis are other potential complications. Therefore, the safety and the efficacy of the coronary sinus approach in the treatment of mitral regurgitation are yet to be determined.

In surgical contexts, Alfieri et al. previously demonstrated that suturing of the free mitral valve leaflet edges of the midpart of the line of mitral coaptation creates a double-orifice mitral valve.[62,63] This technique also has had mixed clinical results[64,65] as a way of reducing mitral regurgitation. However, in selected patients, isolated edge-to-edge mitral valve repair may be durable, with 5-year 90% freedom from reoperation and mitral regurgitation greater than 2+.[66]

A percutaneously delivered device under investigation (MitraClip) duplicates the Alfieri edge-to-edge repair (Evalve, San Francisco, CA). Following a transatrial-septal puncture, the clip is positioned in the center of the mitral valve orifice. The mitral valve leaflets are grasped by opening the clip, passing it into the left ventricular cavity, and drawing it back to come in contact with the mitral valve leaflets. The clip is closed to create a double-orifice mitral valve.[67,68] A phase 1 clinical trial demonstrated 2-year freedom from death, mitral valve surgery, or recurrent mitral regurgitation greater than 2+ in up to 80% of patients receiving successful clip deployment.[69] This phase 1 trial success of the Evalve clip procedure has led to a randomized trial comparing this procedure to mitral valve surgery in selected patients, the EVEREST II trial.[57] General anesthesia, fluoroscopy, and TEE to help guide placement of the device are part of the Evalve procedure.[26]

Percutaneous Aortic Valve Replacement

Anderson and Pavcnik performed the initial animal work in the development of percutaneous aortic valve replacement, and Cribier developed the first percutaneous heart valve for humans.[70,71] Percutaneous aortic valve replacement trials were previously open only for patients with severe aortic stenosis, New York Heart Association (NYHA) class IV symptoms related to their aortic stenosis, and comorbidities excluding them from cardiac surgery due to excessive risk.[72] However, ongoing randomized controlled clinical trials are in progress comparing surgical aortic valve replacement (SAVR) to percutaneous aortic valve replacement in patients who are candidates for cardiac surgery using newer generation percutaneous aortic prosthetic valves.[73] Depending on the trial results and future technological advances, some experts in this field believe that percutaneous aortic valve replacement may be a viable option for a patient in need of a prosthetic aortic valve to avoid the concomitant complications inherent in open heart surgery.[73]

The Cribier-Edwards valve (Cribier-Edwards aortic valve, Edwards Lifesciences, Irvine, CA) has three bovine pericardial leaflets sutured to a stainless steel balloon expandable stent. This valve is crimped on an aortic valvuloplasty balloon that is expandable to 23 or 26 mm (NuMed, Inc., Hopkinton, NY). An antegrade approach using a transatrial septal puncture delivers this system through a 24-French (8-mm) sheath. The percutaneous valve is then positioned across the native aortic valve and delivered with rapid inflation and deflation of a balloon. High-rate pacing temporarily minimizes antegrade aortic flow.[72] In a recently reported series of 35 patients undergoing this procedure, 27 patients underwent a successful implantation with improvement of aortic valve area and left ventricular function.[74] Moderately severe aortic insufficiency developed in five patients, and no patients developed a device-related death in 9 to 26 months of follow-up.[74]

Technological advances are rapidly occurring in this domain. A self-expanding percutaneous aortic valve consisting of a bioprosthetic pericardial tissue valve sutured into a Nitinol metal stent is in development (CoreValve, Paris, France).[72] Preliminary results indicated that one advantage of a self-expanding stent-valve system is lack of significant aortic regurgitation.[72] The AorTx (Redwood City, CA), another percutaneously delivered aortic valve, can be retrieved after deployment. Technological advancement will improve delivery systems so that valves are easier and safer to deploy.[72]

Edwards Lifesciences Corporation announced European approval for commercial release of the Edwards Sapien transcatheter aortic valve technology with the Retroflex transfemoral delivery system on September 5, 2007.[75] The profile of this bovine pericardial tissue valve constructed with a cobalt chromium alloy stent reduces the profile of the system by 4 to 5 French as compared to the other systems described previously. This system allows easier access into and within the patient's vasculature, potentially reducing the risk of procedural complication.[76] This valve is presently being studied in the PARTNER Trial: Placement of AoRTic TranNscathetER Valve Trial in high-risk symptomatic patients with severe aortic stenosis.[76] This valve may also be placed in the aortic position via a transapical approach with the Ascendra delivery system, which is also being studied in the PARTNER Trial.[76]

The initial clinical experience for transapical transcatheter aortic valve implantation was first reported in 2006.[77] An anterolateral intercostal incision is used to expose the left ventricular apex. Direct needle puncture of the left ventricular apex allows introduction of a hemostatic sheath into the left ventricle. The prosthetic valve is placed into the left ventricular cavity after being crimped onto a valvuloplasty balloon and passed over a wire. Proper positioning is confirmed by fluoroscopy, aortography, and echocardiography. Rapid ventricular pacing is utilized to decrease cardiac output while the balloon is inflated and the prosthesis is deployed within the annulus. The initial experience was reported on seven patients. There were no procedural deaths. However, one death occurred within 87 ± 56 days.[76] More recently, other reports in the literature have demonstrated safety, with good early results in high-risk patients.[78,79]

The final 5-year outcomes PARTNER I trial results, comparing SAVR to transcatheter aortic valve replacement (TAVR), were published in 2015. TAVR was found to be noninferior to SAVR in all-cause mortality, cardiovascular mortality, all stroke, and mortality at 1 year.[80] The 2-year results of the CoreValve US Pivotal Trial of patients with extreme risk for surgery found TAVR to be noninferior or superior to SAVR, with low rates of perivalvular leaks and improvement in NYHA classifications by at least one or two levels.[81] The 3-year CoreValve US Pivotal Trial for extreme- or high-risk surgical patients found a superiority of TAVR over SAVR, and the NOTION Trial of all comers found no significant difference between TAVR and SAVR in death, stroke, and myocardial infarction in both low- and intermediate-risk patients.[82,83] The SAPIEN XT PARTNER II 2-year results of patients with intermediate risk for surgery found TAVR to be superior to SAVR for intermediate-risk patients, and the SAPIEN 3 PARTNER II trial 1-year results showed TAVR to be noninferior *and* superior to SAVR for intermediate-risk patients.[84,85] The authors concluded that "TAVR might be the preferred treatment alternative in intermediate-risk patients." It is too soon to tell if these early results will hold in the future; however, TAVR appears to be a viable alternative that is not going away any time soon for the treatment of aortic valve disease.

Although all of these procedures are investigational, they represent the changing paradigm of interventional cardiology procedures; procedures are more complex with increased patient acuity. Experts increasingly are recommending that the care of these patients requires the same level of expertise as anesthesiology in cardiac surgery, and that anesthesia departments are responsible for training and assigning dedicated anesthesiologists to these cases.[86,87] The 2014 AHA/ACC Guidelines for the Management of Patients With Valvular Heart Disease state that the clinical team should consist of "a multi-disciplinary, collaborative group of caregivers, including cardiologists, structural valve interventionalists, cardiovascular imaging specialists, cardiovascular surgeons, *anesthesiologists* [emphasis added], and nurses, all of whom have expertise in the management and outcomes of patient with complex valvular heart disease."[88] Medical and surgical approaches to complex cardiac patient care are now sharing common ground. Anesthesiologists must be prepared for this new and changing patient population.

All percutaneous mitral valve repairs are performed under general anesthesia with fluoroscopic and TEE guidance. Patients typically have moderate-to-severe mitral regurgitation. The type of device and approach should be communicated prior to the procedure.[57,79]

During percutaneous valve replacements/repairs, the procedure room is very crowded. Planning for equipment deployment can be difficult for anesthesiologists. It is well worth taking time to look the room over before the case. Sometimes, two anesthesiologists are needed because TEE guidance is often critical. Two peripheral intravenous lines should be placed for infusions and boluses. Endotracheal intubation is required if TEE is used, and arterial monitoring is important because noninvasive blood pressure cuffs will not work when the patient goes into a fast rhythm. Communication during the procedure is vital to successful placement of the device, as the case can be long and multiple attempts may be needed to ensure proper device placement with an acceptable result.

Percutaneous aortic valve replacement involves patients who are extremely ill. Patients have severe aortic stenosis, NYHA class IV symptoms, and comorbidities excluding them from cardiac surgery due to excessive risk.[72] Fluoroscopy and TEE are used to guide device placement. Patients frequently become hemodynamically unstable during the case and can develop myocardial ischemia and significant arrhythmias. Many patients receive general endotracheal anesthesia and invasive monitoring. Central intravenous access may be preferable for infusion of necessary medications.

EVOLUTION IN THE MAKING: THE PEDIATRIC CARDIAC CATHETERIZATION LABORATORY

A description of anesthetic care in 1954 in the pediatric CCL[90] instructs the anesthetist and anesthesiologist to consider the following:

- The type of patients who will undergo this procedure
- The details of the procedure itself and how to provide ideal conditions
- The potential complications of the procedure
- The challenges produced by the environment (remote access to patient, exposure to radiation, etc.)

Over half a century later, while these tenets still hold true, the increasing complexity of the patient population and the transition from diagnostic to transcatheter or combined surgical and transcatheter (hybrid) interventions have drastically changed the landscape of the pediatric CCL.[91,92]

THE PATIENTS

First, consider the profile of the patients who will be selected for cardiac catheterization: With advances in echocardiography, magnetic resonance imaging/angiography, and computed tomographic angiography, diagnosis of congenital heart disease and presurgical evaluation are accomplished noninvasively in the majority of patients. Patients are small and have a complex anatomy. They often present for preoperative stabilization or transcatheter interventions to correct postoperative defects.[93] For example, the neonate with parallel circulation and inadequate mixing of systemic and pulmonary venous returns may present to the catheterization laboratory for balloon atrial septostomy in cardiogenic shock associated with profound hypoxemia and lactic acidosis.[94] Hybrid palliation is often used to stabilize the tenuous parallel circulation of the critically ill neonate with hypoplastic left heart syndrome. Table 22.1 demonstrates the complexity of this particular patient population who may present to the catheterization suite for a combined surgical and transcatheter intervention.[95]

The patient with a failing Fontan circulation may present moribund for diagnostic catheterization in anticipation of possible Fontan revision or transcatheter fenestration of the Fontan pathway. Ventricular dysfunction, arrhythmias, hepatic and renal insufficiency, marginal cerebral perfusion pressure, thromboembolic complications, and poor vascular access are frequent sequelae of the failing cavopulmonary circulation. Positive pressure ventilation, often a supportive modality in the patient with biventricular circulation, may cause acute deterioration of hemodynamics in these patients.

TABLE 22.1. Characteristics of Neonates With Hypoplastic Left Heart Syndrome (HLHS) for Hybrid Versus Norwood Palliation

VARIABLE	HYBRID (N = 14)	NORWOOD (N = 19)	P VALUE
Age (days)	4.3 ± 3.4	3.5 ± 1.6	.96
Weight (kg)	2.6 ± 0.6	2.7 ± 0.04	.77
ACS	19.3 ± 3.1	18.3 ± 2.6	.46
Asc Ao (mm)	3.2 ± 1.7	2.7 ± 1.0	.13
Lowest pH	7.14 ± 0.2	7.29 ± 0.05	.040
Ao atresia	6 (43%)	12 (63%)	.15
Additional cardiac factors	3 (21.4%)	13 (68.4%)	.009
Organ dysfunction	9 (64%)	5 (26%)	.03
Genetic/ chromosomal	3 (21.4%)	4 (21.8%)	.78
LBW (<2.5 kg)	5 (35.7%)	6 (31.5%)	.54
Prematurity (<36 weeks)	4 (28.5%)	4 (21%)	.46

ACS, Aristotle comprehensive score; Asc, ascending; Ao, aorta; LBW, low birth weight.

SOURCE: Information taken from the US Department of Health and Human Services, Agency for Healthcare Research and Quality. Healthcare Cost and Utilization Project (HCUP). http://hcupnet.ahrq.gov.

Pediatric patients ranging from neonates to adolescents present with hypertrophic, dilated, or restrictive cardiomyopathies for diagnostic evaluation for transplant and endomyocardial biopsy. Careful titration of anesthetics and sedatives is paramount in these patients with limited hemodynamic reserve.

THE PROCEDURE

Second, the clinician providing sedation or general anesthesia should be familiar with the objectives and technical aspects of the catheter procedure. This is often easy to obtain by reviewing the medical history of the patient and interviewing the family, but a preprocedural discussion with the interventional cardiologist will often determine whether the case can be accomplished best with sedation, a natural airway, a general anesthetic, and so forth. Although complications are infrequent, a candid discussion about the worst-case scenario will allow the anesthetist or the clinician responsible for sedation to be better prepared.

Diagnostic catheterizations typically involve three processes: obtaining multiple blood samples for saturation data used in the Fick equation; pressure measurements to evaluate ventricular function, gradients across stenotic valves and vessels, and as variables in calculating pulmonary and systemic vascular resistance; and angiography of the cardiac chambers, pulmonary architecture, and outflow tracts. Alveolar oxygen content and arterial pH markedly affect pulmonary vascular resistance, and maintaining a consistent FIO_2 (often 21%) and normal pH is paramount to obtaining accurate and reliable data. Achieving this with a natural airway and spontaneous ventilation can be challenging. Even in the older, cooperative child, a skilled anesthesia provider may opt for a general anesthetic, endotracheal intubation, and controlled ventilation. The cardiologist may prefer that respirations are "held" during critical hemodynamic data so that various ventilation modalities and their influence on venous return and ventricular wall tension are trivial.

Challenging vascular access is not uncommon in children presenting to the catheterization laboratory. Multiple factors contribute to this, such as prolonged intensive care unit stays, long-term indwelling central venous and arterial lines, and thromboembolic complications associated with congenital heart disease. Thrombosis of femoral veins and arteries may make routine femoral access impossible. Transhepatic access to the hepatic venous system and inferior vena cava may be used in these cases and is remarkably safe in skilled hands.[96–99]

Nitric oxide is often used as a provocative agent to determine whether elevated pulmonary vascular resistance is reversible. The anesthesia/sedation provider should be familiar with the delivery system, pharmacology, and pharmacokinetics of this agent in the pediatric cardiac catheterization lab.

Transcatheter interventions in the pediatric population typically require general anesthesia. The interventionalist must have a motionless patient, and the anesthetist must be prepared for hemodynamic instability and hemoptysis. With the increasing use of intracardiac (ICE) versus TEE, transcatheter closure of a PFO can be accomplished using general anesthesia with a natural airway or LMA in the older cooperative child (femoral venous sheaths for the intensive care unit probe are still fairly large).[100,101]

The types of catheter interventions commonly performed in the pediatric catheterization laboratory can be grouped as shown in Table 22.2.[102] Hybrid procedures combine surgical and transcatheter interventions in a single maneuver or in a short succession of maneuvers to overcome the limitations of each modality. For example, the percutaneous approach in low-birth-weight infants can be challenging and risk vascular damage and hemodynamic instability. These infants may also be at an increased risk with prolonged cardiopulmonary bypass times. Therefore, combining both the transcatheter and surgical venue may avoid complications. For instance, muscular VSDs can be very difficult for surgeons to adequately visualize and repair without a left ventriculotomy. In the small infant, deploying a septal occlusive device requires a relatively large introducer sheath, and the transcatheter procedure is often complicated by valvular insufficiency, blood loss requiring transfusion, and arrhythmias. Sternotomy and perventricular insertion of an introducer into the right ventricular wall followed by deployment of a septal occluder under fluoroscopic guidance have been described.[103,104] Both cardiopulmonary bypass and insertion of large catheters in small vessels are avoided.

An alternative strategy for neonatal palliation of the infant with hypoplastic left heart syndrome is well described and avoids the complex arch reconstruction in the first 1–2 weeks of life[91,95,105,106] (Figure 22.1). An alternative hybrid "bailout" for palliation of a failed biventricular repair of critical congenital aortic stenosis has recently been described and adds another layer to the complexity of the patients in the pediatric CCL.[107]

Hybrid procedures present the greatest challenges to the anesthesia provider, who is often the individual most familiar with the requirements of both the surgical and the interventional teams. This is a truly collaborative effort that can easily become chaotic when competing interests (space, sterile setups, visibility, etc.) collide. The anesthetist's ability to help coordinate and align these two medical services can mean the difference between success and failure. Detailed planning and constant communication among the surgical, interventional, and anesthesiology services are paramount.

Anesthetizing critically ill patients for catheter procedures becomes daunting when median sternotomies and cardiac procedures are done in an environment designed for fluoroscopic procedures. Today, more and more medical facilities are designing and building "hybrid" suites that have the capacity to accommodate the electrical and physical requirements of these procedures.

THE COMPLICATIONS

In a prospective study of over 4000 pediatric cardiac catheterizations at a single institution from 1987 to 1993, investigators found a mortality rate of 0.14% among diagnostic, interventional, and electrophysiologic (EP) studies performed in the pediatric CCL[108] (Table 22.3). Complications occurred in 8.8% of procedures. Independent risk factors for major complications (death, life-threatening instability, need

TABLE 22.2. Indications for Transcatheter Interventional Procedures

INTERVENTION	INDICATION
Opening of atrial communications	Transposition of the great arteries with inadequate venous return mixing
	Tricuspid atresia with restrictive ASD
	Pulmonary atresia with intact ventricular septum
Occlusion of septal defects	Secundum ASD with adequate septal rims
	Patent foramen ovale[a]
	Muscular VSD
	Fenestration closure in Fontan patients
Balloon dilation of cardiac valves	Pulmonary valve stenosis
	Aortic valve stenosis (congenital)
Balloon angioplasty	Coarctation of the aorta (native and recoarctation)
	Branch pulmonary artery stenosis
	Systemic vein stenosis
Endovascular stents	Pulmonary artery stenosis
	Superior or inferior vena caval stenosis
	Systemic venous obsturction at the superior or inferior baffle limb after atrial repair of transposition
	Stenotic right ventricle-to–pulmonary artery conduit[a]
	Aortic coarctation[a]
	PDA in infants with ductal dependent circulations[a]
Coil occlusion	Aortopulmonary collaterals with dual supply
	Small patent ductus arteriosus
	Surgical aortopulmonary shunts
	Intrapulmonary arteriovenous fistulas
	Anomalous venovenous or venoatrial connections
	Post bidirectional Glenn or Fontan patients
	Coronary arteriovenous fistulas[a]

ASD, atrial septal defect; PDA, patent ductus arteriosus; VSD, ventricular septal defect.

[a]Condition for which the procedure may be indicated.

SOURCE: Allen HD, Beekman RH 3rd, Garson A Jr, et al. Pediatric therapeutic cardiac catheterization: a statement for healthcare professionals from the Council on Cardiovascular Disease in the Young, American Heart Association. *Circulation.* 1998;97(6):609–625.

for surgical intervention) were interventional procedures and age less than 6 months. In a similar study examining complication rates from 1993 to 2007, investigators found the incidence of adverse events to be 9.3%. Interventional catheterizations had an adverse event rate of 11.7%. Infants (<1 year of age) had a complication rate of 13.9%.[109]

Frequent complications in the pediatric CCL are bleeding and hematoma formation at the catheter sites.[108] The anesthetic must provide a smooth emergence, devoid of coughing and delirium, while maintaining airway patency and adequate ventilation. This calm state must continue in the early recovery period so that the infant, toddler, or uncooperative child can remain in the supine position for anywhere from 30 minutes to 2 hours (depending on introducer sheath size and activated clotting time) to avoid bleeding at puncture sites.

Arterial injury and potential limb ischemia can occur, particularly in transcatheter procedures that require large arterial sheaths, such as balloon angioplasty of congenital aortic

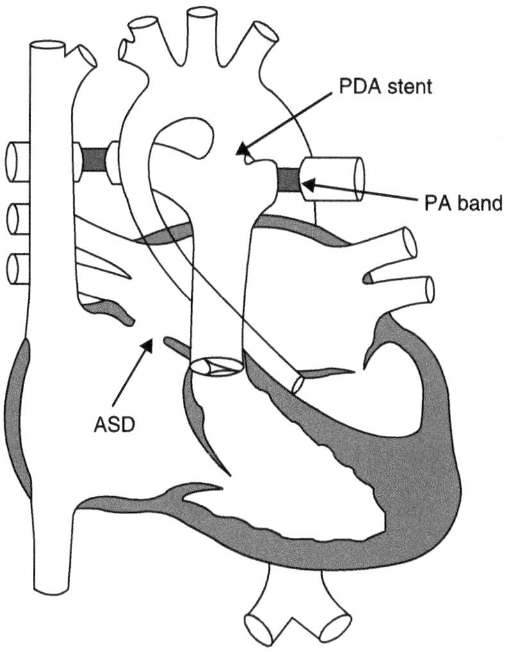

Figure 22.1. *Key features of hybrid palliation for hypoplastic left heart syndrome (HLHS). Note the bilateral pulmonary artery (PA) bands are surgically placed. The patent ductus arteriosus (PDA) patency is maintained by a transcatheter ductal stent, and the atrial septal defect (ASD) is made nonrestrictive by either a septostomy or a transcatheter stent. (From Langeron O, Masso E, Huraux C, et al. Prediction of difficult mask ventilation. Anesthesiology. 2000;92:1229.)*

stenosis or aortic coarctation. Heparin therapy, thrombolytic therapy, or surgical intervention may be required to prevent significant morbidity.[108,110]

Thermal injuries from forced air warming systems can occur and have been described in the lower extremity where arterial and venous sheaths were placed (personal communication). Patients with low cardiac output states may be at particular risk. Precautions include avoiding the highest temperature setting and preventing direct contact of the warming blanket with the patient's skin.[111,112]

Device embolization is always a possibility in interventional procedures. Embolization to the systemic circulation is generally an indication for emergent surgical retrieval. Embolization of devices or ruptured balloons into the pulmonary circulation can often be retrieved by transcatheter approaches. Arrhythmias, valvular obstruction or insufficiency, or vascular obstruction/ischemia may require escalating pharmacologic or mechanical support until the device can be removed.

Pulmonary hemorrhage ranging from trivial to life threatening can occur in patients who undergo balloon angioplasty of pulmonary arteries, a common intervention in the pediatric CCL. Angioplasty is unlikely to be successful unless there is disruption of the intima extending into the media.[113] Cutting balloons are often employed to achieve this intimal tear. Extension of the vascular disruption past the media and adventitia may result in massive hemoptysis and cardiovascular instability. Cuffed endotracheal tubes are a must and will allow the anesthetist to escalate ventilator parameters and add positive end-expiratory pressure.

TABLE 22.3. Mortality Data in the Pediatric Cardiac Catheterization Laboratory

	AGE	CARDIAC LESION	NOTES	PROCEDURE	EVENT LEADING TO DEATH	LOCATION
1	1 day	Pulmonary atresia with intact ventricular septum	On PGE_1	Diagnostic	Perforation of the left atrium	Catheterization lab
2	3 days	Pulmonary atresia with intact ventricular septum	On PGE_1	Pulmonary valve dilation	Ductal thrombosis	OR
3	14 days	Double-outlet right ventricle with transposition of the great arteries		Balloon atrial septostomy	Cardiac perforation	Catheterization lab
4	4 years	Complete AV canal with right ventricular hypoplasia	POD 4 Fontan	Branch PA stent	Cardiac tamponade	ICU
5	5 years	Double-inlet LV with transposed great arteries	POD 1 Fontan	Atrial defect dilation	Desaturation and bradycardia	Catheterization lab
6	4 months	Pulmonary atresia with intact ventricular septum	Cyanotic	Diagnostic	Desaturation and bradycardia	Catheterization lab
7	3 days	Aortic valve stenosis and aortic coarctation		Diagnostic	Bleeding from perforation of paraductal area	OR

AV, atrioventricular; ICU, intensive care unit; LV, left ventricle; OR, operating room; PA, pulmonary artery; PGE_1, prostaglandin E_1; POD, postoperative day.

SOURCE: Reprinted from Vitiello R, McCrindle BW, Nykanen D, Freedom DM, Benson LN. Complications associated with pediatric cardiac catheterization. *J Am Coll Cardiol.* 1998;32(5):1433–1440, with permission from Elsevier.

Perforation of thin atrial walls, calcified conduits, and hypertensive pulmonary arteries can occur during diagnostic or interventional catheterizations. Cardiac tamponade and massive hemoptysis require the skills of both the interventional and the anesthesia teams. The cardiologist can place a covered stent at vessel rupture sites and emergently place a drainage catheter in the pericardial space. The anesthetist must be prepared to start inotropic support, transfuse blood products, and provide care while transitioning onto mechanical support in the catheterization lab.[114] Surgical intervention may be urgently required and may occur in the catheterization suite or involve transfer to an operating room.[115] Unlike the adult catheterization laboratories, which may be in freestanding facilities or hospitals without cardiac surgical services, cardiac surgical support is mandatory for any institution performing diagnostic or therapeutic pediatric cardiac catheterizations.[116]

The clinician providing anesthetic care of children in the pediatric catheterization laboratory must have a working knowledge of the wide spectrum of congenital heart defects, their pre- and postrepair physiology, the various transcatheter procedures and their concomitant risks, and the challenges of resuscitation in an environment that may be remote from the operating room. The anesthetist must remain engaged in the procedure, alert to any signs of potential cardiovascular compromise. As in all non–operating room areas where sedation and general anesthesia are performed, the clinician's ability to effectively communicate with other services is requisite to providing safe and effective care.

THE ELECTROPHYSIOLOGY LAB

OVERVIEW OF ELECTROPHYSIOLOGY INTERVENTIONS

Since the 1960s, modern clinical EP has undergone a transformative evolution from simple diagnostic procedures to major, life-saving, therapeutic interventions. As technology has advanced and the demand has significantly increased, there has been exponential growth in the number of EP procedures. Additionally, the complexity and length of these procedures has dramatically increased.

The performance of these procedures now frequently mandates administration of moderate sedation or general anesthesia. Consultation with a cardiac anesthesiologist may be necessary because many patients frequently have comorbidities such as advanced heart failure and multisystem disease. Optimal conscious sedation/general anesthesia requires the anesthesiologist to understand EP procedures to maximize potential for desired outcomes and to avoid complications. This section reviews the most commonly performed EP procedures.

ELECTROPHYSIOLOGY STUDIES

Diagnostic EPSs are presently commonly performed in conjunction with therapeutic procedures to evaluate and treat specific arrhythmias. Currently, an EPS is performed to determine the electrophysiologic etiology of specific symptoms or events, such as syncope or palpitations.[89] Intracardiac recordings are made from catheters that are commonly placed via femoral venous access into the high right atrium (HRA), His bundle, coronary sinus, and right ventricular apex (RVA) or right ventricular outflow tract (RVOT). Ventricular or supraventricular tachycardias are induced by programmed stimulation performed from the HRA, RVA, or RVOT. The etiology of bradyarrhythmias may also be assessed from intracardiac recordings. For these studies, sedation with benzodiazepines and short-acting analgesic medication such as fentanyl is usually sufficient. Drugs that may affect inducibility of certain arrhythmias should be avoided. These include sympathetic and parasympathetic modulating agents because they commonly influence the function of the AV node and sinus node and thus may influence the outcome of the study.

CATHETER ABLATION

Catheter ablation is commonly used to treat supraventricular tachyarrhythmias such as AV nodal reentry tachycardia; Wolf-Parkinson-White syndrome–related tachycardias; atrial flutter; atrial fibrillation; and ventricular arrhythmias in selected patients. Recent ACC/AHA atrial fibrillation guidelines state that in patients with little or no left atrial enlargement, catheter ablation is a "reasonable alternative to pharmacologic therapy" to help prevent recurrence of atrial fibrillation. These guidelines have categorized catheter ablation for atrial fibrillation as II-A, level of evidence C.[117]

Although other energies, such as focused ultrasound, laser, microwave, and cryotherapy, have been employed in cardiac ablation procedures, RF is the energy most commonly utilized.[118] However, regardless of the energy source delivered to specific targets, the patient may experience pain and may require deep sedation or general anesthesia.

Radio-frequency catheter ablation has been used as a treatment for arrhythmias that are refractory to pharmacologic therapy as well as a first-line treatment for other arrhythmias.[89] The following arrhythmias have been treated with RF ablation: AV reentrant tachycardia, supraventricular arrhythmias associated with the Wolf-Parkinson-White syndrome; atrial ventricular reentrant tachycardia; atrial tachycardia; atrial flutter; idiopathic ventricular tachycardia; bundle branch reentrant ventricular tachycardia; right ventricular outflow tachycardia; atrial fibrillation with an uncontrollable rapid ventricular response (RF ablation of the atrial ventricular node and placement of a permanent pacemaker); and atrial fibrillation. Radio-frequency is also used as adjunctive therapy for recurrent ventricular tachycardia due to coronary artery disease or arrhythmogenic right ventricular dysplasia.[118] During the ablation procedure, catheters are placed in different cardiac chambers, and programmed stimulation is performed from different sites to induce tachyarrhythmias. In addition, different medications, such as isoproterenol, epinephrine, dopamine, aminophylline, atropine, adenosine, β-blockers, ibutilide, verapamil, and procainamide are used to induce as well as terminate tachyarrhythmias.[89]

Complex mapping techniques are utilized to identify the source of the arrhythmia to specify the exact intracardiac location to which the RF energy must be applied. Mapping techniques include activation mapping; pace mapping; entrainment mapping; anatomic fluoroscopy-based, three-dimensional (3D) electroanatomical mapping; 3D noncontact mapping; and intracardiac echo-guided anatomical mapping. Because of the precision needed to identify and apply the RF energy to the intracardiac site of an arrhythmia, the patient must lie still during the procedure. Therefore, deep sedation or general anesthesia is necessary to ensure patient comfort and to optimize mapping. Thus, the role of the anesthesiologist becomes crucial during the procedure in order to maintain the patient's airway and ensure hemodynamic stability with minimal movement of the patient's body. A multidisciplinary team approach, including both anesthesiologists and electrophysiologists, is necessary to efficiently facilitate ablation procedures while optimizing patient safety.

Radio-frequency ablation procedures are becoming more tedious and more time consuming. Patients with atrial fibrillation often require a procedure time of at least 4–6 hours, followed by a prolonged observation time after ablation with repeat EP testing to ensure success of the procedure.[89]

Patients can be young and essentially healthy or have extensive comorbidities. Coughing, snoring, and partial airway obstruction can be problematic during intracardiac mapping because they precipitate a swinging motion of the intra-atrial septum and make transeptal catheter placement difficult. Deep sedation is sometimes necessary to keep the patient comfortable during ablations, and ventilatory control with general anesthesia may be needed for obese patients, those with sleep apnea, or those with potential pulmonary problems. Drugs that affect the sympathetic nervous system should be avoided, if possible, during mapping of ectopic foci and tracts. Local anesthetics that are of moderate or long duration should be avoided during intubation. In patients with ventricular dysfunction, inotropic and vasoactive agents may be necessary in order to both sedate and maintain hemodynamic stability during arrhythmia induction.[26] Communication with the cardiologist is necessary in these situations to maintain patient safety and still allow the mapping process to proceed. Frequently, electrical cardioversion is necessary during the case, which may require at least transient general anesthesia for the patient to tolerate the delivered shock. Usually, 20–40 mg of propofol is all that is needed to accomplish temporary deep sedation.

ELECTROPHYSIOLOGIC DEVICES

Devices for the control or eradication of arrhythmias have diminished in size and increased in sophistication over the past 15 years. As a result, more patients qualify for device implants, and the number of procedures for implantation and upgrade of devices has increased enormously. The two most common types of devices are ICDs and pacemakers.

IMPLANTABLE CARDIOVERTER/DEFIBRILLATORS

Implantable cardioverter/defibrillators have been demonstrated to be efficacious and safe in a number of large, prospective, multicenter, randomized trials in patients with coronary and noncoronary heart diseases. Benefits accrue mainly in patients with depressed left ventricular ejection fractions of 35% or less.[119] Indications for ICD implantation as listed in the 2008 ACC, AHA, and the Heart Rhythm Society (HRS) guidelines (seven class I indications) have clearly been shown to prolong life and decrease the risk of sudden cardiac death for both primary and secondary ventricular tachycardia or ventricular fibrillation.[119] With the advent of smaller biphasic, transvenous ICDs and the experience gained over the years, it is now feasible for electrophysiologists to implant ICDs safely in the pectoral under general anesthesia in the operating room. However, currently only local anesthesia combined with conscious sedation is utilized. The role of anesthesiologist is crucial during defibrillation threshold (DFT) testing when general anesthesia is required. This is especially true in patients who generally have significant comorbidities and significant left ventricular dysfunction.

Many electrophysiologists consider DFT testing to be the most critical part of the ICD implantation procedure. Serious complications may occur during DFT, although the risk is usually low. Complications may include transient ischemic attack, stroke, cardiopulmonary arrest due to refractory ventricular fibrillation, pulseless electrical activity, cardiogenic shock, embolic events, and death.[119,120] DFT testing is commonly omitted due to the potential life-threatening risks of the procedure in unstable patients or patients with untreated coronary artery disease.

BIVENTRICULAR PACING AND DEFIBRILLATION LEAD PLACEMENT

Cardiac resynchronization therapy with and without defibrillation systems is prescribed for both primary and secondary prevention of sudden cardiac death in patients with heart failure associated with both an ischemic and a nonischemic etiology. In 2008, the ACC/AHA/HRS guidelines gave cardiac resynchronization therapy with or without an ICD a class I indication for those with a left ventricular ejection fraction less than or equal to 35% with a QRS duration greater than or equal to 120 milliseconds and drug-refractory NYHA functional class III or ambulatory class IV heart failure who are receiving optimal medical therapy.[119–121]

Because of advanced heart failure, these patients may be unable to lie flat on the EP table despite optimal medical therapy. Therefore, close monitoring of the patient's vital signs and oxygenation is extremely important. The skill of an anesthesiologist is needed to successfully administer conscious sedation and avoid cardiac decompensation during these long procedures. The procedure is frequently complex and lengthy due to positioning the left ventricular lead via the coronary sinus and great cardiac vein in the setting of distorted ventricular anatomy resulting from cardiac dilation and advanced heart failure. In addition, valvular regurgitation may potentially further complicate lead positioning. Finally, lead dislodgement may occur immediately after lead placement, further prolonging these procedures.

Because implantation of biventricular pacing/ICD systems may precipitate development of refractory heart failure, the need for airway protection is critical, and the ability to intubate the patient is crucial to the success of the procedure and survival of the patient. Pneumothorax and coronary sinus perforation related to lead placement are also possible. Coronary sinus perforation can immediately be recognized by contrast extravasation. Perforation of the coronary sinus or cardiac perforation related to ventricular or atrial lead placement may lead to the development of cardiac tamponade. This necessitates immediate intraprocedure pericardiocentesis.

ANESTHETIC ISSUES: IMPLANTABLE CARDIOVERTER/DEFIBRILLATORS AND BIVENTRICULAR PACEMAKERS

Many patients who qualify for ICDs and biventricular pacemakers have multiple comorbidities, including a history of ventricular tachycardia/fibrillation, ejection fraction less than 30%, and coronary artery disease (these are indications for ICD placement).[119,122] Other indications include arrhythmogenic right ventricular dysplasia, long QT syndrome, and hypertrophic cardiomyopathy.[119]

Most of these devices are placed with mild-to-moderate sedation and standard monitors. Testing the device requires deep sedation or general anesthesia. ICD placement and testing can be accomplished without an arterial line. External cardioverter/defibrillator pads are placed on the patient at the beginning of the procedure. When testing ICDs, they are used to induce ventricular fibrillation and to serve as backup if the implanted device fails.

Typically, an implanted ICD is tested twice at the end of the procedure. Repeated testing is usually well tolerated without deterioration of ventricular function even in patients with ejection fractions below 35%.[123,124] In patients with evidence of untreated coronary disease, recent stent placement, or evidence of atrial or ventricular thrombus, testing is sometimes omitted. Significant coronary artery disease is a concern when testing with prolonged hypotension as a possible complication. It is important to remember that ICD testing is always an elective procedure should the patient demonstrate deterioration during implantation.[26]

Some patients needing ICDs are also having biventricular pacemakers placed for cardiac resynchronization therapy. Any patient scheduled for a biventricular pacemaker has extensive cardiac morbidity, including low ejection fractions, valvular heart disease, pulmonary hypertension, and right ventricular dysfunction. Patients may not be able to lie flat comfortably and can easily become hemodynamically unstable with sedation. Oversedation can lead to hypercapnia, which is problematic in patients with pulmonary hypertension or right ventricular dysfunction. The anesthesiologist must be ready to convert to general anesthesia at any time during the case. Coronary sinus lead placement for biventricular pacing can be difficult, making the procedure much longer than dual-chamber pacemaker and ICD placements. Complications from these procedures include possible cardiac injury (perforation/tamponade), myocardial infarction, stroke, and pneumothorax from the subclavian venous access.

RADIATION

Anesthesiologists need lead in procedure rooms where radiation is utilized. Unfortunately, it is all too common that they come to the CCL or EPL and have to dig through the available lead aprons usually worn by others because anesthesiologists are not considered part of the team. Yet, many of the cases described involve significant radiation exposure during the procedure.

All radiation exposure should be "as low as reasonably achievable" during the procedure.[125] Reductions in radiation time, distance from the source of radiation, and barriers to radiation are the three mechanisms to reduce exposure. Radiation time is under the control of the cardiologist performing the procedure. Many of the new and more complex procedures (device placement, percutaneous valves, biventricular pacemakers, ablations) require prolonged exposure to radiation.

Distance from the source of radiation and barriers to radiation are under the control of the anesthesiologist. The radiation beam attenuates based on the inverse square law ($1/d^2$).[125] The strength of the beam decreases exponentially the farther away the anesthesiologist is from the radiation source. Barriers such a lead aprons and thyroid collars should be worn at all times. Even with proper leaded apparel, 18% of active bone marrow is still exposed to the effects of radiation.[126] Lead shields should be used for additional protection. It is highly recommended to wear leaded eyeglasses to reduce the risk of cataracts. Every anesthesiologist spending time in the CCL or EPL should wear a dosimeter to track cumulative radiation exposure. A study by Katz in 2005 demonstrated that radiation exposure to those in an anesthesia department doubled after the introduction of an EPL.[127]

CONCLUSION

The anesthesiologist's patient safety record in the operating room is well documented. As procedures become more complex and the acuity of patients increases, safe and efficient care for the growing patient population in the CCL and EPL is now a concern for all anesthesiologists and cardiologists. Anesthesiologists are uniquely trained to care for this complicated patient population, allowing the cardiologist to focus on successfully completing the interventional procedure. Anesthesiologists, in collaboration with cardiologists, must establish guidelines for their involvement in patient care and procedure planning in the CCL and EPL. We are in many ways victims of our own success. Increased numbers of more complicated patients, an ever-expanding arsenal of technologically sophisticated tools, and an aging population make it likely that the demand for CCL and EPL services will continue to grow. Collaboration between cardiologists and anesthesiologists is increasingly necessary. Reframing the boundaries between disciplines is the likely pathway to success. The goal is to improve patient safety and procedural efficiency while advancing the frontiers of medical care in an expanding and exciting new venue.

REFERENCES

1. Fleisher LA, Beckman JA, Brown KA, et al. ACC/AHA 2007 guidelines on perioperative cardiovascular evaluation and care for noncardiac surgery: executive summary: a report of the American College of Cardiology/ American Heart Association Task Force on Practice Guidelines (Writing Committee to Revise the 2002 Guidelines on Perioperative Cardiovascular Evaluation for Noncardiac Surgery). *Anesth Analg.* 2008;106:685.
2. Langeron O, Masso E, Huraux C, et al. Prediction of difficult mask ventilation. *Anesthesiology.* 2000;92:1229.
3. American Society of Anesthesiologists Task Force on Sedation and Analgesia by Non-Anesthesiologists. Practice guidelines for sedation and analgesia by non-anesthesiologists. *Anesthesiology.* 2002;96:1004.
4. Paris A, Tonner PH. Dexmedetomidine in anaesthesia. *Curr Opin Anaesthesiol.* 2005;18:412.
5. Petronio AS, Giannini C, De Carlo M, et al. Anaesthetic management of transcatheter aortic valve implantation: results from the Italian CoreValve registry. *Eurointervention.* 2016;12(3):381–388.
6. American Society of Anesthesiologists. Statement on nonoperating room anesthetizing locations, last amended 2008. Available at: http://www.asahq.org/quality-and-practice-management/standards-guidelines-and-related-resources/statement-on-nonoperating-room-anesthetizing-locations. Accessed on March 1, 2018.
7. US Department of Health and Human Services, Agency for Healthcare Research and Quality. Healthcare Cost and Utilization Project (HCUP). Available at: http://hcupnet.ahrq.gov. Accessed on July 20, 2010.
8. Kushner FG, Hand M, Smith SC, et al. 2009 focused updates: ACC/AHA guidelines for the management of patients with ST-elevation myocardial infarction (updating the 2004 guideline and 2007 focused update) and ACC/AHA/SCAI guidelines on percutaneous coronary intervention (updating the 2005 guideline and 2007 focused update). *J Am Coll Cardiol.* 2009;54(23):2205–2241.
9. Smith SC Jr, Feldman TE, Hirshfeld JW Jr, et al. ACC/AHA/SCAI 2005 guideline update for percutaneous coronary intervention: a report of the American College of Cardiology/American Heart Association Task Force on Practice Guidelines (ACC/AHA/SCAI Writing Committee to Update the 2001 Guidelines for Percutaneous Coronary Intervention). *J Am Coll Cardiol.* 2006;47(1):e1–e121.
10. Boden WE, O'Rourke RA, Teo KK, et al. Optimal medical therapy with or without PCI for stable coronary artery disease. *N Engl J Med.* 2007;356:1503.
11. The TIMI II B Investigators. Effects of tissue plasminogen activator and a comparison of early invasive and conservative strategies in unstable angina and non-Q-wave myocardial infarction. Results of the TIMI IIIB Trial. Thrombolysis in myocardial ischemia. *Circulation.* 1994;89(4):1545–1556.
12. Anderson HV, Cannon CP, Stone PH, et al. One-year results of the Thrombolysis in Myocardial Infarction (TIMI) IIIB clinical trial. A randomized comparison of tissue-type plasminogen activator versus placebo and early invasive versus early conservative strategies in unstable angina and non-Q wave myocardial infarction. *J Am Coll Cardiol.* 1995;26(7):1643–1650.
13. Cannon C, Weintraub WS, Demopoulos LA, et al. Comparison of early invasive and conservative strategies in patients with unstable coronary syndromes treated with the glycoprotein IIb/IIIa inhibitor tirofiban. *N Engl J Med.* 2001;344:1879–1887.
14. Seung KB, Park DW, Kim YH, et al. Stents versus coronary-artery bypass grafting for left main coronary artery disease. *N Engl J Med.* 2008;358:1781–1792.
15. Buszman PE, Kiesz SR, Bocenek A, et al. Acute and late outcomes of unprotected left main stenting in comparison with surgical revascularization. *J Am Coll Cardiol.* 2008;51:538–545.
16. Brener SJ, Galla JM, Bryant R 3rd, et al. Comparison of percutaneous versus surgical revascularization of severe unprotected left main coronary stenosis in matched patients. *Am J Cardiol.* 2008;101:169–172.
17. Serruys PW, Morice MC, Kappetein AP, et al. Percutaneous coronary intervention versus coronary-artery bypass grafting for severe coronary artery disease. *N Engl J Med.* 2009;360:961–972.
18. Huang HW, Brent B, Shaw R. Trends in percutaneous versus surgical revascularization of unprotected left main coronary stenosis in the drug-eluting stent era—a report from the American College of Cardiology-national cardiovascular data registry. *Catheter Cardiovasc Interv.* 2006;68:867–872.
19. Biondi-Zoccai GGl, Lotrionte M, Morett C, et al. A collaborative systematic review and meta-analysis on 1278 patients undergoing percutaneous drug-eluting stenting for unprotected left main coronary artery disease. *Am Heart J.* 2008;155:274–283.
20. Jones RH. Percutaneous intervention vs. coronary artery bypass grafting in left main coronary artery disease. *N Engl J Med.* 2008;358(17):1851–1853.
21. Kar B, Adkins LE, Civitello AB, et al. Clinical experience with the TandemHeart® percutaneous ventricular assist device. *Tex Heart Inst J.* 2006;33(2):111–115.
22. Siegenthaler MP, Brehm K, Strecher T, et al. The Impella Recover microaxial left ventricular assist device reduces mortality for postcardiotomy failure: a three-center experience. *J Thorac Cardiovasc Surg.* 2004;127:812–822.
23. Windecker S, Meier B. Impella assisted high-risk percutaneous coronary intervention. *Karddiovaskulare Medizin.* 2005;8:187–189.
24. Henriques JP, Remmelink M, Baan J Jr, et al. Safety and feasibility of elective high-risk percutaneous coronary intervention procedures with left ventricular support of the Impella Recover LP 2.5. *Am J Cardiol.* 2006;97:990.
25. Pretorius M, Hughes AK, Stahlman MB, et al. Placement of the TandemHeart percutaneous left ventricular assist device. *Anesth Analg.* 2006;103:1412.
26. Shook DC, Gross W. Offsite anesthesiology in the cardiac catheterization lab. *Curr Opin Anaesthesiol.* 2007;20:352.
27. AMPLATZER® Septal Occluder. Available at: https://www.fda.gov/ohrms/dockets/ac/01/briefing/3790b1_03_sponsorss&e.pdf. Accessed on March 1, 2018.
28. Bayard YL, Ostermayer SH, Hein R, et al. Percutaneous devices for stroke prevention. *Cardiovasc Revascular Med.* 2007;8:216–225.
29. Pinto Slottow TL, Steinberg DH, Waksman R. Overview of the 2007 Food and Drug Administration circulatory system devices panel meeting on patent foramen ovale closure devices *Circulation.* 2007;116:677–682.
30. AGA Medical Corporation. AMPLATZER® septal occluder for atrial septal defect closure. Available at: https://www.sjm.com/en/professionals/featured-products/structural-heart/structural-heart-occluders/asd-closure-devices/amplatzer-septal-occluder. Accessed on July March 1, 2018.
31. Wiegers SE, St John Sutton MG. Devices for percutaneous closure of a secundum atrial septal defect. Available at: http://www.uptodate.com/patients/content/topic.do?topicKey=~OqyyJUSBGuod2c. Last updated December 9, 2015. Accessed on July 20, 2010.
32. Pedra CA, Pihkla J, Lee KJ, et al. Transcatheter closure of atrial septal defects using the Cardio-Seal implant. *Heart.* 2000;84:320.
33. Carminati M, Chessa M, Butera G, et al. Transcatheter closure of atrial septal defects with the STARflex device: early results and follow up. *J Interv Cardiol.* 2001;14:319.
34. Valente AM, Rhodes JF. Current indications and contraindications for transcatheter atrial septal defect and patent forman ovale device closure. *Am Heart J.* 2007;153(suppl 4):81–84.
35. Butera G, Chessa M, Carminati M. Percutaneous closure of ventricular septal defects. *Cardiol Young.* 2007;17:243–253.
36. Delaney JW, Li JS, Rhodes JF. Major complications associated with transcatheter atrial septal occluder implantation: a review of the medical literature and the manufacturer and user facility device experience (MAUDE) database. *Congenit Heart Dis.* 2007;2(4):256–264.
37. Chessa M, Carminati M, Walsh K, et al. Early and late complications associated with transcatheter occlusion of secundum atrial septal defect. *J Am Coll Cardiol.* 2002;39:1061.
38. Krumsdorf U, Ostemayer S, Billinger K, et al. Incidence and clinical course of thrombus formation on atrial septal defect and patent foramen ovale closure devices in 1000 consecutive patients. *J Am Coll Cardiol.* 2004;43(2):302–309.
39. LaRosee K, Krause D, Becker M, et al. Transcatheter closure of atrial septal defects in adults. Practicality and safety of four different closure systems used in 102 patients. *Dtsch Med Wochenschr.* 2001;126(38):1030–1036.
40. Carroll JD, Dodge S, Groves BM. Percutaneous patent forman ovale closure. *Cardiol Clin.* 2005;23:13–33.
41. Martinez MW, Mookadam F, Sun Y, et al. Transcatheter closure of ischemic and post-traumatic ventricular septal ruptures. *Catheter Cardiovasc Interv.* 2007;69:403.

42. Garay F, Cao QL, Hjazi ZM. Percutaneous closure of post-myocardial infarction ventricular septal defect. *J Interv Cardiol.* 2006;19:S67.
43. Nugent AW, Britt A, Gauvreau K, et al. Device closure rates of simple atrial septal defects optimized by the STARFlex device. *J Am Coll Cardiol.* 2006;48:538.
44. Boccalandro F, Baptista E, Muench A, et al. Comparison of intracardiac echocardiography versus transesophageal echocardiography guidance for percutaneous transcatheter closure of atrial septal defect. *Am J Cardiol.* 2004;93:437.
45. Thom T, Hasse N, Rosamond W, et al. Heart disease and stroke statistics—2006 update: a report from the American Heart Association Statistics Committee and Stroke Statistics Subcommittee. *Circulation.* 2006;113:e85.
46. Selvin E, Erlinger TP. Prevalence of and risk factors for peripheral arterial disease in the United States: results from the National Health and Nutrition Examination Survey, 1999–2000. *Circulation.* 2004;110:738.
47. Hirsch AT, Haskal ZJ, Hertzer NR, et al. ACC/AHA 2005 guidelines for the management of patients with peripheral arterial disease (lower extremity, renal, mesenteric, and abdominal aortic): a collaborative report from the American Association for Vascular Surgery/Society for Vascular Surgery, Society for Cardiovascular Angiography and Interventions, Society for Vascular Medicine and Biology, Society of Interventional Radiology, and the ACC/AHA Task Force on Practice Guidelines (Writing Committee to Develop Guidelines for the Management of Patients with peripheral arterial disease, 2005). *Circulation.* 2006;113:e463.
48. Creager MA, Libby P. Peripheral arterial diseases. In: Libby P, Bonow RO, Mann DL, Zipes DP, eds. *Braunwald's Heart Disease: A Textbook of Cardiovascular Medicine.* 8th ed. New York, NY: Elsevier; 2007:1491–1514.
49. Norgen L, Hiatt WR, Dormandy JA, et al. Inter-society consensus for the management of peripheral arterial disease (TASC II). *J Vasc Surg.* 2007;45(suppl S):S5.
50. Pell JP. Impact of intermittent claudication on quality of life. The Scottish vascular audit group. *Eur J Vasc Endovasc Surg.* 1995;9:469.
51. Tuman KJ, McCarthy RJ, March RJ, et al. Effects of epidural anesthesia and analgesia on coagulation and outcome after major vascular surgery. *Anesth Analg.* 1991;73(6):696–704.
52. Vandermeulen EP, Van Aken H, Vermylen J. Anticoagulants and spinal-epidural anesthesia. *Anesth Analg.* 1994;79:1165–1177.
53. Onishchuk JL, Carlsson C. Epidural hematoma associated with epidural anesthesia: complications of anticoagulant therapy. *Anesthesiology.* 1992;77:1221–1223.
54. Vassiliades TA, Block PC, Cohn LH, et al. The clinical development of percutaneous heart valve technology: a position statement of the Society of Thoracic Surgeons, the American Association for Thoracic Surgery and the Society for Cardiovascular Angiography and Interventions Endorsed by the American College of Cardiology Foundation and the American Heart Association. *J Am Coll Cardiol.* 2005;45:1554–1560.
55. Cribier A, Eltchanioff H, Bash A, et al. Percutaneous transcatheter implantation of an aortic valve prostheses for calcific aortic stenosis: first human case description. *Circulation.* 2002;106:3006–3008.
56. Cribier A, Eltchanioff H, Tron C, et al. Percutaneous implantation of aortic valve prosthesis in patients with calcific aortic stenosis: technical advances, clinical results and future strategies. *J Interv Cardiol.* 2006;19:S87–S96.
57. Feldman T. Percutaneous mitral valve repair. *J Int Cardiol.* 2007;20(6):488–494.
58. Byrne MJ, Power JM, Alferness CA, et al. Percutaneous mitral annular reduction. A novel approach to the management of heart failure associated mitral regurgitation. *Circulation.* 2003;108:1795–1799.
59. Maniu CV, Patel JB, Reuter DG, et al. Percutaneous mitral annular reduction provides continued benefit in an ovine model of dilated cardiomyopathy. *Circulation.* 2004;110:3088–3092.
60. Liddicoat JR, MacNeill BD, Gillinov AM, et al. Percutaneous mitral valve repair: a feasibility study in an ovine model of acute ischemic mitral regurgitation. *Catheter Cardiovasc Interv.* 2003;60:410–416.
61. Maselli D, Guarracino F, Chiaramonti F, et al. Percutaneous mitral annuloplasty: an anatomic study of human coronary sinus and its relation with mitral valve annulus and coronary arteries. *Circulation.* 2006;114:377–380.
62. Alfieri O, Maisano F, DeBonis M, et al. The edge-to-edge technique in mitral valve repair: a simple solution for complex problems. *J Thorac Cardiovasc Surg.* 2001;122:674–681.
63. Alfieri O, Elefteriades JA, Chapolini RJ, et al. Novel suture device for beating-heart mitral leaflet approximation. *Ann Thorac Surg.* 2002;74:1488–1493.
64. Bhudia SK, McCarthy PM, Smedira NG, et al. Edge-to-edge (Alfieri) mitral repair: results in diverse clinical settings. *Ann Thorac Surg.* 2004;77:1598–1606.
65. Kherani AR, Cheema FH, Casher J, et al. Edge-to-edge mitral valve repair: the Columbia Presbyterian experience. *Ann Thorac Surg.* 2004;78:73–76.
66. Maaisano F, Vigano G, Blasio A, et al. Surgical isolated edge-to-edge mitral repair without annuloplasty—clinical proof of principle for an endovascular approach. *Eurointervention.* 2006;2:181–186.
67. St. Goar FG, James FI, Komtebedde J, et al. Endovascular edge-to-edge mitral valve repair: short-term results in a porcine model. *Circulation.* 2003;108:1990–1993.
68. Fann JI, St Goar FG, Komtebedde J, et al. Off-pump edge-to-edge mitral valve technique using a mechanical clip in a chronic model. *Circulation.* 2003;108(suppl 4):493.
69. Feldman T, Wasserman H, Herrmann HC, et al. Edge-to-edge mitral valve repair using the Evalve MitraClip: one year results of the EVEREST phase I clinical trial. *Am J Cardiol.* 2005;96:49H.
70. Pavcnik D, Wright KC, Wallace S. Development and initial experimental evaluation of a prosthetic aortic valve for transcatheter placement. Work in progress. *Radiology.* 1992;183:151–154.
71. Cribier A, Elchanioff H, Bash A, et al. Percutaneous transcatheter implantation of an aortic valve prosthesis for calcific aortic stenosis: first human case description. *Circulation.* 2002;106:3006–3008.
72. Rajagopal V, Kapadia SR, Tuzcu EM. Advances in the percutaneous treatment of aortic and mitral valve disease. *Minerva Cardioangiol.* 2007;55:83–94.
73. Webb JG. New treatment options in aortic stenosis. *ACCEL.* 2008;40:4 disc 1.
74. Cribier A, Eltchanioff H, Tron C, et al. Treatment of calcific aortic stenosis with the percutaneous heart valve: mid-term follow-up from the initial feasibility studies: the French experience. *J Am Coll Cardiol.* 2006;47:1214–1223.
75. Edwards Lifesciences Corporation. Edwards Lifesciences receives CE Mark for Edwards SAPIEN Transcatheter Heart Valve. Available at: https://www.edwards.com/fr/newsroom/Pages/ShowPR.aspx?PageGuid=%7B252fa581-d645-4c47-a20c-44e03fe6c8f3%7D. Published 2007. Accessed on March 1, 2018.
76. Edwards Lifesciences Corporation. Edwards Sapien Transcatheter Aortic Valve makes human debut. Available at: http://medgadget.com/archives/2008/03/edwards_sapien_transcatheter_aortic_valve_makes_human_debut.html. Published 2008. Accessed on July 20, 2010.
77. Lichenstein SV, Cheung A, Ye J, et al. Transapical transcatheter aortic valve implantation in humans: initial clinical experience. *Circulation.* 2006;114:591–596.
78. Walther T, Simon P, Dewey T, et al. Transapical minimally invasive aortic valve implantation multicenter experience. *Circulation.* 2007;116(suppl I):I-240–I-245.
79. Walther T, Falk V, Borger MA, et al. Minimally invasive transapical beating heart aortic valve implantation—proof of concept. *Eur J Cardiothorac Surg.* 2007;31:9–15.
80. Kapadia SR, Leon MB, Makkar RR, et al. 5-year outcomes of transcatheter aortic valve replacement compared with standard treatment for patients with inoperable aortic stenosis (PARTNER I): a randomized controlled trial. *The Lancet.* 2015;385(9986):2485–2491.
81. Yakubov SJ, Adams DH, Watson DR, et al. 2-year outcomes after iliofemoral self-expanding transcatheter aortic valve replacement in patients with severe aortic stenosis deemed extreme risk for surgery. *J Am Coll Cardiol.* 2015;66(12):1327–1334.
82. Deeb GM, Reardon MJ, Chetcuti S, et al. 3-year outcomes in high-risk patients who underwent surgical or transcatheter aortic valve replacement. *J Am Coll Cardiol.* 2016;67(22):2565–2574.
83. Sondergaard L, Steinbruchel DA, Ihleemann N, et. al. Two-year outcomes in patients with severe aortic valve stenosis randomized to transcatheter versus surgical aortic valve replacement: The All-Comers Nordic Aortic Valve Intervention Randomized Clinical Trial. *Circ Cardiovasc Interv.* 2016;9(6). pii:e003665.
84. Castrodeza J, Amat-Santos IJ, Blanco M, et. al. Propensity score matched comparison of transcatheter aortic valve implantation versus conventional surgery in intermediate and low risk aortic stenosis patients: a hint of real-world. *Cardiol J.* 2016;23(5):541–551.
85. Thourani V, Kodali S, Makkar RR, et al. Transcatheter aortic valve replacement versus surgical valve replacement in intermediate-risk patients: a propensity score analysis. *The Lancet.* 2016;387(10034):2218–2225. doi 10.1016/S0140-6736(16)30073-3.
86. Saroul C, Keller G, Benaissa M, Lehot JJ. Anesthesia for minimally invasive cardiac procedures [in French]. *Ann Fr Anesth Reanim.* 2011;30(suppl 1):S38–S43.
87. Hamid A. Anesthesia for cardiac catheterization. *Heart Lung Vessel.* 2014;6(4):225–231.
88. Nishimura RA, Otto CM, Bonow RO, et al. 2014 AHA/ACC guideline for the management of patients with valvular heart disease. A report of the

American College of Cardiology/American Heart Associate Task Force on Practice Guidelines. *J Am Coll Cardiol.* 2014;63(22):2438–2488. doi:10.1016/j.jacc.2014.02.536.
89. Block PC. Percutaneous transcatheter repair for mitral regurgitation. *J Interv Cardiol.* 2006;19:547.
90. ACC/AHA/HRS Writing Committee. ACC/AHA/HRS 2006 key data elements and definitions for electrophysiological studies and procedures: a report of the American College of Cardiology/American Heart Association Task Force on Clinical Data Standards (ACC/AHA/HRS Writing Committee to Develop Data Standards on Electrophysiology). *Circulation.* 2006;114:2534–2570.
91. Inglis JM. Anaesthesia for cardiac catheterisation in children. *Anaesthesia.* 1954;9(1):25–30.
92. Gutgesell HP, Lim DS. Hybrid palliation in hypoplastic left heart syndrome. *Curr Opin Cardiol.* 2007;22(2):55–59.
93. Shim D, Lloyd TR, Crowley DC, Beekman RH 3rd. Neonatal cardiac catheterization: a 10-year transition from diagnosis to therapy. *Pediatr Cardiol.* 1999;20(2):131–133.
94. Lalwani K. Demographics and trends in nonoperating-room anesthesia. *Curr Opin Anaesthesiol.* 2006;19(4):430–435.
95. Lee C, Mason LJ. Pediatric cardiac emergencies. *Anesthesiol Clin North Am.* 2001;19(2):287–308.
96. Pizarro C, Derby CD, Baffa JM, Murdison KA, Radtke WA. Improving the outcome of high-risk neonates with hypoplastic left heart syndrome: hybrid procedure or conventional surgical palliation? *Eur J Cardiothorac Surg.* 2008;33(4):613–618.
97. Shim D, Lloyd TR, Beekman RH 3rd. Transhepatic therapeutic cardiac catheterization: a new option for the pediatric interventionalist. *Catheter Cardiovasc Interv.* 1999;47(1):41–45.
98. Emmel M, Sreeram N, Pillekamp F, Boehm W, Brockmeier K. Transhepatic approach for catheter interventions in infants and children with congenital heart disease. *Clin Res Cardiol.* 2006;95(6):329–333.
99. Johnston TA, Donnelly LF, Frush DP, O'Laughlin MP. Transhepatic catheterization using ultrasound-guided access. *Pediatr Cardiol.* 2003;24(4):393–396.
100. Book WM, Raviele AA, Vincent RN. Transhepatic vascular access in pediatric cardiology patients with occlusion of traditional central venous sites. *J Invasive Cardiol.* 1999;11(6):341–344.
101. Cao QL, Zabal C, Koenig P, Sandhu S, Hijazi ZM. Initial clinical experience with intracardiac echocardiography in guiding transcatheter closure of perimembranous ventricular septal defects: feasibility and comparison with transesophageal echocardiography. *Catheter Cardiovasc Interv.* 2005;66(2):258–267.
102. Hijazi Z, Wang Z, Cao Q, Koenig P, Waight D, Lang R. Transcatheter closure of atrial septal defects and patent foramen ovale under intracardiac echocardiographic guidance: feasibility and comparison with transesophageal echocardiography. *Catheter Cardiovasc Interv.* 2001;52(2):194–199.
103. Allen HD, Beekman RH 3rd, Garson A Jr, et al. Pediatric therapeutic cardiac catheterization: a statement for healthcare professionals from the Council on Cardiovascular Disease in the Young, American Heart Association. *Circulation.* 1998;97(6):609–625.
104. Bacha EA, Hijazi ZM, Cao QL, et al. New therapeutic avenues with hybrid pediatric cardiac surgery. *Heart Surg Forum.* 2004;7(1):33–40.
105. Bacha EA, Cao QL, Starr JP, Waight D, Ebeid MR, Hijazi ZM. Perventricular device closure of muscular ventricular septal defects on the beating heart: technique and results. *J Thorac Cardiovasc Surg.* 2003;126(6):1718–1723.
106. Bacha EA, Daves S, Hardin J, et al. Single-ventricle palliation for high-risk neonates: the emergence of an alternative hybrid stage I strategy. *J Thorac Cardiovasc Surg.* 2006;131(1):163–171.e162.
107. Pizarro C, Murdison KA, Derby CD, Radtke W. Stage II reconstruction after hybrid palliation for high-risk patients with a single ventricle. *Ann Thorac Surg.* 2008;85(4):1382–1388.
108. Pizarro C, Bhat MA, Derby CD, Radtke WA. Bailout after failed biventricular management of critical aortic stenosis: another application of the hybrid approach. *Ann Thorac Surg.* 2009;87(5):e40–e42.
109. Vitiello R, McCrindle BW, Nykanen D, Freedom RM, Benson LN. Complications associated with pediatric cardiac catheterization. *J Am Coll Cardiol.* 1998;32(5):1433–1440.
110. Bennett D, Marcus R, Stokes M. Incidents and complications during pediatric cardiac catheterization. *Paediatr Anaesth.* 2005;15(12):1083–1088.
111. Rothman A. Arterial complications of interventional cardiac catheterization in patients with congenital heart disease. *Circulation.* 1990;82(5):1868–1871.
112. Siddik-Sayyid SM, Abdallah FW, Dahrouj GB. Thermal burns in three neonates associated with intraoperative use of Bair Hugger warming devices. *Paediatr Anaesth.* 2008;18(4):337–339.
113. Truell KD, Bakerman PR, Teodori MF, Maze A. Third-degree burns due to intraoperative use of a Bair Hugger warming device. *Ann Thorac Surg.* 2000;69(6):1933–1934.
114. Latson L. Pulmonary artery stenosis. In: Sievert H, Qureshi SA, Wilson N, Hijazi Z, eds. *Percutaneous Interventions for Congenital Heart Disease.* London, England: Informa; 2007:447–460.
115. Allan CK, Thiagarajan RR, Armsby LR, del Nido PJ, Laussen PC. Emergent use of extracorporeal membrane oxygenation during pediatric cardiac catheterization. *Pediatr Crit Care Med.* 2006;7(3):212–219.
116. Schroeder VA, Shim D, Spicer RL, Pearl JM, Manning PJ, Beekman RH 3rd. Surgical emergencies during pediatric interventional catheterization. *J Pediatr.* 2002;140(5):570–575.
117. Bashore TM, Bates ER, Berger PB, et al. American College of Cardiology/Society for Cardiac Angiography and Interventions Clinical Expert Consensus Document on cardiac catheterization laboratory standards. A report of the American College of Cardiology Task Force on Clinical Expert Consensus Documents. *J Am Coll Cardiol.* 2001;37(8):2170–2214.
118. Fuster V, Ryden LE, Cannom DS, et al. ACC/AHA/ESC 2006 guidelines for the management of patients with atrial fibrillation-executive summary: a report of the American College of Cardiology/American Heart Association Task Force on Practice Guidelines (Writing Committee to Revise the 2001 Guidelines for the Management of Patients With Atrial Fibrillation): developed in collaboration with the European Heart Rhythm Association and the Heart Rhythm Society. *Circulation.* 2006:114;700–752.
119. Ganz L. Catheter ablation of cardiac arrhythmias: overview and technical aspects. Available at: http://www.uptodate.com/patients/content/topic.do?topicKey=~z7.zDl5gb599mrR. Last updated January 23, 2017. Accessed on July 20, 2010.
120. Epstein AE, DiMarco JP, Ellenbogen KA, et al. ACC/AHA/HRS 2008 guidelines for device-based therapy of cardiac rhythm abnormalities: a report of the American College of Cardiology/American Heart Association Task Force on Practice Guidelines (Writing Committee to Revise the ACC/AHA/NASPE 2002 Guideline Update for Implantation of Cardiac Pacemakers and Antiarrhythmia Devices) developed in collaboration with the American Association for Thoracic Surgery and Society of Thoracic Surgeons. *J Am Coll Cardiol.* 2008;51:e1.
121. Brignole M, Raciti G, Bongiorni MG, et al. Testing at the time of implantation of cardioverter defibrillator in clinical practice: a nation-wide survey. *Europace.* 2007;9(7):540–543.
122. McAlister FA, Ezekowitz JA, Wiebe N, et al. Systematic review: cardiac resynchronization in patients with symptomatic heart failure. *Ann Intern Med.* 2004;141:381–390.
123. Moss AJ, Zareba W, Hall WJ, et al. Prophylactic implantation of a defibrillator in patients with myocardial infarction and reduced ejection fraction. *N Engl J Med.* 2002;346:877.
124. Meyer J, Mollhoff T, Seifert T, et al. Cardiac output is not affected during intraoperative testing of the automatic implantable cardioverter defibrillator. *J Cardiovasc Electrophysiol.* 1996;7:211.
125. Gilbert TB, Gold MR, Shorofsky SR, et al. Cardiovascular responses to repetitive defibrillation during implantable-cardioverter-defibrillator testing. *J Cardiothorac Vasc Anesth.* 2002;16:180.
126. Bashore TM, Bates ER, Berger PB, et al. American College of Cardiology/Society for Cardiac Angiography and Interventions Clinical Expert Consensus Document on cardiac catheterization laboratory standards. A report of the American College of Cardiology Task Force on Clinical Expert Consensus Documents. *J Am Coll Cardiol* 2001;37:2170.
127. Katz JD. Radiation exposure to anesthesia personnel: the impact of an electrophysiology laboratory. *Anesth Analg.* 2005;101:1725.

23 | ANESTHESIA FOR ASSISTED REPRODUCTIVE TECHNOLOGIES

VESELA KOVACHEVA, MD, PHD, PATRICIA M. SEQUEIRA, MD

INTRODUCTION

In vitro fertilization (IVF) is a broad term used to describe the process of obtaining an oocyte, uniting it with sperm in a laboratory setting, and subsequently placing the fertilized oocyte or embryo into the uterus in hopes of achieving a live birth. In terms of anesthesiology, IVF primarily means oocyte retrieval. Historically, the oocytes were retrieved laparoscopically. With the introduction of the transvaginal ultrasound, the method of retrieval changed to a less invasive and costly procedure. Transvaginal ultrasound-guided oocyte aspiration changed the requirements for anesthesia. In this chapter, the anesthesia for oocyte retrieval and related IVF procedures is described.

CAUSES OF INFERTILITY

Infertility is defined as the inability to conceive for a given period of time, usually 1 year. The causes of infertility include (fallopian) tubal factors, ovulatory dysfunction, diminished ovarian reserve, endometriosis, uterine factors, male factors (very low sperm count or abnormal sperm motility), other factors (not treatable by current available methods), and unknown factors. Female infertility causes account for approximately one-third of the infertility cases; male infertility causes account for another one-third, and the remaining one-third of cases are caused by a mixture of female and male problems or by idiopathic factors.[1]

ASSISTED REPRODUCTIVE TECHNOLOGIES

Assisted reproductive technologies (ARTs) refer to all techniques involving the direct extraction of oocytes from the ovaries.[2] Advances in endocrine assays, controlled ovarian stimulation (COH), hormonal manipulation, cryopreservation, ultrasonography, and procedures on eggs, sperm, and embryos have transformed IVF. The ART physician is a gynecologist subspecialty trained in reproductive endocrinology and infertility. IVF usually refers to the process of oocyte retrieval and fertilization in the laboratory with subsequent embryo transfer to the uterus. Intrauterine insemination (IUI) is the placement of prepared sperm into the endometrial cavity via a small catheter. Intracytoplasmic sperm injection (ICSI) is an ART procedure where a single sperm is injected into the retrieved ovum. IVF also refers to other ART techniques, such as gamete intrafallopian transfer (GIFT) and zygote intrafallopian transfer (ZIFT). The GIFT procedure involves the transfer of retrieved oocytes and washed sperm into the fallopian tube by laparoscopy. The ZIFT procedure involves transfer of one or more embryos laparoscopically into the fallopian tube. Since the introduction of the transvaginal ultrasound probe for oocyte retrieval, these technologies are rarely used. IVF–embryo transfer (IVF-ET) is a widely used term for transvaginal ultrasound–guided oocyte aspiration and the subsequent transcervical embryo transfer.

THE IVF CYCLE

The IVF cycle consists of several ART steps over a period of approximately 2 weeks. The cycle is considered a series of treatments rather than a single procedure. The IVF cycle starts when a woman begins taking hormonal medications to stimulate oocyte production or starts ovarian monitoring with the intention of having embryos transferred. A successful IVF cycle starts either naturally or with medication and is followed by the production of oocytes. Next is oocyte retrieval. If fertilization is successful, then the next step is incubation and subsequent embryo transfer. If the embryo implants within the uterus, then pregnancy is achieved. This is followed by the delivery of one or more live births. The absence of oocyte production, excessive ovarian hyperstimulation, or other medical reasons may require the discontinuation of the cycle.

CONTROLLED OVARIAN HYPERSTIMULATION

Controlled ovarian hyperstimulation (COH) is an ART process through which the ovaries are purposely stimulated to develop more than one dominant follicle. This is considered the start of an IVF cycle. Having multiple dominant follicles will increase the number of oocytes retrieved and the likelihood of successful pregnancy from transferred embryos. The goal of COH is to promote the development of a relatively synchronous cohort of ovarian follicles so that the oocyte retrieval can be performed at a specified time. A typical COH protocol uses a combination of a gonadotropin-releasing hormone agonist (GnRH-a), human menopausal gonadotropin (hMG), and human chorionic gonadotropin (hCG). Ovarian suppression and follicular variation are achieved with GnRH-a. The ovaries are monitored by serial ultrasound examinations. Ovarian stimulation is begun with hMG administration. Serial follicular diameters and estrogen levels guide the timing of the administration of hCG. Oocyte retrieval is usually approximately 36 hours after the start of hCG. COH also achieves the development of the proper endometrial environment for the subsequent embryos to be transferred.[3] The hormonal protocols vary by clinic, endocrinologist, and patient and adjustments can be done to account for the individual hormonal response. COH is always carefully monitored with serial ultrasound examination to evaluate the follicle size and progression of hormonal blood levels.

OVARIAN HYPERSTIMULATION SYNDROME AND IVF SURGICAL RISKS

The ART of COH is not without adverse effects. Ovarian hyperstimulation syndrome (OHSS) is an iatrogenic, potentially life-threatening complication of COH. Symptoms begin with abdominal bloating and progress to nausea, vomiting, and diarrhea. Lethargy and loss of appetite follow. Shortness of breath and decreased urine output may indicate accumulating ascites and increasing morbidity. The patient with moderate or severe OHSS may have signs of rapid weight gain, oliguria, hemoconcentration, leukocytosis, hypovolemia, electrolyte imbalance, ascites, pleural and pericardial effusions, adult respiratory distress syndrome, hypercoagulability and thromboembolic events, and multiorgan failure. OHSS should be self-limiting, and regression takes place as long as prompt and appropriate supportive care is provided. Exogenous and endogenous hCG will worsen OHSS.[4]

Surgical risks for IVF transvaginal ultrasound-guided oocyte retrieval may include bleeding, infection, and injury to pelvic or abdominal organs. These surgical complications may require hospitalization or subsequent surgery. Oskowitz et al.[5] reported on a series of 6776 procedures performed in a freestanding surgical facility dedicated to ART. Of the 4199 patients who had vaginal oocyte retrieval procedures, seven required hospital admission during the first 24 hours after surgery. Two patients had serious morbidity, defined as requiring major intervention, such as a repeat surgery. Nausea and vomiting, syncope, hemoperitoneum, and ovarian hematoma were included in the admitting diagnoses.

ANESTHESIA FOR TRANSVAGINAL OOCYTE RETRIEVAL

Ultrasound-guided oocyte retrieval can be performed under a paracervical block, intravenous sedation, or general, spinal, and epidural anesthesia. The literature concerning the choice of anesthesia on the success of IVF should be interpreted with caution. Specific anesthetic drugs and techniques must be evaluated for their compatibility. Animal data may not reflect the human experience.[6]

UK AND US IVF ANESTHESIA PRACTICE EVALUATIONS

According to Elkington's questionnaire of ART centers in the United Kingdom, there are significant variations in the personnel present during the procedure, the choice of medications, the degree of monitoring, and the availability of emergency drugs.[7] Eighty-four percent of the ART centers used intravenous sedation, and 16% used general anesthesia for transvaginal oocyte retrieval.

Results from a Ditkoff et al.[8] telephone survey in the United States of 278 ART programs revealed that 91 private (68%) and 41 academic (56%) programs used personnel from the Department of Anesthesiology. A large number of ART programs used their own trained personnel to provide sedation. Ninety-five percent of the transvaginal oocyte retrievals and transcervical embryo transfers were performed under conscious sedation. For the remaining 5%, general, regional, or local anesthesia was used. The majority of the IVF personnel typically used meperidine and midazolam. Ninety percent of the anesthesiology personnel used midazolam or propofol with fentanyl.

IVF PATIENT DEMOGRAPHICS

Although the majority of IVF patients are healthy adult women, overweight and morbidly obese patients are sometimes encountered. Other medical conditions common in this population include asthma and hypertension. Psychosocial disorders such as anxiety, depression, and stress secondary to the infertility status may be present. The women typically range in age from the late 20s to mid-40s.

THE IVF FACILITIES

According to a questionnaire by Yasmin and colleagues,[9] 69% of the responding IVF centers performed oocyte retrieval outside of the general operating room environment. A typical IVF procedure room may be located within a university-based or freestanding fertility clinic. The embryology and andrology laboratories are usually adjacent to the procedure room for immediate processing of the oocytes and sperm. The IVF anesthesiologist is required to be familiar with the IVF procedures, the fertility center's choice of sedation/analgesia and anesthesia, the individual surgeon's needs, and the needs of the IVF patient.

ANESTHESIA FOR IVF

GOALS

The anesthetic goals for IVF oocyte retrieval and related procedures are effective pain relief and sedation, together with minimal postoperative nausea and vomiting (PONV). These goals should be executed in a safe manner. IVF goals also include the ease of administering intravenous medications and patient monitoring. The medications should be short acting and easily reversible. These drugs should minimally affect the oocytes, the embryos, and the endocrine and the immune systems. It is important to keep in mind that these procedures are costly, and economic factors should be considered.[10]

CONSIDERATIONS

The foremost anesthetic considerations for the IVF patient in the preprocedural period are patient anxiety management. This unique population of patients may have stress, anxiety, and depression due to their infertile status. They may arrive with varying degrees of anxiety from the expectant wait of the oocyte or sperm retrieval. Empathy from all those involved in their care, such as the IVF nursing staff, the procedure room staff, the embryologist, the reproductive medicine physician, and the anesthesiologist, is invaluable.

Preprocedural anesthesia concerns are minor due to the general health of the IVF patient. On occasion, airway issues can arise from patients who have a history of loud snoring, sleep apnea, or obesity. The patients with a history of asthma or hypertension are usually medically compliant, and most commonly their conditions are well controlled. A history of PONV or motion sickness should be elicited and reduction of baseline risks planned for and initiated. Pain management should be discussed with the patient. Patients who did not adhere to the instructions to take nothing by mouth represent a unique challenge because the oocyte retrieval is a carefully timed procedure, and postponing it for more than 30 minutes puts the patients at risk for spontaneous ovulation. In those patients, full aspiration precautions are needed, and spinal anesthesia should be considered.

Once in the procedure room, any airway issues should be communicated to the surgeon because the sedation level or anesthetic may be different from usual. Care and vigilance should be taken during the placement of the patient in the dorsal lithotomy position. Positioning while awake and not sedated ensures proper padding for comfort of the patient. Adequate anesthesia and sedation should ensure an immobile patient to help avoid injury to pelvic vessels or organs.

RISKS

When administering intravenous anesthetic agents, attention should be directed to avoiding apnea. Recognition and immediate treatment are therefore essential. Reducing the dose of intravenous agents and providing a greater stimulus (chin lift or a jaw thrust) may help overcome the apnea. In a case of airway obstruction, oral or nasal airway insertion may be necessary. Bag/mask ventilation may become necessary if the patient experiences prolonged apnea. Opioid or benzodiazepine reversal should not be routinely used. Instead, the desired anesthetic level is achieved by careful titration of the intravenous agents to proper effect.

Patients at risk for aspiration should be identified during the preoperative consultation. Aspiration needs to be recognized quickly, and suction should be readily available. Laryngospasm is a risk in the anesthetized and obtunded patient. Successful laryngospasm management includes early recognition followed by positive pressure ventilation and deepening of the anesthetic level, possible intubation, or waking up the patient. Hypotension from an anesthetic agent such as propofol is treated with generous fluid hydration. Vasopressors are rarely needed. PONV can be seen in this patient population, and appropriate prophylaxis strategies should be employed.

IVF PROCEDURES

The most common procedure that requires anesthesia during an IVF cycle is oocyte retrieval. On occasion, an embryo transfer procedure will be scheduled with anesthesia. The dilation and curettage (D&C) procedure is sometimes scheduled in the IVF suite. Additionally, the urologist may request anesthesia services for microscopic epididymal sperm aspiration (MESA) and testicular sperm extraction (TESE) procedures.

OOCYTE RETRIEVAL

The reproductive medicine surgeon selectively retrieves oocytes from the individual ovarian follicles, which have been stimulated via COH. Because the patient has been given hormonal drugs to induce ovulation, there is a small time window in which the oocytes can be retrieved. As oocyte retrieval is a specially scheduled and timed procedure, the anesthesia service should be available to accommodate these patients 7 days a week. The surgeon may request a dose of antibiotics for the patient with a history of tubal disease to prevent a pelvic infection.

The patient is positioned in the dorsal lithotomy position. Once the patient is sterilely prepped and draped, the surgeon places a transvaginal ultrasound probe equipped with a long needle to aspirate the ovarian follicles. The aspirating needle is usually of a 16 or 17 gauge and is guided through the posterior vaginal wall to the ovary, where each follicle is aspirated. Follicular fluid is aspirated into a test tube with culture medium. These test tubes are given to the embryologist, who then examines and counts the oocytes. The oocyte retrieval is then continued on the contralateral ovary. The duration of this procedure is usually 5–10 minutes.

EMBRYO TRANSFER

Embryo transfer is a short IVF procedure. The process consists of transferring one or several embryos from the laboratory to the patient's uterus. The patient is placed in the dorsal lithotomy position with stirrups. The vagina is sterilely prepped. A small, semirigid catheter containing the embryos is placed into the uterine cavity via the cervix. When the uterine anatomy is difficult or abnormal, an abdominal ultrasound may aid in this process. The catheter is then returned to the embryology lab to ensure the embryos are no longer in the catheter. Patients with difficult, or abnormal, cervical or uterine anatomy and those who are extremely anxious may require anesthesia.

DILATION AND CURETTAGE

The IVF patient is at a higher risk for miscarriage. The D&C procedure in the outside of the operating room (OOOR) environment, such as the IVF suite, should be done only on carefully selected patients. A healthy patient of normal weight and normal coagulation who is not excessively bleeding and is less than 12 weeks' pregnant is ideal for D&C in the OOOR setting. D&Cs for obese patients, those with a full stomach, and patients with second-trimester pregnancies should be reserved for the operating room.

The patient is placed in a dorsal lithotomy position with stirrups. The vagina is sterilely prepped and draped. The surgeon examines the uterus with the vaginal ultrasound to reconfirm the miscarriage. A vaginal speculum is inserted, and the cervix is grasped with a clamp. The cervical canal is then dilated with progressively larger dilators. Utmost care is taken not to perforate the uterine cavity. The endometrial lining and products of conception are removed with the curette and the suction aspirate.

SPERM RETRIEVAL TECHNIQUES

Microscopic epididymal sperm aspiration, percutaneous epididymal sperm aspiration (PESA), and TESE are a few of the different sperm retrieval procedures that take place at an infertility center. These methods refer to certain cases of male infertility. These procedures are done by the urologist and are tailored to the individual couple's needs. The sperm that is obtained is then used for intracytoplasmic sperm injection. The MESA technique utilizes microsurgical techniques to obtain sperm from the epididymis. The TESE technique involves removal of a small sample of testis tissue for extraction of sperm by the andrology laboratory. During the PESA technique, a needle is used to draw sperm from the epididymis.

The male patient is in the supine position. The scrotum is sterilely prepped and draped. Local anesthesia is used. If the procedure is an open one, the urologist will use the operating microscope. The sperm retrieval usually lasts approximately 1 hour. The urologist may request anesthesia services.

CRITERIA FOR SELECTION OF ANESTHETIC TYPE

The selection of anesthesia type will depend on the IVF center and the surgeon's preference. This is seen by the variation in personnel and drugs used. The anesthesia provider can modify those choices, especially in select patients who may have a difficult airway, are obese, or have a history of PONV.

ANESTHESIA FOR EGG RETRIEVAL: MODERATE SEDATION

Intravenous moderate sedation for transvaginal ultrasound-guided oocyte retrieval is the most commonly used anesthetic type.[8] This is usually accomplished by the IVF center's dedicated anesthesia group or its own personnel who are specially trained in administering moderate sedation. The personnel may include nursing staff or medical doctors who are trained and experienced in IVF procedures.

According to the American Society of Anesthesiologists (ASA), moderate ("conscious") sedation is defined as follows:

> *A drug-induced depression of consciousness during which patients respond purposefully to verbal commands, either alone or accompanied by light tactile stimulation. No interventions are required to maintain a patent airway, and spontaneous ventilation is adequate. Cardiovascular function is usually maintained.*[11]

Keeping in mind the goals of moderate sedation, oocyte retrieval can be safely accomplished. The patient's chart is reviewed, including the nursing staff's preoperative assessment. This includes the medical and surgical history and the patient's medications and allergies. The height, weight, and baseline vital signs are noted.

The patient interview includes the status of nothing taken by mouth, medical and anesthesia history, as well history of PONV or motion sickness. After the physical examination, the sedation plan and the expectations are explained to the patient. This explanation helps alleviate some of the anxiety associated with the procedure.

The discussion should include the information that the patient will be sedated yet responsive to tactile touch or voice commands for the evaluation of pain or discomfort. The patient should be reassured that comfort and pain control are the goals of moderate sedation. The anesthesia consent is obtained. The IVF procedure team readiness is checked so that the patient can be brought into the procedure room. This is necessary because the embryology laboratory also participates in this procedure by accepting the collected oocytes and reports the oocyte count intraprocedurally. Once in the procedure room, the nursing staff, surgeon, embryologist, and anesthesiologist will identify the patient and perform a safety checklist.

The patient is positioned supine on the operating room table. The routine monitors and an intravenous catheter are placed. Oxygen is usually provided via a nasal cannula. As soon as the intravenous line is in place, the patient is repositioned to the dorsal lithotomy position with perineum positioned at the edge of the operating room table.

Once the patient reports no discomfort in this position, the sedation is started. The opioid is usually the first agent given because the goal of sedation is pain management during oocyte retrieval. The opioid most frequently used is fentanyl. The usual dose of fentanyl is in the range of 50 to 100 μg IV.[7] Once fentanyl titration is begun, then the anxiolytic is administered. The most common agent is a benzodiazepine, such as midazolam or diazepam. This agent is also titrated to the desired effect: The patient is relaxed and sedated yet responsive to light tactile touch and voice.

When the desired sedation level is achieved, the surgeon places the ultrasound probe into the vagina. Both ovaries are examined, and the physician reports a gross estimate of the oocytes to be retrieved. This report helps gauge the length of time expected for the procedure. The placement of the probe can be very stimulating when the ovaries are difficult to visualize and maximal pressure is applied into the posterior vaginal wall. The next stimulus is the puncture through the vaginal wall into the ovary and follicles. A 16- or 17-gauge needle is used alongside the vaginal probe. Each follicle that is visualized is aspirated until there are no follicles left in the ovary. This procedure is then repeated on the contralateral ovary. Once the retrieval is complete, the probe is used to evaluate the ovaries for possible bleeding or surrounding vessel and tissue injury. Finally, the probe is withdrawn. A vaginal speculum is then placed to evaluate for bleeding or vaginal wall injury. Pressure is typically held at the vaginal wall puncture sites for a short time. Usually, no additional medication is needed at this point because the inspection of the vagina may not be uncomfortable or painful. If the surgeon needs to place a suture or hold extensive vaginal pressure, additional opioids may be needed as well as further verbal reassurance. Once there is no bleeding, the patient is brought to a more awake state. The patient is then transferred to a gurney and transported to the adjacent postprocedure room.

GENERAL ANESTHESIA

Anesthesiologists use general anesthesia (most commonly total intravenous anesthesia) extensively during IVF procedures. The most commonly used drug for general anesthesia is propofol, as reported by Ditkoff and coworkers.[8] This type of anesthesia may need airway support, but it rarely requires endotracheal intubation. The support of the airway is generally assisted with minimally invasive maneuvers, such as a chin lift or jaw thrust. On occasion, a nasopharyngeal airway may be needed in the patient who is obstructing his or her airway, has a small chin, or is obese. The goals of this type of anesthetic are an immobile, or nearly immobile, patient who is unconscious. Associated risks such as apnea, aspiration, laryngospasm, or hypotension need to be considered. Therefore, the specially trained anesthesiologist is required, and expert airway management is essential. In this anesthetic, plans for emergency management of the airway include having equipment available in the procedure room. A laryngoscope, various sizes of blades and endotracheal tubes, and a self-inflating type of bag-mask should be present.

After careful review of the IVF patient chart and checking status of having nothing by mouth, the interview focuses on medical and anesthesia issues, and a focused airway examination is performed. A past history of PONV, pain management, and any vasovagal events are noted.

The goals of the anesthetic are discussed, and a brief description of the procedure and postprocedure anesthesia plan are outlined. This overview is very much appreciated by the patient receiving IVF and may alleviate some of the preprocedural anxiety. The oocyte retrieval anesthesia consent is obtained. Once the procedure team, which includes the embryologist, is ready to proceed, the patient is brought into the procedure room. The patient identifications are obtained by the IVF nursing staff and the embryologist, and a safety pause is performed. The patient is placed supine on the operating room table. The routine monitors that are placed include a continuous electrocardiogram, pulse oximetry, noninvasive blood pressure, and CO_2 analysis. An intravenous catheter is placed. The patient is repositioned into the dorsal lithotomy with the perineum at the edge of the table. Pressure points and any discomfort are checked and relieved. Oxygen is administered by a nasal cannula or face mask.

Once the patient positioning is complete, the anesthetic is begun with the opioid. Fentanyl is titrated along with the hypnotic agent propofol by boluses or continuous infusion. The usual required doses of fentanyl range from 75 to 150 µg, with the most common total being 100 µg. A small dose of lidocaine is usually administered along with the start of the propofol when the intravenous catheter is in place. Lidocaine is usually not needed when the intravenous catheter is located at the antecubital area in a large vein.

The surgeon is allowed to start once the patient has been rendered unconscious and immobile. There are two potentially stimulating portions of the IVF-oocyte retrieval. The first stimulus is the placement of the vaginal probe deep into the vagina to examine the ovaries. The second stimulus is the puncture of the vaginal wall and ovarian follicle with the 16- or 17-gauge aspirating needle. This procedure is repeated until all the follicles have been aspirated, and then it is continued on the contralateral ovary. Once the aspiration is completed, the ovaries and surrounding tissue and vessels are examined by ultrasound for bleeding or injury. The probe is removed and replaced with a vaginal speculum for inspection of the posterior vaginal wall for bleeding or injury. On occasion, a bleeding puncture site may need a suture or maximal tamponade with pressure. If this is the case, the patient is kept sedated until the vaginal wall examination is completed.

The patient is awakened at the end of the procedure and asked to move to the awaiting gurney. The patient is transported to the adjacent recovery room. The dedicated recovery room nursing staff is given a report and monitors the patient until discharge.

INTRAVENOUS GENERAL ANESTHESIA FOR EMBRYO TRANSFER

Occasionally, the patient receiving IVF will request anesthesia for the transcervical embryo transfer. The main reason is to alleviate the procedural anxiety and discomfort of the vaginal speculum and cervical stimulation. Usually, the IVF center will administer an oral benzodiazepine for those with mild-to-moderate anxiety because the patient is kept "awake" for this very short, yet anxiety-provoking, event. The reproductive medicine physician may request anesthesia for the patient with a difficult cervical or uterine anatomy. Having the patient under a brief period of deep anesthesia will facilitate the maneuvering of the small plastic catheter containing the embryos into the uterus. The embryo transfer is facilitated by the simultaneous use of the abdominal ultrasound by an assistant to visualize the uterine cavity. This ultrashort procedure is not very stimulating or painful; therefore, the use of short-acting agents is encouraged.

The patient chart is reviewed, and the history and physical exam are obtained. The goal of the anesthetic is discussed with the patient. Patient safety, comfort, and anxiolysis are emphasized. Describing the anesthetic/IVF procedure helps ease some of the preprocedure anxiety.

In the procedure room, the patient's identification is verified by the nurse and again by the embryologist. The patient is positioned supine on the operating table. The routine monitors and an intravenous catheter are placed. Then, the patient is repositioned into the dorsal lithotomy position. Pressure points are padded and checked. The anesthesia is started during the vaginal preparation, which also includes the placement of a vaginal speculum by the proceduralist. Deep sedation/general anesthesia can be accomplished with a combination of fentanyl and propofol. Approximately 50 μg of fentanyl are titrated along with 75 to 150 mg of propofol. Care is taken to keep the patient breathing spontaneously and deeply and in an immobile state for the embryo transfer.

ANESTHESIA FOR DILATION AND CURETTAGE

From time to time, the IVF anesthesiologist will be scheduled to administer an intravenous deep sedation or general anesthesia for a missed abortion. This is not unusual because the IVF patient has a higher risk for a missed abortion. The ideal patient for a D&C in the OOOR environment is a healthy patient of normal weight. This should not include the morbidly obese individual or a patient with a coagulation abnormality or difficult airway. Additionally, the patients should not be past 12 weeks' gestational age and should adhere to the guidelines for nothing by mouth. The more challenging patients, the morbidly obese, or those with a difficult airway or coagulation abnormalities should be scheduled in an operating room facility equipped to handle these situations. They may need general anesthesia with an endotracheal tube, a regional anesthetic, or blood products available. Few reproductive medicine surgeons may elect to do the D&C without the anesthesiologist's presence. In these instances, the surgeon may provide moderate intravenous sedation together with a paracervical block.

The patient's chart is reviewed with emphasis on the reason for the D&C and the approximate gestational age. The laboratory work is reviewed for the hematocrit, platelet count, and blood type. When an Rh-negative woman carries an Rh-positive pregnancy, RhoGAM® is given to prevent the woman's immune system from reacting to Rh-positive blood of any subsequent pregnancy.

The goals of the anesthetic are reviewed with the patient. Safety and comfort are emphasized. Empathy and reassurance help with the preprocedural anxiety.

The anesthesia setup should include an emergency intubation kit and vasoactive drugs. Major surgical risks include uterine bleeding and perforation. A dose of antibiotic will likely be requested by the reproductive medicine surgeon. The most stimulating part of the D&C is the serial dilation of the cervical os and canal.

In the procedure room, the nursing staff, surgeon, and anesthesiologist should perform a safety pause. The patient is positioned supine onto the operating room table. The routine monitors are placed. A minimum of a 20-gauge intravenous catheter is placed. The patient is then repositioned in the dorsal lithotomy position with the perineum at the lateral edge of the table. Pressure points are checked for any discomfort. Oxygen is administered via a nasal cannula or face mask. A small dose of midazolam is given for anxiolysis and amnesia. A few minutes later, fentanyl is titrated in doses of 25 μg. The usual required doses of fentanyl range from 50 to 100 μg, with the most common total a 100-μg dose. Propofol is usually administered in a bolus (250–500 μg/kg) followed by an infusion (25–75 μg/kg/min) to induce hypnosis yet keep the patient spontaneously breathing with minimal airway assistance. The duration of the D&C procedure is usually short, lasting from 10 to 20 minutes.

IVF POSTANESTHESIA CARE UNIT CONSIDERATIONS

After IVF, the care of the patient in the postanesthesia care unit (PACU) or recovery room has a few, yet very important, considerations. In the designated recovery area, patient care is transferred to the assigned recovery room nurse. The patient care transfer begins with proper patient identification, followed by a description of the procedure, the anesthetics used, drug allergies, antiemetics, antibiotics, and fluids administered. Anesthesia or surgery-related complications encountered are communicated. Pertinent patient details for the patient receiving IVF, such as history of PONV, extreme preprocedural anxiety, large amounts of anesthetics required intraprocedurally, and approximate oocyte count, should be communicated. This information will help patient management. A young patient or egg donor with many oocytes retrieved will most probably require additional analgesic care in the PACU.

On arrival in the PACU, attention is focused on the oxygenation, ventilation, and circulation by monitoring the pulse oximetry, respiratory frequency, airway patency, systemic blood pressure, and heart rate. Supplemental oxygen and suction should be readily available. The vital signs are recorded at the very least every 15 minutes while in the recovery room. Initially in the PACU, care may be directed toward the need for airway support for a sedated patient. This is treated by patient stimulation and a chin lift. Initial hypotension is usually secondary to the propofol anesthesia and is self-limiting. Continuing the intravenous fluids and awakening the patient usually will resolve the hypotension. Moderate-to-severe pain on admission should be immediately treated with intravenous fentanyl; discharge may be otherwise delayed secondary to increasing pain or PONV.

Patients who have received IVF usually stay in the PACU from 90 to 120 minutes.[8] Typical causes for a delay in the discharge from the recovery room are abdominal cramping or pain, PONV, a vasovagal event, or delay in urination.

The approach to the treatment and relief of abdominal or pelvic pain in the IVF patient is to first identify what type of pain the patient is experiencing and where it is located. It is also important for the anesthesiologist to quantify the amount of pain experienced in order to achieve treatment success. Moderate-to-severe pain is treated with opioids, while mild pain is treated with nonopioids such as acetaminophen. Any unrelenting pain should be evaluated by the reproductive medicine surgeon. The evaluation involves talking to the patient, a physical examination, and possibly a pelvic ultrasound. A full bladder also may be responsible for ongoing abdominal pain. If this is the case, the patient is encouraged to urinate; otherwise, the patient may undergo straight catheterization of the bladder.

Considerations for PONV actually start during the preprocedure period. The recognition that the IVF population is at risk is the first step.[12] Furthermore, the identification of the individual at high risk for PONV is extremely important for patient safety, satisfaction, and efficiency. By identifying the individual in need of prophylactic antiemetic therapy, patient care and satisfaction can significantly improve. According to Apfel and colleagues,[13] the four primary risk factors for PONV are female gender, nonsmoking status, a history of PONV, and opioid use. The typical patient receiving IVF has at least three of the four risk factors. A history of PONV and motion sickness can be specifically determined during the patient interview. The PONV risk reduction strategies include preprocedural anxiolysis, aggressive intravenous hydration, supplemental oxygen, and total intravenous anesthesia with propofol. PONV antiemetic prophylaxis coupled with these strategies is known as a multimodal approach.[12]

The PONV risk reduction begins with a calming and reassuring interview and plan. Intravenous hydration is started intraprocedurally and continued in the PACU. Oxygen is administered during the procedure, and prophylactic antiemetics are given to select patients, such as those with a history of PONV and motion sickness. Additionally, a patient with many aspirated follicles and an increased opioid requirement will benefit from prophylactic antiemetics.

When PONV occurs in the PACU and the patient has not received prophylaxis, a 5-hydroxytryptamine (serotonin) receptor 3 (5-HT_3) antagonist such as ondansetron should be administered. Aggressive intravenous fluid administration should be verified as ongoing, and a vasovagal event eliminated. In the event that PONV prophylaxis with a 5-HT_3 antagonist is found to be inadequate, an additional dose of a 5-HT_3 antagonist should not be used as a rescue agent because it does not give additional benefit when used within the first 6 hours after surgery.[14] Prochlorperazine, droperidol, dexamethasone, or metoclopramide have been used for PONV rescue.

On occasion, a patient may experience lightheadedness and nausea as a result of becoming bradycardic and hypotensive. This vasovagal event should be immediately identified and treated. Placing the patient in the supine position and administering a bolus of crystalloid fluid should suffice. Symptoms usually resolve quickly. If bradycardia accompanied by hypotension persists, a dose of atropine should be administered. Cramping pain may be responsible for the vasovagal event and should be treated.

Rarely, brisk vaginal bleeding is observed in the PACU. If this is the case, the reproductive medicine surgeon should evaluate the patient. This may involve a trip back to the procedure room for a thorough vaginal examination. Persistent hypotension is rarely seen but should be evaluated as well by the reproductive medicine surgeon.

The IVF nursing staff documents the patient's PACU course. Once the PACU criteria for discharge are met, the patient and the adult escort are given written discharge instructions. A postprocedure follow-up call is made the following morning by the nursing staff.

CONCLUSION

Oocyte retrieval is a very important part of the IVF cycle. Transvaginal oocyte retrieval is increasingly being performed OOOR. Moderate sedation is most commonly used for oocyte retrieval in the United States and the United Kingdom, although the trend is toward greater involvement of anesthesia professionals and more cases performed under deep sedation and general anesthesia. There is variability in personnel and medications used. A significant number of IVF centers are providing their own sedation team. The best sedation and anesthetic practices have yet to be proven.

REFERENCES

1. US Department of Health and Human Services Centers for Disease Control and Prevention. Assisted Reproductive Technology Success Rates. Available at: https://www.cdc.gov/art/Archived-PDF-Reports/2006ART.pdf. Accessed on January 15, 2018.
2. Bokhari A, Pollard BJ. Anaesthesia for assisted conception. *Eur J Anaesth.* 1998;15:391–396.
3. Wallach EE, Zacur HA. *Reproductive medicine and surgery.* Saint Louis, MO: Mosby; 1995.
4. Schenker JG, Ezra Y. Complications of assisted reproductive techniques. *Fertil Steril.* 1994;61:411–422.
5. Oskowitz SP, Berger MJ, Mullen L, et al. Safety of a freestanding surgical unit for the assisted reproductive technologies. *Fertil Steril.* 1995;63:874–879.
6. Tsen LC. From Darwin to Desflurane? Anesthesia for assisted reproductive technologies. *Anesth Analg.* 2002;94(suppl):109–114.
7. Elkington N, Kehoe J, Acharya U. Intravenous sedation in assisted conception units: a UK Survey. *Hum Fertil.* 2003;6:74–76.
8. Ditkoff EC, Plumb J, Selick A, et al. Anesthesia practices in the United States common to in vitro fertilization (IVF) centers. *J Assist Reprod Genet.* 1997;14:145–147.
9. Yasmin E, Dresner M, Balen A. Sedation and anaesthesia for transvaginal oocyte collection: an evaluation of practices in the UK. *Hum Reprod.* 2004;19(12):2942–2945.
10. Trout SW, Vallerand AH, Kemmann E. Conscious sedation for in vitro fertilization. *Fertil Steril.* 1998;69:799–808.
11. American Society of Anesthesiologists. Continuum of depth of sedation: definition of general anesthesia and levels of sedation/analgesia, last amended October 2014. http://www.asahq.org/quality-and-practice-management/standards-guidelines-and-related-resources/continuum-of-depth-of-sedation-definition-of-general-anesthesia-and-levels-of-sedation-analgesia. Last amended: October 2014. Accessed on January 15, 2018.
12. Gan TJ, Meyer T, Apfel CC, et al. Consensus guidelines for managing postoperative nausea and vomiting. *Anesth Analg.* 2003;97:62–71.
13. Apfel CC, Laara E, Koivuranta M, et al. A simplified risk score for predicting postoperative nausea and vomiting. *Anesthesiology.* 1999;91:693–700.
14. Kovac AL, O'Connor TA, Pearman MH, et al. Efficacy of repeat intravenous dosing of ondansetron in controlling postoperative nausea and vomiting: a randomized, double-blind, placebo-controlled multicenter trial. *J Clin Anesth.* 1999;11:453–459.

24 | ANESTHESIA FOR UROLOGIC PROCEDURES

CHRISTOPHER V. MAANI, MD, GAELEN HORNE, DO

INTRODUCTION

Thirty years ago, extracting a kidney stone was an extensive procedure that required a large incision, necessitated a 4- to 7-day hospitalization, and carried significant risk of morbidity.[1] However, advances in technology accompanied the development of new and less-invasive surgical techniques, and procedures that once required a traditional operating room could now be accomplished in smaller outpatient settings. In fact, procedures performed in offices tripled from 400,000 to 1.2 million per year from 1984 to 1990.[2,3] Maximizing efficiency and improving patient outcomes while minimizing hospitalization and recovery time became a focus of many anesthetic practices throughout the United States.

Because more procedures are being performed in outpatient and outside of the operating room (OOOR) settings, it is increasingly important for the anesthesiologist to ensure patient and personnel safety in addition to providing an optimal anesthetic for the patient.[4–7] This chapter discusses anesthesia for common urologic outpatient/OOOR procedures, including cystourethroscopy, ureteroscopy, transurethral procedures except transurethral resection of the prostate (TURP), laser use, percutaneous renal procedures, and extracorporeal shock wave lithotripsy (ESWL).

PREOPERATIVE CONSIDERATIONS

Urologic procedures comprise 10%–20% of most anesthetic practices and include patients of all ages. Particularly high-risk individuals (i.e., known difficult airway, severe aortic stenosis, morbid obesity) may not be candidates for outpatient surgery or off-site anesthesia and should have their procedures performed in a more controlled environment. Patients of any age undergoing urologic procedures should be evaluated preoperatively for renal insufficiency.

Some specific patient populations frequently present for outpatient or OOOR urologic procedures and require special anesthetic considerations that are discussed here. Elderly patients must be evaluated for coexisting diseases, including coronary artery disease, pacemaker or automatic implantable cardioverter/defibrillator (AICD) history, peripheral vascular disease, cerebrovascular disease, congestive heart failure, and chronic obstructive pulmonary disease. The risk of acute renal dysfunction is amplified by certain patient characteristics often associated with advancing age (Box 24.1), specifically after shock wave lithotripsy (SWL). These conditions should be evaluated, documented, and optimized if possible.

Paraplegics and quadriplegics have a high rate of recurrent nephrolithiasis and instrumentation[8,9] and require special consideration. Preoperatively, the anesthesia team must have a high suspicion for autonomic hyperreflexia, spastic contractures, and chronic infections, including pressure sores, recurrent urinary tract infections, and pneumonia. If muscle relaxants are to be used, resistance to nondepolarizing muscle relaxants may be present secondary to denervated muscle containing an increased number of extrajunctional acetylcholine receptors. Patients with denervated muscle are at higher risk for hyperkalemia and subsequent risk of cardiac arrest when succinylcholine is used. In addition, renal insufficiency may worsen after succinylcholine use due to increased myoglobin release from atrophied muscle.

Pediatric patients may also present for outpatient/OOOR urologic procedures. Effective and safe use of percutaneous lithotripsy and nephrolithotomy, holmium laser, and even SWL has been demonstrated for each in the pediatric and infant populations.[10] Cystoscopy is often performed in children with vesicoureteral reflux and patients with congenital kidney malformations; these patients may have associated syndromes or genetic defects.[11,12] A history of associated congenital anomalies should be pursued, even though the external features may be subtle; this is particularly true for cardiac and craniofacial abnormalities because of the potential for cardiac complications or a difficult airway in the OOOR environment. If a complicated medical history or suspected difficult airway is anticipated, the anesthesiologist should rethink the benefit/risk ratio of performing the procedure in the outpatient/OOOR milieu.

Therapies started by the urology team for most nonobstructed patients prior to the procedure include a high fluid intake (2–3 L), as well as pain medications and antibiotics. Certain patients should receive intravenous prophylactic antibiotics[13,14] before endourologic procedures (Box 24.2) or may already be receiving scheduled antibiotics. Percutaneous nephrolithotomy (PCNL) is considered clean-contaminated, and prophylactic antibiotics are recommended in all patients.[15] Typically, cephalosporins are given for PCNL

BOX 24.1. RISK FACTORS FOR ACUTE RENAL SIDE EFFECTS AFTER SHOCK WAVE LITHOTRIPSY

Age
Obesity
Coagulopathies
Thrombocytopenia
Diabetes mellitus
Coronary artery disease
Peripheral vascular disease
Preexisting hypertension

SOURCE: This table was published in *Campbell-Walsh Urology*. 9th ed., Vol. 2. Copyright Elsevier 2007.

BOX 24.2. DIAGNOSES THAT WARRANT PROPHYLACTIC INTRAVENOUS PREOPERATIVE ANTIBIOTICS

Proximal or impacted stone
Preoperative stent, catheter, nephrostomy tube
High-risk comorbidities

- *Immunosuppression*
- *Diabetes*
- *Presence of urinary stasis*
- *HIV*
- *Malignancy*
- *Malnourishment*

SOURCE: This table was published in *Campbell-Walsh Urology*. 9th ed., Vol. 2. Copyright Elsevier 2007.

to cover *Staphylococcus epidermidis*. Patients requiring subacute bacterial endocarditis (SBE) prophylaxis typically receive gram-positive and gram-negative coverage, most often with gentamycin and ampicillin.[16]

PREOPERATIVE PAIN CONTROL

Renal colic is a phenomenon caused by increased ureteral peristalsis in the setting of a partial obstruction. It is characterized by intense flank pain with radiation to the groin. Prostaglandins are often released to aid in stone passage, along with bradykinins, which sensitize nociceptors to stimuli. These induce pain and visceral responses such as nausea and vomiting.[17] Parenteral opioids, particularly meperidine, have been the mainstay of treatment. Morphine has been traditionally avoided because of its propensity to increase smooth muscle tone and peristaltic activity of the ureter, whereas meperidine has been the agent of choice secondary to its mild, atropine-like antispasmodic effect. However, recent studies have shown no difference in analgesic efficacy between the two agents.[18] Nonsteroidal anti-inflammatory agents such as ketorolac have been shown to be equal in efficacy to narcotics in these patients.[19,20] There have been studies to support the use of anticholinergics to reduce pain with renal colic.[21] Studies have been mixed regarding the efficacy of calcium channel blockers.[22]

EMERGENCY EQUIPMENT

When called to administer anesthesia in the lithotripsy suite, office, or other off-site location, it is prudent to have all emergency equipment available, including a crash cart, emergency medications, and airway equipment. Airway equipment should include appropriate size laryngeal mask airways (LMAs), oral airways, laryngoscopes, endotracheal tubes, and suction as well as an oxygen supply and manual ventilation equipment. Should complications arise, the anesthesia provider should realize that many outpatient surgery centers and OOOR environments may lack certain facilities, such as a laboratory, blood bank, and inpatient care. In addition, the outpatient/OOOR staff may need more direction regarding complicated patient care, especially in a crisis situation.

PATIENT POSITIONING

The most common position for patients undergoing outpatient/OOOR urologic procedures is supine; however, lithotomy position is also commonly encountered. In lithotomy position, however, there are physiologic changes and dangers to the patient that the anesthesiologist needs to consider. While positioning the patient, two persons should move the legs simultaneously, securing the ankles into position with a strap. Ensure that the lateral or medial thigh does not rest on the strap because this may result in injury to the common peroneal or saphenous nerve,[23,24] respectively. If the thigh is excessively flexed at the groin, obturator and femoral nerve injury may result. There is a risk of compartment syndrome of the lower extremity if prolonged time is spent in lithotomy position.[23,25] It is important to pay careful attention to the patient's fingers because they are in danger of being crushed between the lower and center sections of the mechanical operating room table. Physiologic alterations with lithotomy position include decreased functional residual capacity (FRC), resulting in atelectasis and hypoxia. Increased venous return and preload and increase in mean arterial pressure can be anticipated in lithotomy as well; these effects dissipate once the legs are lowered.

For PCNL, nephrostomy, nephroscopy, and lithotripsy procedures, the patient may be in prone or flank position. Ensure that pressure points are padded, extremities are not hyperextended, and adequate eye care is given because injury to these structures not only is harmful to the patient but also will delay patient discharge from the recovery room. Other physiologic changes and specific risks pertaining to supine, prone, and flank positions can be reviewed in other sources.[24]

UROLITHIASIS

The most common indication for a majority of these procedures is urolithiasis. The incidence is estimated to be 10%–15% of all people during their lifetime[26,27]; men are three times more likely to be affected than women.[28-30] Although any age can be affected, urolithiasis is most likely to occur in the fourth to sixth decade.[27,28,31] Pediatric incidence is approximately one-tenth that of adult incidence, but it is thought to be increasing in prevalence.[32] Decision for type of surgical intervention is dependent on stone composition, size, and location.

Anesthetic requirements may be influenced by stone composition. Because stones composed of cystine, calcium oxalate, brushite, and uric acid are hard, they are more likely to require re-treatment and higher levels of shock wave energy during lithotripsy. Higher levels of energy may cause more pain, leading to increased anesthetic requirements in these individuals. Stone composition, occurrences, and associated conditions can be reviewed in Table 24.1.

UROENDOSCOPIC PROCEDURES

The most commonly performed outpatient/OOOR urologic procedure is cystoscopy. Often, transurethral procedures may be performed via cystoscope or ureteroscope. A resectoscope may be used for some transurethral procedures. A resectoscope is a cystoscope that has both cutting and cauterizing functions and is capable of resecting tumor. Commonly encountered procedures include bladder biopsy, retrograde pyelograms, extraction or laser lithotripsy of renal stones, as well as stent placement for stricture or tumor. We do not discuss TURP in this section. If additional transurethral procedures are planned, procedure time and morbidity increase significantly (Table 24.2). Specifically, bladder perforation is a serious complication of this procedure, and the anesthesiologist should be aware of its presentation. Bladder perforation in the awake patient will present as shoulder pain. Under general anesthesia, bladder perforation may initially present as hypertension and tachycardia. Hypotension has also been a described phenomenon in bladder perforation.

TABLE 24.1. Composition of Renal Stones and Anesthetic Implications

TYPE	OCCURRENCE	NOTES
Calcium oxalate	60%	Associated with primary hyperparathyroidism, hypercalciuria, sarcoidosis, cancer; resistant to fragmentation
Calcium phosphate (hydroxyapatite)	20%	Associated with chronic UTIs and alkalemic urine
Uric acid	7%	Associated with acidic urine, gout; radiolucent
Cystine	1%–3%	Associated with cystinuria, higher risk for renal loss with procedures; resistant to fragmentation
Struvite	7%	Associated with UTIs due to urea-splitting bacteria; may release endotoxin if fragmented[34,35]
Brushite	2%	Resistant to fragmentation

UTI, urinary tract infection.

Note: Other rare causes of stones include 2,8-dihydroxyadenine, silica, triamterene.

SOURCE: From Pearle MS, Pak YC. Renal calculi: a practical approach to medical evaluation and management. In: Andreucci VE, Fine LG, eds. *International Yearbook of Nephrology*. New York, NY: Oxford University Press; 1996:69.[33]

ANESTHESIA FOR ENDOUROLOGIC PROCEDURES

Local anesthesia alone is the typical agent used for simple cystoscopy and ureteroscopy, particularly in office settings. However, a few recent studies have shown no benefit in using lidocaine gel over simple lubricant.[36–40] If the patient requires additional sedation, preferred agents include midazolam, nitrous oxide,[41] propofol, and short-acting opioids. If interventions such as tumor resection are planned in addition to uroendoscopy, often local with light sedation will be inadequate. If so, general anesthesia is performed, often with short-acting agents and a LMA. Children typically require general anesthesia for all urologic procedures depending on age and developmental level, and mask technique or LMA is generally satisfactory. Please note that it is important, particularly in children, to maintain a relatively deep plane of anesthesia prior to insertion of the cystoscope because urethral stimulation may precipitate laryngospasm (Breuer-Lockhart reflex).[42]

Although rarely necessary, regional anesthesia and neuraxial techniques may be chosen for this procedure. Most recent studies have shown that neuraxial techniques prolong recovery time and delay time to discharge when compared to intravenous sedation or general anesthesia.[43,44] However, these may still be used if a patient is a poor candidate for sedation or general anesthesia, transurethral procedures are to be performed, or patient intolerance prevents adequate analgesia with local anesthesia. A transrectal periprostatic block alone has recently been shown to be inadequate analgesia as a lone anesthetic for transurethral manipulations.[45] For neuraxial anesthesia, a T10 sensory level is necessary to provide analgesia for bladder manipulations (cystoscopy), while a T8 level is required to provide analgesia to the ureters (ureteroscopy). Please note that if a neuraxial technique is chosen, the obturator reflex is not abolished; this reflex is characterized by external rotation and adduction of the thigh after stimulation of the obturator nerve by electrocautery through the bladder wall.

PERCUTANEOUS RENAL PROCEDURES

Percutaneous nephrolithotomy, nephrostomy, or nephroscopy may be infrequently performed in the OOOR setting. These patients are often admitted for at least 24 hours postoperatively. Typically, PCNL or percutaneous nephrostomy is performed for relief of renal obstruction, particularly when it involves the renal pelvis or calyx. Surgical time, blood loss, morbidity, and mortality for this procedure are listed in Table 24.3. Urologists may use electrocautery, shock wave or laser

TABLE 24.2. Indications, Surgical Time, Blood Loss, Morbidity, and Mortality for Cystoscopy and Transurethral Procedures (Except TURP)

	INDICATIONS	SURGICAL TIME	BLOOD LOSS	MORBIDITY	MORTALITY
Without transurethral intervention	Hematuria, hemorrhagic or interstitial cystitis, recurrent UTI, renal calculi, hydronephrosis, BPH, cancer, stricture	15–30 min	Minimal	5% infection, < 5% ureteral perforation	<1%
With transurethral intervention	Same	1 hour	100 mL	10% bleeding, 5% infection, 2% bladder perforation	<1%

BPH, benign prostatic hyperplasia; TURP, transurethral resection of the prostate; UTI, urinary tract infection.

SOURCE: From Harcharan S, Freiha FS, Deem SA, Pearl RG. Diagnostic transurethral (endoscopic) procedures. In: Jaffe RA, Samuels SI, eds. *Anesthesiologist's Manual of Surgical Procedures.* 3rd ed. Philadelphia, PA: Lippincott Williams & Wilkins; 2004:696–699.

TABLE 24.3. Indications, Surgical Time, Blood Loss, Morbidity, and Mortality Associated with Percutaneous Nephrolithotomy

INDICATIONS	SURGICAL TIME	BLOOD LOSS	MORBIDITY	MORTALITY
Renal obstruction	2–3 hours	500 mL	10% bleeding, 5% infection, 2% bladder perforation, 2% retained stones	<1%

SOURCE: From Harcharan S, Freiha FS, Deem SA, Pearl RG. Diagnostic transurethral (endoscopic) procedures. In: Jaffe RA, Samuels SI, eds. *Anesthesiologist's Manual of Surgical Procedures.* 3rd ed. Philadelphia, PA: Lippincott Williams & Wilkins; 2004:697–698.

lithotripsy, and ultrasound or fluoroscopy for guidance. A stab wound incision is made, and a nephrostomy tube may be placed. Typically, a high volume of irrigant, usually 0.9% saline, is used to disperse heat, remove stone fragments, and prevent obstruction. If a nephrostomy tube or bladder catheter is placed, the patient may require flushing of the Foley catheter or nephrostomy tubes postoperatively to prevent obstruction and clear blood clots.

Complications other than those listed in Table 24.3 may include trauma to the spleen, kidney, liver, or colon, so one must be aware of the potential for acute blood loss. If access above the 12th rib or a cephalad kidney is necessary, pleural injury is possible. If irrigant is absorbed intravenously, a TURP-like syndrome, including fluid overload and electrolyte abnormalities, may be observed.[46,47] Fluid may be extravasated into the pleural space, leading to pleural effusion and hydropneumothorax, or into the retroperitoneal or intraperitoneal spaces. Monitoring fluid intake in comparison to output is particularly important, and the anesthesiologist should have a high index of suspicion for these complications once the discrepancy is greater than 500 mL.

Anesthetic choice for PCNL is often general anesthesia with an endotracheal tube, particularly if prolonged time in the prone position or need for paralysis is anticipated. Local anesthesia, an intercostal block, or a paravertebral block may be used as an adjunct for pain control. Neuraxial techniques are a viable option, but again, they may delay discharge and will require a relatively high sensory level, approximately T6. Of note, regional and neuraxial anesthesia may not attenuate the vasovagal reaction associated with distention of the renal pelvis.

LASER USE IN UROLOGY

Light amplification by stimulated emission of radiation (LASER or, more commonly, laser) use is also frequently encountered in urologic surgery. Specifically, it is used in treating the following conditions: renal calculi; condyloma acuminatum of external genitalia and urethra; ureteral strictures or bladder neck contractures; interstitial cystitis; benign prostatic hyperplasia (BPH); and superficial carcinomas of the penis, bladder, ureter, and renal pelvis. There are several advantages to laser therapy, including minimal blood loss, decreased postoperative pain, and tissue denaturation. Several common types of laser and their indications can be found in Table 24.4. The anesthesiologist's role during laser surgery is to ensure that all personnel and the patient are safe to proceed with laser use.

Between January 1989 and June 1990, there were 21 injuries related to laser use reported to the US Food and Drug Administration (FDA): 2 were minor, 12 were serious, and 7 were fatal.[48] The hazards associated with laser use can be divided into four major categories:

1. Atmospheric contamination
2. Perforation of vessel or structure[49]
3. Embolism (associated with hysteroscopic surgeries)[50]
4. Inappropriate energy transfer

With regard to inappropriate energy transfer, there have been case reports of lasers igniting fires and causing thermal injury to patients, personnel, surgical drapes, and endotracheal

TABLE 24.4. Commonly Used Lasers in Urologic Surgery: Advantages and Special Notes

LASER TYPE	ADVANTAGES	NOTES
CO_2	Useful in cutaneous lesions; minimal tissue penetration	Unable to penetrate water
Argon	Used for coagulation of bleeding	Poorly absorbed by water, absorbed by hemoglobin and melanin
Holmium:YAG (pulsed dye)	Photothermal mechanism, works via vaporization of water, good cutting effect with poor hemostasis; used often to fragment calculi	Safe, effective; capable of cutting through metal (e.g., endoscopes, guidewires)
Nd-YAG (neodymium-yttrium-aluminum-garnet)	Little heat generation, good deep-tissue penetration, and protein denaturation	Beam carried over bare wire through rigid ureteroscope; risk of ureteral perforation; general anesthesia preferred to stop patient movement
KTP-532 (potassium-titanium-phosphate)	Frequency doubled Nd-YAG; better at cutting with less-deep tissue penetration	Can be used in water or urine without loss of effectiveness

SOURCE: Data taken from Fitzpatrick JM. Minimally invasive and endoscopic management of benign prostatic hyperplasia. In: Wein AJ, Kavoussi LR, Novick AC, Partin AW, Peters CA, eds. *Campbell-Walsh Urology*. 9th ed. Philadelphia, PA: Saunders; 2007.

tubes.[51,52] Risk of airway fire exists in any procedure room where oxygen is in use. Appropriate caution in avoiding direct laser contact and minimizing oxygen concentrations when possible are of paramount importance.

Direct and reflected laser beams can cause eye injury. CO_2 lasers cause corneal ulcerations and pass no energy to the fundus,[54] while argon, neodymium-yttrium-aluminum-garnet (Nd-YAG), and potassium-titanium-phosphate 532 (KTP-532) pass through the anterior chamber of the eye and damage the retina.[55] Therefore, the anesthesia team should ensure that all operating room personnel and the patient wear wavelength-specific goggles prior to laser activation. All windows in the operating room should be covered, and specific warning signs should be posted. The patient's eyes should be taped closed and then padded with an opaque, saline-soaked knit or metal shield[56,57] and wavelength-specific goggles applied. Lasers can also cause inadvertent thermal injury to the skin; put the laser in standby mode when not in operation.

If the CO_2 laser is being used to excise condyloma acuminatum, laser masks should be used to prevent small particles from being inhaled. Ordinary surgical masks efficiently filter particles only to 3.0 μm, while laser particulate was found to be an average size of less than 0.8 μm.[58] Atmospheric contamination associated with laser particulate has been shown to cause interstitial pneumonia, bronchiolitis, reduced mucociliary clearance, inflammation, and emphysema in animal models.[59,60] The laser plume has also been shown to be mutagenic, teratogenic, and a vector for viral infection,[61–64] and it is most safely managed with a smoke evacuation system.

EXTRACORPOREAL SHOCK WAVE LITHOTRIPSY

Removal of renal calculi prior to the 1980s involved an invasive, lengthy surgery with significant morbidities. The introduction of ESWL via the Dornier HM-3 in Munich, Germany, in 1984 revolutionized the treatment of ureteral calculi. As lithotripter technology advanced, ESWL was transformed into an outpatient procedure. Of patients harboring "simple" renal calculi, 80% to 85% can be treated satisfactorily with SWL.[65–67]

LITHOTRIPTER STRUCTURE AND FUNCTION PRINCIPLES

In ESWL, repetitive high-energy shocks or sound waves are generated and focused on the calculus, which fragments as tensile and shear forces develop inside the stone and cavitations are formed outside the surface. There are four components to a shock wave lithotripter (Figure 24.1):

1. *Energy source*, most commonly an electrohydraulic, or "spark plug" type; also electromagnetic and piezoelectric types
2. *Focusing device*, either ellipsoid or reflecting mirrors
3. *Acoustic coupler or coupling medium*, usually water or conducting gel; links the energy source to the patient
4. *Stone localization system*, usually ultrasound or fluoroscopy

During stone fragmentation, a "spark plug" capacitor is discharged within the shock wave generator, generating a loud noise and intense heat, which vaporizes surrounding water. A gaseous water bubble is created and subsequently collapses, generating a shock wave. Shock waves are perpetuated to the stone by the coupling medium (deionized water, warmed to 36°C–37°C) and focused on the stone by a hyperbolic reflector mirror. The focus point (F2) is the point of maximum energy, and beyond this point energy is dissipated.[65,68,69] F2 can be matched to the stone location via fluoroscopy and avoid damage to surrounding tissues. It is important,

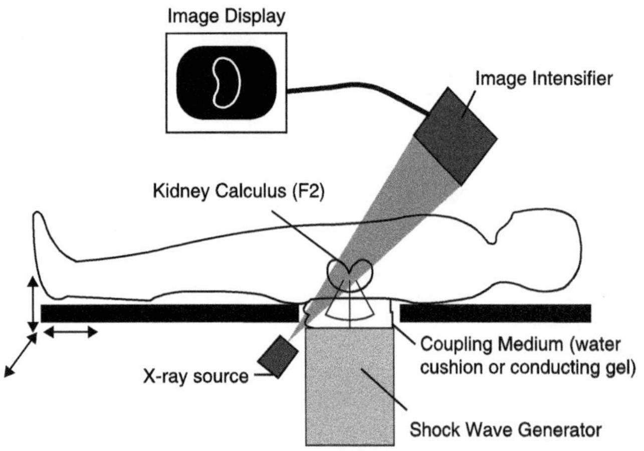

Figure 24.1. Components of a shock wave lithotripter, shown as second- or third-generation lithotripter. In first-generation lithotripters, the patient was strapped to a gantry chair and immersed to the clavicles in a metal tub filled with warmed water (coupling medium). (Courtesy of Ronald G. Frank, MD. http://www.urologistnewjersey.com)

if possible, to avoid movement of the stone. Therefore, respiratory variations and patient movement should be minimized.

Very little energy loss or tissue damage occurs as the shock waves move from the coupling medium, usually water cushion or conducting gel, to the patient because the acoustic impedance is similar. As the shock wave enters the stone's surface, a change in acoustic impedance occurs, releasing compressive energy on the stone approximately several atmospheres in magnitude. As the wave exits on the opposite side of the stone, a change in acoustic impedance is again encountered, and energy is released in a blast. Repetition of this process causes the stone to disintegrate; typically, 1000–2000 shocks are required. The limits to avoid tissue injury are 3000 shocks at a maximum voltage of 24,000; if the stone is in a ureter, the limit is 2400 shocks at 30,000 V.

CONTRAINDICATIONS TO EXTRACORPOREAL SHOCK WAVE LITHOTRIPSY

Contraindications to ESWL include pregnancy, bleeding disorders, urinary obstruction below the stone, and untreated infection. Relative contraindications, more relevant to first-generation lithotripters, include calcified abdominal aortic aneurism, which may rupture or embolize distally; gas/tissue interfaces, such as pneumothorax or dilated bowel loops; orthopedic prosthetic devices; or pacemaker/AICD in the path of the shock waves. If the pacemaker/AICD is in the path of the shock waves, it is recommended to check with the manufacturer if the device should be reprogrammed or if use of a magnet is recommended.

SAFE USE OF SHOCK WAVE LITHOTRIPSY

Shock wave lithotripsy has been used safely in the pediatric population, including infants.[10] The higher water concentration in pediatric tissue compared with adults is thought to increase resistance to tissue damage.[70,71] Special precautions with SWL in infants include using lower energy levels on the lithotripter and the use of foam tape to protect their lungs from contusion.[72]

Using ESWL safely includes limiting exposure to ionizing radiation by providing staff with lead shields, radiation badges, and keeping physical distance from fluoroscopy equipment. Total radiation exposure per ESWL is approximately the same as a barium enema.[73] Second, if using immersion lithotripsy, headphones or earphones should be utilized by lithotripsy suite personnel and the patient.[74–76] With the most current lithotripters, the use of hearing protection by staff and the patient is optional by Occupational Safety and Health Administration (OSHA) standards (exposure > 90 dB for 8 hours daily).[76]

COMPLICATIONS

There are several problems specific to the first-generation lithotripters. These devices were located on a separate lithotripsy unit, separate from the operating suite and available resuscitation equipment. If additional interventions such as stent or cystoscopy needed to be performed, the patient had to be removed from the water bath and placed onto another operating table. With regard to the device itself, the calculus and patient must be moved to align the shock wave generator with the target F2 focus, which varies with the patient's respirations. There are several hemodynamic and physiologic changes associated with the immersion water bath (Box 24.3). Vasodilation

BOX 24.3. PHYSIOLOGIC CHANGES WITH IMMERSION EXTRACORPOREAL SHOCK WAVE LITHOTRIPSY

PULMONARY

Decreased FRC, VC, TV
Increased intrathoracic blood volume 30%–60%
Increased RR, work of breathing; promotes atelectasis

CARDIAC

Increased preload secondary to compression of submerged veins
Increased central venous, right atrial, and pulmonary artery pressures
Increase in systemic MAP and CO
If LV failure, may see decreased MAP & CO

TEMPERATURE

Cold water: vasoconstriction, shivering, hypothermia
Warm water: Vasodilation, decreased blood pressure, hyperthermia
Sitting position: Decreased RAP, PCWP, CO

FRC, functional residual capacity; LV, left ventricle; MAP, mean arterial pressure; PCWP, pulmonary capillary wedge pressure; RAP, right atrial pressure; RR, respiratory rate; TV, tidal volume; VC, vital capacity.

SOURCE: From Malhotra V, Sudheendra V, Diwan S. Anesthesia and the renal and genitourinary systems. In: Miller R, ed. *Miller's Anesthesia*. 6th ed. Philadelphia, PA: Churchill Livingstone; 2005:2105–2134.

associated with the warm water bath was exacerbated by epidural or spinal anesthesia, often requiring a fluid preload of 1000–2000 mL. Additionally, immersion requires waterproof monitors and occlusive dressings over epidural and intravenous sites.

Unfortunately, cardiac arrhythmias are encountered up to 80% of the time with first-generation lithotripters.[77] This is primarily thought to be due to two mechanisms: irritation of the myocardium by the shock wave *or* the 10- to 20-kV discharge prior to each shock could evoke premature electrical stimulation of the atria, most frequently resulting in supraventricular tachycardia.[78,79] This can be reduced by coupling shock wave delivery to the electrocardiogram (ECG) so that shocks are delivered 20 milliseconds after the R wave, corresponding to the ventricular refractory period. However, once coupled, the length of the procedure is directly correlated to the heart rate. This became an issue if regional anesthesia was undertaken and a sympathectomy with a resultant bradycardia occurred. Some practitioners used atropine or isoproterenol to alleviate the bradycardia, but these drugs can significantly increase cardiac workload and oxygen demand.

SECOND- AND THIRD-GENERATION LITHOTRIPTERS

Some of the difficulties encountered with the first-generation lithotripters were avoided in the development of the second- and third-generation lithotripters. The water bath was replaced with a water cushion or conductive gel,[80,81] thereby avoiding problems specific to immersion. Furthermore, newer models incorporated a cardiac simulator and reduced energy delivered to improve treatment times and reduce the rate of arrhythmia to approximately 20%.[82] However, even with the lowest-energy lithotripters, arrhythmias have been encountered.[83] If observed, the internal simulator can be deactivated and ECG triggered mode can be utilized.[84] Stone localization is still frequently performed with fluoroscopy; however, ultrasound may also be used with these devices.

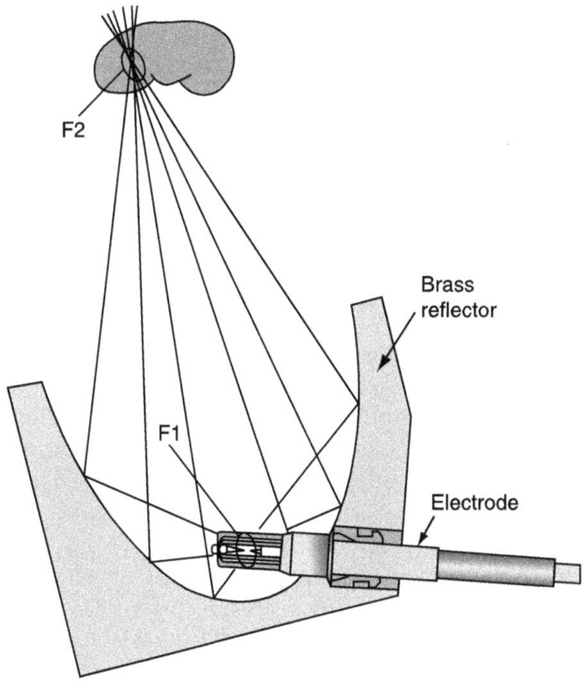

Figure 24.2. Schematic for an electrohydraulic generator. (This figure was published in Campbell-Walsh Urology. 9th ed, Vol. 2. Copyright Elsevier 2007.)

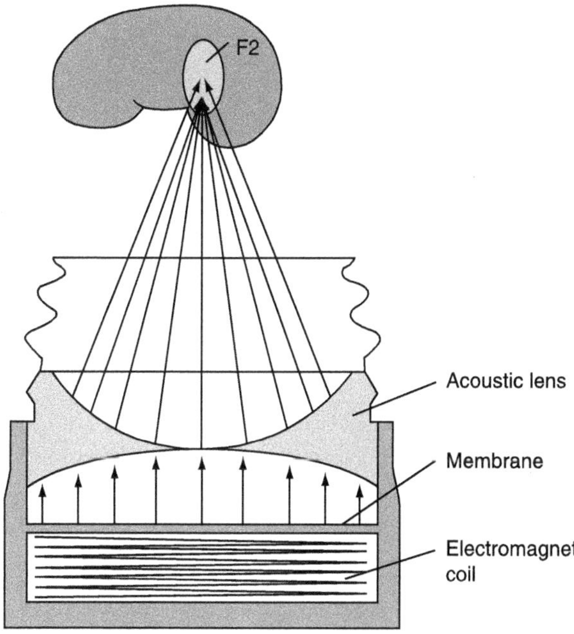

Figure 24.3. Schematic for electromagnetic generator with acoustic lens-focusing mechanism (not shown: parabolic reflector). (This figure was published in Campbell-Walsh Urology. 9th ed, Vol. 2. Copyright Elsevier 2007.)

Because pain at the entry site was linked to the increased voltage and energy density,[85,86] an effort was made to decrease the energy necessary to produce adequate stone fragmentation. However, with decreased energy density and voltage, the total number of shocks delivered was increased to compensate. Shock wave generators are still commonly electrohydraulic (Figure 24.2), as in the Dornier HM3, but currently lower-energy lithotripters with more focused beams are used. Other lithotripters use electromagnetic or piezoelectric sources in efforts to decrease energy needs. Electromagnetic generators vibrate a metallic plate over an electromagnet, generating shock waves in a water-filled "shock tube" (Figure 24.3). The advantage of electromagnetic lithotripters is that they provide more controllable and reproducible shock waves than electrohydraulic sources; however, the energy is introduced over a larger skin area, which may cause decreased pain.[3] Because a small focal region with increased energy density is being utilized, patients are at an increased risk for subcapsular hematoma.[87]

Piezoelectric generators apply electrical current to a crystal, whose external dimensions change when electric current is applied. Once applied to many crystals in a spherical dish, this results in shock waves (Figure 24.4). Piezoelectric lithotripters are the lowest-energy lithotripters and have focusing accuracy, low energy at the skin, and the least amount of pain, allowing for an "anesthetic-free" treatment.[80]

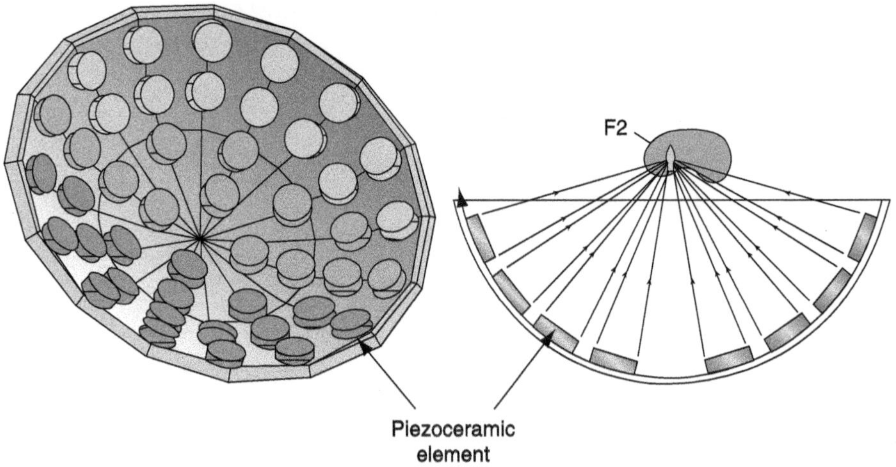

Figure 24.4. Schematic view of a piezoelectric shockwave generator. Numerous polarized polycrystalline ceramic elements are positioned on the inside of a spherical dish. (This figure was published in Campbell-Walsh Urology. 9th ed, Vol. 2. Copyright Elsevier 2007.)

Laser lithotripters are also used instead of SWL, particularly in stones that are low in the ureter or if SWL has failed or cannot be used.

ANESTHESIA FOR EXTRACORPOREAL SHOCK WAVE LITHOTRIPSY

Pain associated with ESWL is cutaneous, somatic, and visceral in nature.[84,88] Patients may experience shock wave– and cavitation-mediated irritation of the renal capsule, lumbar muscles, rib periosteum, vertebrae, and skin; upper calyx stones may be more painful than middle and lower caliceal stones.[89–91] The use of subdermal infiltration with local anesthesia or use of EMLA Cream has been described to mediate the cutaneous pain.

Local anesthesia with sedation is the preferred method for nonimmersion SWL.[92] Even the low-energy, anesthesia-free lithotripters still require supplemental analgesia.[84,88] Local anesthesia does reduce total anesthetic requirements, but it is inadequate for analgesia as SWL energy is increased.[90,93–95]

Shock wave lithotripsy is stimulating and painful during shock wave delivery; however, postoperatively patients are fairly comfortable. The use of short-acting opioids, nonsteroidal anti-inflammatory drugs (NSAIDs), and tramadol is recommended. Intravenous opioids are well known to cause hypoventilation, apnea, and nausea[88,96–98] and therefore may prolong recovery time. Alternatively, analgesia with diclofenac and tramadol has been shown in several studies to have a lower side-effect profile.[99]

General anesthesia may be the modality of choice if a secure airway is necessary. One must consider whether an OOOR setting is appropriate for the patient requiring a secure airway. Alternatively, the patient might be better suited for a more controlled environment where additional help is available. The risk/benefit ratio of the alternate site environment should be continuously reassessed. Recovery from general anesthesia has been shown to be faster than from regional.[44] Shorter-acting agents are preferred, and nitrous oxide has been shown to provide effective analgesia in SWL.[100] General anesthesia allows tidal volume control and improves control over stone movements that may vary with respiration during regional anesthesia.[96] If stone movement with respiration is anticipated, despite minimizing tidal volumes, this may cause difficulty with stone targeting. In such a scenario, it may be necessary to move this procedure in advance to a center where high-frequency jet ventilation (HFJV) is available. HFJV has been described as superior over conventional ventilation in controlling stone movement and improving ease of stone targeting.[101–104]

Occasionally, regional or neuraxial techniques will be chosen if the patient is unable to tolerate sedation or general anesthesia. If regional anesthesia is chosen, intercostal nerve blocks and paravertebral blocks have been described with adequate analgesic results.[105,106] If neuraxial anesthesia is chosen, achieving a sensory level to T8 will provide analgesia for renal structures and ureters; however, if immersion lithotripsy is being used, T6 sensory levels bilaterally should be achieved. If epidural anesthesia is chosen, note that the onset time for analgesia will take approximately 10–20 minutes. Injection with air should be avoided; this provides a theoretical air-fluid interface or change in impedance that may lead to damage to surrounding structures.[107] The use of foam tape should be avoided because this can dissipate shock waves.

In the past, a spinal with lidocaine was preferred, and it is still used at some institutions. If chosen, a lower dose of lidocaine may improve return of motor function and decrease time to discharge.[43] However, lidocaine is now being avoided at most institutions for spinal anesthesia because there has been a higher risk of transient neurologic syndrome, particularly associated with lithotomy position.[108] Many combinations of lidocaine, multiple other local anesthetics,[109–111] and various opioids have been studied to delineate a combination with the fewest side effects and fastest time to recovery. Of note, sufentanil is comparable to lidocaine with regard to analgesia. Patients receiving sufentanil have a lower incidence of hypotension[112] and earlier discharge[113] than patients receiving lidocaine, and sufentanil has a beneficial effect in conjunction with bupivacaine and other agents.[112,114]

SUMMARY AND CONCLUSIONS

Over the last 25 years, the number and diversity of urologic procedures performed in the outpatient/OOOR setting have increased substantially. As such, the variety of patients requiring anesthesia in these remote locations has increased as well. Some patients may have special needs that must be evaluated with considerable scrutiny. It is paramount that the anesthesiologist, in consultation with the surgical team, decides whether the patient is suited to an OOOR setting or if the procedure must be performed in the operating room. In order to provide a safe, timely, and effective anesthetic, the anesthesiologist must also be aware of potentially dangerous situations involving the patient, staff, or surgical equipment and be familiar with what resources are available in these potentially challenging environments.

REFERENCES

1. Gil-Vernet J. New surgical concepts in removing renal calculi. *Urologia Internationalis.* 1965;20:255–288.
2. Patterson P. Office surgery is gaining market share. *OR Manager.* 1996;12(2):1, 12.
3. Lazarov SJ. Office-based surgery and anesthesia: where are we now? *World J Urol.* 1998;16(6):384–385.
4. Nagrebetsky A, Gabriel RA, Dutton RP, Urman RD. Growth of nonoperating room anesthesia care in the United States: a contemporary trends analysis. *Anesth Analg.* 2017;124(4):1261–1267.
5. Chang B, Kaye AD, Diaz JH, Westlake B, Dutton RP, Urman RD. Complications of non-operating room procedures: outcomes from the national anesthesia clinical outcomes registry. *J Patient Saf.* 2015. [Epub ahead of print].
6. Chang B, Urman RD. Non-operating room anesthesia: the principles of patient assessment and preparation. *Anesthesiol Clin.* 2016;34(1):223–240.
7. Woodward ZG, Urman RD, Domino KB. Safety of non-operating room anesthesia: a closed claims update. *Anesthesiol Clin.* 2017;35(4):569–581.
8. Kilciler M, Sumer F, Bedir S, Ozgok Y, Erduran D. Extracorporeal shock wave lithotripsy treatment in paraplegic patients with bladder stones. *Int J Urol.* 2002;9(11):632–634.
9. Deliveliotis C, Picramenos D, Kostakopoulos A, Stavropoulos NI, Alexopoulou K, Karagiotis E. Extracorporeal shock wave lithotripsy in paraplegic and quadriplegic patients. *Int Urol Nephrol.* 1994;26(2):151–154.
10. Durkee CT, Balcom A. Surgical management of nephrolithiasis. *Pediatr Clin North Am.* 2006;53:465–477.
11. Canning DA, Nguyen MT. Evaluation of the pediatric urology patient. In: Wein AJ, Kavoussi LR, Novick AC, Partin AW, Peters CA, eds. *Campbell-Walsh Urology.* 9th ed., Vol. 4. Philadelphia, PA: Saunders Elsevier; 2007.
12. Barakat AY, Seikaly MG, Der Kaloustian VM. Urogenital abnormalities in genetic disease. *J Urol.* 1986;136(4):778–785.
13. Grabe M. Controversies in antibiotic prophylaxis in urology. *Int J Antimicrob Agents.* 2004;23(suppl 1):S17–S23.
14. Grabe M. Perioperative antibiotic prophylaxis in urology. *Curr Opin Urol.* 2001;11:81–85.
15. Inglis JA, Tolley DA. Antibiotic prophylaxis at the time of percutaneous stone surgery. *J Endourol.* 1988;2:59–62.
16. Santucci RA, Krieger JN. Gentamicin for the practicing urologist: review of efficacy, single daily dosing and "switch" therapy. *J Urol.* 2000;163:1076–1084.
17. Selmy GI, Hassouna MM, Khalaf IM, et al. Effects of verapamil, prostaglandin F2 alpha, phenylephrine, and noradrenaline on upper urinary tract dynamics. *Urology.* 1994;43:31–35.
18. OConnor S, Cardwell HA. Comparison of the efficacy and safety of morphine and pethidine as analgesia for suspected renal colic in the emergency setting. *J Accident Emerg Med.* 2000;17:261–264.
19. Sandhu DP, Iacovou JW, Fletcher MS, et al. A comparison of intramuscular ketorolac and pethidine in the alleviation of renal colic. *Br J Urol.* 1994;74:690–693.
20. Stein A, Ben Dov D, Finkel B, et al. Single dose intramuscular ketorolac versus diclofenac for pain management in renal colic. *Am J Emerg Med.* 1996;14:385–387.
21. Fornapiero E, Barone A, Francolini G, Pupita F. Clinical experience with an anticholinergic spasmolytic cimetropium bromide in the treatment of patients with renal colic [in Italian]. *Clin Ter.* 1990;135(6):465–468.
22. Capecchi S, Pignatelli R, Alegiani F. Emergency treatment of ureteral colic with nifedipine [in Italian]. *Minerva Urol Nefrol.* 1991;43(4):287–291.
23. Battillo JA, Hendler MA. Effects of patient positioning during anesthesia. In: Lebowitz RW, ed. *Anesthesia for Urologic Surgery.* Boston, MA: Little, Brown; 1993:67.
24. Warner MA. Patient positioning. In: Barash PG, Cullen BF, Stoelting RK, eds. *Clinical Anesthesia.* 5th ed. Philadelphia, PA: Lippincott, Williams & Wilkins; 2006:643–665.
25. Warner ME, LaMaster LM, Thoerning AK, Shirk Marienau ME, Warner MA. Compartment syndrome in surgical patients. *Anesthesiology.* 2001;94(4):705–708.
26. Norlin A, Lindell B, Granberg PO, Lindvall N. Urolithiasis: a study of its frequency. *Scand J Urol Nephrol.* 1976;10:150–153.
27. Johnson CM, Wilson DM, O'Fallon WM, et al. Renal stone epidemiology: a 25-year study in Rochester, Minnesota. *Kidney Int.* 1979;16:624–631.
28. Hiatt RA, Dales LG, Friedman GD, Hunkeler EM. Frequency of urolithiasis in a prepaid medical care program. *Am J Epidemiol.* 1982;115:255–265.
29. Soucie JM, Thun MJ, Coates RJ, et al. Demographic and geographic variability of kidney stones in the United States. *Kidney Int.* 1994;46:893–899.
30. Pearle MS, Calhoun, EA, Curhan GC. Urologic diseases in America project: urolithiasis. *J Urol.* 2005;173:848–857.
31. Marshall V, White RH, Chaput de Saintonage M, et al. The natural history of renal and ureteric calculi. *Br J Urol.* 1975;47:117–124.
32. Stapleton FB. Nephrolithiasis in children. *Pediatr Rev.* 1989;11:21–30.
33. Pearle MS, Pak YC. Renal calculi: a practical approach to medical evaluation and management. In: Andreucci VE, Fine LG, eds. *International Yearbook of Nephrology.* New York, NY: Oxford University Press; 1996:69.
34. McAleer IM, Kaplan GW, Bradley JS, et al. Staghorn calculus endotoxin expression in sepsis. *Urology.* 2002;59:601.
35. McAleer IM, Kaplan GW, Bradley JS, et al. Endotoxin content in renal calculi. *J Urol.* 2003;169:1813–1814.
36. Chitale S, Hirani M, Swift L, Ho E. Prospective randomized crossover trial of lubricant gel against an anaesthetic gel for outpatient cystoscopy. *Scand J Urol Nephrol.* 2008;42(2):164–167.
37. Cho JH, Kwak KW, Hong JH, Lee HM. Efficacy of lidocaine spray as topical anesthesia for outpatient rigid cystoscopy in women: a prospective, randomized, double blind trial. *Urology.* 2008;71(4):561–566.
38. Clayman R. Ureteroscopic lithotripsy under local anesthesia: analysis of effectiveness and patient tolerability. *J Urol.* 2005;173(6):2022–2023.
39. Kobayashi T, Nishizawa K, Mitsumori K, Ogura K. Instillation of anesthetic gel is no longer necessary in the era of flexible cystoscopy: a crossover study. *J Endourol.* 2004;18(5):483–486.
40. Patel AR, Jones JS, Babineau D. Lidocaine 2% gel versus plain lubricating gel for pain reduction during flexible cystoscopy: a meta-analysis of prospective, randomized, controlled trials. *J Urol.* 2008;179(3):986–990.
41. Calleary JG, Masood J, Van-Mallaerts R, Barua JM. Nitrous oxide inhalation to improve patient acceptance and reduce procedure related pain of flexible cystoscopy for men younger than 55 years. *J Urol.* 2007;178(1):184–188.
42. Stehling LC, Furman EB. Anesthesia for congenital anomalies of the genitourinary system. In: Stehling LC, Zauder HL, eds. *Anesthetic Implications of Congenital Anomalies in Children.* New York, NY: Appleton-Century-Crofts; 1980:162–163.
43. Rushmer J, Miles W, Jones RD, Ho JY, Cheung CK, Chan SS. Motor power pharmacodynamics of subarachnoid hyperbaric 5% lidocaine in the sitting position. *Acta Aneaesthesiol Scand.* 1997;41(5):557–564.
44. Richardson MG, Dooley JW. The effects of general versus epidural anesthesia for outpatient extracorporeal shock wave lithotripsy. *Anesth Analg.* 1998;86(6):1214–1218.
45. Mutener M, Fatzer M, Praz V, Straumann U, Strebel RT, John H. Local anesthesia for transurethral manipulations: is a transrectal perprostatic nerve block effective? *World J Urol.* 2005;23(5):349–352.

46. Fellahi JL, Richard JP, Bellezza M, Antonini A, Thouvenot JP, Chathala B. The intravascular transfer of glycine during percutaneous kidney surgery [in French]. *Cah Anesth*. 1992;40(5):343–347.
47. Cariou G, Le Duc A, Serrie A, Cortesse A, Teillac P, Ziegler F. Reabsorption of the irrigation solute during percutaneous nephrolithotomy [in French]. *Ann Urol (Paris)*. 1985;19(2):83–86.
48. US Food and Drug Administration. Special report: laser safety. *Laser Nurs*. 1990;4:3.
49. D'Hallewin MA, Clays K, Persoons A, et al. Large-bowel perforation: a rare complication of intravesical Nd-YAG laser irradiation of bladder tumors. *Urol Int*. 1989;44:373.
50. Baggish MS, Daniell JF. Catastrophic injury secondary to the use of co-axial gas-cooled fibers and artificial sapphire tips for intrauterine surgery: a report of five cases. *Lasers Surg Med*. 1989;9:581.
51. Bauman N. Laser drape fires: how much of a risk? *Laser Med Surg News Adv*. 1989;7:2.
52. Berg P. Laser starts fire in operating room. *Washington Post*. 1988;A5.
53. Liebowitz HM, Peacock GR. Corneal injury produced by carbon dioxide laser radiation. *AMA Arch Opthalmol*. 1980;52:993.
54. Wolbarski M, Fligster KE, Hayes JR. Pathology of neodymium and ruby laser burns. *Science*. 1965;150:1453.
55. Garry BP, Bivens HE. Anesthetic technique for safe laser use in surgery. *Sem Surg Oncol*. 1990;6:184.
56. Keon TP. Anesthetic considerations for laser surgery. *Int Anesthesiol Clin*. 1988;26:50.
57. Nezhat C, Winer WK, Nezhat F, et al. Smoke from laser surgery: is there a health hazard? *Lasers Surg Med*. 1987;7:376.
58. Baggish MS, Elbakry M. The effects of laser smoke on the lungs of rats. *Am J Obstet Gynecol*. 1987;156:1260.
59. Freitag L, Chapman G, Sielczak M. Laser smoke effect on the bronchial system. *Lasers Surg Med*. 1987;7:283.
60. Kukosa J, Eugene J. Chemical composition of laser-tissue interaction smoke plume. *J Laser Appl*. 1989;2:59.
61. Tomita Y, Mihashi S, Nagata K, et al. Mutagenicity of smoke condensates induced by CO_2-laser and electrocauterization. *Mutat Res*. 1981; 89:145.
62. Ferenczy A, Bergeron C, Richart RM. Human papillomavirus DNA in CO_2 laser-generated plume of smoke and its consequences to the surgeon. *Obstet Gynecol*. 1990;75:114.
63. Ferenczy A, Bergeron C, Richart RM. Carbon dioxide laser energy disperses human papillomavirus deoxyribonucleic acid onto treatment fields. *Am J Obstet Gynecol*. 1990;163:1271.
64. Chaussy CG, Fuchs GJ. World experience with extracorporeal shock wave lithotripsy for the removal of urinary stones: an assessment of its role after 5 years of clinical use. *J Endourol*. 1986;1:7.
65. Krings F, Tuerk C, Steinkogler I, et al. Extracorporeal shock wave lithotripsy retreatment ("stir-up") promotes discharge of persistent caliceal stone fragments after primary extracorporeal shock wave lithotripsy. *J Urol*. 1992;198:1040–1041.
66. Wickham JE, Miller RA, Kellett MJ, et al. Percutaneous nephrolithotomy: one stage or two? *Br J Urol*. 1984;56:582–585.
67. Drach DW, Dretler S, Fair W, et al. Report of the United States cooperative study of extracorporeal shock wave lithotripsy. *J Urol*. 1986;135:1127.
68. Chaussy W, Brendel W, Schmiedt E. Extracorporeally induced destuction of kidney stones by shock waves. *Lancet*. 1980;2(8207):1265–1268.
69. Lottman HB, Archambaud F, Traxer OB. The efficacy and parenchymal consequences of extracorporeal shock wave lithotripsy in infants. *Br J Urol Int*. 2000;85(3):311–315.
70. Orsola A, Diaz I, Caffaratti J, et al. Staghorn calculi in children: treatment with monotherapy and extracorporeal shock wave lithotripsy. *J Urol*. 1999;162(3, part 2):1229–1233.
71. Shukla AR, Hoover DL, Homsey YL, et al. Urolithiasis in the low birth weight infant: the role and efficacy of extracorporeal shock wave lithotripsy. *J Urol*. 2001;165(6, part 2):2320–2323.
72. Bush WH, Jones D, Gibbons RP. Radiation dose to patient and personnel during extracorporeal shock wave lithotripsy. *J Urol*. 1987;138:716–719.
73. Lusk RP, Tyler RS. Hazardous sound levels produced by extracorporeal shock wave lithotripsy. *J Urol*. 1987;137:1113–1114.
74. Kraus S, Weidner W. Prolonged exposure to extracorporeal shock wave lithotripsy and noise induced hearing loss. *J Urol*. 2001;165:1984.
75. Dawson C, Chilcott-Jones A, Corry DA. Does lithotripsy cause hearing loss? *Br J Urol*. 1994;73:129–135.
76. Ganem JP, Carson CC. Cardiac arrythmias with external fixed rate signal generators in shock wave lithotripsy with the Medstone lithotripter. *Urology*. 1998;51:548–552.
77. Billbote DB, Challapalli RM, Nadler RB. Unintended supraventricular tachycardia induced by extracorporeal shock wave lithotripsy. *Anesthesiology*. 1998;88:830–832.
78. Walts LF, Atlee JL. Supraventricular tachycardia associated with extracorporeal shock wave lithotripsy. *Anesthesiology*. 1986;65:521–523.
79. Lingeman JE. Extracorporeal shock wave lithotripsy: development, instrumentation and current status. *Urol Clin North Am*. 1997;24:185–211.
80. Wilson WT, Preminger GM. Extracorporeal shock wave lithotripsy: an update. *Urol Clin North Am*. 1990;17:231–242.
81. Greenstein A, Kaver I, Lechtman V, et al. Cardiac arrythmias during nonsynchronized extracorporeal shock wave lithotripsy. *J Urol*. 1995;154:1321–1322.
82. Kataoka H. Cardiac dysrythmias related to extracorporeal shock wave lithotripsy using a piezoelectric lithotripter in patients with kidney stones. *J Urol*. 1995;153:1390–1394.
83. Gravenstein D. Extracorporeal shock wave lithotripsy and percutaneous nephrolithotomy. *Anesthesiol Clin North Am*. 2000;18(4):953–971.
84. Bromage PR, Husain I, El-Faqih SR, et al. Critique of the Dornier HM3 lithtripter as a clinical algesimeter. *Pain*. 1990;40:255–265.
85. Allman DB, Richlin DM, Ruttenberg M, et al. Analgesia in anesthesia free extracorporeal shock wave lithotripsy: a standardized protocol. *J Urol*. 1991;146:718–720.
86. Piper NY, Dalrymple N, Bishoff JT. Incidence of renal hematoma formation after ESWL using the new Dornier Doli-S lithotriptor. *J Urol*. 2001;165:377.
87. Irwin MG, Campbell RGH, Siu Lun T, et al. Patient maintained alfentanil target-controlled infusion for analgesia during extracorporeal shock wave lithotripsy. *Can J Anaesth*. 1996;43:919–924.
88. Schelling G, Weber W, Mendi G, et al. Patient-controlled analgesia for shock wave lithotripsy: the effect of self administered alfentanil on pain intensity and drug requirement. *J Urol*. 1996;155:44–47.
89. Tiselius H. Cutaneous anesthesia with lidocaine-prilocaine cream: a useful adjunct during shock wave lithotripsy with analgesic sedation. *J Urol*. 1993;149:6–11.
90. Vandeursen H, Pittomvils G, Matura E, et al. Anesthetic requirements during electromagnetic extracorporeal shock wave lithotripsy. *Urol Int*. 1991;47:77–80.
91. Hosking MP, Morris SA, Klein FA, Dobmeyer-Ditrich C. Anesthetic management of patients receiving calculus therapy with a third generation extracorporeal lithotripsy machine. *J Endourol*. 1997;11:309–311.
92. Ganapathy S, Razvi H, Moote C, et al. Eutectic mixture of local anesthesia is not effective for extracorporeal shock wave lithotripsy. *Can J Anaesth*. 1996;43:1030–1034.
93. Honnens de Lichtenberg M, Miskowiak J, Mogensen P, et al. Local anesthesia for extracorporeal shock wave lithotripsy. *J Urol*. 1992;148:1034–1035.
94. Monk TG, Boure B, While PF, et al. Comparison of intravenous sedative-analgesic techniques for outpatient immersion lithotripsy. *Anesth Analg*. 1991;72:616–621.
95. Bromage PR, Bonsu AK, el-Faquih SR, et al. Influence of Dornier HM3 system on respiration during extracorporeal shock wave lithotripsy. *Anesth Analg*. 1990;68:363–367.
96. Chin CM, Tay KP, Lim PHC, et al. Use of patient-controlled analgesia in extracorporeal shock wave lithotripsy. *Br J Urol*. 1997;79:302–307.
97. Dawson C, Vale JA, Corry DA. Choosing the correct pain relief for extracorporeal lithotripsy. *Br J Urol*. 1994;74:302–307.
98. Ozcan S, Yilmaz E, Buyukkocak U, Basar H, Apan A. Comparison of three analgesics for extracorporeal shock wave lithotripsy. *Scand J Urol Nephrol*. 2002;36(4):281–285.
99. Mazdak H, Abazari P, Ghassami F, Najafipour S. The analgesic effect of inhalational Entonox for extracorporeal shock wave lithotripsy. *Urol Res*. 2007;25(6):331–334.
100. Carlson CA, Boysen PG, Banner MJ, et al. Stone movement in extracorporeal shock wave lithotripsy: conventional and high frequency jet ventilation. In: Gravenstein JSP, ed. *Extracorporeal Shock Wave Lithotripsy for Renal Stone Disease: Technical and Clinical Aspects*. Stoneham, MA: Butterworth; 1986:77–86.
101. Cormack JR, Hui R, Olive D, Said S. Comparison of two ventilation techniques during general anesthesia for extracorporeal shock wave lithotripsy: high-frequency jet ventilation versus spontaneous ventilation with a laryngeal mask. *Urology*. 2007;70(1):7–10.
102. Zeitlin GL, Roth RA. Effect of three anesthetic techniques on the success of extracorporeal shock wave lithotripsy in nephrolithiasis. *Anesthesiology*. 1988;68:272–276.

103. Warner MA, Warner ME, Buck CF. Clinical efficacy of high frequency jet ventilation during extracorporeal shock wave lithotripsy of reanl and ureteral calculi: a comparison with conventional mechanical ventilation. *J Urol.* 1988;139:486–487.
104. Malhotra V, Long CW, Meister MJ. Intercostal block with local infiltration anesthesia for extracorporeal shock wave lithotripsy. *Anesth Analg.* 1987;66:85–88.
105. Jameison BD, Mariano ER. Thoracic and lumbar paravertebral blocks for outpatient lithotripsy. *J Clin Anesth.* 2007;19(2):149–151.
106. Abbott MA, Samuel JR, Webb DR. Anesthesia for extracorporeal shock wave lithotripsy. *Anaesthesia.* 1985;40:1065–1072.
107. Panadero A, Monedero P, Fernandez-Liesa JI, Percaz J, Olavide I, Iribarren MJ. Repeated transient neurological symptoms after spinal anaesthesia with hyperbaric 5% lidocaine. *Br J Anaesth.* 1998;81(13):471–472.
108. Cook RJ, Neerhut R, Thomas DG. Does combined epidural lignocaine and fentanyl provide better anaesthesia for extracorporeal shock wave lithotripsy than lignocaine alone? *Anaesth Intensive Care.* 1991;19:357–364.
109. Terai T, Tegul S, Bakkaloglu M, et al. A double-blind comparison of lidocaine and mepivicaine during epidural anesthesia. *Acta Anaesthesiol Scand.* 1993;37:607–610.
110. Kopacz DJ, Mulroy MF. Chloroprocaine and lidocaine decrease hospital stay and admission rate after outpatient epidural anesthesia. *Reg Anesth.* 1990;15:19–25.
111. Eaton MP, Chhibber AK, Green DR. Subarachnoid sufentanil versus lidocaine spinal anesthesia for extracorporeal shock wave lithotripsy. *Reg Anesth.* 1997;22(6):515–520.
112. Lau WC, Green CR, Faerber GJ, Tait AR, Golembiewski JA. Intrathecal sufentanil for extracorporeal shock wave lithotripsy provides earlier discharge of the outpatient than intrathecal lidocaine. *Anesth Analg.* 1997;84(6):1227–1231.
113. Shenkman Z, Eidelman LA, Cotev S. Continuous spinal anaesthesia using a standard epidural set for extracorporeal shock-wave lithotripsy. *Can J Anaesth.* 1997;44(10):1042–1046.

25 | ANESTHESIA FOR PROCEDURES IN THE EMERGENCY DEPARTMENT

JAMES E. ANDRUCHOW, MD, MSC, FRCPC, ABEM, BENJAMIN EASTER, MD

INTRODUCTION

The practice of emergency medicine has changed significantly over the past several decades, having evolved into a separate and distinct specialty with a unique knowledge base and training program. As the specialty has evolved, so has the complexity of patients being cared for in the emergency department (ED), as well as the range of tests and treatments being performed. For many of these patients, the acute management of pain and anxiety is an essential component of their ED care and fundamental to the performance of diagnostic and therapeutic interventions. Consequently, possessing an arsenal of anesthesia techniques is essential to the safe and effective practice of modern emergency medicine. This chapter reviews the provision of such anesthesia in the ED setting.

SPECIAL CONSIDERATIONS

Practice in the ED poses special challenges to anesthesia providers. Unlike the typically controlled environment of the operating room, where most patients have been optimized and scheduled for a given procedure, ED patients, by definition, present unexpectedly, are undifferentiated, and may be critically ill. Moreover, they may be in acute distress, have unclear past medical and surgical histories, or have a limited ability to communicate with health care providers. Despite this, many of these patients may require immediate diagnostic or therapeutic interventions to prevent serious morbidity or mortality. In such situations, there is no option to "cancel a case," and ED anesthesia providers are often forced to proceed with limited time and information on patients with acute medical issues that may make performing anesthesia more risky and complicated.

Fortunately, the ED environment also possesses a unique array of resources not necessarily present in the operating room. One of the biggest assets of the ED (particularly at larger centers) is the presence of a highly skilled multidisciplinary health care team with experience rapidly assessing and stabilizing undifferentiated patients. In addition to physicians and nurses, the team often includes other skilled personnel, including physician assistants, nurse practitioners, respiratory therapists, orthopedic technicians, physical therapists, and clinical assistants. In fact, the ability to rapidly mobilize additional human resources as required for an individual scenario is a hallmark of ED care. Provider teams performing anesthesia in the ED also generally have advanced airway assessment and management skills, as well as comfort in resuscitating and performing procedures in critically ill patients. Moreover, most EDs have a wide array of monitoring, supportive, and rescue equipment to both prevent complications and rapidly address them should they arise. Thus, while the ED environment often necessitates performing procedures in higher-risk clinical scenarios, it is also resource rich and well equipped for such situations.

RIGHT PATIENT, RIGHT PLACE, RIGHT TIME: THE CHOICE TO PERFORM ANESTHESIA IN THE ED

When considering performing a procedure potentially requiring anesthesia for a patient in the ED, the health care provider must ask two important questions. First, is this the right time and place for this procedure to be performed for this patient? Second, are there better alternatives to both the procedure and its timing? The answers to these questions will depend on patient, procedural, and departmental factors.

Patient factors relate to the patient's acute clinical condition as well as underlying medical comorbidities. Complex laceration repair or wound debridement in a hemodynamically unstable trauma patient is best deferred until more acute medical issues have been stabilized. Hip dislocation reduction for a morbidly obese patient with a serious cardiovascular history may be best performed urgently under general anesthesia in the operating room given the significant potential for complications.

Procedural factors relate to both the complexity and the urgency of the procedure being considered. For example, reduction of a fracture-dislocation resulting in a pulseless limb or cardioversion of a hemodynamically unstable dysrhythmia are both true medical emergencies that should be addressed immediately unless clear contraindications exist. In contrast, incision and drainage of an abscess or reduction of a wrist fracture without neurovascular compromise should be performed urgently but may be safely delayed somewhat if conditions for the procedure are suboptimal. Physicians must also consider if alternative procedural approaches exist; for example, can the stable dysrhythmia be cardioverted chemically instead of electrically, obviating the need for anesthesia entirely?

Departmental factors are also a unique consideration of EDs. Given that most health care providers in the ED are responsible for many (often critically ill) patients at any point in time, it may not be feasible or in the best interest of the department to perform a procedure requiring anesthesia if it may compromise the care of other patients and can safely be deferred. These issues are particularly common in smaller EDs, which may be staffed by a single provider or have limited resources available, particularly overnight. Health care providers must weigh the potential harms and benefits of immediately performing the procedure originally planned versus delaying the procedure until more resources can be mobilized or the patient can be transferred to a more resource-rich setting.

RIGHT TECHNIQUE: SELECTING THE BEST ANESTHESIA OPTION

When discussing anesthesia in the ED, many individuals immediately think of procedural sedation and analgesia (PSA). While indeed PSA is the major focus of this chapter, it is important for ED anesthesia providers to consider all options available to them, as many excellent, lower-risk, and less-resource-intensive anesthesia alternatives to PSA exist for many procedures (Table 25.1). For details on how to safely perform the procedures discussed, please see one of the excellent emergency procedural textbooks available, such as *Clinical Procedures in Emergency Medicine*[1] or *Emergency Medicine Procedures*.[2]

PROCEDURAL SEDATION AND ANALGESIA

DEFINITION

Procedural sedation and analgesia, formerly known as "conscious sedation" or "intravenous conscious sedation," is a technique of administering sedatives, analgesics, and/or dissociative agents to induce a state that allows patients to tolerate unpleasant procedures while maintaining cardiorespiratory function.[3] Mastering this technique is essential to the performance of many procedures that would otherwise be impossible in the ED setting, including long-bone fracture and large-joint dislocation reductions, electrical cardioversion, and painful minor surgical procedures, especially in the pediatric population. Effective PSA increases the success rate of the procedure and also enhances patient and provider experience.[4]

While predefined levels of sedation exist based on the degree of suppression of consciousness, airway and respiratory status, and cardiovascular function (also see Chapter 4), it is important to recognize that sedation actually represents a continuum of depth. Accordingly, the levels of sedation represent a conceptual framework and should not be considered determinant of a given patient's response.[5] The first level is minimal sedation or anxiolysis, in which patients are in a state of drug-induced relaxation but respond normally to verbal commands.

TABLE 25.1. Procedural Sedation and Analgesia Alternatives Commonly Available in the Emergency Department (ED)

TYPE	SUBTYPE	CLINICAL APPLICATIONS
Local	Topical anesthesia For example, lidocaine-prilocaine, lidocaine-epinephrine-tetracaine	• Pediatric venipuncture • Pediatric laceration repair • Pediatric lumbar puncture
	Field block	• Abscess incision and drainage • Epidermoid (sebaceous) cyst excision
	Hematoma block	• Wrist fracture/dislocation • Ankle fracture/dislocation
Regional	Common nerve blocks by region Facial blocks • Forehead • Supraorbital • Infraorbital • Ear • Lip • Mental • Dental Upper extremity • Radial • Median • Ulnar Lower extremity • Femoral • Ankle Digits • Digital (ring) block • Metacarpal head	• Laceration repair • Tendon repair • Wound exploration • Foreign body removal • Digit fracture or dislocation reduction • Digit amputation revision • Analgesia for extremity fractures • Dental pain
	Intravenous regional anesthesia (Bier block)	• Extremity fracture reduction • Wound exploration/debridement
Intra-articular	• Shoulder	• Shoulder dislocation reduction

Airway, ventilation, and cardiovascular function are unaffected. Moderate sedation refers to a drug-induced, depressed level of consciousness where patients are still able to respond purposefully to verbal commands and airway, respiratory, and cardiovascular functions are usually preserved. Deep sedation is a drug-induced, depressed level of consciousness from which patients cannot be easily aroused but will respond purposefully after noxious or repeated stimuli. In this state, patients may need support in maintaining airway patency and may require mild respiratory support to maintain adequate ventilation. This contrasts with general anesthesia, in which patients experience total loss of consciousness as a consequence of drug administration, are not arousable, and may have significant impairments to both respiratory and cardiovascular function.

A separate, but related, sedation state produced by certain agents, such as ketamine, is dissociative sedation, in which patients are in a trance-like state, maintaining respiratory and cardiovascular function but experiencing deep analgesia and amnesia. Dissociation refers to the disruption of communication between sensory processing areas of the brain in the cortex and association areas in the limbic system, which leads to a loss of normal processing of sensory inputs, effectively "dissociating" the patient from his or her environment.[6]

The goal of most procedural sedations performed in the ED on adult patients is to reach a state of moderate or deep sedation in order to facilitate performance of a diagnostic or therapeutic intervention. A dissociative state is more often achieved in children because of the proven efficacy and favorable side-effect profile of ketamine in pediatric procedural sedation, although the use of this method in adults is increasing.

Procedural sedation and analgesia is commonplace in both adult and pediatric EDs around the country, and the American College of Emergency Physicians (ACEP) supports its practice by emergency physicians. Accordingly, ACEP has developed its own clinical policy, updated in 2014, regarding PSA in the ED.[4] Practice guidelines for sedation and analgesia for nonanesthesiologists have also been approved by the American Society of Anesthesiologists.[7] In addition, many facilities have local guidelines governing this practice.

REQUIRED RESOURCES AND CREDENTIALING

Safe and effective performance of PSA in the ED requires significant departmental resources. As previously described, most EDs are well-resourced environments with staff experienced in caring for critically ill patients. Emergency physicians' knowledge of advanced airway techniques and experience with resuscitation of hemodynamically unstable patients provides a safety margin in administering PSA, particularly in rescuing patients who experience higher levels of sedation than intended. Nevertheless, a number of departmental factors are necessary to the safe and effective performance of PSA.

First, the ED and hospital should have clear policies related to credentialing of providers who perform PSA, including initial training, scope of practice, and maintenance of certification. In many facilities, emergency medicine residency training and board certification are sufficient for this privilege, but providers should be sure to comply with local guidelines.

Second, EDs should consider the use of clinical pathways or checklists for the administration of PSA. In general, clinical pathways have been shown to improve adherence to guidelines, enhance outcomes, and reduce costs across a range of conditions and patient populations.[8] While no data specifically examining a clinical pathway for PSA in the ED are currently available, it is reasonable to assume that similar benefits would exist.

Third, every ED should possess mandatory equipment to provide PSA. In addition to standard airway equipment such as high flow oxygen, pulse oximetry, suction, nasal and/or oral airways and bag-valve mask equipment, ED providers should have the equipment and training to provide rescue airways (e.g., supraglottic airways and/or endotracheal intubation) immediately during PSA should the need arise. The ability to achieve intravenous access (and rapidly re-establish access if lost) is also essential in order to provide intravenous fluids and vasoactive medications. Knowledge of multiple techniques beyond standard peripheral intravenous access, such as ultrasound-guided, central venous or intraosseous access is also advantageous. Finally, ED providers performing PSA should have a "crash cart" or equivalent immediately available with the ability to quickly provide advanced life support if required.

All patients undergoing PSA require ongoing monitoring. Patient monitoring should begin with vital signs, including blood pressure, oxygen saturation, and heart rate and rhythm, prior to the administration of medications. Patient monitoring to detect possible respiratory depression, hypotension, or other adverse effects should continue at regular intervals throughout PSA and into the recovery period.

When it has been determined that the patient is a good candidate for procedural sedation, the health care provider performing the procedure must obtain an informed consent from the patient or health care proxy after explaining in detail the rationale for the procedure as well as the potential risks and benefits.

PRESEDATION ASSESSMENT

Past Medical History and Precipitating Events

Procedural sedation is an advanced anesthesia technique in which the patient may experience total loss of consciousness, diminished protective airway reflexes, and serious complications, such as apnea or hypotension[9]; therefore, it is essential that a thorough assessment of the patient occurs prior to initiating the procedure. This should include an AMPLE (i.e., allergies, medications, past medical history, last oral intake, events leading to the present situation) history. Allergies to medications or medications related to those planned for use in the procedure, or the concurrent use of medications with known drug interactions, may necessitate different medications than originally planned. Past medical history of asthma or lung disease, sleep apnea, heart disease, trauma, or substance use/abuse may necessitate significant modifications to the procedural sedation method, agents used, or dosing or may result in abandoning PSA entirely and opting for definitive airway control in an operating room setting.

Because there is a theoretical increased risk of aspiration during PSA, some published guidelines recommend that the last oral intake of solids should ideally be 6 hours before the procedure and 2 hours for liquids.[7] However, preprocedure fasting has not been shown to decrease aspiration risk,[10–13] and recent oral intake is not an absolute contraindication to PSA. In fact, the most recent ACEP clinical policy recommends against delaying PSA in adults or children based on fasting time.[4] Still, given the theoretical concern, it may be prudent to avoid PSA for nonemergent procedures in patients who have recently eaten a large meal.

Finally, the acute and unscheduled nature of ED visits, and hence the need for ED PSA, may lead to complicating factors not typically present in elective anesthesia. These may include intoxication with drugs or alcohol; ingestion of toxic substances; traumatic injuries (particularly to the head, face, neck or chest); lack of medical optimization or preparation for a procedure; and more general lack of information about the patient's history or medical status.

PHYSICAL EXAM AND AIRWAY ASSESSMENT

A physical exam of relevant systems and a formal airway assessment must also be completed in all patients undergoing procedural sedation. At a minimum, the physical exam should include vital signs, mental status, and examination of the cardiovascular and respiratory systems. Airway assessment should include an evaluation of the likelihood of difficulty with spontaneous respiration during PSA, as well as the difficulty of bag-mask ventilation and intubation[7] (Box 25.1). Mnemonics such as MOANS© (Box 25.2) and LEMON© (Box 25.3) may be helpful in anticipating difficult bag-valve mask ventilation and difficult intubation, respectively.[14] Finally, an accurate patient weight should be obtained in order to appropriately dose the PSA agents.

If the patient has markers of a difficult airway, then providers must anticipate a significant risk of failed bag-valve mask ventilation or intubation in the event that significant respiratory depression or apnea occurs. Providers should consider modifying their sedation plan to minimize the risk of complications and have rescue devices prepared where appropriate in order to avoid serious adverse outcomes.

BOX 25.1. AIRWAY ASSESSMENT PROCEDURES FOR SEDATION AND ANALGESIA

Positive pressure ventilation, with or without tracheal intubation, may be necessary if respiratory compromise develops during sedation-analgesia. This may be more difficult in patients with atypical airway anatomy. In addition, some airway abnormalities may increase the likelihood of airway obstruction during spontaneous ventilation. Some factors that may be associated with difficulty in airway management are as follows:

History

Previous problems with anesthesia or sedation
Stridor, snoring, or sleep apnea
Advanced rheumatoid arthritis
Chromosomal abnormality (e.g., trisomy 21)

Physical examination

Habitus
Significant obesity (especially involving the neck and facial structures)

Head and neck

Short neck, limited neck extension, decreased hyoid-mental distance (<3 cm in an adult), neck mass, cervical spine disease or trauma, tracheal deviation, dysmorphic facial features (e.g., Pierre-Robin syndrome)

Mouth

Small opening (<3 cm in an adult); edentulous; protruding incisors; loose or capped teeth; dental appliances; high, arched palate; macroglossia; tonsillar hypertrophy; nonvisible uvula

Jaw

Micrognathia, retrognathia, trismus, significant malocclusion

SOURCE: Reprinted with permission from American Society of Anesthesiologists Task Force on Sedation and Analgesia by Non-Anesthesiologists. Practice guidelines for sedation and analgesia by non-anesthesiologists. *Anesthesia*. 2002;96(4):1004–1017.

BOX 25.2. MOANS© MNEMONIC FOR ANTICIPATING DIFFICULT BAG-VALVE MASK VENTILATION (BMV)

M—*Mask Seal/Male Sex/Mallampati:* Beards, facial trauma, abnormal anatomy or debris on the face may make mask seal difficult. Male sex and Mallampati 3 or 4 are also associated with difficult BMV.
O—*Obesity/Obstruction:* Patients with body mass index greater than 26 or a gravid uterus are often difficult to ventilate with BMV secondary to resistance of diaphragmatic excursion, redundant airway soft tissues, and more rapid oxygen desaturation.
A—*Age > 55 years:* Older patients tend to be more difficult to bag, often because of decreased muscle and tissue tone.
N—*No Teeth:* Adequate mask seal may be difficult to achieve in the edentulous patient. Where possible, dentures should be left in when BMV is being performed.
S—*Stiff/Snoring:* Patients with increased airway resistance secondary to obstructive lung disease, acute respiratory distress syndrome, diminished chest wall elasticity, or a history of obstructive sleep apnea (often manifest by snoring) may require increased airway pressures to ventilate adequately, and thus BMV may be challenging.

SOURCE: Adapted from Walls RM, Murphy MF. Identification of the difficult and failed airway. In: Walls RM, Murphy M, eds. *Manual of Emergency Airway Management*. 4th ed. Philadelphia, PA: Lippincott, Williams & Wilkins; 2012:8–21.

BOX 25.3. LEMON© MNEMONIC FOR ANTICIPATING A DIFFICULT INTUBATION

L—*Look* externally for signs of a difficult airway or ventilation, including facial trauma, a beard, large tongue, abnormal facies, and so on.
E—*Evaluate* for the 3:3:2 rule, which states that a difficult airway may occur if the mouth cannot open three finger breadths, the distance from the hyoid bone to the chin is less than three finger breadths, or the distance from the thyroid bone to the floor of the mouth is less than two finger breadths.
M—*Mallampati*. Determine the patient's Mallampati score.
O—*Obstruction*. Determine if upper airway obstruction could be present from a foreign body, blood, inflammation in the upper airway (epiglottitis), and so on.
N—*Neck*. Is there sufficient mobility in the patient's neck to allow for airway manipulation?

SOURCE: Adapted from Walls RM, Murphy MF. Identification of the difficult and failed airway. In: Walls RM, Murphy M, eds. *Manual of Emergency Airway Management*. 4th ed. Philadelphia, PA: Lippincott, Williams & Wilkins; 2012:8–21.

INFORMED CONSENT

When it has been determined that the patient is a good candidate for procedural sedation, the health care provider performing the procedure must obtain an informed consent from the patient or health care proxy after explaining in detail the rationale for the procedure as well as the potential risks and benefits. However, it is reassuring that a recent meta-analysis has demonstrated a very low incidence of serious adverse events during ED PSA[15] (Table 25.2). Finally, providers should ensure they take the time to address any questions or concerns the patient or family members may have. If informed consent cannot be obtained because of altered mental status or other limitations but the procedure is deemed emergent, caregivers should adhere to local waiver of consent guidelines or policy and document accordingly.

MEDICATION CHOICES FOR PSA

Many medications have been used with varying degrees of success in EDs for PSA, with midazolam combined with fentanyl being one of the earliest used regimens. However, propofol, ketamine, and etomidate have demonstrated safety in ED PSA, and newer agents such as alfentanil, remifentanil, and dexmedetomidine are being explored. The dose, pharmacologic profile, and side effects differ among the drugs considerably, making some agents particularly advantageous in some situations and contraindicated in others (Table 25.3).[16] However, the formularies of some hospitals are restrictive and do not permit the use of certain medications outside of the operating room or in the hands of nonanesthesiologists.[17] As such, the widespread adoption of new medications with potentially better efficacy and side-effect profiles has been delayed in many instances.

The clinician must take into account many factors when selecting agents for PSA, including the patient's age, past medical history and comorbidities, the type and duration of the procedure being performed, adjunctive pain control therapies, and elements of the patient's presentation that could complicate PSA. Therefore, it is essential to have a detailed understanding of the commonly used PSA agents, their advantages, disadvantages, and contraindications.

TABLE 25.2. Adverse Event Rates With Emergency Department Procedural Sedation and Analgesia

ADVERSE EVENT	EVENTS PER SEDATIONS	ESTIMATE PER 1000	95% CI
Agitation	137/6631	9.8	6.1–13.5
Apnea	68/3264	12.4	7.9–16.9
Aspiration	1/2370	1.2	0.0–2.6
Bradycardia	11/837	6.5	1.1–11.8
Hypotension	122/5801	15.2	10.7–19.7
Hypoxia	373/7116	40.2	32.5–47.9
Intubation	2/3636	1.6	0.3–2.9
Laryngospasm	1/883	4.2	0.0–8.5
Vomiting	100/3319	16.4	9.7–23

SOURCE: Adapted from Bellolio MF, Gilani WI, Barrionuevo P, et al. Incidence of adverse events in adults undergoing procedural sedation in the emergency department: a systematic review and meta-analysis. *Acad Emerg Med.* 2016;23:119–134.

SEDATIVES AND ANALGESICS

MIDAZOLAM

Midazolam belongs to the benzodiazepine class of drugs and is well known for its anxiolytic, sedative, and anticonvulsant properties. Because it acts rapidly, has a short half-life, and has amnestic properties, it is the most commonly used benzodiazepine for PSA. The most common adverse effects of midazolam are hypotension when rapidly administered and, especially when used in combination with an opioid such as fentanyl, respiratory depression. The benzodiazepine antagonist flumazenil can be useful for reversing respiratory depression associated with midazolam administration, but it can provoke seizures in long-term benzodiazepine users or alcoholics, so it should be used cautiously. While midazolam is used for PSA in many EDs, newer drugs with shorter durations of action and better side-effect profiles are now widely available and have largely supplanted midazolam as a first-line agent for PSA in adults.

PROPOFOL

Propofol is a nonbenzodiazepine, nonbarbiturate drug that has long been favored in the operating room for induction of general anesthesia because of its extremely fast onset and short duration of action. Hospitals have been slow to adopt the use of propofol in the ED, however, because of concerns over difficulty titrating the medication outside the operating room and the risk of respiratory depression, aspiration, and oversedation. These concerns persist despite extensive evidence supporting the use of propofol in the ED setting,[18–22] and there are still EDs that do not have access secondary to administrative barriers to propofol for PSA.[23] However, the most recent ACEP clinical policy provides a level A recommendation for propofol use for ED PSA.[4] In fact, propofol has become the drug of choice in many clinical scenarios.

ETOMIDATE

Etomidate is a nonbarbiturate sedative-hypnotic that has gained widespread adoption in EDs because of its demonstrated efficacy and safety in induction for rapid sequence intubation. It has many theoretical advantages for use in PSA because of its rapid onset, short duration of action, and well-documented preservation of hemodynamic stability, and there is a growing body of literature suggesting that etomidate can be used safely for PSA in the ED.[24–28] Side effects, such as vomiting and myoclonus, which can occur in 20%–72% of people undergoing PSA with etomidate,[29,30] may limit its widespread adoption as a first-line agent for PSA.

FENTANYL

A highly lipid-soluble synthetic opioid, fentanyl is a rapid acting and highly potent analgesic that has been used extensively for PSA when combined with a sedative. Fentanyl causes less respiratory depression and histamine release than other opioids, leading to a very favorable side-effect profile. Because of its rapid onset, short duration of action, and demonstrated respiratory and hemodynamic stability, it is currently the analgesic of choice for PSA in the ED. Its respiratory depressant effects are synergistic with benzodiazepines such as midazolam, and hypotension can occur in the presence of ethanol, so caution must be demonstrated when using fentanyl in patients who already have either of the above agents on board. Rapid administration of high-dose fentanyl has been associated with chest wall and glottic rigidity requiring intubation, so care must be taken to administer boluses of the drug slowly, over 3 to 5 minutes. It is important to note that, in analgesic doses, fentanyl alone has little if any sedative properties; because of this, it is commonly used in combination with a sedative-hypnotic agent such as midazolam.

DISSOCIATIVE AGENTS

Ketamine

Ketamine, a phencyclidine derivative and dissociative anesthetic, is a first-line agent for pediatric PSA.[31] In the past, it has been used less frequently among adults, largely for concerns over "emergence phenomena," which can include hallucinations and intense dysphoric experiences.[32] Administration of a benzodiazepine such as midazolam can attenuate these side effects. Ketamine, which results in release of endogenous catecholamines, is well known for its maintenance of hemodynamic stability and bronchodilatory effects, making it an ideal agent in patients with borderline hypotension or pulmonary disease. Importantly, ketamine does not demonstrate the same dose-response curve as other agents reviewed here; once the dissociative threshold is reached, additional dosing of ketamine has no effect on the level of sedation.[33] The catecholamine release can induce tachycardia and hypertension, but previous reports of ketamine increasing intracranial pressure have been largely unsubstantiated.[34,35] Hypersalivation is another known side effect of ketamine administration, and it can be mitigated by pretreatment with glycopyrrolate or atropine.

Ketofol (Ketamine-Propofol Combination)

The combination of ketamine and propofol (administered 1:1 from the same syringe as ketofol or simply concomitantly during a sedation) has the potential to attenuate the negative effects of either drug. The opposing physiologic effects produce adequate sedation and analgesia while theoretically reducing the adverse effects of either drug administered alone. While the hypothesized decrease in adverse events has not been borne out in the literature,[36] sedation effectiveness appears to be high with a low rate of adverse events.[37–39] While it is clear that ketofol is safe and effective for ED PSA, there does not appear to be clear superiority over either ketamine or propofol individually (though this may exist for as yet undefined subpopulations), and the complexity of administering two agents, and accounting for both sets of side effects, should be considered.[40]

OTHER AGENTS

Other medications have been successfully used in ED PSA, including methohexital and nitrous oxide. Methohexital is a short-acting barbiturate that has been used in general anesthesia for many years, and more recently it was applied to ED PSA with good results.[41,42] Because of side effects, including hypotension and respiratory depression, the drug has fallen out of favor with the advent of newer agents. Nitrous oxide is a colorless gas long used in general anesthesia and has both sedative and analgesic properties. Because it is a known teratogen and requires a well-ventilated room with a dedicated scavenging system to prevent inhalation by health care providers, it was never broadly adopted for ED PSA in the United States, although it is widely accepted in other countries. The use of dexmedetomidine, a central-acting α_2-agonist, has also been reported in PSA. While it has the advantage of minimal respiratory depression, its drawbacks, including dosing via infusion, a lack of significant amnestic properties, and potential for hypotension and bradycardia, may limit its widespread adoption in the ED.[43]

REVERSAL AGENTS

While rarely required in carefully performed PSA, reversal agents should be readily available when performing PSA, and clinicians should be aware of their presence should the need arise.

Naloxone

Naloxone is an opioid antagonist readily available in most EDs. It is usually administered intravenously, but it can also be given subcutaneously, intramuscularly, or via an endotracheal tube. It has a rapid onset of action and can reverse opiate-induced sedation and respiratory depression within a minute or less. However, the drug's short half-life means that patients receiving long-acting opioids can become resedated as the naloxone effect diminishes. This is not normally an issue in PSA because relatively small amounts of short-acting opiates (such as fentanyl) are usually used. Nonetheless, patients receiving naloxone should be observed for at least 1 hour following administration of the drug to ensure resedation does not occur. Naloxone may precipitate acute opioid withdrawal in patients with a history of chronic opiate use.

Flumazenil

Flumazenil is a competitive antagonist of the benzodiazepine γ-aminobutyric acid (GABA) receptors in the central nervous system. The drug is rapidly acting, reversing benzodiazepine effects within 1–2 minutes, but like naloxone, it has a short duration of action, and patients can become resedated following a single administration. As such, patients should be observed for at least 1 hour following flumazenil administration. Flumazenil can also precipitate acute benzodiazepine withdrawal and seizures, particularly in long-term benzodiazepine users. Flumazenil should be used cautiously and at the lowest possible doses whenever required.

PREPROCEDURE PREPARATION

EQUIPMENT

It is essential that all necessary PSA and reversal medications, monitoring equipment, health care providers, and rescue airway equipment are prepared prior to administration of medication. An oxygen supply and basic face mask should be available prior to and throughout the procedural

TABLE 25.3. Medications Commonly Used in Adult Procedural Sedation

MEDICATION	ROUTE	INITIAL IV DOSE	USUAL TOTAL DOSE	TIME OF ONSET	DURATION OF ACTION	ADVANTAGES	SERIOUS ADVERSE EFFECTS	COMMENTS
Sedative-hypnotic agents								
Midazolam (benzodiazepine)	IV	0.05 mg/kg	0.02–0.1 mg/kg	1–2 min	30 min	Rapid onset Short duration Easily titrated Low incidence of pain on injection and phlebitis Multiple routes	Respiratory depression Hypotension	Respiratory depression more severe in elderly patients, those with COPD, and when coadministered with other respiratory depressants Reduce dosage in patients with COPD or older than 60 years of age
	IM		0.1 mg/kg	10–15 min	60–120 min			
	Oral		0.5 mg/kg	15–30 min	60–90 min			
	PR		0.5 mg/kg	10–30 min	60–90 min			
Propofol (alkylphenol)	IV	0.5 mg/kg	1.0 mg/kg	<1 min	8–10 min	Rapid onset Short duration; antiemetic	Respiratory depression Hypotension Injection pain	Procedures lasting longer than 8–10 min will require repeat boluses or infusion
	INF		25–125 μg/kg/min					
Etomidate (imidazole derivative)	IV	0.1 mg/kg	0.1–0.2 mg/kg	<1 min	5–10 min	Rapid onset Short duration Minimal cardiovascular effects Cerebral protective	Respiratory depression Myoclonus Vomiting	Adrenal suppression not clinically relevant with one-time administration
Dissociative agents								
Ketamine (phencyclidine derivative)	IV	1 mg/kg	1–2 mg/kg	1 min 15 min	Rapid onset Short duration No respiratory depression Multiple routes Predictable given IM	Hypertension Tachycardia May cause laryngospasm	Associated with emergence phenomena and emesis	
	IM		4–5 mg/kg	5 min 15–30 min				
	Oral		5–10 mg/kg	30–45 min 120–240 min				
	PR		5–10 mg/kg	5–10 min 15–30 min				

Analgesics								
Fentanyl (opiate)	IV	1.0 μg/kg	2–3 μg/kg	1–2 min	30–40 min	Rapid onset, short duration, titratable Minimal cardiovascular effects	Respiratory depression Muscle rigidity	Respiratory depression more pronounced when administered with other respiratory depressants Causes minimal histamine release May cause transient chest wall rigidity
Reversal agents								
Naloxone (opiate antagonist)	IV/IM	0.1–0.2 mg	0.1–1mg	<1 min	15–30 min	Rapid-acting reversal	Opiate withdrawal	Short duration; monitor for resedation
Flumazenil (benzodiazepine antagonist)	IV	0.2 mg	1.0 mg	1–2 min	45 min	Rapid-acting reversal	Benzodiazepine withdrawal	Short duration; monitor for resedation Use cautiously in patients with a history of benzodiazepine or ethanol use; can precipitate withdrawal and seizures

CNS, central nervous system; COPD, chronic obstructive pulmonary disease; ICP, intracranial pressure; IV, intravenous; IM, intramuscular; PR, rectal; INF, infusion; TBI, traumatic brain injury.

NOTE: All dosing provided is for adult patients.

SOURCE: Adapted from Burbulys DB. Procedural sedation and analgesia. In: Marx JA, Hockberger RS, Walls RM, eds. *Rosen's Emergency Medicine: Concepts and Clinical Practice*. 8th ed. New York, NY: Elsevier; 2014:50–60.

sedation to preoxygenate the patient prior to sedation and maintain oxygen saturation throughout the procedure, especially during periods of depressed respiratory drive. Basic airway equipment should include, at a minimum, a bag-mask, suction, and nasopharyngeal or oropharyngeal airway. Other equipment that should be located nearby and easily accessible should include rescue airway devices such as laryngeal mask airways (LMAs), a working laryngoscope with multiple sizes of laryngoscope blades and endotracheal tubes, and any other equipment necessary to facilitate a successful intubation or rescue airway or Acute Cardiac Life Support (ACLS) should cardiorespiratory failure occur.

PATIENT MONITORING

Basic monitoring equipment must include a pulse oximeter and blood pressure cuff, as some of the most common side effects of procedural sedation are respiratory depression and hypotension. It is therefore essential that both oxygen saturation and blood pressure can be monitored throughout the induction, procedure, and recovery phases.

Monitoring of exhaled carbon dioxide can also provide valuable information about a patient's respiratory status. This can take the form of capnometry, a numeric display of the end-tidal CO_2 ($ETCO_2$) level, or capnography, a waveform of the CO_2 concentration over time. $ETCO_2$ > 50 mm Hg, absent $ETCO_2$ waveform, or an absolute change in $ETCO_2$ greater than 10 mm Hg recorded on capnography during PSA have been shown to correlate with respiratory depression not detected by pulse oximetry.[44] While the benefits of capnography at reducing hypoxia and respiratory depression are clearly established, it has not been demonstrated to reduce related adverse events, such as neurologic injury, perhaps because of the very rare nature of such outcomes.[4] Nevertheless, as a relatively cheap, noninvasive form of monitoring that provides early warning of PSA complications, it is likely that capnography will continue to assume a greater role in PSA in the future as it has in the intensive care unit and the operating room.

Finally, the bispectral index, a tool based on electroencephalography (EEG) well established for measuring depth of sedation in the operating room during general anesthesia, also has been applied to PSA in the ED[45–47] and has shown some benefit in preventing respiratory depression.[48] However, there is insufficient evidence at this point to recommend its routine use in PSA.[49]

PERSONNEL

Several guidelines recommend that a minimum of two health care providers should be involved in any procedural sedation. The first provider should be wholly dedicated to monitoring the patient, documenting vital signs, and administering medications, and the second should be the provider performing the procedure for which the procedural sedation is being administered. In ideal circumstances, the team would also include an experience nurse, respiratory therapist and any other support staff the clinical scenario may warrant (e.g., orthopedic technician for fracture reduction and immobilization).

DRUG ADMINISTRATION

When appropriate agents have been selected for the indication, drug administration should proceed in a weight-based and stepwise fashion to ensure effectiveness and patient safety. The physician performing the PSA should feel comfortable in his or her knowledge of the drug's weight-based dosing, contraindications, adverse effects, and reversal agents (if any).

Aside from ketamine, most commonly used PSA agents do not have significant analgesic properties; consequently, most PSA strategies involve a combination of fentanyl and a sedative-hypnotic agent. Because effective analgesia is a cornerstone of PSA, and respiratory depression and excessive sedation are adverse effects primarily associated with the administration of sedative-hypnotic agents, it is recommended that the analgesic agent be administered first in any PSA. Therefore, when using fentanyl and sedative-hypnotic agents, fentanyl should be administered first, observed for effect, and then the sedative-hypnotic agents should be titrated slowly and incrementally until the desired level of sedation is reached.

It is important to remember that constant painful stimuli during procedures such as fracture or dislocation reduction can result in a higher level of consciousness than would be expected in the absence of painful stimuli; thus, one must be careful not to overtitrate medications. It is not uncommon for a patient who is actively moving and moaning in pain while undergoing fracture reduction to become completely unconscious and apneic within seconds of removal of the painful stimulus.

POSTPROCEDURE CARE

Patients should be monitored in an adequately staffed and monitored area of the ED following completion of the procedural sedation until the patient has regained normal mental status, is no longer at risk of cardiorespiratory depression, and has normal vital signs. On discharge, patients should be given written instructions detailing postprocedure diet, medications and level of activity and be alerted to seek medical attention for concerning signs and symptoms. Patients should be discharged in the care of family members or friends and should be instructed to avoid driving a vehicle and avoid other potentially dangerous activities for the remainder of the day given the risk of ongoing functional impairment.

CONCLUSION

Practice in the ED provides many unique challenges and opportunities for the anesthesia provider. As the number and complexity of patients presenting to EDs continue to increase, anesthesia providers must be aware of their growing scope of practice, as well as the tools and techniques available to them outside of the operating room.

REFERENCES

1. Roberts JR, Hedges JR, eds. *Clinical Procedures in Emergency Medicine.* 6th ed. Philadelphia, PA: Saunders; 2014.

2. Reichman EF, ed. *Emergency Medicine Procedures*. 2nd ed. New York, NY. McGraw-Hill Education; 2013.
3. Green SM, Krauss B. Procedural sedation terminology: moving beyond "conscious sedation." *Ann Emerg Med*. 2002;39:433–435.
4. Godwin SA, Burton JH, Gerardo CJ, et al. American College of Emergency Physicians (ACEP) clinical policy: procedural sedation and analgesia in the emergency department. *Ann Emerg Med*. 2014;63(2):247–258.
5. American Society of Anesthesiologists. Continuum of depth of sedation: definition of general anesthesia and levels of sedation/analgesia. Amended 2014. Available at: http://www.asahq.org/quality-and-practice-management/standards-guidelines-and-related-resources/continuum-of-depth-of-sedation-definition-of-general-anesthesia-and-levels-of-sedation-analgesia. Last accessed March 1, 2018.
6. Haas DA, Harper DG. Ketamine: a review of its pharmacologic properties and use in ambulatory anesthesia. *Anesth Prog*. 1992;39:61–68.
7. American Society of Anesthesiologists Task Force on Sedation and Analgesia by Non-Anesthesiologists. Practice guidelines for sedation and analgesia by non-anesthesiologists. *Anesthesia*. 2002;96:1004–1017.
8. Rotter T, Kinsman L, James EL, et al. Clinical pathways: effects on professional practice, patient outcomes, length of stay and hospital costs. *Cochrane Database Syst Rev*. 2010;(3):CD006632. doi:10.1002/14651858.CD006632.pub2.
9. Miller MA, Levy P, Patel MM. Procedural sedation and analgesia in the emergency department: what are the risks? *Emerg Med Clin North Am*. 2005;23:551–572.
10. Molina JA, Lobo CA, Goh HK, et al. Review of studies and guidelines on fasting and procedural sedation at the emergency department. *Int J Evid Based Healthc*. 2010;8:75–78.
11. Thorpe RJ, Benger J. Pre-procedural fasting in emergency sedation. *Emerg Med J*. 2010;27:254–261.
12. Green SM, Roback MG, Miner JR, et al. Fasting and emergency department procedural sedation and analgesia: a consensus-based clinical practice advisory. *Ann Emerg Med*. 2007;49:454–461.
13. Roback MG, Bajaj L, Wathen JE, et al. Preprocedural fasting and adverse events in procedural sedation and analgesia in a pediatric emergency department: are they related? *Ann Emerg Med*. 2004;44:454–459.
14. Walls RM, Murphy MF. Identification of the difficult and failed airway. In: Walls RM, Murphy M, eds. *Manual of Emergency Airway Management*. 4th ed. Philadelphia, PA. Lippincott Williams & Wilkins; 2012:8–21.
15. Bellolio MF, Gilani WI, Barrionuevo P, et al. Incidence of adverse events in adults undergoing procedural sedation in the emergency department: a systematic review and meta-analysis. *Acad Emerg Med*. 2016;23:119–134.
16. Burbulys DB. Procedural sedation and analgesia. In: Marx JA, Hockberger RS, Walls RM, eds. *Rosen's Emergency Medicine: Concepts and Clinical Practice*. 8th ed. New York, NY: Elsevier; 2014:50–60.
17. Sacchetti A, Harris RH, Packard D. Emergency department procedural sedation formularies. *Am J Emerg Med*. 2005;23:569–587.
18. Hohl CM, Sadatsafavi M, Nosyk B, Anis AH. Safety and clinical effectiveness of midazolam versus propofol for procedural sedation in the emergency department: a systematic review. *Acad Emerg Med*. 2008;15(1):1–8.
19. David H, Shipp J. A randomized controlled trial of ketamine/propofol versus propofol alone for emergency department procedural sedation. *Ann Emerg Med*. 2011;57:435–441.
20. Mallory MD, Baxter AL, Yanosky DJ, et al. Emergency physician-administered propofol sedation: a report on 25,433 sedations from the Pediatric Sedation Research Consortium. *Ann Emerg Med*. 2011;57:462–468.
21. Black E, Campbel SG, Magee K, et al. Propofol for procedural sedation in the emergency department: a qualitative systematic review. *Ann Pharmacother*. 2013;47(6):856–868.
22. Wakai A, Blackburn C, McCabe A, et al. The use of propofol for procedural sedation in emergency departments. *Cochrane Database Syst Rev*. 2015;(7):CD007399. doi:10.1002/14651858.CD007399.pub2.
23. Green SM, Krauss B. Barriers to propofol use in emergency medicine. *Ann Emerg Med*. 2008;52(4):392–398.
24. Ruth WJ, Burton JH, Bock AJ. Intravenous etomidate for procedural sedation in emergency department patients. *Acad Emerg Med*. 2000;8:13–18.
25. Hunt GS, Spencer MT, Hays DP. Etomidate and midazolam for procedural sedation: prospective, randomized trial. *Am J Emerg Med*. 2005;23:299–303.
26. Miner JR, Danahy M, Moch A, Biros M. Randomized clinical trial of etomidate versus propofol for procedural sedation in the emergency department. *Ann Emerg Med*. 2007;49(1):15–22.
27. Falk J, Zed PJ. Etomidate for procedural sedation in the emergency department. *Ann Pharmacother*. 2004;38:1272–1277.
28. Disel NR, Yilmaz HL, Sertdemir Y, et al. Etomidate vs ketamine: effective use in procedural sedation for pediatric orthopedic injuries. *Pediatr Emerg Care*. 2106;32(12):830–834.
29. Van Keulen SG, Burton JH. Myoclonus associated with etomidate for ED procedural sedation and analgesia. *Am J Emerg Med*. 2003;21:556–558.
30. Yates AM, Wolfson AB, Shum L, Kehrl T. A descriptive study of myoclonus associated with etomidate procedural sedation in the ED. *Am J Emerg Med*. 2013;31(5):852–854.
31. Green SM, Krauss B. Clinical practice guideline for emergency department ketamine dissociative sedation in children. *Ann Emerg Med*. 2004;44:460–471.
32. Strayer RJ, Nelson LS. Adverse events associated with ketamine for procedural sedation in adults. *Am J Emerg Med*. 2008;26:985–1028.
33. Green SM, Roback MG, Kennedy RM, et al. Clinical practice guideline for emergency department ketamine dissociative sedation: 2011 update. *Ann Emerg Med*. 2011;57(5):449–461.
34. Zeiler FA, Teitelbaum J, West M, Gilman LM. The ketamine effect on ICP in traumatic brain injury. *Neurocrit Care*. 2014;21(1):163–173.
35. Cohen L, Athaide V, Wickham ME, et al. The effect of ketamine on intracranial and cerebral perfusion pressure and health outcomes: a systematic review. *Ann Emerg Med*. 2015;65(1):43–51.
36. Andolfatto G, Abu-Laban RB, Zed PJ, et al. Ketamine-propofol combination (ketofol) versus propofol alone for emergency department procedural sedation and analgesia: a randomized double-blind trial. *Ann Emerg Med*. 2012;59(6):504–512.
37. Willman EV, Andolfatto G. A prospective evaluation of ketofol (ketamine/propofol combination) for procedural sedation in the emergency department. *Ann Emerg Med*. 2007;49(1):23–30.
38. Andolfatto G, Willman E. A prospective case series of pediatric procedural sedation and analgesia in the emergency department using single syringe ketamine-propofol combination (ketofol). *Acad Emerg Med*. 2010;17:194–201.
39. Nejati A, Moharari RS, Ashraf H, et al. Ketamine/propofol versus midazolam/fentanyl for procedural sedation and analgesia in the emergency department: a randomized, prospective, double blind trial. *Acad Emerg Med*. 2011;18(8):800–806.
40. Green SM, Andolfatto G, Krauss B. Ketofol for procedural sedation? Pro and con. *Ann Emerg Med*. 2011;57(5):444–448.
41. Zink BJ, Darfler K, Salluzzo RF, Reilley KM. The efficacy and safety of methohexital in the department. *Ann Emerg Med*. 1991;20:1293–1298.
42. Lerman B, Yoshida D, Levitt MA. A prospective evaluation of the safety and efficacy of methohexital in the emergency department. *Am J Emerg Med*. 1996;14:351–354.
43. Parashchanka A, Schelfout S, Coppens M. Role of novel drugs in sedation outside the operating room: dexmedetomidine, ketamine and remifentanil. *Curr Opin Anaesthesiol*. 2014;27(4):442–447.
44. Miner JR, Heegaard W, Plummer D. Endtidal carbon dioxide monitoring during procedural sedation. *Acad Emerg Med*. 2002;9(4):275–280.
45. Gill M, Green SM, Krauss B. A study of the bispectral index monitor during procedural sedation and analgesia in the emergency department. *Ann Emerg Med*. 2003;41:234–241.
46. Miner JR, Biros MH, Heegaard W, Plummer D. Bispectral electroencephalographic analysis of patients undergoing procedural sedation in the emergency department. *Acad Emerg Med*. 2003;10:638–643.
47. Agrawal D, Feldman HA, Krauss B, Waltzman ML. Bispectral index monitoring quantifies depth of sedation during emergency department procedural sedation and analgesia in children. *Ann Emerg Med*. 2004;43:247–255.
48. Miner JR, Biros MH, Seigel T, Ross K. The utility of the bispectral index in procedural sedation with propofol in the emergency department. *Acad Emerg Med*. 2005;12:190–196.
49. Conway A, Sutherland J. Depth of anaesthesia monitoring during procedural sedation and analgesia: a systematic review and meta-analysis. *Int J Nurs Stud*. 2016;63:201–212.

26 | OFFICE-BASED ANESTHESIA

LAURENCE M. HAUSMAN, MD

INTRODUCTION

Over the past several decades, surgery has become less invasive. This change has led to a shift from the inpatient hospital-based paradigm of surgery to an ambulatory surgery model.[1] It was estimated that even by 1998, 60%–70% of all surgical procedures were done on an ambulatory basis.[2] Further improvements in anesthetic drugs have enabled this shift. Newer anesthetic agents are generally associated with quicker onsets, shorter durations of action, and fewer hemodynamic side effects.[3,4] These combined advances in both surgery and anesthesia have allowed surgical procedures to be performed not only in hospitals or freestanding ambulatory surgery centers (ASCs) but also in private offices. It is now estimated that approximately 16% of all ambulatory surgery—approximately 12 million procedures—is performed in private offices annually.[5]

There are many advantages to office-based procedures for both patients and practitioners. The patient is afforded more privacy with a more personal experience, as well as a decreased facility fee if paying out of pocket and less risk of exposure to nosocomial infections. The practitioner will generally have improved ease in scheduling cases and the convenience of being able to perform surgery within the same office as preoperative and postoperative care; in some cases, the practitioner will receive an enhanced professional fee.[6]

An office practice cannot provide the same level of care as a tertiary care medical center or even a small community hospital. For this reason, not all surgical procedures or patient populations are appropriate for this venue. For example, procedures associated with large fluid shifts, blood loss, excessive postoperative pain, or respiratory compromise should continue to be performed in the hospital setting. Likewise, patients with significant comorbidities, potentially difficult airways, or at risk for aspiration should not be considered suitable candidates for an office-based procedure. The American Society of Anesthesiologists (ASA) has published specific recommendations regarding what types of surgery and patient populations should be excluded from this venue.[7] Generally, ASA physical status (ASA-PS) 1 and 2 patients are ideal patients for this surgical venue.[7] ASA-PS 3 patients should be evaluated by an anesthesiologist prior to scheduling a surgical procedure requiring anesthesia, and patients at ASA-PS 4 and 5 are generally not appropriate. Special attention should be paid to the patient with suspected or diagnosed obstructive sleep apnea syndrome.[8]

SAFETY IN THE OFFICE

Anesthetic care performed in a private office must be as safe as that performed within a hospital or freestanding ASC. In this regard, the ASA has taken the position that office-based practitioners must adhere to the same perioperative guidelines as the more traditional hospital-based caregivers.[9]

Almost since its inception, the safety record for office-based surgery and anesthesia has been reported and debated.[10,11] It was not long ago considered the "Wild West" of medicine.[12] Reports of injuries and deaths were seen in the lay press and covered by national news organizations.[13] Vila et al. reported that there is as much as a 10% increase in morbidity and mortality associated with surgery performed in this remote location.[14] There have, however, been several conflicting published studies highlighting the fact that office-based surgery and anesthesia are safe.[15,16]

The reason for this discrepancy is multifactorial. A major problem with any study investigating adverse patient outcomes starts with the accuracy of data collection. Most analysis of office-based morbidity and mortality relies on self-reporting of these outcomes by the private offices. Moreover, even in states where adverse event reporting is mandated and enforced, the anesthesia care delivery model for the individual surgical offices will vary. For example, in one office, the anesthetic may be performed by a board-certified anesthesiologist, while in another it is performed by a nurse anesthetist supervised by the surgeon; in yet another, a dental anesthetist, who may be simultaneously doing the procedure, gives the anesthetic. The training and qualifications of the caregiver may in fact have more of an effect on safety than the location of the operating room suite. Because of advances in anesthetic agents, perioperative monitoring, and provider training, modern-day anesthesia has an impressive safety record. The risk of injury during an anesthetic is quite small. Thus, the calculation of any true anesthetic-related morbidity or mortality rate will require sample sizes much larger than those presently reported.

There has been a move toward mandatory reporting of adverse outcomes during office-based surgery and anesthesia.[17] Some states have made it mandatory to report any deaths or hospital admissions following an office-based surgical procedure. Starling et al. have recently analyzed and reported 10 years of Florida and 6 years of Alabama data.[18] Analysis of these data revealed that in Florida there were a total of 263 hospital transfers and 46 deaths. Of these, 49.8% (131/263) of the hospital transfers were for cosmetic procedures. Cosmetic procedures also accounted for 56.5% (26/46) of the deaths.

Further, of these transfers and deaths, 74% of the transfers and 67% of the deaths were for patients who had undergone general anesthesia. Liposuction or liposuction in association with another cosmetic procedure accounted for 34 hospital admissions and 10 deaths. Plastic surgeons accounted for 45% of all reported complications, and 38% of the offices reporting complications were accredited by a nationally recognized accrediting agency. It is also important to note that 98% of all complications were performed by board-certified surgeons. Alabama had a similar breakdown during its 6 years of recorded data. Over that period, there were 49 reported hospital transfers and 3 mortalities. Of all hospital transfers, 42% were following cosmetic procedures, and of these 86% were under general anesthesia. Plastic surgeons again accounted for 42.3% of all hospital admissions.[18]

Recently, the Society for Ambulatory Anesthesia published outcomes from seven practices providing office-based anesthesia between 2008 and 2009. Overall complication rate in this study was less than 1%. Of the 37,669 cases reported, 24 resulted in an unplanned hospital transfer. The mortality rate was 0. Other complications noted were laryngospasm, aspiration, medication errors, narcotic overdose, and wrong-side surgery.[19]

The ASA, along with other medical societies such as the American Society of Plastic Surgeons (ASPS), has been an active patient safety advocate. Both these organizations have released guidelines and recommendations for office-based practitioners. The ASPS has mandated that, as of 1996, all of its members must only operate in accredited office facilities.

OFFICE ACCREDITATION

One way of attempting to standardize quality of patient care within and among private offices is office accreditation. Hospitals have long had governmental oversight into the way they are run and managed. Hospitals have strict rules and regulations regarding all aspects of care, ranging from infection control, fire safety, administration, patient records, staffing, and so on. The Joint Commission (TJC) has been the organization responsible for hospital accreditation. Participation with TJC is required for most private and governmental insurance reimbursements. There can be no doubt that this has helped lead to the tremendous safety record in hospitals within the United States.

As office-based surgery has expanded as a viable venue for patient care, there has been much attention placed on the creation of a similar type of regulatory agency or accreditation bodies to oversee and standardize patient care. Three such organizations have emerged. Currently, the organizations that can accredit an office to perform surgery are the TJC, American Association of Ambulatory Surgical Facilities (AAAASF), and Accreditation Association for Ambulatory Health Care (AAAHC). All three agencies, although unique, have similar requirements for office accreditation. This chapter begins by looking at some of the important aspects required for accreditation.

Many states now regulate office-based surgery and anesthesia (presently approximately 30 states have specific regulations on the books regarding this surgical arena); some require accreditation.[20] It is thus important to categorize these surgical offices regarding the type of anesthesia and surgery being performed. Surgical offices are presently classified as level I, II, or III (Box 26.1). As mentioned, these levels are based on the types of surgery performed as well as the depth of anesthesia. This classification system varies a bit from state to state, but the fundamentals remain constant. For the most part, the office-based anesthesiologist will have more involvement with level III facilities, and the regulations are generally more stringent as the level of the office increases.

GOVERNANCE AND ADMINISTRATION

The office should be a legally constituted entity with a medical director and governing body. This governing body should be responsible for creating the mission statement of the organization, establishing and enforcing all policies and procedures, and ensuring that all applicable local laws and regulations are adhered to. It is also responsible for determining patients' rights within the facility and the credentialing and privileging process of caregivers.

The governing body must work in conjunction with the administrative arm of the organization to ensure that quality health care is administered in a uniform fashion in accordance with the mission statement. There must be policies in place for hiring and training of all new employees. The administrative responsibilities include care of private patient information and records in accordance with state, local, and federal laws; patient satisfaction data collection; and employee occupational safety.

BOX 26.1. LEVELS OF SURGICAL OFFICES AND SURGERY

Level I (class A). Office surgery includes minor procedures performed under topical or local anesthesia not involving drug-induced alteration of consciousness other than minimal preoperative antianxiety medications.

Level II (class B). Office surgery includes any procedure that requires administration of minimal or moderate sedation/analgesia making postoperative monitoring necessary. The surgical procedures are limited to those in which there is only a small risk of surgical and anesthetic complications, and hospitalization as a result of these complications is unlikely. (Many states limit this type of facility to ASA physical status [ASA-PS] 1 or 2 patients and some ASA-PS 3 patients if the patients' physical status would not be affected by the procedure.)

Level III (class C). Office surgery is a procedure that requires or reasonably should require the use of deep sedation/analgesia, general anesthesia, or major conduction blockade. The known complications of the surgical procedure may be serious or life threatening. (Many states limit this type facility to ASA-PS 1, 2, or 3.)

ASA, American Society of Anesthesiologists.

SOURCE: Mississippi State Board of Medical Licensure.

There must be a printed or electronic policy and procedures manual readily available. This manual must address staff conduct and responsibilities during all medical emergencies, including fire, bomb threat, malignant hyperthermia (MH; when triggering agents are stocked), emergency admissions, and hospital transfers. To assist office workers in familiarizing themselves with individual responsibilities during such emergencies, drills must be conducted regularly throughout the year. There must be identified sentinel events that would trigger a chart review. Policies must be in place that specify how all drugs, controlled and noncontrolled, will be purchased, stored, dispensed, and disposed.

QUALITY IMPROVEMENT AND OUTCOME MONITORING

Every surgical office should have a continuous quality improvement program built into its policies and procedures.[7] The program should constantly assess and document outcomes and should include corrective actions. The quality improvement committee should meet on a regular basis and include members of the surgical team, nursing staff, and anesthesia providers.

The ASA task force on office-based anesthesia has published a list of outcome indicators that should be examined at each office site.[21] Examples of sentinel events that should trigger a chart review would include events such as cardiopulmonary arrest, reintubation, return to the operating room, intractable nausea and vomiting, nerve injury, prolonged postanesthesia care unit (PACU) stay, equipment malfunction, medication error, infection, or uncontrolled pain.

PHYSICIAN QUALIFICATIONS

All practicing physicians must hold an active state medical license and registration, and a current Drug Enforcement Administration (DEA) certificate. They should have the education and training commensurate with their responsibilities within the office and have current curriculum vitae (CV) on file. Board certification or board eligibility within the American Board of Medical Specialties (ABMS) or its equivalent is preferable. All training and qualifications must be verified independently by the office administration. The National Practitioner Database and the American Medical Society are helpful resources for primary source verification. Physicians should carry the amount of malpractice insurance mandated by state and local law, and the presence or absence of such insurance must be communicated to patients.

All practitioners must be properly credentialed and privileged by the organization. Although it may be helpful to ensure that a practitioner has privileges to perform the intended procedures in a community hospital, it is not usually a requirement. However, the physician should have admitting privileges in a local hospital. There should be a process in place to provide peer review, performance improvement, and ensure continued medical education (CME).

All physicians should hold an active certificate in basic life support (BLS). There should be at least one physician with advanced cardiac life support (ACLS) certification (or pediatric advanced life support [PALS] certification in the case of pediatric patients) present in the office until the last patient is physically discharged from the facility.

THE OFFICE FACILITY

Much information can be garnered during a brief walkthrough of a surgical office. The anesthesia provider must have an idea of what to look for when evaluating a potential new office practice site (Box 26.2). The office should be clean, well lit, and properly ventilated, with well-marked emergency and fire exits. Doors and hallways should have been designed in such a way that would allow for the safe egress of a sedated patient on a stretcher during an emergency evacuation. Arm rails in hallways should have been designed to not inadvertently "catch" on clothing. There must be proper firefighting equipment available and inspected regularly. The operating suite must be large enough not only to perform the intended procedure but also to allow room at the head of the bed for the

BOX 26.2. OFFICE CHECKLIST

1. Size of surgical suite and recovery area
2. Hallway width and turns to maneuver a stretcher with an anesthetized patient
3. Lighting
4. Ventilation
5. Monitors in surgical suite with battery backup
6. Monitors in recovery area with battery backup
7. Adequate oxygen supply with backup
8. Source of suction
9. Defibrillator, "crash cart"
10. Double-lock narcotic cabinet
11. Backup generator
12. Firefighting equipment
13. Policy and procedure manual
    a. Emergency transfer plan
    b. Office governance and administration
    c. Infection control
    d. Disaster planning
14. Accreditation status
    a. Proceduralists
        i. Curriculum vitae
        ii. License and registration
        iii. Drug Enforcement Administration certificate
        iv. Postgraduate training record
        v. Continuing medical education, peer review, performance improvement, admitting privileges
    b. Basic life support/advanced cardiac life support/pediatric advanced life support certificates of clinical staff
    c. Fire marshal report

anesthesia provider to secure the patient's airway if need be. There must also be adequate room on both sides of the stretcher to allow health care workers patient access should there be the need for cardiopulmonary resuscitation. There must be a "crash" cart with a defibrillator, equipped with backup battery power, and appropriate emergency drugs, which are checked and documented on a regular basis. This cart should have age- and size-appropriate defibrillator paddles and emergency airway equipment.

If volatile anesthetics or succinylcholine are being used or stocked, it is necessary to have on hand the supplies and equipment needed to perform the initial treatment of MH. These supplies are best organized in a designated MH cart. The cart must include at least dantrolene with its dilutant (sterile water), bicarbonate, glucose, calcium, and insulin. There must be ice available as well as cooled intravenous fluids. A complete up-to-date listing of all necessary supplies and equipment for the initial treatment of MH can be found online (http://www.mhaus.org). There must be a transfer agreement with a local hospital in place for this medical emergency, and the office staff should have an MH drill at least annually.

The office must have reliable sources of both supplemental oxygen and suction. There must be a means of delivering the oxygen to the sedated patient both passively (i.e., nasal cannula or face mask) and actively, via positive pressure ventilation (i.e., manual self-inflating resuscitation device or anesthesia machine). If an anesthesia machine is present, it need not, and often will not, be a state-of-the-art machine. However, it must not be obsolete, and the ASA has published guidelines on anesthesia machine obsolescence that must be followed.[22] The machine must be routinely maintained and serviced in accordance with the manufacturer's specification and have battery backup.

Physiologic patient monitors, to be used throughout the perioperative period, also must be present. They must be serviced in accordance with the manufacturer's recommendation and have a battery backup. At a minimum, there must be a continuous electrocardiogram (ECG) monitor, as well as monitors to measure noninvasive blood pressure, oxygen saturation, and exhaled carbon dioxide (CO_2). A device to measure patient temperature also must be available. The anesthesia provider must adhere to the ASA monitoring standards perioperatively.[23,24]

Medical gases must be transported and stored in accordance with state and local regulations, and waste gases must be adequately scavenged in accordance with Occupational Safety and Health Administration (OSHA) regulations. Controlled substances must be purchased, stored, and dispensed in accordance with federal, state, and local law.

There must be an adequately staffed area for patient recovery. This is usually a separate room outside the operating suite. If space is an issue, it is acceptable to recover the patent in the operating room. Like the operating room, the recovery area must be of adequate size to allow for resuscitation of the patient should the need arise. The patient must be monitored postoperatively in accordance with the ASA guidelines.[25] Although this seems intuitive, a review of the closed claims data revealed it is not uniformly done. In this study, Domino reported that 100% of respiratory events leading to patient morbidity in the PACU after an office-based anesthetic would have been prevented by the use of an oxygen saturation monitor.[26]

SUPPLIES AND EQUIPMENT

There are complex federal and state laws that deal with monopolies, antitrust issues, self-referrals, and "kickbacks." It would be unusual for a health care provider to be conversant with all of the nuances of these laws. It would be even more uncommon for a health care provider to be adept enough to arrange a business agreement that does not inadvertently violate them. It is a tenet of the US legal system that ignorance of the law is not an excuse. Therefore, before providing anesthesia services it would be advisable for the office-based practitioner to engage outside legal counsel to draft the requisite agreement(s). This contract should cover insurance participation, global fees, fee-for-service arrangements, liability, and termination of services. Additionally, it should clearly delineate responsibility for the purchasing and storage of drugs and supplies associated with the anesthetic care. This is of particular importance with Medicare as well as privately insured patients, for whom either an enhanced surgical fee or a facility fee is paid to the office. These additional fees pay for the associated costs of many, if not all, of the drugs and supplies utilized on the patient. Therefore, the party collecting these fees should be required to purchase the associated drugs and supplies.

THE FLORIDA OFFICE-BASED EXPERIENCE

The trend within this country is one of increasing governmental oversight of the office-based practitioner. The history of this medical field within the state of Florida teaches many lessons. The Florida Medical Board has long been an outspoken advocate for patient safety as it relates to office-based surgery and anesthesia. Between March and July 2000, there were nine adverse outcomes associated with office-based surgery reported to their office. Of these injuries, five were patient deaths. On August 10, 2000, the Florida Medical Board placed an emergency 90-day moratorium on all level III surgeries within surgical offices.[22] During this moratorium, the board looked at all aspects of office-based surgery safety. At the expiration of the moratorium, the board allowed resumption of office-based level III surgery, but with several stipulations. Surgeons were no longer permitted to perform liposuction in combination with abdominoplasty or any other surgical procedure. The new law required that offices performing level II and III procedures submit surgical logs to the department of health and implement a risk management program. It also forbade ASA-PS 3 and greater patients to undergo a level III office-based procedure, and it required that all patients 40 years of age and older or patients of an ASA-PS 2 or greater have a complete medical workup prior to undergoing level III surgery. Finally, the law mandated compliance with the ASA guidelines for perioperative monitoring.[27]

As more states adopt regulations overseeing office-based surgery and anesthesia, many have implemented requirements similar to those of Florida. It is imperative that any office-based practitioner consult with the state and local health departments in his or her area to ensure that all laws are adhered to. Failure to do so can result in civil or even criminal prosecution.

OFFICE-BASED SURGERY AND PLASTIC SURGERY

Many medical and surgical disciplines regularly utilize private offices to perform surgery and invasive procedures. These specialties include plastic surgery, urology, otolaryngology, gynecology, dentistry, general surgery, and gastroenterology. Plastic surgeons have long been in the forefront of office-based surgery, and their society, the ASPS, regularly publishes statistics on cosmetic surgery frequency and outcomes. According to recent (for 2007) ASPS statistics, 11.8 million cosmetic procedures were performed. This represents a 59% increase from 2000. Of these procedures, 59% were performed in private offices throughout the United States.[28] The top five procedures according to this publication were liposuction, breast augmentation, eyelid surgery, abdominoplasty, and breast reduction.

Both plastic surgeons and dermatologists routinely perform liposuction, currently the most common office-based cosmetic procedure.[29] The procedure is initiated by inserting hollow rods into small incisions in the skin and suctioning subcutaneous fat into an aspiration canister. Superwet and tumescent techniques were introduced into the practice of liposuction in the mid-1980s. These techniques involve utilizing large volumes (1–4 mL) of infiltrate solution (0.9% normal saline with 1:1,000,000 epinephrine and 0.025%–0.1% lidocaine) for each 1 mL of fat to be removed. Blood loss of approximately 1% of the aspirate should be anticipated.[30] With this technique of liposuction, the peak serum levels of lidocaine will occur 12–14 hours after injection and decline over the next 6–14 hours.[31,32] Although the maximum dose of lidocaine is usually limited to approximately 7 mg/kg, we consider dosages of 3.5–5.5 mg/kg safe because this technique results in a single-compartment clearance of lidocaine similar to that of a sustained-release medication.[32,33]

One of the important lessons from the Florida moratorium is that liposuction should not be considered a procedure without risk. In 2000, Grazer and deJong published a report that revealed an overall mortality rate of 19.1 per 100,000 after liposuction.[34] A common cause of death was pulmonary embolism (PE; 28.5%). Other reported causes included fat embolism, abdominal viscus perforation, infection, hemorrhage, and anesthesia-related causes. Several risk factors associated with morbidity and mortality were also documented (Box 26.3).

Perioperative anesthetic care of the patient undergoing liposuction should include careful attention to fluid management. The patient's preexisting fluid deficit, as well as physiologic maintenance, intraoperative loss, and third spacing, should guide fluid replacement. In addition to pain control, during the postoperative period, fluid and electrolyte balance should continue to be given special attention. It is recommended that office-based liposuction be limited to 5 L of total aspirant (supernatant fat and fluid).[35] Large-volume liposuction (greater than 3 L) should not be done in conjunction with other procedures in an office. In 2002, Iverson and Lynch, in conjunction with ASPS, published specific considerations for practitioners performing office-based liposuction[30,36] (Box 26.4).

BOX 26.3. CONSIDERATIONS AND RECOMMENDATIONS REGARDING OFFICE-BASED LIPOSUCTION

1. Plastic surgeons should follow current ASA guidelines for sedation and analgesia.
2. General anesthesia can safely be used in the office setting.
3. General anesthesia has advantages for more complex liposuction procedures, including precise dosing, airway management, and controlling patient movement.
4. Epidural and spinal anesthesia are discouraged because of their association with vasodilation, hypotension, and fluid overload.
5. Moderate sedation/analgesia augments the patient's comfort and is an effective adjunct to local infiltration.

ASA, American Society of Anesthesiologists.

SOURCE: Reprinted with permission from Iverson RE, Lynch DJ, American Society of Plastic Surgeons Committee on Safety. Practice advisory on liposuction. *Plast Reconstr Surg.* 2004;113:1478–1490.

DEEP VEIN THROMBOSIS

The development of deep vein thrombosis (DVT) and ultimately PE is a common cause of death after liposuction and other cosmetic procedures. It accounts for a significant number of deaths among office-based surgical patients in general.[37,38] Reinish reported a 0.39% rate of DVT formation in patients who underwent rhytidectomy (37/9493).[39] Of these patients, 15 of 37 (40.5%) went on to develop a PE. It was also reported that although general anesthesia accounted for only 43% of the anesthetics used in this patient population, this anesthetic technique accounted for 83.7% of the embolic events. Grazer reported a 1.2% incidence of DVT formation among abdominoplasty patients and a 0.8% incidence of developing a PE.[40]

The development of DVT is related to both the procedure[41] and the underlying medical conditions of the patient. Patient-related risk factors appear in Box 26.5.[42,43] It has been established that the risk of developing DVT can be decreased by the use of either mechanical or pharmacologic methods.[44,45] Mechanical compression can be accomplished via intermittent pneumatic compression of the leg or through graduated elastic compression of the leg. Contraindications to this type of mechanical DVT prevention would include skin lesions or peripheral artery occlusive disease. Pharmacologic interventions include

BOX 26.4. RISK FACTORS ASSOCIATED WITH LIPOSUCTION

1. Use of multiliter wetting solution infiltrate
2. Megavolume (greater than 5 L) aspiration causing massive third spacing
3. Multiple concurrent procedures
4. Anesthetic sedative effects causing hypoventilation
5. Permissive discharge policies (discharge criteria not based on peer-reviewed and accepted discharge parameters)

SOURCE: Reprinted with permission from Grazer FM, deJong RH. Fatal outcome from liposuction: census survey of cosmetic surgeons. *Plast Reconstr Surg*. 2000;105:436.

Box 26.5. RISK FACTORS ASSOCIATED WITH THE DEVELOPMENT OF DEEP VEIN THROMBOSIS

1. Age greater than 40 years
2. Previous history of deep vein thrombosis
3. Family history of deep vein thrombosis
4. Malignancy
5. Obesity
6. Antithrombin III deficiency
7. Central nervous system disease
8. Estrogen-containing oral contraceptive use or hormone replacement therapy, tamoxifen
9. Previous miscarriage
10. Severe infection or trauma
11. Venous insufficiency
12. Heart failure or respiratory failure
13. Presence of lupus anticoagulant
14. Polycythemia
15. Radiation therapy for pelvic neoplasms
16. Inflammatory bowel disease
17. Smoking
18. Immobilization or limb paralysis
19. Idiopathic or acquired thrombophilia

three types of anticoagulants: heparins (both unfractionated and low molecular weight), vitamin K antagonists, and the newer oral antithrombotic agents (anti-IIa, anti-Xa). The ASPS recommends stratifying patients according to their risk of development of DVT and guiding therapy based on this stratification[46,47] (Table 26.1).

FIRE SAFETY

The office-based anesthesia provider must be knowledgeable regarding the issue of operating room fires. The ASA has published an advisory on the prevention and management of such an emergency.[48]

Fire requires three components known as the "fire triad": an oxidizer (oxygen and nitrous oxide); an ignition source (electrocautery, laser, drill, etc.); and fuel (sponges, drapes, endotracheal tubes, solutions containing alcohol or other volatile compounds, etc.). The modern operating room contains all three in great supply.

The first step in fire prevention is education. All members of the surgical and anesthesia team must be educated on how fires are started, maintained, and prevented. There must be regularly scheduled fire drills that include all employees, even those with nonclinical duties. These drills should highlight the responsibilities of each staff member.

Fire prevention is of the utmost importance. The ASA recommends that if flammable materials are used to prep the skin, they should be allowed to completely dry prior to draping the surgical field. The field should then be draped in a manner that does not allow for oxygen to accumulate. This is important because these accumulated pockets of oxygen may flow into the surgical field where there is a source of ignition, such as electrocautery. There must be communication between the surgeon and anesthesiologist when an oxygen-rich environment is being created near a surgical site. This is particularly relevant during procedures with monitored anesthesia care (MAC)—utilizing deeper sedation in and around the face. This scenario is common during facial plastic surgery. The surgeon and anesthesiologist must decide on the depth of sedation required throughout different points of the procedure, and the need for supplemental oxygen must be determined. The inspiratory oxygen flow rate should be kept at a minimum, as guided by the oxygen saturation, and nitrous oxide should be avoided. The surgeon must be made aware of the inspiratory oxygen concentration, and the anesthesiologist must keep the oxygen concentration as low as clinically possible. Medical air insufflations or suctioning can be used to reduce oxygen accumulation. When using an ignition source in an oxygen-rich environment, the ASA recommends reducing the oxygen flow as low as possible without creating hypoxia and waiting several minutes to allow the oxygen to dissipate.[48]

The management of a fire will require recognizing the early signs, stopping the procedure and ignition source, extinguishing the fire, and delivering care to the patient. It may even be necessary to evacuate the building. In any case, it is imperative that all these steps be reviewed regularly and drills performed.

CONCLUSIONS

Surgery and anesthesia performed within an office provide a viable alternative to care within a hospital or freestanding ASC. This unique venue offers a multitude of benefits to both the patient and the practitioner. However, like all new innovations, it is not without its own possible risks.

Safety concerns are legitimate. The relative lack of governmental oversight in many areas of the country shifts the responsibility of ensuring patient and location safety to the physicians and related health care workers. The ASA has long been a politically active advocate of patient safety within the hospital. They along with other medical societies, such as the ASPS, have continued to be outspoken advocates for safety within this new venue for providing surgical and anesthetic care. It

TABLE 26.1. Stratification of Risk and Treatment for the Development of Deep Vein Thrombosis

	PATIENT RISK FACTORS	TREATMENT
Low risk (one factor)	No risk factors Uncomplicated surgery Short duration of surgery	Comfortable position Knees flexed 5° Avoid constriction and external pressure
Moderate risk (two factors)	Any age, uncomplicated surgery, other risk factors Age 40–60 with no other risk factors Major surgery, age less than 40, no other risk factors Oral contraceptive use	Proper positioning Intermittent pneumatic compression of calf or ankle (before sedation and continued postoperatively) Frequent alterations of the operating room table
High risk (three factors)	Age greater than 60 with other risk factors and uncomplicated surgery Major surgery and older than 40 or additional risk factors	Treatment identical to moderate-risk patients Preoperative hematology consultation to consider pharmacologic intervention

would be recommended that any anesthesia providers or even surgeons/proceduralists planning to shift their medical practice to include this remote area review the recommendations and guidelines of these societies (available online at http://www.ASAHQ.org and http://www.ASPS.org). Additionally, because state and local regulations are in a constant state of flux, it is recommended that all practitioners regularly check local state medical boards for any new regulations or statutes.

As with health care delivered in a traditional hospital or freestanding ASC, patient safety must always be a priority. This entails ensuring that all safety mechanisms, often with areas of redundancy, are in place, before the first patient is anesthetized. As other chapters in this text have pointed out, any depth of sedation can be safely performed in many remote locations, including the private office. However, it is imperative that the operative and perioperative location is properly staffed, equipped, and stocked. Staffing must take into account not only the qualifications of the surgeon or proceduralist but also the training and qualifications of the anesthesia provider(s), nursing staff, and office staff.

REFERENCES

1. Cullen KA, Hall MJ, Golosinsky A. *Ambulatory Surgery in the United States, 2006*. Hyattsville, MD: National Center for Health Statistics; 2009. National Health Statistics Report, no 11. Revised.
2. Owings MF, Kozac LJ. Ambulatory and inpatient procedures in the United States 1996. *Vital Health Stat*. 1998;13:1–119.
3. White PF, Song D. New criteria for fast-tracking after outpatient anesthesia: a comparison with the modified Aldrete's scoring system. *Anesth Analges*. 1999;88(5):1069–1072.
4. Tang J, White PF, Wender RH, et al. Fast-track office-based anesthesia: a comparison of propofol versus desflurane with antiemetic prophylaxis in spontaneously breathing patients. *Anesth Analg*. 2001;92(1):95–99.
5. American Hospital Association. Chart 2.5: percent of outpatient surgeries by facility type, 1981–2005. Available at: http://www.aha.org/aha/trendwatch/chartbook/2007/07chapter2.ppt#265, 8 Published 2007. Accessed on June 5, 2009.
6. Byrd HS, Barton FE, Orenstein HH, et al. Safety and efficacy in an accredited outpatient plastic surgery facility: a review of 5316 consecutive cases. *Plast Reconstr Surg*. 2003;112(2):636–641.
7. American Society of Anesthesiologists. *Office-Based Anesthesia: Considerations for Anesthesiologists in Setting Up and Maintaining a Safe Office Anesthesia Environment*. 2nd ed. Park Ridge, IL: ASA; 2008.
8. Patient Safety Authority. Obstructive sleep apnea may block the path to a positive postoperative outcome [reprint]. *PA-PSRS Patient Safety Advisory*. 2007;4:1–8.
9. American Society of Anesthesiologists. Guidelines for office-based anesthesia. Available at: https://www.google.com/url?sa=t&rct=j&q=&esrc=s&source=web&cd=1&cad=rja&uact=8&ved=0ahUKEwjlycyEgazaAhVGT98KHXj4A3gQFggnMAA&url=https%3A%2F%2Fwww.asahq.org%2F~%2Fmedia%2Fsites%2Fasahq%2Ffiles%2Fpublic%2Fresources%2Fstandards-guidelines%2Fguidelines-for-office-based-anesthesia.pdf&usg=AOvVaw0_NLfoGkqC1aw2Yfe-API1, Oct 14, 2014. Accessed on April 8, 2018.
10. Shapiro FE, Punwani N, Rosenberg NM, Valedon A, Twersky R, Urman RD. Office-based anesthesia: safety and outcomes. *Anesth Analg*. 2014;119(2):276–285. doi:10.1213/ANE.0000000000000313.
11. Gaulton TG, Shapiro FE, Urman RD. Administrative issues to ensure safe anesthesia care in the office-based setting. *Curr Opin Anaesthesiol*. 2013;26(6):692–697. doi: 10.1097/ACO.0000000000000005.
12. Quattrone MS. Is the physician office the wild, west of health care? *J Ambul Care Manage*. 2000;23:64.
13. Jones, L. Death follows breast implant : medicine: a laguna beach mother just wanted to improve her bust line. She sank into a coma and died four days later. Los Angeles Times, March 22, 1990. Available at: https://www.google.com/url?sa=t&rct=j&q=&esrc=s&source=web&cd=8&cad=rja&uact=8&ved=0ahUKEwiYk5u2gazaAhWkdd8KHd7sBYAQFgh8MAc&url=http%3A%2F%2Farticles.latimes.com%2F1990-03-22%2Flocal%2Fme-1152_1_laguna-beach&usg=AOvVaw34s8mK7DrA5Y5gokZ7lg94, Accessed on April 8, 2018.
14. Vila H, Soto R, Cantor AB, Mackey D. Comparative outcomes analysis of procedures performed in physician offices and ambulatory surgery centers. *Arch Surg*. 2003;138:991–995.
15. Morello DC, Colon GA, Fredericks S, Iverson RE, Singer R. Patient safety in accredited office surgical facilities. *Plast Reconstr Surg*. 1997;99:1496–1499.
16. Keyes GR, Singer, Iverson RE, et al. Mortality in outpatient surgery. *Plast Reconstr Surg*. 2008;122:245–250.
17. Urman RD, Punwani N, Shapiro FE. Patient safety and office-based anesthesia. *Curr Opin Anaesthesiol*. 2012;25(6):648–653. doi:10.1097/ACO.0b013e3283593094.
18. Starling J, Thosani MK, Coldiron BM. Determining the safety of office-based surgery: what 10 years of florida data and 6 years of Alabama data reveal. *Dermatol Surg*. 2012;38:171–177.
19. Walsh MT, Kurrek MM, Desai M. Anesthesia outcomes in office based surgery. Paper presented at: American Society of Anesthesiologists Annual Meeting, A798; October 16–20, 2010; San Diego, CA.
20. Shapiro FE, Punwani N, Rosenberg NM, ct al. Office-based anesthesia: safety and outcomes. *Anesth Analg*. 20014;119(2);276–285.
21. American Society of Anesthesiologists. Outcome indicators for office-based and ambulatory surgery. Available at: https://www.google.com/url?sa=t&rct=j&q=&esrc=s&source=web&cd=1&cad=rja&uact=8&ved=0ahUKEwjamuH-gazaAhVwg-AKHVUdDYEQFggnMAA&url=http%3A%2F%2Fwww.asahq.org%2F~%2Fmedia%2FSites%2FASAHQ%2FFiles%2FPublic%2FResources%2Fstandards-guidelines%2Foutcome-indicators-for-office-based-and-ambulatory-surgery.pdf&usg=AOvVaw2GfJAIT0w-kXeekH5-AyGt. October 16, 2013, Accessed on April 8, 2018.

22. American Society of Anesthesiologists. Guidelines for determining anesthesia machine obsolescence. Available at: https://www.google.com/url?sa=t&rct=j&q=&esrc=s&source=web&cd=1&cad=rja&uact=8&ved=0ahUKEwjpyoWcgqzaAhXKct8KHT3lC3YQFggnMAA&url=https%3A%2F%2Fwww.asahq.org%2F~%2Fmedia%2Fsites%2Fasahq%2Ffiles%2Fpublic%2Fresources%2Fasa%2520committees%2Fasa%2520publications%2520anesthesia%2520machine%2520obsolescence%252020041.pdf%3Fla%3Den&usg=AOvVaw2Ox2SSEYQAZqYrgxt0rI-Z. June 22, 2004, Accessed on April 8, 2018.
23. American Society of Anesthesiologists. Standards for basic anesthetic monitoring, last amended 2005. Available at: https://www.google.com/url?sa=t&rct=j&q=&esrc=s&source=web&cd=1&cad=rja&uact=8&ved=0ahUKEwib08i5gqzaAhVSneAKHaS6AH4QFggnMAA&url=https%3A%2F%2Fwww.asahq.org%2F~%2Fmedia%2FSites%2FASAHQ%2FFiles%2FPublic%2FResources%2Fstandards-guidelines%2Fstandards-for-basic-anesthetic-monitoring.pdf&usg=AOvVaw0qgwg44MfdisQUoRF_wo79. Last affirmed October 28, 2015, Accessed on April 8, 2018.
24. American Society of Anesthesiologists. Practice guidelines for postanesthetic care. Available at: https://www.google.com/url?sa=t&rct=j&q=&esrc=s&source=web&cd=1&cad=rja&uact=8&ved=0ahUKEwjlz-LZgqzaAhUMSN8KHafjCXoQFggsMAA&url=http%3A%2F%2Fanesthesiology.pubs.asahq.org%2Farticle.aspx%3Farticleid%3D1918686&usg=AOvVaw3yXngKGju1JhjbBYXLSXj4. February 2013, Accessed April 8, 2018.
25. American Society of Anesthesiologists. Standards for postanesthesia care, last amended 2009. Available at: https://www.google.com/url?sa=t&rct=j&q=&esrc=s&source=web&cd=1&cad=rja&uact=8&ved=0ahUKEwjFwsODg6zaAhWIVt8KHWx7D38QFggnMAA&url=http%3A%2F%2Fwww.asahq.org%2F~%2Fmedia%2FSites%2FASAHQ%2FFiles%2FPublic%2FResources%2Fstandards-guidelines%2Fstandards-for-postanesthesia-care.pdf&usg=AOvVaw1VsKZek2FVPyqDTbheeyUL. October 15, 2014, Accessed on April 8, 2018.
26. Domino KB. Office-based anesthesia: lessons learned from the closed-claims project. *ASA Newsletter.* 2001;65:9.
27. Federation of State Medical Boards. Office-based surgery regulation overview by state. Available at: http://www.fsmb.org/pdf/GRPOL_Regulation_Office_Based_Surgery.pdf. Accessed on July 21, 2010.
28. American Society of Plastic Surgeons. Largest review of office-based plastic surgery confirms safety in accredited facilities. Available at: http://www.plasticsurgery.org/Media/Press_Releases/Largest_Review_of_Office-Based_Plastic_Surgery_Confirms_Safety_in_Accredited_Facilities.html. Published 2008. Accessed on July 21, 2010.
29. American Society of Plastic Surgeons. Information on procedural statistics. Available at: http://www.plasticsurgery.org.
30. Iverson RE, Lynch DJ, American Society of Plastic Surgeons Committee on Safety. Practice advisory on liposuction. *Plast Reconstr Surg.* 2004;113:1478.
31. Fodor PB, Watson JP. Wetting solutions in ultra-sound assisted lipoplasty: a review. *Clin Plast Surg.* 1999;26:289.
32. Klein JA. Tumescent technique for regional anesthesia permits lidocaine doses of 35 mg/kg. *J Dermatol Surg Oncol.* 1990;16:248.
33. Ostad A, Kageyama N, Moy RL. Tumescent anesthesia with lidocaine dose of 55 mg/kg is safe for liposuction. *Dermatol Surg.* 1996;22:921.
34. Grazer FM, deJong RH. Fatal outcome from liposuction: census survey of cosmetic surgeons. *Plast Reconstr Surg.* 2000;105:436.
35. Iverson R, ASPS Task Force on Patient Safety in Office-Based Surgery Facilities. Patient safety in office-based surgery facilities: I. Procedures in the office-based surgery setting. *Plast Reconstr Surg.* 2002;110:1337.
36. Iverson RE, Lynch DJ, ASPS Task Force on Patient Safety in Office-Based Surgery Facilities. Patient safety in office-based surgery facilities: II. Patient selection. *Plast Reconstr Surg.* 2002;110:1785.
37. Coldiron B, Shreve E, Balkrishnan SD. Patient injuries from surgical procedures performed in medical offices: three years of Florida data. *Dermatol Surg.* 2004;30:1435–1443.
38. Claymen MA, Seagle BM. Office surgery safety: the myths and truths behind the Florida moratorium—six years of Florida data. *Plast Reconstr Surg.* 2006;118:777–785.
39. Reinish JF, Russo RF, Bresnick SD. Deep vein thrombosis and pulmonary embolism following face lift: a study of incidence and prophylaxis. *Plast Surg Forum.* 1998;21:159.
40. Grazer FM, Goldwyn RM. Abdominoplasty assessed by survey, with emphasis on complications. *Plast Reconstr Surg.* 1977;59:513.
41. Samana CM, Albaladejo P, Benhamou D, et al. Venous thromboembolism prevention in surgery and obstetrics: clinical practice guidelines. *Eur J Anaesthesiol.* 2006;23(2):95–116.
42. Davison SP, Venturi ML, Attenger CE, et al. Prevention of venous thromboembolism in the plastic surgery patient. *Plast Reconstr Surg.* 2004;114:43e–51e.
43. Hill J, Treasure T. Reducing the risk of venous thromboembolism (deep vein thrombosis and pulmonary embolism) in patients having surgery: summary of NICE guidelines. *BMJ* 2007;334:1053–1054.
44. Sachdeva A, Dalton M, Amarigi SV, Lees TA. Elastic compression stockings for prevention of deep vein thrombosis. *Cochrane Database Syst Rev.* 2010;(3):CD001484.
45. Hirsh J, Raschke R. Heparin and low-molecular-weight heparin: the sevent ACCP conference on antithrombotic and thrombolytic therapy. *Chest.* 2004;126(3)(suppl):188S–203S.
46. Davison SP, Venturi ML, Attinger CE, Baker SB, Spear SL. Prevention of venous thromboembolism in the plastic surgery patient. *Plast Reconstr Surg.* 2004;114:43e.
47. Most D, Koslow J, Heller J. Thromboembolism in plastic surgery. *Plast Reconstr Surg.* 2005;115:20e–30e.
48. American Society of Anesthesiologists Task Force on Operating Room Fires. Practice advisory for the prevention and management of operating room fires. *Anesthesiology.* 2008;108:786–801.

27 | PEDIATRIC ANESTHESIA OUTSIDE OF THE OPERATING ROOM

MOHAMED MAHMOUD, MD, ROBERT S. HOLZMAN, MD, KEIRA P. MASON, MD

INTRODUCTION

Over the past several decades, recent advances in technological innovation have led to an increased demand for invasive and noninvasive pediatric procedures and imaging modalities. This clinical demand has resulted in tremendous growth in pediatric procedural sedation (PS) in in non–operating room anesthesia (NORA) locations.[1] Currently, anesthesiologists play a critical role in guiding the practice of pediatric sedation among all providers in these locations. Providing anesthesia in NORA locations challenges us to gain a familiarity with the procedures, tailor an anesthesia plan to the procedure and location, as well as to plan for the management of life-threatening situations. Anesthesia providers are the final arbiter of whether the child is optimized for the procedure or not in a NORA location with potentially limited access to backup help. This chapter reviews the different NORA locations and discusses the unique aspects of patient management associated with each area. Typical locations are outlined in Table 27.1.

TABLE 27.1. Typical Off-Site Anesthetizing Locations

Gastroenterology suite
Epilepsy service
Radiology suite
Computed tomography
Magnetic resonance imaging
Nuclear medicine
Interventional radiology
Radiation oncology
Dental and oral surgery
Emergency Department
Cardiac catheterization laboratory

A TOUR OF THE DIFFERENT OFF-SITE LOCATIONS AND PROCEDURES

THE GASTROENTEROLOGY SUITE: ENDOSCOPIC PROCEDURES

Gastrointestinal (GI) endoscopy has become an essential modality for evaluation and treatment of GI diseases, and as such it constitutes the bulk of procedures performed by a pediatric gastroenterologist.[2] To date, there has been no validated protocol of sedation and consequent airway management standardized to the endoscopic procedure for the pediatric population.[3]Children may tolerate this procedure with various levels of sedation (moderate or deep), monitored anesthetic care (MAC), or general anesthesia (GA).[4] Aside from GA, other intravenous agents have been explored as an alternative to an inhalational anesthetic. Propofol is the most commonly used intravenous agent employed for adult endoscopies. It is considered by the American Society for Gastrointestinal Endoscopy (ASGE) to be an acceptable sedative for gastroenterologist administration. A major setback to the use of propofol for sedation by nonanesthesiologists is a result of the directive released by the American Society of Anesthesiologists (ASA) and the Royal College of Anesthetists (Great Britain) that "propofol must only be used by healthcare provider with specialized training in airway management."[5–10] Despite this concern, propofol has been the backbone of sedation in GI endoscopy, and gastroenterologists have demonstrated that they also are able to safely administer sedation.[11–18]

Regardless of who administers propofol, its success for providing acceptable conditions for lower endoscopy with an unsecured airway has been described.[19]Alternative agents, which include opioids, benzodiazepines, and more recently, dexmedetomidine (DEX), have been described as an acceptable alternative to propofol.[6,19] Increased awareness of the complications associated with sedation during GI endoscopy in children, and involving the anesthesiologists in caring for these children, may be optimal for safety. Upper endoscopies are prone to respiratory complications, which include apnea, laryngospasm, bronchospasm, and airway obstruction. These complications may persuade some anesthesiologists to secure the airway with an endotracheal tube (ETT). Particular consideration should be given to smaller children and infants who undergo these esophagogastroduodenoscopies. Insufflation of air during the upper endoscopy can lead to distension of the stomach, small intestine, and sometimes even large intestine. Abdominal distension may impair diaphragmatic excursion and lead to hypoventilation, hypercarbia, and possibly oxygen desaturation. Recognizing these risks, some experts suggested that infants less than 6 months of age should undergo GA with endotracheal intubation.[15,18]

There is no consensus on which airway technique can offer the best balance of minimizing respiratory complications and maximizing efficiency during esophagogastroduodenoscopy (EGD). Insufflation of sevoflurane through a nasopharyngeal airway has been associated with an increase in airway complications without benefitting efficiency.[20] Maintenance of anesthesia with propofol using the native airway and without administration of adjuncts in children undergoing EGD was associated with a significantly higher incidence of respiratory complications compared to techniques including endotracheal intubation, without any improvement in efficiency.[21] On the other hand, other studies have shown that using propofol without airway intervention during EGD is feasible without increasing the risk of respiratory complications.[22] A recent study examined the safety and efficacy of a laryngeal mask airway (LMA), compared with an ETT, for 84 ASA patients, status 1 to 3, undergoing elective EGD; they concluded that the LMA appears to be an acceptable and safe alternative for otherwise-healthy children undergoing routine EGD.[23]

THE EPILEPSY SERVICE: ELECTROENCEPHALOGRAMS

Performing electroencephalograms (EEGs) in infants and children can be challenging. These children often present with intractable seizures, aberrant behavior, and sleep disturbances. Children affected are often neurologically and developmentally challenged and pose a challenge. Even the process of applying the electrodes to the scalp can be difficult, and not infrequently patient movement makes these studies difficult to interpret. Common anesthetic agents (both inhalational and intravenous) that are used for GA are known to suppress brain electrical activity by stimulating the γ-aminobutyric acid A (GABA-A) receptors in the cerebral cortex. In general, GA, opioids, and propofol disrupt the EEG.[24,25] Chloral hydrate has been the mainstay agent administered to children who require sedation for EEG.[26] In clinical use for almost a century, chloral hydrate is generally safe and effective but with a disadvantage of a long half-life of up to 24 hours.

Dexmedetomidine (Precedex®, Hospira, Lake Forest, IL; and Dexdor, Orion Corp., Espoo, Finland) is a 2-adrenoceptor agonist that has been shown to offer a beneficial pharmacological profile, with sedation that parallels natural sleep, sympatholysis, and anesthetic-sparing effect without relevant respiratory depression. Currently, it is approved by the Food and Drug Administration (FDA) for the provision of sedation for adult patients via bolus and continuous infusion for up to 24 hours on intubated adults as well as for adult PS in areas outside the intensive care unit (ICU) and operating room settings. To date, there are no FDA-approved indications for its use in the pediatric population.[27,28] DEX acts on subcortical areas of the brain and does not bind to the GABA receptors. It preserves epileptiform activity in children with seizure disorders, facilitating localization and identification of seizure foci.[29,30] In a recent prospective study, the ECG was monitored during DEX infusion in 34 adult patients undergoing anterior temporal lobe resection with amygdalo-hippocampectomy for drug-resistant mesial temporal lobe epilepsy. The authors concluded that DEX is useful during intraoperative electrocorticogram recording in epilepsy surgery as it enhances or does not alter the spike rate in most of the cases, without any major adverse effects.[31]

Magnetoencephalography (MEG) is increasingly used in the presurgical evaluation of epileptic children with a seizure focus. Many pediatric patients require sedation or anesthesia to tolerate these exams. Anesthetic agents, such as propofol or inhalational volatile agents, may produce adverse effects on interictal activity. In our experience, a DEX-based technique presents a suitable alternative to a propofol-based technique for anesthesia/sedation of pediatric patients with seizure disorders presenting for MEG scanning.[32]

DEPARTMENT OF RADIOLOGY

COMPUTED TOMOGRAPHIC SCAN

Perhaps the most important cause of a suboptimal computed tomographic (CT) study is the lack of understanding of the anesthetic requirement for the different CT image studies. Understanding the goal of each imaging study allows the anesthesiologist to choose the safest and most effective regimen to allow a meaningful study. As an example, the goal of dynamic airway imaging in patients is to evaluate airway changes during spontaneous respiration. Utilizing an inhalational agent such as sevoflurane or intravenous propofol is safe and has the advantage of fast induction and recovery times. When a CT scan is performed to evaluate lung parenchymal detail (a "high-resolution" CT), motion-free images at full inspiration and usually at expiration are required.

The majority of actual scanning sequences are short and can range from 10 to 80 seconds. With distraction techniques and scheduling these examinations around naptime, many children are able to complete a CT scan without adjuvant sedation or anesthesia. When an anesthesia is required, it is commonly for those children who are medically compromised, complicated, or fragile. CT scans for evaluation of craniofacial anomalies or choanal atresia may be particularly challenging because of the head manipulation that is required: extreme head extension, sometimes with the head suspended below the neck. This positioning enables better visualization of the sinuses, ears, inner auditory canal, and temporomandibular bones.

Three-dimensional airway and cardiac studies have evolved and pose unique anesthetic requirements. The airway studies require breath holding during image acquisition on both inspiration and expiration to visualize potential areas of airway collapse.[33] To minimize motion artifact and ensure immobility on inspiratory pause and full expiration, anesthesiologists usually intubate these children for the study. Cardiac studies pose an added challenge because the anesthesiologist is asked to administer adenosine during the study to briefly pause heart function so that image quality is maximized.[34]

Neck imaging with CT or magnetic resonance imaging (MRI) may be requested to evaluate neck stability in those patients with Down syndrome and possible atlantoaxial instability. In these patients with Down syndrome, the reported risk of subluxation is between 12% and 32%.[35] Cervical spine films should not be referred to as an indication of neck stability or to indicate whether there is a risk for dislocation.[36] Rather, the clinical exam and history are the best determinants to distinguish those necks that are stable from those that are at risk. Those children who exhibit neurological signs or symptoms such as abnormal gait, increased clumsiness, fatigue with ambulation, or a new preference for sitting games are at risk. In these patients, anesthetic management should be guided only after direct consultation and evaluation by orthopedics or neurosurgery.

Angiography and venography using CT imaging are part of an evolving and useful imaging technique. These patients require motionless conditions and often breath holding to minimize motion artifact and are administered contrast to map the vasculature. The timing of the image acquisition is critical, and imaging must be obtained during contrast injection. Any patient movement during this time will render the imaging study uninterpretable. In these cases, reinjection of contrast for image reacquisition is not possible because the children will have already received their maximum allowable amount of iodine contrast for that 24-hour period.

In infants and children, CT studies of the abdomen and pelvis may require the administration of oral contrast. The Gastrograffin® contrast is required to be present in the areas for which imaging is requested, thus rendering these children with contrast in their upper GI system at the time of an anesthetic induction. Diluted to a concentration of 1.5%, many anesthesiologists and radiologists consider Gastrograffin to be a clear liquid. The volume that is administered orally can vary. Newborns less than 1 month of age receive 60 to 90 mL, infants between 1 month and 1 year of age may receive up to 240 mL, and children between the ages of 1 and 5 years receive between 240 and 360 mL. Some institutions administer the contrast on a weight basis to reduce the probability of patients with large gastric fluid volume. Gastrografin typically requires no more than a 2-hour window after ingestion until actual CT imaging. The scan must be completed while the Gastrografin is still in the GI tract. There are no published data citing an increased aspiration risk in this population. Rather, a large review of children who received oral contrast prior to receiving pentobarbital or chloral hydrate sedation indicated that there was no significant risk of aspiration.[31] Full-strength (3%) Gastrografin is hyperosmolar and hypertonic and should be diluted to an isomolar and isotonic 1.5% concentration at neutral pH prior to oral or nasogastric tube administration. There is one case report of 1.5% Gastrografin aspiration in a child with no adverse sequelae; therefore, the risk of using a 1.5% concentration of neutral of Gastrografin seems low.[37,38]

It is important to note that most of the patients who present for abdominal CT and need enteric contrast material have coexisting diseases that might affect GI mobility. The ideal fasting intervals for these patients are still unknown. The management of children who require oral contrast for a tomographic scan is controversial. Our institutional protocol begins contrast administration 2 hours and ends 1 hour prior to PS. The challenge lies in balancing technical factors governing the image quality of the study with safety concerns related to sedating a child with a potentially full stomach for an elective CT. There is considerable variation in sedation/anesthesia practices and in airway management techniques. Currently, there is no consensus among institutions. Different anesthetic plans include rapid sequence induction of GA with tracheal intubation, deep sedation without airway protection, and oral contrast given 2 hours before the study or administered through an oral gastric tube after placement of an ETT.[39,40]

Computed tomographic imaging of the chest is needed when more routine imaging modalities, such as the standard chest radiograph, are insufficient for either the diagnosis or the management of children with respiratory disease. An important reason for a poor-quality CT chest study is the lack of appreciation of how much lung atelectasis can be associated with GA in the absence of a standardized anesthesia, lung recruitment, and controlled-ventilation technique. Atelectasis in the dependent regions of lungs appears within 5 minutes of induction of anesthesia.[41] Opening collapsed lungs can be done by applying sufficient levels of peak inspiratory pressure and maintaining alveoli open by using sufficient levels of positive end-expiratory pressure.[42] This recruitment maneuver has been shown to improve arterial oxygenation and lung compliance.[43]

MAGNETIC RESONANCE IMAGING

Magnetic resonance imaging is employed for the evaluation of neoplasms, trauma, skeletal abnormalities, vascular anatomy,[44] developmental delay, behavioral disorders, seizures, failure to thrive, apnea/cyanosis, hypotonia, and mitochondrial/metabolic disorders. Magnetic resonance angiography (MRA) and magnetic resonance venography (MRV) are especially helpful for evaluating vascular flow, generally do not require the administration of intravenous contrast, and can sometimes replace invasive catheterization studies for follow-up or initial evaluations of vascular malformations, interventional treatment, or radiotherapy.[45]

Gadolinium diethylenetriaminepentaacetic acid (DTPA) is a low osmolar ionic contrast medium used for MRI; it has slower clearance in neonates and young infants than adults, yielding longer windows for imaging.[46] Free gadolinium is quite toxic and is therefore chelated to another structure that restricts the ion and decreases its toxicity. Transient elevations in serum bilirubin (3%–4% of patients) have been reported, and a transient elevation in iron for Magnevist and Omniscan (15%–30% of patients) tends to reverse spontaneously within 24–48 hours.[47] Anaphylactoid reactions occur on the order of 1:100,000 to 1:500,000 and are more rare (<1:100,000 doses) in children.

Functional MRI (fMRI) is an evolving technology that measures the hemodynamic or even metabolic response related to neural activity. Currently, the clinical use of fMRI in children is primarily presurgical. The two major clinical scenarios are (1) presurgical evaluation of language and memory function prior to surgery for intractable epilepsy and (2) preoperative assessment of cortex in patients with brain lesions (tumors, cavernous malformations).[48] Some fMRI studies require cognitive facility and interaction with a responsive patient.[49] All-digital audiovisual stimulation technology (Resonance Technology, Inc., Los Angeles, CA) employs MRI-safe goggles that are worn by the child and useful for fMRI. Even with these audiovisual stimulating goggles, there may be the added challenge if a 3-tesla magnet is used rather than a 1.5 tesla: the noise of the 3 tesla can interfere with the acoustic stimulation generated for purposes of obtaining the fMRI.[50,51] It is recommended that earplugs or MRI-compatible headphones be offered to all pediatric patients. They are required for all patients imaged in the 3-tesla magnet. Functional MRI studies are challenging in children who are unable to respond appropriately because of age or cognitive compromise. The advent and introduction of the MRI-safe video goggles, introduced in 1993, have revolutionized our ability to perform fMRI studies as well as provide distraction to the child and avoid sedation in some.

Even motivated children and adolescents may suffer from claustrophobia and have difficulty cooperating when in the confined bore of the magnet. In adults, anxiety reactions can occur in 4% to 30%.[52,53] The MRI-safe video goggles are equipped with headphones and enable patients to watch favorite videos or listen to music while in the MRI scanner. These goggles can offer children an alternative to sedation or anesthesia and are particularly useful in those patients between the ages of 5 and 7 years who are motivated but require distraction. Alternatively, some patients, although motivated, may not be able to complete a MRI scan without adjuvant sedation or anesthesia. For example, patients with extreme skeletal abnormalities, such as advanced scoliosis or flexion contractures, although motivated, may be unable to lie motionless or supine on the solid, uncushioned MRI table for the extended duration of a spine MRI. These patients may require GA for positioning and comfort or may need adjunctive pain medication.

With newer sedatives, it is possible that immobility in some children may be achieved without a general anesthetic. Propofol may be used to maintain spontaneous ventilation without airway intervention. The risk of respiratory complications, albeit small, must be anticipated with propofol. DEX, although not FDA approved for usage in children, presents another alternative. It has been successfully used as a sole sedative agent for MRI.[1,54] Those children who are not appropriate for sedation will require GA. Over the past decade, the ability to provide anesthesia in the MRI suite has evolved, paralleling the development of MRI-compatible and safe anesthesia machines, equipment, and monitors. Historically, anesthetic management of children in the MRI suite has been highly dependent and somewhat limited by the availability of MRI-compatible monitors and anesthesia gas machines.[55–57]

In 2007, the American College of Radiology established guidelines to minimize the risk of MRI-related mishaps, but it did not address the anesthesiologist's needs.[58] These guidelines were written in response to fatalities that had occurred when loose, nonferrous oxygen cylinders became projectiles when brought inadvertently into the MRI suite.[59] In 2008, the ASA assembled a task force composed of anesthesiologists and a radiologist with MRI expertise to create the "Practice Advisory on Anesthetic Care for Magnetic Resonance Imaging."[60] This document, updated in 2014, established important recommendations for safe practice as well as consistency of anesthesia care in the MRI environment.[61] The purpose of this advisory was to promote safety in the magnetic resonance (MR) and postanesthetic care environment, avoid MR-associated mishaps, optimize patient care and decrease adverse events associated with MR anesthesia, identify and discuss physiologic monitors and anesthesia equipment available in the MR suite, and identify health-related concerns with exposure to the MR environment. Important to this advisory was the need for MRI-safe/conditional physiological monitors that adhere to ASA standards as well as the preference for MR-safe/conditional anesthesia machines. The practice of using non–MRI-safe anesthesia machines outside of the MRI suite (zone III) with elongated ventilator tubing threaded through a waveguide in the scanner wall was cited as posing an added risk of adverse events as compared to the use of the MRI-safe anesthesia machines within the suite.

Unique risks occur in MRI. Magnetic field strength creates a risk environment where mishaps with ferromagnetic objects can potentially happen with disastrous consequences. Clipboards, pens, watches, scissors, clamps, credit cards, eyeglasses, paper clips, and even stethoscopes are just some of the objects that can become projectiles.[55–57] During emergency situations, quenching of the magnet could be necessary to remove a ferromagnetic object. The magnet is made of coils of superconducting wire that requires constant cooling by helium. During quenching, there is significant risk of hypoxic mixtures due to escape of helium and risk of hearing impairment due to the extremely noisy levels. The use of MRI-compatible infusion pumps is highly recommended. Non–MRI-compatible pumps must remain distant from the MRI magnetic field or be mounted outside the MRI scanner and fitted with appropriately long extension tubing. Ferromagnetic tracheostomies in children must be changed to nonferromagnetic tracheostomies.

Physiologic monitoring can also be distorted in the MR suite, regardless of modifications to the equipment. Conventional ECG monitoring, similar to that used in the operating room, may not be used in the MR suite. The ECG leads would cause patient burns. Rather, the traditional ECG cables must be replaced with fiber-optic ECG to minimize the risk of burns. Even with fiber-optic cables, it is important to recognize that the connections between the ECG pads and the telemetry box are still hardwired, and careful attention must be paid to prevent frays, overlap, exposed wires, and knots in the cables.[62] To prevent patient injury, no exposed wires or conductors should touch the patient's skin. Similar to the ECG leads, pulse oximeters are also fiber optic. Particularly when inpatients are transported to the MRI suite, the anesthesiologist must uncover the patient and do a thorough search for conventional leads, probes, or adhesives (ECG, pulse oximeter probes), which could result in second-and third-degree burns if not removed.[62,63]

When MRI-safe/conditional anesthesia machines are available in the MRI suite, anesthesiologists may elect to perform the anesthetic induction and subsequent management in the MRI suite itself. As in the operating room, some anesthesiologists may offer parent-present inductions in these situations. However, the biologic effect of MRI should be considered when offering parent-present induction, although to date there are no conclusive reports implicating chromosomal aberrations in humans to the MR environment. Amphibians exposed to a high-tesla magnet field have been shown to be free of any defects in embryologic development.[64] Most hospital MRI machines are 1.5 tesla. Despite these studies, many institutions still prohibit pregnant patients or family members from accompanying the child into the MRI suite. Unless fetal imaging is required or the MRI is necessary for emergent medical care, MRI during the first and second trimesters is discouraged by the American College of Radiology.[34]

A 1.5-tesla MRI reaches on average noise levels of 95 dB. Exposure to this level of noise has not been considered hazardous if it is limited to less than 2 hours per day.[65] There are case reports, however, of both temporary and permanent hearing loss after an MRI scan.[66,67] Therefore, patients and relatives who stay in the MRI room must wear earplugs to protect against the high-intensity sound.

Neonates and infants are at risk of hypothermia in the MRI due to continuous cooling of the room, which is necessary to guarantee the function of the magnet and the noncompatibility of air-forced warming systems in the MRI. Therefore, use of warm blankets in the neonates is imperative.

Finally, MRI technology continues to evolve, introducing new scanning methods that continue to change diagnostic imaging standards of practice. Anesthesia providers need to adapt to these technological advances and have in-depth understanding of each new imaging study. MRI sleep studies and MR enterography are examples of these relatively new imaging studies.

Magnet resonance enterography, a nonradiation method of examining the bowel, has recently emerged as a highly effective method of assessing inflammatory bowel disease (including Crohn disease and ulcerative colitis) in children. This technique requires oral ingestion of contrast. Appropriate timing of the study after oral contrast agent administration is crucial in order to opacify the bowel and optimize the study image. We administer enteric contrast through an oral gastric tube after placement of an ETT and extubate these patients awake after suctioning the stomach.[68]

Magnetic resonance imaging cine sleep studies have become a useful tool to identify the anatomic and dynamic causes of persistent obstructive sleep apnea (OSA) in children. It provides evaluation of the airway during sleep without radiation exposure. The ideal sleep MRI allows assessment of the native airway free of artificial airway adjuncts. Maintaining spontaneous ventilation and avoiding upper airway collapsibility-associated significant oxygen desaturation in patients with OSA under anesthesia can be a challenge. DEX possesses sedative properties that more closely parallel natural sleep. The ability to maintain spontaneous ventilation and upper airway tone makes DEX an attractive choice for dynamic airway evaluation during imaging of children with OSA.[69–71]

NUCLEAR MEDICINE

Single-photon emission computed tomographic (SPECT) scans and positron emission tomographic (PET) scans are commonly utilized nuclear medicine imaging studies in children. SPECT scans produce three-dimensional brain images and involve the use of radiolabeled technetium-99 (half-life, 6 hours).[72] The technetium radionuclide is trapped intracellularly, in proportion to regional blood flow. When injected immediately following a seizure, the technetium can identify areas of increased blood flow, potentially identifying areas of recent seizure activity. Ideally, the imaging should be performed within 1–6 hours of the seizure. PET scans use positron emission tomography and radionuclide tracers of metabolic activity, such as oxygen or glucose metabolism.[73,74] Unlike SPECT scans, PET scans should be performed during the seizure itself. Because of the short half-life of the glucose tracer (110 minutes), the scan is best completed during the seizure or within 1 hour thereafter. These children do not commonly require GA, particularly because many are postictal and naturally sedated in this state. However, those who are unable to undergo the imaging alone can frequently receive moderate-to-deep sedation to induce motionless conditions. These children may be resistant to some anesthetics and barbiturates, particularly because they may already be on a multitude of antiepileptic medications.

Currently, there is no consensus on the best protocol for the sedation of children presenting for these studies. The choice of drugs and route of administration depend on the patient's age and medical history. In 2003, the Society of Nuclear Medicine updated its 1997 "Procedure Guideline for Pediatric Sedation in Nuclear Medicine." The guideline cites the rectal, oral, nasal, and parenteral routes for administration of chloral hydrate, pentobarbital, meperidine, fentanyl, valium, midazolam, chlorpromazine, promethazine, and ketamine.[75] DEX[76] or propofol may offer reasonable intravenous sedation, MAC, or intravenous anesthesia for these children.

RADIATION ONCOLOGY

Pediatric radiation oncologists use ionizing photons to destroy lymphomas, acute leukemias, Wilm tumor, retinoblastomas, and tumors of the central nervous system. Repeat sessions are typical, requiring reliable motionlessness to precisely aim the beam at malignant cells while sparing healthy cells. Radiation oncology requires anesthesia involvement for procedures ranging from daily radiology therapy to stereotactic radiosurgery. Radiation therapy—whether it occurs once, daily, or as a fractionated or hyperfractionated (multiple sessions per day) session—is challenging for the anesthesiologist. The procedures, albeit brief, require absolute immobility. The anesthesiologist and all other personnel remain outside the suite during the therapy. Remote video monitoring along with remote monitoring of physiological vital signs are essential. Most of these patients present with a central line for easy access. A small core group of anesthesiologists is appreciated by family and patients, enabling the child to develop a nonthreatening, consistent, positive relationship with the anesthesiologist.

Stereotactic radiosurgery (gamma knife) is a major advance in the treatment of selected intracranial arteriovenous malformations (AVMs) and tumors in children and usually requires coordination between the departments of radiology, radiation therapy, neurosurgery, and anesthesiology.[77] Typically, the stereotactic procedure begins in either CT or MRI, during which a stereotactic head frame is applied. Although most adults tolerate this with local anesthesia or sedation, pediatric patients (including most adolescents) typically require a general anesthetic.

Following the MRI or CT scan, these images are reviewed and calculations for dose and the three-dimensional coordinates for the focused single large-fraction radiation beam may take several hours. During this time, the younger patient usually remains intubated and sedated to avoid untoward airway incidents while the heavy, cumbersome head frame is still in place. The most common perioperative problems for this procedure are nausea and vomiting, probably due to radiation sensitivity of the chemoreceptor trigger zone. The actual radiosurgery occurs in the radiosurgery suite, following which the patient is typically extubated after removal of the head frame.[77]

Total body irradiation (TBI) is generally performed twice a day over a 6-week period. As these patients progress with their TBI treatment, vomiting, respiratory illness, poor nutrition, and hypovolemia are all possible. Although anesthesiologists are wary of the risks of aspiration, both sedation and general endotracheal anesthesia have been found to be equally safe.[78,79] Anesthesiologists should be reluctant and resistant to cancel a child's TBI session, as consistent repeat treatment is necessary for a favorable chance of positive outcome.

INTERVENTIONAL RADIOLOGY

Over the past two decades, recent advances in interventional radiology (IR) procedures have led to an increased demand for GA and PS of infants and children.[1,80] Anesthesia and sedation are often needed for pediatric image-guided diagnostic and therapeutic procedures in order to provide anxiolysis, analgesia, amnesia, sedation, and immobility.[81] Anesthesia providers should be familiar with the nature and technical demands of each procedure, along with the challenges and associated risks in IR. The majority of interventional procedures are nonvascular and include biopsies, insertion or repositioning of drainage catheters, and insertion of catheters for central intravenous access. Airway management is dictated by the imaging needs: endotracheal intubation when the radiologist requires controlled ventilation, breath holding during angiography sequences, and hypercarbia to promote vasodilation. Regional anesthesia, rarely administered outside the pediatric operating room, nevertheless remains a valid choice in some circumstances. Intercostal nerve blocks may be very useful for lung or rib biopsies, chest tubes, biliary or subphrenic drainage procedures, and insertion of biliary stents.

VASCULAR INTERVENTIONS

The vascular interventions can range from straightforward angiography to complex procedures. Embolization and sclerotherapy are important and often complex interventional vascular procedures used in the management of vascular malformations, aneurysms, fistulas, and hemorrhage and to accomplish renal ablation. Percutaneous transluminal angioplasty and fibrinolytic therapy are gaining popularity even for small babies. Vascular malformations are congenital aberrant connections between vessel, lymphatic, arterial, or venous connections. Vascular malformations may be high-flow or low-flow lesions. Particularly with large lesions, high-output cardiac failure and congestive heart failure with the potential for pulmonary edema should be anticipated. Stainless steel coils, absorbable gelatin pledgets and powder, polyvinyl alcohol foam, glues, thread, and ethanol may be used for sclerotherapy or embolization.

Absolute ethanol is unique and has special safety considerations of which the anesthesiologist should be aware. Ethanol can elicit denaturation of blood proteins and may produce a coagulum of blood with endothelial necrosis along with a postprocedure coagulopathy[82] marked by positive d-dimers, elevated prothrombin time, and decreased platelets.[83] The use of ethanol for sclerosis or embolization can elicit a coagulation disturbance that resembles disseminated intravascular coagulation (DIC). Ethanol also denatures blood proteins and can result in hematuria, for which generous fluid replacement can avoid potential renal failure. During procedures that involve lower extremity lesions and tourniquets, hemoglobinuria should be anticipated as soon as the tourniquet is released. Generous hydration and furosemide (0.5 to 1.0 mg/kg) facilitate the resolution of gross hematuria. At our institution, in the event of persistent hemoglobinuria, in the recovery room, the radiologists request that sodium bicarbonate (75 mEq/L in 5% dextrose and water) be administered at two times the maintenance rate to alkalinize the urine and minimize precipitation of hemoglobin in the renal tubules.[84]

Administration of ethanol has the potential for cardiovascular collapse. Most reported cases of cardiovascular collapse involved lower extremity malformations.[85]

Ethanol can produce a state of intoxication. The ethanol used for embolization and sclerotherapy is 95% to 98% pure. Patients who receive more than 0.75 mL/kg can be clinically intoxicated and display extremes of behavior (Figure 27.1).[83] Hypothermia is a risk in IR because these suites are kept cool to maintain the equipment. Heating lamps and forced-air heaters may be used when safe and appropriate.

Anesthesia providers require in-depth understanding of the physiology of the cerebral lesions to be treated, the requirements for successful treatment, and the potential effects of the proposed treatment. Cerebral angiograms, although often short and straightforward, typically require endotracheal intubation in the pediatric population to provide hypercarbia and breath-holding conditions. Anesthesia providers must pay attention during induction of anesthesia to avoid hypotension, which can put patients with a vasculopathy such as Moyamoya at risk of cerebral hypoperfusion.[86] On the other hand, acute hypertension should also be avoided due to potential catastrophic bleeding in an unstable aneurysm or AVM. An arterial line for this short procedure is generally not required. Normocapnia is desirable in the vast majority of cases, and any proposed acute

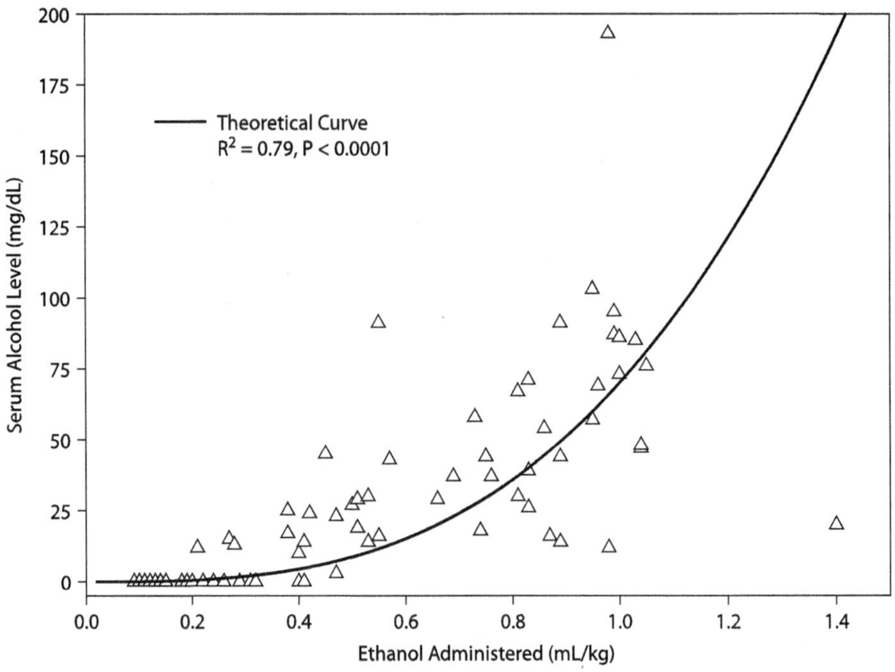

Figure 27.1 Graph shows the positive relationship between serum ethanol level and amount of ethanol administered in all 71 patients. Solid line indicates the theoretic curve based on the nonlinear exponential power model y =70x³, where x is the amount of ethanol administered, and y is the predicted serum ethanol level. Triangles represent empirical values. Theoretic curve demonstrates the most accurate fit compared with all other linear and nonlinear models tested.

hypocapnia should be discussed with the proceduralist. While the risk of significant bleeding is extremely rare, adequate intravenous access should be obtained immediately after anesthesia induction. Orogastric and nasogastric tubes, esophageal stethoscopes, and esophageal temperature probes should be avoided for cerebral angiography because they create artifacts on the angiographic images. Lying flat for several hours after the femoral arterial sheath is removed can be a challenge for a child. Noninterventional techniques that can distract an older or more cooperative child can be helpful; medications have a role for younger or less-cooperative children. Deep extubation when feasible and a period of quiet sleep in the recovery area with opioids or α_2-agonists as adjuncts can be helpful in this scenario.[87]

The vein of Galen aneurysmal malformation (VGAM) is a congenital anomaly of intracranial circulation that constitutes 1% of all intracranial vascular malformations.[88] Cardiac failure occurs as the large flow volume of the VGAM shunt is unloaded into the right atrium and pulmonary circulation, with pulmonary vasoconstriction and pulmonary hypertension resulting in right ventricle failure. Early identification and staged embolization of both the feeding arteries and draining veins can result in reduction of blood flow and a greater survival rate in these patients.[89] Anesthetic management of these patients poses multiple challenges to the anesthesiologist in view of its complex pathophysiology and must be tailored to address heart failure and pulmonary hypertension.[90]

Angiographic imaging of the abdomen or pelvis may be enhanced with glucagon (0.25–1 mg IV), which carries the risks of hyperglycemia, vomiting (particularly when given rapidly), gastric hypotonia with postprocedure vomiting, anaphylaxis with rapid administration, and physiologic signs (tachycardia and hypertension) that mimic pheochromocytoma.[91–93] Antiemetics may be considered prophylactically or as a treatment in the recovery room.

BIOPSIES

Pediatric percutaneous biopsy image-guided procedures include soft tissue and bone biopsy, organ (renal and hepatic) biopsy, and intra-articular steroid injections. Because of the need for patient immobility and the potential risk of morbidity with patient movement during the procedure, GA rather than deep sedation is usually recommended. Nursing-administered ketamine sedation, however, has been successfully used for solid-organ biopsy without significant morbidity.[94]

Ultrasound-guided biopsies of anterior mediastinal masses may be used to diagnose and guide management. These procedures pose serious challenges for the anesthesiologist because of the absolute necessity of ensuring minimal smooth muscle relaxation and preventing airway collapse. Furthermore, positive pressure ventilation may be difficult or impossible and may also pose fatal cardiopulmonary events and dramatic respiratory and cardiovascular complications, including progressive airway obstruction, loss of lung volume, pulmonary artery or cardiac compression, and superior vena caval (SVC) obstruction.[95] These procedures should be approached with caution, with multidisciplinary involvement, the least-invasive diagnostic techniques, careful preoperative evaluation, and avoidance of GA for diagnostic procedures. Maintenance of spontaneous breathing in these procedures is recommended because the initiation of positive pressure ventilation can compromise blood flow in the pulmonary vessels, which are already narrowed by the tumor mass. In the event of ventilatory difficulties or cardiac compromise, turning the patient prone or lateral may alleviate the symptoms. In preparation for these procedures, access to an otolaryngologist with rigid bronchoscope, and, in some cases, ability to initiate cardiopulmonary bypass should be immediately available. DEX in combination with ketamine may be a successful combination in this challenging scenario, with relatively fast onset and amnesia, sedation, analgesia, and hemodynamic stability.[96,97]

PROCEDURES THAT REQUIRE PATIENT COOPERATION

The carotid occlusion test is primarily used to test the adequacy of the cerebrovascular collateral circulation before electing to occlude the carotid artery; the test shows whether the patient can tolerate temporary or permanent occlusion. During such a test, the patient has to be awake and alert so neurological examinations can be conducted as the carotid artery is occluded with a balloon catheter deployed from a transfemoral arterial access site. It is necessary to provide an adequate level of sedation during groin access and carotid catheterization and ensure that the patient is alert and cooperative once the balloon is inflated, so neurological examinations can be conducted.

Diskography is a diagnostic modality used to determine whether the intervertebral disk is the cause of pain. It allows clinicians to determine whether diskogenic pain is the source of the patient's back pain and to identify the levels related to the pain.[98,99] The patients need to cooperate when asked the questions during the procedure. Our experience with DEX as a sole sedative agent enabled us to effectively sedate four patients with stable hemodynamics and no adverse outcomes.[100]

Wada testing is performed to identify areas of cortical language and memory representation and may provide important information for surgical planning in pediatric patients with medically refractory epilepsy. The test requires that the patient be "awake" to respond when a barbiturate (usually sodium amobarbital) is introduced into one of the internal carotid arteries via a cannula or intra-arterial catheter from the femoral artery. The barbiturate, injected one hemisphere at a time, is designed to "sedate" one hemisphere so that the other hemisphere may remain "active" and responsive to tests of memory and language. The patient must be able to engage in and respond to tests designed to evaluate language and memory function in the areas that remain unaffected by the barbiturate. The angiographic portion of this procedure may be difficult to perform in children without sedation or anesthesia, the aftereffects of which may confound the results of neuropsychological testing. Carefully administered titration of opioids is usually a preferred technique for maintaining sedation while sparing cortical function. Propofol is also an acceptable anesthetic choice for this test due to a rapid return to baseline neuropsychological function after discontinuing the infusion.[101]

Popliteal artery entrapment syndrome is a rare limb-threatening disease seen predominantly in young athletes. Clinical examination and laboratory data may not helpful for diagnosis. Diagnostic angiography can be used to demonstrate the focal narrowing of popliteal arteries only on active flexion and extension while these patients are sedated.

Cooperation required during these procedures is not always easily achieved with traditional sedatives such as fentanyl, midazolam, or propofol. In addition, these agents have well-known respiratory depressant effects. The unique sedative properties of DEX has led to its evaluation in a variety of pediatric procedures requiring cooperation and response due to its beneficial pharmacological profile, with sedation that parallels natural sleep, sympatholysis, and an anesthetic-sparing effect without relevant respiratory depression.[27,28]

DENTAL AND ORAL SURGERY

Anesthesia for dentistry includes the full spectrum of anesthetic/sedative care ranges from orally administered sedatives to nitrous oxide inhalation, parenteral moderate or deep sedation, and general ETT anesthesia. Most of the pediatric dental studies reported in the literature focused on oral benzodiazepines and nitrous oxide, either alone or in combination for PS in patients requiring mild-to-moderate levels of sedation.[102] Moderate or deep sedation or GA are required for patients who have special needs or when the dental or surgical requirements become more complex.[103]

Midazolam alone can result in insufficient sedation to allow the dental procedure, and the addition of an opioid may increase the risk of respiratory depression or vomiting in these procedures. DEX appears to provide the desirable properties for successful dental sedation compared to traditional sedatives because of its analgesic property, antisalivatory properties, anxiolytic and sympatholytic effects, and lack of respiratory depression. A recent study compared the efficacy and safety of DEX and midazolam for dental outpatient procedures; the study showed that DEX works as well as midazolam for outpatient dental procedures and can be used as an alternative to midazolam.[104] Conversely, a Japanese study compared intravenous sedation with DEX and propofol for minor oral surgery and reported hypotension and bradycardia with DEX but no difference in respiratory response.[105]

Recent studies examined morbidities and mortalities associated with dental treatment of children; they showed that the majority of children were less than 6 years of age and being cared for by a general dentist.[106,107] The deaths described in these reports suggested that some pediatric deaths related to dental anesthesia are preventable, through improved knowledge of or compliance with standard-of-care guidelines for those who must have GA for dental procedures. No single sedative was implicated in these reports. These deaths also raise many concerns, including risk-benefit threshold for sedation versus GA in pediatric dentistry, training skills for providers using sedation, and finally equipment requirements in NORA locations.

The equipment requirements for dental surgery in NORA locations closely mimic those of the operating room environment. Supplies, drugs, and equipment necessary for the administration of anesthesia and emergency management may be immediately available in a designated cart in these locations. The ASA issued a statement on NORA locations in October 2003; it was last amended in October 2013.[108] The statement identified that the standards for delivering anesthesia in these locations should be almost identical to those set for the operating room. Specifically, a reliable source of oxygen must be available. If a central fresh gas supply is not available, portable cylinders may be used. At a minimum, a portable oxygen source should be available for emergency use. Suction apparatus that meets the operating room standards, illumination (inclusive of a battery-operated device such as a flashlight), and scavenging. Many dental anesthetics are performed without the use of an anesthesia machine. In these instances, intravenous agents are utilized, and oxygen is delivered via a nasal cannula or mask. Positive pressure ventilation is available through the use of a bag-valve-mask device. These sites are expected to have immediate access to emergency supplies, such as a cart, defibrillator, drugs, and resuscitation equipment and to communication in the event of an emergency.

Potential risks of adverse events during the recovery period mandate accessibility to basic monitoring, suction equipment, oxygen source, devices (Mapleson or Ambu bag) to provide positive pressure ventilation, and specific antagonists of opioids and benzodiazepines. If the administration of an antagonist is necessary, continuous and prolonged monitoring is necessary. The ASA statement on NORA locations issued in the October 2013 update recognized the importance of the recovery period, with the expectation that there will be a designated postanesthetic recovery area with qualified personnel for the transport and recovery of these patients.[108]

PREPARING FOR EMERGENCIES IN AREAS DISTANT TO THE OPERATING ROOM

CARDIOPULMONARY RESUSCITATION

The ASA issued a statement on NORA locations in October 2003, last amended in October 2013.[108] Each NORA location is unique with regard to logistics, planning, and equipment necessary to conduct airway or cardiopulmonary resuscitation. Redundancy of monitoring devices and equipment is important in all NORA locations. Areas with restricted access, MRI in particular, should have designated adjacent locations equipped with wall oxygen, suction, and full monitoring and resuscitation capability. A self-inflating silicone bag (no ferromagnetic working parts) or nonferrous Jackson Rees circuit should always be kept inside the MRI suite to initiate resuscitation while transporting the child outside the MRI suite. Codes should never be conducted in the MRI scanner for multiple safety reasons. First, there is a risk of morbidity or mortality from ferrous objects. As support personnel rush inside to assist, unremoved ferrous materials will become projectiles and create an even more hazardous situation. Quenching a magnet should not be an alternative because it requires a minimum of 3 minutes to eliminate the magnetic field. To date, there are no MRI-compatible defibrillators, and those that have been brought in have demonstrated lack of adequate function.[109] To reiterate, in an emergency, the patient should be removed from the scanner to an area outside of the magnetic field that is equipped with a wall oxygen source for a self-inflating bag and access to appropriate monitors.

DIFFICULT AIRWAY MANAGEMENT

The unrecognized difficult airway is particularly challenging in any area that is remote to the operating room. If a child with a known difficult airway requires endotracheal intubation, a conservative approach is to perform the anesthetic induction in the operating room. Airway management in the operating room environment provides the comfort and security of having backup expertise and equipment in the event of a difficult airway. Following intubation, the child may then be transported to the NORA location. Anesthesia providers should confirm that appropriate airway management instruments, including different size face masks, oral airway, nasopharyngeal airways, ETTs, laryngoscope blades and handles, and appropriate size LMA that has successfully managed children with craniofacial anomalies associated with difficult airways.[110–112] It is extremely important for the anesthesiologist to jointly discuss the plan for management of the airway in these patients and have a clear plan before anesthesia induction. The availability of a fiber-optic bronchoscope, video laryngoscope, and a difficult airway cart should be confirmed. Upper airway obstruction during sedation can be relieved by head tilt, chin lift, jaw thrust, and the application of continuous positive airway pressure.[113]

SUMMARY

The demand for anesthesia and sedation services for the pediatric patient in NORA locations, both within the hospital and in freestanding ambulatory centers, are increasing. Over half of most NORA pediatric anesthetics are performed in the Department of Radiology. As technology advances, the anesthesiologist must also maintain an understanding of the procedures in order to tailor the anesthetic appropriately. A collaborative relationship between extramural and anesthesiology departments is critical to create and maintain a safe, productive, and efficient environment for sedation in these locations. As more experience with the procedures, risks, and newer sedation alternatives is gathered, the anesthesiologist will be better able to care for the pediatric patient in settings distant to the operating room.

REFERENCES

1. Mason KP. Sedation trends in the 21st century: the transition to dexmedetomidine for radiological imaging studies. *Paediatr Anaesth.* 2010;20(3):265–272.
2. Fox V. Clinical competency in pediatric endoscopy. *J Pediatr Gastroenterol Nutr.* 1998(26):200.
3. Lightdale JR, Mahoney LB, Schwarz SM, Liacouras CA. Methods of sedation in pediatric endoscopy: a survey of NASPGHAN members. *J Pediatr Gastroenterol Nutr.* 2007;45(4):500–502.
4. American Society of Anesthesiologists Task Force on Sedation and Analgesia by Non-anesthesiologists. Practical guidelines for sedation and analgesia by non-anesthesiologists. *Anesthesiology.* 2002;96:1004.
5. American Society for Gastrointestinal Endoscopy. Guidelines for the use of deep sedation and anesthesia for GI endoscopy. *Gastrointest Endosc.* 2002;56(5):613–617.
6. Abu-Shahwan I, Mack D. Propofol and remifentanil for deep sedation in children undergoing gastrointestinal endoscopy. *Paediatr Anaesth.* 2007;17(5):460–463.
7. Perera C, Strandvik GF, Malik M, Sen S. Propofol anesthesia is an effective and safe strategy for pediatric endoscopy. *Paediatr Anaesth.* 2006;16(2):220–221.

8. Rex DK. Review article: moderate sedation for endoscopy: sedation regimens for non-anaesthesiologists. *Aliment Pharmacol Ther.* 2006;24(2):163–171.
9. Rex DK, Heuss LT, Walker JA, Qi R. Trained registered nurses/endoscopy teams can administer propofol safely for endoscopy. *Gastroenterology.* 2005;129(5):1384–1391.
10. Walker JA, McIntyre RD, Schleinitz PF, et al. Nurse-administered propofol sedation without anesthesia specialists in 9152 endoscopic cases in an ambulatory surgery center. *Am J Gastroenterol.* 2003;98(8):1744–1750.
11. Bouchut J, Godard J, Lachaux A. Deep sedation for upper gastrointestinal endoscopy in children. *J Pediatr Gastroenterol Nutr.* 2001;32:108.
12. Dillon M, Brown S, Casey W. Colonoscopy under general anesthesia in children. *Pediatarics.* 1998;102:381.
13. Hassall E. Should pediatric gastroenterologists be IV drug users? *J Pediatr Gastroenterol Nutr.* 1993;16:370–372.
14. Hassall E. Who should perform pediatric endoscopic sedation? *J Pediatr Gastroenterol Nutr.* 1994;18:114.
15. Koh J, Black D, Leatherman I. Experience with an anesthesiologist interventional model for endoscopy in a pediatric hospital. *J Pediatr Gastroenterol Nutr.* 2001;33:314.
16. Paspatis GA, Charoniti I, Manolaraki M, et al. Synergistic sedation with oral midazolam as a premedication and intravenous propofol versus intravenous propofol alone in upper gastrointestinal endoscopies in children: a prospective, randomized study. *J Pediatr Gastroenterol Nutr.* 2006;43(2):195–199.
17. Saint-Maurice C, Hamza J. Sedation techniques in pediatric anesthesia. *Curr Opin Anesthesiol.* 1992;5:392–397.
18. Wolfe T, Rao C. Anesthesia for selected procedures. *Semin Pediatr Surg.* 1992;1:74.
19. Hammer GB, Sam WJ, Chen MI, Golianu B, Drover DR. Determination of the pharmacodynamic interaction of propofol and dexmedetomidine during esophagogastroduodenoscopy in children. *Paediatr Anaesth.* 2009;19(2):138–144.
20. Hoffmann CO, Samuels PJ, Beckman E, et al. Insufflation versus intubation during esophagogastroduodenoscopy in children. *Paediatr Anaesth.* 2010;20(9):821–830.
21. Patino M, Glynn S, Soberano M, et al. Comparison of different anesthesia techniques during esophagogastroduedenoscopy in children: a randomized trial. *Paediatr Anaesth.* 2015;25(10):1013–1019.
22. Rajasekaran S, Hackbarth RM, Davis AT, et al. The safety of propofol sedation for elective nonintubated esophagogastroduodenoscopy in pediatric patients. *Pediatr Crit Care Med.* 2014;15(6):e261–e269.
23. Acquaviva MA, Horn ND, Gupta SK. Endotracheal intubation versus laryngeal mask airway for esophagogastroduodenoscopy in children. *J Pediatr Gastroenterol Nutr.* 2014;59(1):54–56.
24. Olofsen E, Dahan A. The dynamic relationship between end-tidal sevoflurane and isoflurane concentrations and bispectral index and spectral edge frequency of the electroencephalogram. *Anesthesiology.* 1999;90(5):1345–1353.
25. Ebrahim ZY, Schubert A, Van Ness P, Wolgamuth B, Awad I. The effect of propofol on the electroencephalogram of patients with epilepsy. *Anesth Analg.* 1994;78(2):275–279.
26. Olson DM, Sheehan MG, Thompson W, Hall PT, Hahn J. Sedation of children for electroencephalograms. *Pediatrics.* 2001;108(1):163–165.
27. Mason KP, Lerman J. Review article: dexmedetomidine in children: current knowledge and future applications. *Anesth Analg.* 2011;113(5):1129–1142.
28. Mahmoud M, Mason KP. Dexmedetomidine: review, update, and future considerations of paediatric perioperative and periprocedural applications and limitations. *Br J Anaesth.* 2015;115(2):171–182.
29. Mason KP, O'Mahony E, Zurakowski D, Libenson MH. Effects of dexmedetomidine sedation on the EEG in children. *Paediatr Anaesth.* 2009;19(12):1175–1183.
30. Souter MJ, Rozet I, Ojemann JG, et al. Dexmedetomidine sedation during awake craniotomy for seizure resection: effects on electrocorticography. *J Neurosurg Anesthesiol.* 2007;19(1):38–44.
31. Chaitanya G, Arivazhagan A, Sinha S, et al. Dexmedetomidine anesthesia enhances spike generation during intra-operative electrocorticography: a promising adjunct for epilepsy surgery. *Epilepsy Res.* 2015;109:65–71.
32. Konig MW, Mahmoud MA, Fujiwara H, Hemasilpin N, Lee KH, Rose DF. Influence of anesthetic management on quality of magnetoencephalography scan data in pediatric patients: a case series. *Paediatr Anaesth.* 2009;19(5):507–512.
33. Lee EY, Mason KP, Zurakowski D, et al. MDCT assessment of tracheomalacia in symptomatic infants with mediastinal aortic vascular anomalies: preliminary technical experience. *Pediatr Radiol.* 2008;38(1):82–88.
34. Woodard PK, Bluemke DA, Cascade PN, et al. ACR practice guideline for the performance and interpretation of cardiac magnetic resonance imaging (MRI). *J Am Coll Radiol.* 2006;3(9):665–676.
35. Blankenberg F, Loh N, Bracci P, et al. Sonography, CT, and MR imaging: a prospective comparison of neonates with suspected intracranial ischemia and hemorrhage. *Am J Neuroradiol.* 2000;21(1):213–218.
36. Davidson RG. Atlantoaxial instability in individuals with Down syndrome: a fresh look at the evidence. *Pediatrics.* 1988;81(6):857–865.
37. Friedman B, Hartenberg M, Mulroy J, Tong T, Mickell J. Gastrografin aspiration in a 3-3/4-year-old girl. *Pediatr Radiol.* 1986;16(6):506–507.
38. Wells H, Hyrnchak M, Burbridge B. Direct effects of contrast media on rat lungs. *Can Assoc Radiol J.* 1991;42(4):261–264.
39. Mahmoud M, McAuliffe J, Kim HY, et al. Oral contrast for abdominal computed tomography in children: the effects on gastric fluid volume. *Anesth Analg.* 2010;111(5):1252–1258.
40. Mahmoud M, McAuliffe J, Donnelly LF. Administration of enteric contrast material before abdominal CT in children: current practices and controversies. *Pediatr Radiol.* 2011;41(4):409–412.
41. Hedenstierna G, Lundquist H, Lundh B, et al. Pulmonary densities during anaesthesia. An experimental study on lung morphology and gas exchange. *Eur Respir J.* 1989;2(6):528–535.
42. Lachmann B. Open up the lung and keep the lung open. *Intensive Care Med.* 1992;18(6):319–321.
43. Tusman G, Bohm SH, Vazquez de Anda GF, do Campo JL, Lachmann B. "Alveolar recruitment strategy" improves arterial oxygenation during general anaesthesia. *Br J Anaesth.* 1999;82(1):8–13.
44. Barnes P. Imaging of the central nervous system in pediatrics and adolescence. *Pediatr Clin North Am.* 1992;39:743.
45. Edelman RR, Warach S. Magnetic resonance imaging (Part I). *N Engl J Med.* 1993;328:708–716.
46. Ledneva E, Karie S, Launay-Vacher V, Janus N, Deray G. Renal safety of gadolinium-based contrast media in patients with chronic renal insufficiency. *Radiology.* 2009;250(3):618–628.
47. Van Wagoner M, Worah D. Gadodiamide injection. First human experience with the nonionic magnetic resonance imaging enhancement agent. *Invest Radiol.* 1993;28:S44–S48.
48. Leach JL, Holland SK. Functional MRI in children: clinical and research applications. *Pediatr Radiol.* 2010;40(1):31–49.
49. Engstrom M, Ragnehed M, Lundberg P. Projection screen or video goggles as stimulus modality in functional magnetic resonance imaging. *Magn Reson Imaging.* 2005;23(5):695–699.
50. Ravicz ME, Melcher JR, Kiang NY. Acoustic noise during functional magnetic resonance imaging. *J Acoust Soc Am.* 2000;108(4):1683–1696.
51. Menendez-Colino LM, Falcon C, Traserra J, et al. Activation patterns of the primary auditory cortex in normal hearing subjects: a functional magnetic resonance imaging study. *Acta Otolaryngol.* 2007;127(12):1283–1291.
52. Granet RB, Gelber LJ. Claustrophobia during MR imaging. *NJ Med.* 1990;87:479–482.
53. Melendez JC, McCrank E. Anxiety-related reactions associated with magnetic resonance imaging examination. *JAMA.* 1993;270:745–747.
54. Koroglu A, Teksan H, Sagir O, Yucel A, Toprak HI, Ersoy OM. A comparison of the sedative, hemodynamic, and respiratory effects of dexmedetomidine and propofol in children undergoing magnetic resonance imaging. *Anesth Analg.* 2006;103(1):63–67.
55. Karlik SJ, Heatherley T, Pavan F, et al. Patient anesthesia and monitoring at a 1.5 T MRI installation. *Magn Reson Med.* 1988;7:210–221.
56. Menon DK, Peden CJ, Hall AS, Sargentoni J, Whitwam JG. Magnetic resonance for the anaesthetist. Part I: physical principles, applications, safety aspects. *Anaesthesia.* 1992;47:240–255.
57. Tobin JR, Spurrier EA, Wetzel RC. Anaesthesia for critically ill children during magnetic resonance imaging. *Br J Anaesth.* 1992;69:482–486.
58. Chaljub G, Kramer L, Johnson RR, Johnson RJ, Singh H, Crow W. Projectile cylinder accidents resulting from the presence of ferromagnetic nitrous oxide or oxygen tanks in the MR suite. *AJR Am J Roentgenol.* 2001;177(1):27–30.
59. Kanal E, Barkovich A, Bell C, et al. ACR Guidance document for safe MR practices: 2007. *AJR Am J Roentgenol.* 2007;188:1–27.
60. American Society of Anesthesiologists Task Force on Anesthetic Care for Magnetic Resonance Imaging, Ehrenwerth J, Singleton MA, et al. Practice advisory on anesthetic care for magnetic resonance imaging: a report by the american society of anesthesiologists task force on anesthetic care for magnetic resonance imaging. *Anesthesiology.* 2009;110(3):459–479.
61. Practice advisory on anesthetic care for magnetic resonance imaging: an updated report by the American Society of Anesthesiologists Task Force on Anesthetic Care for Magnetic Resonance Imaging. *Anesthesiology.* 2015;122(3):495–520.

62. Shellock FG. Biological effects and safety aspects of magnetic resonance imaging. *Magn Reson Q.* 1989;5:243–261.
63. Brow TR, Goldstein B, Little J. Severe burns resulting from magnetic resonance imaging with cardiopulmonary monitoring. Risks and relevant safety precautions. *Am J Phys Med Rehabil.* 1993;72:166–167.
64. Prasad N, Wright D, Ford J, Thornby J. Safety of 4-T MR imaging: study of effects on developing frog embryos. *Radiology.* 1990;174(1):251–253.
65. Gangarosa RE, Minnis JE, Nobbe J, Praschan D, Genberg R. Operational safety issues in MRI. *Magn Reson Imaging.* 1987;5:287–292.
66. Brummett R, Talbot J, Charuhas P. Potential hearing loss resulting from MR imaging. *Radiology.* 1988;169(2):539–540.
67. Kanal E, Shellock FG, Talagala L. Safety considerations in MR imaging. *Radiology.* 1990;176:593–606.
68. Ngamprasertwong P, Mahmoud M. Anesthesia for MRI enterography in children. *J Clin Anesth.* 2014;26(3):249.
69. Mahmoud M, Gunter J, Donnelly LF, Wang Y, Nick TG, Sadhasivam S. A comparison of dexmedetomidine with propofol for magnetic resonance imaging sleep studies in children. *Anesth Analg.* 2009;109(3):745–753.
70. Mahmoud M, Radhakrishman R, Gunter J, et al. Effect of increasing depth of dexmedetomidine anesthesia on upper airway morphology in children. *Paediatr Anaesth.* 2010;20(6):506–515.
71. Mahmoud M, Jung D, Salisbury S, et al. Effect of increasing depth of dexmedetomidine and propofol anesthesia on upper airway morphology in children and adolescents with obstructive sleep apnea. *J Clin Anesth.* 2013;25:529–541.
72. Chiron C, Raynaud C, Dulac O, Tzourio N, Plouin P, Tran-Dinh S. Study of the cerebral blood flow in partial epilepsy of childhood using the SPECT method. *J Neuroradiol.* 1989;16(4):317–324.
73. Chugani H. PET in preoperative evaluation of intractable epilepsy. *Pediatr Neurol.* 1993;9(5):411–413.
74. Griffeth L, Rich K, Dehdashti F, et al. Brain metastases from noncentral nervous system tumors: evaluation with PET. *Radiology.* 1993;186(1):37–44.
75. Mandell GA MM, Shalaby-Rana EI, Gordon I. Society of Nuclear Medicine procedure guideline for pediatric sedation in nuclear medicine: version 3.0. Available at: http://interactive.snm.org/index.cfm?PageID=809. Approved January 25, 2003. Accessed on October 4, 2016.
76. Mason KP, Robinson F, Fontaine P, Prescilla R. Dexmedetomidine offers an option for safe and effective sedation for nuclear medicine imaging in children. *Radiology.* 2013;267(3):911–917.
77. Loeffler J, Rossitch EJ, Siddon R, Moore M, Rockoff M, Alexander ER. Role of stereotactic radiosurgery with a linear accelerator in treatment of intracranial arteriovenous malformations and tumors in children. *Pediatrics.* 1990;85(5):774–782.
78. Westbrook C, Glaholm J, Barrett A. Vomiting associated with whole body irradiation. *Clin Radiol.* 1987;38:263–266.
79. Whitwam JG, Owen JR, Spiers ASD, Morgan M, Goolden AW, Gordon-Smith EC. General anaesthesia for high-dose total-body irradiation. *Lancet.* 1978;1(8056):128–129.
80. Wachtel RE, Dexter F, Dow AJ. Growth rates in pediatric diagnostic imaging and sedation. *Anesth Analg.* 2009;108(5):1616–1621.
81. Krauss B, Green SM. Procedural sedation and analgesia in children. *Lancet.* 2006;367(9512):766–780.
82. Mason KP, Neufeld EJ, Karian VE, Zurakowski D, Koka BV, Burrows PE. Coagulation abnormalities in pediatric and adult patients after sclerotherapy or embolization of vascular anomalies. *AJR Am J Roentgenol.* 2001;177(6):1359–1363.
83. Mason KP, Michna E, Zurakowski D, Koka BV, Burrows PE. Serum ethanol levels in children and adults after ethanol embolization or sclerotherapy for vascular anomalies. *Radiology.* 2000;217(1):127–132.
84. Burrows PE, Mason KP. Percutaneous treatment of low flow vascular malformations. *J Vasc Interv Radiol.* 2004;15(5):431–445.
85. Yakes WF, Baker R. Cardiopulmonary collapse: sequelae of ethanol embolotherapy. *Radiology.* 1993;189:145–147.
86. Iwama T, Hashimoto N, Yonekawa Y. The relevance of hemodynamic factors to perioperative ischemic complications in childhood moyamoya disease. *Neurosurgery.* 1996;38(6):1120–1125; discussion 1125–1126.
87. Dahmani S, Stany I, Brasher C, et al. Pharmacological prevention of sevoflurane- and desflurane-related emergence agitation in children: a meta-analysis of published studies. *Br J Anaesth.* 2010;104(2):216–223.
88. Gupta AK, Varma DR. Vein of Galen malformations: review. *Neurol India.* 2004;52(1):43–53.
89. Jones BV, Ball WS, Tomsick TA, Millard J, Crone KR. Vein of Galen aneurysmal malformation: diagnosis and treatment of 13 children with extended clinical follow-up. *AJNR Am J Neuroradiol.* 2002;23(10):1717–1724.
90. Ashida Y, Miyahara H, Sawada H, Mitani Y, Maruyama K. Anesthetic management of a neonate with vein of Galen aneurysmal malformations and severe pulmonary hypertension. *Paediatr Anaesth.* 2005;15(6):525–528.
91. Chernish SM, Maglinte DD. Glucagon: common untoward reactions—review and recommendations. *Radiology.* 1990;177(1):145–146.
92. Jehenson PM. Reducing doses of glucagon used in radiologic examinations. *Radiology.* 1991;179(1):286–287.
93. McLoughlin MJ, Langer B, Wilson DR. Life-threatening reaction to glucagon in a patient with pheochromocytoma. *Radiology.* 1981;140(3):841–845.
94. Mason KP, Padua H, Fontaine PJ, Zurakowski D. Radiologist-supervised ketamine sedation for solid organ biopsies in children and adolescents. *AJR Am J Roentgenol.* 2009;192(5):1261–1265.
95. Dilworth KE, McHugh K, Stacey S, Howard RF. Mediastinal mass obscured by a large pericardial effusion in a child: a potential cause of serious anaesthetic morbidity. *Paediatr Anaesth.* 2001;11(4):479–482.
96. Char D, Drover DR, Motonaga KS, et al. The effects of ketamine on dexmedetomidine-induced electrophysiologic changes in children. *Paediatr Anaesth.* 2013;23(10):898–905.
97. Tobias JD. Dexmedetomidine and ketamine: an effective alternative for procedural sedation? *Pediatr Critical Care Med.* 2012;13(4):423–427.
98. Cohen SP, Larkin TM, Barna SA, Palmer WE, Hecht AC, Stojanovic MP. Lumbar discography: a comprehensive review of outcome studies, diagnostic accuracy, and principles. *Reg Anesth Pain Med.* 2005;30(2):163–183.
99. Bogduk N. The innervation of the lumbar spine. *Spine.* 1983;8(3):286–293.
100. Furstein J, Patel M, Sadhasivam S, Mahmoud M. Use of dexmedetomidine for monitored anesthesia care for diskography in adolescents. *AANA J.* 2011;79(5):421–425.
101. Masters LT, Perrine K, Devinsky O, Nelson PK. Wada testing in pediatric patients by use of propofol anesthesia. *AJNR Am J Neuroradiol.* 2000;21(7):1302–1305.
102. Houpt MI, Kupietzky A, Tofsky NS, Koenigsberg SR. Effects of nitrous oxide on diazepam sedation of young children. *Pediatr Dent.* 1996;18(3):236–241.
103. Caputo AC. Providing deep sedation and general anesthesia for patients with special needs in the dental office-based setting. *Spec Care Dentist.* 2009;29(1):26–30.
104. Fan TW, Ti LK, Islam I. Comparison of dexmedetomidine and midazolam for conscious sedation in dental surgery monitored by bispectral index. *Br J Oral Maxillofac Surg.* 2013;51(5):428–433.
105. Taniyama K, Oda H, Okawa K, Himeno K, Shikanai K, Shibutani T. Psychosedation with dexmedetomidine hydrochloride during minor oral surgery. *Anesth Prog.* 2009;56(3):75–80.
106. Chicka MC, Dembo JB, Mathu-Muju KR, Nash DA, Bush HM. Adverse events during pediatric dental anesthesia and sedation: a review of closed malpractice insurance claims. *Pediatr Dent.* 2012;34(3):231–238.
107. Lee HH, Milgrom P, Starks H, Burke W. Trends in death associated with pediatric dental sedation and general anesthesia. *Paediatr Anaesth.* 2013;23(8):741–746.
108. American Society of Anesthesiologists. Statement on nonoperating room anesthetizing locations. Available at: http://www.asahq.org/~/media/Sites/ASAHQ/Files/Public/Resources/standards-guidelines/statement-on-nonoperating-room-anesthetizing-locations.pdf. Last amended October 16, 2013. Accessed on February 12, 2015.
109. Snowdon S. Defibrillator failure in a magnetic resonance unit [letter]. *Anaesthesia.* 1989;44:359.
110. Fan S, Lee T, Chen L. Long-term propofol infusion and airway management in a patient with Goldenhar's syndrome. *Acta Anaesthesiol Sin.* 1995;33:233–236.
111. Hansen T, Joensen H, Henneberg S. Laryngeal mask airway guided tracheal intubation in a neonate with the Pierre Robin syndrome. *Acta Anaesthesiol Scand.* 1995;S39:129.
112. Haxby E, Liban J. Fiberoptic intubation via a laryngeal mask in a infant with Goldenhar syndrome. *Anaesth Intensive Care.* 1995;23:753.
113. Meier S, Geiduschek J, Paganoni R, Fuehrmeyer F, Reber A. The effect of chin lift, jaw thrust, and continuous positive airway pressure on the size of the glottic opening and on stridor score in anesthetized, spontaneously breathing children. *Anesth Analg.* 2002;94(3):494–499

28 | PROCEDURES IN THE ADULT AND NEONATAL INTENSIVE CARE UNITS

MATTHEW READ, MD, CHRISTOPHER V. MAANI, MD

INTRODUCTION

Bedside procedures in the intensive care unit (ICU) are an integral component of critical care medicine. Anesthesiologists who are assigned to provide anesthesia for operations in the ICU must adapt principles of safe and effective anesthesia practice to this novel outside of the operating room environment. Among the reasons to perform surgical procedures at the bedside in the ICU is the avoidance of transporting an unstable, critically ill patient from the ICU to the operating room (OR),[1] as critically ill patients are at an increased risk for morbidity and mortality during transport.[2] Also, the urgency of the procedure may not allow adequate time to mobilize resources to perform the procedure in the OR. Therefore, patients who need anesthesia care and undergo surgical procedures in the ICU can present a major challenge. The types of procedures performed in the ICU are listed in Table 28.1. Essential to care of the critical patient outside of the OR is to ensure readiness of the entire team, without compromising care due to production pressure or lack of standards routine to the OR environment.

THE ENVIRONMENT

Although an ICU does not qualify as an austere anesthetizing location, it presents significant challenges to the anesthesiologist. Unless surgical nurses accompany the surgeons, the anesthesiologist will have to work with nurses who are unfamiliar with the pace of the operation and the needs of the anesthesiologist. Identifying the roles of involved personnel is imperative to allow quick identification of qualified staff members to assist in case of emergency. It is important to gather needed equipment and supplies prior to commencing anesthetic care for the surgical procedure. If the anesthesiologist has the necessary equipment and supplies conveniently at hand, he or she will be able to remain near the patient and concentrate on those necessary anesthetic tasks instead of being frustrated by lack of cooperation from naïve assistants. Table 28.2 lists anesthetic equipment typically needed in an ICU.

Although the monitoring standards for critically ill patients in the ICU are similar to the monitoring standards for anesthetized patients in the OR, subtle differences exist between monitoring systems in the two areas.[3] Anesthesiologists should familiarize themselves with the bedside monitoring system in the ICU prior to initiating anesthesia. It is especially important that the anesthesiologist understand how to change the monitor display in order to follow the needed frequency of measurements for monitoring the anesthetized patient.

Space allocation in the typical ICU room frequently cramps the anesthesiologist in an awkward position. This space limitation may also interfere with maintenance of sterile fields necessary for surgery.[4] The anesthesiologist should take a few minutes to plan for the positions of personnel and equipment.

Fluid management of the ICU patient can present challenges, just as for an anesthetized patient with ongoing surgical fluid losses. Many critically ill patients have only a few small-gauge peripheral intravenous lines or small-bore ports in relatively high-resistance central venous catheters. Therefore, if rapid intravenous volume replacement is anticipated for the bedside surgical procedure, the anesthesiologist should place appropriate vascular access. If blood replacement is anticipated, the anesthesiologist must verify availability of appropriate blood products before becoming ensnared with continually managing the ICU patient undergoing a surgical procedure.

Nutritional requirements of critically ill patients are increased from baseline metabolic requirements, and these patients' increased needs are rarely met, increasing risk of morbidity and mortality.[5] For these reasons, it is imperative to minimize interruptions in nutrition administration. The American Society of Anesthesiologists (ASA) guidelines for perioperative fasting are intended to decrease the risk of pulmonary aspiration of gastric contents.[6] However, these guidelines are intended to be applied to healthy patients undergoing elective procedures, not critically ill patients. In the presence of a secured airway, risk of aspiration is decreased, especially when enteral nutrition is administered via a postpyloric tube.[7,8] In one of the most at-risk bedside procedures for aspiration, tracheostomy, fasting times as short as 45 minutes were not associated with increased incidence of aspiration.[9] As with all interventions, the benefits and risks must be considered to make the most appropriate decision.

MONITORING REQUIREMENTS

Table 28.3 lists basic monitors required during ICU anesthesia. Managing general anesthesia in the critical care unit

TABLE 28.1. Surgical Procedures Performed at the Bedside in the Adult Intensive Care Unit

I. Under Local Anesthesia
Chest tubes/thoracentesis
Diagnostic peritoneal lavage/paracentesis
Pericardiocentesis
II. Under General Anesthesia
A. Common procedures
Percutaneous tracheostomy
Percutaneous endoscopic gastrostomy (PEG)
Esophagogastroduodenoscopy (EGD) and/or colonoscopy
Inferior vena cava (IVC) filter placement
Transesophageal echocardiogram (TEE)
Ventriculostomy or intracranial pressure (ICP) monitor placement
Wound dressing changes
B. Uncommon procedures
Thoracotomy
Laparotomy
Amputation/fasciotomy
Extracorporeal membrane oxygenation (ECMO) cannulation

TABLE 28.2. Anesthetic Equipment for the Intensive Care Unit

Airway:	Laryngoscope
	Endotracheal tube
	Stylet
	Self-inflating ventilation bag (for patient intubated prior to procedure, only needed in case of emergency extubation)
Hemodynamic:	Intravenous fluid Blood products
	Pumps as needed
Pharmaceuticals:	Hypnotics—propofol/ketamine
	Analgesics—opioids/dexmedetomidine
	Muscle relaxants (nondepolarizing) Hemodynamic agents—vasopressors/inotropes/vasodilators
	Antibiotics
	Miscellaneous—diuretics/corticosteroids

TABLE 28.3. Monitoring Requirements for Anesthesia in the Intensive Care Unit

Oxygenation:	Pulse oximetry
Ventilation:	Capnometry/capnography
	Chest excursion
Circulation:	ECG/HR monitor
	BP, noninvasive
Body temperature:	Core temperature

BP, blood pressure; ECG, electrocardiogram; HR, heart rate.

requires the same standards of monitoring used in the OR.[3] Cardiopulmonary monitoring includes continuous pulse oximetry for oxygen saturation and heart rate; continuous electrocardiography for heart rate and rhythm; noninvasive blood pressure to monitor cardiac performance and intravascular volume status; continuous capnography to monitor endotracheal tube position, respiratory rate, and metabolic function; and body temperature monitoring to assess metabolic state.

Invasive hemodynamic monitors provide useful information about cardiovascular performance and are frequently indwelling in unstable ICU patients who require bedside procedures. Arterial catheters provide a route to monitor beat-to-beat arterial pressure as well as ready access for blood sampling to assess glycemic control, gas exchange, and acid-base status. Central venous pressure or pulmonary artery pressure monitoring provides information about a patient's blood volume and myocardial performance. Either systolic pressure variation or pulse oximeter plethysmographic volume variation with respiration suggests hypovolemia correctable by volume infusion.[10,11]

Cardiac output is an important metabolic variable that can be monitored in the critically ill patient.[12] Pulse wave contour analysis via an intra-arterial catheter provides measurements of cardiac stroke volume and cardiac output. Either intermittent or continuous thermodilution via a pulmonary artery catheter can also be used to measure cardiac output. A pulmonary artery catheter has the added advantage of providing a route to sample mixed venous blood gases that are used to monitor a critically ill patient's metabolic demand for oxygen and the cardiopulmonary system's ability to supply that demand.

Other techniques to measure cardiac output and additionally assess cardiovascular structure and monitor adequacy of cardiovascular responses are transthoracic echocardiography (TTE) and transesophageal echocardiography (TEE).[13,14] However, these techniques require advanced training.

CHOICE OF ANESTHETIC DRUGS

Anesthesia vaporizers are rarely fitted to critical care ventilators; therefore, the anesthesiologist must rely on total intravenous anesthesia (TIVA) in the ICU.[15] Besides the lack of vaporizers in the ICU, ability to scavenge waste anesthetic gases is compromised in this setting. Therefore, TIVA has significant environmental advantages in the ICU. Another advantage of TIVA in the ICU is the fact that most of the patients are managed with sedation and analgesia similar to the analgesics and hypnotics used with TIVA.[16]

Opioids continue to be an important component of critical care unit sedation. Opioid infusions, most commonly fentanyl and hydromorphone, are often used for critical care sedation and analgesia.[17] Patients who are receiving opioid infusions as part of their ICU sedation may need a bolus to supplement their infusion prior to commencing the surgical procedure. Further, the anesthesiologist can titrate the opioid infusion to blunt the physiologic responses to surgical procedures. Other useful opioids include sufentanil, remifentanil, and morphine, although these are less commonly used for ICU patients.[17–19] Nonopioid analgesics and regional anesthetic techniques are an especially important component to consider in order to achieve optimal pain management in critically ill patients.[20]

Sedation is frequently provided by a propofol infusion, which is an excellent hypnotic to continue for a bedside procedure.[17–19] However, extended use of propofol can be problematic in the ICU because of the propofol infusion syndrome. Infusions of propofol at greater than 50 μg/kg per minute for longer than 24 hours puts the patient at risk of developing metabolic acidosis and muscle necrosis secondary to a defect of mitochondrial fatty acid metabolism.[21–23] However, propofol continues to be safe and efficacious for short-term use in ICU patients undergoing surgical procedures. Patients who have already developed propofol infusion syndrome should be managed with alternative hypnotics.

Other hypnotics include benzodiazepines, etomidate, and ketamine. Although hemodynamic stability is more easily achieved with benzodiazepines, compared to propofol, the recovery from sedation is slower. Additionally, benzodiazepines are deliriogenic and have been shown to increase morbidity and mortality, except in limited circumstances.[16,24,25] Etomidate has a short half-life, but its use is associated with significant adrenal cortical suppression,[26,27] and alternative agents are more suitable for care of the critically ill, especially those with sepsis or septic shock.[28] Ketamine, on the other hand, can be hemodynamically stable and has the added benefit of analgesia via NMDA (*N*-methyl-D-aspartate) receptor antagonism, making it an excellent adjunct for sedation of critically ill patients.[29] However, ketamine can precipitate delirium and hallucinations.[30]

The specific α_2-adrenergic agonist dexmedetomidine is a useful addition to balanced multidrug TIVA for ICU patients undergoing surgical procedures[31] and is a recommended strategy.[16] Stimulation of central α_2 receptors causes sedation and mild analgesia without depressing brainstem respiratory centers. The main side effects arise from modulation of the sympathetic nervous system, leading to bradycardia and hypotension, especially with high-dose boluses or infusions. Patients may also display a hypertensive response to rapid bolus administration, which should be avoided. However, a modest infusion rate of dexmedetomidine will reduce the requirements of hypnotics and analgesics required for surgical anesthesia.[32] Neuromuscular blocking drugs are frequently needed for anesthesia for patients who require bedside surgical procedures. Succinylcholine may be useful for intubation of patients who are not ventilator dependent with a native airway, in absence of prolonged immobility. Succinylcholine should also be avoided in patients who have significant body surface area burned; upper or lower motor neuron paralysis, including spinal cord injury; or significant crush injury with rhabdomyolysis, who are at risk for extreme hyperkalemia and cardiac arrest from succinylcholine.[33] There seems to be little pharmacologic reason to choose one nondepolarizing neuromuscular blocking drug over another in the setting of an established secured airway. Vecuronium, cisatracurium, and rocuronium all have devotees among critical care anesthesiologists.[34] The presence of impaired hepatic drug clearance or renal failure may favor cisatracurium, which spontaneously degrades in the plasma, thus providing a route of elimination. Vecuronium and rocuronium are associated with cardiovascular stability, which may make them the drug of choice in hemodynamically labile patients.[35]

SURGICAL PROCEDURES IN THE CRITICAL CARE UNIT

TRACHEOSTOMY

Although formal open tracheostomies can be performed on a patient in an ICU bed, percutaneous tracheostomy is especially adapted for the critical care unit.[36] The anesthesiologist will place a bronchoscope near the tip of the endotracheal tube to view the trachea during transtracheal needle puncture at the first or second tracheal ring. The needle puncture is followed by passing a flexible guidewire through the needle, which is exchanged for a tracheal dilator over the wire, similar to the Seldinger technique used for vascular cannulation. Prior to the surgeon inserting the needle into the trachea, the anesthesiologist must partially withdraw the endotracheal tube and bronchoscope so that the tip of the endotracheal tube is not punctured by the needle. The anesthesiologist's observations through the bronchoscope ensure that the needle does not traverse the posterior membranous trachea before the guidewire is inserted. Further observations via the bronchoscope document the correct positioning of the wire distally in the center of the tracheal lumen. After the dilator prepares a track for the tracheostomy, an appropriate size tracheostomy tube is rapidly advanced through the stoma, and the ventilator circuit is attached to the tracheostomy tube to reestablish mechanical ventilation.[37]

The procedure is ideally monitored via a video tower attached to the bronchoscope so that all members of the surgical and anesthesia team can observe. The bronchoscope rapidly identifies needle malposition so that the guidewire, dilator, and tube will not be forced into a false passage. Anesthesia needs to be calibrated to prevent the patient from coughing during the procedure.

GASTROSTOMY

Similar to percutaneous tracheostomy, a percutaneous endoscopic gastrostomy (PEG) combines a percutaneous needle entry into an internal hollow organ and guidewire exchange of the needle for a tube under endoscope guidance. PEG placement is also safely performed at bedside in the ICU and often is performed in conjunction with percutaneous tracheostomy.[38]

In this procedure, an endoscope placed in the gastric antrum identifies the proper position of a needle pushed through the left upper quadrant of the abdomen into the stomach. A long, flexible guidewire advanced through the needle into the gastric lumen is snared by the endoscope and pulled out through the patient's mouth. The gastrostomy tube is attached to the wire and pulled by its distal end through the esophagus and out through the abdominal wall, where a flange on the end of the tube holds it in the gastric lumen.[37]

The anesthesiologist must ensure adequate gas exchange throughout the procedure as well as analgesia for the stimulation of passing the endoscope into the esophagus and the needle puncture through the anterior abdominal wall. The anesthesiologist must be especially vigilant that the endoscope does not dislodge the endotracheal tube during these manipulations.

EXTRACORPOREAL MEMBRANE OXYGENATION CANNULATION

In many centers, the implementation of emergency bedside extracorporeal membrane oxygenation (ECMO) has been established in patients who fail conventional therapies for cardiogenic or pulmonary failure.[39,40] There are multiple strategies for cannulation: peripheral versus central, venovenous (VV), venoarterial (VA), and venovenoarterial (VVA), dependent on the indication for initiation of ECMO.[41] In presence of a potentially reversible cardiac arrest, with quality chest compressions, good perfusion, and metabolic support, extracorporeal cardiopulmonary resuscitation (E-CPR) may be deployed to aid resuscitative efforts.[42] Certainly, this patient population is extremely critical, and the anesthesiologist may be called on to assist with management.

MAJOR SURGICAL PROCEDURES

Occasionally, unstable ICU patients require emergency thoracotomies, laparotomies, fasciotomies, or amputations to be performed in the ICU because of lack of OR time or inability to transport the patient to the OR. These procedures require a full OR crew with a circulating nurse, a scrub nurse, a surgeon and assistants, and an anesthesiologist. Because these patients are often bleeding, it is imperative to have adequate venous access and blood products available before draping the patient for the procedure.

Many surgical ICUs have built-in lighting that can illuminate a surgical procedure; however, in many ICUs portable lighting must be brought in to illuminate the surgical field. Adequate suction for the surgical field also has to be ensured prior to starting the surgical procedure. Electrosurgical cautery units are also among the necessary equipment brought to the ICU before commencing major surgery.

OTHER PROCEDURES

Many of the surgical procedures performed in an ICU, such as for thoracostomy tubes, paracentesis, wound dressing changes, EGD, colonoscopy, ventriculostomy, and TEE, can be performed with local anesthesia and minimal sedation. These procedures rarely require an anesthesiologist to manage the patient; however, if the patient is unstable, an anesthesiologist may be requested.

NEONATAL INTENSIVE CARE

The neonatal period, encompassing the first 30 days of extrauterine life, is filled with many anatomic, physiologic, and pharmacologic changes to maintain hemodynamics, which are necessary for infant survival.[43] Varying pathologic states, anesthesia, or surgery can alter the necessary developmental changes and even threaten neonatal survival. The anesthesiologist and surgeon must understand normal neonatal development and the pathophysiology of these neonatal disease processes to develop a logical, effective anesthetic and surgical plan.

In the past decade, tremendous advances have been made in the field of neonatology, particularly managing severe prematurity, respiratory failure, sepsis, and congenital heart disease, thus improving neonatal morbidity and mortality. Therefore, as anesthesiologists, we are caring for more and more premature infants with critical issues, many of which require some form of surgical intervention. Typically, the neonatal intensive care unit (NICU) is not in close proximity to the OR, thus requiring a fragile, often critically ill, newborn to be transported a significant distance. Transports can be extremely cumbersome for maintaining the necessary intravenous lines, respiratory support, and monitoring equipment.[2,43–45] If any of these interventions are disrupted for even a moment in a neonate, the results can be disastrous. With critically ill neonates, it may be safer to move the OR to the infant, rather than transporting the infant to the OR.[44,45] This change in surgical locale takes tremendous planning and anticipation

TABLE 28.4. Surgical Procedures Performed at the Bedside in the Neonatal Intensive Care Unit

Thoracotomy
Patent ductus arteriosus (PDA) ligation
Congenital diaphragmatic hernia (CDH) repair Tracheoesophageal fistula (TEF) repair
Laparotomy
Necrotizing enterocolitis (NEC)
Gastroschisis
Malrotation reduction
Abdominal wall defect repair
Tracheostomy
GastrostomyVentriculostomy
Broviac catheter insertion
Laser therapy for retinopathy of prematurity (ROP) Urinary diversion
Extracorporeal membrane oxygenation (ECMO) cannulation

of problems by the surgeon, anesthesiologist, OR nurses, and NICU staff. Table 28.4 lists procedures often performed in the NICU. Indications for surgery outside the OR are based on the specific diagnosis and the underlying medical condition of the neonate.

Performing surgery and anesthesia in the NICU provides several logistical challenges. Space for equipment and patient access is very limited. This space must be shared with the surgeon, scrub nurse, ventilator, and any other medical equipment.[43] A direct route to the neonate must be identified prior to the start of surgery in the case of an emergency requiring intravenous drugs or an inadvertent disconnection of a vital monitor or respiratory equipment. Most NICUs have several patients and related personnel sharing one large community-style room. Infection control is a concern because of the nature of the room, including the exposure from multiple patient areas.[46] Thus, a sterile radius must be set up before the start of the procedure. Finally, the NICU nursing staff has very different roles than the OR staff, and the NICU nurse's role during the procedure must be clarified before the start of the case for all to work well as one cohesive team.

NEONATAL THERMOREGULATION

The neonatal body habitus favors heat loss. The large surface area of the body relative to the mass of a newborn enhances radiant heat loss.[47] Heat loss is further exacerbated in the setting of an open abdomen with exposed bowel. Covering the head can significantly reduce heat loss,[48,49] as does covering the entire body. Neonates also have a very thin layer of subcutaneous fat, increasing thermal convective heat loss. Evaporative heat loss is increased due to the reduced keratin content of neonatal skin. Neonates do not shiver or sweat effectively to maintain body temperature and rely primarily on brown fat metabolism to maintain body heat.[50] Brown fat cells begin to develop between 26 and 30 weeks of gestation and thus may not be present in severely premature infants.[51]

Normally in the OR environment, one would use radiant warming lights or convective air warming blankets or raise the ambient temperature in the OR, although in the NICU these modalities may not be as easily obtainable. Radiant warming lights will not be effective when the infant is under the drapes, a convective warming blanket may be too forceful for a low-birth-weight neonate, and the temperature of the entire NICU cannot be adjusted as easily as a single OR. Thus, thermoregulation during surgery in the NICU may be difficult, but careful attention to temperature regulation is imperative to decrease the neonatal stress response and adverse effects associated with hypothermia, such as hypoglycemia and hypoxemia.[47]

DRUG CHOICE

Anesthetic management in the NICU is not the same as that in the OR. As an anesthesia machine is not usually present, volatile agent–based anesthesia is seldom used, making TIVA the anesthetic modality of choice.[15] Evidence has shown that the neonatal response to pain is similar to the response in adults.[52] The basis of most anesthetics given in the NICU is high-dose fentanyl, for analgesia and amnesia, with nondepolarizing muscle relaxation. Fentanyl is used frequently because of its ability to provide rapid analgesia, maintain cardiovascular stability, block the endocrine response, and prevent pain-induced increases in pulmonary vascular resistance.[53–56] Drawbacks of fentanyl include vagal bradycardia, chest wall rigidity, and opioid tolerance after prolonged therapy.[56] With NMDA antagonists and γ-aminobutyric acid (GABA) agonists implicated in neuroapoptotic neurotoxicity, they may be best avoided.[53]

SURGICAL PROCEDURES IN THE NEONATAL INTENSIVE CARE UNIT

PATENT DUCTUS ARTERIOSUS

The ductus arteriosus is a vascular connection between the left pulmonary artery and the descending thoracic aorta. This connection allows shunting of blood past the fetal lungs in utero. The ductus arteriosus typically closes from increased arterial oxygen exposure shortly after birth. If the ductus arteriosus does not close, the neonate can develop increased pulmonary circulation from left-to-right shunting across the ductus, leading to possible congestive heart failure, hemodynamic instability, or respiratory failure.[57] First-line therapy for a patent ductus arteriosus (PDA) is medical management with indomethacin or ibuprofen.[58] If medical management fails or is contraindicated, as in cases of renal dysfunction or bleeding abnormalities, surgical correction is warranted.[59] Equally safe and effective surgical approaches include thoracotomy and video-assisted thoracoscopy (VATS).[60]

For either approach, the neonate is placed in the right lateral decubitus position, with specific attention to positioning of fragile extremities, manipulation of the airway, and location of vascular access and emergency equipment prior to draping the patient. Due to increased pulmonary blood flow from the PDA, the diagnosis of heart failure is not uncommon. Hypovolemia is often present, due to treatment with fluid restriction and diuretics, making anesthetic management that much more challenging.[61] Blood loss is typically minimal, but blood products and albumin must be available in case of an emergency.

EMERGENCY LAPAROTOMY FOR NECROTIZING ENTEROCOLITIS

The most common surgical emergency in the premature neonate is necrotizing enterocolitis (NEC). The cause of NEC is unclear, but the result is ischemic damage to the intestinal mucosa, leading to full-thickness necrosis or perforation.[62] Early clinical signs of NEC may be apnea, bradycardia, and feeding intolerance, progressing to signs of abdominal distention and bloody stools. The diagnosis can be confirmed with an abdominal radiograph showing pneumatosis intestinalis, small pockets of gas in the bowel wall. NEC can rapidly progress to sepsis, with hemodynamic instability, respiratory failure, and coagulopathy. Medical management should be ongoing, with fluid resuscitation and antibiotics. If there are any signs of peritoneal air or perforation of the gastrointestinal tract, surgical intervention is certainly indicated. However, extensive necrosis or perforation can occur without evidence of free air on the radiograph. As a result, other signs that indicate bowel necrosis must be considered, including unremitting clinical deterioration, the presence of an abdominal mass, ascites, or intestinal obstruction.[63]

The removal of perforated or necrotic intestine is accomplished via emergency laparotomy. If a significant portion of the intestine is affected, the resection can be extensive, predisposing the infant to short-gut syndrome. As sepsis associated with NEC causes some degree of coagulopathy, neuraxial anesthesia is contraindicated. Fluid requirements may be excessive secondary to fluid loss into the bowel wall causing massive third spacing of fluid.[63] Thus, adequate vascular access needs to be established prior to surgical incision. Blood loss is usually minimal, but blood products and 5% albumin should be available prior to the start of the operation.

RETINOPATHY OF PREMATURITY

Retinopathy of prematurity (ROP) is a proliferative vitreoretinopathy of preterm infants. The precise pathways that regulate apoptosis of normal neuronal and vascular development of the retina and subsequent aberrant retinal vascularization in ocular development remain uncertain. Low birth weight, gestational age, and hyperoxia are significant risk factors for the development of ROP. Other risk factors include respiratory distress, bradycardia, PDA, sepsis, transfusion, multiple births, white race, jaundice, and intraventricular hemorrhage (IVH).[64] Premature infants born prior to 30 weeks' gestation or less than 1500 g are at risk of developing ROP. These at-risk neonates should have a complete ocular examination starting at 4 to 6 weeks after delivery and at biweekly intervals thereafter until retinal vascular maturation. If threshold ROP is identified, laser treatment with peripheral retinal ablation should be instituted within 72 hours of diagnosis.[65,66]

Laser treatment for ROP in the NICU requires general anesthesia, again, likely with a TIVA. To complete the procedure in the NICU, an environment is needed where the lights can be dimmed to facilitate the ocular exam. Additionally, appropriate eye protection must be provided to all health care providers in proximity to the laser. Heart rate decelerations and apnea with oxygen desaturations are frequent complications, which often resolve with cessation of eye manipulation. However, the vital signs may not recover spontaneously, thus requiring pharmacologic intervention and bag-mask ventilation. Often, the apneas and bradycardias may continue into the postoperative period, requiring additional monitoring and interventions.[67]

SUMMARY

Unstable critically ill patients frequently need surgical interventions for either diagnostic or therapeutic purposes. These procedures may often be performed at the bedside within the ICU, based on the principle of relocating OR resources to the patient in order to provide a safe environment for the unstable patient.

Total intravenous anesthesia is the anesthetic technique of choice, and patients should be monitored to the same standards as patients undergoing anesthesia in the OR. The anesthesiologists must familiarize themselves with the bedside monitors in the ICU, gather drugs and supplies into a convenient place prior to starting the anesthetic, and ensure readiness of all personnel. When one is prepared to provide complex anesthetic care in the ICU to the most critically ill of patients, it is a satisfying and rewarding experience.

REFERENCES

1. Warren J, Fromm RE, Orr RA, et al. Guidelines for the inter- and intrahospital transport of critically ill patients. *Crit Care Med.* 2004;32:256–262.
2. Schwebel C, Clec'h C, Magne S, et al. Safety of intrahospital transport in ventilated critically ill patients: a multicenter cohort study. *Crit Care Med.* 2013;41:1919–1928.
3. American Society of Anesthesiologists. Standards for basic anesthetic monitoring, 2015. Available at: http://www.asahq.org/quality-and-practice-management/standards-guidelines-and-related-resources/standards-for-basic-anesthetic-monitoring. Accessed on March 1, 2018.
4. Sidi A, Yusim Y. Anesthesia in the ICU. In: Gabrielli A, Layon AJ, Yu M, eds. *Civetta, Taylor and Kirby's Critical Care.* 4th ed. Philadelphia, PA: Lippincott Williams and Wilkins; 2009:575–608.
5. Cahill NE, Dhaliwal R, Day AG, et al. Nutrition therapy in the critical care setting: what is "best achievable" practice? An international multicenter observational study. *Crit Care Med.* 2010;38:395–401.
6. American Society of Anesthesiologists Committee. Practice guidelines for preoperative fasting and the use of pharmacologic agents to reduce the risk of pulmonary aspiration: application to healthy patients undergoing elective procedures: an updated report by the American Society of Anesthesiologists Committee on Standards and Practice Parameters. *Anesthesiology.* 2011;114:495–511.
7. Alkhawaja S, Martin C, Butler R, et al. Post-pyloric versus gastric tube feeding for preventing pneumonia and improving nutritional outcomes in critically ill adults. *Cochrane Database Syst Rev.* 2015;(22):CD008096.
8. Jiyong J, Tiancha H, Huiqin W. Effect of gastric versus post-pyloric feeding on the incidence of pneumonia in critically ill patients: observations from traditional and Bayesian random-effects meta-analysis. *Clin Nutr.* 2013;32:8–15.
9. Gonik N, Tassler A, Ow TJ, et al. Randomized controlled trial assessing the feasibility of shortened fasts in intubated ICU patients undergoing tracheotomy. *Otolaryngol Head Neck Surg.* 2016;154:87–93.
10. Michard F. Changes in arterial pressure during mechanical ventilation. *Anesthesiology.* 2005;103:419–428.
11. Cannesson M, Desebbe O, Rosamel P, et al. Pleth variability index to monitor the respiratory variations in the pulse oximeter plethysmographic waveform amplitude and predict fluid responsiveness in the operating theatre. *Br J Anaesth.* 2008;101:200–206.
12. McGuinness S, Parke R. Using cardiac output monitoring to guide perioperative haemodynamic therapy. *Curr Opin Crit Care.* 2015;21:364–368.
13. Spencer KT, Kimura BJ, Korcarz CE, et al. Focused cardiac ultrasound: recommendations from the American Society of Echocardiography. *J Am Soc Echocardiogr.* 2013;26:567–581.
14. Field LC, Guldan GJ III, Finley AC. Echocardiography in the intensive care unit. *Semin Cardiothorac Vasc Anesth.* 2011;15:25–39.
15. Soifer BE. Procedural anesthesia at the bedside. *Crit Care Clin.* 2000;16:7–28.
16. Barr J, Fraser GL, Puntillo K, et al. Clinical practice guidelines for the management of pain, agitation, and delirium in adult patients in the intensive care unit. *Crit Care Med.* 2013;41:263–306.
17. Gill KV, Volis SA, Chenault GA, et al. Perceived versus actual sedation practices in adult intensive care unit patients receiving mechanical ventilation. *Ann Pharmacother.* 2012;46:1331–1339.
18. Yassin SM, Terblanche M, Yassin J, et al. A web-based survey of United Kingdom sedation practice in the intensive care unit. *J Crit Care.* 2015;30:436.e1–e6.

19. Payen JF, Chanques G, Mantz J, et al. Current practices in sedation and analgesia for mechanically ventilated critically ill patients. *Anesthesiology.* 2007;106:687–695.
20. Ehieli E, Yalamuri S, Brudney CS, et al. Analgesia in the surgical intensive care unit. *Postgrad Med J.* 2017;93:38–45.
21. Krajčová A, Waldauf P, Anděl M, et al. Propofol infusion syndrome: a structured review of experimental studies and 153 published case reports. *Crit Care.* 2015;19:398.
22. Feng AY, Kaye AD, Kaye RJ, Belani K, Urman RD. Novel propofol derivatives and implications for anesthesia practice. *J Anaesthesiol Clin Pharmacol.* 2017;33(1):9–15.
23. Diaz JH, Prabhakar A, Urman RD, Kaye AD. Propofol infusion syndrome: a retrospective analysis at a level 1 trauma center. *Crit Care Res Pract.* 2014;2014:346968. doi: 10.1155/2014/346968.
24. Pandharipande P, Shintani A, Peterson J, et al. Lorazepam is an independent risk factor for transitioning to delirium in intensive care unit patients. *Anesthesiology.* 2006;104:21–26.
25. Steiner LA. Postoperative delirium. Part 1: pathophysiology and risk factors. *Eur J Anaesthesiol.* 2011;28:628–636.
26. Annane D. ICU physicians should abandon the use of etomidate. *Intensive Care Med.* 2005;31:325–326.
27. Tanious MK, Beutler SS, Kaye AD, Urman RD. New Hypnotic Drug Development and Pharmacologic Considerations for Clinical Anesthesia. *Anesthesiol Clin.* 2017;35(2):e95–e113. doi: 10.1016/j.anclin.2017.01.017.
28. Cuthbertson BH, Sprung CL, Annane D. The effects of etomidate on adrenal responsiveness and mortalitiy in patients with septic shock. *Intensive Care Med.* 2009;35:1868–1876.
29. Umunna BP, Tekwani K, Barounis D. Ketamine for continuous sedation of mechanically ventilated patients. *J Emerg Trauma Shock.* 2015;8:11–15.
30. Vadivelu N, Schermer E, Kodumudi V, Belani K, Urman RD, Kaye AD. Role of ketamine for analgesia in adults and children. *J Anaesthesiol Clin Pharmacol.* 2016;32(3):298–306.
31. Martin E, Ramsay G, Mantz J, Sum-Ping STJ. The role of the alpha2-adrenoceptor agonst dexmedetomidine in postsurgical sedation in the intensive care unit. *J Intensive Care Med.* 2003; 18:29–41.
32. Aydogan MS, Korkmaz MF, Ozgul U, et al. Pain, fentanyl consumption and delirium in adolescents after scoliosis surgery: dexmedetomidine versus midazolam. *Pediatr Anaesth.* 2013;23:446–452.
33. Blanié A, Ract C, Leblanc PE. The limits of succinylcholine for critically ill patients. *Anesth Analg.* 2012;115:873–879.
34. Greenberg SB, Vender J. The use of neuromuscular blocking agents in the ICU: where are we now? *Crit Care Med.* 2013;41:1332–1344.
35. Warr J, Thiboutot Z, Rose L, et al. Current therapeutic uses, pharmacology, and clinical considerations of neuromuscular blocking agents for critically ill adults. *Ann Pharmacother.* 2011;45:1116–1126.
36. Díaz-Regañón G, Miñambres E, Ruiz A, et al. Safety and complications of percutaneous tracheostomy in a cohort of 800 mixed ICU patients. *Anaesthesia.* 2008;63:1198–1203.
37. Jaffe RA, Samuels SI, Schmiesing CA, Golianu B, eds. *Anesthesiologist's Manual of Surgical Procedures.* 4th ed. Philadelphia, PA: Lippincott Williams and Wilkins; 2009.
38. Yarmus L, Gilbert C, Lechtzin N. Safety and feasibility of interventional pulmonologists performing bedside percutaneous endoscopic gastrostomy tube placement. *Chest.* 2013;144:436–440.
39. Anselmi A, Flécher E, Corbineau H, et al. Survival and quality of life after extracorporeal life support for refractory cardiac arrest: a case series. *J Thorac Cardiovasc Surg.* 2015;150:947–954.
40. Extracorporeal Life Support Organization. *ELSO Guidelines for Cardiopulmonary Extracorporeal Life Support.* Ver. 1.3. Ann Arbor, MI: Extracorporeal Life Support Organization; 2013.
41. Annich GM, Lynch WR, MacLaren G, Wilson JM, Bartlett RH, eds. *Extracorporeal Cardiopulmonary Support in Critical Care.* 4th ed. Ann Arbor, MI: Extracorporeal Life Support Organization; 2012.
42. Cardarelli MG, Young AJ, Griffith B. Use of extracorporeal membrane oxygenation for adults in cardiac arrest (E-CPR): a meta-analysis of observational studies. *ASAIO J.* 2009;55:581–586.
43. McKee M. Operating on critically ill neonates: the OR or the NICU. *Semin Perinatol.* 2004;28:234–239.
44. Beckmann U, Gillies DM, Berenholtz SM, et al. Incidents relating to the intra-hospital transfer of critically ill patients. An analysis of the reports submitted to the Australian incident monitoring study in intensive care. *Intensive Care Med.* 2004;30:1579–1585.
45. Hall NJ, Stanton MP, Kitteringham LJ, et al. Scope and feasibility of operating on the neonatal intensive care unit: 312 cases in 10 years. *Pediatr Surg Int.* 2012;28:1001–1005.
46. Hooven TA, Polin RA. Healthcare-associated infections in the hospitalized neonate: a review. *Early Hum Dev.* 2014;90(suppl 1):S4–S6.
47. Chitty H, Wyllie J. Importance of maintaining the newly born temperature in the normal range from delivery to admission. *Semin Fetal Neonatal Med.* 2013;18:362–368.
48. Marks KH, Devenyi AG, Bello ME, et al. Thermal head wrap for infants. *J Pediatr.* 1985;107:956–959.
49. Stothers JK. Head insulation and heat loss in the newborn. *Arch Dis Children.* 1981;56:530–534.
50. Lunze K, Hamer DH. Thermal protection of the newborn in resource-limited environments. *J Perinatol.* 2012;32:317–324.
51. Knobel R, Holditch-Davis D. Thermoregulation and heat loss prevention after birth and during neonatal intensive-care unit stabilization of extremely low-birthweight infants. *J Obstet Gynecol Neonatal Nurs.* 2007;36:280–287.
52. Carbajal R, Rousset A, Danan C, et al. Epidemiology and treatment of painful procedures in neonates in intensive care units. *JAMA.* 2008;300:60–70.
53. McCann ME, Soriano SG. Progress in anesthesia and management of the newborn surgical patient. *Semin Pediatr Surg.* 2014;23:244–248.
54. Brusseau R, McCann ME. Anaesthesia for urgent and emergency surgery. *Early Hum Dev.* 2010;86:703–714.
55. Brett C, Davis PJ. Anesthesia for general surgery in the neonate. In: Davis PJ, Cladis FP, Motoyama EK, eds. *Smith's Anesthesia for Infants.* 8th ed. Philadelphia, PA: Elsevier; 2011:554–588.
56. Pacifici GM. Clinical pharmacology of fentanyl in preterm infants. A review. *Pediatr Neonatol.* 2015;56:143–148.
57. Clyman RI. Ibuprofen and patent ductus arteriosus. *N Engl J Med.* 2000;343:728–730.
58. Sivanandan S, Agarwal R. Pharmacological closure of patent ductus arteriosus: selecting the agent and route of administration. *Pediatr Drugs.* 2016;18:123–138.
59. Mandhan P, Brown S, Kukkady A, et al. Surgical closure of patent ductus arteriosus in preterm low birth weight infants. *Congenit Heart Dis.* 2009;4:34–37.
60. Stankowski T, Aboul-Hasssan SS, Marczak J, et al. Is thoracoscopic patent ductus arteriosus closure superior to conventional surgery? *Interact Cardiovasc Thorac Surg.* 2015;21:532–538.
61. Janvier A, Martinez JL, Barrington K, et al. Anesthetic technique and postoperative outcome in preterm infants undergoing PDA closure. *J Perinatol.* 2010;30:677–682.
62. Niño DF, Sodhi CP, Hackman DJ. Necrotizing enterocolitis: new insights into pathogenesis and mechanisms. *Nat Rev Gastroenterol Hepatol.* 2016;13:590–600.
63. Papillon S, Castle SL, Gayer CP, et al. Necrotizing enterocolitis: contemporary management and outcomes. *Adv Pediatr.* 2013;60:263–279.
64. Hellström A, Smith LE, Dammann O. Retinopathy of prematurity. *Lancet.* 2013;382:1445–1457.
65. Fierson WM; American Academy of Pediatrics Section on Ophthalmology; American Academy of Ophthalmology; American Association for Pediatric Ophthalmology and Strabismus; American Association of Certified Orthoptists. Screening examination of premature infants for retinopathy of prematurity. *Pediatrics.* 2013;131:189–195.
66. Houston SK, Wykoff CC, Berrocal AM, et al. Laser treatment for retinopathy of prematurity. *Lasers Med Sci.* 2013;28:683–692.
67. Eipe N, Kim J, Ramsey G, et al. Anesthesia for laser treatment for retinopathy of prematurity—all clear now? *Pediatr Anaesth.* 2008;18:1103–1105.

29 | ELECTROCONVULSIVE THERAPY

LISA ROSS, MD, MBA

INTRODUCTION

Electroconvulsive therapy (ECT) is used in the United States for the treatment of major depression and a limited number of other psychiatric disorders. Patients require general anesthesia and airway management for these procedures, which are most often performed on psychiatric wards or in outpatient facilities. Because many of these patients are elderly and often have comorbidities, the sudden stimulus to the cardiovascular and cerebrovascular systems during this brief procedure creates the potential for several cardiac and neurological complications. Despite this, ECT remains a very safe and well-tolerated procedure for inpatients as well as outpatients, as long as proper preoperative evaluation is performed and there is adherence to safe anesthesia practice guidelines.

EPIDEMIOLOGY

At any given time, 6.7% to 7.6% of the US population above 12 years of age meets the criteria of the Diagnostic and Statistical Manual of Mental Disorders (fifth edition; *DSM-5*) for moderate-to-severe depressive symptoms.[1,2] It is a leading cause of disability, carries an increased mortality risk (primarily as a result of suicide), and in 2000 cost the United States $83 billion, two-thirds of which was related to decreased productivity in and absence from the job site.[3,4] Ohayon published a study in 2006 where 6694 individuals in New York State and California were randomly interviewed by phone and asked questions pertaining to sleep habits and symptoms of depression. Their findings, similar to those published in the National Comorbidity Survey (NCS), indicated depression was more prevalent in women, the unemployed, the less educated, and those divorced or separated and significantly higher in those who were obese. The incidence was overall lower in the nonwhite population.[5] And, although depression is found to be less common in the elderly population, these patients undergo ECT therapy more frequently because it is tolerated better than the side effects of most antidepressants and because it tends to be diagnosed in this group more frequently because such patients are followed by physicians for related and unrelated medical illnesses.[6]

In the 1990s, there was increased focus on the diagnosis and treatment of depression; in fact, the number of patients diagnosed and prescribed medication doubled between 1987 and 1997.[6] Even with such a high prevalence of depression in the general population, the Centers for Disease Control and Prevention/National Center for Health Statistics (CDC/NCHS) study found that only 35.3% of those with the condition actually sought help from a mental health professional. Explanations for this include the continued stigma attached to mental illness, failure to recognize the condition, and medical expenses for therapy and medication.[1] Antidepressant medications, psychotherapy, and ECT are methods of treating this disease, with ECT being the one of the most successful and safest modalities to date.

HISTORY

Electroconvulsive therapy was first used in 1937 in Italy by Cerletti and Bini[7] and then introduced into the United States in the early 1940s. Initially, it was used to treat several types of psychiatric disorders and to subdue unruly inpatients on psychiatric wards, regardless of diagnosis. At that time, ECT was performed by the "unmodified" technique in which patients were conscious and muscle relaxants were not used; the incidence of musculoskeletal complications was as high as 40%. In the 1970s, the treatment began to be considered abusive. Its use declined not only due to an anti-ECT movement, but also due to the advancement in pharmacotherapy, development of better neuroleptics, and the institution of judicial and regulatory restrictions.[8]

Currently, antidepressants are the first line of therapy for those diagnosed with major depression. The first of these drugs were the monoamine oxidase inhibitors (MAOIs), followed by the tricyclic antidepressants (TCAs), and then most recently by the new generation selective serotonin reuptake inhibitors (SSRIs) and the serotonin-norepinephrine reuptake inhibitors (SNRIs). The success rate in the treatment of depression using antidepressants alone is between 65% and 70%; however, none of these medications is without side effects. The TCAs have anticholinergic and cardiac effects that make them difficult to tolerate, especially within the elderly population. The MAOIs often cause orthostatic hypotension, require a tyramine-free diet, and are associated with hypertensive crises and malignant neurolept syndrome. The SSRIs have undesirable sexual side effects, often requiring additional medication to offset these effects.[9] And, antidepressants can take anywhere from 2 weeks to 2 months to demonstrate their efficacy.

Once guidelines for ECT were defined by the American Psychiatric Association (APA) and the procedure was administered safely, the practice regained popularity, and it was discovered to be very successful and well tolerated. A meta-analytic review published in 2004 found ECT alone to be statistically favorable when compared to simulated ECT, placebo, antidepressants in general, and TCAs and MAOIs specifically.[10] Gagne et al. found that the continuation of ECT and long-term antidepressant therapy helped prevent relapse of depression when compared to patients who discontinued ECT and were maintained on antidepressants alone.[11] It is estimated that 100,000 patients receive ECT each year in the United States, and 1 million receive it worldwide. Even though there have not been studies comparing ECT to the SSRIs or SNRIs to date, no trials with these medications have proven them to be better than ECT in the treatment of depression.[12]

INDICATIONS FOR ECT

Indications for ECT are clearly outlined by the APA and are as follows: major depression (unipolar or bipolar) with lack of response to medications; intolerance to medication due to side effects or coexisting conditions; a need for a rapid response in conditions, such as catatonia, psychosis, suicidal ideations, or clinically significant dehydration or malnutrition. Schizophreniform and schizoaffective manic disorders are also treated with ECT[12] (Table 29.1). ECT has also been indicated in patients who previously demonstrated a positive response to ECT. A course of ECT comprises two or three treatments per week, with a usual course of 6–12 treatments over a 3- to 4-week period of time.[12]

MECHANISM OF ACTION

There are many theories regarding the mechanism by which ECT works. One hypothesis is that the seizure itself leads to a flood of neurotransmitters (specifically dopamine and serotonin) into the brain. These neurotransmitters are known to play a role in depression and schizophrenia.[13] Another hypothesis suggests that the seizure activity affects the rate of glucose metabolism and cerebral blood flow to specific regions of the brain.[14] Still others suggest that treatment changes the way in which brain cells communicate at the synaptic level and may even promote the generation of new brain cells.[15] The understanding about why ECT creates a positive reaction is far from clear, and research is ongoing.

TABLE 29.1. Indications for Electroconvulsive Therapy

Major depression (unipolar or bipolar)
Lack of response to medications
Intolerance to medications due to side effects or coexisting conditions
Need for rapid response due to conditions such as catatonia, psychosis, suicidal ideations, or significant dehydration or malnutrition
Mania
Schizophreniform disorder
Schizoaffective disorder

CARDIOVASCULAR RESPONSES

There are significant hemodynamic changes that occur during ECT. Initially, there is a predictable decrease in heart rate and sometimes brief asystole resulting from the parasympathetic outflow. Following this is an increase in both the systolic and diastolic blood pressures by 25 mm Hg and a 52% increase in heart rate due to sympathetic outflow. Most of these changes resolve within the first 20 minutes following treatment, but in those who remain hypertensive or tachycardic, β-blockers, calcium channel blockers, hydralazine, and sodium nitroprusside have been used successfully to return the blood pressure to normal values.[16] Increased myocardial consumption of oxygen is expected due to the increase in heart rate and inconsequential electrocardiographic (ECG) changes similar to those seen surrounding an intracranial event have been seen and sometimes misdiagnosed as acute subendocardial infarctions.[17]

CEREBRAL RESPONSES

During the induced seizure, cerebral metabolic activity increases, which in turn increases the cerebral blood flow 100%–400% above baseline, leading to an acute rise in cerebral oxygen consumption and resultant increased intracranial pressure (ICP). In the presence of an intracranial lesion, there will be increased edema. For patients with a cerebral aneurysm, hydralazine, sodium nitroprusside, and β-blockers have been used to control swings in blood pressure.[16,18]

NEUROENDOCRINE RESPONSES

Epinephrine, norepinephrine, corticotropin (adrenocorticotropin hormone), arginine vasopressin, and cortisol levels all increase following ECT to varying degrees and peak at different times. The catecholamines that are released from the adrenal medulla and sympathetic nerve endings cause the hypertensive response. Blood samples have shown norepinephrine levels to increase 3-fold and epinephrine levels to increase 15-fold. Norepinephrine levels remain elevated longer than the epinephrine levels.[19] Corticotropin is immediately released from the pituitary during the seizure itself.[20] Attempts have been made to attenuate these neuroendocrine and cardiovascular responses by pretreatment with fentanyl, labetalol, and esmolol. It was found that fentanyl and esmolol significantly decreased the norepinephrine peak that followed the seizure, but only esmolol decreased the epinephrine secretion. Fentanyl was found to decrease the levels of corticotropin after therapy.[19]

ADMINISTRATION OF THERAPY

In order for ECT to be performed safely, the patient must be rendered unconscious and have the appropriate degree of muscle relaxation. In the past when the "unmodified" technique was employed, there was a significant incidence of vertebral and long-bone fractures. The role of unconsciousness is 2-fold: to prevent the feeling of suffocation after the administration of the muscle relaxant before the stimulus is applied and to prevent recall of the procedure in patients who do not have a seizure and therefore are not amnestic. A generalized seizure is necessary for the ECT to exert its antidepressant effects.[21]

After monitors have been applied, baseline vital signs are obtained, and intravenous access is established. An induction agent is administered followed by a short- to intermediate-acting muscle relaxant after unconsciousness is confirmed. The patient is ventilated or hyperventilated with 100% oxygen, usually administered by mask, until muscle relaxation is confirmed; then, a bite block is inserted to prevent damage to the teeth. Several techniques have been employed to track the point of maximal muscle relaxation. A nerve stimulator can be used to follow the train-of-four ratio; one can use the cessation of fasciculations as a sign of relaxation (more difficult to determine in the elderly patient) or decrease of the knee, ankle, or plantar withdrawal reflexes.

The goal is to induce a generalized motor seizure that lasts at least 25 seconds and a central electroencephalogram (EEG) seizure that lasts at least 40 seconds at a stimulus dose of approximately 50–100 joules of energy with approximate voltage of 150–200 V.[22] The therapeutic seizure involves the entire brain, from the point of contact on the scalp, deep into the brain, and then spreading to both cortices. It is delivered either unilaterally on the nondominant hemisphere or bilaterally. Contrary to previous beliefs, the success of the therapy is not directly related to the length of the seizure; however seizures lasting less than 25 seconds are considered subtherapeutic. ECT is administered by either a brief pulse stimulus or a sine wave. Although the efficacy has been found to be equivalent, administering a sine wave stimulus causes more cognitive dysfunction.[12] Thymatron DGx (Somatics, Inc., Lake Bluff, IL) is a commonly used machine that administers the stimulus and records the EEG.

If a seizure of desirable length is not elicited, the stimulus can be increased for the subsequent treatment, or, providing the patient is still anesthetized and relaxed, an additional stimulus can be applied immediately. In the past, caffeine was used to increase seizure length,[23] but with more recent review of the issue, evidence of its efficacy is lacking, and most psychiatrists have abandoned this practice. When using the "cuff" technique, a blood pressure cuff is inflated above the systolic blood pressure just prior to the administration of the intravenous medications. If a limb is isolated (cuff technique) prior to the administration of the muscle relaxant, that limb can be used as a guide to determine when the motor seizure begins and ends. Recording of the EEG is more reliable and is usually longer than the motor seizure. Blood pressure, oxygen saturation, and ECG are recorded at regular intervals.

Once it is established that the seizure is complete, the patient is again ventilated by mask until spontaneous respirations resume. Only after the patient is hemodynamically stable, has a clear patent airway, and does not appear unusually restless or disoriented is intravenous access discontinued. The patient is recovered by a registered nurse either in the same room or in a separate postanesthesia care unit (PACU). The PACU is equipped as mandated by American Society of Anesthesiologists (ASA) guidelines. Although there might be some postprocedure confusion, the patient should be able to answer basic questions correctly before discharge from the PACU.

SIDE EFFECTS

Side effects include loss of retrograde memory (recall of events before treatment) or anterograde memory (inability to retain new memories), cognitive dysfunction, headache, and nausea and vomiting. The incidence of memory loss is affected by the placement of the electrodes, the type of stimulus administered, and the age of the patient. Fasciculations that occur from the administration of succinylcholine can lead to myalgias.[12]

CONTRAINDICATIONS

The most recent APA guidelines of 2001 state that there are no absolute contraindications to ECT. It had been previously stated that an increase in ICP was a contraindication; however, most recently it is among those conditions that only present an increased risk of complications. It can be performed safely with tight control of blood pressure and the appropriate monitoring and anesthetic management. ECT has been administered safely in patients with Parkinson disease, seizure disorders, and pacemakers and is the treatment of choice for depressed or psychotic patients when in the first trimester of pregnancy. There are conditions that place patients at increased risk for ECT, such as recent myocardial infarction, recent cerebrovascular accident, ASA 4 classification, unstable or severe cardiovascular disease (severe valvular or uncompensated congestive heart failure), cerebral aneurysm, or atrioventricular (AV) malformation.[12]

ECT SETTING

Electroconvulsive therapy is administered usually to inpatients in psychiatric wards and occasionally to outpatients who receive maintenance less frequently. Inpatients are fasted overnight, and the procedures usually take place in the morning to prevent violations of the nothing by mouth restriction with patients who are impaired or have difficulty with memory.[12] There is usually a separate procedure or treatment room on the inpatient ward designated for the administration of ECT. The room is equipped with stretcher, oxygen source, continuous suction, positive pressure ventilation device, standard ASA monitors, medications, and an EEG stimulus machine, which often has an incorporated EEG monitor. ECT is performed only by a psychiatrist.

Electroconvulsive therapy has been regulated by the Food and Drug Administration only to the extent that the device itself is regulated and categorized as "medical equipment." Early in 2016, there were proposals put forth to regulate the procedure more closely. ECT is not a required subject in medical schools in the United States but is a required skill in accredited psychiatric residency training programs. Privileging for ECT practice at institutions is a local option; no national certification standards are established, and no ECT-specific continuing training experiences are required of ECT practitioners,[23] and ECT clinical training is not a required rotation in anesthesia residency programs.[12]

PREPROCEDURE EVALUATION

The role of the anesthesiologist in the evaluation and treatment of the patient for ECT is the same as that for any patient who will undergo general anesthesia. The anesthesiologist interviews the patient; performs an appropriate physical examination, concentrating on airway assessment; and reviews the medical history and pertinent laboratory data.[16] Any patient at increased risk for ECT should be identified and the appropriate consultations performed. ECGs are advisable in patients over the age of 50 as this group is most at risk for major cardiac complications.

MONITORING

Standard monitors include ECG, a manual or automatic blood pressure device, and a pulse oximeter throughout the procedure and into the recovery stage. Additionally, the ASA, in its "Standards for Basic Monitoring," states that the adequacy of ventilation must be evaluated in all patients receiving general anesthesia. Because patients receiving ECT are usually ventilated by mask, qualitative clinical signs such as chest excursions are acceptable. However, in cases where an endotracheal tube or laryngeal device is inserted, proof of adequate ventilation must be measured quantitatively with a continuous end-tidal carbon dioxide monitor.[24] Table 29.2 lists the required and recommended equipment and medications that should be available when performing ECT. In the event of a complication that would require intubation and transport to another location for continued care, a long-acting sedative and an intermediate-acting muscle relaxant are included.

Use of a laryngeal airway for ECT has been suggested as it reduces hypercarbia when compared to mask ventilation and provides a viable alternative when mask fit is difficult. ASA monitoring standards recommend quantitative CO_2 monitoring when using an endotracheal tube or supraglottic airway device, in which case a portable monitor or CO_2 detector is adequate.[25]

TABLE 29.2. Required and recommended equipment and medications that should be available when performing ECT

Required Equipment
Ambu bag with oxygen supply
Device that administers positive pressure ventilation via mask (this can be the Ambu bag)
Either heparin lock or infusing intravenous bag for intravenous access
Continuous electrocardiography monitor
Pulse oximeter
Automatic or manual blood pressure cuff
Continuous suction
Laryngoscope
Oral airway
Endotracheal tube
Bite block
Resources to maintain the airway for prolonged period of time if necessary
Required Medications
Induction agent
Muscle relaxant
Anticonvulsant
Sympathomimetic (atropine or glycopyrrolate)
Suggested Equipment
Laryngeal mask airway/King airway
Nerve stimulator
Suggested Medications
Beta-Blocker
Long-acting sedative appropriate for intramuscular injection
Intermediate-acting muscle relaxant

PREMEDICATION AND MEDICATION INTERACTIONS

The initial parasympathetic discharge can cause severe bradycardia and even asystole. Glycopyrrolate is often administered intramuscularly in a dose of 0.2–0.4 mg as a premedication at least 30 minutes before the scheduled procedure or can be given intravenously just prior to the induction agent in the dose of 0.2–0.4 mg. Its antisialogogue properties are also advantageous as the parasympathetic outflow causes increased salivation.[12] Some criticize the routine use of an anticholinergic before treatment as it may lead to an increased heart rate, which could lead to myocardial ischemia in those with cardiac disease. Glycopyrrolate causes less heart rate increase than atropine and is preferable.

Medications that should be held prior to ECT include the anticonvulsants and benzodiazepines as they increase the seizure threshold and lithium as it is associated with increased confusion post-ECT. It was previously recommended that MAOIs be discontinued 2 weeks before the first treatment due to concerns about wide fluctuations in blood pressure, especially if pressors are needed during therapy. More recently, patients have been maintained on MAOIs without adverse reactions. One should continue dosing of antidepressants and antipsychotics as they decrease the seizure threshold. Cardiac and antihypertensive medications should be continued as well.[26]

INDUCTION AGENTS

Ideally, the induction agent should be short acting, impart hemodynamic stability, cost little, have few side effects, and maintain or lower the seizure threshold. However, almost all general anesthetics impart some antiepileptic activity. Currently, the barbiturate methohexital is the medication against which all others are compared. Sodium pentothal, ketamine, etomidate, propofol, and the inhalational agent sevoflurane have all been used with varying results. Table 29.3 shows the different induction agents and recommended doses. Sodium pentothal was the first medication used as it was the only intravenous induction agent. When methohexital, a newer barbiturate, was developed, it became more popular because it had slightly less anticonvulsant activity than sodium pentothal.[21] Unfortunately, drug shortages, especially in the United States, have made it difficult to acquire methohexital or sodium pentothal.

Propofol, which is used frequently, is associated with reduced cardiovascular response due to its direct myocardial depression and vasodilator properties.[27] Although the seizures were found to be shorter and the threshold increased, the efficacy was similar to the barbiturates. It has been suggested that propofol is the medication of choice in patients who experience prolonged seizures with methohexital or in patients who suffer with postprocedure nausea and vomiting.[28] Propofol has demonstrated an earlier return to cognitive function when compared to methohexital while allowing comparable seizure quality.[29]

TABLE 29.3. *Intravenous sedative and analgesic agents used for ECT.*

INDUCTION AGENT	DOSAGE
Methohexital	0.5–1.0 mg/kg
Propofol	1.0–1.5 mg/kg
Pentothal	2–3 mg/kg
Etomidate	0.15–0.30 mg/kg
Ketamine	2–3 mg/kg
Remifentanil + methohexital or propofol	1 μg/kg + methohexital 0.5–0.75 mg/kg or propofol 0.5–1 mg/kg
Fentanyl	1.5 μg/kg + methohexital 0.5–0.75 mg/kg or propofol 0.5–1 mg/kg
Alfentanil	10–25 μg/kg + methohexital 0.5–0.75 mg/kg or propofol 0.5—1 mg/kg
Remifentanil alone	4–8 μg/kg[42]

In a double-blind comparison of etomidate, propofol, and sodium pentothal in patients without previous cardiovascular disease, Rosa et al. found that the three had similar cardiovascular effects with respect to blood pressure and heart rate.[30] Grati et al. had similar findings when they compared propofol and etomidate.[31] The conclusion is that all three can be used safely in patients without preexisting myocardial disease as the hemodynamics are similar.[30,31]

Opioids are known to blunt autonomic responses to noxious stimuli, and they lack anticonvulsant activity. Remifentanil has been studied alone and in combination with methohexital and propofol to compare hemodynamic effects, seizure length, and cognitive function. In a study of 110 ECT treatments, Irefin et al. showed that when remifentanil was added to a hypnotic dose of methohexital, the hemodynamic effects of the sympathetic discharge was reduced significantly when compared to methohexital alone.[32] Current evidence shows that remifentanil alone or in combination with another agent might even lower the seizure threshold, therefore allowing for lower absolute electrical doses, imparting longer seizures, leading to comparable recovery times, and when given in appropriately large doses, blunting the hemodynamic response. It is the medication recommended in patients who when treated with methohexital remain refractory despite maximum stimulus.[21,33] Unlike methohexital, there is no increase in seizure threshold from treatment to treatment with remifentanil.[33] To date, there have not been extensive prospective studies on the efficacy and cognitive side effects when using the opioid regimen.[21]

In recent years, there has been interest in neuroprotection, which is equated with improved cognitive function post-ECT. Ketamine has been known for its cognitive-sparing properties and is a "proconvulsant," but because it causes transitory psychotic episodes, it is an undesirable choice for ECT.[21] Ketamine, which had been used in the past and fell out of favor, has made a resurgence in both the area of pain management and anesthesia in general. In its current clinical usage, ketamine is administered as an intravenous racemic mixture; however, the development of the (S) isomer, which has fewer psychomimetic affects and is more potent,[21,34,35] has led to renewed interest in this drug on many fronts. Research on ketamine and its neuroprotective quality in preliminary studies demonstrated shorter reorientation times posttreatment when compared to methohexital.[36] There has been discussion regarding the use of ketamine with ECT to enhance the antidepressant effects of ECT as ketamine is an NMDA receptor antagonist. However, studies have not supported this theory.[37]

Sevoflurane in concentrations of 5%–8% has been evaluated as an induction agent for ECT. This method is particularly useful in patients who are agitated or uncooperative, making intravenous access a great challenge. Sevoflurane has been compared to sodium pentothal, methohexital, etomidate, and propofol, with varying and conflicting results. Rasmussen et al. compared hemodynamic changes, seizure length, and postictal recovery between sodium pentothal and sevoflurane. They found that although the hemodynamics were similar, the postictal orientation 20 minutes after therapy was superior with sevoflurane. Furthermore, even though patients who received sevoflurane had shorter motor and EEG-recorded seizures when compared to those receiving sodium pentothal, the length still remained within the therapeutic range of seizures seen with the more commonly used medication methohexital.[21,38,39] In another study where the hemodynamics of sevoflurane and sodium pentothal were compared, the rate pressure product increased for both but was attenuated the most with 2MAC sevoflurane.[40] The overall conclusions support sevoflurane as a comparable alternative to sodium pentothal. Propofol and sevoflurane have been compared, with findings inconsistent with respect to seizure length.[41,42] But, with respect to hemodynamics, two studies found that the pulse and heart rate increased more with sevoflurane than with propofol, emphasizing cautious use in patients with ischemic heart disease.[41,43]

MUSCLE RELAXATION

During ECT, the appropriate degree of muscle relaxation is required in order to minimize the motor component of the seizure. Like the induction agent, a short-acting medication that imparts hemodynamic stability and has few side effects is ideal. Because of its desirable properties, succinylcholine in a dose of 0.5–1.0 mg/kg IV is the most frequently used muscle relaxant. For those patients in whom succinylcholine is contraindicated—those with pseudocholinesterase deficiency, a history of malignant hyperthermia, or concerns of hyperkalemia—an intermediate-acting muscle relaxant administered in doses that can easily be reversed is used. However, it is imperative that consciousness is not regained prior to complete reversal.

To ensure maximum muscle relaxation, an accelomyography device is the most reliable instrument available. Less-sophisticated clinical signs include the cessation of muscle fasciculations or the ablation of deep tendon reflexes.

SPECIAL CONDITIONS

PREGNANCY

Electroconvulsive therapy is safe for both the pregnant patient and the fetus. In most cases, it is the treatment of choice, especially during the first trimester when organogenesis occurs. However, it is not without complications. In 300 cases of pregnant patients who received ECT, 28 had complications, consisting of transient fetal arrhythmias, abdominal pain, mild vaginal bleeding, and self-limited contractions. As pregnancy progresses, there is increased risk of aspiration, hypotension due to aortocaval compression, and respiratory alkalosis.[44] Therefore, preparations should include hydration, aspiration prophylaxis and rapid sequence induction and intubation (if indicated), uterine tilt, and vigilance in avoiding hyperventilation. In the third trimester, one should consider tocodynamometry and pelvic examination.[44,45]

OBESITY

A retrospective review looked at ECT performed on obese patients (body mass index [BMI] > 29) in two major medical centers. Fifty obese patients received 660 ECT treatments using methohexital and succinylcholine. Patients were supine with the back elevated 15°–30° and were fasted overnight. No clinical cases of aspiration were recorded, leading to the conclusion that it is safe to anesthetize obese patients for ECT without aspiration prophylaxis or tracheal intubation.[46]

A study by Folk and coworkers in 2000 suggested that aspiration prophylaxis should be considered in obese patients undergoing ECT.[47] If one is to strictly follow the guidelines for patients with a full stomach, then a rapid sequence induction with cricoid pressure and tracheal intubation must follow. This would subject the patient to laryngoscopy and intubation two to three times per week, possibly leading to the associated sore throat, swelling, and other forms of airway trauma. As well, the stimulation during laryngoscopy and intubation would produce a greater cardiovascular response.[46] This remains a controversial issue that deserves further investigation.

PACEMAKERS

There is a lack of consensus when it comes to the management of patients with pacemakers. There is concern that during administration of the electrical stimulus itself or the fasciculations that result from succinylcholine there could be malfunctioning of the device. Two retrospective studies suggested that these concerns are unwarranted. Despite this, there is no common agreement regarding how to program pacemakers so function is maintained. The American College of Cardiology/American Heart Association (ACC/AHA) have specific recommendations for patients with pacemakers who will undergo ECT: determine the reason for pacemaker insertion, assess the comorbidities, and interrogate the device before the procedure.[48]

In one retrospective study, 10 patients with pacemakers had undergone 147 treatments. All had dual-chamber pacemakers, and nine had a rate-responsive device. Sodium pentothal or propofol and succinylcholine were used for all treatments, and none of the pacemakers was reprogrammed or disabled beforehand. In 146 of the 147 treatments, there was no malfunction of the pacemaker or instability hemodynamically. One treatment resulted in asystole as recorded on the ECG and was later attributed to artifact.[49]

Although magnets are used frequently during surgery, pacemaker response can be unreliable and often depends on the age of the battery. In a retrospective study by Dolenc et al., 493 treatments were administered to patients with pacemakers and implantable cardioversion/defibrillators undergoing ECT. None of the pacemaker settings was altered preprocedure, yet there was no disturbance in pacemaker function. It should be noted that all patients had evaluation of the pacemaker or defibrillator device before and after each treatment.[50]

Therefore, studies have borne out that ECT can be administered safely to patient with pacemakers or defibrillator devices if evaluated by a cardiologist beforehand and there is verification of a properly functioning pacemaker.

MORBIDITY AND MORTALITY

When ECT was first introduced, it had a mortality rate of 0.1% (1 per 1000 treatments) and a complication rate as high as 40%. Complications included laryngospasm, circulatory insufficiency, tooth damage, vertebral compression fractures, status epilepticus, peripheral nerve palsy, skin burns, prolonged apnea, and arrhythmias.[8] Today, the mortality-related death rate is 1 per 10,000 patients or 1 per 80,000 treatments. The majority of complications fall into three categories (cardiac, respiratory, or prolonged seizure activity) and occur either during treatment or immediately following treatment. The majority of deaths involve cardiovascular events.[12]

In a retrospective study of 2279 patients who underwent 17,394 ECT treatments, 0.92% of the patients (21 patients) had some type of complication during their first series of treatments, the vast majority of complications being arrhythmias. There were no permanent or irreversible complications, and none of the deaths that occurred within 30 days following treatment was directly related to the therapy itself. When prolonged seizure was removed from the statistics, the complication rate fell to 0.6% per series and 0.08% per treatment. Patients ranged in age from 43 to 74 years, with the majority being ASA classification 3. As well, all of the patients who had cardiac-related events had underlying heart disease.[51]

Arrhythmias are the most common complications seen with ECT. These arrhythmias are benign and most often resolve spontaneously. One must evaluate the degree of risk relative to the potential benefits of ECT (Table 29.4), even in those ASA class 4 patients.[12] Huuhka et al. used Holter monitoring 24 pre- and 24 hours post-ECT treatment to record the incidence of arrhythmia. They observed the most common arrhythmias postprocedure (described as nonmalignant or transient) were as frequent as those observed preprocedure.[52]

Case reports have documented pulmonary embolism, acute embolic stroke, complications in a patient with severe aortic stenosis, and negative pressure pulmonary edema following ECT.[53–56] Table 29.5 indicates the physiological consequences of ECT. However, these complications are rare and can be maintained at a minimum provided there is (1) adequate preprocedure evaluation and recognition of medical conditions that, when possible, are optimized; (2) recognition of comorbidities in the population treated; (3) maintenance of safe anesthetic techniques; and (4) the ability to transfer patients or have backup services if a complication does occur. Because of its short procedure time, low incidence of major cardiac complications, and absence of fluid shifts, ECT remains a "low-risk" procedure according to the 2007 guidelines issued by the ACC/AHA.[48]

TABLE 29.4. Those at Increased Risk During ECT

Recent myocardial infarction
Recent cerebrovascular accident
Increased intracranial pressure
Valvular heart disease
Uncompensated congestive heart failure
Pheochromocytoma
Angina
Intracranial mass
Recent intracranial surgery

TABLE 29.5. Physiologic Consequences of Electroconvulsive Therapy

Cerebral effects
Increased cerebral oxygen consumption
Increased cerebral blood flow
Increased intracranial pressure
Cardiovascular effects
Immediate parasympathetic stimulation
Bradycardia
Hypotension
Possible asystole
Late (after 1 minute): sympathetic stimulation
Tachycardia
Hypertension
Dysthymias
Increased cardiac output
Increased myocardial consumption
ST and T wave changes on electrocardiogram
Neuroendocrine effects
Elevated levels of corticotropin, cortisol
Elevated levels of catecholamines
Effect on plasma glucose level
Miscellaneous
Musculoskeletal pain and trauma
Increased intragastric pressure
Increased intraocular pressure

SOURCE: From Russell GB. *Alternate-Site Anesthesia*. New York, NY: Elsevier; 1997.

INFORMED CONSENT

Electroconvulsive therapy is unique in that one consent is obtained for a series of treatments that will be administered over an undetermined period of time. This practice is more feasible especially when a health care proxy is involved. It is imperative that the patient or health care proxy understand that consent can be withdrawn at any time. In institutions where separate anesthesia consents are the practice, permission must be obtained by a privileged or authorized anesthesia provider and should encompass the series of treatments planned.[12]

REFERENCES

1. Pratt LA, Brody DJ. *Depression in the United States Household Population, 2009-2012.* Hyattsville, MD: National Center for Health Statistics; 2014. NCHS Data Brief, Number 172..
2. National Institute of Mental Health. Major depression among adults. Available at: https://www.nimh.nih.gov/health/statistics/prevalence/major-depression-among-adults.shtml. n.d. Accessed on December 19, 2016.
3. Cuijpers P, Smit F. Excess mortality in depression: a meta-analysis of community studies. *J Affect Disord.* 2002;72:227–236.
4. Greenberg PE, Kessler RC, Birnbaum HG, et al. The economic burden of depression in the United States: how did it change between 1990 and 2000? *J Clin Psychiatry.* 2003;64(12):1465–1475.
5. Ohayon MM. Epidemiology of depression and its treatment in the general population. *J Psychiatr Res.* 2007;41:207–213.
6. Olfson M, Marcus SC, Druss B, Elinson L, Tanielian T, Pincus HA. National trends in the outpatient treatment of depression. *JAMA.* 2002;287:203–209.
7. Abrams R. *Electroconvulsive Therapy.* New York, NY: Oxford University Press; 1997.
8. National Institutes of Health, National Institute of Mental Health. *Electroconvulsive Therapy: Consensus Development Conference Statement.* Washington, DC: National Institutes of Health; June 1985.
9. Cipriana A, Furukawa TA, Salanti G, et al. Comparative efficacy and acceptability of 12 new-generation antidepressants: a multiple-treatments meta-analysis. *Lancet.* 2009;373:746–758.
10. Pagnin D, Queiroz V, Pini S, et al. Efficacy of electroconvulsive therapy in depression: a meta-analytic review. *J ECT.* 2004;20:13–20.
11. Gagne G, Furman M, Carpenter L, Price LH. Efficacy of continuation ECT and antidepressant drugs compared to long-term antidepressants alone. *Am J Psychiatry.* 2000;157:1960–1965.
12. Jaffe E. *The Practice of Electroconvulsive Therapy: Recommendations for Treatment, Training and Privileging: A Task Force Report of the American Psychiatric Association.* 2nd ed. Washington, DC: American Psychiatric Association; 2001.
13. Grover S, Mattoo SK, Gupta N. Theories on mechanism of action of electroconvulsive therapy. *German J Psychiatry.* 2005;8:70–84.
14. Sackheim H. The anticonvulsant hypothesis of the mechanisms of action of ECT: current status. *J ECT.* 1999;15(1):5–26.
15. O'Connor MK. Hypotheses regarding the mechanism of action of electroconvulsive therapy, past and present. *Psychiatry Ann.* 1998;23:15.
16. Tess AV, Smetana GV. Medical evaluation of patients undergoing electroconvulsive therapy. *N Engl J Med.* 2009;306:1437–1444.
17. Burch GE, Meyers R, Abildskov JA. A new electrocardiographic pattern observed in cerebrovascular accidents. *Circulation.* 1954;9:719.
18. Gaines GY, Rees D, Ian MD. Anesthetic considerations for electroconvulsive therapy. *South Med J.* 1993;85:5.
19. Weinger MB, Partridge BL, Hauger R, et al. Prevention of cardiovascular and neuroendocrine response to electroconvulsive therapy: II. Effects of pretreatment regimens on catecholamine, ACTH, vasopressin and cortisol. *Anesth Analg.* 1991;73:563–569.
20. Allen J, Denney D, Kendall J, et al. Corticotropin release during ECT in man. *Am J Psychiatry.* 1974;131:1225–1228.
21. MacPherson RD, Loo CK. Cognitive impairment following electroconvulsive therapy—does the choice of anesthetic agent make a difference? *J ECT.* 2008;24(1):52–56.
22. Abrams R. *Electroconvulsive Therapy.* 4th ed. New York, NY: Oxford University Press, USA; 2002.
23. Coffey CE, Figiel GS, Weiner RD, et al. Caffeine augmentation of ECT. *Am J Psychiatry.* 1990;147:579–585.
24. Fink M, Taylor AM. Electroconvulsive therapy: evidence and challenges. *JAMA.* 2007;298(3):330–332.
25. Standards for Basic Anesthetic Monitoring. Committee of Origin: Standards and Practice Parameters. (Approved by ASA House of Delegates on October 21, 1986, last amended on October 20, 2010 and last affirmed on October 28, 2015).
26. Fumio N, Makio O, Haruhiko H, et al. Benefits of the laryngeal mask for airway management during electroconvulsive therapy. *J ECT.* 2003;19(4):211–216.
27. Swartz CM, Abrams R. *ECT Instruction Manual.* Lake Bluff, IL: Somatics; 1993.
28. Bailine SH, Petrides G, Doft M, et al. Indications for the use of propofol in electroconvulsive therapy. *J ECT.* 2003;19(3):129–131.
29. Geretsegger C, Nickel M, Judendorfer B, et al. Propofol and methohexital as anesthetic agents for electroconvulsive therapy: a randomized, double-blind comparison of electroconvulsive therapy seizure quality, therapeutic efficacy, and cognitive performance. *J ECT.* 2007;23(4):239–243.
30. Rosa MA, Rosa MO, Marcolin MA, et al. Cardiovascular effects of anesthesia in ECT: a randomized, double-blind comparison of etomidate, propofol and thiopental. *J ECT.* 2007;23(1):6–8.
31. Grati L, Louzi M, Nasr K, et al Compared effects of etomidate and propofol for anaesthesia during electroconvulsive therapy. *Presse Med.* 2005;34:282–284.
32. Irefin SA, Cywinski JB, Samuel SW, et al. The comparative hemodynamic effects of methohexital and remifentanil in electroconvulsive therapy. *Anesthesiology.* 2004;101:A197.
33. Hossain A, Sullivan P. The effects of age and sex on electroconvulsive therapy using remifentanil as the sole anesthetic agent. *J ECT.* 2008;24(3):232–235.
34. Krystal AD, Weiner RD, Dean MD, et al. Comparison of seizure duration, ictal EEG, and cognitive effects of ketamine and methohexital anesthesia with electroconvulsive therapy. *J Neuropsychiatry Clin Neurosci.* 2003;15:27–34.
35. White PF, Schuttler J, Horai Y, et al. Pharmacology of the ketamine isomers. *Br J Anesth.* 1985;57:197–203.
36. Sullivan PM, Sinz EH, Gunel E, et al. A retrospective comparison of remifentanil versus methohexital for anesthesia in electroconvulsive therapy. *J ECT.* 2004;20:219–224.
37. Abdallah CG, Fasula M, Kelmendi B, et al. The rapid antidepressant effect of ketamine in the electroconvulsive therapy setting. *J ECT.* 2012;28(3):157–161.
38. Rasmussen KG, Laurila DR, Brady BM, et al. Anesthesia outcomes in a randomized double-blind trial of sevoflurane and thiopental for induction of general anesthesia in electroconvulsive therapy. *J ECT.* 2007;23(4):236–238.
39. Rasmussen KG, Laurila DR, Brady BM, et al. Seizure length with sevoflurane and thiopental for induction of general anesthesia in electroconvulsive therapy: a randomized double-blind trial. *J ECT.* 2006;22(4):240–242.
40. Tanaka N, Saito Y, Hikawa Y, et al. Effects of thiopental and sevoflurane on hemodynamics during anesthetic management of electroconvulsive therapy. *Masui.* 1997;46(12):1575–1579.
41. Wajima Z, Shiga T, Yoshikawa T, et al. Propofol alone, sevoflurane alone, and combined propofol-sevoflurane anesthesia in electroconvulsive therapy. *Anesth Intensive Care.* 2003;31:396–400.
42. Hodgson RE, Dawson P, Hold AR, et al. Anesthesia for electroconvulsive therapy: a comparison of sevoflurane with propofol. *Anesth Intensive Care.* 2004;32:241–245.
43. Loughnan T, McKenzie G, Leong S. Sevoflurane versus propofol for induction of anesthesia for electroconvulsive therapy: a randomized crossover trial. *Anesth Intensive Care.* 2004;32:236–240.
44. Miller LJ. Use of electroconvulsive therapy during pregnancy. *Hosp Community Psychiatry.* 1994;45(5):444–450.
45. Ferrill MJ, Kehoe WA, Jacisin JJ. ECT during pregnancy: physiologic and pharmacologic considerations. *Convuls Ther.* 1992;8(3):186–200.
46. Kadar AG, Caleb HT, Ing MS, et al. Anesthesia for electroconvulsive therapy in obese patients. *Anesth Analg.* 2002;94:360–361.
47. Folk JW, Kellner CH, Beale MD, et al. Anesthesia for electroconvulsive therapy: a review. *J ECT.* 2000;16:157–1570.
48. Fleisher LA, Beckman JA, Brown KA, et al. ACC/AHA 2007 guidelines on perioperative cardiovascular evaluation and care for noncardiac surgery: executive summary: a report of the American College of Cardiology/American Heart Association Task Force on Practice Guidelines developed in collaboration with the American Society of Echocardiography, American Society of Nuclear Cardiology, Heart Rhythm Society, Society for Cardiovascular Angiography and Interventions, Society for Vascular Medicine and Biology, and Society for Vascular Surgery. *J Am Coll Cardiol.* 2007;50:1707–1732.
49. MacPherson RD, Loo CK, Barrett N. Electroconvulsive therapy in patients with cardiac pacemakers. *Anaesth Intensive Care.* 2006;34(4): 470–474

50. Dolenc T, Barnes R, Hayes D, et al. Electroconvulsive therapy in patients with cardiac pacemakers and implantable cardioverter defibrillators. *PACE*. 2004;27:1257–1263.
51. Nuttall GA, Bowersox MR, Douglass SR, et al. Morbidity and mortality in the use of electroconvulsive therapy. *J ECT*. 2004;20(4):237–241.
52. Huuhka M, Seinela L, Reinikainen P, et al. Cardiac arrhythmias induced by ECT in elderly psychiatric patients: experience with 48-hour Holter monitoring. *J ECT*. 2003;19:22–25.
53. Mamah D, Lammle M, Isenberg KE. Pulmonary embolism after ECT. *J ECT*. 2005;21(1):39–40.
54. Lee K. Acute embolic stroke after electroconvulsive therapy. *J ECT*. 2006;22(1):67–69.
55. Sutor B, Mueller PS, Rasmussen KG. Bradycardia and hypotension in a patient with severe aortic stenosis receiving electroconvulsive therapy dose titration for treatment of depression. *J ECT*. 2008;24(4):281–282.
56. Myers CL, Gopalka A, Glick D, et al. A case of negative-pressure pulmonary edema after electroconvulsive therapy. *J ECT*. 2007;23(4):281–283.

30 | PAIN MANAGEMENT PROCEDURES

CHRISTOPHER V. MAANI, MD, LT COL EDWARD M. LOPEZ, MD

INTRODUCTION

Pain management is the right of every patient and the responsibility of every health care provider. Nowhere is that more obvious than with pain management specialists and with patients seeking assistance at pain clinics across the nation. Often, the patients referred are those with the most severe pain who have failed more conservative approaches or strictly medical (noninterventional) modalities. In other instances, the patients are referred for concerns of comorbidities or lack of pain management resources such as a clinic and procedure room with fluoroscopic capabilities. While the goal for these percutaneous interventions is improved pain control, they should be considered adjuncts and not replacements for a comprehensive pain management strategy. Most patients benefit from multimodal pain medication strategies,[1] physical therapy, stress management and relaxation training, occupational therapy, acupuncture, or other treatment therapies.

This chapter will prove useful to anesthesiologists and nonanesthesiologists alike in providing an overview and discussion of several of the most common pain procedures encountered in clinical pain management practices today. These procedures are listed in Box 30.1. Each procedure is discussed with an initial description of the strategy, including technical aspects, medical indications, and relevant complications important for the pain management physician to understand. This is followed by a section on considerations for anesthetic management. While every attempt will be made to ensure thoroughness, readers are referred to sources such as *Principles and Practice of Pain Medicine, Practical Management of Pain*, or *Pain Medicine: An Essential Review*—all excellent textbooks that provide more information for interventional pain management procedures.[2–4]

BOX 30.1. PAIN PROCEDURES

1. Epidural steroid injections
   a. Cervical
   b. Thoracic
   c. Lumbar
   d. Transforaminal
2. Facet interventions
   a. Diagnostic facet blocks
   b. MBBs
   c. Intra-articular facet injections
   d. Radio-frequency ablation
3. SIJ interventions
   a. SIJ injection
   b. Lateral branch nerve blocks of sacral nerves
4. Sympathetic blocks
   a. Stellate
   b. LSB
5. Spinal cord stimulator
   a. Trial
   b. Implantation (in OR)
6. Neuraxial pumps (briefly)
   a. Intrathecal
   b. Epidural

LSB, lumbar sympathetic block; MBBs, medial branch nerve blocks; OR, operating room; SIJ, sacroiliac joint.

EPIDURAL STEROID INJECTIONS

Epidural steroid injections (ESIs) for radicular complaints have become quite commonplace in the setting of pain management practices. The typical indications are related to signs of irritation and compression of the spinal cord and nerve roots. Symptoms include pain, numbness, tingling, or weakness localized to a dermatomal distribution indicative of the vertebral level where lesions such as inflammation or compression of neural structures may be found. Typically, diagnostic studies such as computed tomographic (CT) scans, magnetic resonance images (MRIs), and electromyograms (EMGs) are used to localize and characterize the lesion.

Cervical, thoracic, and lumbar ESIs may be performed at practically any level depending on where the nerve irritation or compression is taking place. The intervention targets the epidural space Because all spinal nerves must travel through this space prior to exiting the spine. By bathing the spinal cord and proximal nerve roots with a solution of long-acting depot steroid such as triamcinolone 40–60 mg (with or without dilute local anesthetic), the goal is to minimize inflammation and thereby severity of symptoms. While epidural administration of steroids is off-label use of the drug and there is no evidence that ESIs serve to improve simple back pain (musculoskeletal pain), there is abundant medical literature to support use of ESIs for the management of radicular pain.[5]

After proper patient positioning and placement of monitors, a local anesthetic skin wheal will be applied to the insertion site. Further local anesthetic may be used to numb the projected tissue track between skin entry and the vertebrae. An epidural needle is then passed through the skin and directed to the interlaminar space of interest. Fluoroscopic guidance and contrast dye may be used during the procedure to help confirm proper placement. Preprocedure counseling and verbal reassurance at the time of injection often help allay concerns brought on by transient sensations of pressure or reproduction of symptoms.

With respect to lateral spread of injectate, the dorsal median epidural septum may be an anatomical cause for limitation. With fluoroscopic guidance and contrast dye, it can be reliably overcome by use of a transforaminal approach in lieu of the traditional interlaminar approach. In spite of lower drug volumes, transforaminal ESIs (TFESIs) allow for higher concentrations of drug to penetrate at the site of lesion by utilizing laterality and promoting more ventral spread. Indications include unilateral radiculopathy secondary to herniated nucleus pulposus, disk prolapse, foraminal stenosis, shingles/acute herpes zoster, and occipital headaches.

Transforaminal ESIs do carry their own risks, such as greater exposure to radiation. They rely more on digital subtraction angiography (DSA), which utilizes real-time fluoroscopy to reduce risk of intravascular and subarachnoid injection and to ensure proper location for delivery. Contrast dye is placed and expected to outline the proximal end of the exiting nerve root and spread centrally toward the epidural space (Figures 30.1 and 30.2). This can be performed with patients in the supine, oblique, or lateral decubitus position, depending on provider preference and patient comfort. Regardless of patient position, symptoms may take up to 2 weeks to improve when injecting steroid only and deferring on local anesthetic.

FACET INTERVENTIONS

There are 25 paired facet joints located in the spinal column, and they are involved in movement between adjacent vertebrae. They play a larger role in the cervical and lumbosacral spine, where there is greater freedom for vertebral movement. When facet joints are the etiology of the pain, a facet block injection should be considered. These injections are a diagnostic tool used to isolate and confirm the lesion. These blocks also serve as a therapeutic option given their analgesic and anti-inflammatory effects for the patient. Like ESIs, facet blocks may be used to manage pain associated with moderate-to-severe degenerative arthritis of the spine. It is important to remember, however, that the presence of damaged facet joints does not assure the clinician that the facet joint itself is the pain generator of concern. On the other hand, immediate resolution of pain may serve to confirm facet pathology as the source of the pain.

Once diagnostic facet blocks confirm symptomatic facet joints, they may be followed by radio-frequency (RF) ablation or neurotomy of respective medial branch nerves for longer lasting, but not necessarily permanent, relief. It is worth noting that because of the increased likelihood of osteoporosis (poor visualization on x-ray/fluoroscopy) and osteophytic growths in people over 65 years of age, facet blocks can quickly become very challenging. When the facet joint cannot be entered due to anatomical constraints, practitioners may choose to perform diagnostic MBBs and RF ablations instead. Regardless, facet joint rhizolysis may afford analgesia from months to years.

Procedurally, diagnostic MBBs and RF ablations (Figures 30.3 and 30.4) are similar with addition of electrical testing and then RF lesioning of nerves that innervate the facet joint for 60–90 seconds at 80°C with the ultimate goal being more

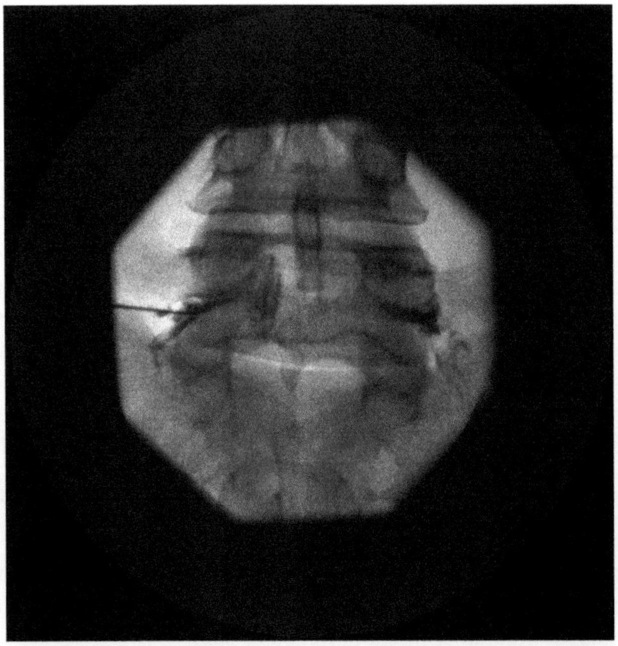

Figure 30.1. Anteroposterior view of a left L5/S1 transforaminal epidural steroid injection with spread along the L5 nerve root and central epidural spread.

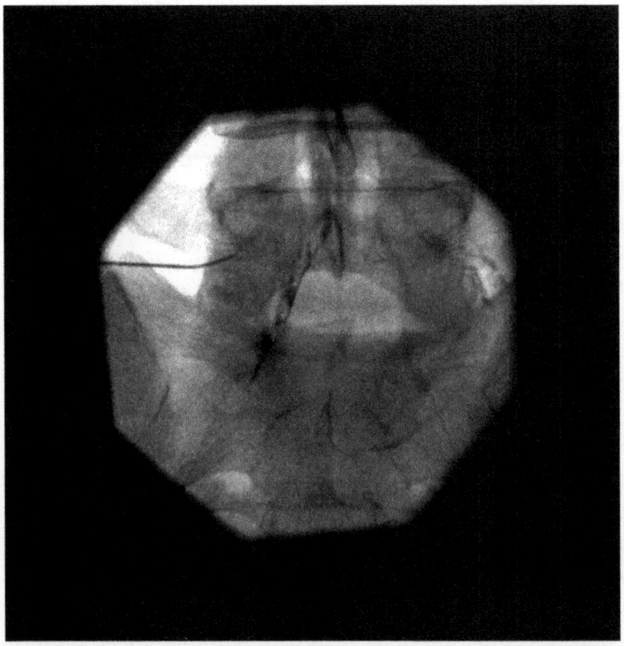

Figure 30.2. Anteroposterior view of a left L5/S1 transforaminal epidural steroid injection with spread along the L5 and left S1 nerve root.

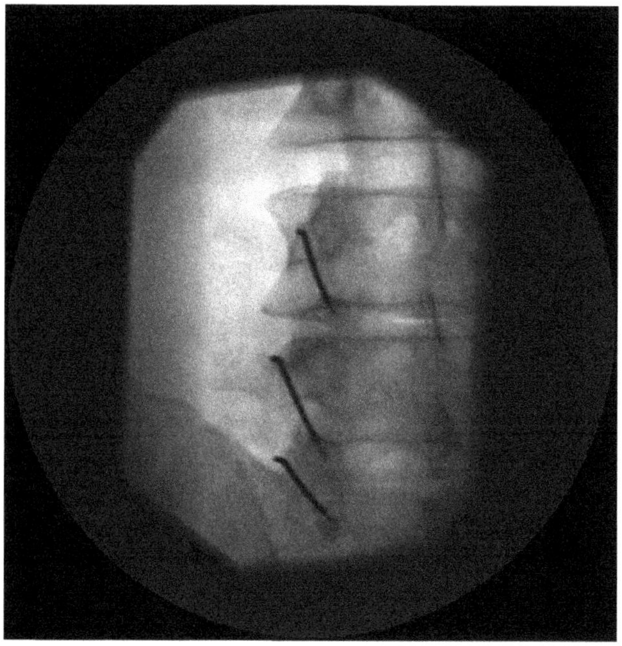

Figure 30.3. Left anterior oblique view of needle placement for radio-frequency ablation of the L3 and L4 medial branch nerves and the L5 posterior primary ramus on the L3 and L4 transverse process and sacral ala, respectively.

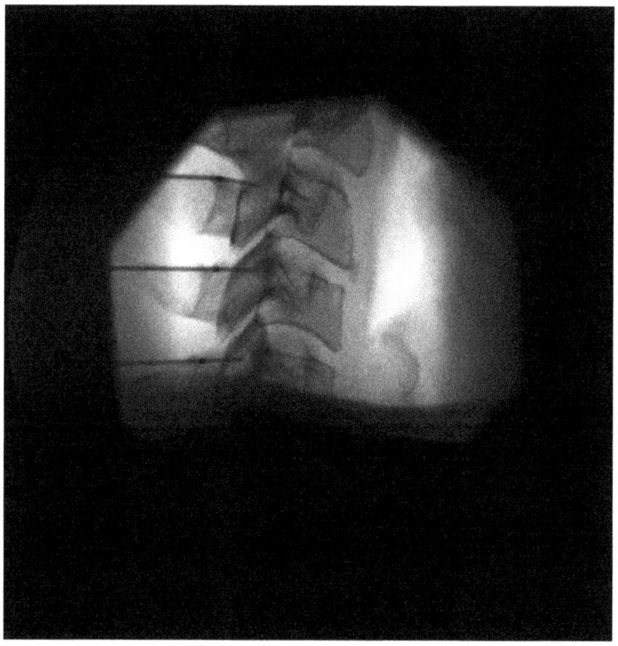

Figure 30.4. Lateral view of the upper C-spine with needle tips placed for radio-frequency ablation of medial branch nerves of C3, C4, and C5.

permanent interruption of the pain signals to the brain. For patient safety, electrical grounding pads must be applied during the ablations. For MBBs, physicians utilize fluoroscopy to guide 25-gauge, 3.5-inch spinal needles (typical diameter and length) toward the junction of the transverse process and the superior articular process for the desired medial branch nerve. Injectate for the diagnostic block is composed of a small volume of contrast dye, followed by 0.5 mL of local anesthetic directed toward to the desired medial branch nerve. Injectate following ablations is usually a mixture of local anesthetic and steroid. Because each facet joint has dual innervations from two vertebral levels, coverage of a single facet joint implies targeting the medial branch nerves above and below that joint. Common practice is to limit oneself to no more than six facet joint interventions per visit for bilateral pain or three facet joint interventions if the complaint is unilateral.

Because of the frequent use of sedatives/anxiolytics to help patients tolerate the confirmatory electrical testing and the electrocautery lesioning of the medial branch nerves during RF ablations, longer postprocedure observations may be required. On the other hand, following diagnostic MBBs, patients are quickly discharged as the procedure is less painful and short in duration and usually requires no sedation medications. After these diagnostic blocks, patients must be counseled to carefully take note of their presenting symptoms and severity during this time. Use of a pain diary facilitates this documentation as well. A greater number of interventions per visit confers a greater likelihood of patients noting postprocedure soreness after the local anesthetic wears off. This is associated with bruising or tissue trauma of the local back muscles. A short course of oral nonsteroidal anti-inflammatory drugs (NSAIDs) or acetaminophen, in combination with ice packs and rest, often relieves symptoms quickly; however, complaints of exacerbated back pain and increased analgesic consumption may last for 1–2 weeks, especially after ablations. Swelling around the lesioned nerves may even last 6 weeks.

SACROILIAC JOINT INTERVENTIONS

The sacroiliac (SI) joint connects the sacrum and the iliac bone of the pelvis. Inflammation of this joint may lead to low back pain and referred lower extremity pain, classically starting over the buttocks and extending laterally to the hip and thigh. Investigation of SI joint dysfunction, much like facet joint intervention, usually starts with diagnostic blocks. Diagnostic injections may be used to investigate low back and leg pain suspected to be due to pathology in the SI joint. If positive, interventional pain specialists may move on to the permanent/semipermanent RF ablation of the lateral branches of the sacral nerves, which innervate the SI joint. Typical indications include inflammation of the synovial lining of the SI joint, traumatic injury, rheumatoid arthritis, and other osteodegenerative or arthritic conditions, such as ankylosing spondylitis. Being a difficult clinical diagnosis, SI joint dysfunction is commonly a diagnosis of exclusion.[6]

The technique for SI joint injection is very similar to that for facet joint injection, with the exception of the anatomical target and fluoroscopy-guided visualization. Local anesthesia with or without light intravenous sedation is used with the patient prone and the x-ray tube perpendicular to the fluoroscopy table. Skin markings are made to denote the distal portion of the joint, where it is the widest and will allow easiest penetration of delivered drugs. This is followed by a 20°–30° rotation of the x-ray tube in the cephalad direction to make the posterior and caudal aspect of the SI joint more visible. Next, a small-diameter needle (i.e., 22-gauge, 3.5- or 5-inch spinal needle) is manipulated into the joint in question using fluoroscopy. Radiopaque dye is then used to confirm proper needle placement. Typical injectate is 2–3 mL of local anesthetic and steroid mixture (usually 1–2 mL of 0.5% ropivacaine plus methylprednisolone 40–80 mg). This is often repeated up to three times per year, but to be optimized each injection should be followed by a physical therapy regimen and rehabilitation.

Sacroiliac joint injections present some special considerations worth noting. These interventions are known to be much more difficult in the absence of fluoroscopic guidance.[5] The degree of difficulty often is a marker for number of attempts and remanipulations. Like other percutaneous procedures, though, there may also be an exacerbation of pain or no noted change in pain afterward. Other similarities also exist between SI and facet interventions. For RF ablations, patient safety and use of an electrical grounding pad (Bovie pad) is again paramount when using high-frequency energy. Alternating current creates precisely controlled heat, which is then delivered by narrow electrode needles to the affected area, resulting in destruction of pain-sensing nerves. Subsequently, patients should expect the likely ache associated after the ablation-induced tissue trauma. Also, because of proximity of the sciatic nerve as it runs anterior to the SI joint, leg weakness for several hours may be seen due to diffusion of local anesthetic.

SYMPATHETIC BLOCKS

Sympathetic blocks are now commonly performed in outpatient settings such as medical offices and ambulatory surgery centers (ASCs). In an effort to control certain pain syndromes, these blocks target disruption of the sympathetic pathways.[7] The most common indication for sympathetic blocks is for complex regional pain syndrome (CRPS).[7] This diagnosis is divided into three parts: CRPS I (formerly reflex sympathetic dystrophy, or RSD); CRPS II (formerly causalgia); and CRPS NOS (not otherwise specified). All three parts may have a component of sympathetically mediated pain and thus potentially be suitable for sympathetic blocks. These are primarily limited to stellate ganglion blocks (SGBs) and lumbar sympathetic blocks (LSBs) because they are commonly performed to help diagnose and treat CRPS. RF ablation may be used after diagnostic blocks when the indication is either sympathetically mediated chronic pain of the upper extremity (stellate ganglionotomy) or sympathetically mediated chronic pain of the lower extremity (lumbar sympathectomy). Patients with lower extremity neuropathy or peripheral vascular disease may also benefit from LSBs. Celiac plexus blocks, on the other hand, may be used to manage a variety of chronic abdominal pains by interfering with sensory transmission from much of the abdomen. While these blocks may be guided by endoscopic ultrasound (EUS), CT, or MRI, the most common image guidance is via fluoroscopy.

For SGBs, an obliqued C-arm is used to provide ipsilateral fluoroscopic guidance, and the C7 uncinate process is visualized. A 25- or 21-gauge spinal needle is then advanced through a lidocaine skin wheal toward the vertebral body junction and the base of the uncinate process. Using DSA to confirm an appropriate nonvascular spread pattern on injection of contrast, the practitioner can verify correct position of the needle (see Figure 30.5). In the absence of vascular flow patterns (i.e., rapid arterial washout) of the contrast, one can exclude improper needle placement within the vertebral artery located anteriorly and the common carotid artery located posteriorly. Approximately 5–10 mL of local anesthetic is administered for the diagnostic block.

Lumbar sympathetic blocks are performed using fluoroscopy with the patient again in the prone position and having routine physiological monitors (electrocardiogram, blood pressure, and SpO_2) applied. Placement of an abdominal pillow will lessen thoracolumbar curvature and facilitate performance of the LSB, as it does the SGB. Entering through a lidocaine skin wheal over the L2 transverse body, a 22-gauge, 5-inch spinal needle is advanced until contacting the vertebral body. The needle is then retracted and "walked off" the lateral border of the vertebral body. Proper placement is confirmed by fluoroscopy with the needle tip at the anterior edge of the vertebral body on the lateral view and at the medial border of the ipsilateral pedicle on the anterior/posterior view. In this position, the needle tip is expected to be adjacent to the lumbar sympathetic chain, and an aliquot of contrast is delivered to confirm a prevertebral location. Then, approximately 10 mL of local anesthetic or lytic solution are injected. Following removal of the needle, the patient must be continually monitored for hypotension and reflex tachycardia.

Albeit especially useful for malignant pains such as pancreatic cancer or severe chronic visceral pains, neurolytic celiac plexus blocks still have not found widespread use outside of tertiary care centers and more highly specialized pain centers. Suffice it to say that even with the advent of EUS, the

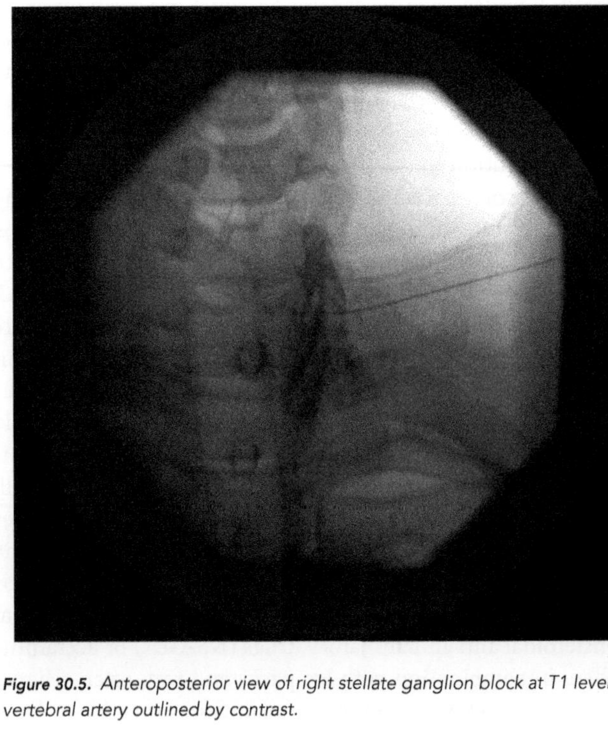

Figure 30.5. Anteroposterior view of right stellate ganglion block at T1 level; vertebral artery outlined by contrast.

performance of celiac plexus blocks is still frequently reserved for tertiary care centers and more highly specialized interventional pain management centers.[7,8]

Sympathetic blocks carry with them specific clinical concerns that should be discussed with the patient as part of the informed consent process prior to the start of the procedure. SGBs may cause Horner syndrome, with ipsilateral face and eyelid droop as well as hoarseness. LSBs may cause one or both of the patient's legs to become warmer than baseline. While relatively common, both these are self-resolving within a few hours. Although rare, other complications include inadvertent needle placement into the vertebral artery or adjacent tissues; vertebral disks; gastrointestinal tract (esophagus); cerebrospinal fluid (CSF); pleura; or neural structures. These complications have resulted in intravascular injection, hematoma formation, seizures, spinal anesthesia, cervical epidural abscess, brachial plexus block, pneumochylothorax, pneumothorax, temporary blindness, hoarseness, dysphagia, and death.[5] The unusual cardiac complication of left ventricular dysfunction can be seen after left SGB due to disrupted autonomic balance to the heart. When right-sided SGBs disrupt sympathetic outflow to the heart, parasympathetic predominance may be overwhelming, resulting in a dysrhythmic heart rate or even asystolic cardiac arrest.

SPINAL CORD STIMULATORS

Spinal cord stimulators (SCSs) are implantable medical devices used to treat chronic pain of neurologic origin, such as sciatica, intractable back pain (such as failed back surgery syndrome or failed laminectomy syndrome), and diabetic neuropathy.[9] Over the past four decades, they have been used successfully in many of the most challenging pain management cases. These stimulators function by generating an electric pulse near the dorsal surface of the spinal cord, providing a paresthesia sensation that alters the perception of pain by the patient. Recent developments in SCS technology now provide the patient with three choices for stimulation. The first option is the traditional low-frequency (40- to 60-hertz) or tonic stimulation that supplies a continuous paresthesia sensation. The second possibility is burst frequency (varied, with 40- to 500-hertz) stimulation that delivers little-to-no paresthesia sensation. The third choice is high-frequency (10,000-hertz) stimulation that provides no sensation. They are typically used in conjunction with continued conventional medical management.

Increasingly, SCSs are permanently implanted to supply a low-intensity impulse to a location in the spinal cord in an attempt to disrupt native pain transmission signals that are being transmitted to the brain. Being an invasive and permanent intervention, this is usually performed after an SCS trial. After a successful SCS trial with marked improvement in pain relief, implantation usually occurs as a scheduled case within the operating room. As such, it is not discussed in this chapter. Figures 30.6 and 30.7 provide examples of SCS lead placement.

INTRATHECAL/EPIDURAL PUMPS

Both intrathecal pumps and epidural pumps are meant to function as continuous drug infusion systems. They are usually reserved for patients who have severe, debilitating chronic pain that has not responded adequately to traditional treatments. The most common drug delivered is morphine.[7,8] The infusion catheter is inserted midline at the low back, terminating in the spinal space and the epidural space, respectively. The infusion

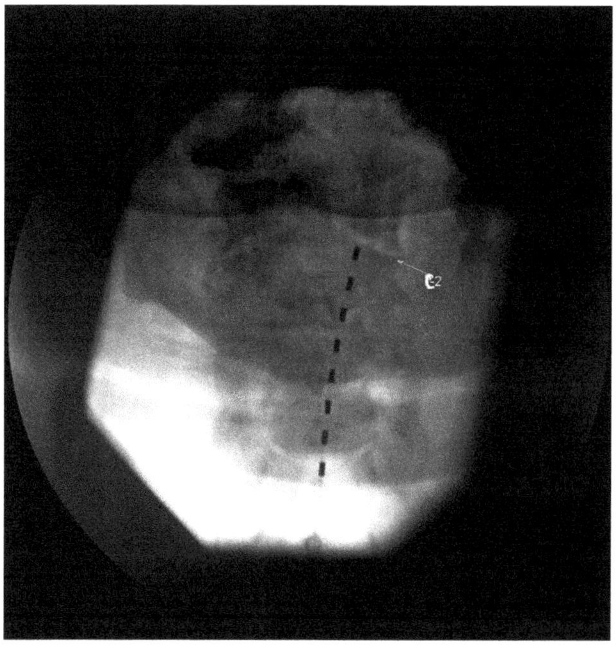

Figure 30.6. Anteroposterior view of a right octrode spinal cord stimulator lead at the C2 level, right of midline.

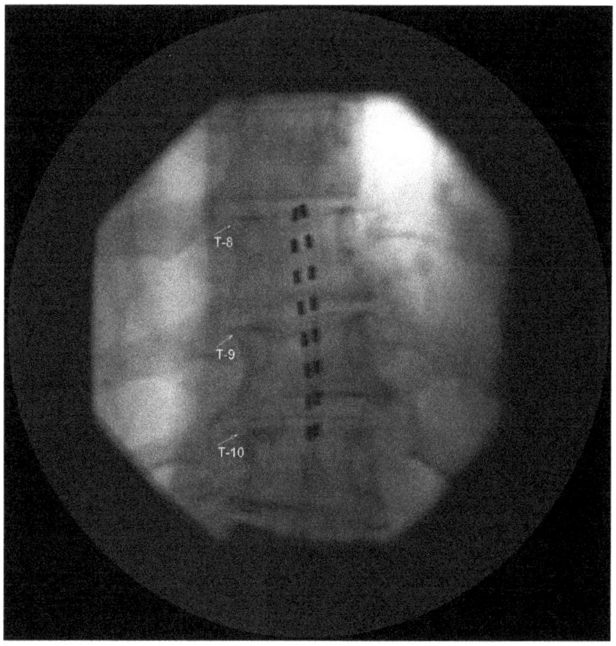

Figure 30.7. Anteroposterior view of two octrode leads with the first contact at the top of T8. This position will typically cover leg pain.

pump is placed on either side of the abdomen, upper posterior gluteal region (buttocks), or in the midflank areas (below the inferior ribs) in a pocket under the subcutaneous skin. Typical indications include refractory chronic pain secondary to failed back syndrome, postlaminectomy syndrome, cancer pain, reflex sympathetic dystrophy, and severe osteoporosis or end-stage arthritis.

Consideration of intrathecal and epidural pumps has traditionally been restricted to malignant pain (chronic pain related to underlying cancer). The expected equipment life span is about 5–7 years before anticipating replacement.[10] Recent developments have led to the consideration of utilizing these pumps in other patient cohorts as well, but these procedures themselves are still primarily performed in the operating room. As such, we do not discuss them at length here for the purposes of this chapter.

COMMON ANESTHETIC CONSIDERATIONS FOR PAIN PROCEDURES OUTSIDE OF THE OPERATING ROOM

While sedation and analgesic options are plentiful for utilization during percutaneous pain techniques, many, if not most, of these procedures can be done without sedating the patient. In fact, it is not uncommon for some providers to typically rely on only light sedation for SCSs, implantable pumps, and sympathetic blocks (however, some of these procedures may require deep sedation or general anesthesia and may need to be performed in the operating room). Most providers, however, will use sedation for facet procedures, and many will use sedation for both epidural and facet injections. Ultimately, individual provider comfort, clinical discretion, patient health, and patient disposition often come together in deciding whether to use sedation. Thorough preprocedure history and examination are crucial in recognizing and avoiding clinical pitfalls, such as preexisting coagulopathies and potentially difficult airways. Other pertinent patient disposition traits include individual pain tolerance and availability of a responsible adult to assist with postprocedure management and transport home. Postintervention care and discharge instructions will be influenced by the degree of sedation achieved (as opposed to the level of sedation targeted) and the potential for altered sensory and motor baselines following the procedure.[11]

The most common anesthesia concerns and pitfalls are important for all interventional pain management specialists. Vagal responses are the most commonly encountered concern following percutaneous pain procedures.[12] While variances are expected for the vast array of techniques and anatomical locations involved, the incidence may range from less than 1% to over 10% even when limiting inclusion to just interlaminar epidural injections.[13] Several important factors must be considered when trying to explain such disparity. Factors such as typical patient body habitus, procedural experience and interoperator variability, selection of needle type and needle placement, use of fluoroscopy or image guidance with or without radiopaque contrast dyes, and use of sedation may be involved. Avoidance of sedation, lesser degree of patient anatomic variation, and clinical experience may all decrease the incidence significantly. Oversedation may also be concurrent with loss of airway. When pharmacological sedation is planned, guidelines for nothing by mouth should be enforced in accordance with departmental or institutional standards.

With the exception of SGBs, all the procedures discussed are likely performed in the prone position. This can complicate airway management and rescue in case of oversedation. This is especially evident when procedures such as cervical MBBs and TFESIs are complicated by seizures; similarly when cervical epidurals utilizing local anesthetic are complicated by occurrence of a total spinal anesthetic. While rare, clinicians also must be aware of the potential for stroke and paralysis with interventions such as cervical or lumbar TFESIs. On the other hand, management of pneumothorax, if seen with thoracic procedures, is not significantly altered by the prone position.[14]

As with all anesthesia care plans, patient safety and monitoring remain top priorities for the pain interventionalist to minimize problems.[6,12] Standard American Society of Anesthesiology monitors, such as electrocardiogram, noninvasive blood pressure, oxygen saturation, when combined with radiographic monitoring, are used to aid in percutaneous procedures. It is important to note, however, that despite reports that fluoroscopically guided interventions prove safer, they are not fail-safe. Many pain procedures have been shadowed by complications despite image guidance.[5] There is no substitute for proper training, clinical expertise, and cautious patient monitoring to ensure patient safety and improve outcomes.

When the improved outcome means less pain and a definite increase in a patient's quality of life, it is easy to see why interventional pain management is so rewarding. This must be tempered by the unarguable reality that while an improvement in symptoms is expected, pain relief is not always immediate or permanent. Analgesic effects may be immediate and last for several weeks. On the other hand, the pain symptoms may be worse postprocedure, with improvements coming later and lasting for several weeks. There also may be no change for several days and then a slow improvement that lasts for several weeks. Sadly, the pain may also be worsened or exacerbated by the procedure, with no improvement perceived by the patient.

More commonly, the patients will complain of local soreness and bruising at the injection site. This is usually self-resolving within a few days. Infection, bleeding, and scarring are all commonly counseled against, but they are also unlikely given close monitoring and precise injections.[7] Patients with known clotting abnormalities or who are taking anticoagulants should let their physicians know prior to having any percutaneous interventions performed. Epidural hematomas or any neuraxial hematoma/infection poses significant concern and warrants longer observation times with possible admission to the hospital. This is especially worrisome with diabetic, septic, and immunocompromised patients.

Post–dural puncture headache (PDPH) is a low spinal fluid pressure headache that occurs if the procedure needle (or other instrument) penetrates the dural membrane and results in a persistent CSF leak. Management options include oral hydration, oral caffeine, an epidural blood patch, intravenous fluids, and analgesics. In most instances, the dural puncture seals with spontaneous resolution of the headache in less than 2 weeks.[5] Should the needle tip deliver injectate directly into the CSF, one must observe for a total spinal anesthetic. Damage to the nerve itself could arise via needle trauma and result in permanent neuralgic pain, numbness, and weakness in variable parts of the body. However, most paresthesias resolve within hours and almost all within 2 weeks.

More rare complications include arachnoiditis, allergic reaction, and intravascular penetration or injection.[5,14] Arachnoiditis is a very painful condition caused by the inflammation of the arachnoid membrane. It is associated with injection of medication into the CSF. Allergic reaction is rare and more often than not is a reaction to the preservative or the contrast and not to the local anesthetic or steroid. Symptomatic and supportive care is the principal management technique. With the use of contrast dyes, vascular puncture is becoming extremely rare. Using less than 1 mL of contrast, improper needle placement may be confirmed whether arterial (rapid washout), venous (slow washout), or even intrathecal (dilution of contrast).

Ultimately, there is no substitute for large, randomized, controlled clinical trials to answer the remaining questions regarding interventional pain management. Until those answers are afforded us, providers must continue to optimize pain management using all available resources, including multimodal therapeutics; diagnostic studies such as EMG, CT, or MRI; interventional pain procedures; reassessment visits with thorough history and serial physical exams; documentation of findings; and clinical acumen with a multidisciplinary approach to patient care. The pain interventionalist will continue to engage a detailed understanding of anatomy and judicious use of real-time fluoroscopy.

REFERENCES

1. Abrecht CR, Brovman EY, Greenberg P, Song E, Rathmell JP, Urman RD. A contemporary medicolegal analysis of outpatient medication management in chronic pain. *Anesth Analg.* 2017;125(5):1761–1768.
2. Bajwa ZH, Wootton RJ, Warfield CA, eds. *Principles and Practive of Pain Medicine.* 3rd ed. New York: McGraw-Hill; 2016.
3. Benzon H, Rathmell JP, Wu CL, eds. Practical Management of Pain. 5th ed. New York: Mostby; 2013.
4. Yong RJ, Nguyen M, Nelson ER, Urman RD, eds. *Pain Medicine: An Essential Review.* New York: Springer Press; 2017.
5. Robbertze R, Psner KL, Domino KB. Closed claims review of anesthesia for procedures outside the operating room. *Curr Opin Anaesthesiol.* 2006;19(4):436–442.
6. Pino RM. The nature of anesthesia and procedural sedation outside of the operating room. *Curr Opin Anaesthesiol.* 2007;20(4):347–351.
7. Leak JA. Hospital-based anesthesia outside the operating room. *ASA Newsl.* 2003;67:10.
8. American Society of Anesthesiologists. Statement on nonoperating room anesthetizing locations. Available at: http://www.asahq.org/quality-and-practice-management/standards-guidelines-and-related-resources/statement-on-nonoperating-room-anesthetizing-locations. Amended 2013. Last accessed March 1, 2018.
9. Abrecht CR, Greenberg P, Song E, Urman RD, Rathmell JP. A contemporary medicolegal analysis of implanted devices for chronic pain management. *Anesth Analg.* 2017;124(4):1304–1310.
10. Dexter F, Xiao Y, Dow AJ, et al. Coordination of appointments for anesthesia care outside of operating rooms using an enterprise-wide scheduling system. *Anesth Analg.* 2007;105:1701–1710.
11. Joint Commission. Pain Management-Leadership Responsiblity: Patient Monitoring Following Sedation or Anesthesia- LD.04.03.13 EP 7. https://www.jointcommission.org/standards_information/jcfaqdetails.aspx?StandardsFaqId=1567&ProgramId=46. Last accessed May 23, 2018.
12. Cote CJ, Wilson S. The Work Group on Sedation: guidelines for monitoring and management of pediatric patients during and after sedation for diagnostic and therapeutic procedures: an update. *Pediatrics.* 2006;118:2587–2602.
13. Gross JB. The American Society of Anesthesiologists Task Force on Sedation and Analgesia by Non-Anesthesiologists: practice guidelines for sedation and analgesia by non-anesthesiologists. *Anesthesiology.* 2002;96:1004–1017.
14. Parfrey PS, Griffith SM, Barrett BJ, et al. Contrast-induced renal failure. *N Engl J Med.* 1989;320:143–149.

31 | ANESTHESIA IN THE MILITARY SETTING

CRAIG McFARLAND, MD, ROBERT H. BURCH III, MD, CHRISTOPHER V. MAANI, MD

INTRODUCTION

Students of anesthesia history are well aware of the medical contributions of pioneers such as Joseph Priestley, Crawford Long, Horace Wells, William T. G. Morton, and John Snow; however, numerous events in the development of military anesthesia also deserve mention. In fact, it is fair to say that the practices of military and civilian anesthesia have existed symbiotically. Except where otherwise noted, these considerations are summarized from Condon-Rall's "A Brief History of Military Anesthesia."[1] These advances in military anesthetic care have often mirrored more global advances in combat casualty care, as shown in Box 31.1.[2]

In 1847, during the Mexican War, Edward H. Barton, a surgeon, provided the first-known "modern" American military anesthetic. Using diethyl ether, Dr. Barton anesthetized a soldier in order to amputate both of his legs. An observer commented, "The unfortunate man was soon rendered completely insensible to all pain, and indeed, to everything else, and the limb was removed without the quiver of a muscle." It

BOX 31.1. ADVANCES IN COMBAT CASUALTY CARE: 1914–2007

I. World War I
   A. Use of intravenous fluids and blood transfusions
   B. Motorized ambulances
   C. Laparotomy for penetrating abdominal wounds
   D. Use of surgical specialists
   E. Effective topical antisepsis: Carrel-Dakins wound irrigation system
   F. Antitetanus serum
   G. Radiologic localization of foreign bodies
   H. Neurosurgical trauma databank
II. World War II
   A. General availability of whole blood and plasma
   B. Formulaic resuscitation of burn patients
   C. Availability of "well-trained" surgeons and use of specialty-specific auxiliary surgical groups
   D. Hierarchical organization of trauma care
   E. Use of antibiotics
   F. Use of fixed-wing aeromedical evacuation
   G. Identification of "wet lung in war casualties"
III. Korean Conflict
   A. Fluid resuscitation adequate to correct shock and prevent organ failure
   B. Availability of board-certified surgical specialists
   C. Forward availability of definitive surgery
   D. Use of helicopters for patient transport
   E. Primary repair and vascular grafts for injured vessels
   F. Use of hemodialysis in theater of operations
   G. Identification of high-output renal failure
IV. Vietnam Conflict
   A. General use of helicopters for patient transport
   B. Monitoring of organ function in theater of operations
      1. Blood gas measurements
      2. Serum chemistries
   C. Portable radiology equipment
   D. Use of mechanical ventilators in theater of operations
   E. Effective topical antimicrobial chemotherapy for burns
   F. Staged intercontinental aeromedical transport of burn patients
   G. Identification of acute respiratory distress syndrome
V. Operation Desert Shield/Storm
   A. Burn team augmentation of evacuation hospitals to provide theater-wide burn care
   B. Reactivation of intercontinental burn patient transport system
VI. Operation Enduring Freedom and Operation Iraqi Freedom
   A. Development of a military trauma registry
   B. "Low-volume" resuscitation fluids—colloids and red blood cells
   C. Hemostatic agents
      1. Systemic
      2. Topical
   D. Use of "damage control" initial surgery
   E. Use of endovascular stents
   F. Common use of external fixators
   G. Improved tourniquets
   H. CAD/CAM limb prostheses

CAD/CAM, computer-aided design and manufacturing.

SOURCE: Reprinted with permission from Pruitt BA. The symbiosis of combat casualty care and civilian trauma care: 1914–2007. *J Trauma.* 2008;64:S4–S8.

was another 2 years before ether gained the widespread surgical support within the American military community that it was earning among civilian surgeons, due predominantly to an incomplete understanding of the agent. In the late 1840s, chloroform also gained widespread use, primarily among British surgeons. American military surgeons began using both agents shortly thereafter.

The American Civil War witnessed significant growth in the role of battlefield anesthesia. Jonathan Letterman, the medical director of the Army of the Potomac, recommended an assistant surgeon be responsible for anesthesia at the 18 division hospitals, which ultimately helped to improve the standardization of military anesthesia. It was estimated that the Union Army provided anesthesia for at least 80,000 surgical cases. Chloroform was the chosen agent in 76% of these cases, its popularity attributed to a favorable smell, nonflammability, and a decreased incidence of vomiting and excitability relative to ether. Chloroform was considered generally safe when used for short durations and in the presence of appropriate levels of room air relative to the concentration of chloroform. Orally administered alcohol and opiates gained widespread use due to their perceived ability to alleviate pain. Cannabis was also occasionally used, particularly for the treatment of tetanus and head injury.

The practice of military anesthesiology as a medical subspecialty came into its own during World War I, though not without significant growing pains. Immediately preceding WWI, specialized training in anesthesia became more prominent, directing the development of both physician and nurse anesthetists. However, during the early years of WWI, anesthetics were often delivered by inexperienced individuals and were attributed to otherwise-preventable deaths. To help counter this, the British army began sending anesthesiologists forward in 1916. At this same time, anesthesiologists were first accepted into the Medical Corps of both the US Army and Navy, and the Army began to send nurses to specialized anesthesia training programs. By 1917, the United States was fighting in WWI, and most American anesthetists were reserve civilian surgeons, nurses, and dentists. The Army also began to send medical officers to civilian medical institutions, where they received intense training in war surgery and administration of anesthetics. Anesthetists remained in short supply throughout the war, and they were commonly overworked and undersupplied. True to historical military fashion, the charge to military anesthetists was to make the most of what was available. A variety of new anesthetic delivery systems were developed; the most popular anesthetizing agent was nitrous oxide, followed by ether, chloroform, and ethyl chloride. According to the British, a nitrous oxide-oxygen mixture "in experienced hands . . . was the ideal anesthetic for such patients, since it fulfilled the three essential conditions—safety, speed, and rapid recovery." Intravenous morphine, spinal anesthesia, or local anesthesia was often used in conjunction with, or in place of, general inhalational anesthesia. Additionally, a better understanding of the mechanisms underlying shock allowed for the initial development of blood transfusion therapy.

During World War II, the US military again suffered a shortfall of specialized anesthesia providers despite offering anesthesiology residency training beginning in 1939. Nonetheless, medical, nursing, and dental officers all provided successful anesthetic care. Endotracheal intubation and closed-circuit anesthesia delivery systems soon gained wide acceptance, and a variety of portable systems were introduced. Commonly used agents included ether, chloroform, ethyl chloride, nitrous oxide, sodium thiopental, procaine, tetracaine hydrochloride, and cocaine. Reversing the preference for nitrous oxide–oxygen seen during WWI, ether was more commonly used in severely injured and shock patients because of its overall tolerance. Spinal and intravenous anesthetics were also employed in the critically injured, particularly when inhalational anesthesia was not available or, more commonly, experienced anesthesia providers were not available. Transfusion therapy continued to gain acceptance, primarily with plasma and whole blood. As the war progressed, whole blood became favored over plasma for the treatment of shock. Other advances included the use of splints to minimize hemorrhage, body heat conservation, gastric emptying to minimize the risk of aspiration, and supplemental oxygen. By the end of WWII, combat deaths attributable to anesthesia had declined considerably versus earlier conflicts. Additionally, the recognition of anesthetists as highly skilled and specialized medical and nursing providers ushered in an era of appreciation for the specialty not previously seen in military medicine.

The Korean War demonstrated more numerous and better trained personnel, as well as more readily available equipment and supplies, though shortfalls were still apparent. The evacuation system was considered worse than in WWII, and medical officers rarely had field medical experience. Much of the standardization in anesthetic care seen in WWII was forgotten by the Korean War, and practitioners often used their personal favored techniques, frequently with their own personal equipment. Intravenous fluid resuscitation and blood transfusion continued to be used successfully, and whole-blood transfusion became more prominent. In 1954, the US Army initiated its first 3-year postinternship residency program in anesthesiology. The Army also offered greater training opportunities for nurse anesthetists in the years following the Korean War.

During the Vietnam War, the role of the combat anesthesiologist continued to increase, including specific advances in critical care that were later extended to the civilian sector. An improved evacuation system, continued efforts at better understanding shock and resuscitation, and better availability of whole blood led to a 10-fold improvement in delay from the POI to appropriate care in Vietnam relative to WWI. Advanced airway management also became more prominent, including tracheal intubation in 76% of patients receiving general anesthesia. Muscle relaxants were more commonly used, and halothane and methoxyflurane gained increasing acceptance. After 1970, techniques utilizing nitrous oxide–oxygen with muscle relaxants, opioids, and intravenous sedatives were favored, partially due to concerns with halothane hepatitis. Morphine, meperidine, fentanyl, ketamine, and droperidol were also commonly administered. Neuromuscular reversal with neostigmine and atropine gained acceptance. Neuraxial anesthesia, upper extremity regional nerve blockade, and intravenous regional anesthesia were also employed successfully.

Combat anesthetic care continued through Operations Desert Storm and Desert Shield. Major advances during this conflict primarily involved in-theater care of severely burned patients as well as improved intercontinental evacuation of these patients.[2]

OPERATION IRAQI FREEDOM/OPERATION ENDURING FREEDOM

Anesthetic care in the current Global War on Terror (GWOT) has mirrored the broad range of injuries seen and has sought to meet the surgical and critical care needs for these wounded patients. In the civilian population, trauma deaths are largely blunt in nature (84%–90%), whereas in Operation Iraqi Freedom (OIF)/Operation Enduring Freedom (OEF), penetrating trauma has been the mechanism of death in 83% of cases.[3] A range of historically less-conventional methods for attack by enemy combatants has been employed, complicated further by unclear battleground and front-line demarcations. Blast injuries associated with enemy improvised explosive devices (IEDs) and explosively formed projectiles (EFPs) have contributed significantly to major burns, polytrauma, multiextremity amputation, and traumatic brain injury, each presenting unique challenges to the anesthesia provider.

Holcomb et al. demonstrated that relative to World War II and Vietnam, OIF/OEF has seen a substantial decrease in those killed in action (KIA), died of wounds (DOW), and overall case fatality rates.[4] These data offer some reassurances regarding military personal protective gear, including improved combat body armor. However, as demonstrated in Table 31.1, the DOW rate relative to the case fatality rate is higher in the current conflict relative to WWII and Vietnam, indicating that more American military personnel are surviving long enough to reach medical care. Among potentially survivable injuries, hemorrhage is the primary cause of death, representing 83% of cases.[3] This presents significant surgical and anesthetic challenges not previously seen.

The US military currently supports five different levels of integrated patient care, termed Roles I through V. These designations differ from trauma designations used in American civilian hospitals. The Department of Defense describes these levels of care in the *Emergency War Surgery* textbook.[5] Inherent to these levels of care is consideration for the combat evacuation system. Casualty evacuation (CASEVAC) begins at the point of injury (POI) and involves movement of the wounded to a site where they can receive a higher level of care. These patients typically have only received basic life-saving strategies as provided under tactical combat casualty care (TCCC) at the POI and do not receive specialized care during transport. Medical evacuation (MEDEVAC) also allows for movement of the wounded, though care is provided en route. Aeromedical evacuation (AE) provides fixed-wing transport of wounded patients and health care providers within a combat theater of operations as well as between the combat theater and supporting areas outside of the combat zone. A critical care air transport team (CCATT) provides a higher level of AE, including a physician intensivist (commonly an anesthesiologist), a critical care or emergency room nurse, and a cardiopulmonary technician.

Role I care is that care provided closest to the POI. This care is typically qualified as either first-aid or life-saving measures and may be provided by the injured individual, a buddy ("buddy aid"), or a combat lifesaver. Alternatively, a combat emergency medical technician–basic (EMT-B) may be available from an affiliated medical platoon. These soldiers are commonly called combat medics, although a variety of different titles may be applicable depending on the service branch and unit. Role I medical treatment facilities (MTFs), also known as battalion aid stations (BASs), offer triage, immediate first-aid or life-saving treatment, and evacuation capabilities. They are commonly staffed by a single primary care physician or a physician assistant in addition to combat medics and rarely have any surgical capabilities. The Marine Corps offers a similar Role I facility called a shock trauma platoon, which has surgical capabilities limited to life- and limb-saving procedures.[6,7]

Role II facilities have capabilities unique to the respective branch of service and bridge patients between the POI and a Role III facility. Generally, they offer broader care options compared to Role I care, commonly including surgical

TABLE 31.1. Comparison of Proportional Statistics for Battle Casualties, US Military Ground Troops, World War II, Vietnam, Afghanistan/Iraq

	WWII	VIETNAM	TOTAL IRAQ/AFGHANISTAN	AFGHANISTAN	IRAQ
% KIA	20.2[a]	20[b]	13.8[c]	18.7	13.5*
% DOW	3.5[a]	3.2[b]	4.8[c]	6.7	4.7*
CFR	19.1[a]	15.8[b]	9.4[c]	16.4	9.1*

CFR, case fatality rate; DOW, died of wounds; KIA, killed in action; RTD, return to duty; WIA, wounded in action.

[a,b,c] Comparisons between WWII, Vietnam, and total Iraq/Afghanistan, $p < .05$.

*Comparison between Iraq and Afghanistan, $p < .05$.

% KIA = 100 × KIA/[(WIA–RTD) + KIA].

% DOW = 100 × DOW/(WIA–RTD).

CFR = 100 × (KIA + DOW)/(WIA + KIA).

SOURCE: Reprinted with permission from Holcomb JB, Stansbury LG, Champion HR, Wade C, Bellamy RF. Understanding combat casualty care statistics. *J Trauma.* 2006;60:397–401.

capabilities and limited inpatient options. In the Army, Role II MTFs continue basic and life-saving care, including packed red blood cell (PRBC) transfusion and limited radiographic, laboratory, and dental options. The forward surgical team (FST) can be mobilized to provide emergency life-saving damage control surgery (DCS); it employs 20 personnel, including general and orthopedic surgeons, anesthesia providers, and nursing staff. The FST works in conjunction with the supporting medical company to support two operating room (OR) beds capable of providing 72 hours of continuous surgery and an intensive care unit (ICU) capable of supporting eight patients for up to 6 hours. An FST anesthetic environment is shown in Figure 31.1. As shown in this particular photo, supplies are frequently limited to absolute necessities; in this instance, a Narkomed M anesthesia machine was used for the first OR bed, while an Ohmeda draw-over vaporizer was used for the second. Typically, only draw-over vaporizers are available. The Air Force, Navy, and Marine Corps offer branch-specific variations of the FST, each maintaining different levels of mobility, surgical and holding care, and personnel. Each, however, maintains at least one surgeon to support a temporary surgical mission.

Role III facilities are the pinnacle of in-theater combat patient care. They are the ultimate destination of in-theater patient evacuation and serve to further triage patients. Ultimately, wounded American military personnel are either treated and returned to duty or evacuated to a Role IV facility. In the Army, the combat support hospital (CSH) maintains

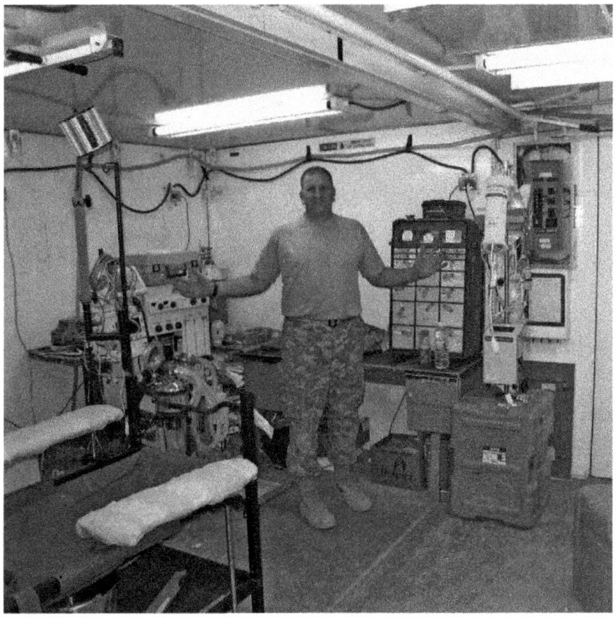

Figure 31.1. Anesthesia setup for 102nd Forward Surgical Team, Forward Operating Base (FOB) Normandy, Iraq. A typical forward surgical team (FST) operating table is partially viewed in the foreground. In the left background is a Narkomed M (Dräger Medical, Germany) anesthesia machine and Propaq model 106 EL (Welch Allyn, Skaneateles Falls, NY) patient monitor. To the right is a Belmont FMS 2000 (Belmont Instrument Corp., Billerica, MA) rapid fluid infusion device. The second operating bed (not pictured) utilized the Ohmeda U-PAC for delivery of draw-over general anesthesia. (Photo by Clinkscales CP, 2008.)

a variety of medical and surgical personnel, including multiple surgical subspecialties, anesthesiologists, and nurse anesthetists to support a broad array of surgical missions. Most surgical patients present with trauma-related concerns requiring life- or limb-saving intervention, though urgent and elective care may be offered according to the operations tempo. Relative to a Role II facility, a CSH also confers greater radiographic and laboratory capabilities, as well as a comprehensive blood bank and a variety of ancillary support personnel, including pharmacists, nutritionists, and respiratory and physical therapists. Again, the Air Force and Navy offer branch-specific variations of a CSH, each with higher levels of care provided relative to a Role II facility.

Role IV facilities exist outside of the combat zone and offer more definitive medical and surgical care as well as enhanced inpatient and outpatient support. Role IV facilities may serve for longer durations of patient care and rehabilitation prior to a patient's return to duty, or they may serve as yet another stop for continued care prior to ultimate disposition to a Role V facility located in the continental United States or Hawaii. Once at a Role V facility, patients have access to the entirety of military resources, including medical, rehabilitative, and administrative support.

Formal training in anesthesia remains a focus for today's military. Presently, Army, Air Force, and Navy anesthesiology residencies exist, often training residents from multiple branches concurrently. Residents and attending anesthesiologists alike have opportunities to participate in humanitarian medical missions around the globe, where they often encounter anesthetic challenges unique to austere environments. These opportunities serve dual purposes in that they extend goodwill between the US military and host nations as well as prepare anesthesiologists for future combat deployments. The Uniformed Services Society of Anesthesiologists (USSA), a component society within the American Society of Anesthesiologists (ASA), was founded in 2003 by COL Paul D. Mongan, MD (Ret.). The USSA meets yearly during the annual ASA meeting to further the mission of continued education relevant to the military anesthesiologist. Nurse anesthesia training programs also exist in the Army, Air Force, and Navy, with training sites throughout numerous military medical hospitals. Because of their historical and continued contributions to combat anesthesia, military student nurse anesthetists are exposed to a unique curriculum with specific focus on combat-relevant anesthesia practices.

An important consideration for the practice of deployed combat anesthesia is the recognition that the delivery of care is only as good as the supply line. Combat anesthesia providers often practice without many of the conveniences of a civilian practice, particularly in the early stages of a conflict and as they approach the front lines of combat. Many of the standards of anesthetic care are nonetheless maintained, and in this respect, experienced anesthesia providers can make easy adjustments to the combat environment. For instance, airway management remains crucial to the combat anesthesia provider much as it does the civilian practitioner.

In one of our recent experiences with the 86th CSH in Baghdad, Iraq, many standard and adjunctive airway devices were available, though fewer than were available at home. Nonetheless, appropriate care was provided at all times, and sufficient equipment was available to support the ASA's difficult airway algorithm. Monitoring devices were similarly limited, though adequate, and included the ability to perform arterial pressure waveform transduction and transesophageal echocardiography. Of paramount importance to the combat anesthesia provider is the ability to provide rapid, life-saving resuscitation measures while prompt DCS is performed.

The practice of trauma anesthesia, discussed briefly under Damage Control Resuscitation, is very similar in the combat environment relative to the civilian environment, and the two undoubtedly continue to provide a useful symbiotic relationship. For instance, the recognition of the lethal triad (also known as the "bloody vicious cycle" or "triad of death") seen in major trauma, comprising acidosis, hypothermia, and coagulopathy, was reported in 1981 by the trauma group at the Denver Health Medical Center.[8] This continues to be a source of significant interest within the military combat and civilian trauma communities alike, and considerable energy is currently being expended to identify ideal modalities for fluid resuscitation, particularly where blood and blood product transfusion is concerned.[9] As the body of literature and evidence grows, so will the practice of combat anesthesia. The focus of the remainder of this chapter is topics of current interest to the combat anesthesia provider.

DRAW-OVER ANESTHESIA

Combat anesthesia providers commonly employ draw-over vaporizers for delivering general anesthesia, particularly in forward environments. Unfortunately, formal training with the draw-over vaporizer is not a common focus of either military or civilian anesthesiology residencies or civilian certified registered nurse anesthetists (CRNA) programs. Army CRNA programs in particular, however, provide both didactic and clinical training of this nature. Anesthetic care at Role II combat facilities is routinely provided by nurse anesthetists and occasionally by anesthesiologists who may not have received formal training with draw-over anesthesia, making an understanding of the equipment and physiologic considerations pertinent to any combat anesthesia provider. Role III and above facilities commonly utilize late-model anesthesia machines that should be familiar to any experienced anesthesia provider.

Draw-over general anesthesia provides many advantages over standard machine-driven general anesthesia: It is light and portable; equipment can be put together rapidly by a single individual; delivery of anesthetic gases is dependent on the patient's spontaneous ventilatory drive; compressed air or oxygen is not mandatory but can be accommodated easily; and electricity is not necessary unless supplemental ventilator support is desired. Additionally, rapid induction and emergence can be achieved easily because the system is nonrebreathing and has a small circuit volume, and scavenging of waste gases is easy to achieve.[10] Presently, the US military uses the Ohmeda Universal Portable Anesthesia Complete (U-PAC) system (Figure 31.2) with or without an Impact Uni-Vent Eagle 754 portable ventilator (Figure 31.3). In its basic configuration (Figure 31.4), the U-PAC includes an inspiratory prevaporizer limb of reservoir tubing, a universal vaporizer, an outlet adapter, a length of postvaporizer tubing connected to a self-inflating bag, and a second length of postvaporizer tubing connected to a face mask and preceded by a unidirectional nonrebreathing valve. A bacteriostatic gas humidifier can be added between the nonrebreathing valve and face mask, and the face mask can be replaced by a direct connection to an endotracheal tube or similar airway device. In its simplest explanation, draw-over anesthesia allows the patient's spontaneous (or assisted) breaths to "draw" fresh gas from the reservoir tubing into the vaporizer and "over" the selected volatile anesthetic, ultimately delivering a mixture of this volatile anesthetic and fresh gas to the patient.

The vaporizer is temperature compensated, and variable-bypass mechanics allow for precise delivery of anesthetic concentrations. The draw-over vaporizer is demand driven; hence, if the patient's ventilation is not spontaneous or

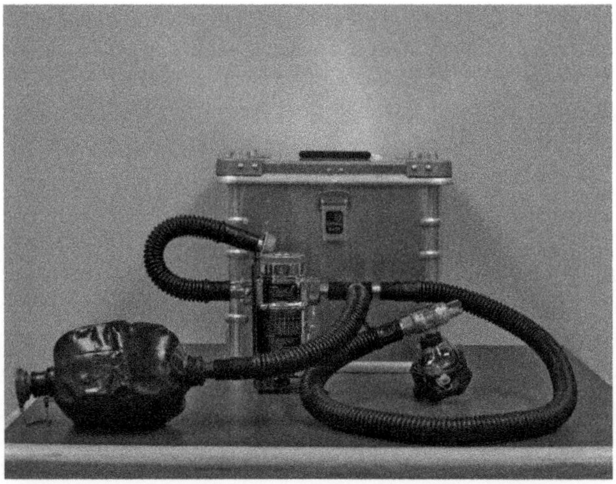

Figure 31.2. Standard Ohmeda Universal Portable Anesthesia Complete (U-PAC) system. Foreground: Unmodified Ohmeda U-PAC ready for use. Background: The Ohmeda U-PAC container is compact and lightweight. Dimensions: approximately 15" wide × 15" tall × 10" deep. Weight: approximately 6 kg. (Photo by Clinkscales CP, 2009.)

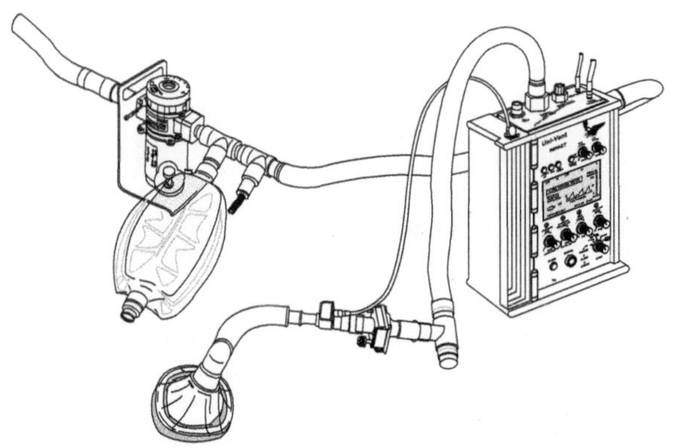

Figure 31.3. Draw-over apparatus in combination with ventilator. (From Emergency War Surgery, Third United States Revision. Department of Defense, United States of America, 2004.)

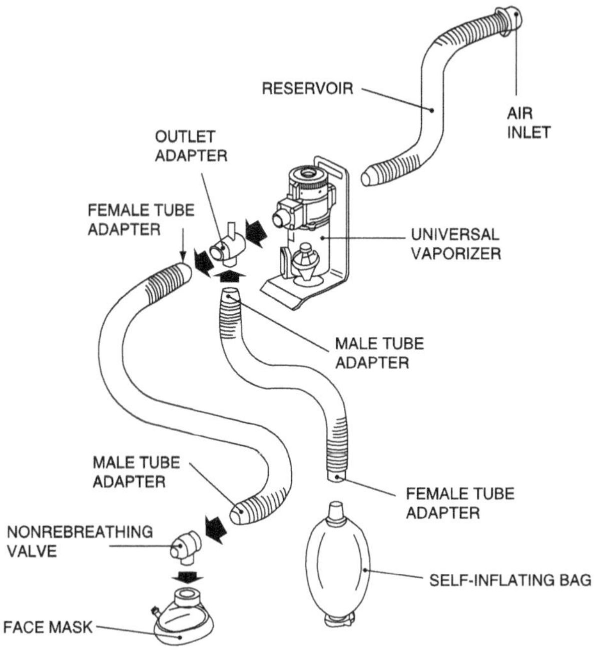

Figure 31.4. *Breakout view of the Universal Portable Anesthesia Complete Draw-Over Anesthetic System. (Reprinted with permission from Gegel BT. A field-expedient Ohmeda Universal Portable Anesthesia Complete Draw-over Vaporizer setup. AANA J. 2008;76:185–187.)*

supported, no anesthetic gas will be delivered. The universal vaporizer can support a variety of different inhalational agents, though isoflurane and halothane are most commonly used in today's forward deployed environment. When selecting an agent, it should be recalled that halothane carries the added risk of hepatic damage and sensitization of the myocardium to catecholamines, whereas isoflurane is associated with greater vasodilation. Isoflurane preserves cardiac index better, likely due to an associated increase in heart rate. Additionally, halothane is associated with a greater increase in cerebral blood flow compared to isoflurane, while both agents contribute to a reduction in the cerebral metabolic rate for oxygen.[11] These characteristics should be considered in the forward combat environment, where patients are likely hypovolemic and potentially have head trauma. Whatever agent is used, anticipate the consumption of approximately 40 mL of anesthetic per hour of vaporizer use, recognizing that delivery may actually need to be far less in the setting of significant hemorrhage and hemodynamic instability.[12]

While oxygen is not necessary to provide ventilation using the draw-over apparatus, it can and should be utilized when readily available. Supplementary oxygen can be provided by either pipeline or tank sources or by an oxygen concentrator; a nipple on the vaporizer allows for oxygen entrainment into the inspiratory limb. An oxygen reservoir tube on the prevaporizer end of the apparatus allows for further increases in oxygen concentration when attached to a supplementary source.

Gegel described increasing the length of the oxygen reservoir tubing from the standard 18 inches, or 46 cm (130 mL), to 36 inches, or 91 cm (260 mL), using 22-mm plastic tubing (Figure 31.5). This further concentrated oxygen supply to the patient and provided an increased margin of safety. Additionally, the factory oxygen reservoir tube was added to the standard length of tubing between the outlet adapter and self-inflating bag to allow the bag to rest on the floor and be used as a foot pump, freeing the anesthesia provider's hand to perform other functions.[13] This modification is commonly used in the forward combat environment among American anesthesia providers.

Eales et al. described yet another method for providing more efficient oxygen delivery to patients under draw-over general anesthesia, utilizing a variety of prevaporizer modifications along the inspiratory limb: an oxygen reservoir tube of 300 mL with an end-capped, one-way valve, a volume-increasing reservoir bag, and an adjustable pressure-limiting valve set to deliver 5 cm H_2O continuous positive airway pressure (CPAP). This was specifically demonstrated in the setting of high minute ventilation.[14]

Scavenging waste gases is important in any anesthetic delivery system, and draw-over anesthesia is no exception. Tubing can be easily connected to the nonrebreathing valve and extended outside of the operating arena, whether that arena is a tent or other temporary facility or a fixed structure.

The Impact Uni-Vent Eagle 754 portable ventilator can be added to the Ohmeda U-PAC when controlled ventilation is desired. The ventilator sits between the vaporizer and the patient and contains a nonreturn valve that inhibits dangerous back pressure on the vaporizer; it contains another nonreturn valve on the patient side that prevents back pressure into the

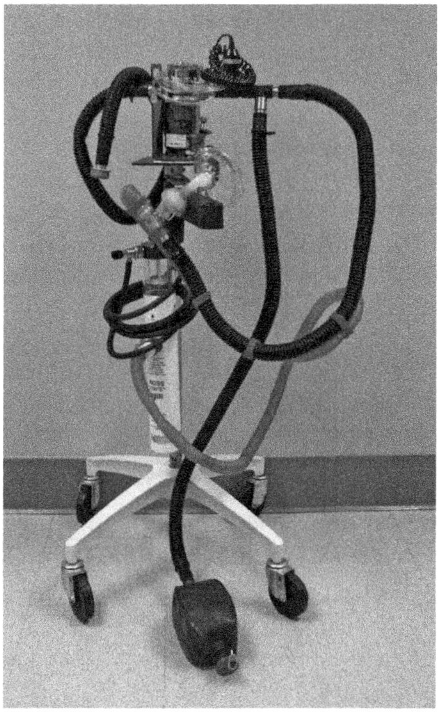

Figure 31.5. *Gegel-Mercado modification to the Ohmeda U-PAC. Note the increased length of reservoir tubing on the inspiratory end, or left, of the vaporizer. This configuration is equipped with an oxygen analyzer and scavenging apparatus (termination of light blue tubing, extending from face mask). It can be further configured to accommodate gas sampling and spirometry. (Photo by Clinkscales CP, 2009.)*

ventilator. Either the induction circuit or the ventilator circuit can support the scavenging of waste gases.[5]

TOTAL INTRAVENOUS ANESTHESIA

Total intravenous anesthesia (TIVA) has gained recent attention from American combat anesthesia providers due to its many inherent advantages. Among these advantages, TIVA is versatile and applicable in a variety of different clinical scenarios, it is accommodating to different drugs and their inherent pharmacologic profiles, it does not require electricity or significant manpower or delivery support, and there is a lower risk of redistribution hypothermia when ketamine is added to the solution.[15] TIVA is conducive to natural or artificial airways, spontaneous or assisted ventilation, and a breadth of operative cases ranging from minor and elective to traumatic and emergent. In the combat environment, the major disadvantage regarding TIVA is a lack of familiarity with the practice for many anesthesia providers.[15]

The Tri-service Anesthesia Research Group Initiative (TARGIT) on TIVA, formed at Brooke Army Medical Center in 2004, was instrumental in bringing TIVA to the forefront of American combat anesthesia. In 2003, Dr. Mark Meeks was the first anesthesiologist to enter Iraq. As a member of the 86th CSH, Dr. Meeks successfully performed many combat anesthetics using ketamine as a sole anesthetic. Dr. Joel McMasters was also deployed to Iraq in 2003 as an anesthesiologist with the 28th CSH. During his deployment, Dr. McMasters employed many of the first combined TIVAs utilizing propofol, ketamine, and fentanyl, also with great success. Dr. Kurt Grathwohl was the first Army anesthesiologist to utilize combat TIVA on a large scale, performing over 100 anesthetics using the technique during his deployment with the 359th neurosurgical team, 31st CSH in Baghdad, Iraq, in 2004–2005. As an anesthesiologist with the 10th CSH in Iraq in 2006, Dr. Craig McFarland performed an estimated 400 anesthetics using TIVA. Figure 31.6 shows Dr. McFarland performing TIVA on a spontaneously ventilating Iraqi patient undergoing surgery on a traumatically amputated lower extremity. The patient maintained a natural airway and did not require a regional anesthetic (personal communication between McMasters, Grathwohl, and McFarland.) A multitude of different TIVA techniques have been utilized with great success as well, by both civilian and combat anesthesiologists. As a result of this growing body of evidence and experience, military anesthesiologists and nurse anesthetists, as well as their civilian counterparts, are becoming increasingly aware of the applicability and benefits of TIVA.

Of the multitude of TIVA formulations available for clinical practice, one of the most commonly employed in the US military environment is a solution containing propofol, ketamine, and fentanyl. In stateside military hospitals, this solution is often administered with ketamine 100 mg (50 mg/mL, 2 mL) and fentanyl 100 µg (50 µg/mL, 2 mL) added to propofol 1000 mg (10 mg/mL, 100 mL). This solution, commonly referred to as $P_{10}K_1F_1$ (reflecting the concentrations of the individual drugs in the solution as milligrams per milliliter for propofol

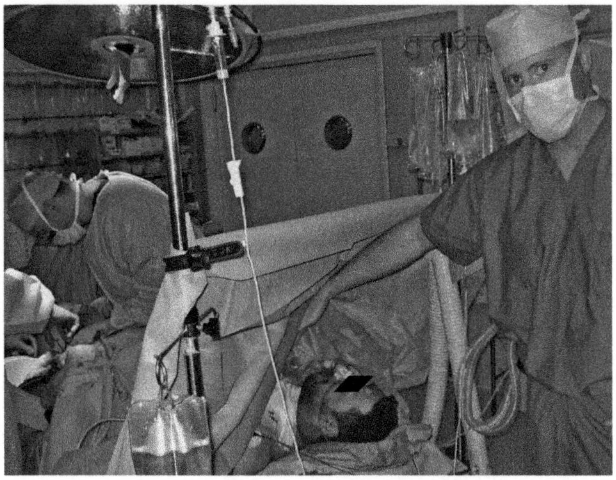

Figure 31.6. Application of total intravenous anesthesia (TIVA) in the deployed environment. The patient, a member of the Iraqi military who served alongside American military forces, is breathing spontaneously via his natural airway with only supplemental oxygen via nonrebreathing face mask. He does not have a regional anesthetic despite having surgery on a traumatically amputated lower extremity. The TIVA mixture is propofol, ketamine, and fentanyl administered from a single bag, 100 mL via a dripper at 20 drops/mL. (Photo by McFarland CC, 2006. Used with permission.)

and ketamine and micrograms per milliliter for fentanyl), is then infused to the patient using a standard infusion pump at rates of 75–150 µg/kg per minute of propofol to maintain general anesthesia. Infusion rates may be lowered to maintain sedation when general anesthesia is not desired. Additionally, the amount of ketamine and fentanyl may be tailored to meet specific anesthetic needs. Ketamine is often discontinued after the first 100 mg are delivered to facilitate emergence. Sufentanil and remifentanil have been successfully substituted for fentanyl in equipotent doses.

In the deployed environment, equipment and supplies are often at a premium, so it has become common practice to exchange lower concentrations of propofol for higher concentrations of ketamine and fentanyl, as described by Mahoney and McFarland.[15] This solution is then administered to the patient using a standard intravenous (IV) dripper, thus negating the need for large quantities of 100-mL vials of propofol as well as mechanical infusion pumps. To establish this solution of $P_4K_{2.5}F_{2.5}$, 400 mg of propofol (10 mg/mL, 40 mL), 250 mg of ketamine (50 mg/mL, 5 mL), and 250 µg of fentanyl (50 µg/mL, 5 mL) are added to 50 mL of normal saline. When a 20-drop/mL intravenous dripper is used, and assuming an 80-kg patient, 1 drop every 3 seconds equates to an infusion of 50 µg/kg per minute of propofol. Using this information, 1 drop every 2 seconds establishes an infusion of 75 µg/kg per minute of propofol, 1 drop every second establishes an infusion of 150 µg/kg per minute of propofol, and so forth. Further adjustments can be made based on the individual patient's weight as well as surgical and anesthetic needs. Figure 31.7 demonstrates the equipment necessary to perform this anesthetic technique.

Continuous infusions of intravenous agents offer many advantages over intermittent boluses of the same medications, namely by establishing better control of plasma drug levels

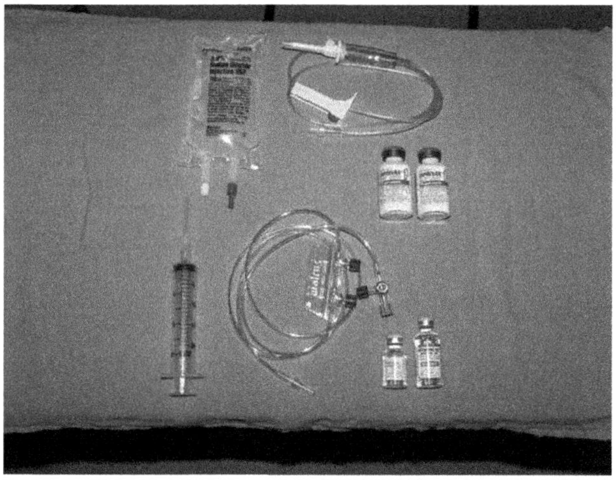

Figure 31.7. Equipment and medications needed for suggested combat total intravenous anesthesia (TIVA) setup. From the upper left and working clockwise: 100-mL normal saline bag with 50 mL removed, 20 drops/mL IV dripper, two propofol 10 mg/mL 20-mL vials, ketamine 50 mg/mL 10-mL vial, fentanyl 50 μg/mL 2-mL vial, intravenous extension tubing, and 20-mL syringe with 18-gauge needle for drawing medications. (Photo by McFarland CC, 2006. Used with permission.)

within the therapeutic range rather than oscillations above and below the desired levels. This has been long understood particularly in regard to the administration of fentanyl and ketamine.[16] Clinically, this is demonstrated by reliable titration of anesthesia and analgesia, as well as rapid emergence from general anesthesia versus easy maintenance of sedation for transfer to a critical care ward.

In recent years, TIVA has demonstrated itself to be at least equivalent to a volatile-based anesthetic in terms of reliability and reproducibility. Recent studies, however, have potentially conferred an advantage on TIVA that is particularly relevant in the combat environment. In patients experiencing head trauma, further increases in cerebral blood flow and intracranial pressure (ICP) associated with volatile anesthetics may be undesirable despite the associated reductions in cerebral metabolic rate. Cole et al. reviewed numerous prospective studies regarding the use of TIVA in elective intracranial procedures and found that, relative to volatile anesthetics in elective intracranial operations, TIVA offered decreased ICP in the setting of increased cerebral perfusion pressure.[17] The extension of these findings to the traumatically injured brain in the combat environment is lacking. Grathwohl et al. retrospectively evaluated neurologic outcome in patients with operative traumatic brain injury and found no benefit with TIVA relative to volatile-based anesthesia; however, by their own estimation there were many confounding variables and limitations to their study, not the least of which was the inability to adequately power and perform a prospective analysis.[18]

In addition to propofol's hypnotic and amnestic properties and fentanyl's analgesic properties, the addition of ketamine offers further hypnotic, dissociative, amnestic, and analgesic properties. Also, the sympathomimetic properties of ketamine may offset the vasodilating effects of propofol, potentially allowing for greater hemodynamic stability. The utility of ketamine in a combat environment has been recognized for many years.[19,20] In a swine model, a ketamine-based TIVA model was shown to produce less-pronounced hypotension in the setting of uncontrolled hemorrhagic shock relative to an isoflurane anesthetic, albeit at the potential expense of end-organ perfusion.[21] It is noted, however, that Englehart et al. used doses of ketamine (as well as midazolam) significantly beyond that typically used in TIVA, so the true effect of ketamine on blood pressure and end-organ perfusion in a hemorrhagic shock model remains unknown. Additionally, historical concerns regarding the use of ketamine in the setting of central neurologic injury has been challenged. Himmelseher and Durieux demonstrated Level II clinical evidence in stating that ketamine is not associated with increases in ICP when coadministered in the setting of controlled mechanical ventilation and a γ-aminobutyric acid (GABA) receptor agonist, given the avoidance of nitrous oxide.[22] Counterintuitively, the use of perioperative ketamine may also be associated with a reduced incidence of posttraumatic stress disorder (PTSD) in wounded service members, as demonstrated in a recent study by McGhee et al.[23]

ACUTE PAIN MANAGEMENT

Combat anesthesia providers are commonly faced with wounded personnel presenting with myriad traumatic injuries. Significant perioperative acute pain is expected, allowing anesthesia providers to have a significant positive effect on patient outcome. Unlike the civilian population, where operative intervention is commonly expected and planned, combat surgery rarely avails itself to preemptive analgesia. Anesthesia on the battlefield often begins at the POI and is either provided by the casualty, a fellow soldier (battle buddy or buddy aid), or a combat medic within the group. Wounded American military personnel may have the opportunity to ingest a "Combat Pill Pack," which includes acetaminophen, a nonsteroidal anti-inflammatory drug (NSAID) (i.e., celecoxib or meloxicam), and an antibiotic (i.e., gatifloxacin) at the POI, prior to evacuation and medical evaluation. Medics are also equipped with opioid medications for escalating pain requirements. Intramuscular morphine autoinjector pens have found use on the battlefield for acute pain as well and oral transmucosal fentanyl citrate (OTFC) to provide alternate routes for analgesia in the combat setting.[42] Patients wounded in theater are commonly evacuated to successive levels of higher care rapidly, potentially inhibiting methodical evaluation and subsequent and ongoing treatment of acute pain. Additionally, significant pain can result from non–combat-related accidents and injuries.[24] As such, combat anesthesia providers face unique challenges. A complete discussion of acute pain management is beyond the scope of this chapter, though the following provides some generic considerations that are applicable in the combat environment.

Although definitive outcome studies evaluating the merits of acute pain management are lacking,[25] various physiologic and psychologic benefits associated with adequate pain control are appreciated and can intuitively be assumed to improve patient morbidity and mortality. Specifically, in the presence of poorly controlled pain, oxygenation and ventilation become impaired; myocardial oxygen consumption increases; the stress response is increased, resulting in a catabolic state; hypercoagulability develops, which predisposes patients to thromboembolic events; and immune function is impaired.[26] Psychologically, patients feel helpless and experience needless suffering.[25] Additionally, poorly controlled acute pain may contribute to the development of PTSD and chronic pain,[27–29] both of which are currently areas of significant concern within the American military medical community.

Noxious stimuli activate nociceptors, leading to the release of numerous local chemical mediators, including substance P, glutamate, aspartate, prostaglandins, serotonin, leukotrienes, bradykinin, and histamine. These nociceptors communicate with the dorsal horn of the spinal cord via Aδ and C first-order pain fibers, where additional chemical mediators are released, including glutamate, aspartate, vasoactive intestinal peptide, calcitonin gene–related peptide, neuropeptide Y, and substance P. At this level, inhibitory mechanisms also exist and may be modulated by GABA, glycine, enkephalins, β-endorphins, norepinephrine, dopamine, adenosine, somatostatin, and acetylcholine. Second-order neurons then transmit these data to the brainstem and thalamus via the contralateral spinothalamic tract. Finally, third-order neurons extend from the thalamus to the sensory cortex.[26,30]

Based on this understanding, there is much interest currently in a multimodal approach to the treatment of acute pain, in both the civilian and the deployed combat environments. Hartrick described multimodal pain therapy as the use of multiple pharmacologic and nonpharmacologic analgesic therapies utilizing varying mechanisms of action.[31] Furthermore, multimodal pain management is believed not only to improve postoperative analgesia but also to reduce the incidence of analgesia-related deleterious side effects.[32] Historically, postoperative pain has been treated by a model similar to the World Health Organization's pain ladder for the relief of cancer pain, which begins with nonopioid management with or without an adjuvant, advancing then to the addition of opioid medications and additional adjuvants as pain severity increases.[33] This remains an appropriate response to acute postoperative pain, though in the combat environment, health care providers often rely heavily on opioid medications while underutilizing adjuvant therapies. This may be an incomplete treatment strategy considering the frequent presentation of pain from somatic, visceral, and neuropathic origins.

Classic analgesics that can be useful in a multimodal approach include nonopioid and opioid medications alike. Acetaminophen and NSAIDs exert their action via the inhibition of central prostaglandin synthesis in the case of acetaminophen and a combined inhibition of peripheral and central prostaglandin synthesis in the case of NSAIDs.[30] Cyclooxygenase 2 (COX-2)–selective NSAIDs can also be employed, and they generally have a more favorable side-effect profile.[25] Each of these classes exerts opioid-sparing effects in the treatment of acute pain. However, as acute pain increases in severity, the addition of opioids often becomes necessary.

Activation of the μ-receptor primarily accounts for the analgesic effect of opioids as well as many of their deleterious side effects, whereas κ-receptor agonism accounts for analgesia with less respiratory depression.[30] In the combat environment, opioids are typically administered by the parenteral route, often by patient-controlled analgesic (PCA) devices. There are many advantages of PCA delivery, as pointed out by Malchow and Black, including patient self-empowerment and satisfaction. However, they continued that studies of PCA delivery provided conflicting data regarding efficacy and patient safety.[25] Nonetheless, PCA delivery remains a viable option, and the American Society of Regional Anesthesia and Pain Medicine (ASRA) has released a consensus statement identifying PCA as superior to nurse-administered parenteral opioids in regard to patient outcomes.[32] Table 31.2 shows various starting points for an opioid PCA regimen.

Numerous opioid medications also exist for enteral dosing. Of these, methadone deserves special mention because of its antagonism of NMDA receptors and inhibition of serotonin reuptake in addition to opioid receptor activation.[25] Because of these unique properties among opioids, methadone can be invaluable in a multimodal treatment regimen. Also unique to methadone, though, is its variable pharmacologic profile, which can contribute to delayed onset of side effects due to gradual accumulation of the drug, including a peak risk of mortality 5 days after starting the medication in previously opioid-näive patients.[25]

Among nonopioid adjuvant medications, many can be utilized successfully in the combat environment. Ketamine exerts its action via antagonism of the excitatory neurotransmitter glutamate by binding to and modifying the *N*-methyl-D-aspartate (NMDA) receptor and can be given as an adjunctive analgesic during operative analgesia or in the postoperative period.[34] Ketamine can be bolused in 10- to 20-mg IV doses to provide rapid analgesia; due to the potential development of psychomimetic effects, however, it is prudent to consider coadministration with a benzodiazepine. Alternatively, ketamine can be combined with a morphine PCA delivery system

TABLE 31.2. Recommendations for Opioid Delivery by Patient-Controlled Analgesia (PCA)

DRUG	MG/ML	LOAD (MG)	BASAL (MG/H)	PCA DOSE (MG)	LOCKOUT (MIN)
Morphine	1	5–10	0–1	1–3	6–12
Hydromorphone	0.2	1–2	0–0.2	0.2–0.6	6–10
Fentanyl (μg)	25	100–200	0–25	20–30	6–10

SOURCE: Reprinted with permission from Malchow RJ, Black IH. The evolution of pain management in the critically ill trauma patient: emerging concepts from the global war on terrorism. *Crit Care Med.* 2008;36:S346–S357.

(morphine 1 mg + ketamine 1 mg per demand bolus) to provide safe and ongoing analgesia.[35]

Clonidine functions in acute pain management via its actions at the α_2-receptor in the locus ceruleus as well as via its inhibitory actions at the spinal cord level.[25] Clonidine is quite versatile and can be administered orally, transdermally, intravenously, neuraxially, and as an adjunct to peripheral nerve blockade. Oral and transdermal routes are most common; orally, 0.1–0.2 mg given once or twice daily versus a 0.1- or 0.2-mg transdermal patch is a reasonable starting point. Sedation and hemodynamic instability are potential concerns, particularly in predisposed patients.

Gabapentin and pregabalin are anticonvulsants that can be used as analgesic adjuvants; their mechanism of action is not completely understood, though they may regulate excitatory neurotransmitters at the spinal cord level by activating noradrenergic receptors.[25,36] Both agents are given by the oral route. Gabapentin is commonly started at 300 mg three times daily, with gradual escalation to a maximum dose of 1200 mg three times daily. Pregabalin is commonly started at 75 mg twice daily and increased to 150 mg twice daily. Clinically, pregabalin may be associated with less sedation than gabapentin.

Tricyclic antidepressants (TCAs) block the reuptake of norepinephrine and serotonin, which are active mediators of spinal inhibitory pathways. Additionally, they provide sedation and are useful as a sleep aid. As such, they can be a valuable addition to a multimodal plan. Amitriptyline is typically started at 10–25 mg orally at bedtime and gradually increased to 50 mg. TCAs present a broad side-effect profile, necessitating close follow-up by prescribing health care providers.

Mexiletine is an oral analogue to lidocaine; in addition to its antiarrhythmic properties, it can be beneficial in acute pain treatment due to blockade of sodium channels and action at the spinal NMDA receptors.[25,37] Intravenous lidocaine and oral mexiletine are thus potentially useful agents in the treatment of acute pain, particularly of neuropathic origin. Side-effect limitations include sedation, fatigue, nausea, and dizziness.[38] There may also be concerns about the introduction of cardiac conduction abnormalities.[25] Mexiletine can be started orally at 150 mg twice daily and gradually increased to 300–450 mg twice daily. Malchow and Black suggested an intravenous lidocaine test prior to beginning oral treatment with mexiletine, ostensibly to assess for expected continued response.[25]

REGIONAL ANESTHESIA AND ANALGESIA

Regional anesthesia has been utilized in combat situations throughout the 20th century and continues to be utilized in the current GWOT. Though used by American military anesthetists in combat as early at WWI, spinal anesthesia did not emerge as an accepted and common practice until the Vietnam War. Similarly, epidural anesthesia and peripheral nerve blockade in the combat environment also emerged at that time.[1] These techniques remain valuable adjuncts in today's combat environment. In the words of Schulz-Stübner et al., "Regional analgesia using single-injection regional blocks and continuous neuraxial and peripheral catheters can play a valuable role in a multimodal approach to pain management in the critically ill patient to achieve optimum patient comfort and to reduce physiologic and psychological stress."[39] In their review of pain management for the critically ill patient, Malchow and Black identified numerous measures of improved patient outcomes with regional analgesia, including lessened lengths of stay, improved physiologic performance, and decreased mortality in addition to improved pain scores.[25]

There is evidence that epidural analgesia eases management and improves comfort, without necessarily reducing mortality, in the critical care population. Specific surgical populations encountered in the combat environment that this statement applies to include chest trauma and thoracic, abdominal, major vascular, and major orthopedic surgery.[39] Neuraxial techniques can be employed in the combat environment, though concerns with hemorrhage-induced hypotension and hemodynamic instability as well as coagulopathy associated with trauma may impede the use of these techniques. In the combat trauma patient, it is often prudent to allow the initial surgical course to proceed utilizing a general anesthetic; on completion of DCS, initial resuscitation, and complete evaluation of the patient's presentation and expected hospital course, reassessment for continual epidural analgesia might be considered. One of us frequently placed thoracic and lumbar epidural catheters in trauma patients utilizing this formula. Bolus injections of local anesthetics into the epidural space may not be desirable in the setting of recently completed or ongoing fluid resuscitations, although infusions of local anesthetics are likely to be better tolerated. Opioids may be added to the epidural solution as allowed by the patient's ventilatory and mental states.

In 2003, while deployed with the 21st CSH in Balad, Iraq, COL Chester "Trip" Buckenmaier III, MD, placed the first successful in-theater continuous peripheral nerve block catheter in a wounded soldier. Soon thereafter, the Army Regional Anesthesia and Pain Management Initiative (ARAPMI) was founded at Walter Reed Army Medical Center in Washington, D.C., to advance the practice of regional anesthesia and acute pain management in both the military and civilian environments. Additionally, the ARAPMI maintains the Regional Anesthesia Tracking System (RATS), which allows anesthesia providers to track a patient's pain control from the POI, often in theater, to a stateside military hospital. ARAPMI, now known as Defense and Veterans Pain Management Initiative (DVPMI), also works in conjunction with the triservice collaborative group Military Advanced Regional Anesthesia and Analgesia (MARAA) to provide combat acute pain management support. The MARAA handbook (available for free online download http://www.dvcipm.org/clinical-resources/dvcipm-maraa-book-project/) is an excellent resource for acute pain management in the combat environment.[40]

Peripheral nerve blockade can be provided by a single-shot technique or continuous infusion via an indwelling catheter. In the combat environment, wounded American military personnel often do not stay in theater for prolonged periods of time, as evacuation to a higher echelon of care proceeds quickly after initial surgical intervention. As such, time constraints may make placement of an indwelling catheter more challenging, so a single-shot technique may be preferred. Figure 31.8

demonstrates the equipment needed for a single-shot peripheral nerve block, as well as a block being performed by one of us on a sedated pediatric patient. Ultrasound capabilities are presently available throughout the combat theater, though machines may be older and thus less "user friendly" compared to newer models.

Table 31.3 lists local anesthetic considerations for peripheral nerve blocks, including recommendations for infusion rates and PCA demand options when indwelling catheters are placed. Indwelling catheters unquestionably have a role in perioperative combat analgesia provided the additional time necessary for placement is allowed by the surgical and evacuation time-frame.[41] In Figure 31.9, an ultrasound-guided brachial plexus catheter is placed utilizing the supraclavicular approach in a sedated Iraqi woman admitted to the hospital for contracture releases resulting from full-thickness burns. These catheters should be placed under strict sterile conditions, and adequate patient education and follow-up are mandatory. When sufficient time is not available, a prolonged block can be achieved by administering bupivacaine 0.5% and a vasoconstrictor such as 1:400,000 epinephrine. It should be recalled that the cardiotoxicity of bupivacaine is greater than ropivacaine, so appropriate preparation is necessary. The addition of tetracaine to this solution can prolong the single-shot block further when added to this bupivacaine/epinephrine solution. Some providers commonly added lyophilized tetracaine 10 mg to every 20 mL of solution. The goal was to safely establish peripheral nerve blockade for sufficient duration to allow the patient to be evacuated to Landstuhl Regional Medical Center in Germany, where more definitive acute pain management could be started.

When providing peripheral nerve blockade for combat patients, the same risks exist as those for noncombat patients. However, there might be a greater likelihood of undiagnosed injuries and comorbidities, necessitating close attention and care by the anesthesia provider. Additionally, considering the common "dirty" nature of combat injuries, particular attention should be paid to sterile technique in recognition of the potential for increased risk of infection. Also, prompt recognition and treatment of local anesthetic toxicity should be available. In Baghdad, Iraq, intralipid 20% solution was readily available for lipid rescue, although it was not needed during the author's deployment.

DAMAGE CONTROL RESUSCITATION

Paramount to modern combat casualty care is recognizing injuries with high mortality (penetrating, blast, burn, etc.), initiating life-saving maneuvers, and evacuating casualties to escalated care facilities. As previously discussed, hemorrhagic blood loss remains the most common cause of preventable death on the battlefield. Although treatments with tourniquets and hemostatic dressings are fundamental during initial care of a casualty with uncontrolled hemorrhage, evacuation to the rear is imperative. These casualties require a treatment facility with a surgical team to initiate DCS concurrently with anesthesia providers to perform damage control resuscitation (DCR). DCR begins at the POI and continues throughout patient care. The NATO Life and Limb Saving Timeline was adopted in June 2011 with the rule of "10-1-2," which provides a expected timeline for care of wounded with life-saving maneuvers in the first 10 minutes, initiating DCR efforts by medical personnel within the first hour, and providing DCS within 2 hours of wounding.[43]

TABLE 31.3. Recommendations for Infusion Volumes for Peripheral Nerve Blockade

TECHNIQUE	ADULT SINGLE INJECTION (ML, 0.5% ROPIVACAINE)[a,b]	CONTINUOUS INFUSION (ML/H, 0.2% ROPIVACAINE)	PCA BOLUS RATE (ML/BOLUS, 0.2% ROPIVACAINE, 20-MIN LOCKOUT)
Interscalene	30–40 mL	8–10 mL	2–3 mL
Supraclavicular	30–40 mL	8–10 mL	2–3 mL
Infraclavicular	30–40 mL	8–10 mL	2–3 mL
Paravertebral	3–5 mL per level	8–10 mL	2–3 mL
Lumbar plexus	25–30 mL	6–8 mL	2–3 mL
Femoral	20–25 mL	6–8 mL	2–3 mL
Sciatic (anterior or posterior approach)	20–25 mL	6–8 mL	2–3 mL
Sciatic (lateral or posterior popliteal approach)	35–40 mL	8–10 mL	2–3 mL

[a] Consider adding a vasoconstrictor as a vascular marker; prolongation of the block is an added benefit. One of the authors adds 1:400,000 epinephrine (2.5 μg epinephrine/mL local anesthetic solution).

[b] For a longer-lasting block, 0.5% bupivacaine can be substituted for ropivacaine. The block can be prolonged further by adding tetracaine to the solution; one of the authors typically adds lyophilized tetracaine 10 mg per 20 mL existing solution.

SOURCE: Reprinted with permission from Chapter 3: Local Anesthetics. *The Military Advanced Regional Anesthesia and Analgesia Handbook*, Army Regional Anesthesia and Pain Management Initiative. Copyright 2008 The Henry M. Jackson Foundation for the Advancement of Military Medicine, Inc.

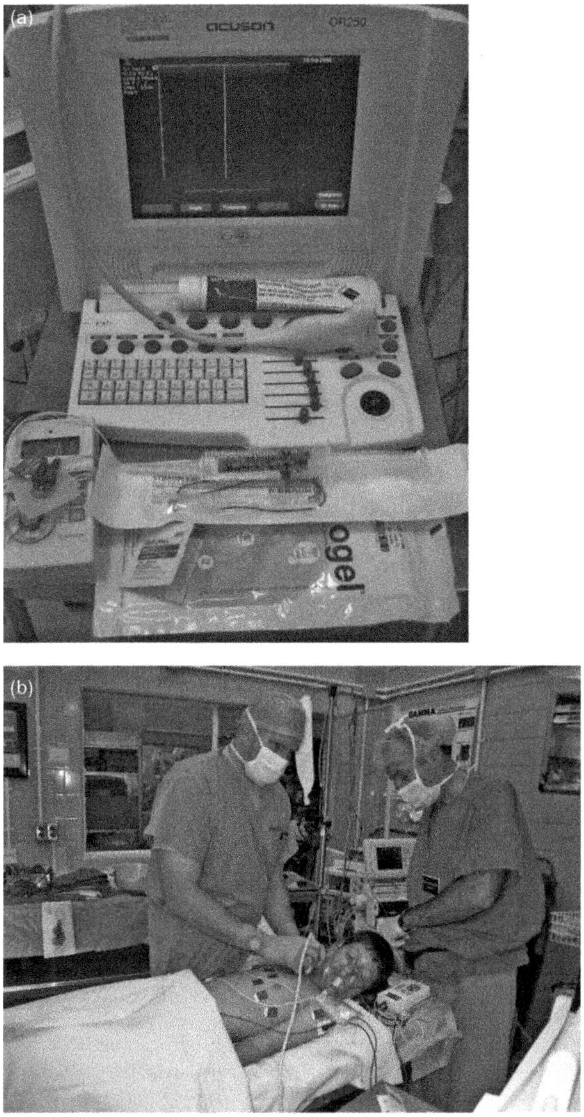

Figure 31.8. Placement of single-shot peripheral nerve blocks in theater is quick, easy, and beneficial. (a) The photo on the left shows the equipment that may be used for a peripheral nerve block, including ultrasound, a nerve stimulator, an appropriate size insulated beveled stimulating needle, local anesthetic mixture, skin prep, and sterile gloves. (b) An ultrasound-guided interscalene brachial plexus block is placed in a noncombatant Iraqi pediatric patient who underwent upper extremity fasciotomies after a snake bite. The patient was sedated with ketamine and midazolam. (Photos by Clinkscales CP, 2008. Permission obtained for inclusion in photo from LTC Joseph O'Sullivan, CRNA, PhD.)

Damage control resuscitation focuses on treatment or prevention of the "lethal triad" of hypothermia, coagulopathy, and acidosis. These factors have been associated with an increased rate of mortality in the setting of trauma.[44] Early goal-directed therapy for correction of hypothermia include active warming of the patient, increasing room temperature as well as convection therapy and warm irrigation by the surgical team. Aggressive correction of hypothermia prevents worsening coagulopathy and helps circumvent alterations in drug metabolism. In DCR, resuscitation with blood products is used in lieu of aggressive crystalloid in an effort to treat any underlying coagulopathy while preventing dilutional anemia.

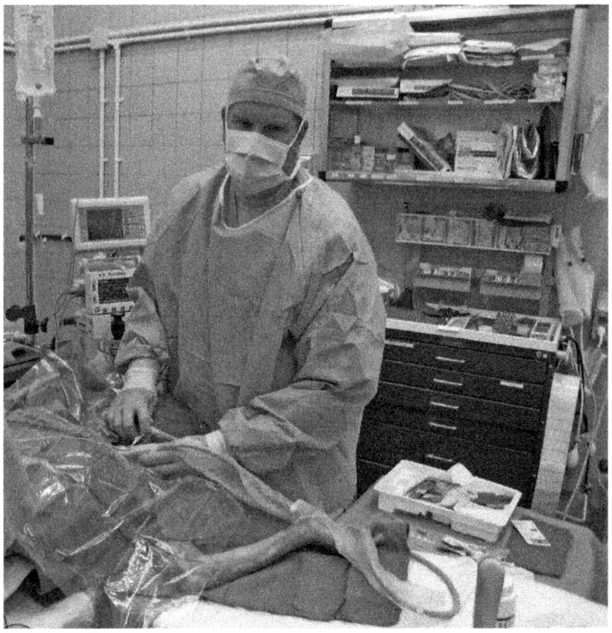

Figure 31.9. Placement of an ultrasound-guided supraclavicular brachial plexus catheter in a sedated patient; a brachial plexus catheter is placed utilizing the supraclavicular approach. The patient was a burned noncombatant Iraqi civilian female. She received her burn care at Ibn Sina Hospital in Baghdad, Iraq, and was later readmitted for contracture release. (Photo by Clinkscales CP, 2008.)

Common practice using a 1:1:1 transfusion ratio of PRBCs to plasma to platelets ratio has been adopted; however, conflicting studies have failed to definitively prove this strategy increases survival.[45–47] Transfusion of whole blood is another possibility in the trauma setting, but it requires planning and specialized training. Treatment of coagulopathy with tranexamic acid (TXA) in an effort to circumvent trauma-induced hyperfibrinolysis has been adopted into TCCC after multiple studies demonstrating its benefit in decreasing mortality in both civilian and military settings.[48,49]

The principles of DCS revolve around surgical intervention to stabilize the wounded in an effort to salvage life, limb, or function.[43] They are not meant as definitive treatment as the physiologic limits may be at capacity.[50] Primary surgical interventions in DCS involve attempts to control bleeding via exploratory laparotomies, thoracotomies, and surgical airways and attempts to preserve or restore blood flow to distal limbs. There are essentially three phases to DCS. The initial phase involves controlling hemorrhage and contamination and maintaining an airway. The second stage involves continuing DCR in an attempt to correct any hemodynamic derangements. Last, the third aspect of DCS focuses on definitive treatment after normal physiology has been restored.[50,51]

CONCLUSION

Military anesthesia provides many unique and challenging situations, particularly in the current age of unconventional warfare. The role of the anesthesia provider has been redefined throughout American warfare and will certainly continue to evolve alongside the US military machine and its global involvement. Providers learn to adapt to their environments and improvise care according to the conveniences available, all the while maintaining standards of care that ensure the best possible care to American military personnel and others. As emerging data and technologies become available, the practice of combat anesthesia will almost certainly change in order to continue providing high-level care to the very deserving military community.

REFERENCES

1. Condon-Rall ME. A brief history of military anesthesia. In: *Textbook of Military Medicine, Part IV, Surgical Combat Casualty Care: Anesthesia and Perioperative Care of the Combat Casualty*. Washington, DC: Office of the Surgeon General, Department of the Army; 1995:855–896.
2. Pruitt BA. The symbiosis of combat casualty care and civilian trauma care: 1914–2007. *J Trauma*. 2008;64:S4–S8.
3. Kelly JF, Ritenour AE, McLaughlin DF, et al. Injury severity and causes of death from operation Iraqi freedom and Operation Enduring Freedom: 2003–2004 versus 2006. *J Trauma*. 2008;64:S21–S27.
4. Holcomb JB, Stansbury LG, Champion HR, et al. Understanding combat casualty care statistics. *J Trauma*. 2006;60:397–401.
5. *Emergency War Surgery, Third United States Revision*. Washington, DC: Department of Defense; 2004.
6. Lewis R. 2/7 Marine shock trauma platoon saves lives. Combined Security Transition Command–Afghanistan News 2008;2:1–2. Available at: http://www.cstc-a.com/News/cstc-a%20newsletters/2008%20newsletters/080503-newsletter.pdf. Accessed on May 11, 2009.
7. McGuire JD, Compeggie ME. Walking blood bank in combat trauma resuscitation. *ASA Newsletter*. 2005. Available at: https://www.asahq.org/Newsletters/2005/12-05/mongan12_05.html. Accessed on May 13, 2009.
8. Kashuk J, Moore EE, Millikan JS, Moore JB. Major abdominal vascular trauma—a unified approach. *J Trauma*. 1982;22:672–679.
9. Kashuk JL, Moore EE, Johnson JL, et al. Postinjury life threatening coagulopathy: is 1:1 fresh frozen plasma: packed red blood cells the answer? *J Trauma*. 2008;65:261–271.
10. Olson KW, Kingsley CP. Drawover anesthesia: a review of equipment, capabilities, and utility under austere conditions. *Anesth Rev*. 1990;17:19–29.
11. McKay RE, Sonner J, McKay WR. Inhaled anesthetics. In: Stoelting RK, Miller RD, eds. *Basics of Anesthesia*. 5th ed. Philadelphia, PA: Churchill Livingstone Elsevier; 2007:77–96.
12. US Army Medical Department, Walter Reed Army Medical Center. Drawover familiarization training guidelines. Available at: http://www.wramc.amedd.army.mil/Patients/healthcare/surgery/anesthesiology/Pages/trainingguidelines.aspx. Accessed on May 7, 2009.
13. Gegel BT. A field-expedient Ohmeda Universal Portable Anesthesia Complete Draw-over Vaporizer setup. *AANA J*. 2008;76:185–187.
14. Eales M, Rowes P, Tully R. Improving the efficiency of the drawover anaesthetic breathing system. *Anaesthesiology*. 2007;62:1171–1174.
15. Mahoney PF, McFarland CC. Field anesthesia and military injury. In: Smith CE, ed. *Trauma Anesthesia*. Cambridge, England: Cambridge University Press; 2008:343–359.
16. White PF. Use of continuous infusion versus intermittent bolus administration of fentanyl or ketamine during outpatient anesthesia. *Anesthesiology*. 1983;59:294–300.
17. Cole CD, Gottfried ON, Gupta DK, Couldwell WT. Total intravenous anesthesia: advantages for intracranial surgery. *Neurosurgery*. 2007;61(operative neurosurgery supplement):369–378.
18. Grathwohl KW, Black IH, Spinella PC, et al. Total intravenous anesthesia including ketamine versus volatile gas anesthesia for combat-related operative traumatic brain injury. *Anesthesiology*. 2008;109:44–53.
19. Restall J, Tully M, Ward PJ, Kidd AG. Total intravenous anesthesia for military surgery. A technique using ketamine, midazolam, and vecuronium. *Anaesthesia*. 1989;44:533–534.
20. Mellor AJ. Anaesthesia in austere environments. *J R Army Med Corps*. 2005;151:272–276.
21. Englehart MS, Allison CE, Tieu BH, et al. Ketamine-based intravenous anesthesia versus isoflurane anesthesia in a swine model of hemorrhagic shock. *J Trauma*. 2008;65:901–909.
22. Himmelseher S, Durieux ME. Revising a dogma: ketamine for patients with neurological injury? *Anesth Analg*. 2005;101:524–534.
23. McGhee LL, Maani CV, Garza TH, et al. The correlation between ketamine and posttraumatic stress disorder in burned service members. *J Trauma*. 2008;64:S195–S199.
24. Cohen SP, Griffith S, Larkin TM, et al. Presentation, diagnoses, mechanisms of injury, and treatment of soldiers injured in Operation Iraqi Freedom: an epidemiological study conducted at two military pain management centers. *Anesth Analg*. 2005;101:1098–1103.
25. Malchow RJ, Black IH. The evolution of pain management in the critically ill trauma patient: emerging concepts from the global war on terrorism. *Crit Care Med*. 2008;36:S346–S357.
26. Lubenow TR, Ivankovich AD, Barkin RL. Management of acute postoperative pain. In: Barash PG, Cullen BF, Stoelting RK, eds. *Clinical Anesthesia*. 5th ed. Philadelphia, PA: Lippincott Williams & Wilkins; 2006:1405–1440.
27. Zatzick DF, Rivara FP, Nathens AB, et al. A nationwide US study of post-traumatic stress after hospitalization for physical injury. *Psychol Med*. 2007;37:1469–1480.
28. Perkins FM, Kehlet H. Chronic pain as an outcome of surgery. A review of predictive factors. *Anesthesiology*. 2000;93:1123–1133.
29. Reuben SS, Buvanendran A. Preventing the development of chronic pain after orthopaedic surgery with preventive multi-modal analgesic techniques. *J Bone Joint Surg Am*. 2007;89:1343–1358.
30. Strassels SA, McNicol E, Suleman R. Postoperative pain management: a practical review, part 1. *Am J Health-Syst Pharm*. 2005;62:1904–1916.
31. Hartrick CT. Multimodal postoperative pain management. *Am J Health-Sys Pharm*. 2004;61:S4–S10.
32. Rathmell JP, Wu CL, Sinatra RS, et al. Acute post-surgical pain management: a critical appraisal of current practice. *Reg Anesth Pain Med*. 2006;21:1–42.
33. WHO's Pain Relief Ladder. Available at: http://www.who.int/cancer/palliative/painladder/en/. Accessed on May 12, 2009.
34. Himmelseher S, Durieux ME. Ketamine for perioperative pain management. *Anesth Analg*. 2005;102:211–220.
35. Sveticic G, Gentilini A, Eichenberger U, et al. Combinations of morphine with ketamine for patient-controlled analgesia: a new optimization method. *Anesthesiology*. 2003;98:1195–1205.
36. Mao J, Chen LL. Gabapentin in pain management. *Anesth Analg*. 2000;91:680–687.
37. Gray P. Acute neuropathic pain: diagnosis and treatment. *Curr Opin Anaesth*. 2008;21:590–595.
38. Tremont-Lukats IW, Challapalli V, McNicol ED, et al. Systemic administration of local anesthetics to relieve neuropathic pain: a systematic review and meta-analysis. *Anesth Analg*. 2005;101:1738–1749.
39. Schulz-Stübner S, Boezaart A, Hata S. Regional analgesia in the critically ill. *Crit Care Med*. 2005;33:1400–1407.
40. Army Regional Anesthesia and Pain Management Initiative website. Available at: http://www.arapmi.org/index.html. Accessed on June 4, 2009.
41. Army Regional Anesthesia and Pain Management Initiative. Local anesthetics. In: *The Military Advanced Regional Anesthesia and Analgesia Handbook*. Available at: http://www.arapmi.org/maraa-book-project/Chapt3.pdf. Accessed on May 13, 2009.
42. Wedmore, IS; Kotwal R, McManus JG, et al. Safety and efficacy of oral transmucosal fentanyl citrate for prehospital pain control on the battlefield. *J Trauma*. 2012;73:490–495.
43. North Atlantic Treaty Organization. Allied Joint Publication 4-10(A) Allied Joint Medical Doctrine; 2011.
44. Jansen JO, Thomas R, Loudon MA, et al. Damage control resuscitation for patient with major trauma. *BMJ*. 2009;338:b1778.
45. Spinella PC, Perkins JG, Grathwohl KW, et al. Effect of plasma and red blood cell transfusion on survival in patients with combat related traumatic injuries. *J Trauma*. 2008;64:S69–S77; discussion S77.
46. del Junco DJ, Holcomb JB, Fox EE, et al. Resuscitat early with plasma and platelets or balance blood products gradually: findings of the PROMMTT study. *J Trauma Acute Care Surg*. 2013;75:S24–S30.
47. Nascimento B, Callum J, Tien H, et al. Effect of a fixed-ratio (1:1:1) transfusion protocol versus laboratory-results-guided transfusion in patients with severe trauma: a randomized feasibility trial. *CMAJ*. 2013;185:E583–E589.
48. CRASH-2 trial collaborators, Shakur H, Roberts I, et al. Effects of tranexamic acid on death, vascular occlusive events, and blood transfusion in trauma patient with significant haemorrhage (CRASH-2): a randomized, placebo-controlled trial. Lancet 2010; 376:23–32.
49. Morrison JJ, Dubose JJ, Rasmussen TE, et al. Military applications of tranexemic acid in trauma emergency resuscitation (MATTERs) study. *Arch Surg*. 2012;147:113–119.
50. Tien H, Beckett A, Garraway N, et al. Advances in damage control resuscitation and surgery: implication on the organization of future military field forces. *Can J Surg*. 2015;58(3)(suppl 3):S91–S97.
51. Blackbourne LH. Combat damage control surgery. *Crit Care Med*. 2008;36(suppl):S304–S310.

32 | ANESTHETIC CONSIDERATIONS IN HOMELAND DISASTERS

ROBERT PERELMUT, MD, ERNESTO A. PRETTO JR., MD, MPH

INTRODUCTION

A disaster is the result of the adverse interaction between a human-made or natural hazard and the environment, resulting in widespread human and/or structural damage that exceeds local capacity to respond in a timely and adequate manner, primarily due to chaos and uncertainty. A health or medical disaster refers to the extent of human injury, illness, or death caused by a disaster and the damage sustained by medical facilities; consequently, the needs of surviving injured or ill and of uninjured survivors will determine the types and quantities of resources required to provide necessary emergency health and medical services to prevent further morbidity and mortality. Depending on the magnitude of human or health system damage, a disaster can be classified as either a mass (involving hundreds) or catastrophic (involving thousands) casualty event. A casualty of a disaster is not only the person who suffers physical trauma or illness but also the person who experiences psychological trauma or interruption in the access to medical care or a breakdown in the provision of basic societal services such as food, water, shelter, electricity, and so on, all of which define the disaster-affected population.

One of the important principles of disaster medicine is that no two disasters are alike. Consequently, the character of medical disaster response will vary depending on the causes, circumstances, types of injury and illness (i.e., traumatic vs. nontraumatic), as well as the quantity and severity of injuries and illnesses generated by the disaster. Therefore, to provide effective emergency medical services response, health care workers and the health care system as a whole must be prepared to respond to a variety of disaster scenarios, to do it quickly, and to be able to adapt to constantly changing circumstances during the event. This requires special training in disaster medicine and disaster management competencies.[1]

Health and medical disaster response differs depending on whether the crisis occurs in a civilian or military context. In war, planning, preparation, and organization for medical care of wounded but otherwise healthy young soldiers (combat casualty care) is different from the care of injured or sick civilians of all ages, many with preexisting comorbidities, observed in homeland disasters. Moreover, military medical operations are strategically planned well in advance of the initiation of hostilities, and combat casualty care is executed at various echelons (levels of care) by well-trained military medics and mobile medical and surgical teams. US armed forces surgical teams operate in well-equipped and staffed modern field hospitals, providing a level of care nearly equivalent to a level 1 trauma center in the United States. The latter is certainly not the case in homeland disasters, which are sudden-impact events managed in an ad hoc manner by civilian responders, many of whom have never worked or trained as a team, let alone in a disaster. Additionally, civilian responders are often physically present in the disaster-affected area and become or fear becoming victims themselves or fear for their families. Nevertheless, modern field anesthesia and surgical techniques, procedures, and equipment in combat casualty care and in civilian disasters are similar.

Based on these assumptions and in keeping with the theme of this book, this chapter focuses primarily on anesthetic considerations in homeland disasters likely to require the presence of the anesthesiologist in the out-of-hospital or prehospital environment. Although most anesthesiologists are adept at handling multiple trauma casualties in the familiar setting of the operating room (OR), even during disasters, this fact does not necessarily apply to anesthesiologists' expertise in the management of casualties of earthquakes or chemical or biological incidents outside the operating room (OOOR).[2] In order to understand the context within which anesthesiologists might be asked to function in the OOOR setting during disaster response, we devote a part of this chapter to a brief review of the disaster management functions of prehospital emergency medical services (EMS)/trauma systems. We also describe the reorganization of hospital and intensive care services necessary to handle a surge of incoming critically injured or ill casualties. Our focus is the role of the anesthesiologist, working in partnership with community or local EMS/trauma system and its network of hospitals, because the local EMS/ambulance system constitutes the basic functional unit of disaster medical response in the United States. We end with a brief description of the major challenges we face in the delivery of intensive care services in mass and catastrophic casualty disasters.

In a medical disaster, mass casualty management requires a series of medical activities or functions that are quantitatively and qualitatively different from in the everyday emergency situation or multicasualty incident (MCI), such as a bus or train accident, which by definition does not overwhelm the local EMS/trauma system. Ideally, these disaster medical management functions are most effective for life-saving when they are implemented in a timely manner by well-organized, experienced EMS/trauma services systems consisting of trained bystanders (e.g., community emergency response teams [CERTs]); first responders; ground and air ambulance EMT/paramedic units; trauma teams/hospitals; and a network of community hospitals preexisting in the community. However, it is important to note that the standard of care in mass casualty and catastrophic disaster events will differ markedly from everyday EMS/trauma care. In a disaster, the objective is no longer to achieve emergency care within the "golden hour" but instead to do so within the "golden 24 hours." As a result, "preventable" deaths may occur. What follows is a detailed description of the organizational framework for EMS/trauma systems and the specific disaster management functions that further define the differences between the medical response to multicasualty events and disasters.

PREHOSPITAL DISASTER MANAGEMENT FUNCTIONS

BASIC FUNCTIONAL COMPONENTS

LEADERSHIP, MANAGEMENT, AND COMMUNICATION (INCIDENT MANAGEMENT SYSTEM)

The incident management system (ICS) and the National Incident Management System (NIMS) are comprehensive organizational structures designed to enable effective command and control (leadership), and coordination and communication (management) of a crisis situation requiring emergency response. It attempts to do this by integrating the facilities, equipment, personnel, procedures, and communications used for the response into a common hierarchical administrative framework.[3] The main advantage of NIMS is that it is used to manage both short- and long-term field disaster operations for a broad spectrum of emergencies by all levels of government in the United States, and has been adopted by many private-sector businesses and nongovernment organizations (NGOs), including EMS trauma systems and hospitals.

In terms of leadership, at the community level, the mayor or the mayor's designee assumes the role of decision-maker in a disaster, in coordination with county emergency managers, fire, police, and EMS, as well as county health officials. In a mass casualty (i.e., 9/11) or catastrophic (i.e., Hurricane Katrina), disaster in the homeland the National Response Framework is activated, in which case one of the federal agencies (Department of Homeland Security [DHS], Department of Health and Human Services (DHHS), Centers for Disease Control and Prevention (CDC) or Department of Defense (DoD) assumes "lead agency" status for command and control.[4] According to this plan, emergency operations centers (EOCs) are activated, thus becoming the epicenters of leadership and management within each jurisdiction (local, state, and federal).

An EOC is a location or "bunker" equipped with high-tech telecommunications and information technology gear such as satellite telephones and reconnaissance, computers, Internet, television monitors, and integrated geospatial information systems designed to maintain "situational awareness" of the event.[5] Agency coordinators present at the EOC relieve on-scene commanders of the burden of external coordination, such as the time consuming logistics of procuring and transporting resources to the disaster zone. In a nutshell, the actions of coordinators at the EOC include decision-making, resource allocation and tracking, data analysis, and dissemination of information to responders and the public at large.

The effectiveness, robustness, and integrity of the communication system infrastucture is essential to alert local and, if judged necessary, regional, state, or federal civilian authorities to the fact that a disaster situation is unfolding. It includes the telecommunications backbone and redundant communication systems (e.g., ham radio, satellite phones, etc.) needed to ensure the uninterrupted flow of information on the disaster situation to all decision-makers (situation reports or sitreps).

Once information on the types and numbers of injured with estimated times of arrival of casualties to hospitals is received, external disaster and plans to cope with a surge of casualties can be activated (see the discussion of the hospital disaster plan). If the number of casualties exceeds hospital capacity, area-wide alerts are sent out to the network of hospitals, based on mutual aid agreements. In major sudden-impact disasters such as earthquakes that strike without warning, communications may be interrupted, requiring federal assets to be deployed to the disaster zone.

In hazards such as severe hurricanes (category greater than 3 on the Saffir-Simpson scale), early warning of wind intensity, flood surge potential, the geographic location of landfall, and instructions on evacuation from seaside areas must be conveyed in a timely manner. In these types of events, the broadcast of emergency alerts to the population at risk is the single most important element to prevent injury and death.

NEEDS IDENTIFICATION

Damage assessment is the process by which authorities become informed of the extent and severity of the disaster. *Needs identification* refers to the amount of materiel and manpower resources required to effectively meet demand. In the case of a medical disaster, the health and medical "needs" (in the form of emergency care, food, adequate clothing, and shelter) of the injured and the uninjured survivors must be met within the shortest time period to avoid collateral damage or secondary disasters. One of the major problems in the technical field of needs identification is the development of methods, procedures, and technology to rapidly and accurately determine the following critical information: total affected population, total number of killed and seriously injured and their locations, number of hospitals destroyed or disabled, as well as those still operating, type and severity of injuries, and types and quantities of medical and surgical services, medical supplies, and pharmaceuticals needed. It is essential to determine whether local resources are exceeded or exhausted, thereby requiring outside support and supplies.[6,7]

These decisions are critical for life-saving efforts because time is a risk factor for death and disability. They are usually the responsibility of local authorities (i.e., the mayor, governor, or their designees, usually made in conjunction with the incident commander and local health and EMS officials). Delays or inaccuracies of needs identification are major causes of delays in response and recovery. This was a major failure in the recent Hurricane in Puerto Rico and after Hurricane Katrina.[8]

SEARCH AND RESCUE AND CASUALTY COLLECTION

Search and rescue is the process whereby specialized teams perform detection and extrication of casualties trapped or pinned in collapsed structures (i.e., extrication from under rubble). During or immediately following extrication victims are transported to nearby staging areas or casualty collection points within the tactical area of operations, where further harm is avoided and patients are initially stabilized, prepared for transport, and loaded onto emergency transport vehicles. In the event of terrorist release of chemical or infectious biological agents, victims are transported by chemical or biological (HazMat) teams equipped with personal protective gear to designated treatment facilities for decontamination or isolation (Figure 32.1), thus protecting rescuers and other individuals from lethal exposure.

TRIAGE

Once casualties are rescued, identified and cleared from the immediate disaster area, and transported to a casualty collection point or to a medical facility, triage and stabilization are performed. *Triage* is the method by which the type, extent, and severity of injury or illness sustained by a disaster victim is prioritized for treatment.[9,10] While the severity of illness is typically the most important factor in the prioritization of standard medical care, the goal of care during a mass casualty incident is to maximize overall patient survival. In order to accomplish this goal, critically ill or moribund victims are often given lower priority than less-critical patients who are more likely to survive with treatment.[11] Triage should be carried out by physicians with advanced trauma life support (ATLS) training familiar with triage methods.

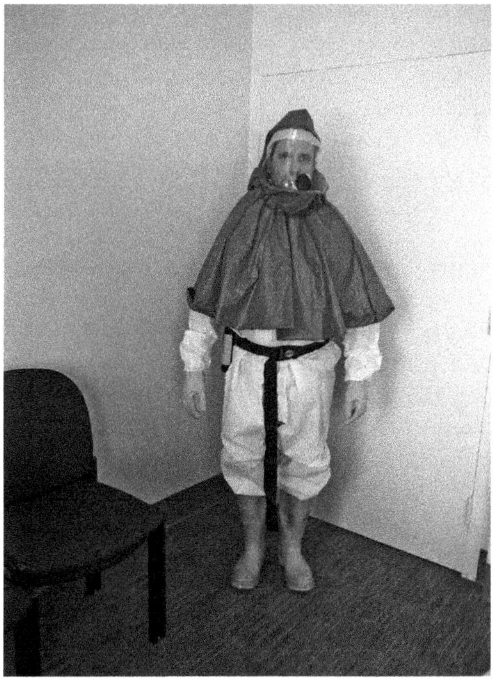

Figure 32.1. Positive air pressure respirator gear.

There have been multiple algorithms developed in order to maximize patient survival in the disaster setting. One such algorithm is the simple triage and rapid treatment (START) algorithm, developed in the 1980s. This was the standard of care until recently, when multiple retrospective studies found a lack of sensitivity and specificity and a tendency to overtriage patients.[12] More recently, a second algorithm was created, known as the sort, assess, life-saving interventions, treatment/transport (SALT) algorithm, which has been endorsed by the American College of Emergency Physicians, American Trauma Society, and American College of Surgeons Committee on Trauma.[13]

Both algorithms sort victims into four groups based on need for timely intervention: green (minimal), yellow (delayed), red (immediate), and black (dead/expectant). The START algorithm sorts victims by ability to walk (green); cannot walk but normal respiratory status, systolic blood pressure (determined by strong radial pulse or normal capillary refill), and mental status (yellow); cannot walk and abnormality of respiratory status, blood pressure, or mental status (red); and cannot walk and apnea despite airway maneuvers (black).

The SALT algorithm is broken down into two steps. First, the victims are sorted into groups based on timing of assessment. If they cannot walk and are unresponsive, they are seen first, followed by victims who cannot walk but can follow commands, and last by those who are able to walk. The second step involves assessment followed by treatment based on color status, and again victims are sorted into four groups: those who are following commands, with normal respiratory status, peripheral pulse, no ongoing hemorrhage, and minor injuries (green); those who meet green criteria but injuries are considered greater than minor (yellow); green criteria not met but patient likely to survive if given life-sustaining intervention, such as hemorrhage control, chest compressions, autoinjector antidotes, and airway management (red); and last, those who are apneic or not likely to survive despite intervention (black).

The ideal triage system would be one that minimizes undertriage (falsely classifying patients as less critical than they are) while also minimizing overtriage.[14] One retrospective study showed both the START and SALT systems correctly triaged patients a majority of the time (55% START and 65% SALT) with high specificity; however, a lack of sensitivity to appropriately identify severity of injury led to a high number of undertriaged victims using either algorithm.[12] The SALT system was found to be less likely to overtriage, while both systems had strong negative and positive predictive values of death.[12] In a disaster scenario, the undertriage of victims is particularly concerning as it may lead to underestimation of the intervention needed and a delay of appropriate care.

FOCUSED ASSESSMENT WITH SONOGRAPHY FOR TRAUMA

Often, the limiting factor to increased sensitivity in triage systems such as the START and SALT algorithms is that they rely solely on information obtained from history and physical exam. One area of possible advancement to patient care in this setting is through the use of ultrasonography. In the trauma setting, ultrasonography has become the standard of care through the use of the focused assessment with sonography for trauma (FAST) examination to detect posttraumatic pericardial tamponade and intraperitoneal hemorrhage.[11] In addition, ultrasound has been shown to detect pneumothoraces and hemothoraces with a sensitivity and specificity of 92% and 100%, respectively.[15] In a recent retrospective study, when the FAST exam was used as an adjunct to the START triage algorithm, an additional 7% of patients originally designated in the yellow category would have been diagnosed with delayed hemoperitoneum.[16]

Although there is not much literature regarding the utility of ultrasonography in the setting of a civilian MCI, military experience has shown ultrasonography to be an extremely useful resource. FAST examinations performed by emergency medical physicians on blunt, blast, and penetrating trauma patients in Kuwait in 2003 revealed a sensitivity and specificity of 100% and 99%, respectively, with a negative predictive value of 100% when compared to operative reports and computed tomographic (CT) scans.[11]

Technological advances have allowed for the development of ultrasound devices that are portable and inexpensive and provide real-time diagnostic information. Studies have shown the ability to transmit ultrasound images remotely for viewing by experts for interpretation and decision-making.[17] This would allow for more efficient utilization of resources and personnel. It is with these advancements that portable ultrasonography will soon be the standard of care for the evaluation of critically ill victims in the disaster setting.

FIELD MEDICAL CARE

Field medical care is the spectrum of emergency medical or surgical life-saving interventions applied in the out-of-hospital setting by bystanders, first responders, and emergency medical personnel on casualties of disaster. The objective is to contain or control damage prior to transport. Usually, field medical care, especially "resuscitative surgery" or "damage control surgery," is performed only when the type and severity of illness or injury threaten life or limb, precluding safe transport to a treatment facility. In general, there are four main types of field medical care or damage control interventions:

Life-supporting first aid (LSFA): This involves the delivery of basic first aid by uninjured survivors or covictims and is aimed at initiating the life support chain.[18] It entails the following basic maneuvers: (1) calling for help; (2) knowing when to approach a victim in a hazardous environment; (3) maintaining a patent airway in an unconscious but breathing patient (triple-airway maneuver); (4) external hemorrhage control; (5) positioning for shock; (6) rescue pull; and (7) cardiopulmonary resuscitation (CPR) (if indicated).

Basic rescue or extrication: This involves the simple extrication of victims from vehicles or of those buried under light rubble. It is usually performed by uninjured covictims within the immediate disaster zone; these individuals are equipped only with bare hands, minimal supplies, or improvised tools.[19]

Basic trauma life support (BTLS): BTLS constitutes the second step in the life support chain involving the application of advanced first aid techniques, such as the following: airway control with or without adjuncts, external hemorrhage control, immobilization of unstable limb fractures, placement of peripheral intravenous lines, wound dressing, initial burn treatment, and other life-saving maneuvers by trained first responders.

Advanced trauma life support (ATLS): ATLS is the application of life-saving emergency medical or surgical treatment to critically injured patients by physicians, usually including the following: definitive airway management with endotracheal intubation or assisted ventilation; central venous line placement for fluid resuscitation; administration of vasoactive medication and antidotes; and in the case of traumatic injuries, chest tube placement, wound suturing, and other life-saving medical/surgical interventions.

Resuscitative surgery: This type of surgery involves the application of major surgical procedures, such as emergency exploratory laparotomy, thoracotomy, craniotomy; and wound debridement, limb amputations, among others, performed in the out-of-hospital setting usually to prevent loss of life or limb due to external or internal bleeding, gangrene, compartment syndrome, and so on.

TRANSPORT

In major disasters, casualties are usually not transported in ambulances. Instead, uninjured or lightly injured covictims carry out this function using whatever means is available for transport. Bystanders are usually the relatives, friends, or neighbors of the injured. Once professional rescuers and emergency medical personnel initiate their operations, transport of critically injured casualties is done by land or air ambulance (helicopters) from casualty collection points close to the disaster zone to bring these victims to treatment facilities outside the tactical area of operations; whenever possible, and especially when extended transport times are anticipated, casualties are accompanied by health care professionals with, at minimum, advanced trauma or cardiac life support expertise. The lack of ambulances, helicopters, and so on and traffic jams or disruption of roads and highways to and from the disaster area are frequent causes of delay in the transport of casualties.

DEFINITIVE MEDICAL/SURGICAL CARE

Definitive medical/surgical care is the delivery of specialized definitive or corrective emergency medical or surgical treatment in a permanent medical facility. These interventions are carried out by physicians, surgeons, nurses, and other health care professionals. The objectives are stabilization of vital signs, reversal of life-threatening illness or injury, and prevention of long-term disability or death.

HOSPITAL DISASTER MANAGEMENT FUNCTIONS

Hospital response during a homeland disaster is driven by the hospital's external disaster response plan, whose organization should incorporate the incident management system as modified for hospital operations.

Today, the majority of hospital external disaster plans, when activated, invariably direct anesthesiologists to report to the familiar environment of the OR, irrespective of the disaster type. These plans are outdated and will need revision to account for the most effective use of anesthesiologists and anesthesia services when operative surgical services are not in great demand, such as in an influenza (H1N1 or H5N1) epidemic or a terrorist chemical or biological attack with mass exposure to toxic agents. Revisions to existing protocols governing disaster response by anesthesia personnel are warranted because of the technical skill set and expertise of anesthesiologists, which are rooted in resuscitation (life support management) and crisis management. Anesthesiologists should be prepared to play a life-saving role in the types of disasters mentioned, which most likely will unfold in the OOOR setting.

The Joint Commission provides some direction but limited detail regarding hospital disaster plans or hospital disaster management functions. However, the hospital incident management system has been developed to organize hospital disaster response activities around a set of specific and measurable objectives that define the hospital's performance in the event of a disaster.[20] In general terms, the following items cover primary objectives/functions:

- Assemble a leadership and management team based on the hospital incident management system to lead and coordinate the hospital's disaster response.
- A plan for the acquisition and deployment of necessary medical equipment, supplies, and pharmaceuticals.
- A plan for emergency backup lifeline (power, gas, water, food) and personnel recall (medical and nonmedical) to allow continuous operations for, at minimum, 24 hours.
- Once activated, rapidly reorganize resources to convert to disaster operations by recalling and reassigning personnel to deal promptly and effectively with a surge of casualties (casualty estimates and surge capacity need to be determined beforehand).
- Establish mutual aid and liaison agreements with neighboring hospitals/EMS systems in the event surge capacity is exceeded.
- Create a communications network to manage information exchange among prehospital EMS systems, hospitals, local and state health authorities, families of casualties, the media, and so on with periodic alerts or situation reports (sitreps).
- A plan for the transfer/discharge of stable inpatients or diversion of disaster casualties to other health care institutions, nursing homes, outpatient facilities, and so on.
- A plan for documentation of admission and care provided to casualties by hospital personnel and a plan for inpatient tracking, both before and after admission.
- Designate triage and treatment areas within the hospital, with prioritization of care, as follows:
- Casualty reception, triage areas (usually the emergency room and adjacent areas), with patients segregated according to infectious disease status.
- Decontamination/isolation areas (in the event of casualties of chemical, biological, radiological attack, or pandemic influenza).
- Areas for the diagnosis, treatment, or stabilization of patients who have life-threatening conditions (red) such as acute respiratory failure (ARF), who require intensive care for immediate and continuous physiologic monitoring, medical or surgical intervention, or mechanical ventilation (Figure 32.2).
- Areas for the diagnosis, treatment, or stabilization of patients having urgent conditions (yellow) who will be referred for follow-up care.
- Areas for the treatment of patients with nonurgent conditions (green), with referral for later definitive diagnosis, treatment, and comprehensive care.
- Areas for the reception of moribund or dead casualties (gray/black) for pain management and pastoral services.
- Selection of alternate treatment areas (outside the hospital) in the event the hospital must be evacuated or cannot provide services. (In some situations, hospital personnel may be compelled to evacuate the facility and to deliver medical and surgical services in the out-of-hospital setting, severely hampering the hospital's ability to function.)
- After the event, perform evaluation of performance.
- Revise external disaster plan and provide training based on knowledge gained through experience, after action reports and evaluation.

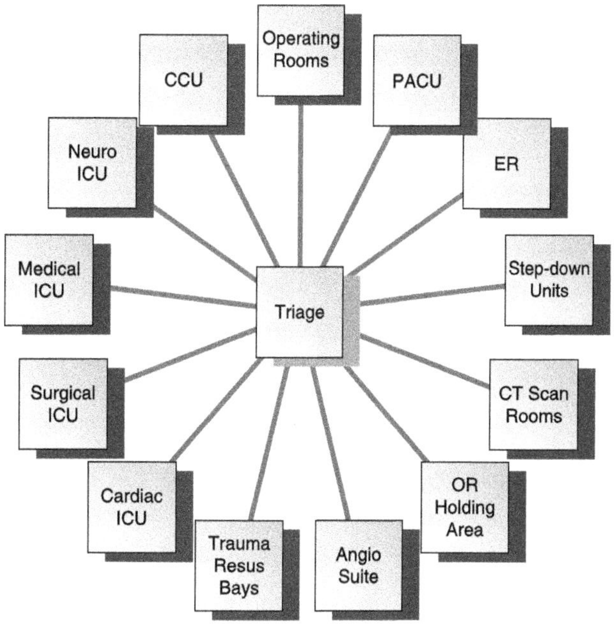

Figure 32.2. *Alternate intensive care treatment areas. CCU, cardiac care unit; CT, computed tomography; ER, emergency room; ICU, intensive care unit; OR, operating room; PACU, postanesthesia care unit.*

SURGE CAPACITY

Hospital external disaster response plans often lack an important component of a hospital's response to a disaster, namely the incorporation of a critical care expansion plan to ensure surge capacity. *Critical care surge capacity* can be defined as the maximal number of patients that can receive adequate critical care for as long as required after recruiting all critical care resources.[21]

When creating a surge capacity plan, it is important to recognize that pharmacy, laboratory, radiology, respiratory therapy, and nutritional services will be relied on to provide adequate critical care during the disaster and thus should be included a priori in all planning measures.[21] Stockpiling of resources, including equipment, supplies, and pharmaceuticals prior to a disaster increases hospital surge capacity. The development and oversight of these stockpiles are integral functions of emergency management programs. Ventilatory support is often limited in a surge capacity scenario, and hospitals working alone are unlikely to be able to provide enough ventilators to support the critically ill. A regional count of ventilators should be performed, with multiple hospitals working together to create a mass disaster critical care operational plan.

Delivery of critical care during a disaster or pandemic not only depends on the allocation of appropriate physical resources, but also hospitals must ensure sufficient numbers of trained medical, nursing, and ancillary staff. A disaster response is likely to consume the available reserves of rested personnel within 24 to 48 hours, and hospitals should use adaptive measures to provide appropriate staffing in these scenarios, such as shorter shifts (i.e., 4–6 hours) to avoid fatigue and exhaustion. While the standard nurse-to-patient ratio in North American ICUs is 1:1 or 1:2, this is not practical during a critical care surge. Strategies used to mitigate the potential for patient harm due to this change in ratio include creation of nursing care teams, with the use of non–critical care nurses to perform tasks within their skill sets in order to offload the demands of the ICU nurses.[21]

POSTDISASTER FUNCTIONS

DISASTER PREPAREDNESS AND EVALUATION

In the broadest sense, disaster preparedness is the development and implementation of a set of disaster prevention, mitigation, and response plans or programs, usually based on hazard risk analysis, vulnerability analysis, casualty estimates, and hospital surge capacity analysis. Disaster preparedness is strengthened by the incorporation of lessons learned through the systematic scientific evaluation of actual events, as well as through exercises and simulation.

Disaster evaluation is a continuum of activities that includes disaster response assessment and research involving evaluation and epidemiologic methodology.[22–24] The short-term aim is the acquisition and translation of knowledge and experience or skill gained by responders in a disaster to other individuals or institutions for the purpose of facilitating the application of a learned set of new facts or adequate performance of a given task or set of practical skills. These become the so-called lessons learned during a disaster event for the purpose of revising/improving disaster planning, preparedness, mitigation, and response programs with the long-term aim of reducing morbidity and mortality in future disasters. Currently, disaster evaluation is the weakest link in the disaster management portfolio because it is not institutionalized or governed by universal standards.

CASE STUDIES IN DISASTER RESPONSE

HAITI

The January 12, 2010, earthquake that struck Port-au-Prince, Haiti, caused over 200,000 deaths, hundreds of thousands of injuries requiring immediate surgical intervention, and a population of 1.5 million internally displaced. The University of Miami Miller School of Medicine Global Institute/Project Medishare, the Jackson Memorial Hospital's Ryder Trauma Center, and the Department of Anesthesia dispatched a surgical scout team within 24 hours to initiate emergency medical response and perform needs assessment.

The primary goal of relief efforts in Port-au-Prince became life-saving surgical care to save life and limb. However, medical facilities were either destroyed or disabled. In the first 72 hours, there was no pressurized oxygen, precluding the sustained delivery of general anesthesia for surgery. The University of Miami surgical team set up a trauma unit in a makeshift tent facility at the airport. Because of the absence of oxygen or the ability to deliver general anesthesia, members of the Division of Regional Anesthesia and Acute Pain Management of the Department of Anesthesia were dispatched to Haiti to provide regional block anesthesia, primarily for extremity surgery.[25] In the first few days following the earthquake, this team performed hundreds of regional nerve blocks for emergency orthopedic surgery, including limb amputations, stump revisions, and wound debridement. This medical team operated out of a storage tent facility until medical supplies, anesthesia equipment, and oxygen arrived and makeshift ORs were organized.

TYPE OF INJURIES

In Haiti, as in other earthquake disasters, the prevalent injury type and cause of death was crush injury from building collapse.[25–29] Casualties with severe crush injury of the head, chest, and abdomen were already dead or in the advanced stages of dying by the time international relief teams arrived. The majority of seriously injured casualties that survived the first 24 hours had crush injury of the limbs, with fractures of the long bones (humerus, femoral, tibia-fibula); pelvic fractures; spine injuries; crush syndrome; extremity compartment syndrome; open fractures with infected and gangrenous wounds; burns; and sepsis. Less-severe injuries included minor blunt head, chest, and abdominal trauma and lacerations, rib fractures, closed fractures of the extremities, burns, and facial and scalp lacerations.

EMERGENCY MEDICAL MANAGEMENT

The type of medical activities and surgical interventions throughout the Haiti relief effort consisted primarily of the following: triage, BTLS and ATLS, improvised medical record keeping, expectant care, first aid, fracture management, placement of intravenous lines, airway management, fluid resuscitation and rehydration, antibiotic and tetanus prophylaxis, orthopedic surgery, open wound and burn care, wound debridement, spine and neurological surgery, disposal of amputated limbs, regional anesthesia and pain management, and preparation and transport of critically ill patients for transport to hospitals in Miami and South Florida.

ANESTHETIC MANAGEMENT

In general, the provision of advanced trauma surgical care in the first 24 hours is extremely difficult in most major earthquake disasters, if not impossible, even in developed nations. Among the limitations are the destruction or disabling of hospital facilities and interruption of lifelines (electricity, water, gas). In our experience in Haiti, besides the nearly complete destruction or disabling of medical facilities, it was the lack of oxygen and general anesthetics that posed the major limiting factor in the delivery of surgical care in the first 24 hours. As an alternative, surgery and acute pain management were achieved with regional block anesthesia combined with the intravenous administration of ketamine and midazolam sedation in a makeshift tent outdoors. This regimen worked extremely well for both adults and children. Moreover, regional block anesthesia (primarily interscalene, axillary, sciatic, and femoral nerve blocks) significantly reduced opioid use and its side effects, thereby markedly reducing the need for postoperative monitoring and nursing care. More important, this approach facilitated rapid deployment of a surgical team for life- and limb-saving surgery when the need was greatest, the first 24–48 hours. As a result, the University of Miami field surgical team was able to do much more in less time with less medical staff.[25]

Our recent experience in Haiti has taught us that a surgical team equipped with the supplies and expertise necessary to perform single-shot block anesthesia is essential for the delivery of surgical anesthesia in the out-of-hospital setting, especially during the early stages of earthquake disasters or in other disasters requiring emergency orthopedic procedures. Mobile surgical teams should incorporate regional anesthesia capability for future disaster response.

NEPAL

A similar disaster experience was seen when a 7.8 magnitude earthquake hit Nepal on April 25, 2015, causing over 9000 deaths and 23,000 injuries. An Israeli disaster team was immediately deployed, opening up a field hospital within 82 hours and remaining open for 11 days, treating over 1600 patients.[30] The Israeli Defense Force Field Hospital consisted of an emergency department, 40 adult beds, 5 pediatric beds, 2 ORs, and a 9-bed intensive care unit (ICU; also serving as a postanesthesia recovery unit). Hospital personnel included both military paramedics and nurses and 42 physicians comprising three anesthesiologists; 15 total surgeons, including orthopedic, general, plastic, ear-nose-throat (ENT), and ophthalmologic specialties; ICU specialists; both internal medicine and pediatric physicians; as well as two obstetricians.

ANESTHETIC MANAGEMENT

Similar to what was seen in Haiti, the majority of surgical procedures performed during this 11-day period were either orthopedic or plastic surgical procedures (84 of 88 total surgeries). Of the 84 operations, 81 (96%) were performed under regional anesthesia, while 2 required general anesthesia and 1 was performed under spinal anesthesia. Peripheral nerve blocks were typically performed in the preoperative holding area, under portable ultrasound guidance using aseptic technique. Lower extremity procedures were performed after femoral block, sciatic block, or a combination of both, while upper extremity procedures were done after interscalene or supraclavicular blocks. Bupivacaine 0.25% or 0.5% was used in dosages of 2–3 mg/kg. All 81 peripheral nerve blocks were noted to have provided adequate anesthesia, and no immediate complications were seen. Postoperative pain was minimal in the first 24 hours postoperatively, occasionally requiring simple supplemental analgesia but rarely requiring additional opioid use.

THE IMPORTANCE OF REGIONAL ANESTHESIA TEAMS

As seen in Haiti and Nepal earthquakes with many severe limb injuries requiring orthopedic and plastic surgical procedures, regional anesthesia was found to be a valuable method of providing rapid and safe anesthesia care in the disaster setting. Patients presenting for operative management are often hypovolemic secondary to dehydration or blood loss.[31] Ketamine combined with regional anesthesia has shown to be an effective and safe option in the hypovolemic earthquake victim. Missair et al. reported over 500 surgeries during the 2010 Haitian earthquake; these surgeries were performed with combined ketamine and monitored anesthesia care (MAC) and single-shot peripheral nerve blocks, with a complication rate of less than 5% and 0 intraoperative deaths.[32] With regional anesthesia, the simplicity of the technique allows for surgeries to be performed in the absence of advanced monitoring devices.[30] Patients often do not require an ICU bed in the immediate postoperative period as would be required during the recovery from general anesthesia, allowing for faster turnover times and better allocation of ICU resources. Performing peripheral nerve blocks also minimizes the need for supplemental oxygen, a resource typically with limited supply during a natural disaster.

AIRWAY INJURY FROM TOXIC CHEMICAL AGENT RELEASE

Chemical weapon agents are classified as persistent or nonpersistent on the basis of the time the agent remains toxic after release (Table 32.1). Chemical agents considered

TABLE 32.1. Types and Clinical Characteristics of Major Chemical Weapon Agents

CLASS	AGENT	MECHANISM OF INJURY	SIGNS AND SYMPTOMS	ONSET	PERSISTENCY
Nerve	Cyclosarin (GF) Sarin (GB) Soman (GD) Tabun (GA) VX	Inactivates acetyl cholinesterase, resulting in accumulation of acetylcholine in the victim's synapses, triggering muscarinic and nicotinic effects.	Miosis Blurred vision Headache Nausea, vomiting, diarrhea Copious secretions/ sweating Muscle twitching/ fasciculation Dyspnea Seizures Loss of consciousness	Vapors: seconds to minutes Skin: 2 to 18 hours	VX is persistent and a contact hazard; other agents in this class are nonpersistent and present mostly inhalation hazards
Cyanide	Most arsines Cyanogen chloride Hydrogen cyanide	Arsine: Causes intravascular hemolysis that may lead to renal failure. Cyanogen chloride/ hydrogen cyanide: Cyanide blocks oxygen utilization. The cells then convert to anaerobic respiration, creating excess lactic acid and metabolic acidosis.	Cherry-red skin Cyanosis Confusion Nausea Air hunger Seizures Metabolic acidosis	Immediate	Nonpersistent and an inhalation hazard
Vesicant	Sulfur mustard (HD, H) Nitrogen mustard (HN-1, HN-2, HN-3) Lewisite (L) Phosgene oxime (CX)	Agents are acid-forming compounds that damage skin and the respiratory system, resulting in airway burns and respiratory complications.	Severe skin, eye, and mucosal pain and irritation Erythema/blisters that heal slowly and may become infected Tearing, conjunctivitis, corneal damage Mild respiratory distress to marked airway compromise	Mustard vapors: 4 to 6 hours, eyes and lungs affected more rapidly; Skin: 2 to 48 hours Lewisite: Immediate	Persistent and a contact hazard
Choking	Chlorine Hydrogen chloride Nitrogen oxides Phosgene	Similar mechanism to blister agents in that the compounds are acids or acid forming, but action is more pronounced in the respiratory system, flooding it and resulting in asphyxiation; survivors often suffer chronic breathing problems.	Airway irritation Eye and skin irritation Dyspnea Cough Sore throat Chest tightness Wheezing Bronchospasm	Immediate to 3 hours	Nonpersistent and an inhalation hazard

nonpersistent are gaseous, such as chlorine, or highly volatile agents such as sarin and most other nerve agents (NAs). These agents dissipate after only a few minutes or hours. Historically, nonpersistent chemical warfare agents were intended for military targets that were to be taken over and controlled quickly. These types of agents pose an inhalation hazard. Persistent agents such as the nonvolatile liquid agent VX and blister agents remain in the environment for as long as several days. VX is an oily liquid that does not easily evaporate. To inflict maximum damage and long-term disruption of a population, terrorists may opt to use persistent agents.

Chemical agents are also organized into several categories according to the manner in which they affect the human body. The names and number of categories vary slightly from source to source, but in general, types and characteristics of chemical weapon agents are illustrated in Table 32.1.

TYPE OF INJURIES

The release of a large quantity of a highly toxic chemical agent in a major city has an immediate and devastating effect on the population of that city and surrounding areas (Table 32.2). In addition to the direct detrimental effects on people and animals, an inadvertent chemical release or intentional attack will overwhelm the city's medical care system. The primary injury is to the respiratory system, requiring urgent airway and respiratory therapy in a monitored environment. The convergence of large numbers of exposed acutely ill, walking

TABLE 32.2. Estimates of Casualties Generated by the Release of Four Tons of Toxic Chemical Agent Two Kilometers Upwind of a City of 500,000 People

AGENT	ESTIMATED CASES	ESTIMATED DEATHS
Sarin	15,000	300
VX	50,000	5000
VX aerosol	120,000	12,000

SOURCE: *Adapted from Health Aspects of Chemical and Biological Weapons.* Report of WHO Group Consultants. Geneva, Switzerland: WHO; 1970.

ill, and moribund victims at hospitals creates demands for hospitalization and intensive care that rapidly exceed medical resources. Types and quantities of medications and supplies needed to treat casualties may not be available in standard medical or pharmaceutical stocks. Medical care providers, nursing personnel, and laboratory personnel require protection against exposure, and autopsy and interment of remains present uncommon hazards.

EMERGENCY MEDICAL MANAGEMENT

Physiological effects of toxic chemicals depend on the agent, route (lung or skin), and duration of exposure.[33] The effects of exposure to vapor are not the same as those from skin contact. Exposure to a small vapor cloud affects the eyes, the nose, and the airways, producing miosis, rhinorrhea, bronchorrhea, and bronchoconstriction. Minute quantities on skin will cause localized sweating and less commonly fasciculations. On initial exposure, if sweating and fasciculations do not occur or are not noticed, gastrointestinal symptoms may develop: nausea and vomiting, with or without diarrhea. Skin exposure to microdroplets floating in a chemical cloud may not be noticed, and its effects may be delayed for hours. Massive or prolonged exposure produces a sudden loss of consciousness, seizures, flaccid paralysis, apnea, and death. The most likely cause of death is from paralysis of the respiratory muscles and severe depression of the central nervous system (CNS).[34]

The immediate life-threatening effects of toxic chemical exposure are found in the respiratory system. Airway injury occurs at all levels of the respiratory tract with varying latency, depending on the circumstances, concentration, and duration of the exposure. Airway reaction to an irritating compound is a massive outpouring of secretions that cause difficulty breathing to complete airway obstruction. There may be laryngeal, bronchial, and bronchiolar spasm; a reduction in compliance; and pulmonary edema. Suction devices are needed to clear secretions and vomitus. Early endotracheal intubation is advisable because it is difficult to assess the level of exposure or the extent of airway or lung injury, and lung injury may progress rapidly to complete obstruction or pulmonary edema.

After securing the airway, 100% oxygen should be administered, unless oxygen and its resupply are limited in the contaminated zone. Initially, manually assisted lung ventilation and oxygenation with filter, bag, and mask are instituted, followed later by mechanical ventilation. Portable mechanical ventilators may be needed for prolonged decontamination or during evacuation and transport from the contaminated zone. A ventilator that filters the toxic ambient atmosphere with an air mix ratio of approximately 50% oxygen should be used in the hazardous zone.

Aggressive monitoring of vital signs is indicated, although equipment limitations will determine the sophistication of monitoring modalities, especially when large numbers of people have been exposed. Inevitably, reliance on basic clinical monitoring modalities, such as mental status (Glasgow Coma Scale, GCS), respiratory and pulse rate, blood pressure, skin color and appearance, and pupil size will guide the response to antidotes. Many chemical agents give rise to toxic pulmonary edema and bronchospasm. It has been suggested that high doses of methylprednisolone should be given as soon as possible after exposure to pulmonary edematogens.[36] However, the use of systemic or inhaled corticosteroids to treat chemical intoxications is somewhat controversial. This is due to the fact that steroids have proved to be of value in the management of severe bronchospasm, but whether they can prevent pulmonary edema is unclear.

Acute respiratory failure due to pulmonary edema may be latent; therefore, special care should be taken to carefully monitor pulmonary function during evacuation and transport to medical facilities or during interhospital transport. Early aggressive respiratory therapy reduces the risk of adult respiratory distress syndrome (ARDS) and ARF.

Nerve agents are potent organophosphate compounds that are similar to but more toxic than insecticides. In 1994, when sarin was released by terrorists in Matsumoto, Japan, and again in 1995 in Tokyo subways, 12 people were killed, and over 4000 sought treatment.[37]

Nerve agents produce biological effects by inhibiting acetylcholinesterase (AChE).[34] This inhibition prevents the hydrolysis of the neurotransmitter acetylcholine and subsequently leads to the overstimulation of end organs with cholinergic receptors.[33] Major affected organs and tissues include the exocrine glands, smooth and striated muscles, and the nerves in the CNS and at ganglia. Other than the severity and extent of signs and symptoms and estimate of red blood cell (RBC) AChE activity,[38,39] there is no quick method to assess the degree of exposure to NAs.

Medical management consists of ventilator support and administration of antidotes and, for severe cases (i.e., seizures), an anticonvulsant.[40] Intense bronchoconstriction may result in high airway pressure with difficulty ventilating. One antidote for mild exposures is atropine 2 mg intramuscular (IM) repeated every 20 minutes until the patient is fully atropinized (atropinization is characterized by the appearance of flushed and dry skin, increased heart rate, and reduced bronchoconstriction and bronchorrhea). The pediatric dose for mild exposures is 0.02 mg/kg IM. In moderate-to-severe cases, the dose of atropine is increased to 2 mg IV every 5–10 minutes for adults and 2.0 mg or 0.02 to 0.1 mg/kg for children. Atropine works by inhibiting the effects of excessive acetylcholine at the synaptic site. Patients exposed to NA may require very large doses of atropine for successful treatment.

While atropine is effective in attenuating many of the symptoms of NA exposure, it does nothing to stop the effects of the NA on the AChE itself.[38] For that, another agent is required, such as the oxime 2-pralidoxime chloride (PAM), which reactivates the AChE by competing with the NA for the active site on the AChE. PAM will allow the AChE to resume almost normal activity.[39] The adult dosage of PAM for mild cases is 1–2 g IM as a single dose. The pediatric dose for mild cases is 15–25 mg/kg IM. For moderate-to-severe exposures, the dose is the same but is usually given intravenously. PAM should be given over 30 minutes; rapid administration may cause significant elevations in blood pressure. PAM doses should be repeated hourly in case of progressive worsening or persistent signs of toxicity.[34]

For reasons other than the obvious need for rapid medical attention, time is of the essence in treating patients exposed to NA. The bonds formed between the NA and AChE will rapidly "age" and become resistant to deactivators, starting right after exposure.[41] Oximes are effective only if the agent-enzyme complex has not aged.[42] Complete aging may take minutes (soman [GD]) to hours (VX). Because in most cases the exact agent is unknown, PAM should be given for any NA exposure regardless of time. Once various AChE are irreversibly inactivated, it must be replaced by cellular production. This occurs at different rates in blood (RBC turnover is 1% per day) and tissue and may take up to 6 weeks in patients who did not receive treatment.[41,43] Due to the inactivation of various AChE, drugs that depend on AChE for breakdown, such as succinylcholine, remifentanyl, esmolol, and mivacurium, should not be used in patients exposed to NA.

Another organ system affected by significant NA exposure is the CNS. Seizures are common and an early sign of significant exposure. Benzodiazepines (Valium 10 mg) and scopolamine (0.25 mg every 4–6 hours for mild cases, and 0.25 mg, repeated in 30 minutes, followed every 4–6 hours for moderate and severe cases) can be used to suppress the CNS effects of NAs. Scopolamine has a sedative effect in addition to a central anticholinergic effect due to its quaternary chemical structure that penetrates the blood-brain barrier. Benzodiazepines stop and can prevent seizures while aiding in mechanical ventilation. Prophylaxis treatment with oral pyridostigmine (30 mg, three times/day for a population at risk) can be an effective partially protective measure against NA intoxication.[34,44,45] There are reports of potential long-term neuromyasthenic injury from chronic pyridostigmine, including its potential role in Gulf War syndrome.[46]

Pulmonary intoxicants are substances that damage the parenchyma of the lung. The damage caused by a gaseous substance usually manifests as pulmonary edema, although there may be some direct tissue damage with some compounds in this category. In contrast, sulfur mustard damages the airway with little parenchymal damage. The best known and most studied of these compounds is phosgene (carbonyl chloride, designated as CG). Phosgene is widely used in industry, with hundreds of thousands of tons manufactured annually.

The first 30 minutes after exposure to low concentrations of phosgene may produce a mild cough, a sense of chest discomfort, and dyspnea. These compounds may also cause minor and transient irritation of the eyes and upper airways on contact. In the lung, they damage the alveolar-capillary membrane and allow fluid to leak through. These effects are often delayed, and coughing (with production of clear, frothy fluid) may begin 2 to 72 hours after exposure. Generally, the shorter the onset time the more severe the illness. The onset of pulmonary edema within 2–6 hours after exposure is predictive of severe injury.[33]

There is no specific antidote for these compounds. Management consists of supportive care, primary pulmonary care, and assisted ventilation and oxygen until the lung parenchyma heals.[47] In some cases, airway injury develops rapidly and progresses to ARDS, requiring prolonged respiratory support. Hypovolemia and hypotension may result from the intravascular fluid loss. Steroids have not been found to be useful in treating phosgene-induced lung damage.[33]

Vesicants are substances that cause vesicles, or blisters, and may be of animal, vegetable, or mineral origin. These agents include sulfur mustard, nitrogen mustard, lewisite (an arsenical agent), and phosgene oxime (CX; this is not a true vesicant because it produces solid lesions). The one of most concern as a chemical weapon is sulfur mustard. This substance was a major casualty producer in World War I; it produced more chemical casualties than all other chemical agents combined and was extensively used in the Iran-Iraq War in the 1980s.[33]

Mustard gas damages and eventually kills cells, probably by disrupting DNA, although its exact mechanism is still unclear. It damages organs, and it especially affects the eyes, skin, and lungs and will cause significant damage in either vapor or liquid form.[33] Absorbed mustard damages bone marrow, lymphoid tissue, and gastrointestinal mucosa, with damage similar to that produced by radiation. At first, contact with mustard causes no effects. After a brief period or mild exposure, erythema may occur, accompanied by pruritus, burning, and tingling. After an onset time of 2 to 24 hours, the characteristic lesions (blisters) appear on the skin. The eyes (the most sensitive organ to mustard) become reddened, with possibly more severe damage to follow, and airway mucosa is damaged beginning in the upper airway with a dose-dependent descent. After a large amount of skin exposure, lesions may be characterized by a central zone of necrosis surrounded by blisters.[48] Bone marrow damage from mustard exposure may lead to reduced resistance to infection. Mustard may be differentiated from other vesicant agents by the fact that other blistering vesicants, such as lewisite, cause pain in minutes after exposure, while mustard will not cause pain until lesions occur. There is no antidote for mustard exposure.[48,49] The only effective means of preventing or decreasing damage after exposure is rapid decontamination within 1–2 minutes. Management consists of relief of symptoms, with emphasis on prevention of infection. Health care workers must wear protective gear to avoid being contaminated.

Cyanide has a reputation as a rapidly acting, toxic substance. The two types in military use are hydrogen cyanide (AC) and cyanogen chloride (CK). To be lethal, the concentration must be high. Cyanide owes its lethal effect to its ability to inhibit oxidative phosphorylation at the mitochondrial level, thus interrupting energy production. Exposures even slightly below lethal doses cause few side effects. Hundreds of thousands of tons of cyanide are manufactured annually for many industrial uses. Cyanide has been used for centuries as an agent for suicide and homicide. The Nazis, in World War II, used Zyklon B, hydrocyanic acid adsorbed onto a dispersible base, to kill millions of civilians and enemy soldiers in its camps as well as on the battlefield.[50,51] In chemical warfare, its use is limited because of its volatility and the amount required to produce biological effects. However, cyanide agents in sufficient concentration can have a devastating effect.

Methyl isocyanide was accidentally released from a Union Carbide plant in Bhopal, India, on December 2 and 3, 1984, killing between 1750 and 2000 people and injuring another 50,000.[52] Cyanide inhibits intracellular enzymes and prevents cells from using oxygen. Effects from cyanide gas or vapor occur quickly. Within seconds of inhalation of a lethal amount of gas or vapor, consciousness is lost; then seizures begin, followed by apnea and death within 8–10 minutes. Antidotes are effective if administered before signs of irreversible damage. Amyl nitrate followed by sodium nitrite converts hemoglobin to methemoglobin, which effectively removes cyanide from the intracellular enzyme. Thiosulfate combines with cyanide to form thiocyanate, a nontoxic compound if liver clearance is normal. Ventilation support is often required while the antidotes begin working.[53]

ANESTHETIC MANAGEMENT

If anesthesia is to be administered to exposed patients at the incident site, specialized equipment is required. The most basic equipment includes apparatus for delivering inhalational, intravenous, and regional anesthetics and for providing oxygenation and ventilation support. Depending on the circumstances, respiratory equipment can be simple and portable or sophisticated and stationary. If necessary, regional anesthesia is preferred because it can be done quickly and limits the need for extensive monitoring equipment. Regional anesthetics can allow anesthesiologists to monitor conscious patients with lesser-trained personnel, thus freeing the anesthesiologist to tend to other patients in the immediate area. Regional anesthesia would, however, only be acceptable for patients with limited agent exposure, especially in the case of an NA. For a more detailed discussion of field anesthesia techniques and equipment, please refer to Chapter 31.

INFECTIOUS DISEASE AGENTS

EBOLA

In December 2013, transmission of the Ebola virus to humans occurred in West Africa, leading to the 2014–2015 epidemic of over 28,000 confirmed cases of Ebola virus disease (EVD) and 11,000 deaths.[54] Transmission occurs through direct contact with body fluids of an infected person, although droplet transmission has also been reported. EVD manifests as a viral hemorrhagic fever leading to nonspecific symptoms, including fever, headache, weakness, vomiting, and diarrhea, with potential for rapid progression to hemodynamic instability, shock, and multiorgan dysfunction.[55]

Due to its high mortality rate and risk of transmission, prevention of nosocomial transmission remained a key component of clinical care throughout the epidemic. In the hospital setting, strict contact precautions (i.e., meticulous hand washing and use of gown and gloves, as well as proper donning and doffing of personal protective equipment [PPE]) is sufficient to prevent viral transmission. However, this was not always the case in the non–climate-controlled West Africa field treatment facilities. The heat and humidity often led to less-than-optimal functioning of PPEs, including collapse of N-95 duckbill respirators, fogging of tight-fitting goggles, and inability to tolerate prolonged periods of time wearing the equipment due to risk of syncope.[54]

Although the mortality rate in Western Europe and the United States is significantly less in comparison to West Africa (18.5% vs. 40%), the ICU will undoubtedly be tasked in providing definitive care to patients with EVD.[54] ICUs taking care of these patients must have a large amount of physical space to accommodate multiple isolation rooms, as well as designated space for the donning and doffing of personal protective equipment. It is advisable to house dedicated diagnostic and therapeutic equipment within the ICU, and there should be specific protocols for the proper pickup and disposal of soiled materials. Although there are no Ebola-specific therapies proven to be effective, treatment will focus on supportive care, including correction of metabolic abnormalities, initiation of antibiotic treatment regimens, and support of renal and respiratory failure that is often seen in the critically ill.

ZIKA

On February 1, 2016, the World Health Organization (WHO) declared a public health emergency due to the rapid spread of Zika virus and its association with congenital microcephaly and Guillain-Barré syndrome (GBS).[56] Zika virus is an arbovirus transmitted by the *Aedes* mosquito and was first discovered in the 1940s in rhesus monkeys of the Zika Rainforest of Uganda.[57] It was believed to be responsible only for an extremely rare, exotic disease of little clinical significance until 2007, when the first of many recent outbreaks occurred, infecting approximately 5000 people of Micronesia, equal to 75% of the population.[57] A second outbreak occurred between 2013 and 2014 in French Polynesia, where Zika infected more than 32,000 people (11% of the population). By 2015, the virus reached the Americas, primarily in Brazil, where it had caused between 500,000 and 1,500,000 cases prior to the February 2016 declaration by the WHO.

Zika virus infection has two main areas of clinical significance: microcephaly in newborns and GBS in adults. Zika virus has been shown to cross the placenta, where it is believed to be responsible for numerous cases of congenital microcephaly, as well as multiple ocular and optic nerve abnormalities.[56] Congenital infection is of particular concern during the first and early second trimester, when its association with microcephaly is the greatest.

Of particular concern to the anesthesiologist is the association between Zika virus infection and GBS. GBS is an autoimmune-mediated neuropathy, characteristically causing progressive weakness in a distal-to-proximal muscle distribution.[56] The association between Zika virus infection and GBS was first reported during the outbreak in French Polynesia, when the incidence dramatically increased from 5 cases per year to 42 cases within 4 months of the initial 2013 outbreak.[57] Over 1700 cases of GBS were documented in Brazil between January and November 2015, an increase in incidence varying from 60% to 526%, depending on the region. Patients with GBS can have profound muscle weakness, often affecting muscles of respiration. Patients should be admitted to the ICU for further management if there is any sign of difficulty swallowing or coughing or if the vital capacity is less than 1.5 L on pulmonary function testing.[56] Patients with bulbar involvement will likely need to be intubated; however, avoidance of succinylcholine is imperative, as cases of hyperkalemic cardiac arrest have been reported. GBS patients may show increased sensitivity to nondepolarizing muscle relaxants, and prolonged paralysis should be expected. In the parturient GBS patient who requires analgesia/anesthesia, neuraxial techniques have been shown to be a safe and effective option. However, it is important to note that a thoracic level of anesthesia, as would be required for cesarean delivery, will likely weaken respiratory muscles of the chest wall and may lead to further respiratory compromise.[56]

BIOLOGICAL WEAPONS

Many bacteria, fungi, viruses, rickettsial agents, and toxins have been mentioned in the literature as possible biological agents. Those mentioned most often include *Bacillus anthracis* (anthrax), botulinum toxin, *Yersinia pestis* (plague), ricin, staphylococcal enterotoxin B (SEB), and Venezuelan equine encephalitis (VEE) virus. All can be dispersed as aerosols, which may remain suspended (in certain weather conditions) for hours. If inhaled, small particles will penetrate into distal bronchioles and terminal alveoli of victims—particles larger than 5 μm are filtered out in the upper airway. Weather conditions are important for the success of these agents. Favorable conditions include inversion conditions with wind speeds of 5 to 10 miles per hour and nighttime or early morning hours. Table 32.3 compares the effects of a chemical or biological attack on a major city.

TABLE 32.3. Estimates of Casualties Generated by Releasing Four Tons of Chemical or Fifty Kilograms of Biological Active Agent Two Kilometers Upwind of a City of 500,000 People

AGENT	CASES	DEATHS
Sarin	15,000	300
VX	50,000	5000
VX aerosol	120,000	12,000
Plague	75,000	41,000
Anthrax	125,000	95,000

SOURCE: Adapted from *Health Aspects of Chemical and Biological Weapons*. Report of WHO Group Consultants. Geneva, Switzerland: WHO; 1970.

TYPE OF INJURIES

The medical response to a biological weapon attack depends on whether preventive measures were taken before exposure and whether the symptoms of exposure are present. Before exposure, active immunization or prophylaxis with antibiotics may prevent illness in those exposed. Active immunization may be effective against several potential biological warfare agents. After exposure, active or passive immunization as well as pretreatment with therapeutic antibiotics or antiviral drugs may attenuate symptoms. After the onset of illness, what remains for medical providers to do is to diagnose the disease and institute general or specific treatment. Several excellent vaccines and antitoxins exist to counteract the agents of bacterial warfare (Table 32.4).

EMERGENCY MEDICAL MANAGEMENT

Signs and symptoms of biological agents are insidious. The first responder will be an alert clinician or public health professional who recognizes an increasing or unusual pattern of illness in the community. The prospect of secondary spread must be considered with many biological agents, and plans to deal with a highly contagious agent must be in place beforehand.

If contamination is suspected but symptoms are unclear, assume the worst. Clues that biological agents have been released include an unexplained increase in respiratory cases or deaths and dead and dying animals. Epidemiological clues include diseases with the wrong mode of transmission in an inappropriate geographic distribution or that infect a new population.

Several biological agents act strictly as toxins. These can often be confused with chemical agents such as NAs. The differential diagnosis of chemical NAs, botulinum toxin, and staphylococcal enterotoxin B intoxication is presented in Table 32.5.

Identification of a patient with anthrax or a confirmed exposure to *B. anthracis* should prompt an epidemiologic investigation. The highest priority is to identify at-risk persons and initiate appropriate interventions to protect them. The exposure circumstances are the most important factors that direct decisions about prophylaxis. Persons with an exposure or contact with an item or environment known or suspected to be contaminated with *B. anthracis*—regardless of laboratory tests results—should be offered antimicrobial prophylaxis. Exposure or contact, not laboratory test results, is the basis for initiating such treatment. Culture of nasal swabs is used to detect anthrax spores. Nasal swabs can occasionally document exposure, but they cannot rule out exposure to *B. anthracis*.[58]

ANTIMICROBIAL TREATMENT

A high index of clinical suspicion and rapid administration of effective antimicrobial therapy are essential for prompt diagnosis and effective treatment of anthrax. Limited clinical experience is available, and no controlled trials in

TABLE 32.4. Types and Characteristics of Biological Warfare Agents

DISEASE	DISSEMINATION MODE	HUMAN-TO-HUMAN ROUTE	INCUBATION	LETHALITY	VACCINE	ANTIBACTERIAL THERAPY
Anthrax	Spores in aerosol	No	1–6 days	High	Yes	Ciprofloxacin, doxycylcine
Brucellosis	Food/supply/aerosol	No	Days to months	Low	Yes	Doxycycline, rifampin
Cholera	Aerosol/food/water	Negligible	1–5 days	Moderate	Yes	Tetracycline
Plague	Aerosol/vectors	High	2–3 days	Very high	Yes	Tetracycline, rifampin
Tularemia	Aerosol	No	2–10 days	Moderate	Yes	Doxycycline, tetracycline
Typhoid	Food/water/aerosol	Negligible	7–21 days	Moderate	Yes	Tetracycline
Smallpox	Aerosol/water	High	7–17 days	High	Yes	Vaccinia/immune globulin

SOURCE: Adapted from NATO Handbook on the Medical Aspects of NBC Defensive Operations, Department of the Army, the Navy, and the Air Force, February 1996.

TABLE 32.5. Differential Diagnosis of Chemical Nerve Agent, Botulinum Toxin, and Staphylococcal Enterotoxin B (SEB) Intoxication

	CHEMICAL AGENT	BOTULINUM TOXIN	SEB
Time to symptoms	Minutes	24–72 hours	3–12 hours
Central nervous system	Convulsions, muscle twitching	Progressive paralysis	Headaches, aches
Cardiovascular	Bradycardia	Normal rate	Normal to fast
Respiratory	Dyspnea	Progressive paralysis	Cough, dyspnea
Gastrointestinal	Pain, diarrhea	Constipation	Nausea, vomiting
Ocular	Miosis	Droopy eyelids	Conjunctival injection
Salivary	Profuse/watery saliva	Difficulty swallowing	Increased salivation
Death	Minutes	2–3 days	Unlikely
Response to atropine/2-pralidoxime chloride (PAM)	Yes	No	Reduction in symptoms

SOURCE: Franz D. *Defense Against Toxin Weapons.* Bethesda, MD: US Army Medical Research and Material Command; 1997.

humans have been performed to validate current treatment recommendations for inhalational anthrax. Based on studies in nonhuman primates and other animal and in vitro data, ciprofloxacin or doxycycline should be used for initial intravenous therapy until antimicrobial susceptibility results are known. Because of the mortality associated with inhalational anthrax, two or more antimicrobial agents predicted to be effective are recommended; however, controlled studies to support a multiple-drug approach are not available. Other agents with in vitro activity suggested for use in conjunction with ciprofloxacin or doxycycline include rifampin, vancomycin, imipenem, chloramphenicol, penicillin and ampicillin, clindamycin, and clarithromycin; but, other than for penicillin, limited or no data exist regarding the use of these agents in the treatment of inhalational *B. anthracis* infection. Cephalosporins and trimethoprim-sulfamethoxazole should not be used for therapy.[58]

Toxin-mediated morbidity is a major complication of systemic anthrax. Corticosteroids have been suggested as adjunct therapy for inhalational anthrax associated with extensive edema, respiratory compromise, and meningitis.[58]

For cutaneous anthrax, ciprofloxacin and doxycycline also are first-line therapy. As for inhalational disease, intravenous therapy with a multidrug regimen is recommended for cutaneous anthrax with signs of systemic involvement, for extensive edema, or for lesions on the head and neck. In cutaneous anthrax, antimicrobial treatment may render lesions culture negative in 24 hours, although progression to eschar formation still occurs.[58,59] Some experts recommend that corticosteroids be considered for extensive edema or swelling of the head and neck region associated with cutaneous anthrax. Cutaneous anthrax is typically treated for 7–10 days. Although infection may produce an effective immune response, a potential for reactivation of latent infection may exist. Therefore, persons with cutaneous anthrax should be treated for 60 days.

Prophylaxis for inhalational anthrax exposure includes the use of either ciprofloxacin or doxycycline as a first-line agent. High-dose penicillin (e.g., amoxicillin or penicillin VK) may be an option for antimicrobial prophylaxis when ciprofloxacin or doxycyclines are contraindicated. The likelihood of β-lactamase induction events that would increase the penicillin minimum inhibitory concentration (MIC) is lower when only small numbers of vegetative cells are present, such as during antimicrobial prophylaxis.

DIFFERENTIAL DIAGNOSIS BETWEEN CHEMICAL AND INFECTIOUS AGENTS

Responses to biological and chemical agents are different. In a biological attack, quick diagnosis of the agent is critical. Most chemical events are acute at onset and are treated as emergencies by the police, fire, emergency medical services personnel, or hazardous materials teams. First responders must be well trained, decontamination procedures must be in place, and a disaster plan should be well practiced. Preventing injury to first responders requires intense training and a high index of suspicion. Differentiating between chemical and biological weapons can be difficult as waves of patients succumb to these agents. An attack with biological weapons, although less likely than a chemical attack, will be much more difficult to identify early and could initiate an epidemic that sickens or kills large numbers of US citizens before medical intervention can be organized. Few physicians have ever seen a case of anthrax, smallpox, or plague, so diagnosis of the epidemic is certain to be delayed. The laboratory capabilities for diagnosis and measuring the antibiotic sensitivity of potential organisms are likewise limited, further delaying diagnosis and the implementation of control measures. An attack would not be obvious for days to weeks depending on the incubation period of the disease. By then, modern transportation would have dispersed widely the population of victims. For contagious agents such as smallpox and plague, this implies ever-widening spread of disease.

If contamination is suspected but symptoms are unclear, assume the worst. Clues that biological agents have been released include an unexplained increase in respiratory cases or deaths.

INTENSIVE CARE SERVICES IN DISASTER

The need for hospital beds—specifically, intensive care beds and especially the personnel and material resources to support the patients in those beds—is one of the most important limiting factors of the emergency medical response, often requiring outside assistance.[60] In each of the disaster scenarios described in this chapter, blunt or penetrating trauma, airway injury, ARF, ARDS, crush syndrome, or acute renal failure from severe crush injury represent the predominant injury or disease mechanisms requiring intensive care. Therefore, life-saving potential will be largely determined by the ability to promptly secure an airway and provide an adequate number of intensive care (monitored) beds, hemodialysis or continuous venovenous hemofiltration, and sufficient mechanical ventilators and respiratory care services.[61] Unfortunately, intensive and respiratory care resources will be quickly overwhelmed in most communities because they are in such limited supply on a daily basis.

It is a major premise of this discussion that anesthesiologists and the anesthesia care team will not be limited to providing traditional OR-based anesthesia services but will also be called on for reserve respiratory and intensive care staffing and services OOOR during a major earthquake, chemical or biological attack on the homeland, or in pandemic influenza. Therefore, anesthesiology education and training programs must include the management of victims of terrorist chemical or biological attack, as well as the ability to function in the out-of-hospital setting in disaster. Likewise, departments of anesthesia should develop contingency plans in the event staff is needed in the field and intensive care areas. As described in this chapter, detailed plans to manage a surge of critically ill or injured patients are an essential component of hospital disaster planning and preparedness.[60–62] Figure 32.2 shows suggested hospital ICU and overflow areas where physiologic monitors are usually found. The establishment of an institutional "critical care crisis team" may aid in the development of such plans.

Because a plan for the provision of critical care services cannot wait until casualty figures become definitive, it is recommended that surge capacity for disaster response be gradated and standardized on a local, citywide, regional, and national basis. This may best be organized by implementing a national registry of intensive care beds, resources, and services, as we do now for general hospital beds among hospitals that are members of the National Disaster Medical System (NDMS). Each institution would report the number of ICU beds; type of ICU bed (i.e., burn, cardiovascular, neurological, etc.); ICU occupancy rates; average length of ICU stay; ICU bed surge capacity; ICU staffing (physicians, nurses, respiratory therapists); and numbers of mechanical ventilators and other supplies and services that could be made available over a specified period of time.

We have already experienced the H1N1 flu epidemic and learned many lessons regarding the provision of intensive care services in these situations. However, a recent study of the H1N1 flu epidemic in Australia and New Zealand estimated a 23%–45% increase in ICU utilization over normal annual use.[63] The lessons learned with the H1N1 epidemic will be applicable also to the intensive care management of casualties of natural disasters, as well as chemical and biological weapon attack.

CONCLUSIONS

As a nation, we face significant challenges in developing the capability to provide health and medical services to casualties of a major earthquake, terrorist use of a chemical or biological weapon, or pandemic flu in the United States. The probability that a major earthquake or a chemical or biological attack will occur in the near future in a densely populated city in the United States causing thousands of critically ill or injured casualties is high. Based on previous disaster events, uninjured survivors (bystanders) will be the first to respond, followed later by emergency personnel from local prehospital EMS systems and hospitals. However, the public at large, first responders, professional rescuers, and their institutions are often unprepared to deal with a surge of casualties. Therefore, mass training of the public in LSFA and basic rescue techniques is essential and has been proven to increase life-saving potential.[27] In order to cover a critical mass of the lay public in the United States, it may be advisable for LSFA training to be linked with driver licensing and renewal and cars equipped with first aid kits.

Anesthesiology residency programs have not systematically incorporated all disaster management competencies into education and training curricula, and they do not require demonstration of ability to function in the OOOR setting under crisis conditions.

In summary, the aim of disaster preparedness and response is to reduce chaos and uncertainty during a disaster. In homeland disaster scenarios that may result in mass injury or illness, as described in this chapter, anesthesiologists will inevitably play a crucial life-saving role not only within the traditional confines of the OR and ICUs, but also in the OOOR setting. Therefore, to broaden disaster response capability among anesthesiologists, it may be prudent for the field of anesthesiology to revise resident education and training curricula to include disaster medicine and management competencies and treatment protocols for chemical and biological agent and to combine simulation-based learning modalities to re-create the OOOR setting and relevant disaster scenarios. The times we are living in behoove us to rethink our traditional role in disaster response and plan for new exigencies.

REFERENCES

1. Hsu DB, Thomas TL, Bois EB, Whyne D, Kelen GD, Green GB. Healthcare worker competencies for disaster training. *BMC Med Educ.* 2006;6:19.
2. Candiotti KA, Kamat A, Barach P, Nhuch F, Lubarsky D, Birnbach D. Emergency preparedness for biological and chemical incidents: a survey of anesthesiology residency programs in the United States. *Anesth Analg.* 2005;101:1135–1140.
3. Molino LN. *Emergency Incident Management Systems: Fundamentals and Applications.* Hoboken, NJ: Wiley; 2006:518.
4. Federal Emergency Management System. National Response Framework resource center. Available at: https://www.fema.gov/media-library/assets/documents/32230. Accessed on April 1, 2018.
5. Chan TC, Killeen J, Griswold W, Lenert L. Information technology and emergency medical care during disasters. *Acad Emerg Med.* 2004;11(11):1229–1236.
6. Anker M. Epidemiological and statistical methods for rapid health assessment: introduction. *World Health Stat Quart.* 1991;44:94–97.
7. Smith GS. Development of rapid epidemiologic assessment methods to evaluate health status and delivery of health services. *Int J Epidemiol.* 1989;18:S2–S15.
8. De Lisi LE. The Katrina disaster and its lessons. *World Psychiat.* 2006;5(1):3–4.
9. Garner A, Lee A, Harrison K, Schultz CH. Comparative analysis of multiple-casualty incident triage algorithms. *Ann Emerg Med.* 2001;38:541–548.
10. Iserson KV, Moskop JC. Triage in medicine, part I: concept, history, and types. *Ann Emerg Med.* 2007;49(3):275–281.
11. Stawicki S, Howard J, Pryor J, Bahner D, Whitmill M, Dean A. Portable ultrasonography in mass casualty incidents: the CAVEAT examination. *World J Orthop.* 2010;1(1):10–19.
12. Bhalla M, Frey J, Rider C, Nord M, Hegerhorst M. Simple triage algorithm and rapid treatment and sort, assess, lifesaving, interventions, treatment, and transportation mass casualty triage methods for sensitivity, specificity, and predictive values. *Am J Emerg Med.* 2015;33(11):1687–1691.
13. SALT mass casualty triage: concept endorsed by the American College of Emergency Physicians, American College of Surgeons Committee on Trauma, American Trauma Society, National Association of EMS Physicians, National Disaster Life Support Education Consortium, and State and Territorial Injury Prevention Directors Association. *Disaster Med Public Health Prep.* 2008;2(4):245–246.
14. Klein K, Burkle F Jr, Swienton R, King R, Lehman T, North C. Qualitative analysis of surveyed emergency responders and the identified factors that affect first stage of primary triage decision-making of mass casualty incidents. *PLoS Curr.* 2016 Aug 19;8. doi:https://dx.doi.org/10.1371%2Fcurrents.dis.d69dafcfb3ad8be88b3e655bd38fba84.
15. Brooks A, Davies B, Smethhurst M, Connolly J. Emergency ultrasound in the acute assessment of haemothorax. *Emerg Med J.* 2004;21(1):44–46.
16. Sztajnkrycer M, Baez A, Luke A. FAST ultrasound as an adjunct to triage using the START mass casualty triage system. *Prehosp Emerg Care.* 2006;10(1):96–102.
17. Strode CA, Rubal BJ, Gerhardt RT, et al. Satellite and mobile wireless transmission of focused assessment with sonography in trauma. *Acad Emerg Med.* 2003;10(12):1411–1414.
18. Angus D, Pretto E, Abrams JI, Safar P. Life supporting first aid training of the lay public for disaster preparedness. *Prehosp Disaster Med.* 1991;6:547.
19. Abrams JI, Pretto E, Angus D, Safar P. Basic extrication training of the lay public for disaster preparedness. *Prehosp Disaster Med.* 1991;6:547.
20. Ricci E, Pretto E. Assessment of prehospital and hospital response in disaster. *Crit Care Clin.* 1991;7(2):471–484.
21. Sandrock C. Care of the critically ill and injured during pandemics and disasters. *Chest.* 2014;146(4):881–883.
22. Ricci E, Pretto E, Safar P, et al. Disaster reanimatology potentials: a structured interview study in armenia II. Method for the evaluation of medical response to major disasters. *Prehosp Disaster Med.* 1991;6(2):159–166.
23. Klain M, Ricci E, Safar P, et al. Disaster reanimatology potentials: a structured interview study in Armenia I. Methodology and preliminary results. *Prehosp Disaster Med* 1989;4(2):135–154.
24. Pretto E, Ricci E, Safar P, et al. Disaster reanimatology potentials: a structured interview study in Armenia III: results, conclusions, and recommendations. *Prehosp Disaster Med.* 1992;7(4):327–338.
25. Missair A, Gebhard R, Pierre E, et al. Surgical care amid the rubble during the January 12, 2010 earthquake in Haiti: the importance of regional anesthesia. *Prehosp Disaster Med.* 2010;25(6):487–493.
26. Pretto E, Angus D, Abrams JI, et al. An analysis of prehospital mortality in an earthquake. *Prehosp Disaster Med.* 1994;9(2):107–117.
27. Angus DA, Pretto E, Abrams JI, et al. Epidemiologic assessment of building collapse pattern, mortality, and medical response after the 1992 earthquake in Erzincan, Turkey. *Prehosp Disaster Med.* 1997;12(3):222–231.
28. Bissell R. Pretto E, Angus D, et al. Post-preparedness disaster response in Costa Rica. *Prehosp Disaster Med.* 1994;9(2):96–106.
29. Aoki N, Murakawa T, Pretto EA, et al. Survival and cost analysis of fatalities of the Kobe earthquake in Japan. *Prehosp Emerg Care.* 2004;8:217–222.
30. Lehavi A, Meroz Y, Maryanovsky M, et al. Role of regional anaesthesia in disaster medicine. *Eur J Anaesthesiol.* 2016;33(5):312–313.
31. Jiang J, Xu H, Liu H, Yuan H, Wang C, Ye J. Anaesthetic management under field conditions after the 12 May 2008 earth- quake in Wenchuan, China. *Injury.* 2010;41(6):e1–e3.
32. Missair A, Gebhard R, Pierre E, et al. Surgery under extreme conditions in the aftermath of the 2010 Haiti earthquake: the importance of regional anesthesia. *Anesth. Analg.* 2013;25(6):487–493.
33. *Health Aspects of Chemical and Biological Weapons.* Report of WHO Group Consultants. Geneva, Switzerland: WHO; 1970.
34. *Medical Aspects of Chemical and Biological Warfare, Textbook of Military Medicine.* Washington, DC: Office of Surgeon General, US Army; 1997.
35. Abraham RB, Rudick V, Weinbroum AA. Practical guidelines for acute care of victims of bioterrorism: conventional injuries and concomitant nerve agent intoxication. *Anesthesiology.* 2002;97:989–1004.
36. Tafuri J, Roberts J. Organophosphate poisoning. *Ann Emerg Med.* 1987;16:193–202.
37. Okumura T, Suzuki K, Fukuda A, et al. The Tokyo subway sarin attack: disaster management. Part 2. Hospital response. *Acad Emerg Med.* 1998;5:618–624.

38. De Bleeker JL. The intermediate syndrome in organophosphate poisoning: an overview of experimental and clinical observations. *J Toxicol Clin Toxicol.* 1995;33:683–686.
39. Milby TH. Prevention and management of organophosphate poisoning. *JAMA.* 1971;216:2131–2133.
40. Shih TM, Duniho SM, McDonough JH. Control of nerve agent induced seizures is critical for neuroprotection and survival. *Toxicol Appl Pharmacol.* 2003;188(2):69–80.
41. Shafferman A, Ordentlich A, Barak D, Stein D, Ariel N, Velan B. Aging of phosphylated human acetylcholinesterase: catalytic processes mediated by aromatic and polar residues of the active center. *Biochem J.* 1996;318(pt 3):833–840.
42. Chemical Casualty Care Office of the USA Army Medical Research Institute of Chemical Defense. *Decontamination, Medical Management of Chemical Casualties Handbook.* 2nd ed. Aberdeen Proving Ground, MD: US Army Medical Research Institute of Chemical Defense; 1995:127–144.
43. Worek F, Backer M, Thiermann H, et al. Reappraisal of indications and limitations of oxime therapy in organophosphate poisoning. *Hum Exp Toxicol.* 1997;16:466–472.
44. Kwong TC. Organophosphate pesticides: biochemistry and clinical toxicology. *Ther Drug Monit.* 2002;24:144–149.
45. Holstege CP, Kirk M, Sidell FR. Chemical warfare. *Crit Care Clin.* 1997;13:923–941.
46. Gronseth GS. Gulf War syndrome: a toxic exposure? A systematic review. *Neurol Clin.* 2005;23(2):523–540.
47. Ellenhorn MJ. Chemical warfare. In: Ellenhorn MJ, ed. *Medical Toxicology: Diagnosis and Treatment of Human Poisoning.* 2nd ed. Baltimore, MD: Williams and Wilkins; 1997:1267–1304.
48. Diller WF. Therapeutic strategy in phosgene poisoning. *Toxicol Ind Health.* 1985;1:93–99.
49. Papirmeister B, Feister AJ, Robinson SI, Ford RD. *Medical Defense Against Mustard Gas: Toxic Mechanisms and Pharmacological Implications.* Boca Raton, FL: CRC Press; 1991.
50. Laurent JF, Richter F, Michel A. Management of the victims of urban chemical attack: the French approach. *Resuscitation.* 1999;42:141–149.
51. Baskin SI. Zyklon. In: La Cleur W, ed. *The Holocaust Encyclopedia.* New Haven, CT: Yale University Press; 1998:717–718.
52. Ayres RU, Rhohatgi PK. Bhopal: lessons for technological decision-makers. *Technol Soc.* 1987;9:19–45.
53. Baker DJ. Management of respiratory failure in toxic disasters. *Resuscitation.* 1999;42:125–131.
54. Leligdowicz A, Fischer W, Uyeki T, et al. Ebola virus disease and critical illness. *Crit Care.* 2016; 20(1):217.
55. Kortepeter M, Bausch D, Bray M. Basic clinical and laboratory features of filoviral hemorrhagic fever. *J Infect Dis.* 2011;204(suppl 3):S810–S816.
56. Padilla C, Pan A, Geller A, Zakowski M. Zika virus: review and obstetric anesthetic clinical considerations. *J Clin Anesth.* 2016;35:136–144.
57. Zammarchi L, Spinicci M, Spinicci M, Bartoloni A, Bartoloni A. Zika virus: a review from the basics to proposed management strategies. *Mediterr J Hematol Infect Dis.* 2016;8(1):e2016056.
58. Reissman DB, Whitney EA, Taylor TH Jr, et al. One-year health assessment of adult survivors of *Bacillus anthracis* infection. *JAMA.* 2004;291:1994–1998.
59. Inglesby TV, O'Toole T, Henderson DA, et al. Anthrax as a biological weapon, 2002. *JAMA.* 2002;287:2236–2252.
60. Shirley PJ, Mandersloot G. Clinical review: the role of the intensive care physician in mass casualty incidents: planning, organization, and leadership. *Crit Care.* 2008;12:214.
61. Nap RE, Andriessen M, Meesen NEL, Miranda D, van der Werf TS. Pandemic influenza and excess intensive care workload. *Emerg Infect Dis.* 2008;14(10):1518–1525.
62. Rubinson L, O'Toole T. Critical care during epidemics. *Crit Care.* 2005;9:311–313.
63. The ANZIC Influenza Investigators. Critical care services and 2009 H1N1 influenza in Australia and New Zealand. *N Engl J Med.* 2009;361:1925–1934.

33 | TELEMEDICINE, TELEANESTHESIA, AND TELESURGERY

W. BOSSEAU MURRAY, MD, SORIN VADUVA, MBA, BENJAMIN W. BERG, MD

INTRODUCTION

This chapter is intended as an overview for the anesthesiologist or administrator who is asking the following questions:

- What changes have occurred since the acceptance of telemedicine[1] practice and technologies in the **Patient Protection and Affordable Care Act (PPACA)**, commonly called the **Affordable Care Act (ACA)**, a US federal statute enacted on March 23, 2010.
- Should I consider using telemedicine in my health care system?
- Can I use aspects of telemedicine in my sites outside of the operating room?
- Are there any dangers?
- What are the advantages?
- If I want to enter the field, what are the implied or expected infrastructure costs at both ends?
- What should I expect in the next 5–10 years?

Implementation of the ACA encouraged and enabled inclusion of telehealth services in health care coverage. The ACA implemented telehealth in selected circumstances through Medicare and delegated the power to determine which, if any, telehealth services are covered by Medicaid as well as through regulation of private payer telehealth reimbursement. Reimbursement and regulation remain largely within the powers of individual states.

Since passage of the ACA, telemedicine services have continued to expand. One example is in North Dakota, where from 2008 to 2014, more than 35% of 3309 trauma patients treated in a North Dakota critical access hospital presented to a facility with telemedicine capabilities. And, among patients presenting to a telemedicine-enabled emergency department, more than 10% were managed with telemedicine consultation.[*] In another application, telemedicine is used to train perioperative nurses in rural settings.[2]

Telemedicine[1] is the result of the information technology (IT) revolution, which is producing major changes in medical practice. Many images are now presented in digital format, including computed tomographic (CT) scans, ultrasound scans, magnetic resonance imaging (MRI), endoscopy, and vital sign waveforms. All these images require highly trained individuals to obtain maximum benefit (information extraction) from this content. For example, graphs of somatosensory evoked potentials (SSEPs) are relatively easy to generate, but the interpretation of "spinal cord being intact, or not" is not that easy, and a "superspecialized" expert is needed for interpretation.

Digital images can be reproduced and presented anywhere in the world in "real time," and support can be provided for analysis and interpretation. Remote assistance (e.g., via telesurgery under teleanesthesia) can help the physician to "dissolve time and space."

Many areas of telehealth (in the broadest sense of the word) have very successfully enabled not only physician-to-physician consultations, but also patient assessment and treatment. Whereas the early emphasis in telemedicine was to provide advanced health care where it was not available (e.g., military and disaster scenarios), thereby overcoming the "tyranny of distance," telemedicine is now also utilized when cost reductions are required. For instance, telemedicine can mean less travel and cost for the patient, reduced need for extra staff and resources at smaller hospitals, and improved mobility and efficiency of health care workers, who can essentially move from patient to patient and "see" the next patient with the switch of a button.

In 2016, twenty-nine states and the District of Columbia had telemedicine parity laws for private insurance coverage, with proposed or pending legislation in eight other states. State telemedicine parity laws require private payers to reimburse telehealth services in the same way they reimburse "in-person" medical treatment. US state Medicaid programs, excepting those of Connecticut and Rhode Island, offer some form of telemedicine coverage. Some state Medicaid programs offer broad coverage for telemedicine, without provider or location restrictions; others have a variety of restrictions.

This chapter encompasses the following:

- The definition and scope of tele–health care (telemedicine in its broadest sense)
- Major recent advances in the field of telemedicine (medical practice and systems technologies)

[*] Mohr NM, Harland KK, Chrischilles E, et al. Telemedicine penetration and consultation among rural trauma patients in critical access hospital emergency departments in North Dakota. Rural Telehealth Research Center. Research & Policy Brief. Available at: http://ruraltelehealth.org/briefs/RTRC-NDTelemedTrauma-Brief-2016-sept.pdf. Published September 2016. Accessed on November 26, 2017.

- State of the art of telemedicine, telesurgery, and teleanesthesia
- Ramifications and implications of technological developments and health care reform for telemedicine
- New directions in anesthesiology practice (including intensive care units [ICUs] based on the use of telemedicine technologies

DEFINITIONS AND TERMINOLOGY

In this chapter, we use the term *telemedicine* to describe the entire range of **tele–health care**. Therefore, we use this term to include distinct disciplines, such as telesurgery, teleanesthesia, tele–internal medicine, **tele–*any discipline*.**

DEFINITIONS

For the US Congress, the term *telemedicine* means

> *a telecommunications link to an end user through the use of eligible equipment that electronically links health professionals or patients and health professionals at separate sites in order to exchange health care information in audio, video, graphic, or other format for the purpose of providing improved health care services. United States Code, 2006 Edition, Supplement V, Title 25 - Indians, page 26*

Historically, there are dozens of definitions of teleanesthesia as found in the academic literature. For instance, Sood et al. presented a compilation of 104 perspectives on definitions.[1] Totten et al.[3] proposed a definition that includes the "time" dimension: "Telehealth is defined as the use of information and telecommunications technology in health care delivery for a specific patient involving a provider across distance or time." Each telemedicine publication and each organization tried to provide its own definition. It is actually complex to produce a comprehensive definition of telemedicine, as any definition will have to encompass at least the three basic elements as outlined by the Index Medicus® definitions in Table 33.1, which includes health occupation aspects, IT principles, as well as aspects of the delivery of health care.

Since 1992, telemedicine has been included in MEDLINE's® MeSH (Medical Subject Headings) under three separate sections (Table 33.1):

1. Health occupations
2. Information science and telecommunications
3. Delivery of health care

While *Remote Consultation, Telepathology, Teleradiology,* and *Telerehabilitation* are the only disciplines that have been included in the Index Medicus listings, it is to be expected that multiple other disciplines will soon be listed (e.g., teleanesthesia, tele–intensive care, teledermatology, telesurgery, and even subspecialties such as teleurology).

TABLE 33.1. Index Medicus Outline

All MeSH Categories
Disciplines and Occupations Category
Health Occupations
Medicine
Telemedicine
Telepathology
Teleradiology
Telerehabilitaion
All MeSH Categories
Information Science Category
Information Science
Communications Media
Telecommunications
Telemedicine
Remote Consultation
Telepathology
Teleradiology
Telerehabilitaion
All MeSH Categories
Health Care Category
Health Services Administration
Patient Care Management
Delivery of Health Care
Telemedicine
Remote Consultation
Telepathology
Teleradiology
Telerehabilitaion
Previous Indexing:
• Telecommunications (1976–1992)
See also:
• Telemetry

The definitions of the other disciplines will most likely be based on, and follow the structure of, the existing definitions as outlined in Index Medicus:

> *Remote Consultation:* Consultation via remote telecommunications, generally for the purpose of diagnosis or treatment of a patient at a site remote from the patient or primary physician.

Teleradiology: The electronic transmission of radiological images from one location to another for the purposes of interpretation or consultation. Users in different locations may simultaneously view images with greater access to secondary consultations and improved continuing education.

Telepathology: Transmission and interpretation of tissue specimens via remote telecommunication, generally for the purpose of diagnosis or consultation, but it may also be used for continuing education.

Telerehabilitation: Delivery of therapeutic rehabilitation at a distance or off site using telecommunication technologies. (https://www.ncbi.nlm.nih.gov/pubmed/)

As intimated in these definitions and the ACA law, it appears that telemedicine will have a major effect on medical education, and medical education will benefit greatly from the telemedicine developments. Expensive simulation laboratories at large universities and institutions can remotely provide robotic simulated patients for rural health care workers to practice common procedures (e.g., advanced cardiac life support [ACLS] and basic life support [BLS]) as well as uncommon crises (e.g., malignant hyperthermia). With such a system, the trainees do not know whether they are working on real patients, images of real patients, or physiology generated by mathematical models (i.e., simulated patients). Therefore, an Index Medicus term for medical education using telemedicine principles and infrastructure will be needed, as this real-time interactive training (using physiologically modeled patients) is totally different from "distance education."

TERMINOLOGY

Terms and definitions related to telemedicine might be unfamiliar and evolve continuously. Table 33.2 therefore provides current terminology and examples as used in telemedicine.

LESSONS FROM PRACTICING TELEMEDICINE PHYSICIANS

Technology-enabled delivery of health care at a distance utilizing telemedicine, telehealth, telepresence, telecare, tele-ICU,[4,5] e-health, decision support systems,[6,7] and myriad other described information technologies have increasingly diffused into American health care.[8] The American Telemedicine Association estimated that over 200 academic medical centers are offering international telemedicine services, in addition to domestic services enabled by the previously mentioned reforms by US domestic private and government payers. There are many examples[3,9] of improved efficiency, enhanced clinical care, and user satisfaction in multiple disciplines, underlying the expanding application of telemedicine methodologies. Previous telehealth initiatives have provided lessons learned at various levels in industry, regulatory bodies,[10] health care organizations, provider groups, and patient experiences that can guide the analysis and implementation of effective processes in health care.

In the quest to improve the efficiency of medical care, leveraging technology to address specific identified "choke points" in the delivery of care remains the cornerstone of successful initiatives. It is essential that those telehealth initiatives should articulate clear and measurable objectives with explicit value-added solutions. Organizational and practitioner factors that have a determinant effect on, and predict, successful program implementation, include (1) technology, (2) acceptance, (3) financing, (4) organization, and (5) policy and legislation.[11] A rich body of literature exists regarding the implementation, value propositions, and practical operation of telehealth solutions across disciplines as diverse as radiology, dermatology, critical care,[12,13] stroke management, cardiology, prehospital care, mental health, disaster medicine, postoperative care, pharmacy services, dentistry, remote patient monitoring in acute and chronic illness, and so on. Practitioner acceptance has been extensively analyzed,[14] and several essential factors have emerged as predictors of successful implementation of enduring telehealth strategies.

APPROACHES TO TELEHEALTH SOLUTIONS

Alignment of available technology with a specific identified need requires knowledge of available core technologies and telehealth implementation strategies.[†] "Best fit" technology solution frameworks consider available methods and workflow models, including asynchronous "store and forward"; synchronous audio/video/data streams; decision support systems; robotics; multipoint versus point to point; and others. Frequently, hybrid solutions are best matched to previously identified needs and capabilities (Table 33.2).

One compilation of reported successful telemedicine programs identified the characteristics of sustainable programs[15]:

1. Local service delivery problems have been clearly stated.
2. Telemedicine has been seen as a benefit.
3. Telemedicine has been seen as a solution to political and medical issues.
4. There was collaboration between promoters and users.
5. Issues regarding organizational and technological arrangements have been addressed.
6. The future operation of the service has been considered.

[†] Additional sources for information: (a) Health Resources and Services Administration Office for the Advancement of Telehealth, Telehealth Resource Centers website: https://www.telehealthresourcecenter.org/, accessed on November 26, 2017; (b) Center for Connected Health Policy website: http://cchpca.org, accessed on November 26, 2017.

TABLE 33.2. Explanation of Terminology of Telemedicine, With Examples

	EXAMPLES	PROS	CONS	ANESTHESIA CONSIDERATIONS
Decision support systems	Drug interaction alerts Clinical guideline alignment	Decrease practice variation	Validated Systems not well developed or widely available	TIVA Pharmacodynamics Automated preoperative triage Ventilator management Closed-loop systems
Networks/multipoint collaboration	Electronic ICU Acute stroke management	VTC widely available and acceptable Coordinated information system integration	Expensive, complex, infrastructure sustainment	Anesthesia surgery preoperative conferences Multipoint outpatient monitoring
Mobile health (m-Health)	Patient text messaging Alerts and education Physiologic monitoring by cell phone	Widely distributed e-technology	Limited content complexity	Remote monitoring Preoperative evaluation Postoperative follow-up Patient education
POTS (plain old telephone service)	Home care monitoring	Familiar, acceptable, and available; low cost	No integrated documentation Slow data transmission	Patient follow-up interviews
Store and forward	International consultation	Flexible scheduling	No interactive queries	Preoperative evaluation
Asynchronous	Austere environments Dermatology Radiology Pathology	Time zone independent	No real-time data	Data and questionnaire information
Synchronous	Critical care	Interactive queries	Scheduling	Preoperative assessment
Audio/video/other	Surgical mentoring Mental health Neurosurgery Preoperative evaluation	Continuous monitoring	Enhanced privacy considerations	Remote monitoring OR/non-OR postoperative care
Robotics/haptics	Surgery Rehabilitation Pharmacy	Remote procedures	Incompletely developed	Medication administration

ICU, intensive care unit; OR, operating room; TIVA, total intravenous anesthesia; VTC, video teleconferencing.

PRACTICAL CONSIDERATIONS FOR TELEMEDICINE PRACTITIONERS

Health care providers who utilize technology solutions, including telemedicine, have well-defined acceptance behaviors.[16] System characteristics that are associated with provider acceptance of newly introduced technology are not surprising. Flexibility and usability, education and training, and goodness of fit between the technology and the clinical workflow and resources are key elements for user acceptance. Technology acceptance is a function of alignment with traditional practice workflow, evidence regarding benefits of IT, organizational support, and system-specific issues such as usability of computer interfaces. Design and introduction of telemedicine practice must carefully consider these factors. Doctors are hesitant to adopt technologies that impose changes in usual practice patterns during implementation, as evidenced by the experience with electronic medical records. The requirement of additional time needed to perform the task with the new technology is a major barrier to physician technology acceptance.[17,18]

The time spent on telemedicine tasks tends to decrease as the health care worker continues to "learn" or request information and support from a remotely located specialist. For instance, after discussing several cases with the remotely located specialist, the on-site physician recognizes and becomes comfortable in diagnosing a specific skin rash. Similarly, the on-site health care worker tends to recognize patterns in the electrocardiogram (ECG), the capnograph, and so on after "seeing" and discussing multiple cases with the specialist. In such cases, *decreased use of telemedicine* is an indication of **success** and not an indication of failure of telemedicine.

Patient acceptance of integrated telemedicine delivery of services cannot be overlooked. Patients are in fact very willing to accept care delivered by remotely located practitioners when there are savings in time, travel, and improved access to specialty services.

Remote delivery of anesthesia services has not been well studied and has proliferated to a lesser degree than other disciplines. However, a number of practical elements learned in telehealth solutions for acute care can be considered for application in teleanesthesia care delivery.

PHYSICIAN FACTORS

- Provide technical personnel to support a physician's seamless use of audio, video, and computer interfaces. This usually requires a dedicated technology facilitator who participates in the episode of care. Such technology facilitators are most effective if they have medical training. Anesthesia technicians, emergency medical technicians (EMTs), respiratory therapy technicians, nurses, and other specialists are often highly effective in these roles. These workers are the glue that holds together all telemedicine programs. A bootstrap program that relies on an enthusiastic motivated individual champion physician for program management and facilitation provides the spark for, but seldom sustains, a successful telemedicine operation.
- Scheduling and coordination of time-efficient telemedicine interactions are one key to physician acceptance and effectiveness. Optimal program performance requires advanced coordination at both the provider and the patient terminus of the telemedicine care system.
- Workflow changes must be minimized, and locating the telemedicine interface (e.g., telemedicine suite, telemedicine computer, telemedicine video telephone conferencing [VTC], etc.) in a location that ensures easy access and rapid return to usual care activities is essential. One strategy is to co-locate telemedicine interfaces in familiar work areas such as the postanesthesia care unit (PACU), PACU care in the ICU,[19] operating room, or preoperative anesthesia clinic.[20–22]
- Telecare requires collaboration between interdisciplinary providers at two or more geographically distinct locations. A fundamental principle of effective collaboration is that of trust and knowledge of mutual capabilities. Collaboration across telehealth interfaces removes interpersonal elements that can facilitate trust and can have an adverse effect on effective collaboration. Periodic face-to-face meetings with collaborating providers and telehealth system personnel are essential for ongoing program review, performance improvement, and maintenance of trust relationships necessary for successful delivery of telecare. Shared health care information systems data (laboratory results, radiology, records) enhance collaborative outcomes.
- Scripted protocols for the delivery of care facilitate effective and efficient telecare. Whether providing routine scheduled comprehensive care (e.g., preoperative evaluation or outpatient endoscopy monitoring) or emergency consultative care (e.g., critical care consultation, remote trauma care), protocol-based communication tools are essential.
- Physician documentation of remotely delivered care is structured to reflect the nature, limitations, and advantages of the remote care episode.

PATIENT FACTORS

- Telecare is presented to patients as a mode of care that is a fully integrated element of total care. Consent to participate is requested by some organizations, but many telecare providers simply provide descriptive information to patients regarding the delivery of specific telehealth services. Some telehealth initiatives, such as home monitoring, require patients to interact directly with the technology. Careful consideration of simplicity, comprehensive support, and user training is required for these systems to provide effective care.

Although becoming less common, skeptics may still ask the following type of question: "How can you possibly provide good care when you cannot examine the patient?"

An appropriate answer is as follows: A majority of health care delivery and decision-making requires cognitive and interpersonal skills, relying on history and data analysis. Specialty-specific decision-making depends on specialty-specific knowledge. Physical examination is but one element of data gathering, which in most instances can be gathered by an on-site provider and in some circumstances can be conducted remotely. Use of a stethoscope and observation of respiratory patterns, gait, neurologic function and many other examination elements can be conducted remotely, using simple tools. Diagnostic monitoring devices can transmit the ECG, cardiac rhythm, vital signs, and a variety of other physiologic signals. For example, an entirely adequate assessment of a patient's Mallampati classification can be directly obtained using simple telemedicine tools. Performance of procedures is developing as an element of telecare (e.g., robotic surgery), although it remains nascent. Telementoring of procedures is well established, and it can safely expand the scope of less experienced and remotely located providers. The telepresence of remotely located practitioners is frequently incorporated in remote specialist consultation services.

In conclusion, telemedicine as a tool for telecare is effective when the tool is optimally matched to the need, when the tool is fully supported by a robust infrastructure envelope, and when providers are an integral element of the implementation of new telemedicine processes.

CURRENT STATE OF THE ART: CLINICAL ASPECTS

Since antiquity, physicians and clinician practitioners have always asked for help from one another. Initially, help was garnered by visiting, personal communication, or writing letters. As hospitals developed and medical practitioners were gathered at one site, help and professional discussions became more immediate. For instance, this included asking each other questions, having discussions, and asking for input/help in the hallway, the coffee lounge, and so on. As technology advanced, the use of a telephone for questions became ubiquitous. As medical knowledge expanded, it became necessary to develop specialization, with the need for even more referrals and communication. However, this occurred in an asynchronous mode, meaning that the referring physician was not "present" when the specialist saw the patient. With the use of physician extenders, especially in underpopulated areas, where a full complement of medical services is not viable, it is becoming necessary to have the local health care worker "see" the patient at the same time as the remote (referred to) physician. Such a consultation is where telemedicine is coming into its own. As video capture technology has become ubiquitous, cheaper, robust, and with increased definition, offline (asynchronous) technology is being replaced with videoconferencing.

Radiology and pathology have been performing via telemedicine because the tasks performed by these specialists were mainly asynchronous. These tasks were accepted as valid by being included in Index Medicus in 1992. As the technology has improved, it is now possible to perform virtually synchronous consultations, as the huge digital files involved can be sent rapidly over the Internet.

On a purely technical and instrumentation level, the telephone has been used for many years to send interactive electronic signals, such as remote checking of an electronic heart pacemaker. Telemetry (wireless monitoring of vital signs at a distance) has been used for ambulatory patients in a hospital setting (e.g., monitoring for arrhythmias in patients after a myocardial infarction), as well as for monitoring patients during transport to a critical care center (e.g., in an ambulance or a helicopter). Telemetry, while still used in its own right, is now also considered to be a subset of the infrastructure of telemedicine.

From this history, it can be seen that telemedicine has been quite successfully employed in a variety of ways. Telemedicine is becoming increasingly acceptable, not only to health care workers but also to the general public. This acceptance has also been approved by politicians and included in the legislative code.

TELEANESTHESIA

The first use of the word *teleanesthesia* in the *title* of a publication that we could find was in a book chapter by Murray and Vaduva[23] in 1997: "Telemedicine, Telesurgery and Teleanesthesia." The first use of the word *teleanesthesia* in an *abstract* listed under the peer-reviewed articles in Index Medicus (https://www.ncbi.nlm.nih.gov/pubmed/), was an article by Sloan in 1967, "An Improved Tele-thermometer."[24]

Several articles since then have described successful uses of various forms of teleanesthesia. For instance, Cone et al. demonstrated the ability to direct an anesthetic in a remote location using satellite communication.[25] Preoperative evaluation at a distance is now offered as a routine service by anesthesia providers.[20–22] Remote critical care services have developed as a widely utilized care model to overcome specialist shortages and enhance clinical and financial outcomes.[4,13,26] Systems have been utilized over vast time zone and geographic distances[26] and are widely used in regional health care systems.[27,28] Tele-ICU services have proliferated in both urban and rural health care over the past 20 years, supported by the publication of guidelines for tele-ICU operations.[29] Demonstrable advantages in clinical processes, worker acceptance, and health care outcomes, health care system performance metrics, and health care costs are variably reported.[30–33] The potential for proliferation of these advantages has driven the development of available commercially scaled comprehensive ICU telehealth systems and solutions. More than 200 US hospitals were using tele-ICU methods in 2016, covering more than 6000 beds, which represent approximately 12% of all American ICU beds.

Anesthesia care in the operating room is a complex, high-reliability endeavor. The multiple elements of care require careful coordination, sequencing, flexibility, data integration, and clinical skill. Reengineering the complex human factors and technology for successful application of telemedicine principles is challenging. Legislative initiatives encouraging increased use of telemedicine have long recognized inherent potential care management advantages (Table 33.3.) Application of telemedicine for anesthesia can be designed to optimize the opportunities for success.

- Not all steps of the anesthesia care processes need necessarily to be performed as "teleanesthesia."
- Only selected steps (pre- or postoperatively) might be used in the telemedicine format.
- For instance, the preoperative visit and evaluation[20–22] and postoperative follow-up could be quite safely performed using telemedicine principles, with potential cost and time savings for the patients and their families, for the physicians, and for the health care system.

TABLE 33.3. Telemedicine Advantages for Health Care Management Services

Telemedicine benefits[3] in care management effectiveness and efficiency[a]
- Cost management of chronic disease
- More consistent and near real-time clinical data
Telemedicine minimizes travel
- Improves quality of care because it "removes barriers of transport"
- Reduces need for costly visits—office, emergency department, hospitalizations
- Results in less missed work
Telemedicine reduces hospitalizations
- Health care provider access to timely clinical data
- Rendering of more timely/appropriate therapeutic interventions
- Key targets for care management outcomes: congestive heart failure, diabetes, cardiac arrhythmias, epilepsy, sleep apnea[34]

[a]The Center for Connected Health Policy. Available at: http://www.cchpca.org/cost-efficiency-studies. Accessed April 4, 2018.

— Combining telemedicine techniques with the standard "physician present in the operating room" anesthesia paradigm may allow delivery of highly efficient comprehensive anesthesia care; pre- and postoperative evaluation and follow-up are "ripe" for increased application of this methodology.

Much of the anesthesia workflow and process (preoperative workup/visit and examination, consent, postoperative follow-up, etc.) can be performed using *standard, existing* telemedicine infrastructure and principles.

Therefore, for our discussion on teleanesthesia, we focus more on the next 5–10 years, that is, on the actual administration and control of the anesthetic agents, monitoring, and depth of anesthesia.

While we are aware of research projects involving robotic placement of an intravenous cannula, autonomous robotic intubation,[‡] and robotic controlled devices to place an endotracheal tube,[35] for the foreseeable future, we envision a trained human ("helper") performing these tasks, most likely under telesupervision of a physician at the controlling base.

Administration of intravenous agents could be accomplished by one or more of several options:

— A trained human locally at the patient's bedside (self-directed, under supervision, or guided by a remote supervisor).

— A digital syringe or infusion pump, autonomously ("computer") controlled,[§] controlled directly by local personnel, or controlled remotely by the main-base physician/advisor.[36]

— Total intravenous anesthesia (TIVA)[37] using target-controlled infusion (TCI) for anesthesia. The digital infusion device runs a pharmacokinetic model and aims to maintain a constant plasma ("blood") concentration of the anesthetic agent(s).

— Close-loop feedback[38] systems. Physiological parameters from the patient, with a fuzzy logic control system, determine the infusion rate(s).

For the pharmacokinetic, model-driven administration schemes, the models will run locally, as well as in the form of a backup, at the supervisory/home base. Should communication be temporarily lost, the two models on the two computers will resynchronize.

MONITORING

Present-day *physiological monitors* mostly handle the data internally as digital data, and the data are presented to the anesthesia personnel in a variety of formats. It is already feasible to present all these data at a distance (anywhere in the world), in near real time. Some *clinical* monitoring signs and symptoms (e.g., signs of shock: cold, clammy, sweaty extremities with poor peripheral perfusion in fingers, etc.) can be provided by additional monitors, for example, peripheral-to-central temperature gradient, skin resistance/impedance monitors (also called "lie detectors") to measure "sweatiness," amplitude of pulsatile oxygen saturation monitors (SPO_2) in the fingers and toes, and so on.[39] However, there are as yet no monitors to replace the overall impression of an experienced clinician ("the patient looks gravely ill"), and a high-definition overall visual image of the patient would still be useful when needed.

DEPTH OF ANESTHESIA

Processed electroencephalogram (EEG) signals would be advisable to monitor the depth of anesthesia. However, such monitoring requires an electrically "clean" environment to reliably and accurately collect and interpret the plus or minus 1-μV signals of the raw EEG. In rural areas, the electrical supply might fluctuate and not be sufficiently stable to provide robust, interpretable signals. Stray currents will tend to "swamp" the low-voltage EEG signal and render the processing algorithms useless. Therefore, backup *clinical* monitoring should be available. For instance, some clinical signs of light anesthesia, such as sweating and forehead furrowing ("frowning"), can be addressed by the telemedicine techniques outlined previously, for example, a high-definition continuous video stream.

CRITICAL CARE: A GROWING ANESTHESIA SUBSPECIALTY

Critical care practice has evolved as a paradigm for successful[3] telemedicine. A deficit of trained critical care specialty providers is nationally recognized. This provider deficit escalates the disparity between rural and urban and between daytime and nighttime critical care services, as well as creates other gaps. The shortage of providers has been addressed successfully in a variety of settings through tele-ICU programs. Such programs have been deployed in large and small health care systems, academic and community hospitals, as well as in general and specialty ICU settings. A hub-and-spoke system most commonly connects a tele-ICU critical care specialist or team with dedicated monitoring and surveillance staffing (a *continuous care model*")[29] to several ICUs staffed with nonspecialists. Staffing by the tele-ICU is provided to either augment (a *responsive or reactive care model*) or replace a critical care specialty presence, for example, using a *scheduled care model*, where the ICU specialist is available for ICU rounds. Tele-ICU services provide direct, immediate, real-time access to a critical care specialist and provide monitoring and early detection of trends and events that may be difficult to monitor due to cognitive, sensory, and task overloading of bedside providers.

‡ Ohio State University, College of Engineering. A better way to open an airway. Available at: https://engineering.osu.edu/news/2015/12/better-way-open-airway. Published December 2, 2015. Accessed on November 26, 2017. The robot uses ultrasound internally and a magnetic target externally on the thyroid cartilage.

§ The SEDASYS® Computer-Assisted Personalized Sedation System was approved by the Food and Drug Administration in 2015 but was withdrawn by the company in the United States due to poor acceptance in the medical community.

In conclusion, all the essential ingredients for teleanesthesia already exist. However, the ingredients need to be combined in a usable and robust configuration. In the meantime, aspects of teleanesthesia such as preoperative evaluation are being implemented[20–22] to test cost and time savings as well as patients' and anesthesiologists' acceptance. Teleanesthesia is eminently available to support other aspects of telemedicine, such as pain therapy and telesurgery. Teleanesthesia will develop hand in hand with, and fulfill the needs of, telesurgery because the patient has to remain motionless for the surgery to proceed expeditiously.

TELESURGERY

The modern era of telesurgery was made possible when endoscopic ("laparoscopic") surgery systems were transformed from analog signals to digitally based ones.

- With early analog devices, the surgeon ("proceduralist") had to view the image through a single eyepiece—only one person at a time could see the image.
- With digital images, the images were displayed on a monitor (or "digital computer screen"). It was an easy further step to duplicate the image on a screen next door, at the local lecture hall for teaching purposes, or with development of the Internet, on a screen anywhere in the world; telementoring became possible.
- With the advent of reliable networks and robotic devices, the distant surgeon could not only advise and tutor but also could actively *participate*; that is, the actions (movements) of the distant surgeon could be faithfully replicated by the robotic device at the patient's side.
- Examples of telerobotic surgery and telesurgery include the following:

- Dr. Rick Satava strongly promoted the concept of telesurgery. In 1994, he enabled remote telementoring for laparoscopic urological surgery.[40] At the Association of the United States Army (AUSA) meeting in Washington, DC, during October 1995, he followed up with another telesurgery project. As a proof of principle, a cholecystectomy was performed in an animal preparation using remote robotic techniques incorporating a fully wired system (solid wire).
- Cheah et al. described the first two international telesurgical, telementored, robot-assisted laparoscopic cholecystectomies performed in the world, between the Johns Hopkins Institute, Baltimore, Maryland, and the National University Hospital, Singapore.[41]
- In an article, "Hands Across the Ocean for World's First Trans-Atlantic Surgery," Kent described Dr. Gagner as the surgeon who performed a cholecystectomy in 2001 from New York City on a patient in Strasbourg, France.[42] Marescaux et al. gave more details about the technology.[43]
- Dr. Tim Broderick, in 2005, performed the first mobile telesurgery (also a cholecystectomy) in the United States. The surgeon was in Ohio, while the patient was in California.[44]

Following the success of the performance of a transatlantic surgery (cholecystectomy), the leader of the team, Jacques Marescaux, said the operation ushered in http://news.bbc.co.uk/2/hi/science/nature/1552211.stm Accessed April 12, 2018[43]

While telesurgery has advanced even past the proof-of-principle stage,[45] there are still several challenges remaining that need to be addressed before telesurgery becomes fully established. One of the surprising limitations is actually the speed of light, which is also the speed of electrons on the Internet. This limitation of the speed of an electrical signal causes a significant delay in the "sense of touch," or haptics, when manipulating a remote object. This will have an influence on remote anesthesia procedures as well, such as placing an intravenous line or remote intubation. Some characteristics of haptics are as follows:

1. Haptics, as generated by a force feedback device, ideally should be rendered at 1-ms intervals (1000 Hz). The average human can readily compensate for a delay of up to 25 ms. Thereafter, it becomes difficult to perform any complex manual task requiring a fine sense of touch. This is in contrast to the eye, which can compensate for delays of up to 125 ms, such as the old 8-mm movies ran at 8–15 frames per second. The movies were a bit jerky, but the eye compensated quite well. Furthermore, the IT infrastructure has a switching overhead, which causes further delays. Anvari and colleagues found that surgeons, with practice, could compensate (albeit with slower performance) for a delay of up to 500 ms, but the error rate increased with greater delays in the feedback speed.[46]
2. Therefore, it is to be expected that surgeries with mainly visual inputs (e.g., with minimal haptic requirements) would be the first operations to be tested and performed (e.g., the cholecystectomy performed from New York to France).[42]
3. Another limitation is financial: The capital investment for the initial setup is quite large. Therefore, telesurgery is expected to be used only where the new technology will save money, thus providing a positive net present value (NPV) at an acceptable return on investment (ROI).
4. Robotics and telesurgery have much in common; in both cases, the operator is working with an image. The operator might be in the same room, might be in the room next door, or might be miles away. In some definitions, "robotic surgery" is equated with "telesurgery"—the operator is removed from the patient (i.e., not touching the patient

but connected to the patient only by IT infrastructure and wires).

Of note is that these haptic characteristics and limitations also apply to manual tasks performed under the rubric of teleanesthesia, such as insertion of intravenous lines and tracheal intubation.

STATE OF THE ART: TECHNOLOGY ASPECTS

Telemedicine is already happening today. In the last several years, the IT industry has improved, and now has well-defined roles of service providers. This enables society to rely more and more on geographically distributed mission-critical applications. Cloud computing has proliferated and become ubiquitous; new data compression protocols make possible transmissions of live audio and video broadcasts; Internet connections are stable, enabling the delivery of reliable services anywhere in the world. Due to the proliferation of high-speed Internet connections close to the point of service, in the office or at home, it is currently possible to have live video conferences across the globe. What is even more remarkable, the Internet penetrated rapidly into third-world countries, making it possible to deliver medical care to any remote location from sites with advanced medical expertise, technology, and available qualified personnel.

Although the required technology is currently available, the telehealth industry is still only at the brink of widespread adoption. We attempt to familiarize the medical practitioner interested in this field with the basic requirements of a telehealth system.

TESTING RELIABILITY OF TELEHEALTH SYSTEMS

What we take for granted in a face-to-face doctor-patient relationship turns out to require a complex set of checks and balances in telemedicine. A telemedicine system must be "robust," with each individual subsystem functioning well. Overall, the system must function properly and should have the ability for self-recovery from exceptional behaviors.

The success of the Internet is mostly based on the fact that regardless of the application, the entire technology that makes the Internet possible is completely transparent and requires no care, input, or even understanding at the user level. The telemedicine practitioners will have to rely on products supported by engineers specializing in testing and maintaining the reliability of several Internet layers. With the help of those experts (e.g., network administrators) and product services like firewalls, antivirus tools, routers, and so on, we have already come to rely on the Internet as a viable and ubiquitous tool. One aspect that still needs to be addressed in special case applications is the nondeterministic nature of Internet infrastructure or the fact that packets of data can travel through different routes before being assembled in the original message. This can add jitter to the communication, an undesirable factor when the application requires predictable and minimal latency, such as in telesurgery.

Yet, as we add telemedicine applications on top of this infrastructure, we need to develop testing equipment and methodologies that will ensure safe usage of the entire system. In this process, there is a need for development of software models to describe the functionality of subsets of the system. Those models will allow the testers to modify parameters that will influence the output of the model, so it behaves as the "real thing." When all the models are combined, the entire system could be tested by varying individual parameters or set points to simulate a desired or undesired behavior for the entire system. Only after those models and subsequent simulators are in place can we develop methodologies for testing the entire system *before* delivering tele-health care to humans.

Depending on the complexity of the telemedicine application, those models, simulators, and testing methodologies will require various complexity levels. The medical practitioners will have to familiarize themselves with the entire system and with methods of testing its functionality.

ETHICAL IMPLICATIONS

An individual rendering medical aid to a needy person is required to stay at the scene until more advanced medical assistance is needed, a rescuer of equal or higher ability takes over, or it is unsafe to continue to give aid. The rules governing those requirements are covered in Good Samaritan laws in countries using an English common law system and duty-to-rescue laws in countries using a civil law system. According to those legal principles, there is a requirement to render medical care until the transfer of responsibility is possible.

In the context of telemedicine, the transfer of responsibility during medical aid is done from the local technician to the remote practitioner, or one remote practitioner to another remote practitioner. Historically, this transfer between caregivers is done routinely and seamlessly. Therefore, not much attention is given to this process. Yet, while providing medical care using telemedicine, technical problems may arise that in turn could create legal implications. Due to Internet infrastructure design, the physical channel may not be available at all times; thus, there are moments during transitions from one channel to another when it is not possible to know if a successful transfer has been made or if the current channel is reliable.

A further point to consider is that the doctor-patient trust relationship is affected. While working with geographically scattered teams during the performance of medical care, using telemedicine technologies, the role of the primary care physician (PCP) is altered. From the patient's perspective, does it need to be an implicit trust from the patient to the "team," or does the trust stay with a single responsible person? Since the physical channel can never be guaranteed to be 100% reliable, should the PCP be at the patient's side? If this is the case, is it then implied that a lesser qualified individual will be in charge during the procedure? Implicit in this question, does the patient need to trust the system? If the patient does need to trust a *technological system*, how could or should this trust be established? While there have been some publications on the ethics of telemedicine,[**] these are questions that will have to be addressed in more depth as telemedicine advances.

BUSINESS MODEL IMPLICATIONS

Any time a new technology is adopted, there is an effect on the way that business is conducted. The penetration of telemedicine technologies in the medical care field is exemplified by tele-ICU. For example, the critical care paradigm has created a new "specialty" of remote critical care providers, has changed the staffing models for ICUs, and has spawned major commercial enterprises and private practices that now comprise standard business practices unheard of 20 years ago. Telemedicine is expected to further affect the current practices and standard operating procedures. The next sections of this chapter are aimed at familiarizing medical practitioners and administrators interested in the value of this field with the basic implications arising from the use of a telehealth system.[47]

MARKET SIZE AND SEGMENTATION

Telemedicine, telesurgery, and teleanesthesia are quite acceptable to most patients as *last resort* options for delivering medical care. For instance, when asked, patients prefer to interact with a human rather than with technology. Yet, if the question is rephrased in terms of an option of last resort, they always say, "Yes, I will accept remote medical care if I have no other options, especially if it is about a life-and-death crisis event." Because of the special situations where telemedicine is a surrogate to face-to-face medical care, an investor who wants to enter this market will want to know how many such systems are needed (market size), what medical situations will require this technology (market segments), where those systems are going to be installed (geographical distribution), and what kind of benefit those systems would bring to the health care industry.

Estimate the Gap Between the Availability of Medical Care in Rural and Metropolitan Areas

The first market segment that comes to mind revolves around geographical distribution of patients and doctors. Although the balance of supply and demand of medical care works in all markets, the high costs related to hospitals create an imperfect geographical distribution of medical centers, with more centers in densely populated areas and fewer in rural areas. The higher the cost of equipment and facilities, the lower the chance that specialized medical care would be available to less populated zones. Telemedicine has the potential of leveling the gap in the availability of medical care between rural areas and metropolitan areas on two dimensions: Distance to state-of-the-art facilities practically vanishes, and the concentration of medical practitioners becomes less acute when using telemedicine techniques. These factors are implicit in Medicare reimbursement policies for telehealth, which continue to require rural geographic criteria.

Although the lower population concentration in rural areas does not justify the capital investment for state-of-the-art facilities and human expertise, due to large numbers of US voters residing in rural areas, there will be continued political pressure to invest in the required IT infrastructure to facilitate telehealth care. This point was confirmed by the legislative language in the ACA legislation regarding telemedicine networks in medically underserved areas to address health care disparities.

Absorb Peak Load During Critical Events

The second market segment that will benefit from telemedicine is related to the capacity of current hospitals and their ability to absorb peak load during critical events. The examples go from accidents involving a large number of people (e.g., train wrecks); to natural disasters (e.g., earthquakes, pandemics, hurricanes, tsunamis); to human-made disasters (e.g., biological disasters from industrial accidents), high-casualty warfare, and limited availability of specialists.

Although not common, such disasters require that current health care facilities have available, at any moment, a certain spare capacity that can absorb the spike in demand for short periods of time. Due to the "golden hour rule," this capacity must be available for triage and first response medical care.

Unfortunately, with the continuous pressure imposed on hospitals to cut costs to survive financially, there is a tendency to reduce the spare capacity to a minimum. The presence of telehealth technologies at the emergency facilities could reduce the need of maintaining a large spare capacity, thus reducing the costs of operation for those hospitals. The legislative language in the ACA legislation awards grants for projects that create telehealth networks to link rural hospitals' health care providers to other hospitals' providers and patients for the health professionals in geographically underserved areas.

Costs for Personnel Overtime Payments

The third market segment that will benefit from the spread of telemedicine is related to the medical facilities that incur high costs for personnel overtime payments. Due to the ability of telemedicine technologies to traverse time zones, there is a new opportunity for health care facilities to balance shift loads and costs by using medical personnel from different time zones in such way that evening and night shifts will be staffed by medical personnel working in daytime shifts. This segment addresses only economic issues, and its outcome is in contradiction with the desire of patients to be treated by a human at the "bedside." We foresee that the pressure from the medical industry will be very strong to overcome the desire of patients. Unless ethical, safety, and legal aspects are opposing it, the practice of outsourcing to different time zones during highly paid shifts (e.g., the pattern of radiology personnel reading x-rays in remote time zones) will continue to expand. The Community Based Collaborative Care Network (CCN) program was authorized by the ACA legislation to provide grants

[**] van Wynsberghe A, Gastmans C. Telesurgery: an ethical appraisal. *J Med Ethics*. 2008;34(10): "Telesurgery will become available to the rest of industrialized society as a treatment option." Available at: http://jme.bmj.com/content/34/10/e22.full. Accessed on November 26, 2017.

to teams of health care providers with joint governance for providing comprehensive and coordinated health care services for low-income populations.

Personnel Cover for Scarce Superspecialization Cases.

The fourth market segment is represented by a lack of superspecialized personnel. Not all hospitals have the patient volume to support the appointment of sufficient personnel to be available around the clock for cases that may occur only occasionally (e.g., neuromonitoring and critical care). Telemedicine incentives to address gaps in specialty services in remote areas and small health care facilities are addressed not only by projecting specialty capabilities, but also by provision of education and training using remote technologies. Legislative intent in the ACA addresses the need for continuing education to reduce professional isolation of health care professionals in underserved communities by enabling the development of infrastructure for collaborative conferences.

MARKET PENETRATION

Like any new technology, telemedicine was initially used by a small group of "early adopters" or "trendsetters" who were motivated by the need to differentiate themselves from the rest of the society, were open to adaptation, were not sensitive to high price costs, and expected high rates of return. Their access to technology infrastructure and application of technical skills validated and built telemedicine into a health care delivery tool with clinical and regulatory standards, as well as commercial successes. Telemedicine has evolved from the domain of early adopters (both individuals and institutions) to the domain of the "early majority." In this accelerating phase of telemedicine technologies, adopters will enjoy a competitive advantage in their medical field, stemming from application of best practices and expertise acquired in early periods, yielding a higher market share. The current early majority are using telemedicine as a solution to current obstacles, such as fragmented legislation, reimbursement, medical coding, licensing, patient acceptance, and so on. The barriers to entry for telemedicine services are diminishing; for example, the *CPT* (*Current Procedural Terminology*) telehealth modifier code GT has been established for telemedicine coding. The medical device industry will attempt to capture a larger share of the market through telemedicine and will establish de facto standards for a variety of required technologies, similar to the digital transition in radiology.

CONCLUSION

The IT support personnel provide services that include around-the-clock ("24/7") support, almost 100% uptime, direct access to the Internet's backbone with consequently very fast communication speeds at higher bandwidth and very good data security. The security includes controlled physical access to the servers, data protection, backups, antivirus software, firewalls, and so on. Delivery of data streams for video and audio channels is a norm, with insignificant transmission lag. We all use web-based conferences with full-duplex ("live" and bidirectional) sound and video images across continents. These technologies and infrastructures are eminently capable of fully supporting telemedicine.

At the time of this writing, Internet "net neutrality" was not definitively clarified. It was established as a principle by the federal administration when the Federal Communications Commission (FCC) published the final rule on its new net neutrality regulations in 2015. As a result, the FCC formalized the concept that online traffic should move freely in an egalitarian fashion. A consequence of this decision is that the general Internet will treat all participants equally, and it will not be able to differentiate and support the very high bandwidth required for telemedicine over regular Internet channels. At the time of this writing, there are ongoing litigations related to violators of net neutrality. Whether net neutrality will survive or not or the debate about constitutional freedom of speech and net neutrality will clarify its future remains to be determined. For this reason, we envision that the businesses providing telemedicine applications will have to lease or own dedicated physical lines to provide the necessary high bandwidth. Early attempts to establish such dedicated networks have already been created by consortiums of business initiatives. In summary, after selecting appropriate technology, telemedicine will be successful if its implementation follows a few important pointers, as discussed in this chapter.

Similar to the general principle of computerizing any process, it is important that telemedicine services be integrated into the way the local organization performs its tasks. It must be easier to perform the tasks with the new technology; otherwise, it will not be accepted. Existing tasks and procedures (scheduling, billing, medical record keeping, preparation for patient encounters, etc.) should be seamlessly integrated into the telemedicine system.

The telemedicine system should not be forced on either the distant site or the local site. Cooperative relationships with providers, administrators, and clinical staff should be developed at both ends.

Highly skilled staff ("technology facilitators") should be immediately available to support the telemedicine infrastructure at both ends. Reliability is absolutely critical—the Internet connection must always be up. Ease of use is critical: There must be a seamless infrastructure. Testing must involve not only clinical testing but also engineering testing of the system and the infrastructure.

In the final instance, physicians and other health care workers adapt well to telehealth technologies that help them do their job more efficiently. From the clinician's point of view, when telehealth is just as easy as providing in-person care, the telemedicine technology will be able to fulfill its great promise.

TELEMEDICINE IN THE AFFORDABLE CARE ACT

Historically, the US health care system was driven by the pressure to provide the best and the newest medical care in the quest to cure and extend life expectancy. In microeconomic terms, this can be characterized as a supply-driven health care system. Because the cost of health care is covered by a third party (the insurer) rather than the patient, the regular supply-and-demand equilibrium is not achieved. This puts an upward pressure on the entire medical system's cost.

If other market forces (financial, political, demographics, ethical, etc.) are going to be used to shift the balance to an equilibrium, then factors such as direct costs, quality of life, distribution of costs per demographic and social groups, society's life expectancy and productivity, and so on will have to be taken into account.

In 2010, ACA legislation intended to transform the US health care system by adding to the mix another factor: access to health care. This is a demand-driven health care approach assuming that increasing the pool of insured people will be enough to balance the microeconomical supply-and-demand equation.

The sociopolitical pressure was not taken into consideration, and as a result, it is possible that it will change. Given the complexity of the health care problem and the large number of people who gained access to health care starting in 2014, it is unlikely that the ACA legislation will be repealed entirely and replaced with a totally new legislation. We foresee that the legislation will be amended over a prolonged period of time, and some aspects of its current form will remain in place, including the provisions relating to telemedicine.

The solution is not easy to find and will have to take into account the social costs of providing health care as well as other social pressures, such as demographic shifts and society's acceptance of limits of quality of care. At any rate, the advantages offered by telemedicine are so significant in the larger picture that it is unlikely this technological aspect of ACA legislation will be eliminated.

At the same time, since the ACA legislation was enacted, progress has been made at the state legislation level to an extent that ensures telemedicine is here to stay. Telemedicine's impact on health care will be seen in the integrative health care delivery across separate facilities and the expansion of quality services across geography.

REIMBURSEMENT

The ACA legislation opened the possibility for reimbursement for practitioners engaging in the delivery of medical care using a telemedicine infrastructure, by allowing agencies that provide off-site interpretation to directly bill Medicare for the services provided and by including the use of telehealth in defining a face-to-face encounter with a patient. Since then, telehealth reimbursement has made progress, with 49 states and the District of Columbia allowing reimbursement for telehealth in their public programs.

ENCOURAGE PARTICIPATION

To encourage the cooperation of providers, the ACA law created a Shared Savings Program that promotes accountability and encourages investment in infrastructure and redesigned care processes for high-quality and efficient service delivery. Under this program, groups of providers of services and suppliers may work together to manage and coordinate care for Medicare fee-for-service beneficiaries through an accountable care organization (ACO[††]) and will be eligible to receive payments for shared savings.

CONTINUING EDUCATION

In its bill, the ACA law created a program to support the continuing education needs for health professionals in underserved communities by making available grants to improve health care, increase retention, increase representation of minority faculty members, enhance the practice environment, and provide information dissemination and educational support to reduce professional isolation through the timely dissemination of research findings using relevant resources through distance learning, continuing educational activities, collaborative conferences, and electronic and telelearning activities.

FUTURE CHANGES IN THE PRACTICE OF ANESTHESIOLOGY

The acceptance of telecommunication technologies as a vehicle to link health professionals and patients at separate geographical sites for the purpose of providing health care services is going to change the playing field for all health care providers.

Anesthesiology as a medical specialty also will be affected. The introduction of telemedicine technologies, combined with the possibility of obtaining reimbursement for services rendered to patients outside of the hospital settings, will increase the "size of the pie" for anesthesia personnel. In some areas, anesthesiologists are ready to start providing telehealth right now without the need for big changes, yet in other areas, such as using teleanesthesia to assist telesurgery, it will take more time to develop reliable technologies, business procedures, and practices that will enable such interventions.

The current legislative efforts for health care reform are driven to a large extent by rapidly escalating costs, which are to a large degree the result of an aging population and increased chronic disease management costs. Furthermore, in the minds of the legislators, chronic disease is a focus area because of its immense social and economic effect and will be increasingly targeted for funding. We see this as an easy-to-penetrate field where anesthesiologists can expand rapidly by providing pain management, anesthesia, analgesia, and sedation through telemedicine infrastructures. In the near future, anesthesiologists will be involved in prescribing home health pain control services and durable medical equipment, such as remotely operated infusion pumps. This will increase the opportunities for anesthesiologists to participate in care of patients in geographically remote and rural locations by supervising the delivery of drugs and conducting required medication reviews without the need for an expensive office visit. The promotion of telenursing initiatives in health care reform legislation could provide opportunities for physician extenders, such as advanced practice nurses and certified registered

[††] "The ACO shall define processes to promote evidence-based medicine and patient engagement, report on quality and cost measures, and coordinate care, such as through the use of telehealth, remote patient monitoring, and other such enabling technologies." http://uscode.house.gov/view.xhtml?req=(title:42%20 section:1395jjj%20edition:prelim). Accessed April 12, 2018.

nurse anesthetists (CRNAs), to support physician outreach through telemedicine. This will have immediate application in perioperative areas such as pre- and postoperative evaluations and other areas, such as chronic pain management and medication reconciliation.

The ACA legislation provides the required legal framework and opens up the possibilities for funding pilot programs that will fulfill the great promise of telemedicine and teleanesthesia. It is up to hospital managers, department chairs, and anesthesiologists to seize the moment and develop new health care models, procedures, and technologies. Teleanesthesia is an area where many successful careers will be made, and we are looking forward in the next few years to see an explosion of academic articles in this field.

REFERENCES

1. Sood S, Mbarika V, Jugoo S, et al. What is telemedicine? A collection of 104 peer-reviewed perspectives and theoretical underpinnings. *Telemed J E Health.* 2007;13(5):573–590.
2. Seibert PS, Reddy T, Whitmore T, Valerio J, DeHaas CJ. The use of telemedicine to train perioperative nurses in rural settings. *Telemed Telecare.* 2013;19(6):311–314.
3. Totten AM, Womack DM, Eden KB, et al. *Telehealth: Mapping the Evidence for Patient Outcomes From Systematic Reviews.* Rockville, MD: Agency for Healthcare Research and Quality (US); June 2016. Technical Briefs, No. 26. Available at: https://www.ncbi.nlm.nih.gov/books/NBK379320/
4. Nannings B, Abu-Hanna A. Decision support telemedicine systems: a conceptual model and reusable templates. *Telemed J E Health.* 2006;12(6):644–654.
5. Holdorf JD, Lilly CM. Intensivist staffing: evolving challenges and solutions. *Semin Respir Crit Care Med.* 2015;36(6):842–850.
6. Hawkins HA, Lilly CM, Kaster DA, Groves RH, Khurana H. ICU telemedicine comanagement methods and length of stay. *Chest.* 2016;150(2):314–319.
7. Mackintosh N, Terblanche M, Maharaj R, et al. Telemedicine with clinical decision support for critical care: a systematic review. *Syst Rev.* 2016;18;5(1):176. Published online 2016 Oct 18. doi:10.1186/s13643-016-0357-7.
8. Jarvis-Selinger S, Chan E, Payne R, Plohman K, Ho K. Clinical telehealth across the disciplines: lessons learned. *Telemed J E Health.* 2008;14(7):720–725.
9. Ekeland AG, Bowes A, Flottorp S. Effectiveness of telemedicine: a systematic review of reviews. *Int J Med Inform.* 2010;79(11):736–771.
10. Marcoux RM, Vogenberg FR. Telehealth: applications from a legal and regulatory perspective. *P T.* 2016;41(9):567–570.
11. Broens TH, Huis in't Veld RM, Vollenbroek-Hutten MM, Hermens HJ, van Halteren AT, Nieuwenhuis LJ. Determinants of successful telemedicine implementations: a literature study. *J Telemed Telecare.* 2007;13(6):303–309.
12. Becker C, Frishman WH, Scurlock C. Telemedicine and tele-ICU: the evolution and differentiation of a new medical field. *Am J Med.* 2016;27;pii:S0002-9343(16)30839-7. doi:10.1016/j.amjmed.2016.05.045.
13. Yoo BK, Kim M, Sasaki T, Melnikow J, Marcin JP. Economic evaluation of telemedicine for patients in ICUs. *Crit Care Med.* 2016;44(2):265–274.
14. Weinstein RS, Lopez AM, Krupinski EA, et al. Integrating telemedicine and telehealth: putting it all together. *Stud Health Technol Inform.* 2008;131:23–38.
15. Obstfelder A, Engeseth KH, Wynn R. Characteristics of successfully implemented telemedical applications. *Implement Sci.* 2007;2:25.
16. Brebner JA, Brebner EM, Ruddick-Bracken H. Experience-based guidelines for the implementation of telemedicine services. *J Telemed Telecare.* 2005;11(suppl 1):3–5.
17. Ward R, Stevens C, Brentnall P, Briddon J. The attitudes of health care staff to information technology: a comprehensive review of the research literature. *Health Info Libr J.* 2008;25(2):81–97.
18. Yarbrough AK, Smith TB. Technology acceptance among physicians: a new take on TAM. *Med Care Res Rev.* 2007;64(6):650–672.
19. Collins TA, Robertson MP, Sicoutris CP, et al. Telemedicine coverage for post-operative ICU patients. *J Telemed Telecare.* 2017;23:360–364. [Epub ahead of print 2016 Jun 30] PMID: 27365321.
20. Boedeker BH, Murray WB, Berg BW. Real-time pre-operative anesthesia at a distance. *J Telemed Telecare.* 2007;13(suppl 3):22–24.
21. Zetterman CV, Sweitzer BJ, Webb B, Barak-Bernhagen MA, Boedeker BH. Validation of a virtual preoperative evaluation clinic: a pilot study. *Stud Health Technol Inform.* 2011;163:737–739.
22. Turabi A, Nessen SC, Boedeker D, Boedeker B. Development of a teleanesthesia preoperative clinic to support distant military treatment facilities for the European regional medical command. *Stud Health Technol Inform.* 2014;196:433–435.
23. Murray WB, Vaduva S. Telemedicine, telesurgery and teleanesthesia. In: Russell GB, ed. *Alternate-Site Anesthesia—Clinical Practice Outside the Operating Room.* Stoneham, MA: Butterworth-Heinemann; 1997:441–450.
24. Sloan IA. An improved tele-thermometer. *Can Anaesth Soc J.* 1967;14(1):62–63.
25. Cone SW, Gehr L, Hummel R, Merrell RC. Remote anesthetic monitoring using satellite telecommunications and the Internet. *Anesth Analg.* 2006;102(5):1463–1467.
26. Berg BW, Vincent DS, Hudson DA. Remote critical care consultation: telehealth projection of clinical specialty expertise. *J Telemed Telecare.* 2003;9(suppl 2):S9–S11.
27. Cummings J, Krsek C, Vermoch K, Matuszewski K. Intensive care unit telemedicine: review and consensus recommendations. *Am J Med Qual.* 2007;22(4):239–250.
28. Thomas EJ, Lucke JF, Wueste L, Weavind L, Patel B. Association of telemedicine for remote monitoring of intensive care patients with mortality, complications, and length of stay. *JAMA.* 2009;302(24):2671–2678.
29. Davis TM, Barden C, Dean S, et al. American Telemedicine Association guidelines for teleICU operations. *Telemed J E Health.* 2016;22(12):971–980.
30. Kleinpell R, Barden C, Rincon T, McCarthy M, Zapatochny Rufo RJ. Assessing the impact of telemedicine on nursing care in intensive care units. *Am J Crit Care.* 2016;25(1):e14–e20.
31. Kahn JM, Cicero BD, Wallace DJ, Iwashyna TJ. Adoption of ICU telemedicine in the United States. *Crit Care Med.* 2014;42(2):362–368.
32. Kohl BA, Gutsche JT, Kim P, Sites FD, Ochroch EA. Effect of telemedicine on mortality and length of stay in a university ICU. *Crit Care Med.* 2007;35(12)(suppl):A22.
33. Kahn JM, Le TQ, Barnato AE, et al. ICU telemedicine and critical care mortality: a national effectiveness study. *Med Care.* 2016;54(3):319–325.
34. Magalang UJ, Arnardottir ES, Chen NH, et al.; S AGIC Investigators. Agreement in the scoring of respiratory events among international sleep centers for home sleep testing. *J Clin Sleep Med.* 2016;12(1):71–77.
35. Hemmerling TM, Taddei R, Wehbe M, Zaouter C, Cyr S, Morse J. First robotic tracheal intubations in humans using the Kepler intubation system. *Br J Anaesth.* 2012;108(6):1011–1016.
36. Hemmerling TM, Arbeid E, Wehbe M, Cyr S, Giunta F, Zaouter C. Transcontinental anaesthesia: a pilot study. *Br J Anaesth.* 2013;110(5):758–763.
37. Rosero E, Joshi GP. Total intravenous anesthesia: present and future. *ASA Monitor.* 2015;79:10–57.
38. Liu N, Chazot T, Hamada S, et al. Closed-loop coadministration of propofol and remifentanil guided by bispectral index: a randomized multicenter study. *Anesth Analg.* 2011;112(3):546–557.
39. Murray WB, Foster PA The peripheral pulse wave: information overlooked. *J Clin Mon.* 1996;12:365–377.
40. Kavoussi LR, Moore RG, Partin AW, Bender JS, Zenilman ME, Satava RM. Telerobotic assisted laparoscopic surgery: initial laboratory and clinical experience. *Urology.* 1994;44(1):15–19.
41. Cheah WK, Lee B, Lenzi JE, Goh PM. Telesurgical laparoscopic cholecystectomy between two countries. *Surg Endosc.* 2000;14(11):1085.
42. Kent H. Hands across the ocean for world's first trans-Atlantic surgery. *CMAJ.* 2001;165(10):1374.
43. Marescaux J, Leroy J, Rubino F, et al. Links transcontinental robot-assisted remote telesurgery: feasibility and potential applications. *Ann Surg.* 2002;235(4):487–492.
44. Lum MJ, Rosen J, King H, et al. Telesurgery via unmanned aerial vehicle (UAV) with a field deployable surgical robot. *Stud Health Technol Inform.* 2007;125:313–315.
45. Anvari M. Remote telepresence surgery: the Canadian experience. *Surg Endosc.* 2007;21(4):537–541.
46. Anvari M, Broderick T, Stein H, et al. The impact of latency on surgical precision and task completion during robotic-assisted remote telepresence surgery. *Comput Aided Surg.* 2005;10(2):93–99.
47. Cusack CM, Pan E, Hook JM, Vincent A, Kaelber DC, Middleton B. The value proposition in the widespread use of telehealth. *J Telemed Telecare.* 2008;14(4):167–168.

34 | ANESTHESIA CONSIDERATIONS IN DENTAL PRACTICE

JANICE A. TOWNSEND, DDS, MS, GABRIEL HERNANDEZ, DDS, LYNDA HARHAD, DDS

INTRODUCTION

The demand for anesthesia providers to deliver sedation and general anesthesia services for dental procedures in nontraditional settings is on the rise.[1,2] This increase may be due to the following:

1. Increased rates of dental disease in young children
2. Rising financial burden of hospitalization with changing insurance landscape
3. Focus on maintaining dentition with complex dental procedures
4. Increasing expectation of anesthesia for dental care
5. Greater scheduling convenience

As a member of the dental care delivery team, one must be aware that a significant portion of the dental population exhibits some level of dental phobia. This inherent level of fear associated with dental treatment does not appear to manifest in other medical procedures that require a similar level of sedation, such as colonoscopy, cosmetic procedures, or other surgical procedures.

Studies showed that approximately 15% of the US population fears the dentist enough to avoid care completely. Among those patients who regularly seek care, as many as 50% report some level of fear and anxiety toward their dental experience and view many of the routine dental procedures in a dental office as frightening.[3,4]

Anesthesia for dental procedures poses unique challenges; this chapter will educate providers on the practice of dentistry and its implications.

LOCAL ANESTHESIA IN DENTISTRY

Local anesthesia is the foundation for the successful delivery of comfortable dentistry. Minimal, moderate, and deep sedation cannot be performed without adequate local anesthesia. The use of profound local anesthesia can assist in preventing any complications secondary to exacerbation of an underlying medical condition that can manifest as a result of pain, such as angina or syncope.

The use of local anesthesia is not required for general anesthesia, but, as with other regional anesthetic techniques, there are advantages. When local anesthesia is used in conjunction with general anesthesia for pediatric dentistry rehabilitations, patients have statistically significant differences in end-tidal carbon dioxide and heart rate when compared to those without, and patients with local anesthesia have fewer interventions by the anesthesiologist.[5] Dentist anesthesiologists also believe it decreases the depth of general anesthesia and avoids activation of deep pain pathways.[6] The impact of local anesthesia in conjunction with general anesthesia on children is more unpredictable than with adults because children and patients with special health care needs may become agitated on awakening with the altered sensation associated with local anesthesia, and this may affect their recovery.[7] A recent meta-analysis concluded that there is no clear benefit to the use of local anesthesia with general anesthesia for children and adolescents.[8]

Contemporary dentistry utilizes a number of local anesthetics, as shown in Table 34.1. Use of a vasoconstrictor is typically indicated to prolong the effects of the anesthetic and prevent systemic redistribution. However, vasoconstrictor should be limited to 0.4 mg in patients with significant cardiovascular impairments, and it should be used with caution in patients taking nonselective β-adrenoreceptor blockers, tricyclic antidepressants, cocaine, and α-adrenergic blockers.[9] Lidocaine and articaine with vasoconstrictor are primarily used for routine restorative and simple surgical procedures. Bupivacaine is useful to provide lasting pain control for patients undergoing significant invasive surgical procedures. Local anesthetics that have minimal vasodilation, such as mepivacaine, are effective without vasoconstrictor and are indicated for patients with significant cardiovascular impairments or an allergy to preservatives used with epinephrine, such as bisulfites.[10]

For children, it is imperative that the maximum recommended dosage of local anesthetic is not is not exceeded. Local anesthetics and sedative agents both depress the central nervous system, and the dose of local anesthesia should be adjusted downward when sedating children with opioids.[11] Adverse outcomes in a recent review of pediatric dental anesthesia and sedation in children are associated with overdose of the local anesthetic 41% of the time.[12]

TABLE 34.1. Common Local Anesthetics Used in Dentistry

AGENT	MAXIUMUM RECOMMENDED DOSAGE (MRD)	DURATION	
		PULPAL ANESTHESIA (MIN)	SOFT TISSUE ANESTHESIA (MIN)
2% Lidocaine with 1:100,000 epinephrine	7 mg/kg, not to exceed 500 mg	60	180–300
4% Articaine with 1:100,000 epinephrine	7 mg/kg, not to exceed 500 mg	60–75	180–360
0.5% Bupivacaine with 1:200,000 epinephrine	1.3 mg/kg, not to exceed 90 mg	>90	240–720
3% Mepivacaine	6.6 mg/kg, not to exceed 400 mg	20 (infiltration) to 40 (nerve block)	120–180
4% Prilocaine	6 mg/kg, not to exceed 400	10–15 (infiltration) 40–60 (nerve block)	90–120 (infiltration) 120–240 (nerve block)

SOURCE: Malamed SF. Clinical action of specific agents. In: *Handbook of Local Anesthesia*. 5th ed. St. Louis, MO: Elsevier Mosby; 2004:55–84.

The maxillary and mandibular divisions (V_2 and V_3, respectively) of the fifth craniofacial nerve or trigeminal nerve provide innervation to the orofacial complex. Local anesthesia is typically administered via infiltration (superperiosteal injections) or nerve block injections. Infiltration is when local anesthetic is delivered near the apices of the teeth and diffuses through cortical bone. It is most effective for pulpal anesthesia of the maxillary teeth and surrounding periodontium (bone and gingiva). Infiltration is less effective for mandibular teeth due to the dense cortical bone. Typically, infiltration has a quick onset and is only adequate for one to two teeth. If local anesthesia is required for multiple teeth or for mandibular molars, block injections are preferred.

Block anesthesia requires the placement of local anesthetic adjacent to nerve trunks and anesthetizes all teeth innervated as shown in Table 34.2. The mandibular inferior alveolar nerve block is the most commonly used block technique in dentistry. This nerve block will provide pulpal anesthesia to all of the teeth in the quadrant. This injection is commonly administered with a lingual nerve block, which provides anesthesia to the anterior two-thirds of the tongue, the floor of the mouth, and the lingual mucous membrane as shown in Figure 34.1 The duration of pulpal anesthesia after nerve blocks is longer than the duration for infiltration.

TABLE 34.2. Innervation of the Teeth

TEETH INNERVATION	NERVE
Maxillary incisors	Anterior superior alveolar (ASA)
Maxillary canines	Anterior superior alveolar
Maxillary premolars	Middle superior alveolar (may have some innervation from ASA and PSA)
Maxillary molars	Posterior superior alveolar (PSA)
Mandibular molars	Inferior alveolar nerve
Mandibular first premolar	Inferior alveolar nerve, mental branch
Mandibular incisors	Inferior alveolar nerve, incisal branch

Because major nerve trunks are often adjacent to vasculature, it is essential that aspiration is used before injection. An aspirating syringe and aspiration are recommended for all dental anesthesia delivery to avoid inadvertent intravascular injections. A detailed description of all dental blocks is beyond the scope of this chapter, but are provided in other dental texts. Accessory injections such as intraligamentary (periodontal ligament) injections, intraosseus injections, and intrapulpal injections are also sometimes indicated.

DENTAL ANXIETY

The presence of dental anxiety among patients can range tremendously, from low to severe, and that anxiety in combination with the pain associated with the patient's dental pathology or perceived pain with its treatment can influence the level of sedation required to have a successful treatment outcome. For those patients with moderate-to-severe dental phobia, the use of nitrous oxide, enteral oral sedation, parenteral intravenous (IV) sedation, and general anesthesia in a dental office have been proven to be several of the most effective ways to successfully treat these patients.

Reduction of anxiety or iatrosedation is fundamental for delivery of dental care. This includes the utilization of verbal and nonverbal communication between the provider and patient to develop a level of comfort that would allow trust and treatment acceptance. The goal is to establish trust and rapport between the clinician and patient, which may take multiple visits and include desensitization. If a patient is still unable to cope with treatment, then sedation should be strongly considered.

PATIENT ASSESSMENT

Regardless of the level of sedation, one of the most critical aspects of preparing a patient for sedation dentistry

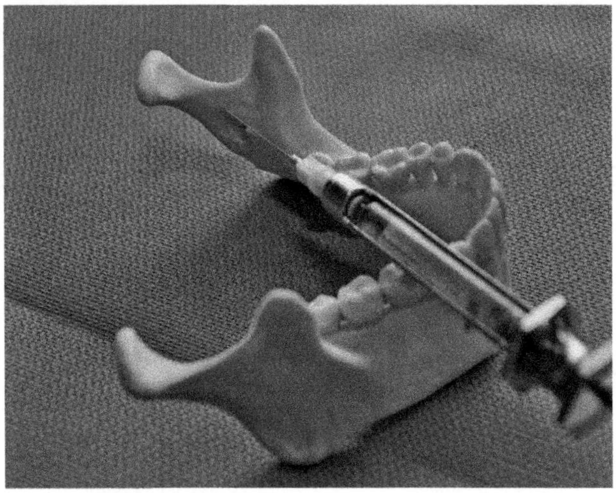

Figure 34.1 Mandibular nerve block.

is to perform a comprehensive physical and psychological assessment to ensure the patient is able to tolerate the dental procedure and the level of sedation being performed. This assessment should be performed by the dentist or anesthesia provider and should consist of the following:

1. Medical history assessment: A thorough medical history, including familial history of surgery complications, should be obtained, and an American Society of Anesthesiologists (ASA) classification system designation should be assigned.[13] It is generally accepted by most clinicians that patients with an ASA 4 classification or above should not be treated in an outpatient dental setting. Appropriateness of ASA 2 and 3 patients may require additional medical information or consultation from a physician prior to performing any level of sedation. Patients who may require postoperative interventions, such as patients with bleeding disorders or sickle cell disease, may best be treated in a hospital setting. Premature children delivered earlier than 37 weeks should be critically assessed due to the increased risk of bronchopulmonary dysplasia and chronic lung disease of prematurity.[14] Patients with a family history of malignant hyperthermia should not receive general anesthesia in the office and should be referred to a hospital.
2. Psychological assessment: The dentists may choose to use an established dental anxiety questionnaire, such as the Corah Anxiety Scale,[15] or to ask a few questions to determine the patient's attitude toward dentistry. Extremely fearful patients should be classified as an ASA 2. Patients with a history of psychiatric disorder may be taking medications that interact with sedation drugs, which should be carefully evaluated.[16] If the use of sedation medications in this phobic population is expected to provoke an adverse paradoxical effect, general anesthesia is indicated.
3. Physical examination: An overall physical examination should be performed, including gathering of height, weight, and vital signs. Obese patients are more prone to sedation complications due to restriction of ventilation, reduced functional residual capacity and expiratory reserve volume, and reduced chest compliance and are more prone to cardiovascular complications.[17] Pediatric patients with a high body mass index (BMI) have been shown to have more adverse sedation events and may be more appropriately treated in a hospital setting.[18]
4. Focused airway examination: A thorough airway assessment, including a Mallampati exam and Brodsky classification, should be performed. Patients with a Mallampati score of 3 or higher are at a high risk for obstruction and other complications in a dental office and should be treated in a hospital setting. Children with enlarged tonsils are at high risk of airway obstruction during sedation.[19] Patients should be screened for obstructive sleep apnea and use of the STOP-Bang questionnaire (**s**noring, daytime **t**iredness, **o**bserved apnea, and high blood **p**ressure, **B**MI, **a**ge > 50 years, **n**eck circumference > 40 cm, and male **g**ender) has been suggested as a screening tool.[20] These patients may not be suitable for sedation or general anesthesia in the dental office. After a comprehensive assessment, the dentist or anesthesia provider can then proceed with the sedation plan.[21] Patients with congenital or acquired pathological conditions of the airway, such as craniofacial anomalies, are poor candidates for office-based anesthesia.

OFFICE PREPAREDNESS

Before sedation or general anesthesia can be administered in a dental office setting, the design must incorporate essential safety equipment and features. At least two oxygen tanks are needed; they should have an audible or visible low-oxygen warning and should be easily accessible by office staff.[22] Operatories must be of sufficient size to accommodate the dentist and anesthesia team, and doorways should be wide enough to allow for passage of wheeled equipment (36 inches).[22] The office should have emergency electricity and backup suction capabilities. A bag-valve-mask (BVM) should be readily available for ventilation in the event of a ventilator failure. Monitoring equipment should comply with regulations and minimally include blood pressure monitor, pulse oximeter, and capnography.[23] Rescue equipment should be available and include airway management equipment and resuscitation drugs.[23] All equipment should be monitored by appropriate specialists every 6 months. If potential triggers of malignant hyperthermia are used, then dantrolene must be immediately available.[24]

Adequate space must be allocated for the pre- and postsedation periods. The recovery area should have access to suction and oxygen.[23] Appropriate personnel trained in adult and/or pediatric advanced life support should be available during the sedation.

NITROUS OXIDE USE IN DENTISTRY

Of all the inhalation anesthetic agents available to produce sedation, nitrous oxide (N_2O) is by far the most commonly used for both medical and dental procedures. The anesthesiologist will likely not use nitrous oxide alone for dental procedures, but it is often combined with sedation regimens for a synergistic effect, so its use in dentistry should be understood. In most states, the dentist and the office require permits for nitrous oxide. It has both anxiolytic and analgesic properties, and it is the safest inhalation anesthetic used today, with a mean alveolar concentration of 105%. This implies it is impossible for N_2O, in even the highest dose, to produce general anesthesia. Nitrous oxide has low solubility in blood, which helps cause a rapid onset of action and, conversely, rapid elimination. The anxiolytic effect involves activation of the γ-aminobutyric acid type A receptor either directly or indirectly through benzodiazepine binding.[25]

Nitrous oxide sedation is indicated for fearful or anxious patients, for patients with a severe gag reflex, when profound local anesthesia cannot be obtained, and for lengthy dental procedures.[26] Patients must breathe through the nitrous hood, and cooperation is necessary. Nitrous oxide sedation is contraindicated in patients with some chronic obstructive pulmonary diseases, severe emotional disturbances or drug-related dependencies, first trimester of pregnancy, receiving treatment with bleomycin sulfate, methylenetetrahydrofolate reductase deficiency, and cobalamin deficiency. Other conditions may require consultation, such as congestive heart failure, sickle cell disease, acute otitis media, recent tympanic membrane graft, and acute severe head injury.[26]

Nitrous oxide sedation can be administered in the dental office via central and portable delivery systems as shown in Figure 34.2. Modern delivery system equipment with an adjustable flowmeter will not allow nitrous oxide administration at more than 70%, ensuring that the patient receives a minimum of 30% oxygen, more than what is in ambient air. This fail-safe system must be checked and calibrated regularly according to regulations.

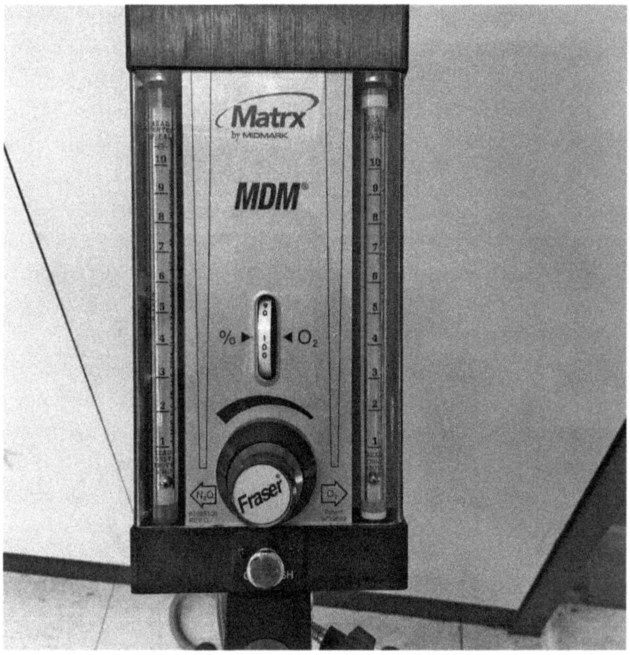

Figure 34.2 Nitrous oxide unit.

Titration technique, as described in the discussion that follows, is the preferred delivery mechanism of nitrous oxide administration for adults in the dental office. The hood is placed over the nose, and the patient is advised to breathe through the mouth and limit talking. Initially, 100% oxygen is delivered, and the flow rate is adjusted to a level where inflation and deflation of the nitrous bag is visible, which is typically 6 L/min in an adult. Nitrous is started at a 10% concentration and titrated in 10% increments each minute until signs of relaxation occur. Typically, nitrous oxide levels exceeding 50% are not used, although studies have shown that nasopharyngeal concentrations in children are 50% lower than the flowmeter settings.[27] In pediatric dentistry, rapid induction at levels of 40%–50% is preferred.

Once signs of relaxation are visible, local anesthesia can be administered. Dentists may choose to reduce nitrous oxide following the completion of demanding or potentially painful parts of the procedure, but frequent fluctuations in concentration should be avoided to prevent nausea. Administration of 100% oxygen for 5 minutes following cessation of nitrous oxide is essential to prevent diffusion hypoxia, which results from the rapid elimination of nitrous oxide from the lungs. Following a return to preoperative state, the patient may be dismissed.

The most common side effects from nitrous oxide are nausea and vomiting, and the incidence is increased when high concentration, long administration, and fluctuations in concentrations are used. One study in children found the incidence in vomiting is 0.5%, and there is no difference in fasting or nonfasting subjects.[28] Use of nitrous oxide in an open system in the dental setting puts office personnel at a high risk of adverse events related to chronic exposure. Scavenger systems limit the environmental exposure to the dentist and staff by venting the gases in the nasal hood outdoors.[27] Nitrous oxide use for the treatment of dental anxiety offers many benefits to the patient and dentist, including safety, quick onset of action and recovery, ease of use, effectiveness, wide acceptance by patients, and very few side effects.

MONITORED ANESTHESIA CARE IN DENTISTRY

Anesthesia staff may be part of the monitored anesthesia care (MAC) team in dentistry. Typically, these procedures will be performed under parenteral sedation, although some offices employ anesthesia staff to monitor enteral sedation cases. Varying levels of licensure or certification may be required, and typically both the office and anesthesia providers need permits.

Patients are assessed to determine if they are an adequate candidate as previously discussed, and the level of sedation indicated is determined. Patients follow the same fasting guidelines as for general anesthesia. At least one responsible adult should accompany the patient to the procedure, and two adults are encouraged to accompany children so that one adult can sit in the back of the car on the ride home and maintain the airway.[23] Patients are encouraged to dress in loose and comfortable clothing and refrain from using fingernail polish. On the day of the sedation appointment, the patient is evaluated to ensure he or she is still a candidate, and the appointment should be canceled if there are any signs of illness.

The determination of drugs to be utilized is based on the medical history of the patient, type of dental treatment required, and length of procedure. Benzodiazepines are usually indicated due to their safety profile and relative lack of side effects. Due to their hypnotic and anterograde amnesic properties, midazolam and diazepam are the two benzodiazepines most frequently used in sedation dentistry for the management of anxiety. They also have muscle-relaxant and anticonvulsant properties that may prove beneficial to patients with seizure disorders.

Opioids are mainly administered for their analgesic properties, which can serve as an adjunct to local anesthesia for painful procedures such as complicated dental extractions. Two of the most frequently utilized opioids in dental sedations are fentanyl and meperidine. Simultaneous use of benzodiazepines and opioids not only enhances the level of sedation but also may lead to respiratory depression. Reversal agents such as naloxone for opioids and flumazenil for benzodiazepines should be available in case of emergency. Typically, the narcotic is reversed first in cases of respiratory depression, followed by the benzodiazepine.

Antihistamines such as hydroxyzine have anxiolytic properties and act synergistically with other sedation medications. Additionally, they have antihistaminic and antinausea properties. They can be especially helpful in combination with narcotics to offset the histamine release and nausea-inducing side effects. The use of promethazine, which has antihistaminic effects, is becoming less popular in sedation dentistry.

During the appointment, patients are monitored with observation, continuous pulse oximetry, precordial stethoscope, and periodic blood pressure readings.[23] Capnography is becoming the standard of care and should be utilized.[23] There is an increased incidence of false-positive readings in the open airway environment, but this is outweighed by the benefits of early detection of hypoxic events. Profound local anesthesia is essential for successful MAC care. During dental procedures, dust and water in the airway should be minimized with aggressive suction and use of a rubber dam as shown in Figure 34.3. The dentistry should be performed efficiently to minimize the amount of time under anesthesia. If a rubber dam is not permitted, an unfolded 4 × 4 gauze should be used to protect the airway from aspiration. The anesthesia staff should be vigilant for any downward force on the mandible while treating the mandibular teeth as this can compromise the airway. Most obstructions can be managed by repositioning the patient with a chin lift maneuver.

Following sedation, patients should be monitored by qualified personnel until they return to their presedation physiological state and vital signs. The patient may recover in a separate recovery area or in the treatment operatory. If the operatory is the site of recovery, then this should be taken into account during scheduling as some patients have prolonged recovery. Patients should be discharged with written and oral postoperative instructions into the care of a responsible adult.

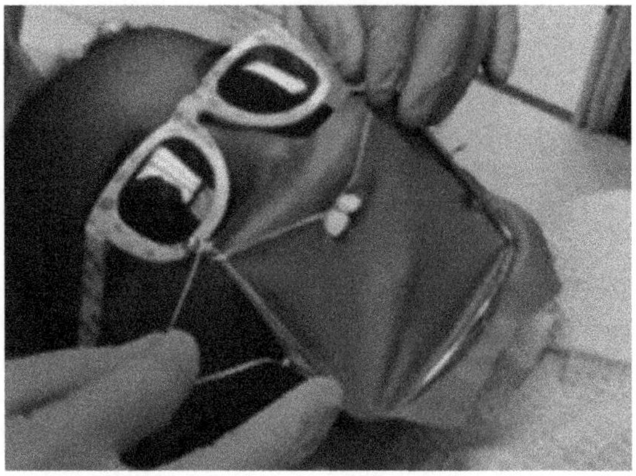

Figure 34.3 Rubber dam.

Enteral sedation may be administered via the oral, sublingual, or rectal routes, but the oral route is most commonly used due to its high acceptance rate among patients. Medications may be dispensed from the office in accordance with Drug Enforcement Administration regulations, or they may be prescribed for the patient to obtain at a pharmacy.

Oral sedation modalities typically range from anxiolysis to moderate sedation.[29] Sedation medication is administered, and there is usually a period of latency for the medications to take effect, which varies for different medications. Placing the patient in a quiet room with dimmed lights that allows for monitoring may encourage a calm state. Titration of oral medications is not recommended, but nitrous oxide may be used concomitantly and titrated to the desired sedation level.

The primary advantage of oral sedation is ease of administration; however, the disadvantage is unpredictable efficacy due to the first-pass effect. In addition, the patient must cooperate with swallowing the medication for effectiveness. If a young child is not expected to cooperate with medication administration, the medication may be slowly syringed into the buccal mucosa while the parent is holding the patient in a knee-to-knee position with the dentist as shown in Figure 34.4. If the child patient spits out the medication, it should not be readministered because it is impossible to determine how much was swallowed.

Typical medications used alone in oral sedation are benzodiazepines such as midazolam or antihistamines such as hydroxyzine. Narcotics are typically administered with an antihistamine to reduce nausea. Antihistamines can be administered with benzodiazepines or narcotics to produce an optimal depth of sedation and working time.

Intravenous sedation is the route of choice for deep and moderate sedation in adults or deep sedation in children. Intravenous sedation is indicated for stressful procedures such as difficult extractions, medically compromised patients, uncooperative patients, patients with a strong gag reflex, those

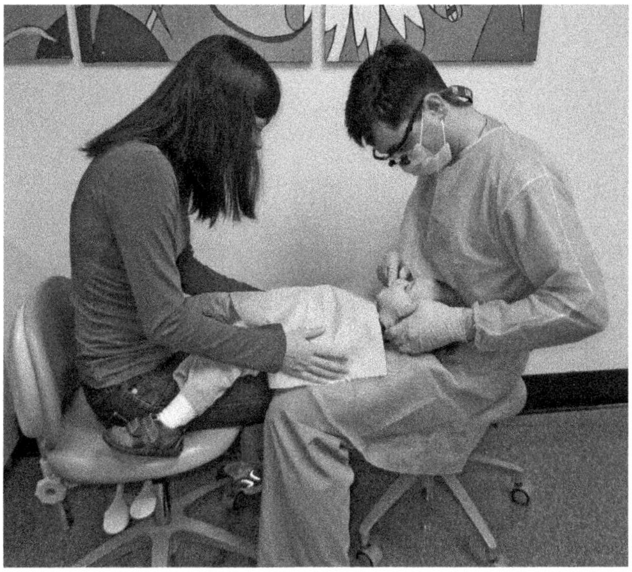

Figure 34.4 Administration of oral medications to a young child in the knee-to-knee position.

who have difficulty achieving proper local anesthesia, or patients with moderate-to-severe anxiety. Advantages of intravenous sedation are rapid onset, ability to titrate the medication quickly, and the effect of a long period of amnesia.[30]

A preoperative oral medication such as midazolam or nitrous oxide inhalation may be indicated to facilitate starting the intravenous line on an anxious or uncooperative patient. The most frequently used medications utilized for intravenous sedation in dentistry are benzodiazepines, opioids, short-acting anesthetics (barbiturates and propofol), ketamine, antihistamines, and anticholinergics. Anticholinergic medications such as glycopyrrolate can also be utilized during intravenous conscious dental sedations because they are competitive antagonists to acetylcholine in the parasympathetic nervous system, which causes dryness of the mouth and makes working in the oral cavity for certain procedures easier.

GENERAL ANESTHESIA FOR DENTISTRY IN NONTRADITIONAL SETTINGS

General anesthesia is necessary to deliver high-quality dental care for patients under the following circumstances:

1. Very young children with extensive dental needs who are unable to cooperate for dental procedures
2. Children who are poor candidates for sedation who are unable to cooperate for treatment
3. Patients with special health care needs who do not have the ability to cooperate for treatment
4. Patients with complex medical needs where treatment under anesthesia is preferred for medical reasons
5. Patients who are unable to obtain profound local anesthesia
6. Patients requiring complex surgical procedures that cannot be performed with local anesthesia alone

Alternative sites such as surgery centers and in-office anesthesia are typically utilized for ASA 1 and select 2 patients. Safe delivery is dependent on rigorous protocols for patient safety. Dental offices must provide a safe environment that complies with local, state, and federal rules and regulations as well as professional guidelines. Anesthesia must be provided by trained individuals, and adequate personnel must be available.[31] The facilities and equipment, monitoring and documentation, and emergency medications and protocols must meet the standards of a hospital setting.[31]

Patients should receive a preoperative evaluation from a qualified medical professional prior to surgery. On the day of the appointment, the history and physical should be updated and the procedure canceled in the event of illness or violation of the nothing by mouth status. A preoperative sedation medication such as midazolam may be administered to improve cooperation and reduce memories of induction.

Anesthesia may be administered utilizing endotracheal intubation or intravenously in an "open-airway" technique. Nasal endotracheal intubation is preferred for most dental cases to allow access to the entire oral cavity. To facilitate atraumatic intubation, a red rubber urethral catheter may be attached to the end of the endotracheal tube to guide it to the oropharynx.[32] It should be noted that these catheters typically have latex and should be avoided in latex-allergic patients. If endotracheal intubation is used, a throat pack with radiopaque material should be utilized to protect the airway. Dexamethasone has been suggested to reduce postoperative pain and swelling following dental extractions.[33]

The oral cavity should be kept clear of debris with aggressive suctioning and use of a rubber dam when permitting. Efficiency should be emphasized to minimize the duration of the anesthesia. Dentists typically perform treatment utilizing quadrant or half-mouth dentistry. Anesthesiologists should communicate with dentists to anticipate stimulating procedures such as extractions as the depth of anesthesia may need to be altered. If local anesthesia is used by the dentist, the anesthesia staff should be informed.

At the end of the case, deep extubation should be avoided to prevent laryngospasm or other airway complications. Dentists should work with anesthesia for a postoperative pain control plan. Typical postoperative agents are intravenous ketorolac, acetaminophen, fentanyl, or morphine. Prolonged monitoring is indicated for patients receiving postoperative narcotics. Patients should be appropriately monitored following the procedure and discharged as in a hospital setting.

POSSIBLE COMPLICATIONS

Complications when performing any of the previously mentioned sedation techniques can be minimized by robust patient assessment, procedure, and emergency protocol. Proper preparation by the dentist and anesthetist could help reduce any patient complications secondary to an underlying medical condition the patient may have or from pain associated with the dental procedure being performed.

Complications with sedation and anesthesia in dentistry are primarily respiratory in nature. These risks are increased by a shared airway, with airway obstruction being a complication more frequently seen in the dental setting when compared with hospital-based practices (2%–4%).[34] The result of possible irritants in the oral cavity and oropharynx such as saliva, blood, and tooth fragments can lead to an increased possibility of laryngospasm. Dentists commonly utilize an oropharynx pack or gauze to prevent as much debris as possible from irritating the patient's airway, but depending on the nature of the dentistry being provided, this may not always be effective. In the conscious or moderately sedated patient, laryngospasm is manifested by the patient trying to expel the debris from their throat by coughing. During deep sedation, laryngospasm may occur due to the anesthetized reflexes. These should be treated immediately with administration of positive pressure through utilization of a BVM. The airway should be suctioned, followed by a head tilt and chin lift or jaw thrust to open the airway, followed by the BVM until ventilations are successful.[35]

Pharmacological reversal of sedative agents is indicated whenever the anesthesia provider is faced with an unconscious patient or when there are airway complications and BVM is unsuccessful. Generally, the pharmacological intervention requires the use of neuromuscular blockers, such as intravenous succinylcholine (0.1–0.2 mg/kg), and should only supplement the use of a positive pressure BVM.[35]

In a critical incident analysis of pediatric adverse sedation events, Cote et al. found that 33.7% of these happened during dental treatment, and that nonhospital-based settings were associated with increased morbidity.[36] However, these adverse events were primarily associated with inadequate physiologic monitoring, and adherence to current guidelines would have likely prevented these outcomes. Perrott et al. evaluated the safety of office-based oral and maxillofacial procedures; the researchers calculated a complication rate that ranged from 0.4% to 1.5% for local anesthesia, conscious sedation, and general anesthesia.[37] Complication types included gastrointestinal (i.e., vomiting, 0.1%–0.3%); laryngospasm, bronchospasm, or other respiratory complications (0.3%); cardiac arrhythmias (0.1%); syncope (0.1%); seizures (<0.1%); neurologic impairment (<0.1%); prolonged recovery (0.2%); and other complications (0.1%). As a result, the authors declared that all three kinds of anesthetics could be used safely in office settings.[37] Though rare, deaths occurring in the dental office and sensationalized in the news media will continue to elicit attempts to reduce anesthesia risk legislatively.[38]

REFERENCES

1. Hicks CG, Jones JE, Saxen MA, et al. Demand in pediatric dentistry for sedation and general anesthesia by dentist anesthesiologists: a survey of directors of dentist anesthesiologist and pediatric dentistry residencies. *Anesth Prog.* 2012;59(1):3–11.
2. Tarver M, Guelmann M, Primosch R. Impact of office-based intravenous deep sedation providers upon traditional sedation practices employed in pediatric dentistry. *Pediatr Dent.* 2012;34(3):e62–e68.
3. Slovin M, Falagario-Wasserman J. Special needs of anxious and phobic dental patients. *Dent Clin North Am. 2009*;53:207–219.
4. Gale E. Fears of the dental situation. *J Dent Res.* 1972;51:964–966.
5. Watts AK, Thikkurissy S, Smiley M, McTigue DJ, Smith T. Local anesthesia affects physiologic parameters and reduces anesthesiologist intervention in children undergoing general anesthesia for dental rehabilitation. *Pediatr Dent.* 2009;31(5):414–419.
6. Townsend JA, Hagan JL, Smiley M. Use of local anesthesia during dental rehabilitation with general anesthesia: a survey of dentist anesthesiologists. *Anesth Prog.* 2014;61(1):11–17.
7. Townsend JA, Ganzberg S, Thikurrisy S. The effect of local anesthetic on quality of recovery characteristics following dental rehabilitation under general anesthesia in children. *Anesth Prog.* 2009;56(4):115–122.
8. Parekh S, Gardener C, Ashley PF, Walsh T. Intraoperative local aneaesthesia for reduction of postoperative pain following general anaesthesia for dental treatment in children and adolescents. *Cochrane Database Syst Rev.* 2014;23(12):CD009742.
9. Moore PA, Hersh EV. Local anesthetics: pharmacology and toxicity. *Dent Clin North Am.* 2010;54(4):587–599.
10. Malamed SF. Clinical action of specific agents. In: *Handbook of Local Anesthesia.* 5th ed. St. Louis, MO: Elsevier Mosby; 2004:55–84.
11. American Academy of Pediatric Dentistry. Guideline on use of local anesthesia for pediatric dental patients. *Pediatr Dent.* 2015;37(special issue):199–205.
12. Chicka MC, Dembo JB, Mathu-Muju KR, Nash DA, Bush HM. Adverse events during pediatric dental anesthesia and sedation: a review of closed malpractice insurance claims. *Pediatr Dent.* 2012;34(3):231–238.
13. Shapiro F, Punwani N, Rosenberg N, Valedon A, Twersky R, Urman R. Office-based anesthesia; safety and outcomes. *Anesth Analg.* 2014;119(2):276–285.
14. Baker S, Parico L. Pathologic paediatric conditions associated with a compromised airway. *Int J Paediatr Dent.* 2010;20(2):102–111.
15. Corah NL, Gale EN, Illig SJ. Assessment of a dental anxiety scale. *J Am Dent Assoc.* 1978;97(5):816–819.
16. Malamed SF. Physical and psychological evaluation. In: *Sedation.* 5th ed. St. Louis, MO: Mosby; 2010:23–37.
17. Baker S, Yagiela JA. Obesity: a complicating factor for sedation in children. *Pediatr Dent.* 2006;28(6):487–493.
18. Kang J, Vann WF, Lee JY, Anderson JA. The safety of sedation for overweight/obese children in the dental setting. *Pediatr Dent.* 2012;34(5):392–396.
19. Fishbaugh DF, Wilson S, Preisch JW, Weaver JM. Relationship of tonsil size on an airway blockage maneuver in children during sedation. *Pediatr Dent.* 1997;19(4):277–281.
20. Ganzberg S. Obstructive sleep apnea and office-based surgery. *Anesth Prog.* 2016;63(2):53–54.
21. Record B, Arribas A. Sedation in Dentistry. In: Urman R, Kaye A, eds. *Moderate and Deep Sedation in Clinical Practice.* Cambridge, England: Cambridge University Press; 2012:254–280.
22. Chung WL. Anesthesia equipment for the oral and maxillofacial surgery practice. *Oral Maxillofac Surg Clin North Am.* 2013;25(3):373–383.
23. Cote CJ. Wilson S. Guidelines for monitoring and management of pediatric patients before, during, and after sedation for diagnostic and therapeutic procedures: update 2016. *Pediatr Dent.* 2016;38(4):13–39.
24. Stronczek MJ. Determining the appropriate oral surgeon anesthesia modality, setting, and team. *Oral Maxillofac Surg Clin North Am.* 2013;25(3):357–366.
25. Emmanouil DE, Quock RM. Advances in understanding the actions of nitrous oxide. *Anesth Prog.* 2007;54(1):9–18.
26. American Academy of Pediatric Dentistry. Guideline on use of nitrous oxide for pediatric dental patients. *Pediatr Dent.* 2015;37(special issue):206–210.
27. Klein U, Bucklin BA, Poulton TJ, Bozinov D. Nitrous oxide concentrations in the posterior nasopharynx during administration by nasal mask. *Pediatr Dent.* 2004;26(5):410–416.
28. Kupietzky A, Shapira J, Ram D. Fasting state and episodes of vomiting in children receiving nitrous oxide for dental treatment. *Pediatr Dent.* 2008;30(5):414–419.
29. American Dental Association. *ADA Guidelines for the Use of Sedation and General Anesthesia by Dentists.* Chicago, IL: American Dental Association; 2016.
30. Harbuz D, O'Halloran M. Techniques to administer oral, inhalational, and IV sedation in dentistry. *Australas Med.* 2016;9(2):25–32.

31. American Academy of Pediatric Dentistry. Guideline on use of anesthesia personnel in the administration of office-based deep sedation/general anesthesia to the pediatric dental patient. *Pediatr Dent.* 2015;37(special issue):246–249.
32. Watt S, Pickhardt D, Lerman J, Armstrong J, Creighton PR, Feldman L. Telescoping tracheal tubes into catheters minimizes epistaxis during nasotracheal intubation in children. *Anesthesiology.* 2007;106(2):238–242.
33. Baxendale BR, Vater M, Lavery KM. Dexamethasone reduces pain and swelling following extraction of third molar teeth. *Anaesthesia.* 1993;48(11):961–964.
34. Boynes SG, Lewis CL, Moore PA, Zovko J, Close J. Complications associated with anesthesia administered for dental treatment. *Gen Dent.* 2010;58;e20–e25.
35. Becker D, Haas D. Management of complications during moderate and deep sedation; respiratory and cardiovascular considerations. *Anesth Prog.* 2007;54(2):59–69.
36. Cote CJ, Notterman DA, Karl HW, Weinberg JA, McCloskey C. Adverse sedation events in pediatrics: a critical incident analysis of contributing factors. *Pediatrics.* 2000;105(pt 1):805–814.
37. Perrot DH, Yuen JP, Andersen RV, Dodson TB. Office-based ambulatory anesthesia; outcomes of clinical practice of oral and maxillofacial surgeons. *J Oral Maxillofac Surg.* 2003;61:983–995.
38. Yagiela J. Office-based anesthesia in dentistry, past, present and future trends. *Dent Clin North Am.* 1999;43(2):201–215.

35 | ULTRARAPID OPIATE DETOXIFICATION

CLIFFORD M. GEVIRTZ, MD, MPH, ELIZABETH FROST, MD,
ALAN D. KAYE, MD, PHD

INTRODUCTION

Drug abuse is at epidemic proportions throughout the United States and the former surgeon general, Dr. Vivek Murthy[1] recently took the unprecedented step of mailing every physician suggestions on how to limit the use of opiates in pain management. The illegal use of opiates, especially prescription drugs, has seen explosive growth in the United States.[2,3] In recent years, opiate-induced deaths have increased in particular because of more potent drugs and easier accessibility. The continuing rise in abuse of opiates has placed greater emphasis on detoxification treatment modalities. Use of prescription pain relievers with or without a doctor's prescription or only for the experience or feeling they cause ("nonmedical" use) is, after marijuana use, the second most common form of illicit drug use in the United States.[4] When used appropriately under medical supervision, hydrocodone (e.g., Vicodin), oxycodone (e.g., OxyContin), morphine, and similar prescription pain relievers provide indispensable medical benefit by reducing pain and suffering, but when taken without appropriate direction and oversight, these medications can cause serious adverse consequences and produce dependence and abuse. Approximately 324,000 emergency department visits in 2006 involved the nonmedical use of pain relievers (including both prescription and over-the-counter pain medications).[5]

When individuals wish to detoxify from opiate dependence, several options are available, including both conventional and newer, more rapid approaches.

CONVENTIONAL DETOXIFICATION

Conventional treatments for opiate abuse include several treatment models, all of which have extremely low success rates. Dose reduction by 10% per week is the simplest approach, but most patients have trouble reducing their daily dose below 60% of their starting point.

Methadone administration involves substitution of a legally accepted opiate for one that is being illegally abused. Methadone is a full opioid agonist at μ-receptor sites. Thus, one negative aspect of methadone is its potential to produce or maintain dependence on opioids, such that patients experience withdrawal if a daily dose is missed, and detoxification can be a lengthy and difficult process, discouraging all attempts.[6] Additionally, because of its full agonist action, there is no ceiling to the level of respiratory depression or sedation that methadone can induce. Methadone overdose can therefore be fatal. Despite its many advantages (legality and cheap availability), methadone maintenance appears to have limited suitability for some patients, including time constraints and continued need for medication and dependence. These factors may restrict the ability of methadone to attract certain users into treatment, and the examination of alternative medications to broaden the range of pharmacotherapies has been the focus of research in recent years.

Buprenorphine is a partial μ agonist and κ antagonist that exerts weaker opioid effects at opioid receptor sites. Buprenorphine and methadone maintenance were compared in a series of impressive studies using fixed doses of the drugs.[7] Results were mixed. Some of the fixed-dose studies showed no difference in efficacy, whereas others showed superiority for methadone, and yet others showed the reverse. The investigators in these fixed-dose studies frequently concluded that the doses of buprenorphine or methadone chosen were too low or that poor induction regimes led to poor retention. A series of variable- (or flexible-) dose studies have been conducted and showed essentially the same results for the two drugs, failing to identify a clearly superior agent.

RAPID OPIATE DETOXIFICATION

Rapid opiate detoxification is a 3-day process involving large amounts of an opiate antagonist, such as naloxone or naltrexone.[7,8] However, there are problems associated with all of these treatments. While methadone treatment has high initial relapse rates, rapid opiate detoxification elicits severe withdrawal symptoms.

ULTRARAPID OPIATE DETOXIFICATION

Ultrarapid opiate detoxification (UROD) entails anesthetizing a patient and precipitating withdrawal during unconsciousness.[9] The procedure, accompanied by appropriate aggressive supportive therapy, shortens the withdrawal period experienced by opiate-dependent patients and diminishes much of the subjective discomfort. One advantage of UROD is that the withdrawal period is markedly shortened to about 4–8 hours versus up to several months for conventional treatments. The patient is anesthetized during the acute withdrawal period and thus does not experience the unpleasant consequences of acute detoxification.

Withdrawal syndrome refers to a constellation of symptoms, including restlessness, rhinorrhea, lacrimation, diaphoresis, myosis, piloerection, and cardiovascular changes due to increased catecholamine release. The catecholamine surge caused by induction of the withdrawal syndrome in UROD has life-threatening implications. Clonidine, an α_2-receptor agonist, reduces these catecholamine surges.[9,10] This drug reduces the severity of the withdrawal syndrome in rats; however, controversy remains in vivo regarding the precise role and effects of clonidine in UROD, perhaps due in part to individual effects of chronic opiate administration.[9–13]

Blum et al. commented on the increasing prescription of high-dose opiate therapy for patients in chronic pain.[14] Noting that a substantial challenge is then rendered on caregivers when these individuals present for surgery, the authors hypothesized that using UROD would rapidly increase the number of opiate receptors and return the patients to a naïve state, making them susceptible to exogenous opiate administration. They validated this hypothesis based on two mechanisms: reports of patients who had undergone UROD for opiate addiction and subsequently suffered respiratory arrest when they began to rapidly abuse opiates shortly after treatment. Also, data demonstrated that tapering of opiates prior to elective surgery allows for substantially better postoperative pain control.

Salimi et al. assessed the long-term efficacy, relapse time, and rate over a 2-year follow-up period in patients who had undergone UROD.[15] They studied a total of 424 patients, and of this number, 303 (75.75%) were successful. The unemployment rate of the relapse group was 76% compared to the successful group (21%). None of the patients in the relapse group continued naloxone maintenance at 6-month follow-up, significantly lower than the successful group (75.8%). The relapse rate was 14% at the first month and 24% at 6 months and thereafter. All patients who relapsed had discontinued oral naltrexone. The authors concluded that UROD could be an effective method of detoxification in addicted patients, but case selection and adhering to the guidelines and maintenance therapy in addition to social support was necessary for continued success.

Naderi-Heiden et al. studied 45 opiate-addicted males who had been detoxified by 6 hours of naloxone infusion under general anesthesia with midazolam, propofol, clonidine, and atracurium.[16] Following UROD, naltrexone 50 mg/d was prescribed for 9 months, with assessments every 4 weeks. Adverse events were recorded in 15 patients (unconscious 1, transient confusion 8, depression 6). Mild withdrawal syndrome was common. Two extreme outliers were found in intravenous and cannabis users. Of the patients, 96% were discharged the following day; 36% continued naloxone therapy for the 9-month period. The authors concluded that UROD and subsequent naloxone maintenance therapy are safe and effective for addicted patients. This study was of Iranian patients and may not correspond to European or American modalities.

Several drugs have been used to induce anesthesia during UROD. Nasr et al. reported on 60 male patients who received a propofol infusion.[17] One group received dexmedetomidine during anesthesia and for 6 days afterward. The control group was treated after anesthesia with lefoxidine 0.2 mg orally three times daily. The group receiving dexmedetomidine had significantly better hemodynamic control and markedly fewer withdrawal symptoms. Patient satisfaction was greater.

The Canadian Agency for Drugs and Technologies conducted a technology review of UROD[18] and concluded that there is some evidence suggesting earlier peaking of, and lower scores for, withdrawal symptoms and higher rates of the commencement and continuation of maintenance treatment in patients receiving UROD compared to patients in control groups (e.g., conventional withdrawal treatment). However, no significant differences were identified between UROD and control groups in the commencement or duration of withdrawal treatment. Mixed results were identified between UROD and control groups in the completion of withdrawal treatment and the incidence of adverse events, depending on which pharmacologic agents were used. One guideline recommended against the use of UROD due to a high risk for adverse events.

THE ALTERED NEUROPHYSIOLOGY OF OPIATE DEPENDENCY

Exogenous administration of opioids in humans reduces the production and release of endogenous opioid substances. Used regularly over a period of months or longer, opioids cause physical dependence and neural adaptation by interaction with central nervous system and systemic opioid receptors. Paradoxically, the treatment of opioid dependence can be carried out with opioid receptor agonists, partial agonists, and antagonists. Methadone is an opioid agonist that meets the needs of opioid-dependent neurons. Methadone has a long half-life and thus occupies receptors longer than agents with shorter half-lives. Partial agonists, such as buprenorphine, may treat opioid dependency by not inducing a full clinical effect when binding to the opioid receptor. Naltrexone, an orally administered opioid antagonist, blocks the opioid receptor and blunts opioid cravings and euphoria. Neural adaptation of the central nervous system due to exogenous opioids may be reversed with naltrexone or other antagonists.[19]

ANCILLARY AGENTS AND AVAILABLE TREATMENTS

A variety of methods have been utilized for the treatment of opioid withdrawal before patients begin long-term opioid-free and naltrexone programs. Most widely accepted is a slow, supervised detoxification process in which methadone is substituted for the abused opiate, as mentioned previously. Methadone maintenance therapy merely replaces an opioid with a short half-life with another that has a longer half-life of approximately 23 hours. This substitution can stabilize general and psychological health and social functioning. Once a patient is on a methadone maintenance program, the drug is slowly tapered to minimize withdrawal and potential complications. Substitution therapy with methadone has a high initial dropout rate (30%–90%) and an early relapse rate.[19,20] Alternative pharmacological detoxification programs include the use of clonidine with or without methadone, midazolam, trazadone, or buprenorphine.[20,21] For those patients who elect to undergo UROD for methadone, a 2-week period of oral hydromorphone with discontinuation of methadone followed by UROD has been completely successful and safe. Placing an individual on methadone under a classic UROD technique of 4–8 hours alone would be illogical in as much as it takes 5–6 half-lives for a drug to be effectively eliminated from the body (e.g., 5–9 days).

Opioid antagonists, such as naloxone, naltrexone, or nalmefene, accelerate the process of detoxification. These substances bind the opioid receptor and block these sites from interacting with the agonists. Once opiate antagonism is established, introduction of an opiate has no effect.[22]

A rapid detoxification protocol allows faster introduction of opioid antagonist maintenance therapy with a subsequent reduction in relapse rates.[22] The acute short-lasting opioid withdrawal syndrome can be more severe than that associated with a more conventional withdrawal. These symptoms are very rarely life threatening but are sufficiently adverse and act as a major deterrent to opioid-dependent patients who want to lose dependency.[23] To mitigate these symptoms, outpatient programs have used α_2 agonists (clonidine, dexmedetomidine); partial agonists (buprenorphine); benzodiazepines (diazepam, midazolam); and antidepressants (trazadone) to assist during detoxification. The process takes place over a week, and patients are then converted to the use of a maintenance antagonist.[24–26]

Symptoms associated with the withdrawal syndrome, such as restlessness, rhinorrhea, lacrimation, diaphoresis, myosis, piloerection, and cardiovascular changes, are mediated through increased sympathetic activity. Thirty-fold increases in the levels of epinephrine and lesser increases in norepinephrine can be observed during withdrawal from opioids.[26,27] During opioid withdrawal, neural activity in the locus ceruleus, the major noradrenergic nucleus in the brain, is greatly increased. This surge is responsible for many of the symptoms seen during withdrawal.[27,28] Clonidine has been effective in suppressing noradrenergic hyperactivity, relieving withdrawal symptoms.[29–31] Without clonidine or an equivalent α_2-agonist agent, UROD would cause large increases in both total and fractionated catecholamine levels, which have the potential to cause unacceptable morbidity and mortality rates.

INDICATIONS FOR DETOXIFICATION

The only indication for detoxification is a proven dependence on opiates demonstrated by sufficient history and by blood, urine, or hair testing. To avoid a Munchausen syndrome, or Munchausen by proxy, positive tests should be documented prior to scheduling the procedure. Drug testing is also useful to identify other drugs that the patient may be using and to evaluate the credibility of the patient (e.g., when supplemental information from friends or relatives indicates that the patient has neglected to inform the physician of cocaine or amphetamine abuse).

In patients with chronic pain, detoxification may be indicated when pain medication use escalates without improving visual analog pain scales or when the patient is having difficulty in weaning off medication. Detoxification may be offered as a safe alternative to complete dismissal from the practice.

CONTRAINDICATIONS

Several situations may exist when UROD is not indicated as the detoxification method of choice. For example, pregnancy, acute hepatitis (greater than five times control values for aspartase aminotransferase [AST] and gamma-glutamyl transferase [GGT]), acute cocaine ingestion, psychosis, lack of informed consent, myocardial infarction within 6 months, and cerebrovascular accident within 2 months are all conditions that constitute at least relative contraindications. If a patient with chronic pain wishes to detoxify and become free from dependence on narcotics, then there must be documented pain-free intervals, or again, the procedure is contraindicated. Detoxification of a pain patient who has no pain-free intervals results in a patient in excruciating pain for whom the only relief mechanism is through nerve block or neurolysis.

Because several of the medications used in the detoxification process may prolong the QTc interval, patients with preexisting prolonged QT syndrome or other conduction abnormality may be at increased risk of developing the Torsade de pointes syndrome and sudden death.

PSYCHIATRIC CLEARANCE

Psychiatric evaluation is an important prerequisite prior to detoxification. The patient must freely express a desire to become detoxified. There must be no evidence of suicidal or homicidal ideation. All other psychiatric illness must be well defined and, in the opinion of the psychiatrist, under good control. Aftercare plans should also be in place before embarking in any detoxification attempt.

It is important that there is a clearly delineated aftercare plan that has been verified in writing. The importance for the patient and the anesthesiologist of outlining a workable postprocedure plan that can be enforced on the part of both the patient and the medical care team and becomes reality cannot be overemphasized.

PREANESTHETIC TESTING

The key issues in preanesthetic preparation are to identify end-organ damage caused by substance abuse. While routine testing may well exclude electrocardiography in a young individual, cocaine abuse can cause myocardial fibrosis and is therefore an appropriate screen with the realization that abnormal findings may be apparent for months after cessation of drug intake. It is, however, important to obtain results of this test as baseline information. Opiate use within 36 hours of the procedure is a contraindication to UROD due to the high level of circulating catecholamines that are stimulated by the detoxification process itself. A well-publicized death in a private hospital in England of a patient undergoing UROD may have been related more to a last-minute "fix" of heroin than to negligent treatment.[32,33] Heroin abuse by the intravenous route is plagued by cross-contamination with other viruses, such as HIV and hepatitis B and C virus, as well as bacteria. Evaluation of liver function and careful cardiac examination are necessary to rule out acute hepatitis and bacterial endocarditis. Tuberculosis is also very common among intravenous drug abusers, and a chest x-ray is indicated.

Routine screening exams such as of a complete blood count and electrolytes are often helpful in evaluation. The finding of a low white cell count without a prior history of HIV infection requires further investigation, or a patient with elevated serum urea nitrogen (BUN) and creatinine levels may have renal damage from heroin nephropathy. Excretion of anesthetic drugs may be impaired, and the dosage should be adjusted accordingly.

THE METHODOLOGY OF ULTRARAPID OPIATE DETOXIFICATION

As noted, the UROD process is designed to detoxify an individual while maintaining cardiovascular stability, a lack of awareness, and analgesia. A review of 20 patients undergoing UROD during general anesthesia detailed successful management.[34]

PREMEDICATION

High-dose clonidine blockade is incrementally introduced to attenuate the systemic effects of withdrawal.[34] This can start the night before the procedure with the application of a transdermal patch of clonidine or by oral dosing. The goal is to reduce the blood pressure to the lower limit of normal. Vitamin C can be utilized, typically in a dose of 1–2 g, to acidify the urine and accelerate opiate elimination from the body. A suppository the night before will reduce the likelihood of diarrhea intraoperatively and postoperatively. Antiemetic medications and sedatives can also be administered. Glycopyrrolate may be added at a dose of 0.2–0.4 mg. Adequate fluid replacement is essential and should exceed the calculated maintenance by three to four times until the deficit is replaced.

MONITORING

Appropriate monitoring includes at a minimum five-lead, two-channel electrocardiography (leads II and V), noninvasive blood pressure, pulse oximetry, neuromuscular blockade, capnography, temperature, and a brain wave monitor to titrate depth of anesthesia. There are currently over a dozen brands of these monitors available throughout the United States. The safest location to perform ultrarapid detoxification is an intensive care unit, although it has been utilized in a variety of settings, including the operating room, the recovery room, and lesser-level units. Postprocedure, patients in an intensive care unit setting, in general, receive the best nursing and superior levels of monitoring, and this location should be considered a prime choice.

INDUCTION AND MAINTENANCE

All narcotics decrease gastric emptying and increase gut transit time. Residual volumes of 300 to 500 mL are not uncommon. Thus, rapid sequence induction with cricoid pressure is indicated. Anesthesia may be induced with propofol (2–3 mg/kg) and succinylcholine or rocuronium. After confirmation of endotracheal tube placement by capnography and auscultation, an orogastric tube is passed to empty the stomach. Metoclopramide should not be used because its effects are antagonized by narcotics; moreover, it is associated with hypertension due to catecholamine release. General anesthesia may be continued with a combination of midazolam, sevoflurane, and isoflurane or propofol infusion, titrated to full general anesthetic depth, for example, a bispectral index (BIS) value between 40 and 60. Indeed, any technique that does not involve drugs to which the patient is addicted is acceptable. Spontaneous ventilation may be used as part of the determination regarding when the patient has completed detoxification. On initial administration of the antagonist, minute ventilation usually doubles. The initial peak minute ventilation is recorded. When the minute ventilation declines to 80% of the peak value, detoxification is usually completed. As with any other anesthetic procedure, monitoring and documentation must be continued for the duration of the process, which is usually 4–6 hours. A procedure is deemed complete when no signs of withdrawal are seen following a final injection of naloxone 0.4 mg IV.

CHOICE OF THE ANTAGONIST

After hemodynamic stability, has been established, a test dose of the antagonist is given (e.g., naloxone 0.4 mg) to determine the degree of hemodynamic stability that has been achieved. Signs of withdrawal such as piloerection, yawning, kicking movements, tearing, hypertension, or tachycardia developing over a 5-minute period indicate the need for deeper anesthesia and additional clonidine.

Any antagonist, such as naloxone (typically up to 20 mg), naltrexone (up to 50 mg), or nalmefene (up to 8 mg) can be used for detoxification. All antagonists have a very high binding coefficient as compared to the agonists; for example, naltrexone binds 34 times more than morphine.

Some questions have arisen regarding the risk of pulmonary edema using naloxone in opiate-dependent patients. The presumed cause of the edema is an adrenergic crisis with a massive surge in catecholamines, an effect elegantly documented in a study by Kienbaum et al.[35] In the presence of clonidine, however, there is no surge in catecholamine plasma levels and no significant cardiovascular changes.[31,36]

POSTOPERATIVE PROBLEMS

Part of the definition of an addictive substance is the presence of a withdrawal syndrome when the substance is abruptly discontinued. Related to opioids, the syndrome consists of drug cravings; piloerection; yawning; sympathetic hyperactivity (tachycardia, diaphoresis); myalgias and bone pain; nausea, vomiting, and diarrhea; and insomnia. A syndrome of "protracted abstinence" is also described that occurs after 3 weeks and lasts until around week 10, which is characterized by restlessness, irritability, insomnia, and hypertension. After detoxification, attention is turned to each component as it occurs.

Naltrexone reduces the feelings of craving. The neuropharmacology is unclear, but reproducibility is marked and suggests that long-term therapy is indicated. It should be noted that with long-term naltrexone therapy, liver function tests need to be monitored.

In general, the patient should be kept warm and be allowed frequent warm soaking showers. Clonidine reduces sympathetic hyperactivity and should be continued through the protracted abstinence syndrome.

Irritability may be managed with psychotherapy, benzodiazepines (in small amounts), and antidepressants such as trazadone or paroxetine.

Immediately following detoxification, patients feel exhausted and extremely weak. They typically describe flu-like symptoms. Other complications related mainly to the gastrointestinal tract follow quickly and may last for days. Slight variations in hemodynamic status or other signs of withdrawal may be treated with small amounts of adjunct medications such as midazolam, ketorolac, or clonidine. Oral naltrexone maintenance may be started as soon as the patient is awake and tolerating fluids, although administration may be delayed because of vomiting. Additional methods of enforced abstinence are discussed further in this chapter.

PROCEDURE-RELATED EMESIS

Emesis is a prominent component of the withdrawal syndrome. The use of prophylactic antiemetic agents such as ondansetron and ranitidine is necessary. In fact, chemotherapy-level prophylaxis is required to prevent intraoperative emesis. Ondansetron is superior in this application because ranitidine in higher doses may be associated with tachycardia, vomiting, insomnia, and elevation of liver enzymes. It should be noted that while the presence of the endotracheal tube prevents large pieces of food from entering the trachea, intubation is not a guarantee against aspiration.

PROCEDURE-RELATED DIARRHEA

Diarrhea should be treated with octreotide, a synthetic polypeptide related to somatostatin. It acts by inhibiting some anterior pituitary hormones, suppressing the exocrine and endocrine functions of the pancreas, inhibiting gastric acid and vasointestinal peptide secretion, suppressing serotonin secretion, and inhibiting gastrointestinal motility. This last function is the most useful in treating the explosive diarrhea that occurs during withdrawal.[37]

Narcotic-based remedies, including loperamide, should be avoided because there is some uptake into the systemic circulation that may increase the signs of withdrawal. Systemic absorption is small but significant and may produce unwanted central nervous system side effects.

INSOMNIA

The number one reason for failure of detoxification in the first 2 weeks postprocedure is insomnia. Narcotics disrupt the normal sleep-wake cycle,[38] and many addicts require narcotics to sleep. The long-term disruption of a normal sleep-wake cycle cannot be corrected rapidly. Melatonin levels and the normal circadian rhythm typically take at least a week to become reestablished. Gabapentin has been utilized for its dual effect of sedation as well as restoring psychological balance.[39]

Orally administered melatonin (3 mg) can help, as can benzodiazepines and antihistamines (diphenhydramine). Hypnosis and alternative relaxation techniques can also be used. Self-hypnosis can be taught easily to addicts.

It is important, however, not to start prescribing large amounts of benzodiazepines because these drugs also have addictive potential and do not lead to a restorative sleep pattern. As part of the preprocedure informed consent, the patient must be made aware of the potential for insomnia.

OTHER COMPLICATIONS

Muscle cramps, bone pain, and low back pain complaints are treated with nonsteroidal anti-inflammatory drugs (NSAIDs) or a cyclooxygenase 2 inhibitor, which has few or no gastrointestinal side effects and does not interfere with coagulation. Many patients describe wide swings of mood, including depression and agitation. It is important to discuss with the therapist this potential issue. Many protocols include starting an antidepressant for 1–3 months postdetoxification procedure. Positioning during general anesthesia can become an issue. It is strongly suggested that an egg crate mattress be utilized and positioning be evaluated at regular intervals, much as in the case of a lengthy operating procedure under a general anesthetic.

ENFORCED ABSTINENCE

Because most relapses occur within the first 2 weeks, removing the patient's ability to choose opiate abuse for several weeks increases the success rate, defined as abstinence for 1 year. Subcutaneous pellets of naltrexone, injectable depot naltrexone, and injections of nalmefene have all been used to this end.

Naltrexone pellets are custom formulated and placed subcutaneously through a small incision.[40] Depending on the formulation and the content of pellets placed, significant plasma levels of naltrexone have been demonstrated for up to 6 months.

In a 3.4-g sustained-release naltrexone preparation produced by GoMedical Industries (Perth, Western Australia), the period of significant plasma antagonist levels was documented to extend to approximately 188 days (plasma levels greater than 2 ng/mL). At least two opiate-dependent addicts tried to overcome the blockade during this period and experienced no effect.

Similar success with naltrexone pellets has been reported by Foster et al.[42] and by Carreno et al.[43] They studied patients for several months post implant and found no relapse. However, Hamilton et al. reported six cases in 2002 where complications arose from this technique, including prolonged opioid withdrawal, drug toxicity, withdrawal from cross-addiction to benzodiazepines and alcohol, aspiration pneumonia, and death.[44]

Injectable depot naltrexone (Vivitrol, Cephalon) was originally developed to provide abstinence in alcohol abuse. As an off-label use, a single monthly injection provides opiate blockade for a month.

The US Food and Drug Administration (FDA) recently warned of the risk of adverse injection site reactions in patients receiving naltrexone (Vivitrol).[45] "Physicians should instruct patients to monitor the injection site and contact them if they develop pain, swelling, tenderness, induration, bruising, pruritus, or redness at the injection site that does not improve or worsens within two weeks. Physicians should promptly refer patients with worsening injection site reactions to a surgeon." The FDA has received 196 reports of injection site reactions, including cellulitis, induration, hematoma, abscess, sterile abscess, and necrosis. Sixteen patients required surgical intervention, ranging from incision and drainage in the cases of abscesses to extensive surgical debridement in cases that resulted in tissue necrosis.

Injectable depot naltrexone should be administered as an intramuscular (IM) gluteal injection and not intravenously, subcutaneously, or inadvertently into fatty tissue. Health care providers should ensure that the naltrexone injection is given correctly with the prepackaged 1½-inch needle that is specifically designed for this drug.

Similarly, nalmefene administered intramuscularly at a dose of 8 mg provides antagonist blockade for a week. However, its use in this manner has only been reported anecdotally.

DOES ULTRARAPID DETOXIFICATION HAVE A FUTURE?

Ultrarapid detoxification is a controversial procedure with many prominent addictionologists in opposition. Unfortunately, they do not have a successful substitute. While buprenorphine has some utility in changing patients from pure agonist addiction, achieving complete detoxification does not occur in a majority of cases.[46]

Collins et al. presented a randomized trial of UROD compared to two other conventional detoxification techniques in heroin addicts.[47] They studied a total of 106 treatment-seeking, heroin-dependent patients, aged 21 through 50 years, who were randomly assigned to one of three inpatient withdrawal treatments (anesthesia-assisted rapid opioid detoxification with naltrexone induction, buprenorphine-assisted rapid opioid detoxification with naltrexone induction, and clonidine-assisted opioid detoxification with delayed naltrexone induction) over 72 hours followed by 12 weeks of outpatient naltrexone maintenance with relapse prevention psychotherapy. Patients were included if the American Society of Anesthesiologists physical status score was 1 or 2, there were no major comorbid psychiatric illnesses, and they were not dependent on other drugs or alcohol. The main outcome measures studied were withdrawal severity scores on objective and subjective scales, proportions of patients receiving naltrexone, completion of inpatient detoxification, and retainment in treatment and the proportion of opioid-positive urine specimens. The authors found that mean withdrawal severities were comparable across the three treatments. Compared with clonidine-assisted detoxification, the anesthesia and buprenorphine-assisted detoxification interventions had significantly greater rates of naltrexone induction (94% anesthesia, 97% buprenorphine, and 21% clonidine), but the groups did not differ in rates of completion of inpatient detoxification. Treatment retention over 12 weeks was not significantly different among groups, with 7 of 35 (20%) retained in the anesthesia-assisted group, 9 of 37 (24%) in the buprenorphine-assisted group, and 3 of 34 (9%) in the clonidine-assisted group. Induction with 50 mg of naltrexone significantly reduced the risk of dropping out (odds ratio, 0.28; 95% confidence interval, 0.15–0.51). There were no significant group differences in proportions of opioid-positive urine specimens. The anesthesia procedure was associated with three potentially life-threatening adverse events. The authors concluded that "these data do not support the use of general anesthesia for heroin detoxification and rapid opioid antagonist induction."

There are several major flaws in the study concerned in the article by Collins et al. For example, there was a failure to pretreat with high-dose antiemetics and high-dose clonidine. By using the antiemetic only as a rescue dose, the objective withdrawal scales were falsely elevated. Similarly, failure to provide adequate high doses of clonidine led to high objective and subjective withdrawal scales. There was also a failure to treat opiate-dependent patients as at risk for aspiration, which apparently resulted in pneumonia in one patient and diabetic ketoacidosis in another. Even though 80% of patients were lost to follow-up, statistical analysis was still performed. However, if just five more anesthesia patients had completed the trial, statistical significance would have been achieved. The other major issue to bear in mind was that this study was conducted in heroin addicts and not in pain patients.

CONCLUSION

The utility of UROD rests in the ability to rapidly detoxify a patient comfortably and using enforced abstinence techniques to ensure sobriety for an extended period of time. The procedure requires a motivated patient with a psychosocial support structure in place. It is not a cure for addiction; however, with the extremely low success rate of conventional treatments for opiate addiction, it is an important therapeutic technique and an important tool for detoxification in selected patients.

REFERENCES

1. Murthy M. Letter to all physicians from the surgeon general of the United States. August 2016. Available at: http://time.com/4468400/surgeon-general-letter-opioid-addiction/
2. Kaye AD, Jones MR, Kaye AM, et al. prescription opioid abuse in chronic pain: an updated review of opioid abuse predictors and strategies to curb opioid abuse (part 1). *Pain Physician.* 2017;20(2S):S93–S109.
3. Kaye AD, Jones MR, Kaye AM, et al. Prescription opioid abuse in chronic pain: an updated review of opioid abuse predictors and strategies to curb opioid abuse (part 2). *Pain Physician.* 2017;20(2S):S111–S133.
4. Manchikanti L. National drug control policy and prescription drug abuse: facts and fallacies. *Pain Physician.* 2007;10:399–424.
5. Manchikanti L. Prescription drug abuse: what is being done to address this new epidemic. *Pain Physician.* 2006;9:287–321.
6. Mattick RP, Breen C, Kinber J, et al. Methadone maintenance therapy versus no opiod replacement therapy for opioid dependence. Cochrane Database Syst Rev. 2009;(3):CD002209.
7. Krabbe PF, Koning JPF, Heinen N, et al. Rapid detoxification from opioid dependence under general anaesthesia versus standard methadone tapering: abstinence rates and withdrawal distress experiences. *Addict Biol.* 2003;8:351–358.
8. McCabe S. Rapid detox: understanding new treatment approaches for the addicted patient. *Perspect Psychiatr Care.* 2000;36:113–119.
9. Kaye AD, Gevirtz C, Bosscher HA, et al. Ultrarapid opiate detoxification: a review. *Can J Anesth.* 2003;50:1–9.
10. Gevirtz C, Frost E. Ultra rapid opiate detoxification. *Curr Concepts Curr Opin Clin Exp Res.* 2000;2:151–168.
11. Ma H, Tang J, White PF, et al. The effect of clonidine on gastrointestinal side effects associated with ultra-rapid opioid detoxification. *Anesth Analg.* 2003;96:1409–1412.
12. White. PF, Wender RH. Convincing effects of clonidine on neurohumoral withdrawal symptoms during antagonist-supported detoxification of opioid addicts. *Anesth Analg.* 2003;97:1542–1551.
13. Kienbaum P, Peters J, Scherbaum N. Convincing effects of clonidine on neurohumoral withdrawal symptoms during antagonist-supported detoxification of opioid addicts. *Anesth Analg.* 2003;97:1542–1551.
14. Blum JM, Biel SS, Hilliard PE, Jutkiewicz EM. Preoperative ultra-rapid opiate detoxification for the treatment of post-operative surgical pain. Med Hypotheses. 2015;84(6):529–531. doi:10.1016/j.mehy.2015.02.008. Epub 2015 Mar 6.
15. Salimi A, Safari F, Mohajerani SA, Hashemian M, Kolahi AA, Mottaghi K. Long-term relapse of ultra-rapid opioid detoxification. J Addict Dis. 2014;33(1):33–40. doi:10.1080/10550887.2014.882727.
16. Naderi-Heiden A, Naderi A, Naderi MM, et al. Ultra-rapid opiate detoxification followed by nine months of naltrexone maintenance therapy in Iran. Pharmacopsychiatry. 2010;43(4):130–137. doi:10.1055/s-0029-1242820. Epub 2010 Jan 25.
17. Nasr DA, Omran HA, Hakim SM, Mansour WA. Ultra-rapid opiate detoxification using dexmedetomidine under general anesthesia. J Opioid Manag. 2011;7(5):337–344.
18. *Rapid and Ultra-Rapid Detoxification in Adults with Opioid Addiction: A Review of Clinical and Cost-Effectiveness, Safety, and Guidelines* [Internet]. Ottawa, Canada: Canadian Agency for Drugs and Technologies in Health; January 15, 2016. Available at: https://www.cadth.ca/.
19. Diaz A, Pazos A, Florez J, et al. Regulation of mu opioid receptors, G-protein-coupled receptor kinases and beta-arrestin 2 in the rat brain after chronic opioid receptor antagonism. *Neuroscience.* 2002;112: 345–353.
20. Jasinski DR. Tolerance and dependence to opiates. *Acta Anaesthesiol Scand.* 1997;41:184–186.
21. Kleber HD, Topazian M, Gaspari J, et al. Clonidine and naltrexone in the outpatient treatment of heroin withdrawal. *Am J Drug Alcohol Abuse.* 1987;13:4–17.
22. O'Brien CP, McLellan AT. Myths about the treatment of addiction. *Lancet.* 1996;347:237–240.
23. Broers B, Giner F, Dumont P, Mino A. Inpatient opiate detoxification in Geneva: follow-up at 1 and 6 months. *Drug Alcohol Depend.* 2000;58:85–92.
24. Fudala PJ, Jaffe JH, Dax EM, Johnson RE. Use of buprenorphine in the treatment of opioid addiction. II. Physiologic and behavioral effects of daily and alternate-day administration and abrupt withdrawal. *Clin Pharmacol Ther.* 1990;47:525–534.
25. Charney DS, Heninger GR. The combined use of clonidine and naltrexone as a rapid safe and effective treatment of abrupt withdrawal from methadone. *Am J Psychiatry.* 1986;143:831–837.
26. Senft RA. Experience with clonidine-naltrexone for rapid opiate detoxification. *J Subst Abuse Treat.* 1991;8:257–259.
27. Kienbaum P, Scherbaum N, Thurauf N, et al. Acute detoxification of opioid-addicted patients with naloxone during propofol or methohexital anesthesia: a comparison of withdrawal symptoms, neuroendocrine metabolic and cardiovascular patterns. *Crit Care Med.* 2000;28:969–976.
28. Gold MS. Opiate addiction and the locus coeruleus. The clinical utility of clonidine, naltrexone, methadone and buprenorphine. *Psychiatr Clin North Am.* 1993;16:61–73.
29. Gevirtz C, Kaye AD. Detoxification techniques for opiates and benzodiazepines. In: Sackheim K, eds. *Pain Management and Palliative Care.* New York: Springer Press; 2016:49–56.
30. Christie MJ, Williams JT, Osborne PB, Bellchambers CE. Where is the locus in opioid withdrawal? *Trends Pharmacol Sci.* 1997;18:134–140.
31. Kienbaum P, Thurauf N, Michel M, et al. Profound increase in epinephrine concentration in plasma and cardiovascular stimulation after μ-opioid receptor blockade in opioid addicted patients. *Anesthesiology.* 1998;88:1154–1161.
32. Langer SZ. Presynaptic regulation of release of catecholamines. *Pharmacol Rev.* 1981;32:337–362.
33. Gold MS, Redmond DE Jr, Kleber HD. Noradrenergic hyperactivity in opiate withdrawal supported clonidine reversal of opiate withdrawal. *Am J Psychiatry.* 1979;136:100–102.
34. Dyer C, Addict died after rapid opiate detoxification. *BMJ.* 1998;316:167–172.
35. Mayor S. Specialists criticize treatment for heroin addiction. *BMJ.* 1997;314:1365.
36. Gold CG, Cullen DJ, Gonzales S, et al. Rapid opioid detoxification during general anesthesia. *Anesthesiology.* 1999:91:1639–1647.
37. Kienbaum P, Thurauf N, Michel M, et al. Profound increase in epinephrine concentration in plasma and cardiovascular stimulation after mu-opiod receptor blockade in opioid addicted patients during barbiturate-induced anesthesia for acute detoxification. *Anesthesiology.* 1998;88:1154–1161.
38. Kaye AD, Banister RE, Hoover JM, et al. Chronic pain and ultra rapid opioid detoxification. *Pain Physician.* 2005;5(1):33–42.
39. Kaye AD, Cornett EM, Helander E, Menard B, Hsu E, Hart B, Brunk A. An update on nonopoids: intravenous or oral analgesics for perioperative pain management. *Anesthesiol Clin.* 2017;35(2):e55–e71.
40. Staedt J, Wassmuth F, Stoppe G, et al. Effects of chronic treatment with methadone and naltrexone on sleep in addicts. *Eur Arch Psychiatry Clin Neurosci.* 1996;246:305–309.
41. Hulse GK, Arnold-Reed DE, O'Neil G. Blood naltrexone and 6-beta-naltrexol levels following naltrexone implant: comparing two naltrexone implants. *Addict Biol.* 2004;9:59–65.
42. Foster J, Brewer C, Steele L. Naltrexone implants can completely prevent early (1-month) relapse after opiate detoxification: a pilot study of two cohorts totaling 101 patients with a note on naltrexone blood levels. *Addict Biol.* 2003;8:211–217.
43. Carreno JE, Alvarez CE, Narciso GI, et al. Maintenance treatment with depot opioid antagonists in subcutaneous implants: an alternative in the treatment of opioids dependence. *Addict Biol.* 2003;8:429–438.
44. Hamilton RJ, Olmedo RE, Shah S, et al. Complications of ultra-rapid opioid detoxification with subcutaneous naltrexone pellets. *Acad Emerg Med.* 2002;9:63–68.
45. United States Food and Drug Administration. Naltrexone (Vivitrol) FDA alert. Available at: https://www.drugs.com/fda/vivitrol-naltrexone-12414.html. Published August 12, 2008. Accessed on August 15, 2010.
46. Duenwald M. Fresh look at a fast way to kick a heroin habit. *New York Times.* December 4, 2001:F6.
47. Collins ED, Kleber HD, Whittington RA, Heitler NE. Anesthesia-assisted vs. buprenorphine-or clonidine-assisted heroin detoxification and naltrexone induction: a randomized trial. *JAMA.* 2005;294: 903–913.

36 | NONELECTIVE CARE ON BOARD AN AIRCRAFT

CHRISTOPHER CONNOR, MD, PHD

BEN O'BRIEN, MD, PHD (HABIL), FRCA, FFICM, MHBA, ATPL

INTRODUCTION

The International Air Transport Association recognizes that "the airline is responsible for carrying its passengers safely and efficiently to the destination," yet "the airline has no real means of ensuring that all passengers are fit to begin their journey."[1] There exists an extensive body of work, including textbooks and guidelines,[2–4] to support prehospital in-flight care. These references deal with the challenges of emergent and elective aeromedical transport and repatriation, as would be confronted by a flight physician or flight nurse. This chapter, on the other hand, aims to support the anesthesia practitioner with a clinic or hospital-based practice, highlighting important factors to consider should he or she be called on to provide medical care and advice incidentally while on an aircraft as a passenger.

As the average age and number of passengers carried on a single flight increase,[5] it becomes increasingly likely that physicians will be called on more frequently to provide assistance to fellow travelers in medical distress. While the cabin crew handle approximately 70% of in-flight requests for medical assistance[6]—the most common problems being diarrhea and nausea[7]—consultation is sought from passengers with some medical training in the remaining 30% of cases.[8] Some airlines, such as Lufthansa, invite and incentivize medical professionals to preidentify themselves by linking frequent flyer data, reservations, and seat numbers. This allows the flight crew to be aware of any medical expertise that might be potentially available to them.

Different legal jurisdictions apply, depending on the country of registration of the aircraft. According to the Tokyo Convention, more formally known as the *Convention on Offences and Certain Other Acts Committed on Board Aircraft*, "the State of registration of the aircraft is competent to exercise jurisdiction over offences and acts committed on board" (p. 222).[9] Medical professionals may worry unnecessarily that they could expose themselves to legal risk when providing medical assistance while off duty. In fact, the law is usually structured to protect, encourage, or even mandate that medical professionals offer their skills when the need arises.

On US registered aircraft, for example, medical professionals who respond to in-flight events are broadly protected against claims for malpractice by "Good Samaritan" legislation,[10] provided that the actions they take are the ones that other competent persons with similar training would take under similar circumstances. The statute covers only those volunteering (making no charge for) their assistance. There is no legal duty under US law to provide medical care to a person with whom there is no preexisting patient-doctor relationship. Judges in the United Kingdom have held a similar position.[11] However, other countries, including France and Australia, do impose a legal obligation to assist even when no prior relationship exists. It is good practice to be clear about one's own background specialty and degree of experience. Regardless of legal obligations, a strong ethical imperative exists to assist a person in extremis.

DeLaune et al.[12] found that when a physician was involved in the decision to divert a flight for medical reasons, the patient was ultimately admitted to a hospital 49% of the time; without physician assistance, admission resulted only 15% of the time. Overall, the most common incidents are gastrointestinal problems, followed by vasovagal syncopal events; cardiac, neurological, respiratory distress; and trauma, with some minor frequency variation across various studies.[13–18] Trauma commonly consists of injuries caused by luggage items falling from overhead storage bins, but it also includes burns from spillage of hot liquids.[7] Cardiac disorders and stroke are the most frequent causes of in-flight deaths.[19]

The type of in-flight treatment can fall into one of three categories, depending on the acuity of the patient. The first category is that of an acutely life-threatening event requiring immediate treatment, such as an acute coronary syndrome or asthma attack. The last category is that of the straightforward, nonthreatening presentation, such as diarrhea or the symptoms of hyperventilation secondary to situational anxiety. In this category, only minimal intervention or reassurance is required. The middle category presents the greatest dilemma in management, as the presentation is more uncertain. The patient may appear acutely unwell and in some distress, for example, the onset of acute abdominal pain in a woman of childbearing age. It may not be possible to provide a definitive diagnosis, and the differential may include conditions that would need urgent intervention in a hospital. In these cases, it is best to determine whether symptomatic treatment can be used safely until definitive care is available. The decision to divert a flight for medical reasons does not lie with the responding physician but rather with the captain of the aircraft; the physician acts solely in an advisory capacity.

When the diagnosis and management of the patient is in doubt, it is helpful to be able to receive a second opinion from another physician. Most airlines provide the capability to contact a ground-based support physician; a large number contract with an independent medical services provider. The largest of these is MedAire's service MedLink, which provides global radio access to consultation with attending emergency physicians based at Good Samaritan Regional Medical Center in Phoenix, Arizona. MedAire maintains a database of medical facilities around the world and assists with planning a diversion or arranging the handoff of continuing patient care to local medical services on arrival. We recommend a low threshold for using radio consultation services unless the diagnosis and management are straightforward and unlikely to require further care.

The environment of the commercial aircraft poses some special challenges to the patient and to the responding medical professional:

1. **Decreased oxygen pressure**: The decrease in atmospheric pressure with altitude is accompanied by a decrease in partial pressure of oxygen and, consequently, in arterial oxygen saturation. Pressurization on commercial flights is not to sea level, but rather to a cabin altitude commonly ranging from 5000 to 8000 feet (1524 to 2438 meters, 632 to 565 mm Hg, 84.3 to 75.3 kPa) above sea level; at 8000 feet, arterial oxygen saturation will be around 90%. The decrease in partial pressure of oxygen during flight may provoke distress in patients with compromised cardiovascular or respiratory function (Figure 36.1); it can also trigger a sickling crisis in susceptible patients.[20]
2. **Decreased barometric pressure**: During ascent, gas expands, while its volume decreases during descent. Therefore, during ascent expanding gas unable to escape from body cavities may exert pressure on surrounding structures. The volume of trapped gas can increase by 30%,[7] which is of particular concern for patients who may have pneumothorax (Figure 36.1),[21] pneumocephalus or ileus. A similar inability to equilibrate pressure during descent is a common cause of ear, nose, and throat (ENT) problems. Changes in barometric pressure may also affect the operation of medical equipment. The reduction in ambient pressure can trigger decompression sickness in patients who have recently been scuba diving. Current recommendations are that divers should allow a surface interval of 12 to 24 hours after diving before flying in a commercial aircraft. In modern commercial passenger aircraft, the cabin pressure can often be brought to sea level by reducing the flight altitude to 22,500 feet or less; the cabin pressurization system can usually correct the internal pressure to sea level up to this flight altitude but not from the more common cruising altitudes above 30,000 feet.[22]
3. **Decreased humidity:** The higher the altitude, the cooler and, consequently, the drier the air. On a commercial aircraft, it typically ranges between 10% and 20%. This may dry secretions and worsen a patient's respiratory status.
4. **Confined space**: The dimensions and crowding compromise both the responding medical professional and the patient. To medical professionals used to practicing within the controlled environment of a clinic or hospital designed for the express purpose of rendering clinical care, the confinement and lack of privacy of a commercial aircraft cabin make it a particularly inhospitable environment in which to care for a patient. Careful consideration needs to be given to bystander safety, for

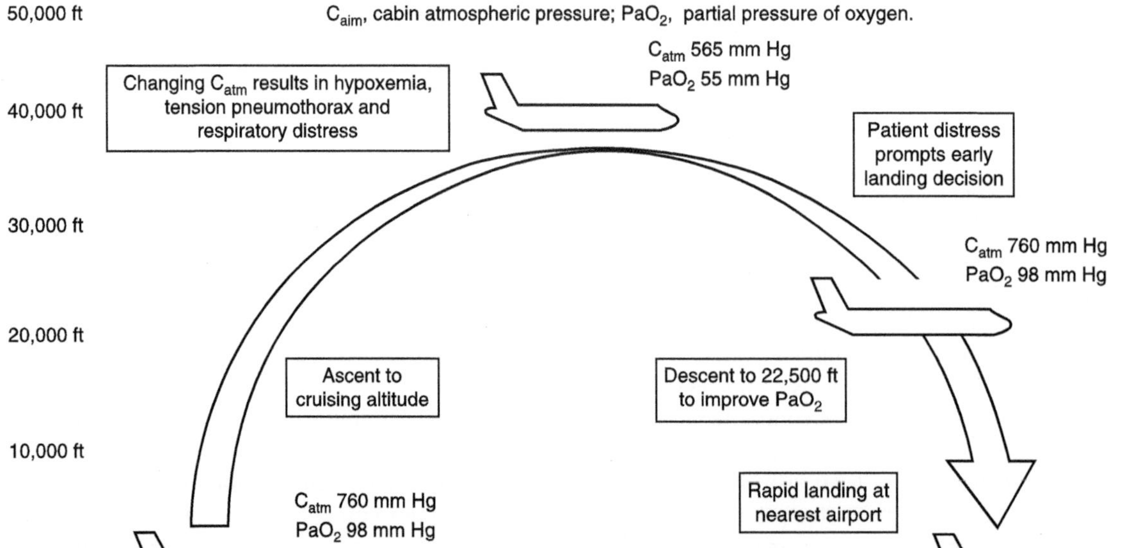

Figure 36.1. A clinical scenario of in-flight hypoxia and tension pneumothorax developing during ascent and responding to a decrease in altitude. Cabin pressure can be maintained at sea level up to 22,500 feet. (Modified from Cheatham ML, Safcsak K. Air travel following traumatic pneumothorax: when is it safe? Am Surg. 1999;65:1160–1164.)

example, the disposal of sharps (e.g., needles, cannulas), electrical safety in defibrillation, and containment of body fluids. Prolonged immobilization may predispose to deep vein thrombosis. Also, it is often difficult to obtain a suitable level of privacy for a physician to perform a thorough history and physical examination, and it may be difficult to lay the patient flat.

5. **Noise**: This may not only prevent a patient's examination (e.g., blood pressure cannot always be determined by auscultation with a stethoscope, and it may have to be palpated), but it can also interfere with effective communication with the patient or crew.
6. **Fatigue**: All the stresses of flight, including jet lag, contribute to fatigue and can worsen a patient's clinical condition and impair the judgment of the physician.
7. **Psychiatric and psychological factors: Anxiety**. Situational anxiety associated with flying is recognized as a clinical disorder as defined by the *International Classification of Diseases, Tenth Revision, Clinical Modification* (*ICD-10-CM* F40.243). Fear of flying appears to be less related to the experience of flight per se, but rather directed against more common psychological triggers embedded within the experience (e.g., heights, confined spaces).[23] The signs and symptoms of acute situational anxiety (e.g., tachycardia, tachypnea, hyperventilation, chest pain, disorientation, altered sensation) can make a differential diagnosis difficult because these symptoms may be shared with significantly more morbid pathologies, such as pulmonary embolism. Among smokers in flight, the enforced nicotine withdrawal[24] can provoke symptoms of "nervousness, craving for tobacco, tension-anxiety, fatigue, difficulty in concentration, decrease in alertness, disorders of fine adjustments, prolonged reaction times, anger-irritability, drowsiness, increase in appetite, and impairment of judgement" (p. 247). The same study found that "all tests recorded an impairment of cognitive functions during abstinence" (p. 247).[25] This can affect medical professionals, potential patients, and even flight crew. **Inebriation**. Availability and social conventions surrounding the consumption of alcohol both in flight and prior to flying may compound and encourage certain passengers to disregard prudent limits on alcohol intake.[26] Contrary to popular belief, however, the cabin pressure altitude itself does not influence the pharmacokinetics or pharmacodynamics of alcohol in the body.[27] Consumption of any given amount of alcohol produces an equivalent blood alcohol level whether at sea level or at cabin pressure altitude. It is true that both high altitude and alcohol consumption do decrease performance on a Multiple Task Performance Battery, but this effect is simply additive rather than synergistic in any physiological sense.[28] **Psychiatric Emergencies.** Most medical professionals do not routinely encounter acute psychiatric decompensation in their clinical practice. Therefore, acute psychiatric emergencies are particularly challenging for the nonpsychiatrist to manage, even within their usual work environment. An aircraft cabin offers no privacy or quiet and no means of segregating the psychiatrically impaired patient. Acutely psychotic patients can pose a hazard to themselves, other passengers, flight crew, and the aircraft. Patients who cause risk and require restraining, either physically or chemically, pose difficult challenges given the layout of an aircraft cabin and the limited availability of drugs and trained assistants.[29]
8. **Vibration**: Particularly in older and smaller aircrafts, vibration may increase the metabolic rate in a patient equivalent to the level of gentle exercise.
9. **Inertial forces**: Acceleration and deceleration along the longitudinal axis during takeoff and landing have the potential to be detrimental to a patient with head or spinal cord trauma. Having the patient's head facing aft during flight, when possible, may help in this regard. Furthermore, a patient needs to be secured with extra padding on vulnerable areas.

The US airlines have been required since 1998 to carry basic first aid kits and also an expanded in-flight medical kit for use by medical professionals.[10] Additionally, an automated external defibrillator (AED) has been required since April 2004 (Reference 1, paragraph 6.2.4). The mandated minimum contents of these kits are shown in Table 36.1. The kits are tailored for use by the general practitioner without training in emergency airway management as there is a concern that mandating medications and equipment that require specialized training may lead to harm.[30] Airlines may provide more than the minimum equipment, and the airline Qantas does provide intubating equipment on long-haul flights.[19]

Of concern to anesthesiologists may be the need to maintain an unprotected airway for a protracted period of time in an unconscious or unresponsive patient when definitive airway management equipment is unavailable. Supplemental oxygen is almost always available for use, although the devices by which it can be administered may be limited to a simple face mask or nasal cannula.

In summary, anesthesiologists responding to an in-flight request for medical assistance should consider the following recommendations (modified from Reference 31):

1. Properly identify yourself and state your medical qualifications. Some airlines require proof of your medical qualifications.
2. Obtain as complete a history as possible, inform the passenger and family members (if present) of your impression, and obtain consent before initiating any form of examination or treatment. Assume implied consent in the case of an incapacitated passenger.
3. If consent has been given, carry out an appropriate physical examination.
4. Request an interpreter if the passenger you are assisting does not speak your language.

(*Continued*)

TABLE 36.1 Mandated Minimum Medical Equipment for US Airlines

FIRST AID KITS

According to the new rule for aircraft registered in the United States, there must be one to four onboard first-aid kits depending on the number of passenger seats. In general, each first-aid kit must contain the following:

CONTENTS	QUANTITY
Adhesive bandage compresses, 1 inch	16
Antiseptic swabs	20
Ammonia inhalants	10
Bandage compresses, 4 inch	8
Triangular bandage compresses, 40 inch	5
Arm splint, noninflatable	1
Leg splint, noninflatable	1
Roller bandages 4 inch	4
Adhesive tape, 1-inch standard roll	2
Bandage scissors	1

EMERGENCY MEDICAL KIT

CONTENTS	QUANTITY
Sphygmomanometer	1
Stethoscope	1
Airways, oropharyngeal (3 sizes): 1 pediatric, 1 small adult, 1 large adult or equivalent	3
Self-inflating manual resuscitation device with 3 masks (1 pediatric, 1 small adult, 1 large adult or equivalent)	3
Cardiopulmonary resuscitation mask (3 sizes): 1 pediatric, 1 small adult, 1 large adult or equivalent	3
Intravenous administration set: tubing with 2 Y connectors	1
Alcohol sponges	2
Adhesive tape, 1-inch standard roll adhesive	1
Tape scissors	1 pair
Tourniquet	1

EMERGENCY MEDICAL KIT

CONTENTS	QUANTITY
Saline solution, 500 mL	1
Protective nonpermeable gloves or equivalent	1 pair
Needles (two 18 gauge, two 20 gauge, two 22 gauge, or sizes necessary to administer required medications)	6
Syringes (one 5 mL, two 10 mL, or sizes necessary to administer required medications)	4
Analgesic, nonnarcotic, tablets, 325 mg	4
Antihistamine tablets, 25 mg	4
Antihistamine injectable, 50 mg (single-dose ampoule or equivalent)	2
Atropine, 0.5 mg, 5 mL (single-dose ampoule or equivalent)	2
Aspirin tablets, 325 mg	4
Bronchodilator, inhaled (metered dose inhaler or equivalent)	4
Dextrose, 50%/50 mL injectable (single-dose ampoule or equivalent)	1
Epinephrine 1:1000, 1 mL, injectable (single-dose ampoule or equivalent)	2
Epinephrine 1;10,000, 2 mL, injectable (single-dose ampoule or equivalent)	2
Lidocaine, 5 mL, 20 mg/mL, injectable (single-dose ampoule or equivalent)	2
Nitroglycerin tablets, 0.4 mg	10
Basic instructions for use of the drugs in the kit	1

SOURCE: 105th US Congress, "Aviation Medical Assistance Act of 1998," HR2843 ed Pub L No 105-170: 1998.

5. Inform the flight crew of your clinical impression.
6. Establish communication with on-ground medical support staff, if available.
7. If the passenger's condition is serious, request that the aircraft be diverted to the nearest appropriate airport. On-ground medical support staff, if available, will help determine the best location for diversion.
8. Respect the ground-based physician's expertise and experience in managing in-flight medical events.
9. Document in writing your findings, impression, treatment, and communication with the flight crew and on-ground medical support.
10. Do not use any treatment that you do not feel confident administering. Keep in mind that Good Samaritan statutes protect you only from liability for actions that other competent persons with similar training would take under similar circumstances.

REFERENCES

1. International Air Transport Association. *Medical Manual.* 9th ed. Montreal, Canada: International Air Transport Association; 2016.
2. Association of Air Medical Services. *Guidelines for Air Medical Crew Education.* Dubuque, IA: Kendall/Hunt; 2004.
3. Hurd WW, Jernigan JG. *Aeromedical Evacuation: Management of acute and Stabilized Patients.* New York, NY: Springer; 2003.
4. Martin T. *Aeromedical Transportation: A Clinical Guide.* 2nd ed. Aldershot, England: Ashgate; 2006.

5. Booth MG, Quasim I, Kinsella J. In-flight medical emergencies: response of anaesthetists who were passengers on commercial flights. *Eur J Anaesthesiol.* 1999;16:840–841.
6. Dowdall N. Is there a doctor on the aircraft? Top 10 in-flight medical emergencies. *BMJ.* 2000;321:1336–1337.
7. Goodwin T. In-flight medical emergencies: an overview. *BMJ.* 2000;321:1338–1341.
8. Hordinsky JR, George MH. *Utilization of Emergency Kits by Air Carriers.* Oklahoma City, OK: Civil Aeromedical Institute; 1991. DOT/FAA/AM-9.
9. *Convention on Offences and Certain Other Acts Committed on Board Aircraft.* Tokyo, Japan: United Nations; 1963. Available as of November 8, 2017 at: https://treaties.un.org/doc/db/terrorism/conv1-english.pdf.
10. Aviation Medical Assistance Act of 1998, Pub L No. 105-170, ed, 1998.
11. *Stovin v. Wise*, ed: 3 WLR 388.
12. DeLaune EF III, Lucas RH, Illig P. In-flight medical events and aircraft diversions: one airline's experience. *Aviat Space Environ Med.* 2003;74:62–68.
13. Cummins RO, Schubach JA. Frequency and types of medical emergencies among commercial air travelers. *JAMA.* 1989;261:1295–1299.
14. Harding RM, Mills FJ. Medical emergencies in the air. In: *Aviation Medicine.* London, England: BMJ; 1993:7–24.
15. Donaldson E, Pearn J. First aid in the air. *Aust N Z J Surg.* 1996;66:431–434.
16. Davies GR, Degotardi PR. Inflight medical facilities. *Aviat Space Environ Med.* 1982;53:694–700.
17. Speizer C, Rennie CJ III, Breton H. Prevalence of in-flight medical emergencies on commercial airlines. *Ann Emerg Med.* 1989;18:26–29.
18. Cottrell JJ, Callaghan JT, Kohn GM, Hensler EC, Rogers RM. In-flight medical emergencies. One year of experience with the enhanced medical kit. *JAMA.* 1989;262:1653–1656.
19. Cocks R, Liew M. Commercial aviation in-flight emergencies and the physician. *Emerg Med Australasia.* 2007;19:1–8.
20. Geva A, Clark JJ, Zhang Y, Popowicz A, Manning JM, Neufeld EJ. Hemoglobin Jamaica plain—a sickling hemoglobin with reduced oxygen affinity. *N Engl J Med.* 2004;351:1532–1538.
21. Wallace TW, Wong T, O'Bichere A, Ellis BW. Managing in flight emergencies. *BMJ.* 1995;311:374–376.
22. Cheatham ML, Safcsak K. Air travel following traumatic pneumothorax: when is it safe? *Am Surg.* 1999;65:1160–1164.
23. Hawkins-Gilligan J, Dygdon JA, Conger AJ. Examining the nature of fear of flying. *Aviat Space Environ Med.* 2011;82:964–971.
24. Allen ME. Nicotine withdrawal at 10,000 m. *CMAJ.* 1986;135:194.
25. Giannakoulas G, Katramados A, Melas N, Diamantopoulos I, Chimonas E. Acute effects of nicotine withdrawal syndrome in pilots during flight. *Aviat Space Environ Med.* 2003;74:247–251.
26. Girasek DC, Olsen CH. Airline passengers' alcohol use and its safety implications. *J Travel Med.* 2009;16:311–316.
27. Higgins EA, Vaughan JA, Funkhouser GE. Blood alcohol concentrations as affected by combinations of alcoholic beverage dosages and altitudes. *Aerosp Med.* 1970;41:1129–1132.
28. Collins WE, Mertens H1, Higgins EA. Some effects of alcohol and simulated altitude on complex performance scores and breathalyzer readings. *Aviat Space Environ Med.* 1987;58:328–332.
29. Wheeler S, Wong B, L'Heureux R. Criteria for sedation of psychiatric patients for air transport in British Columbia. *BC Med J.* 2009;51:346–349.
30. McKenas DK. First, do no harm: the role of defibrillators and advanced medical care in commercial aviation. *Aviat Space Environ Med.* 1997;68:365–367.
31. Newson-Smith MS. Passenger doctors in civil airliners—obligations, duties and standards of care. *Aviat Space Environ Med.* 1997;68: 1134–1138.

37 | THE FUTURE OF NORA

DONALD M. MATTHEWS, MD

INTRODUCTION

Non–operating room anesthesia (NORA) is a very young field of anesthesia practice. The idea of a text concerning NORA would have seemed unlikely as recently as 5 years ago. So, prognosticating about the future of NORA has potential pitfalls. Most particularly, the pace of change in medical practice can be rapid, especially if a disruptive or innovative technology is introduced. Nonetheless, certain predications can be made based on the rapid evolution of NORA. It will be interesting to look back in 30 years to see what percentage of these predications prove to be accurate.

NORA: THE SPECIALTY OF THE FUTURE

Anesthesiologists have been involved in NORA-type care, particularly in the gastrointestinal (GI) area, for a number of years. The understanding that anesthesia practice is different in the NORA areas compared with the traditional operating room has slowly been increasing. This is primarily in response to the growth in the volume of patient care in the disparate areas of NORA care, increases that have been well documented elsewhere in this volume. It is clear that there are administrative, clinical, and educational challenges in the NORA areas that require approaches that differ from traditional thinking. As such, there is a need to identify the best approaches to these challenges instead of expecting each anesthesiologist or group of anesthesiologists to figure this out independently.

Indeed, organized anesthesiology is beginning to take on these challenges. The annual meeting of the American Society of Anesthesiologists (ASA) has an increasing number of NORA-related sessions as has the ASA Practice Management meeting. SAMBA, the Society for Ambulatory Anesthesia, has included NORA topics in its meetings and educational material. Most interesting is the emergence of a new society, SONORIA, the Society of Non OR Intervention and Anesthesia. This group seeks to bring together both the proceduralists and the anesthesiologists to "create and establish interdisciplinary standards, best practice guidelines, educational platforms, and economic constructs which optimize outcome and the safety of patients undergoing Non-OR procedures requiring the collaborative efforts of interventional medical proceduralists and anesthesiologists."[1] The first meeting was held in Knoxville, Tennessee, in May 2016. It is quite likely that this society will grow and exert influential leadership in NORA expansion.

While practicing anesthesiologists have acquired their NORA knowledge "on the fly," today's residents will have a different introduction. That is because the Accreditation Council for Graduate Medical Education Program Requirements for Graduate Medical Education in Anesthesiology were amended in 2016 to include a requirement that "residents must have at least two weeks of experience managing the anesthetic care of patients undergoing diagnostic or therapeutic procedures outside of the surgical suite."[2] This is in addition to a requirement graduating residents "must demonstrate appropriate medical knowledge in the topics related to the anesthetic care of patient management of the specific needs of patients undergoing diagnostic or therapeutic procedures outside of the surgical suite."[2] Residency training programs are meeting the requirements by adding didactic material and by establishing clinical rotations in NORA areas. Interestingly, some programs, such as mine at the University of Vermont College of Medicine, assign residents to directly care for patients (with the required supervision of the faculty of not more than 2:1). Other programs that staff the NORA areas with a ratio greater than 1:2 cannot allow direct patient care by the residents and instead have them help supervise the care by certified registered nurse anesthetists (CRNAs; or anesthesia assistants [AAs]). Both types of experiences are valid learning opportunities. In the future, training programs will evolve to offer more time and research opportunities in the NORA area. Fellowships in NORA will be developed, and as patient complexity increases, NORA subspecialties will evolve, such as in pediatric NORA or NORA/critical care.

Departmental structure will change in the future. In most academic departments, NORA has typically gotten little attention from departmental leadership. Those who have been asked to assume leadership roles have often found it a thankless task with little allotted administrative time. This has started to change as some departments are restructuring to create NORA divisions that are the equivalent of the other academic divisions, and the leadership has received time to administer their responsibilities. This trend will continue. In private practice, groups will be asked to provide more service in more of these areas. As there is usually inefficiency in providing care in NORA areas, groups will have to carefully plan how to provide these services and seek appropriate "capacity" remuneration from their health care facilities.[3,4]

Research opportunities will grow. Operating room management and metrics will be tailored to improve care in the NORA spaces. Large databases will increasingly be used to provide benchmarks for safety, quality, and productivity.[5] Clinical research careers will increasingly focus on the NORA areas providing crucial information about advances in monitoring, airway management, and drug development and delivery devices. We will see the creation of "*The Journal of NORA*," or the current journals will contain a section specifically devoted to NORA research.

NORA FACILITIES OF THE FUTURE

Facilities will have to evolve to accommodate NORA care growth in both the volume and the complexity of the procedures. In most centers, these spaces tend to be retrofitted, squeezing increasing amounts of technology into spaces designed for simpler procedures from the past. Anesthesiologists find that these spaces are not designed with anesthesia care in mind: There is limited room for equipment and no thought about the ergonomics of anesthesia delivery. It is essential that anesthesiologists be involved in the planning of future NORA procedure rooms.

There is also great inefficiency in current NORA space design. NORA sites are typically geographically sited widely across a medical center. This makes it difficult to provide adequate supervision. In addition, it makes no sense to replicate patient intake and recovery areas for various NORA functions in multiple locations of a medical center. It would certainly be much easier (and less expensive) to provide anesthesia services if these areas were consolidated. A blueprint for the future can be found at the University of Chicago Medicine Center for Care and Discovery. There, NORA areas are consolidated on a single floor that contains dedicated areas for bronchoscopy, interventional radiology, cardiac catheterization, magnetic resonance imaging (MRI), radiology, and GI endoscopy (Figure 37.1). There is a common intake/prep and recovery space that can flex between the functions as the day's workload changes (Tom Cutter, oral personal communication, October 26, 2016). This type of combined procedural workspace is very forward thinking and will be emulated in other centers.

Many GI endoscopy centers are free standing. There is a conceptual argument to bring other NORA work out of the hospital and create freestanding, ambulatory NORA centers, such as an interventional radiology ambulatory surgicenter.[6] This will occur if the economics favor such a practice.

THE NORA PATIENTS OF THE FUTURE

Extrapolating from current trends in patients undergoing NORA care, predictions can be made about the patients of the future. First, there will be more of them. They will be older as the population ages, and they will fall into two broad groups. One, with access to resources, such as fresh food and healthy lifestyles, will be increasingly healthy as they age. A second group, particularly those affected by the worsening obesity epidemic, will have more comorbidities and will be more difficult to care for. In fact, NORA centers for the morbidly obese with appropriate size tables, scanners, and equipment may be developed. Patients will live longer with chronic diseases as biologic agents and gene therapies extend longevity. The 80-year-old patient with cystic fibrosis may arrive in your bronchoscopy suite. There will be a continued push to care for the extremes of clinical illness as less-invasive procedures are developed that will be more survivable than the operative procedures they replace. Increases in palliative care will also increase the number of patients in the ASA 4 and 5 categories. All told, these changes will increase the complexity of the "average" NORA patient and will be of increasing challenge to the anesthesiology care team.

THE NORA PROCEDURES OF THE FUTURE

All of the fields that make up current NORA practice are burgeoning with creativity and are seeing rapid development. The trends are toward increased miniaturization of devices and therapeutic agents, such as the use of nanoparticles; new uses of radiation, such as phototherapy; novel uses of ultrasound; and increased reliance on robotics. More and more clinical conditions that previously had surgical indications are now cared for in the NORA area. This trend will accelerate. Consider the combined effect that the development of coronary stent placement and transcatheter aortic valve replacement (TAVR)

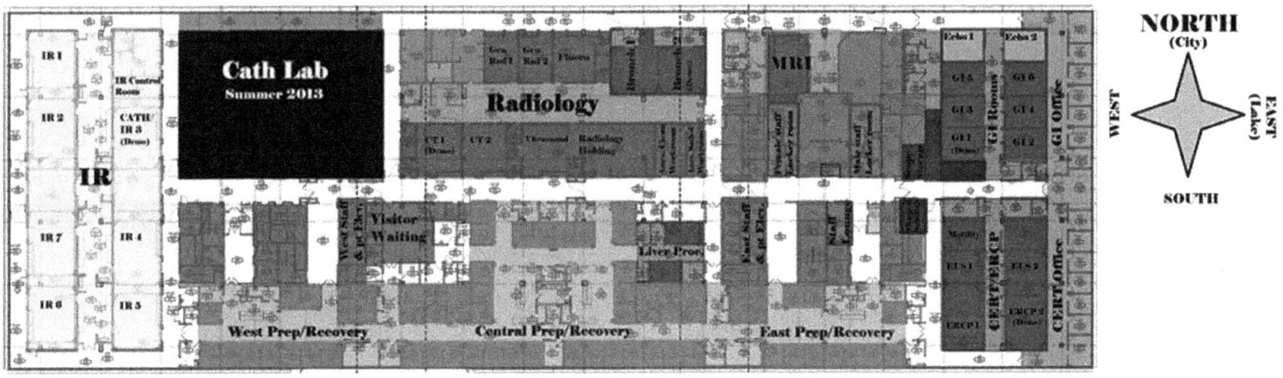

Figure 37.1. The Center University of Chicago Medicine Center for Care and Discovery. The floor contains dedicated areas for bronchoscopy, interventional radiology (IR), cardiac catheterization, magnetic resonance imaging (MRI), radiology, and gastrointestinal (GI) endoscopy. There is a common intake/prep and recovery space. CERT, community emergency response team; ERCP, endoscopic retrograde cholangiopancreatography.

has had on the practice of cardiac surgery. The sternal saw may soon be relegated to the museum shelf. Many lung cancers that previously required a thoracotomy for diagnosis are now being diagnosed in the bronchoscopy suite. Prostate cancer can be treated by cryotherapy in the interventional radiology suite.[7] As these examples demonstrate, the operating room of the future will be fairly empty and will consist of surgeries that the proceduralists have not yet figured out how to bring to the NORA suites.

Endoscopic techniques will continue to evolve. Flexible endoscopes will revolutionize the field of laparoscopic surgery. Small incisions in body cavities will be made and these new endoscopes will be highly maneuverable and will largely replace laparoscopic surgery; these will be done with monitored anesthesia care (MAC) or conscious sedation.[8] Natural orifice transluminal endoscopic surgery (NOTES) will continue to evolve. In this procedure, an incision is made after passing an endoscope through a "natural orifice" (mouth, vulva, urethra, anus), allowing the proceduralist access to the abdominal cavity, where they can perform procedures such as an appendectomy or cholecystectomy. A recent meta-analysis revealed an equivalent complication profile between transvaginal NOTES cholecystectomy compared to a laparoscopic approach.[9] Furthermore, microrobots are being developed that will allow NOTES procedures to be done under sedation.[10]

Gastrointestinal endoscopy will continue to evolve. Endoscopic procedures will render laparoscopic obesity surgery obsolete: An endoscopic sleeve barrier has been developed to replicate the physiologic changes of bariatric surgery with good reported results.[11] Traditionally, achalasia was treated with surgical myotomy. Through per oral endoscopic myotomy (POEM), excellent clinical results are achieved without surgery.[12] Attention is turning to the possibilities offered by endoscopes that can operate in the submucosal space (Figure 37.2). This technique is already being used to remove submucosal lesions, but there are other potential applications, such as drug delivery, biopsy of nerve and muscle, and placement of stimulating and monitoring devices.[8] This will open a whole new field of therapies for motility disorders currently have no endoscopic indications.

The interventional radiology suite will see increased growth with developments in embolization, chemoembolization, gene therapy, tumor ablation, and magnetic resonance guidance.[13] Nano- and microparticle development will lead to revolutionary therapies. These agents can be imaged, can have specific receptor targets, and can carry drugs or genes.[14] Via small capillaries, they can deliver sustained release of an agent directly to the target sites. Or, for stenting procedures, they can be combined with stents to decrease restenosis.[15] Microbubbles or liposomes containing gene therapy–associated viral vectors also hold a great degree of promise. On delivery to the target organ, ultrasound energy is used to disrupt the particles, releasing agent to the target site.[16] Photodynamic therapies are also emerging in clinical practice. Here, a sensitor agent is infused at a target organ and then "activated" by a specific wavelength of light, producing reactive oxygen species and resulting in cell death. Reported uses include the treatment of prostate cancer[17] and cholangiocarcinoma.[18] It is not clear what role the anesthesiologist will have as these procedures develop; however, whenever patient quiescence is essential, anesthesiology care will be required.

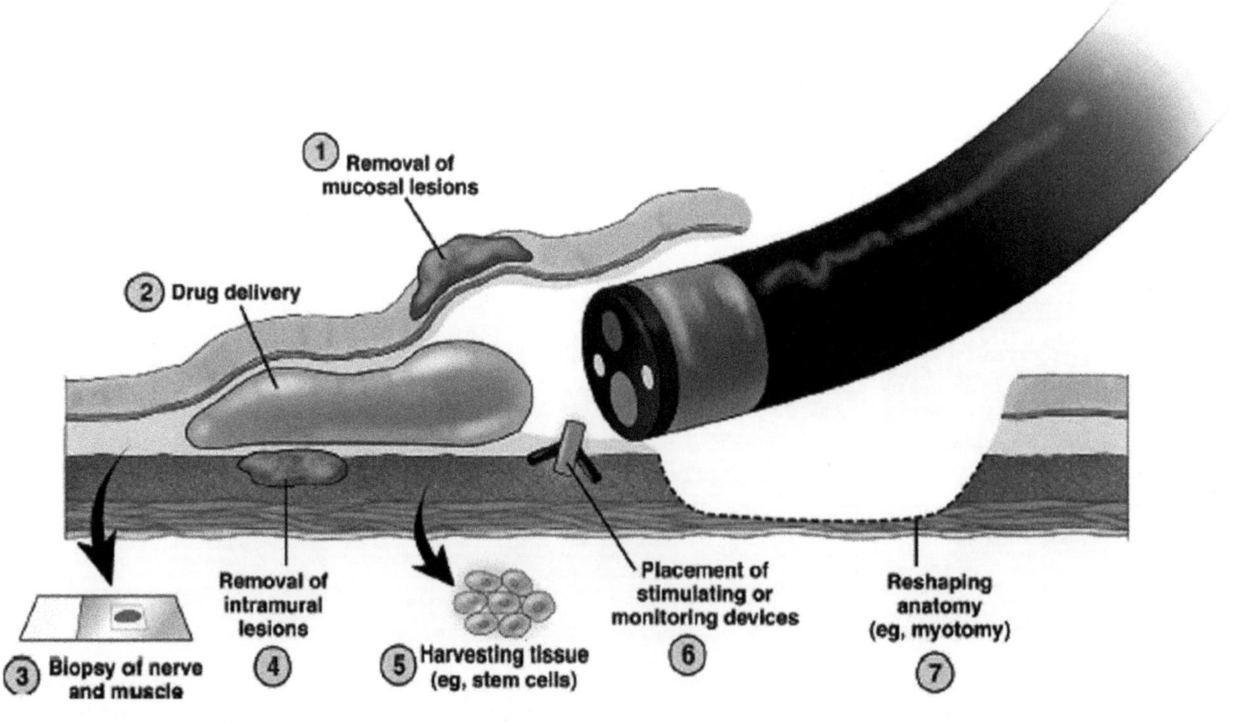

Figure 37.2. Illustration of the possibilities for endoscopic intervention in the submucosal ("third") space. (From reference 8, used with permission.)

All NORA areas will see an increase of robotics. The qualities of maneuverability that have made the da Vinci robot so popular in the operating room will find utility in the NORA suites; the technology has already been employed in the interventional radiology area.[19] Proceduralists of the future will not need to be physically present: combining robotics with the Internet and ultrarapid fiber-optic communications will allow proceduralists to care for patients at distant locations. While not yet widely adopted, "telesurgery" in the operating rooms has been described.[20]

NORA MONITORING OF THE FUTURE

Monitoring for NORA will evolve. When providing sedation, most practitioners rely on clinical signs to judge the adequacy of the state of sedation. However, to really do this properly requires that the patient be stimulated periodically to see if he or she responds to the stimulus. Processed electroencephalography (EEG) monitors might be used instead as continuous information can be provided without the need for stimulation. However, these monitors are not often utilized, partly because there is a lack of correlation between processed EEG index value and the state of sedation.[21] Understanding of the EEG changes associated with general anesthesia is accelerating.[22] Similar understanding about the characteristic EEG changes associated with different depths of sedation will follow. The anesthesiologist of the future will not need a processed EEG index but will be able to observe real-time EEG variables to determine the depth of patient sedation.

Respiratory monitoring will evolve as well. The current controversy between the ASA and the American Gastrointestinal Society in standards for capnography during moderate and deep sedation for endoscopic procedures will be resolved, probably with the adoption of the ASA's standards. Improvements in capnography will continue. Other respiratory monitors will evolve as well. Examples include enhancements in thoracic impedance monitoring[23] and acoustic monitoring of the airway.[24] Combinations of EEG and respiratory monitoring may evolve; such combinations have already been shown to result in fewer alarm events and less respiratory depression.[25]

NORA AIRWAY MANAGEMENT OF THE FUTURE

When one looks closely at current NORA anesthesia practice, many practitioners intend to deliver deep sedation but are, in actuality, delivering general anesthesia with a natural airway (GANA).[26] Patient outcomes are usually positive, as airway management is a core skill set of the specialty. There is some emerging signal, however, that current anesthesia practice has led to complications, such as an increased risk of aspiration pneumonia following colonoscopy.[27] Deep propofol sedation clearly leads to conditions that inhibit airway protection.[28] The risk-benefit evaluation of airway management in NORA will probably evolve. For NORA procedures that require "sedation," GANA will be avoided by maintaining in a state of moderate sedation, perhaps by using evolving EEG technology, thereby allowing patients to protect their own airway. If deeper anesthesia is required, an airway device will be inserted, recognizing the risks associated with each particular device. To decrease the morbidity of endotracheal intubation, videolaryngoscopy will become the standard of care. Supraglottic devices will evolve to allow improved isolation of the respiratory tree from the alimentary canal during upper GI endoscopy. One example is the recently released Gastro™ Airway LMA from Teleflex (Figure 37.3). It includes a port specifically designed to pass a working endoscope.

NORA MEDICATIONS OF THE FUTURE

While propofol has become most utilized medication in NORA sedation, it is not a perfect agent. It can cause significant airway compromise and respiratory depression, there is considerable pain on injection, and its ability to support bacterial growth requires close vigilance for the timing of administration following its withdrawal from sterile containers. There will be continued development of pharmaceutical agents that will have a role in NORA. Some of these new agents will be modifications of current classes of medication, altered to have shorter context-sensitive half-times. Novel agents will be developed as better understanding of the targeted receptors emerge, particularly the γ-aminobutyric acid (GABA) receptor.[29]

Remimazolam is a short-acting midazolam analogue that is rapidly metabolized due to a labile ester linkage allowing

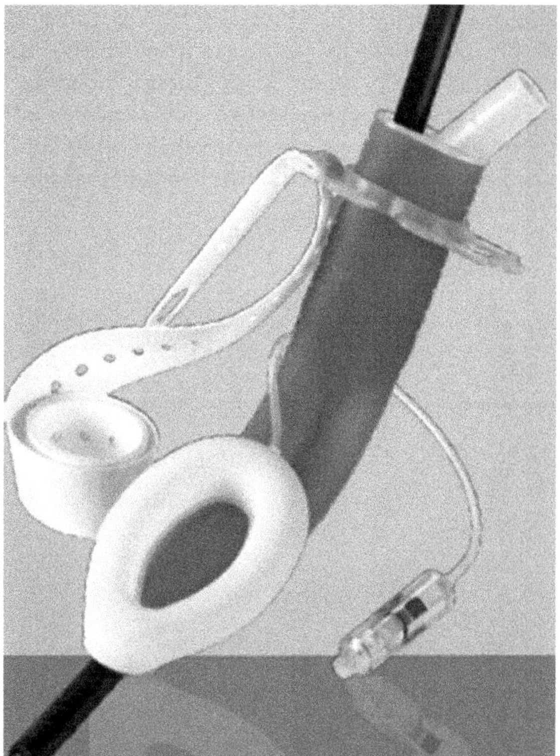

Figure 37.3. The LMA® Gastro™ Airway from Teleflex, Incorporated. It contains a channel for a working endoscope.

degradation by nonspecific esterases.[30,31] Compared with an equipotent dose of midazolam, the recovery time is four times faster, 10 versus 40 minutes.[32] The clinical effect can be reversed with flumazenil within about a minute.[33] The agent has reached phase 2 clinical trials, showing encouraging results: Following 100 μg fentanyl, sedation for colonoscopy was successful with remimazolam in 92% of patients compared with 75% with midazolam (p = .007).[34] Remimazolam will soon be in phase 3 trails and could reach the market within several years. It has the potential to supplant midazolam in a manner similar to the way midazolam replaced diazepam in clinical practice. Its short half-life, however, will require repeated intravenous boluses or delivery by infusion. As such, it will probably be best utilized by anesthesiology personnel.

JM-1232 is a novel nonbenzodiazepine that binds to the $GABA_A$ receptor in a manner similar to classic benzodiazepines and can be reversed by flumazenil. Interestingly, in rats it has been demonstrated to have antinociceptive properties that are reversed by flumazenil but not naloxone.[35] In a 1% aqueous formulation (MR04A3) in healthy male volunteers, it caused rapid sedation and, at higher doses, evidenced a state of general anesthesia (no response to painful stimulation), an effect that lasted up to 50 minutes following a 10-minute infusion.[36] In addition, there was minimal hemodynamic perturbation. Possible antinociceptive properties have not been investigated in humans. This agent could be very useful as, unlike propofol, if does not seem to cause pain on injection, it has a faster clinical onset than midazolam; if indeed it has antinociceptive properties in humans, it could obviate the need for opioid coadministration.

There are several etomidate analogues that are under development and that could emerge as effective NORA agents of the future (Figure 37.4). These are intentionally designed to limit the effect of etomidate's well-known inhibition of 11 β-hydroxylase and suppression of adrenal corticosteroid production.[37] Methoxycarbonyl etomidate (MOC-etomidate) has an ester linkage (like esmolol and remifentanil) that allows for rapid hydrolysis.[38] MOC-etomidate appears to be very favorable compared with etomidate in terms of speed of recovery and lack of adrenal suppression following bolus administration or short infusion.[38] With longer infusions, however, the recovery profile slows, probably due to accumulation of a metabolite that has activity at the GABA receptor.[39]

Further synthetic work has led to the development of other etomidate esters designed to have less effect from metabolites.[40] One of these agents, cyclopropyl MOC-etomidate (CPMM) seems promising: In rats, following a 2-hour infusion, hypnotic recovery occurred in 4.2 minutes compared with 31 minutes for etomidate.[41] Adrenal suppression was significantly less than seen with etomidate, and adrenal responsiveness returned to baseline values within 30 minutes.[42] Clinical trials in humans have begun; it was judged to be safe and well tolerated following a single bolus injection of doses up to 1.0 mg/kg with no evidence of adrenal suppression.[43] It is likely that this agent, currently called ABP-700 and manufactured by the Medicines Company (Parsippany, NJ), will reach clinical practice.

All of the compounds considered thus far are derivatives of known anesthetic agents. Eckenhoff and colleagues have reported their initial success in a novel approach to identifying new compounds that have anesthetic properties.[44] They screened 350,000 compounds for anesthetic potential using the fluorescent anesthetic 1-aminoanthracene and apoferritin as a surrogate anesthetic protein target. One class of compounds, the 6-phenylpyridazin-3(2H)-one chemotype, emerged with great potential. Through medicinal chemistry, four compounds were identified to cause immobility with minimal toxicity in tadpoles. When these four compounds were injected in mice, two had no clinical effect, but two caused loss of righting reflex with no apparent toxicity. If more preclinical studies are favorable, these agents may undergo clinical trials in humans.

Not all the effort in drug development is dedicated to hypnotic agents. Development of opioid and other analgesic drugs is burgeoning, with the goal of creating agents with fewer side

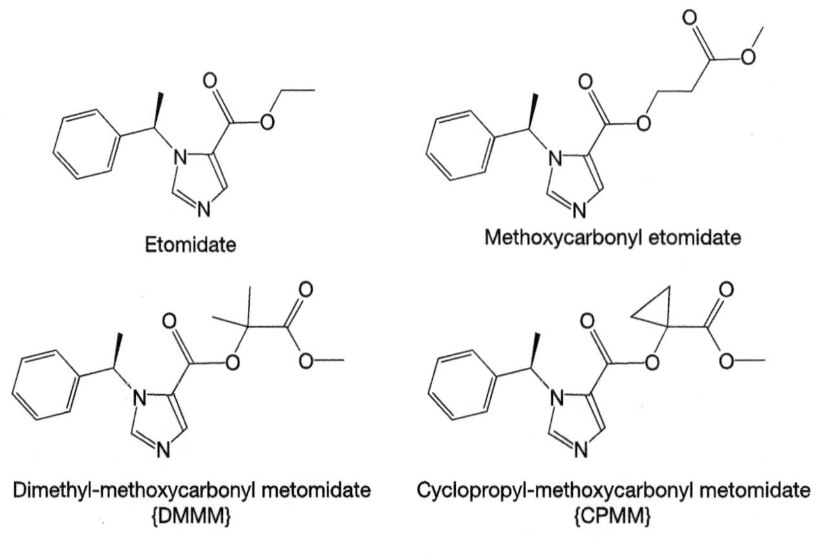

Figure 37.4. Analogues of etomidate, including methoxycarbonyl (MOC) etomidate and cyclopropyl-methoxycarbonyl metomidate (CPMM), being tested commercially as ABV-700. (From ref 37 used with permission.)

effects than current medications. One approach is to develop selective agents that activate the μ-receptor G protein pathway, which conveys analgesia while sparing the β-arrestin pathway, which causes side effects, such as respiratory depression.[45] One such agent, PMZ21, has been recently described with exceptional selectivity for μ-receptor G protein activation and minimal β-arrestin recruitment.[46] Another medication with similar properties, TRV130 (Oliceridine, Trevena Inc., King of Prussia, PA) has reached clinical trials in humans. Following bunionectomy, TRV130 produced significantly greater pain relief than morphine after the first dose of each, with meaningful pain relief occurring in less than 5 minutes, and with no serious adverse events.[47] Another approach is to develop agents that are agonists at the μ receptors as well as the nociceptin/orphanin FQ peptide (NOP) receptor. Cebranopadol (Grünenthal GmbH, Stolberg, Germany) is the first agent of this class to reach human trials. [48] In mice, it produces profound analgesia with fewer side effects and less development of tolerance compared with morphine.[49]

For all of these developmental agents, it remains to be seen which will enter clinical practice and what role they will play in NORA care. It is likely that there will be a role if they provide better control with faster patient throughput and with fewer side effects than our current medications.

NORA MEDICATION DELIVERY OF THE FUTURE

The most revolutionary care in NORA drug delivery will be the ascendance of personalized, genomic medicine.[50,51] Patients will have their entire DNA sequence analyzed. This will allow understanding of the receptor subtypes that they express and about the robustness of their metabolic pathways. Based on this information, caregivers will be able to select the most appropriate medications and dosage for the individual.[52] Population variability will decrease allowing better outcomes, fewer side effects and faster throughput.

It is interesting that all of the new agents listed previously are intravenous medications; there does not seem to be developmental work occurring in the inhalational anesthetic arena. Intravenous medications, obviously, can be delivered by intravenous bolus or by infusions. As newer agents, with shorter half-lives, reach clinical practice, those who prefer to deliver intermittent boluses will find it difficult to maintain a steady level of sedation; infusion techniques will prove to be more stable.

The most sophisticated intravenous delivery system is the target-controlled infusion (TCI) pump. This technology is available in most of the world except in the United States.[53] This will change in the future when one of the TCI pump manufacturers gains approval from the Food and Drug Administration (FDA) and thereby allow US patients the benefits of this technology. TCI pumps contain a library of pharmacokinetic (Pk) models that allows caregivers to select a targeted plasma or, more usefully, a targeted effect site (brain) concentration. One selects a model, enters the model's required demographic information, selects a target concentration, and pushes a button. The pump delivers a bolus and begins an infusion calculated to achieve the targeted concentration and then readjusts the infusion rate, typically every 10 seconds, to maintain the targeted level. Adjustments can be made by the caregiver: When a decrease is selected, the pump suspends the infusion for a calculated period of time and then resumes at a lower rate than previously given. When an increase is selected, a bolus is administered, and a new, higher, infusion rate is instituted. As TCI pump infusions are based on population models, there are inherent inaccuracies between the targeted and actual concentrations. However, when measured, plasma values usually with 20% of targeted level and actually show less variability than seen in bolus techniques.[54]

Target-controlled infusion pump infusions are already being utilized for NORA care. In the GI suite, propofol TCI can be effectively utilized and has been studied compared to manual infusion. During combined upper and lower endoscopy, use of propofol TCI resulted in faster arousal times, less hypotension, and fewer moderate oxygen desaturations.[55] The median effective target concentrations for propofol in the elderly colonoscopy patient were determined to be 3.08, 2.75, and 2.05 μg mL^{-1} following fentanyl boluses of 0, 0.5, and 1.0 μg kg^{-1} fentanyl, respectively (Figure 37.5).[56] In the bronchoscopy suite, propofol TCI has been investigated to titrate sedation for fiber-optic bronchoscopy.[57] Opioids may be delivered by TCI as well: In colonoscopy patients, the addition of remifentanil TCI to a propofol TCI resulted in better clinical outcomes than the addition of manual administration of remifentanil.[58] In the trauma patient undergoing "awake" fiber-optic intubation, remifentanil TCI had better clinical results than manual remifentanil administration.[59] TCI will become a very popular technique to maintain stable states of sedation.

Propofol TCI has been combined with patient-controlled sedation (PCS) in several NORA arenas, demonstrating interesting future uses. In these systems, the patient can increase the targeted level by a preprogrammed increment by pushing a button; some systems require a double button push.[60] There are time lockouts and maximal allowed targeted concentrations. In one study, 16 out of 20 patients successfully underwent endoscopic retrograde cholangiopancreatography (ERCP) with a propofol TCI-PCS system; in three, the maximal target was reached and was inadequate, and one procedure was aborted due to patient confusion.[61] For colonoscopy, propofol TCI-PSC systems demonstrated highly acceptable clinical results.[62,63] While TCI itself has great future promise in the care of the NORA patient, the future of TCI-PCS is less clear. These devices are effective; however, they require that the patient take responsibility for his or her level of sedation, a responsibility that patients may not be willing to assume.

The TCI systems of the future will be more sophisticated. Sensors will be developed that can measure plasma concentrations of the delivered agents in real time, allowing true personalization of the underlying Pk model. Devices that measure end-tidal propofol concentrations are under development.[64] EEG technology will improve to allow close effect site monitoring of the pharmocodynamic effect of anesthetic agents; these will improve model performance as well.

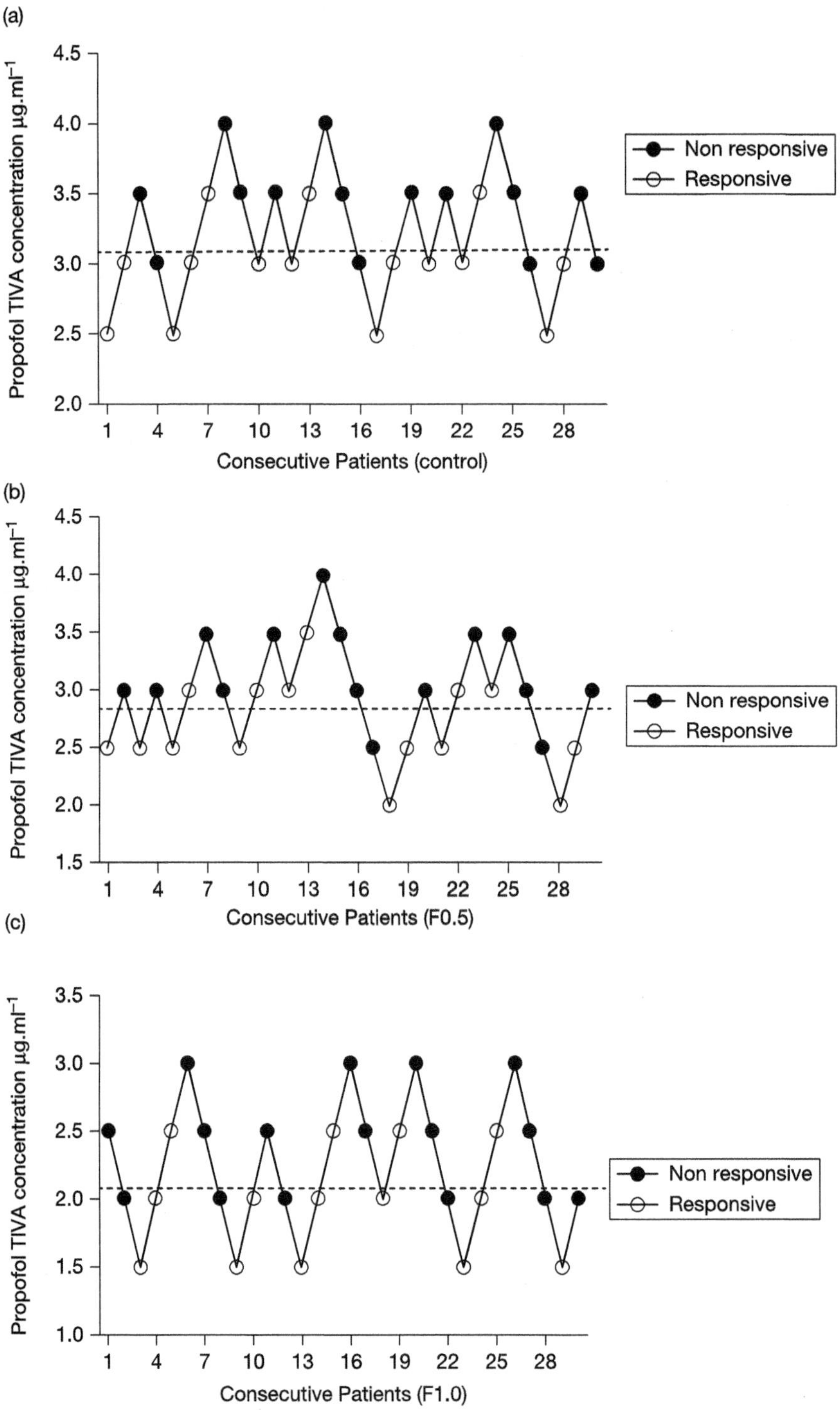

Figure 37.5. *Dixon up-down plots of the median targeted plasma concentration for successful colonoscopy in elderly patients. A, no fentanyl; B, fentanyl 0.5 μg kg^{-1}; C, fentanyl 1.0 μg kg^{-1}. TIVA, total intravenous anesthesia. (From reference 56, used with permission.)*

AUTOMATED NORA CARE OF THE FUTURE

Perhaps the largest potential disrupter of the future of anesthesia care is the creation of an automated anesthesia delivery system, or a closed-loop system. Several have been described in the literature.[65] Typically, they combine a processed EEG monitor, most utilize the bispectral index monitor (BIS; Medtronic, Minneapolis, MN), with a proportional-integral-derivative (PID) algorithm and a TCI pump to deliver propofol. A target BIS index value is chosen, and the system continually monitors how far the measured value deviates from the set point. The PID algorithm determines what adjustments are needed in the TCI delivery of the sedating agent. Multiple investigators have reported clinical outcomes using their technology, including Struys, DeSmet, and coworkers,[66] Liu et al.,[67] Puri et al.,[68] Bibian et al.,[69] and Hemmerling et al.[70] The Liu system is particularly interesting in that it has controllers for both propofol and remifentanil (Figure 37.6), and it has been successfully used in the care of thousands of patients in a research consortium of hospitals in France (Ngai Liu, oral personal communication, October 24, 2016). Clinical results have been reported for "routine" operative patients,[67] obese patients,[71] pediatric patients,[72] and liver[73] and lung[74] transplant patients.

The Sedasys™ system is an automated propofol delivery device that was intended to be operated by the proceduralist. It has recently been withdrawn by Ethicon from the marketplace due to slow sales.[75] The system, however, is interesting in that it combines elements of TCI and closed-loop care without actually being either.[76] A propofol bolus is administered and an infusion is started. The infusion rate is largely determined on how quickly the patient responds to an instruction through an earpiece to push a button on a handheld device.[77] The handheld device vibrates with each command. Should the patient not respond, the system stops the propofol infusion. The system is designed to maintain a state of light-to-moderate sedation. In the one major clinical trial in the literature during colonoscopy and upper GI endoscopy patients, it was reported to do this successfully with fast times to discharge readiness.[78] The reason that the device was unsuccessful in the marketplace is probably multifactorial. Arguably, a device targeted toward moderate sedation might not succeed in an environment where deep sedation is the clinical expectation.[79] Vigorous concerns about the safety of the device from organized anesthesiology concerns certainly created headwinds as well.

It might be tempting to dismiss the potential disruptive threat of closed-loop anesthesia delivery as an interesting research tool that will never reach clinical practice in the NORA arena. Perhaps the withdrawal of the Sedasys system from the marketplace provides solace. Perhaps the difficulty in defining a processed-EEG endpoint that correlates with each level of sedation, mentioned previously, may prove daunting. It should be noted, however, that a closed-loop sedation system has recently been successfully utilized in the care of patients undergoing sedation for transcatheter aortic valve implantation (TAVI).[80] The reality, in my opinion, is that technological progress in inevitable and unstoppable. With well-designed and thoroughly tested safety and ergonomic features, closed-loop systems will bring great benefit to patients and the heath care system. Anesthesiologists will need a new set of skills to understand these systems, to use them properly, and to intervene when appropriate. I would expect, by the year 2047, closed-loop systems for anesthesia delivery will be widespread in the operating rooms and NORA suites around the world.

CONCLUSIONS ABOUT THE FUTURE OF NORA

Predicting the future is probably a fool's errand, and forecasting the state of NORA care 30 years from now is certainly challenging. However, the growth of NORA is reminiscent of the time 30 years ago when ambulatory anesthesia emerged as a field of anesthesiology, prompted by the rapid ascendance of the ambulatory surgery center (ASC). Today, approximately 65% of most anesthesia patient care is for the ambulatory (or short-stay) patient.[81] It is likely that the trends that are moving care from the operating room to the NORA areas will accelerate, creating a disruption as large as the development of the ASC.

By the year 2047, anesthesiologists will care for 60% or more of their patients in the NORA suites of the future. They will care for patients undergoing procedures yet to be created with rapid-acting medications, some of which are currently under development. The medications will be

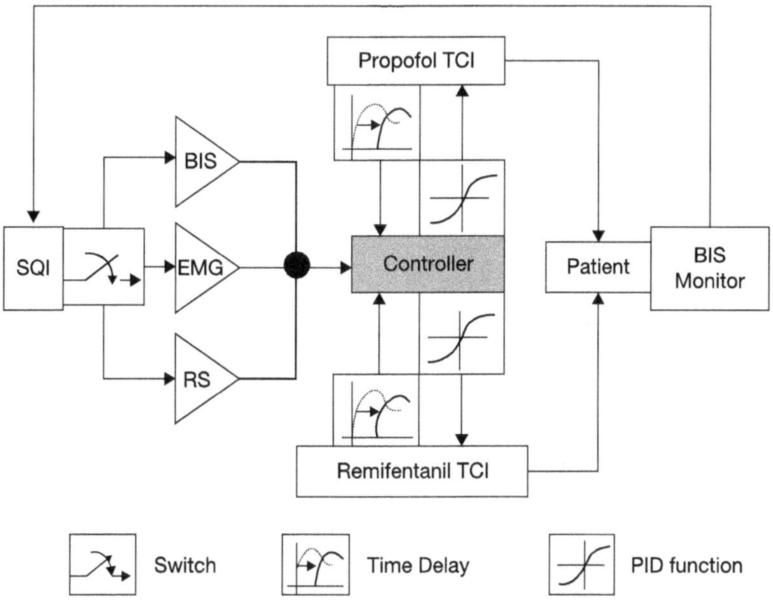

Figure 37.6. *A dual-loop controller for propofol and remifentanil. The operator sets a target bispectral index (BIS) value. The controller, with proportional-integral-derivative (PID) algorithms, adjusts the propofol and remifentanil target-controlled infusion (TCI) levels to maintain the set value. EMG, electromyography. (Details in reference 67, used with permission.)*

specifically selected based on the individual's genetic and metabolic profile. Improved monitoring and enhanced TCI devices with closed-loop delivery systems will be utilized. Technologic developments and robotics will allow the care of multiple patients at the same time, perhaps from a distant location. Despite all of these changes, one thing will remain the same: Anesthesiologists will continue to be vigilant and vigorous defenders of a patient's safety, ensuring that these developments occur in a safe manner.

REFERENCES

1. Society of Non OR Intervention and Anesthesia website. Available at: https://sonoria.org/. Accessed December 22, 2016.
2. Accreditation Council for Graduate Medical Education. Program Requirements for Graduate Medical Education in Anesthesiology. Available at: https://www.acgme.org/Portals/0/PFAssets/ProgramRequirements/040_anesthesiology_2017-07-01.pdf. page 22, Effective July 1, 2016. Revised Common Program Requirements effective July 1, 2017. Accessed on December 22, 2016.
3. Wu A, Sanford JA, Tsai MH, O'Donnell SE, Tran BK, Urman RD. Analysis to establish differences in efficiency metrics between operating room and non-operating room anesthesia cases. *J Med Syst*. 2017;41(8):120.
4. Tsai MH, Huynh TT, Breidenstein MW, O'Donnell SE, Ehrenfeld JM, Urman RD. A system-wide approach to physician efficiency and utilization rates for non-operating room anesthesia sites. *J Med Syst*. 2017;41(7):112.
5 Nagrebetsky A, Gabriel RA, Dutton RP, Urman RD. Growth of nonoperating room anesthesia care in the United States: a contemporary trends analysis. *Anesth Analg*. 2017;124(4):1261–1267.
6. Weiss MF, Kronawitter C. Is there an interventional radiology ASC (irASC) in your future? *Radiol Bus*. April 19, 2016. Available at: http://www.radiologybusiness.com. Accessed on December 23, 2016.
7. Onik G. Percutaneous image-guided prostate cancer treatment: cryoablation as a successful example. *Tech Vasc Interv Radiol*. 2007;10(2):149–158.
8. Pasricha PJ1. Endoscopy 20 years into the future. *Clin Gastroenterol Hepatol*. 2013;11(2):119–122.
9. Peng C1, Ling Y, Ma C, et al. Safety outcomes of NOTES cholecystectomy versus laparoscopic cholecystectomy: a systematic review and meta-analysis. *Surg Laparosc Endosc Percutan Tech*. 2016;26(5):347–353.
10. Forgione A. In vivo microrobots for natural orifice transluminal surgery. Current status and future perspectives. *Surg Oncol*. 2009;18(2):121–129.
11. Schouten R, Rijs CS, Bouvy ND, et al. A multicenter, randomized efficacy study of the EndoBarrier Gastrointestinal Liner for presurgical weight loss prior to bariatric surgery. *Ann Surg*. 2010;251(2):236–243.
12. Chiu PW, Inoue H, Rösch T. From POEM to POET: applications and perspectives for submucosal tunnel endoscopy. *Endoscopy*. 2016;48(12):1134–1142.
13. Tapping CR, Bratby MJ. The changing face of vascular interventional radiology: the future role of pharmacotherapies and molecular imaging. *Cardiovasc Intervent Radiol*. 2013;36(4):904–912.
14. Yang X. Nano- and microparticle-based imaging of cardiovascular interventions: overview. *Radiology*. 2007;243(2):340–347.
15. Kolodgie FD, John M, Khurana C, et al. Sustained reduction of in-stent neointimal growth with the use of a novel systemic nanoparticle paclitaxel. *Circulation*. 2002;106(10):1195–1198.
16. Sirsi SR, Borden MA. Advances in ultrasound mediated gene therapy using microbubble contrast agents. *Theranostics*. 2012;2(12):1208–1222.
17. Swartling J, Axelsson J, Ahlgren G, et al. System for interstitial photodynamic therapy with online dosimetry: first clinical experiences of prostate cancer. *J Biomed Opt*. 2010;15(5):058003. doi: 10.1117/1.3495720.
18. Ortner MA. Photodynamic therapy for cholangiocarcinoma: overview and new developments. *Curr Opin Gastroenterol*. 2009;25(5):472–476.
19. Kassamali RH, Ladak B. The role of robotics in interventional radiology: current status. *Quant Imaging Med Surg*. 2015;5(3):340–343.
20. Marescaux J, Leroy J, Rubino F, et al. Transcontinental robot-assisted remote telesurgery: feasibility and potential applications. *Ann Surg*. 2002;235(4):487–492.
21. Sheahan CG, Mathews DM. Monitoring and delivery of sedation. *Br J Anaesth*. 2014;113(suppl 2):ii37–ii47.
22. Purdon PL, Sampson A, Pavone KJ, Brown EN. Clinical electroencephalography for anesthesiologists: Part I: Background and basic signatures. *Anesthesiology*. 2015;123(4):937–960.
23. Voscopoulos C, Brayanov J, Ladd D, Lalli M, Panasyuk A, Freeman J. Special article: evaluation of a novel noninvasive respiration monitor providing continuous measurement of minute ventilation in ambulatory subjects in a variety of clinical scenarios. *Anesth Analg*. 2013;117(1):91–100.
24. Ramsay MA, Usman M, Lagow E, Mendoza M, Untalan E, De Vol E. The accuracy, precision and reliability of measuring ventilatory rate and detecting ventilatory pause by rainbow acoustic monitoring and capnometry. *Anesth Analg*. 2013;117(1):69–75.
25. Applegate RL 2nd, Lenart J, Malkin M, et al. Advanced monitoring is associated with fewer alarm events during planned moderate procedure-related sedation: a 2-part pilot trial. *Anesth Analg*. 2016;122(4):1070–1078.
26. Goudra B, Singh PM, Gouda G, Borle A, Carlin A, Yadwad A. Propofol and non-propofol based sedation for outpatient colonoscopy-prospective comparison of depth of sedation using an EEG based SEDLine monitor. *J Clin Monit Comput*. 2016;30(5):551–557.
27. Cooper GS, Kou TD, Rex DK. Complications following colonoscopy with anesthesia assistance: a population-based analysis. *JAMA Intern Med*. 2013;173(7):551–556.
28. Gemma M, Pasin L, Oriani A, et al. Swallowing impairment during propofol target-controlled infusion. *Anesth Analg*. 2016;122(1):48–54.
29. Tanious MK, Beutler SS, Kaye AD, Urman RD. New hypnotic drug development and pharmacologic considerations for clinical anesthesia. *Anesthesiol Clin*. 2017;35(2):e95–e113.
30. Kilpatrick GJ, McIntyre MS, Cox RF, et al. CNS 7056: a novel ultra-short-acting benzodiazepine. *Anesthesiology*. 2007;107(1):60–66.
31. Wesolowski AM, Zaccagnino MP, Malapero RJ, Kaye AD, Urman RD. Remimazolam: pharmacologic considerations and clinical role in anesthesiology. *Pharmacotherapy*. 2016;36(9):1021–1027.
32. Antonik LJ, Goldwater DR, Kilpatrick GJ, Tilbrook GS, Borkett KM. A placebo- and midazolam-controlled phase I single ascending-dose study evaluating the safety, pharmacokinetics, and pharmacodynamics of remimazolam (CNS 7056): Part I. Safety, efficacy, and basic pharmacokinetics. *Anesth Analg*. 2012;115(2):274–283.
33. Worthington MT, Antonik LJ, Goldwater DR, et al. A phase Ib, dose-finding study of multiple doses of remimazolam (CNS 7056) in volunteers undergoing colonoscopy. *Anesth Analg*. 2013;117(5):1093–1100.
34. Pambianco DJ, Borkett KM, Riff DS, et al. A phase IIb study comparing the safety and efficacy of remimazolam and midazolam in patients undergoing colonoscopy. *Gastrointest Endosc*. 2016;83(5):984–992.
35. Chiba S1, Nishiyama T, Yamada Y. The antinociceptive effects and pharmacological properties of JM-1232(-): a novel isoindoline derivative. *Anesth Analg*. 2009;108(3):1008–1014.
36. Sneyd JR, Rigby-Jones AE, Cross M, et al. First human administration of MR04A3: a novel water-soluble nonbenzodiazepine sedative. *Anesthesiology*. 2012;116(2):385–395.
37. de Jong FH, Mallios C, Jansen C, Scheck PA, Lamberts SW. Etomidate suppresses adrenocortical function by inhibition of 11 beta-hydroxylation. *J Clin Endocrinol Metab*. 1984;59(6):1143–1147.
38. Cotten JF, Husain SS, Forman SA, et al. Methoxycarbonyl-etomidate: a novel rapidly metabolized and ultra-short-acting etomidate analogue that does not produce prolonged adrenocortical suppression. *Anesthesiology*. 2009;111(2):240–249.
39. Pejo E1, Ge R, Banacos N, Cotten JF, Husain SS, Raines DE. Electroencephalographic recovery, hypnotic emergence, and the effects of metabolite after continuous infusions of a rapidly metabolized etomidate analog in rats. *Anesthesiology*. 2012;116(5):1057–1065.
40. Husain SS, Pejo E, Ge R, Raines DE. Modifying methoxycarbonyl etomidate inter-ester spacer optimizes in vitro metabolic stability and in vivo hypnotic potency and duration of action. *Anesthesiology*. 2012;117(5):1027–1036.
41. Ge R, Pejo E, Husain SS, Cotten JF, Raines DE. Electroencephalographic and hypnotic recoveries after brief and prolonged infusions of etomidate and optimized soft etomidate analogs. *Anesthesiology*. 2012;117(5):1037–1043.
42. Ge R, Pejo E, Cotten JF, Raines DE. Adrenocortical suppression and recovery after continuous hypnotic infusion: etomidate versus its soft analogue cyclopropyl-methoxycarbonyl metomidate. *Crit Care*. 2013;17(1):R20.
43. Meyer P, Sweeney SP, den Daas I, et al. Safety, pharmacokinetics, and pharmacodynamics of ABP-700: a novel intravenous anesthetic. *Anesthesiology*. 2015;123:A3012.
44. McKinstry-Wu AR, Bu W, Rai G, et al. Discovery of a novel general anesthetic chemotype using high-throughput screening. *Anesthesiology*. 2015;122(2):325–333.

45. Burford NT, Traynor JR, Alt A. Positive allosteric modulators of the μ-opioid receptor: a novel approach for future pain medications. *Br J Pharmacol.* 2015;172(2):277–286.
46. Manglik A, Lin H, Aryal DK, et al. Structure-based discovery of opioid analgesics with reduced side effects. *Nature.* 2016;537(7619):185–190.
47. Viscusi ER, Webster L, Kuss M, et al. A randomized, phase 2 study investigating TRV130, a biased ligand of the μ-opioid receptor, for the intravenous treatment of acute pain. *Pain.* 2016;157(1):264–272.
48. Lambert DG, Bird MF, Rowbotham DJ. Cebranopadol: a first in-class example of a nociceptin/orphanin FQ receptor and opioid receptor agonist. *Br J Anaesth.* 2015;114(3):364–366.
49. Linz K, Christoph T, Tzschentke TM, et al. Cebranopadol: a novel potent analgesic nociceptin/orphanin FQ peptide and opioid receptor agonist. *J Pharmacol Exp Ther.* 2014;349(3):535–548.
50. Saba R, Kaye AD, Urman RD. Pharmacogenomics in pain management. *Anesthesiol Clin.* 2017 Jun;35(2):295–304.
51. Saba R, Kaye AD, Urman RD. Pharmacogenomics in anesthesia. *Anesthesiol Clin.* 2017;35(2):285–294.
52. Body SC. Genomics: implications for anesthesia, perioperative care and outcomes. *Adv Anesth.* 2009;27(1):73–94.
53. Absalom AR, Glen JI, Zwart GJ, Schnider TW, Struys MM. Target-controlled infusion: a mature technology. *Anesth Analg.* 2016;122(1):70–78.
54. Hu C, Horstman DJ, Shafer SL. Variability of target-controlled infusion is less than the variability after bolus injection. *Anesthesiology.* 2005;102(3):639–645.
55. Chiang MH, Wu SC, You CH, et al. Target-controlled infusion vs. manually controlled infusion of propofol with alfentanil for bidirectional endoscopy: a randomized controlled trial. *Endoscopy.* 2013;45(11):907–914.
56. Li S, Yu F, Zhu H, Yang Y, Yang L, Lian J. The median effective concentration (EC50) of propofol with different doses of fentanyl during colonoscopy in elderly patients. *BMC Anesthesiol.* 2016;16:24.
57. Lin TY, Lo YL, Hsieh CH, et al. The potential regimen of target-controlled infusion of propofol in flexible bronchoscopy sedation: a randomized controlled trial. *PLoS One.* 2013;8(4):e62744.
58. Moerman AT, Herregods LL, De Vos MM, Mortier EP, Struys MM. Manual versus target-controlled infusion remifentanil administration in spontaneously breathing patients. *Anesth Analg.* 2009;108(3):828–834.
59. Yeganeh N, Roshani B, Azizi B, Almasi A. Target-controlled infusion of remifentanil to provide analgesia for awake nasotracheal fiberoptic intubations in cervical trauma patients. *J Trauma.* 2010;69(5):1185–1190.
60. Irwin MG, Thompson N, Kenny GN. Patient-maintained propofol sedation. Assessment of a target-controlled infusion system. *Anaesthesia.* 1997;52(6):525–530.
61. Gillham MJ, Hutchinson RC, Carter R, Kenny GN. Patient-maintained sedation for ERCP with a target-controlled infusion of propofol: a pilot study. *Gastrointest Endosc.* 2001;54(1):14–17.
62. Campbell L, Imrie G, Doherty P, et al. Patient maintained sedation for colonoscopy using a target controlled infusion of propofol. *Anaesthesia.* 2004;59(2):127–132.
63. Stonell CA, Leslie K, Absalom AR. Effect-site targeted patient-controlled sedation with propofol: comparison with anaesthetist administration for colonoscopy. *Anaesthesia.* 2006;61(3):240–247.
64. Takita A, Masui K, Kazama T. On-line monitoring of end-tidal propofol concentration in anesthetized patients. Anesthesiology. 2007;106(4):659–664.
65. Dumont GA, Ansermino JM. Closed-loop control of anesthesia: a primer for anesthesiologists. *Anesth Analg.* 2013;117(5):1130–1138.
66. Struys MM, De Smet T, Versichelen LF, Van De Velde S, Van den Broecke R, Mortier EP. Comparison of closed-loop controlled administration of propofol using Bispectral Index as the controlled variable versus "standard practice" controlled administration. *Anesthesiology.* 2001;95(1):6–17.
67. Liu N, Chazot T, Hamada S, et al. Closed-loop coadministration of propofol and remifentanil guided by bispectral index: a randomized multicenter study. *Anesth Analg.* 2011;112(3):546–557. doi:10.1213/ANE.0b013e318205680b. Epub 2011 Jan 13.
68. Puri GD, Kumar B, Aveek J. Closed-loop anaesthesia delivery system (CLADS) using bispectral index: a performance assessment study. *Anaesth Intensive Care.* 2007 Jun;35(3):357–362.Links
69. Bibian S, Dumont GA, Black I. Closed-loop target-controlled infusion systems: stability and performance aspects. *Mil Med.* 2015;180(3)(suppl):96–103.
70. Hemmerling TM, Charabati S, Zaouter C, Minardi C, Mathieu PA. A randomized controlled trial demonstrates that a novel closed-loop propofol system performs better hypnosis control than manual administration. *Can J Anaesth.* 2010;57(8):725–735.
71. Liu N, Lory C, Assenzo V, et al. Feasibility of closed-loop co-administration of propofol and remifentanil guided by the bispectral index in obese patients: a prospective cohort comparison. *Br J Anaesth.* 2015;114(4):605–614.
72. Orliaguet GA, Benabbes Lambert F, Chazot T, Glasman P, Fischler M, Liu N. Feasibility of closed-loop titration of propofol and remifentanil guided by the bispectral monitor in pediatric and adolescent patients: a prospective randomized study. *Anesthesiology.* 2015;122(4):759–767.
73. Restoux A, Grassin-Delyle S, Liu N, Paugam-Burtz C, Mantz J, Le Guen M. Pilot study of closed-loop anaesthesia for liver transplantation. *Br J Anaesth.* 2016;117(3):332–340.
74. Liu N, Chazot T, Trillat B, et al. Closed-loop control of consciousness during lung transplantation: an observational study. *J Cardiothorac Vasc Anesth.* 2008;22(4):611–615.
75. J&J to stop selling automated sedation system Sedasys. *Wall Street J.* March 16, 2016. Available at: https://www.wsj.com/articles/j-j-to-stop-selling-automated-sedation-system-sedasys-1457989723, Accessed on December 30, 2016.
76. Urman RD, Maurer WG. Computer-assisted personalized sedation: friend or foe? *Anesth Analg.* 2014;119(1):207–211.
77. Urman RD, Maurer WG. Computer-assisted personalized sedation: friend or foe? *Anesth Analg.* 2014;119(1):207–211.
78. Pambianco DJ, Vargo JJ, Pruitt RE, Hardi R, Martin JF. Computer-assisted personalized sedation for upper endoscopy and colonoscopy: a comparative, multicenter randomized study. *Gastrointest Endosc.* 2011;73(4):765–772.
79. Goudra B, Singh PM. Failure of Sedasys: destiny or poor design? *Anesth Analg.* 2016 Nov 17. [Epub ahead of print]
80. Zaouter C, Hemmerling TM, Mion S, Leroux L, Remy A, Ouattara A. Feasibility of automated propofol sedation for transcatheter aortic valve implantation: a pilot study. *Anesth Analg.* 2016 Dec 22. [Epub ahead of print]
81. Weir LM, Steiner CA, Owens PL. Surgeries in hospital-owned outpatient facilities, 2012. Statistical brief 188. Available at: https://www.hcup-us.ahrq.gov/reports/statbriefs/sb188-Surgeries-Hospital-Outpatient-Facilities-2012.pdf. Published February 2015. Accessed on December 29, 2016.

APPENDIX 1 | PREUSE CHECKING OF ANESTHESIA EQUIPMENT

FRANCIS SPAULDING, MD, CHRISTOPHER V. MAANI, MD

A major contributory cause of anesthesia misadventure has been the use of anesthesia machines or breathing systems that have not been adequately checked by an anesthesiologist before use. The following is the US Food and Drug Administration (FDA) recommended preuse checkout procedure.

ANESTHESIA APPARATUS CHECKOUT RECOMMENDATIONS, ROCKVILLE, MD: US FOOD AND DRUG ADMINISTRATION, 1993

This anesthesia apparatus checkout, or a reasonable equivalent, should be conducted prior to the administration of anesthesia. These recommendations are only valid for an anesthesia system that conforms to current and relevant standards and includes an ascending bellows ventilator and at least the following monitors: capnograph, pulse oximeter, oxygen analyzer, respiratory volume monitor (spirometer), and breathing system pressure monitor with high- and low-pressure alarms. This is a guideline that users are encouraged to modify to accommodate differences in equipment design and variations in local clinical practice. Such local modifications should undergo appropriate peer review. Users should refer to the operator's manual for the manufacturer's specific procedures and precautions, especially the manufacturer's low-pressure leak test (step 5).

EMERGENCY VENTILATION EQUIPMENT

*1. Verify that backup ventilation equipment is available and functioning.

HIGH-PRESSURE SYSTEM

*2. Check oxygen cylinder supply.

a. Open O_2 cylinder and verify at least half full (about 1000 psi).

b. Close cylinder.

*3. Check central pipeline supplies.

a. Check that hoses are connected and pipeline gauges read about 50 psi.

LOW-PRESSURE SYSTEM

*4. Check initial status of low-pressure system.

a. Close flow control valves and turn vaporizers off.

b. Check fill level and tighten vaporizer's filler caps.

* 5. Perform leak check of machine low-pressure system.

a. Verify that the machine master switch and flow control valves are OFF.

b. Attach "suction bulb" to common (fresh) gas outlet.

c. Squeeze bulb repeatedly until fully collapsed.

d. Verify bulb stays fully collapsed for at least 10 seconds.

e. Open one vaporizer at a time and repeat "c" and "d" as above.

f. Remove suction bulb and reconnect fresh gas hose.

*6. Turn on machine master switch and all other necessary equipment.

*7. Test flowmeters.

a. Adjust flow of all gases through their full range, checking for smooth operation of floats and undamaged flowtubes.

b. Attempt to create a hypoxic O_2/N_2O mixture and verify correct changes in flow and/or alarm.

SCAVENGING SYSTEM

*8. Adjust and check scavenging system.

a. Ensure proper connections between the scavenging system and both Adjustable Pressure Limiting (APL) (pop-off) valve and ventilator relief valve.

b. Adjust waste gas vacuum (if possible).

c. Fully open APL valve and occlude Y piece.

d. With minimum O_2 flow, allow scavenger reservoir bag to collapse completely and verify that absorber pressure gauge reads about zero.

e. With the O_2 flush activated, allow the scavenger reservoir bag to distend fully and then verify that absorber pressure gauge reads < 10 cm H_2O.

BREATHING SYSTEM

*9. Calibrate O_2 monitor.

a. Ensure monitor reads 21% in room air.

b. Verify low O_2 alarm is enabled and functioning.

c. Reinstall sensor in circuit and flush breathing system with O_2.

d. Verify that monitor now reads greater than 90%.

10. Check initial status of breathing system.

a. Set selector switch to "bag" mode.

b. Check that breathing circuit is complete, undamaged, and unobstructed.

c. Verify that CO_2 absorbent is adequate.

d. Install breathing circuit accessory equipment (e.g., humidifier, PEEP valve) to be used during the case.

11. Perform leak check of the breathing system.

a. Set all gas flows to zero (or minimum).

b. Close APL (pop-off) valve and occlude Y piece.

c. Pressurize breathing system to about 30 cm H_2O with O_2 flush.

d. Ensure that pressure remains fixed for at least 10 seconds.

e. Open APL (pop-off) valve and ensure that pressure decreases.

MANUAL AND AUTOMATIC VENTILATION SYSTEMS

*12. Test ventilation systems and unidirectional valves.

a. Place a second breathing bag on Y piece.

b. Set appropriate ventilator parameters for next patient.

c. Switch to automatic ventilation (Ventilator) mode.

d. Fill bellows and breathing bag with O_2 flush and then turn ventilator ON.

e. Set O_2 flow to minimum, other gas flows to zero.

f. Verify that during inspiration bellows delivers appropriate tidal volume and that during expiration bellows fills completely.

g. Set fresh gas flow to about 5 L/min.

h. Verify that the ventilator bellows and simulated lungs fill and empty appropriately without sustained pressure at end expiration.

i. Check for proper action of unidirectional valves.

j. Exercise breathing circuit accessories to ensure proper function.

k. Turn ventilator OFF and switch to manual ventilation (Bag/APL) mode.

l. Ventilate manually and ensure inflation and deflation of artificial lungs and appropriate feel of system resistance and compliance.

m. Remove second breathing bag from Y piece.

MONITORS

13. Check, calibrate, and/or set alarm limits of all monitors:

a. Capnometer

b. Oxygen analyzer

c. Pressure monitor with high and low airway alarms

d. Pulse oximeter

e. Expiratory volume monitor (Spirometer)

FINAL POSITION

14. Check final status of machine

a. Vaporizers off

b. APL valve open

c. Selector switch to "Bag"

d. All flowmeters to zero

e. Patient suction level adequate

f. Breathing system ready to use

* If an anesthesia provider uses the same machine in successive cases, these steps (1 to 9) do not need to be repeated or may be abbreviated after the initial checkout.

AUTOMATED CHECKOUT

Clinicians often fail to check their equipment thoroughly, are not successful in detecting machine faults, or do not check their machines at all. Despite extensive instruction, anesthesia residents, at best, could only perform 81% of a checkout procedure. Hence, automated checkout is incorporated in newer machines (Datex-Ohmeda S/5 ADU, Dräger Julian, NM 6000, Fabius GS). They are unique in having a system checkout routine that is electronic and automated. The operator follows instructions to activate flows of gases, occlude the breathing circuit during the leak check, switch from manual to mechanical ventilation, open and close the pop-off valve, or manually check various functions (suction or emergency oxygen cylinder supply). It covers all the steps of the FDA checklist. The system checkout is logged, but it may be bypassed in an emergency.

Despite these automated procedures, not every fault, obstruction, crossed connection, disconnection, or incompetent valve may be detected. It may not be obvious to the clinician regarding what the machine is testing. Hence, in addition to automated checkouts, anesthesiologists must develop appropriate manual checklists to suit the apparatus being used. The anesthesia delivery systems have evolved to the point that one checkout procedure is not applicable to all anesthesia delivery systems currently on the market. Hence, the ASA (American Society of Anesthesiologists) Subcommittee on Equipment and Facilities in 2008 recommended a template for developing checkout procedures that are appropriate for each individual anesthesia machine design and practice setting (Table A1.1 and Table A1.2). Items that are not evaluated by the automated checkout need to be identified and supplemental manual checkout procedures included as needed. Adaptation of the preanesthesia checkout to local needs, assignment of responsibility for the checkout procedures, and training are the responsibilities of the individual anesthesia department. The guidelines also offer suggestions on which tasks must be performed by providers and which may be delegated. These guidelines and examples of institution-specific procedures for current anesthesia delivery systems are available on the ASA website (see listing at the end of this appendix).

In 2012 and 2016, respectively, the Association of Anaesthetists of Great Britain and Ireland (AAGBI) and the Canadian Anesthesiologists' Society released similar checklists, both citing the ASA's updated checklist. Major changes to the AAGBI checklist from 2004 included a recommendation to perform a "two-bag test." This test includes attaching a bag to the patient end of the tubing, setting flows to 5 L/minute, and ventilating manually to ensure both inspiratory and expiratory valves are functioning. Then, both bags are squeezed to test APL valve. Last, fresh gas flows are turned off or set to minimal settings, and each vaporizer is opened and closed while monitoring for a loss in volume in the circuit that may suggest a leak. While newer machines perform leak tests as part of their automated checkout, they will miss leaks at the vaporizer unless each one is opened in turn and the test is repeated. This test allows the provider to manually ensure that they are able to provide positive pressure ventilation.

TABLE A1.1. Summary of Checkout Recommendations by Frequency and Responsible

PARTY (TO BE COMPLETED DAILY).

ITEM TO BE COMPLETED	RESPONSIBLE PARTY
Item 1: Verify auxiliary oxygen cylinder and self-inflating manual ventilation device are available and functioning.	Provider and tech
Item 2: Verify patient suction is adequate to clear the airway.	Provider and tech
Item 3: Turn on anesthesia delivery system and confirm that ac power is available.	Provider or tech
Item 4: Verify availability of required monitors, including alarms.	Provider or tech
Item 5: Verify that pressure is adequate on the spare oxygen cylinder mounted on the anesthesia machine.	Provider and tech
Item 6: Verify that the piped gas pressures are ≥ 50 psig.	Provider and tech
Item 7: Verify that vaporizers are adequately filled and, if applicable, that the filler ports are tightly closed.	Provider or tech
Item 8: Verify that there are no leaks in the gas supply lines between the flowmeters and the common gas outlet.	Provider or tech
Item 9: Test scavenging system function.	Provider or tech
Item 10: Calibrate, or verify calibration of, the oxygen monitor and check the low oxygen alarm.	Provider or tech
Item 11: Verify carbon dioxide absorbent is not exhausted.	Provider or tech
Item 12: Breathing system pressure and leak testing.	Provider and tech
Item 13: Verify that gas flows properly through the breathing circuit during both inspiration and exhalation.	Provider and tech
Item 14: Document completion of checkout procedures.	Provider and tech
Item 15: Confirm ventilator settings and evaluate readiness to deliver anesthesia care. (ANESTHESIA TIME OUT)	Provider

Overall, the ASA guidelines summarize the overarching principles of safe anesthetic delivery as reliable delivery of oxygen to any appropriate concentration up to 100%, reliable means of positive pressure ventilation, reliable backup ventilation equipment (immediately available and functioning), controlled release of positive pressure from breathing circuit,

TABLE A1.2. *Summary of Checkout Recommendations by Frequency and Responsible Party* (TO BE COMPLETED PRIOR TO EACH PROCEDURE)

ITEM TO BE COMPLETED	RESPONSIBLE PARTY
Item 2: Verify patient suction is adequate to clear the airway.	Provider and tech
Item 4: Verify availability of required monitors, including alarms.	Provider or tech
Item 7: Verify that vaporizers are adequately filled and if applicable that the filler ports are tightly closed.	Provider
Item 11: Verify carbon dioxide absorbent is not exhausted.	Provider or tech
Item 12: Breathing system pressure and leak testing.	Provider and tech
Item 13: Verify that gas flows properly through the breathing circuit during both inspiration and exhalation.	Provider and tech
Item 14: Document completion of checkout procedures.	Provider and tech
Item 15: Confirm ventilator settings and evaluate readiness to deliver anesthesia care. (ANESTHESIA TIME OUT)	Provider

anesthesia vapor delivery, adequate suction, and means to conform to standards for patient monitoring. Given that many modern machines have automated checkouts, no universal checkout list is possible. It is ultimately the responsibility of the provider to understand these principles and be able to apply them to any machine they are using.

FURTHER INFORMATION

Association of Anaesthetists of Great Britain and Ireland. Checking anaesthetic equipment. Available at: http://www.aagbi.org/sites/default/files/checking_anaesthetic_equipment_2012.pdf. Published 2012. Accessed on September 26, 2016.

Canadian Anesthesiologists' Society. Guidelines to the practice of anesthesia. *Can J Anesth.* 2016;63. Available at: https://www.cas.ca/English/Page/Files/97_Appendix%203.pdf. Accessed on September 26, 2016.

The Anesthesia Gas Machine. Available at: https://healthprofessions.udmercy.edu/academics/na/agm/11.htm. Accessed on May 24, 2018.

Sub-Committee of ASA Committee on Equipment and Facilities. Recommendations for pre-anesthesia checkout procedures. 2008. Available at: https://www.asahq.org/resources/clinical-information/2008-asa-recommendations-for-pre-anesthesia-checkout. Accessed on May 24, 2018.

US Food and Drug Administration. *Anesthesia Apparatus Checkout Recommendations.* Rockville, MD: US FDA; 1993.

APPENDIX 2 | MALIGNANT HYPERTHERMIA

ANESTHETIC CONSIDERATIONS FOR MALIGNANT HYPERTHERMIA

Malignant hyperthermia (MH) (Figure A2.1) is a rare but life-threatening genetic disorder characterized by hypermetabolic muscle destruction that is precipitated by exposure to inhaled volatile anesthetics and the depolarizing neuromuscular blocking agent succinylcholine. MH has been linked to rare skeletal muscle disorders, including central core disease, multiminicore myopathy, and King-Denborough syndrome.[1] It is important to remember that with the exception of hypokalemic periodic paralysis, neither the dystrophic nor the nondystrophic myotonic syndromes have been definitively associated with true MH.[2] However, the use in these patients of MH-triggering agents, particularly succinylcholine, has been associated with muscle damage and significant metabolic disturbances that mimic MH. Diagnosis of MH susceptibility is made by live muscle biopsy and the caffeine halothane contracture test (CHCT).[3]

The earliest clinical signs of MH are hypercarbia, masseter muscle spasm, and tachycardia.[4] Other symptoms, such as tachypnea, hypertension, hyperthermia, and arrhythmias, are also common and are a result of sympathetic nervous system overactivity. The timing of onset of the first symptom is variable. In a review of 477 cases of MH, Visoiu et al. found that the first symptom was reported within 55 minutes of exposure to MH-triggering agents.[4] However, there have been case reports that describe onset of MH within 1 hour of anesthesia finish time. With progressive muscle tissue damage, laboratory testing often reveals hyperkalemia, hypermagnesemia, mixed metabolic and respiratory acidosis, as well as increased serum myoglobin, creatinine kinase, and lactate dehydrogenase. Sequelae of these metabolic insults can include disseminated intravascular coagulation and hepatic and renal failure.

Early recognition and prompt treatment are paramount in the management of MH. Immediate steps include notifying the surgeon and aborting the procedure if possible, discontinuing all volatile anesthetics and succinylcholine, calling for help as well as the MH cart, and hyperventilating the patient with 100% oxygen. The flow rate through the anesthesia machine should be increased to wash out any residual volatile anesthetic. Once reconstituted, intravenous dantrolene should be bolused at 2.5 mg/kg every 5 minutes until a clinical response is noted. Appropriate responses include decreased muscle rigidity, a decrease in the patient's end-tidal carbon dioxide level, or a decrease in the patient's heart rate. Doses of 10 mg/kg may be required in the setting of persistent muscle rigidity.[5] Dantrium® and Revonto® are dantrolene preparations that consist of 20-mg vials that must be reconstituted in 60 mL of sterile water. The newer agent Ryanodex® comes packaged as a 250-mg vial that is reconstituted in 5 mL of sterile water.[6] Importantly, the former options also contain 3000 mg of mannitol, whereas the latter contains 125 mg mannitol. The differences in mannitol concentration may become important in the management of myoglobinuria-associated renal failure.

Placement of an arterial line should be considered, and serial blood gas analysis should be performed to optimize management of metabolic and respiratory acidosis, as well as hyperkalemia. Management of hyperkalemia includes administration of intravenous calcium chloride or calcium gluconate as well as insulin therapy. In cases of refractory hyperkalemia, dialysis may be required. Urine output should be monitored with a goal of 1 mL/kg per hour and may require augmentation with diuretics such as mannitol and furosemide. Cooling measures should be instituted in those with hyperthermia, with careful monitoring and avoidance of hypothermia. Once stable, the patient should be transferred to an intensive care unit, and intravenous dantrolene should be administered at 1 mg/kg every 6 hours for 24–48 hours to prevent symptom recurrence.

ANESTHESIA AND MACHINE PREPARATION FOR MH-SUSCEPTIBLE PATIENTS

The vaporizers for volatile gas anesthetics should be removed or turned to the "off" position and labeled so volatile anesthetic are not inadvertently introduced to the breathing circuit. A new breathing circuit should be attached in addition to a new reservoir bag. Because of the increasing variety of anesthesia machines, it is recommended that flushing of the anesthesia machine be performed according to the manufacturer's recommendations, which may take greater than 90 minutes in some instances.[7] Alternatively, the system may be flushed with high gas flows greater than 10 L/min for 90 seconds, followed by placement of activated charcoal filters on both the inspiratory and expiratory limbs.[8]

Effective May 2008

MH Hotline
1-800-644-9737
Outside the US:
1-315-464-7079

EMERGENCY THERAPY FOR MALIGNANT HYPERTHERMIA

DIAGNOSIS vs. ASSOCIATED PROBLEMS

Signs of MH:

- Increasing $ETCO_2$
- Trunk or total body rigidity
- Masseter spasm or trismus
- Tachycardia/tachypnea
- Mixed Respiratory and Metabolic Acidosis
- Increased temperature (may be late sign)
- Myoglobinuria

Sudden/Unexpected Cardiac Arrest in Young Patients:

- Presume hyperkalemia and initiate treatment (see #6)
- Measure CK, myoglobin, ABGs, until normalized
- Consider dantrolene
- Usually secondary to occult myopathy (e.g., muscular dystrophy)
- Resuscitation may be difficult and prolonged

Trismus or Masseter Spasm with Succinylcholine

- Early sign of MH in many patients
- If limb muscle rigidity, begin treatment with dantrolene
- For emergent procedures, continue with non-triggering agents, evaluate and monitor the patient, and consider dantrolene treatment
- Follow CK and urine myoglobin for 36 hours.
- Check CK immediately and at 6 hour intervals until returning to normal. Observe for dark or cola colored urine. If present, liberalize fluid intake and test for myoglobin
- Observe in PACU or ICU for at least 12 hours

ACUTE PHASE TREATMENT

1 GET HELP. GET DANTROLENE – Notify Surgeon

- Discontinue volatile agents and succinylcholine.
- Hyperventilate with 100% oxygen at flows of 10 L/min. or more.
- Halt the procedure as soon as possible; if emergent, continue with non-triggering anesthetic technique.
- Don't waste time changing the circle system and CO_2 absorbant.

2 Dantrolene 2.5 mg/kg rapidly IV through large-bore IV, if possible

To convert kg to lbs for amount of dantrolene, give patients 1 mg/lb (2.5 mg/kg approximates 1 mg/lb).

- Dissolve the 20 mg in each vial with at least 60 ml sterile, preservative-free water for injection. Prewarming (not to exceed 39° C.) the sterile water may expidite solublization of dantrolene. However, to date, there is no evidence that such warming improves clinical outcome.
- Repeat until signs of MH are reversed.
- Sometimes more than 10 mg/kg (up to 30 mg/kg) is necessary.
- Each 20 mg bottle has 3 gm mannitol for isotonicity. The pH of the solution is 9.

3 Bicarbonate for metabolic acidosis

- 1-2 mEq/kg if blood gas values are not yet available.

4 Cool the patient with core temperature >39ºC, Lavage open body cavities, stomach, bladder, or rectum. Apply ice to surface. Infuse cold saline intravenously. Stop cooling if temp. <38ºC and falling to prevent drift < 36ºC.

5 Dysrhythmias usually respond to treatment of acidosis and hyperkalemia.

- Use standard drug therapy **except calcium channel blockers, which may cause hyperkalemia or cardiac arrest in the presence of dantrolene.**

6 Hyperkalemia – Treat with hyperventilation, bicarbonate, glucose/insulin, calcium.

- Bicarbonate 1-2 mEq/kg IV.
- For **pediatric,** 0.1 units insulin/kg and 1 ml/kg 50% glucose or for **adult,** 10 units regular insulin IV and 50 ml 50% glucose.
- Calcium chloride 10 mg/kg or calcium gluconate 10-50 mg/kg for life-threatening hyperkalemia.
- Check glucose levels hourly.

7 Follow $ETCO_2$, electrolytes, blood gases, CK, core temperature, urine output and color, coagulation studies. If CK and/or K+ rise more than transiently or urine output falls to less than 0.5 ml/kg/hr, induce diuresis to >1 ml/kg/hr and give bicarbonate to alkalanize urine to prevent myoglobinuria-induced renal failure. (See D below)

- Venous blood gas (e.g., femoral vein) values may document hypermetabolism better than arterial values.
- Central venous or PA monitoring as needed and record minute ventilation.
- Place Foley catheter and monitor urine output.

POST ACUTE PHASE

A Observe the patient in an ICU for at least 24 hours, due to the risk of recrudescence.

B Dantrolene 1 mg/kg q 4-6 hours or 0.25 mg/kg/hr by infusion for at least 24 hours. Further doses may be indicated.

C Follow vitals and labs as above (see #7)

- Frequent ABG as per clinical signs
- CK every 8-12 hours; less often as the values trend downward

D Follow urine myoglobin and institute therapy to prevent myoglobin precipitation in renal tubules and the subsequent development of Acute Renal Failure. CK levels above 10,000 IU/L is a presumptive sign of rhabdomyolysis and myoglobinuria. Follow standard intensive care therapy for acute rhabdomyolysis and myoglobinuria (urine output >2 ml/kg/hr by hydration and diuretics along with alkalinization of urine with Na-bicarbonate infusion with careful attention to both urine and serum pH values).

E Counsel the patient and family regarding MH and further precautions; refer them to MHAUS. Fill out and send in the Adverse Metabolic Reaction to Anesthesia (AMRA) form (www.mhreg.org) and send a letter to the patient and her/his physician. Refer patient to the nearest Biopsy Center for follow-up.

Non-Emergency Information
MHAUS
PO Box 1069 (11 East State Street)
Sherburne, NY 13460-1069
Phone
1-800-986-4287
(607-674-7901)
Fax
607-674-7910
Email
info@mhaus.org
Website
www.mhaus.org

Since 1981
MHAUS
Malignant Hyperthermia Association of the United States
Dedicated to Patient Safety

CAUTION: This protocol may not apply to all patients; alter for specific needs.

Figure A2.1. Emergency therapy for malignant hyperthermia. (Reprinted with permission from the Malignant Hyperthermia Association of the United States [MHAUS]. For more information, go to: http://www.mhaus.org.)

REFERENCES

1. Malignant Hyperthermia Association of the United States. Associated conditions. n.d. Available at: http://www.mhaus.org/healthcare-professionals/be-prepared/associated-conditions. Accessed on December 10, 2016.
2. Parness J, Bandschapp O, Girard T. The myotonias and susceptibility to malignant hyperthermia. *Anesth Analg.* 2009;109:1054–1064.
3. Malignant Hyperthermia Association of the United States. Testing for malignant hyperthermia. n.d. Available at: http://www.mhaus.org/testing. Accessed on December 10, 2016.
4. Visoiu M, Young M, Wieland K, Brandom B. Anesthetic drugs and onset of malignant hyperthermia. *Anesth Analg.* 2014;118:388–396.
5. Malignant Hyperthermia Association of the United States. Managing an MH crisis. Available at: http://www.mhaus.org/healthcare-professionals/managing-a-crisis. Accessed on April 1, 2018.
6. RYANODEX [package insert]. Woodcliff Lake, NJ: Eagle Pharmaceuticals; 2014.
7. Malignant Hyperthermia Association of the United States. Preparation of anesthesia workstations to anesthetize MH susceptible patients. n.d. Available at: http://www.mhaus.org/healthcare-professionals/mhaus-recommendations/anesthesia-workstation-preparation. Accessed on December 10, 2016.
8. Birgenheier N, Stoker R, Westenskow D, Orr J. Activated charcoal effectively removes inhaled anesthetics from modern anesthesia machines. *Anesth Analg.* 2011;112:1363–1370.

APPENDIX 3 | SELECTED AMERICAN SOCIETY OF ANESTHESIOLOGISTS GUIDELINES

Statement of the Anesthesia Care Team is reprinted with permission of the American Society of Anesthesiologists, 520 N. Northwest Highway, Park Ridge, Illinois 60068-2573.

STATEMENT OF THE ANESTHESIA CARE TEAM

Committee of Origin: Anesthesia Care Team
(Approved by the ASA House of Delegates on October 26, 1982, and last amended October 16, 2013)
Anesthesiology is the practice of medicine including, but not limited to, preoperative patient evaluation, anesthetic planning, intraoperative and postoperative care and the management of systems and personnel that support these activities. In addition, anesthesiology includes perioperative consultation, the management of coexisting disease, the prevention and management of untoward perioperative patient conditions, the treatment of acute and chronic pain, and the practice of critical care medicine. This care is personally provided by or directed by the anesthesiologist.

In the interests of patient safety and quality of care, the American Society of Anesthesiologists believes that the involvement of an anesthesiologist in the perioperative care of every patient is necessary. Almost all anesthesia care is either provided personally by an anesthesiologist or is provided by a non-physician anesthesia practitioner directed by an anesthesiologist. The latter mode of anesthesia delivery is called the Anesthesia Care Team and involves the delegation of monitoring and appropriate tasks by the physician to non-physicians. Such delegation should be specifically defined by the anesthesiologist and should also be consistent with state law or regulations and medical staff policy. Although selected tasks of overall anesthesia care may be delegated to qualified members of the Anesthesia Care Team, overall responsibility for the Anesthesia Care Team and patients' safety ultimately rests with the anesthesiologist.

DEFINITIONS

1. CORE MEMBERS OF THE ANESTHESIA CARE TEAM

The Anesthesia Care Team includes both physicians and non-physicians. All members of the team have an obligation to accurately identify themselves and other team members to patients and families. Anesthesiologists should not permit the misrepresentation of non-physician personnel as resident physicians or practicing physicians. The nomenclature below is appropriate terminology for this purpose.

A. PHYSICIANS

ANESTHESIOLOGIST: **Director of the Anesthesia Care Team;** a **physician** licensed to practice medicine who has successfully completed a training program in anesthesiology accredited by the ACGME, the American Osteopathic Association or equivalent organizations.

ANESTHESIOLOGY FELLOW: An **anesthesiologist** enrolled in a training program to obtain additional education in one of the subdisciplines of anesthesiology.

ANESTHESIOLOGY RESIDENT: A **physician** enrolled in an accredited anesthesiology residency program.

B. NON-PHYSICIANS

ANESTHETIST: A **nurse anesthetist** or **anesthesiologist assistant**, as each is defined below. (Note: In some countries where non-physicians do not participate in the administration of anesthesia, a physician who practices anesthesiology is known as an "anaesthetist" or "anesthetist")

NURSE ANESTHETIST: A **registered nurse** who has satisfactorily completed an accredited nurse anesthesia training program and certifying examination (also, "CRNA").

ANESTHESIOLOGIST ASSISTANT: A **health professional** who has satisfactorily completed an accredited anesthesiologist assistant training program and certifying examination (also, "AA").

STUDENT NURSE ANESTHETIST: A **registered nurse** who is enrolled in an accredited nurse anesthesia training program.

ANESTHESIOLOGIST ASSISTANT STUDENT: A **health profession graduate student** who has satisfied all prerequisite coursework typical of an accredited school of medicine and is enrolled in an accredited anesthesiologist assistant training program.

NON-PHYSICIAN ANESTHESIA STUDENT: Student nurse anesthetists, anesthesiologist assistant students, dental anesthesia students and others who are enrolled in accredited anesthesia training programs.

OTHERS: Although not considered core members of the Anesthesia Care Team, other health care professionals make important contributions to the perianesthetic care of the patient (see Addendum A).

2. ADDITIONAL TERMS

ANESTHESIA CARE TEAM: Anesthesiologists supervising resident physicians and/or directing qualified non-physician anesthesia practitioners in the provision of anesthesia care, wherein the physician may delegate monitoring and appropriate tasks while retaining overall responsibility for the patient.

QUALIFIED ANESTHESIA PERSONNEL OR PRACT ITIONERS: Anesthesiologists, anesthesiology fellows, anesthesiology residents, oral surgery residents, anesthesiologist assistants, and nurse anesthetists.

MEDICAL SUPERVISION AND MEDICAL DIRECTION: Terms used to describe the physician work required to oversee, manage and guide both residents and non-physician members of the Anesthesia Care Team. For the purposes of this statement, supervision and direction are interchangeable and have no relation to the billing, payment or regulatory definitions that provide distinctions between these two terms (see Addendum B).

SEDATION NURSE AND SEDATION PHYSICIAN ASSISTANT: A licensed registered nurse, advanced practice nurse or physician assistant who is trained in compliance with all relevant local, institutional, state and/or national standards, policies or guidelines to administer prescribed sedating and analgesic medications and monitor patients during minimal sedation ("anxiolysis") or moderate sedation ("conscious sedation"), but not deeper levels of sedation or general anesthesia. Sedation nurses and sedation physician assistants may only work under the direct supervision of a properly trained and privileged physician (MD or DO).

PROCEDURE ROOM: An operating room or other location where an operation or procedure is performed under anesthesia care.

IMMEDIATELY AVAILABLE: Wherever it appears in this document, the phrase "immediately available" is used as defined in the ASA policy statement "Definition of 'Immediately Available' When Medically Directing" (see Addendum C).

Safe Conduct of the Anesthesia Care Team

In order to achieve optimum patient safety, the anesthesiologist who directs the Anesthesia Care Team is responsible for the following:

1. **Management of personnel**: Anesthesiologists should assure the assignment of appropriately skilled physician and/or non-physician personnel for each patient and procedure.
2. **Preanesthetic evaluation of the patient**: A preanesthetic evaluation allows for the development of an anesthetic plan that considers all conditions and diseases of the patient that may influence the safe outcome of the anesthetic. Although non-physicians may contribute to the preoperative collection and documentation of patient data, the anesthesiologist is responsible for the overall evaluation of each patient.
3. **Prescribing the anesthetic plan**: The anesthesiologist is responsible for prescribing an anesthesia plan aimed at the greatest safety and highest quality for each patient. The anesthesiologist discusses with the patient or guardian, as appropriate, the anesthetic risks, benefits and alternatives, and obtains informed consent. When part of the anesthetic care will be performed by another qualified anesthesia practitioner, the anesthesiologist should inform the patient that delegation of anesthetic duties is included in care provided by the Anesthesia Care Team.
4. **Management of the anesthetic**: The management of an anesthetic is dependent on many factors including the unique medical conditions of individual patients and the procedures being performed. Anesthesiologists will determine which perioperative tasks, if any, may be delegated. The anesthesiologist may delegate specific tasks to qualified non-anesthesiologist members of the Anesthesia Care Team providing that quality of care and patient safety are not compromised, will participate in critical parts of the anesthetic, and will remain immediately available for management of emergencies regardless of the type of anesthetic (see Addendum C).
5. **Postanesthesia care**: Routine postanesthesia care is delegated to postanesthesia nurses. The evaluation and treatment of postanesthetic complications are the responsibility of the anesthesiologist.
6. **Anesthesia consultation**: Like other forms of medical consultation, this is the practice of medicine and should not be delegated to non-physicians.

Safe Conduct of Minimal and Moderate Sedation Utilizing Sedation Nurses and Physician Assistants

The supervising physician is responsible for all aspects of the continuum of care: pre-, intra-, and post-procedure. While a patient is sedated, the responsible physician must be physically present and immediately available in the procedure suite. Although the supervising physician is primarily responsible for pre-procedure patient evaluation, sedation practitioners must be trained adequately in pre-procedure patient evaluation to recognize when risk may be increased, and related policies and procedures must allow sedation practitioners to refuse to participate in specific cases if they perceive a threat to quality of care or patient safety.

The supervising physician is responsible for leading any acute resuscitation needs, including emergency airway management. Therefore, ACLS (PALS or NALS where appropriate) certification must be a standard requirement for sedation practitioners and for credentialing and privileging the non-anesthesiologist physicians who supervise them. However, because non-anesthesia professionals seldom perform controlled mask ventilation or tracheal intubation often enough to remain proficient, their training should emphasize avoidance of excessive sedation over rescue techniques.

Medical Supervision of Nurse Anesthetists by Non-Anesthesiologist Physicians

Note: In this section, the term "surgeon" may refer to any appropriately trained, licensed and credentialed non-anesthesiologist physician who may supervise nurse anesthetists when consistent with applicable law.

General anesthesia, regional anesthesia, and monitored anesthesia care expose patients to risks. Non-anesthesiologist physicians may not possess the expertise that uniquely qualifies and enables anesthesiologists to manage the most clinically challenging medical situations that arise during the perioperative period. While a few surgical training programs (such as oral surgery and maxillofacial surgery) provide some anesthesia-specific education, no non-anesthesiology programs prepare their graduates to provide an anesthesiologist's level of medical supervision and perioperative clinical expertise. However, surgeons and other physicians significantly add to patient safety and quality of care by assuming medical responsibility for perioperative care when an anesthesiologist is not present.

Anesthetic and surgical complications often arise unexpectedly and require immediate medical diagnosis and treatment, even if state law or regulation says a physician is not required to supervise non-physician anesthesia practitioners. The surgeon may be the only physician on site. Whether the need is preoperative medical assessment or intraoperative resuscitation from an unexpected complication, the surgeon may be called upon, as the most highly trained professional present, to provide medical direction of perioperative health care, including nurse anesthesia care. To optimize patient safety, careful consideration is required when a surgeon will be the only physician available, as in some small hospitals, freestanding surgery centers, and surgeons' offices. In the event of an emergency, lack of immediate support from other physicians trained in critical medical management may reduce the likelihood of successful resuscitation. This should be taken into account when deciding which procedures should be performed in settings without an anesthesiologist, and which patients are appropriate candidates.

Medical Supervision of Non-Physician Anesthesia Students

Anesthesiologists who teach non-physician anesthesia students are dedicated to their education and to providing optimal safety and quality of care to every patient. The ASA Standards for Basic Anesthetic Monitoring define the minimum conditions necessary for the safe conduct of anesthesia. The first standard states, "Qualified anesthesia personnel shall be present in the room throughout the conduct of all general anesthetics, regional anesthetics and monitored anesthesia care." This statement does not completely address the issue of safe patient care during the training of non-physician student anesthetists. Further clarification of the issues involved is in the best interests of patients, students, and anesthesia practitioners.

During 1:1 supervision of non-physician anesthesia students, it may become necessary for the supervising anesthesiologist or nurse anesthetist to leave briefly to attend to other urgent needs or duties. This should only occur in circumstances judged to cause no significant increased risk to the patient.

This practice is to be distinguished from that of scheduling a non-physician student as the primary anesthetist, meaning that no fully-trained anesthesia practitioner is also continuously present to monitor the anesthetized patient. Though the brief interruption of 1:1 student supervision may be unavoidable for the efficient and safe functioning of a department of anesthesiology, the use of non-physician students as primary anesthetists in place of fully trained and credentialed anesthesia personnel is not endorsed as a best practice by the ASA. While the education of non-physician anesthesia students is an important goal, patient safety remains paramount. Therefore, the supervision of students at a ratio other than 1:1 must meet criteria designed to protect the safety and rights of patients and students, as well as the best interests of all other parties directly or indirectly involved: anesthesia practitioners, families, and health care institutions.

1. **Delegation**: All delegating anesthesiologists and the department chairperson must deem non-physician student anesthetists fully capable of performing all duties delegated to them, and all students must express agreement with accepting responsibility delegated to them.
2. **Privileging**: An official privileging process must individually deem each student as qualified to be supervised 1:2 by an anesthesiologist who remains immediately available (see Addendum C). Students must not be so privileged until they have completed a significant portion of their didactic and clinical training and have achieved expected levels of safety and quality (if at all, no earlier than the last ~4 months of training). Privileging must be done under the authority of the chair of anesthesiology and in compliance with all federal, state, and professional organization and institutional requirements.
3. **Case Assignment and Supervision**: Students must be supervised at a 1:1 or 1:2 anesthesiologist to student ratio. Assignment of cases to students must be done in a manner that assures the best possible outcome for patients and the best education of students, and must be commensurate with the skills, training, experience, knowledge and willingness of each individual non-physician student. Care should be taken to avoid placing students in situations beyond their level of skill. It is expected that most students will gain experience caring for high-risk patients under the continuous supervision of qualified anesthesia practitioners. This is in the best interest of education and patient safety. The degree of continuous supervision must be at a higher level than that required for fully credentialed anesthesiologist assistants and nurse anesthetists. If an anesthesiologist is engaged in the supervision of non-physician students, he/she must

remain immediately available. This means not leaving the procedure suite to provide other concurrent services or clinical duties that would be considered appropriate if directing fully credentialed anesthesiologist assistants or nurse anesthetists.

4. **Back-up Support**: If an anesthesiologist is concurrently supervising two non-physician students assigned as primary anesthetists (meaning the only anesthesia personnel continuously present with a patient), the anesthesiologist could be needed simultaneously in both rooms. To mitigate this potential risk, one other qualified anesthesia practitioner must also be designated to provide back-up support and must remain immediately available.
5. **Informed Consent**: The chair of anesthesiology is responsible for assuring that every patient (or the patient's guardian) understands through a standardized departmental informed consent process that the patient may be in the procedure room with only a non-physician student physically present, although still directed by the responsible anesthesiologist. In the best interest of all involved parties, documentation of this aspect of informed consent must be included in the informed consent statement.
6. **Disclosure to Professional Liability Carrier**: To be assured of reliable professional liability insurance coverage for all involved (qualified anesthesia practitioners, their employers and the institution), the chair of anesthesiology must notify the responsible professional liability carrier(s) of the practice of allowing non-physician anesthesia students to provide care without continuous direct supervision by a fully trained, credentialed and qualified anesthesia practitioner.

ADDENDUM A

1. Other personnel involved in perianesthetic care:

POSTANESTHESIA NURSE: A **registered nurse** who cares for patients recovering from anesthesia.

PERIOPERATIVE NURSE: A **registered nurse** who cares for the patient in the procedure room.

CRITICAL CARE NURSE: A **registered nurse** who cares for patients in a special care area such as an intensive care unit.

OBSTETRIC NURSE: A **registered nurse** who provides care to patients during labor and delivery.

NEONATAL NURSE: A **registered nurse** who provides care to neonates in special care units.

RESPIRATORY THERAPIST: An **allied health professional** who provides respiratory care to patients.

CARDIOVASCULAR PERFUSIONIST: An **allied health professional** who operates cardiopulmonary bypass machines.

2. **Support personnel for technical procedures, equipment, supply and maintenance:**

ANESTHESIA TECHNOLOGISTS AND TECHNICIANS
ANESTHESIA AIDES
BLOOD GAS TECHNICIANS
RESPIRATORY TECHNICIANS
MONITORING TECHNICIANS

ADDENDUM B

Commonly Used Payment Rules and Definitions

ASA recognizes the existence of commercial and governmental payer rules applicable to payment for anesthesia services and encourages its members to comply with them. Commonly prescribed duties include:

- Performing a preanesthetic history and physical examination of the patient;
- Prescribing the anesthetic plan;
- Personal participation in the most demanding portions of the anesthetic, including induction and emergence, where applicable;
- Delegation of anesthesia care only to qualified anesthesia practitioners;
- Monitoring the course of anesthesia at frequent intervals;
- Remaining immediately available for diagnosis and treatment while medically responsible;
- Providing indicated postanesthesia care;
- Performing and documenting a post-anesthesia evaluation.

ASA also recognizes the lack of total predictability in anesthesia care and the variability in patient needs. In certain rare circumstances, it may be inappropriate from the viewpoint of overall patient safety and quality to comply with all payment rules at every moment in time. Reporting of services for payment must accurately reflect the services provided. The ability to prioritize duties and patient care needs, moment to moment, is a crucial skill of the anesthesiologist functioning safely within the Anesthesia Care Team. Anesthesiologists must strive to provide the highest quality of care and greatest degree of patient safety to all patients in the perioperative environment at all times.

MEDICAL "DIRECTION" by anesthesiologists: A payment term describing the specific anesthesiologist work required and restrictions involved in billing payers for the management and oversight of non-physician anesthesia practitioners. This pertains to situations where anesthesiologists are involved in not more than four concurrent anesthetics.

MEDICAL "SUPERVISION" by anesthesiologists: Medicare payment policy contains a special payment formula for "medical supervision" which applies "when the anesthesiologist is involved in furnishing more than four procedures concurrently or is performing other services while directing the concurrent procedures." [Note: The word "supervision" may also be used outside of the Anesthesia Care Team to describe the perioperative medical oversight of non-physician anesthesia practitioners by the operating practitioner/surgeon. Surgeon-provided supervision pertains to general medical management and to the components of anesthesia care that are physician and not nursing functions (e.g., determining medical readiness of patients for anesthesia and surgery, and providing critical medical management of unexpected emergencies).]

See the Medicare Claims Processing Manual (Chapter 12, Section 50.C-D) and individual payer manuals for additional information.

ADDENDUM C

Definition of "Immediately Available" When Medically Directing (HOD 2012)

A medically directing anesthesiologist is immediately available if s/he is in physical proximity that allows the anesthesiologist to return to re-establish direct contact with the patient to meet medical needs and address any urgent or emergent clinical problems. These responsibilities may also be met through coordination among anesthesiologists of the same group or department.

Differences in the design and size of various facilities and demands of the particular surgical procedures make it impossible to define a specific time or distance for physical proximity. *Standards for Basic Anesthetic Monitoring is reprinted with permission of the American Society of Anesthesiologists, 520 N. Northwest Highway, Park Ridge, Illinois 60068-2573.*

STANDARDS FOR BASIC ANESTHETIC MONITORING

Committee of Origin: Standards and Practice Parameters (Approved by the ASA House of Delegates on October 21, 1986, last amended on October 20, 2010, and last affirmed on October 28, 2015)

These standards apply to all anesthesia care although, in emergency circumstances, appropriate life support measures take precedence. These standards may be exceeded at any time based on the judgment of the responsible anesthesiologist. They are intended to encourage quality patient care, but observing them cannot guarantee any specific patient outcome. They are subject to revision from time to time, as warranted by the evolution of technology and practice. They apply to all general anesthetics, regional anesthetics and monitored anesthesia care. This set of standards addresses only the issue of basic anesthetic monitoring, which is one component of anesthesia care. In certain rare or unusual circumstances, 1) some of these methods of monitoring may be clinically impractical, and 2) appropriate use of the described monitoring methods may fail to detect untoward clinical developments. Brief interruptions of continual† monitoring may be unavoidable. These standards are not intended for application to the care of the obstetrical patient in labor or in the conduct of pain management.

1. STANDARD I

Qualified anesthesia personnel shall be present in the room throughout the conduct of all general anesthetics, regional anesthetics and monitored anesthesia care.

1.1 Objective

Because of the rapid changes in patient status during anesthesia, qualified anesthesia personnel shall be continuously present to monitor the patient and provide anesthesia care. In the event there is a direct known hazard, e.g., radiation, to the anesthesia personnel which might require intermittent remote observation of the patient, some provision for monitoring the patient must be made. In the event that an emergency requires the temporary absence of the person primarily responsible for the anesthetic, the best judgment of the anesthesiologist will be exercised in comparing the emergency with the anesthetized patient's condition and in the selection of the person left responsible for the anesthetic during the temporary absence.

2. STANDARD II

During all anesthetics, the patient's oxygenation, ventilation, circulation and temperature shall be continually evaluated.

2.1 Oxygenation

2.1.1 ObjectiveTo ensure adequate oxygen concentration in the inspired gas and the blood during all anesthetics.

2.2 Methods

2.2.1 Inspired gas: During every administration of general anesthesia using an anesthesia machine, the concentration of oxygen in the patient breathing system shall be measured by an oxygen analyzer with a low oxygen concentration limit alarm in use.*

2.2.2 Blood oxygenation: During all anesthetics, a quantitative method of assessing oxygenation such as pulse oximetry shall be employed.* When the pulse oximeter is utilized, the variable pitch pulse tone and the low threshold alarm shall be audible to the anesthesiologist or the anesthesia care team personnel.* Adequate illumination and exposure of the patient are necessary to assess color.*

3. VENTILATION

3.1 Objective

To ensure adequate ventilation of the patient during all anesthetics.

3.2 Methods

3.2.1 Every patient receiving general anesthesia shall have the adequacy of ventilation continually evaluated. Qualitative clinical signs such as chest excursion, observation of the reservoir breathing bag and auscultation of breath sounds are useful. Continual monitoring for the presence of expired carbon dioxide shall be performed unless invalidated by the nature of the patient, procedure or equipment. Quantitative monitoring of the volume of expired gas is strongly encouraged.*

3.2.2 When an endotracheal tube or laryngeal mask is inserted, its correct positioning must be verified by clinical assessment and by identification of carbon dioxide in the expired gas. Continual end-tidal carbon dioxide analysis, in use from the time of endotracheal tube/laryngeal mask placement, until extubation/removal or initiating transfer to a postoperative care location, shall be performed using a quantitative method such as capnography, capnometry or mass spectroscopy.* When capnography or capnometry is utilized, the end tidal CO_2 alarm shall be audible to the anesthesiologist or the anesthesia care team personnel.*

3.2.3 When ventilation is controlled by a mechanical ventilator, there shall be in continuous use a device that is capable of detecting disconnection of components of the breathing system. The device must give an audible signal when its alarm threshold is exceeded.

3.2.4 During regional anesthesia (with no sedation) or local anesthesia (with no sedation), the adequacy of ventilation shall be evaluated by continual observation of qualitative clinical signs. During moderate or deep sedation the adequacy of ventilation shall be evaluated by continual observation of qualitative clinical signs.

and monitoring for the presence of exhaled carbon dioxide unless precluded or invalidated by the nature of the patient, procedure, or equipment.

4. CIRCULATION

4.1 Objective

To ensure the adequacy of the patient's circulatory function during all anesthetics.

4.2 Methods

4.2.1 Every patient receiving anesthesia shall have the electrocardiogram continuously displayed from the beginning of anesthesia until preparing to leave the anesthetizing location.*

4.2.2 Every patient receiving anesthesia shall have arterial blood pressure and heart rate determined and evaluated at least every five minutes.*

4.2.3 Every patient receiving general anesthesia shall have, in addition to the above, circulatory function continually evaluated by at least one of the following: palpation of a pulse, auscultation of heart sounds, monitoring of a tracing of intra-arterial pressure, ultrasound peripheral pulse monitoring, or pulse plethysmography or oximetry.

5. BODY TEMPERATURE

5.1 Objective

To aid in the maintenance of appropriate body temperature during all anesthetics.

5.2 Methods

Every patient receiving anesthesia shall have temperature monitored when clinically significant changes in body temperature are intended, anticipated or suspected.

† Note that "continual" is defined as "repeated regularly and frequently in steady rapid succession" whereas "continuous" means "prolonged without any interruption at any time."

* Under extenuating circumstances, the responsible anesthesiologist may waive the requirements marked with an asterisk (*); it is recommended that when this is done, it should be so stated (including the reasons) in a note in the patient's medical record.

Statement on Nonoperating Room Anesthetizing Locations is reprinted with permission of the American Society of Anesthesiologists, 520 N. Northwest Highway, Park Ridge, Illinois 60068-2573.

STATEMENT ON NONOPERATING ROOM ANESTHETIZING LOCATIONS

Committee of Origin: Standards and Practice Parameters (Approved by the ASA House of Delegates on October 19, 1994, and last amended on October 16, 2013)

These guidelines apply to all anesthesia care involving anesthesiology personnel for procedures intended to be performed in locations outside an operating room. These are minimal guidelines which may be exceeded at any time based on the judgment of the involved anesthesia personnel. These guidelines encourage quality patient care but observing them cannot guarantee any specific patient outcome. These guidelines are subject to revision from time to time, as warranted by the evolution of technology and practice. ASA Standards, Guidelines and Policies should be adhered to in all nonoperating room settings except where they are not applicable to the individual patient or care setting.

1. *There should be in each location a reliable source of oxygen adequate for the length of the procedure. There should also be a backup supply. Prior to administering any anesthetic, the anesthesiologist should consider the capabilities, limitations and accessibility of both the primary and backup oxygen sources. Oxygen piped from a central source, meeting applicable codes, is strongly encouraged. The backup system should include the equivalent of at least a full E cylinder.*
2. *There should be in each location an adequate and reliable source of suction. Suction apparatus that meets operating room standards is strongly encouraged.*
3. *In any location in which inhalation anesthetics are administered, there should be an adequate and reliable system for scavenging waste anesthetic gases.*
4. *There should be in each location: (a) a self-inflating hand resuscitator bag capable of administering at least 90% oxygen as a means to deliver positive pressure ventilation; (b) adequate anesthesia drugs, supplies and equipment for the intended anesthesia care; and (c) adequate monitoring equipment to allow adherence to the "Standards for Basic Anesthetic Monitoring." In any location in which inhalation anesthesia is to be administered, there should be an anesthesia machine equivalent in function to that employed in operating rooms and maintained to current operating room standards.*
5. *There should be in each location, sufficient electrical outlets to satisfy anesthesia machine and monitoring equipment requirements, including clearly labeled outlets connected to an emergency power supply. In any anesthetizing location determined by the health care facility to be a "wet location"* (e.g., *for cystoscopy or arthroscopy or a birthing room in labor and delivery), either isolated electric power or electric circuits with ground fault circuit interrupters should be provided.**
6. *There should be in each location, provision for adequate illumination of the patient, anesthesia machine (when present) and monitoring equipment. In addition, a form of battery-powered illumination other than a laryngoscope should be immediately available.*
7. *There should be in each location, sufficient space to accommodate necessary equipment and personnel and to allow expeditious access to the patient, anesthesia machine (when present) and monitoring equipment.*
8. *There should be immediately available in each location, an emergency cart with a defibrillator, emergency drugs and other equipment adequate to provide cardiopulmonary resuscitation*
9. *There should be in each location adequate staff trained to support the anesthesiologist. There should be immediately available in each location, a reliable means of two-way communication to request assistance.*
10. *For each location, all applicable building and safety codes and facility standards, where they exist, should be observed*
11. *Appropriate postanesthesia management should be provided (see Standards for Postanesthesia Care). In addition to the anesthesiologist, adequate numbers of trained staff and appropriate equipment should be available to safely transport the patient to a postanesthsia care unit.*

**See National Fire Protection Association. Health Care Facilities Code 99; Quincy, MA: NFPA, 2012.*

Guidelines for Office-Based Anesthesia is reprinted with permission of the American Society of Anesthesiologists, 520 N. Northwest Highway, Park Ridge, Illinois 60068-2573.

GUIDELINES FOR OFFICE-BASED ANESTHESIA

Committee of Origin: Ambulatory Surgical Care (Approved by the ASA House of Delegates on October 13, 1999; last amended on October 21, 2009; and reaffirmed on October 15, 2014)

These guidelines are intended to assist ASA members who are considering the practice of ambulatory anesthesia in the office setting: office-based anesthesia (OBA). These recommendations focus on quality anesthesia care and patient safety in the office. These are minimal guidelines and may be exceeded at any time based on the judgment of the involved anesthesia personnel. Compliance with these guidelines cannot guarantee any specific outcome. These guidelines are subject to periodic revision as warranted by the evolution of federal, state and local laws as well as technology and practice.

ASA recognizes the unique needs of this growing practice and the increased requests for ASA members to provide OBA for health care practitioners* who have developed their own office operatories. Since OBA is a subset of ambulatory anesthesia, the ASA "Guidelines for Ambulatory Anesthesia and Surgery" should be followed in the office setting as well as all other ASA standards and guidelines that are applicable.

There are special problems that ASA members must recognize when administering anesthesia in the office setting. Compared with acute care hospitals and licensed ambulatory surgical facilities, office operatories currently have little or no regulation, oversight or control by federal, state or local laws. Therefore, ASA members must satisfactorily investigate areas taken for granted in the hospital or ambulatory surgical facility such as governance, organization, construction and equipment, as well as policies and procedures, including fire, safety, drugs, emergencies, staffing, training and unanticipated patient transfers.

ASA members should be confident that the following issues are addressed in an office setting to provide patient safety and to reduce risk and liability to the anesthesiologist.

ADMINISTRATION AND FACILITY

Quality of Care

- The facility should have a medical director or governing body that establishes policy and is responsible for the activities of the facility and its staff. The medical director or governing body is responsible for ensuring that facilities and personnel are adequate and appropriate for the type of procedures performed.
- Policies and procedures should be written for the orderly conduct of the facility and reviewed on an annual basis.
- The medical director or governing body should ensure that all applicable local, state and federal regulations are observed.[2]
- All health care practitioners* and nurses should hold a valid license or certificate to perform their assigned duties.
- All operating room personnel who provide clinical care in the office should be qualified to perform services commensurate with appropriate levels of education, training and experience.
- The anesthesiologist should participate in ongoing continuous quality improvement and risk management activities.
- The medical director or governing body should recognize the basic human rights of its patients, and a written document that describes this policy should be available for patients to review.

Facility and Safety

- Facilities should comply with all applicable federal, state and local laws, codes and regulations pertaining to fire prevention, building construction and occupancy, accommodations for the disabled, occupational safety and health, and disposal of medical waste and hazardous waste.
- Policies and procedures should comply with laws and regulations pertaining to controlled drug supply, storage and administration.

CLINICAL CARE

Patient and Procedure Selection

- The anesthesiologist should be satisfied that the procedure to be undertaken is within the scope of practice of the health care practitioners and the capabilities of the facility.
- The procedure should be of a duration and degree of complexity that will permit the patient to recover and be discharged from the facility.
- Patients who by reason of pre-existing medical or other conditions may be at undue risk for complications should be referred to an appropriate facility for performance of the procedure and the administration of anesthesia.

Perioperative Care

- The anesthesiologist should adhere to the "Basic Standards for Preanesthesia Care," "Standards for Basic Anesthetic Monitoring," "Standards for Postanesthesia Care" and "Guidelines for Ambulatory Anesthesia and Surgery" as currently promulgated by the American Society of Anesthesiologists.
- The anesthesiologist should be physically present during the intraoperative period and immediately available until the patient has been discharged from anesthesia care.
- Discharge of the patient is a physician responsibility. This decision should be documented in the medical record.
- Personnel with training in advanced resuscitative techniques (e.g., ACLS, PALS) should be immediately available until all patients are discharged home.[3]

Monitoring and Equipment

- At a minimum, all facilities should have a reliable source of oxygen, suction, resuscitation equipment and emergency drugs. Specific reference is made to the ASA "Statement on Nonoperating Room Anesthetizing Locations."
- There should be sufficient space to accommodate all necessary equipment and personnel and to allow for expeditious access to the patient, anesthesia machine (when present) and all monitoring equipment.
- All equipment should be maintained, tested and inspected according to the manufacturer's specifications.
- Back-up power sufficient to ensure patient protection in the event of an emergency should be available.
- In any location in which anesthesia is administered, there should be appropriate anesthesia apparatus and equipment which allow monitoring consistent with ASA "Standards for Basic Anesthetic Monitoring" and documentation of regular preventive maintenance as recommended by the manufacturer.

- In an office where anesthesia services are to be provided to infants and children, the required equipment, medication and resuscitative capabilities should be appropriately sized for a pediatric population.

Emergencies and Transfers

- All facility personnel should be appropriately trained in and regularly review the facility's written emergency protocols.
- There should be written protocols for cardiopulmonary emergencies and other internal and external disasters such as fire.
- The facility should have medications, equipment and written protocols available to treat malignant hyperthermia when triggering agents are used.
- The facility should have a written protocol in place for the safe and timely transfer of patients to a prespecified alternate care facility when extended or emergency services are needed to protect the health or well-being of the patient.

*defined herein as physicians, dentists and podiatrists

Standards for Postanesthesia Care is reprinted with permission of the American Society of Anesthesiologists, 520 N. Northwest Highway, Park Ridge, Illinois 60068-2573.

STANDARDS FOR POSTANESTHESIA CARE

Committee of Origin: Standards and Practice Parameters (Approved by the ASA House of Delegates on October 27, 2004, and last amended on October 15, 2014)

These standards apply to postanesthesia care in all locations. These standards may be exceeded based on the judgment of the responsible anesthesiologist. They are intended to encourage quality patient care, but cannot guarantee any specific patient outcome. They are subject to revision from time to time as warranted by the evolution of technology and practice.

STANDARD I

ALL PATIENTS WHO HAVE RECEIVED GENERAL ANESTHESIA, REGIONAL ANESTHESIA OR MONITORED ANESTHESIA CARE SHALL RECEIVE APPROPRIATE POSTANESTHESIA MANAGEMENT.[1]

1. A Postanesthesia Care Unit (PACU) or an area which provides equivalent postanesthesia care (for example, a Surgical Intensive Care Unit) shall be available to receive patients after anesthesia care. All patients who receive anesthesia care shall be admitted to the PACU or its equivalent **except** by specific order of the anesthesiologist responsible for the patient's care.
2. The medical aspects of care in the PACU (or equivalent area) shall be governed by policies and procedures which have been reviewed and approved by the Department of Anesthesiology.
3. The design, equipment and staffing of the PACU shall meet requirements of the facility's accrediting and licensing bodies.

STANDARD II

A PATIENT TRANSPORTED TO THE PACU SHALL BE ACCOMPANIED BY A MEMBER OF THE ANESTHESIA CARE TEAM WHO IS KNOWLEDGEABLE ABOUT THE PATIENT'S CONDITION. THE PATIENT SHALL BE CONTINUALLY EVALUATED AND TREATED DURING TRANSPORT WITH MONITORING AND SUPPORT APPROPRIATE TO THE PATIENT'S CONDITION.

STANDARD III

UPON ARRIVAL IN THE PACU, THE PATIENT SHALL BE RE-EVALUATED AND A VERBAL REPORT PROVIDED TO THE RESPONSIBLE PACU NURSE BY THE MEMBER OF THE ANESTHESIA CARE TEAM WHO ACCOMPANIES THE PATIENT.

1. The patient's status on arrival in the PACU shall be documented.
2. Information concerning the preoperative condition and the surgical/anesthetic course shall be transmitted to the PACU nurse.
3. The member of the Anesthesia Care Team shall remain in the PACU until the PACU nurse accepts responsibility for the nursing care of the patient.

STANDARD IV

THE PATIENT'S CONDITION SHALL BE EVALUATED CONTINUALLY IN THE PACU.

1. The patient shall be observed and monitored by methods appropriate to the patient's medical condition. Particular attention should be given to monitoring oxygenation, ventilation, circulation, level of consciousness and temperature. During recovery from all anesthetics, a quantitative method of assessing oxygenation such as pulse oximetry shall be employed in the initial phase of recovery.* This is not intended for application during the recovery of the obstetrical patient in whom regional anesthesia was used for labor and vaginal delivery.

2. An accurate written report of the PACU period shall be maintained. Use of an appropriate PACU scoring system is encouraged for each patient on admission, at appropriate intervals prior to discharge and at the time of discharge.
3. General medical supervision and coordination of patient care in the PACU should be the responsibility of an anesthesiologist.
4. There shall be a policy to assure the availability in the facility of a physician capable of managing complications and providing cardiopulmonary resuscitation for patients in the PACU.

STANDARD V

A PHYSICIAN IS RESPONSIBLE FOR THE DISCHARGE OF THE PATIENT FROM THE POSTANESTHESIA CARE UNIT.

1. When discharge criteria are used, they must be approved by the Department of Anesthesiology and the medical staff. They may vary depending upon whether the patient is discharged to a hospital room, to the Intensive Care Unit, to a short stay unit or home.
2. In the absence of the physician responsible for the discharge, the PACU nurse shall determine that the patient meets the discharge criteria. The name of the physician accepting responsibility for discharge shall be noted on the record.

1 Refer to Perianesthesia Nursing Standards, Practice Recommendations and Interpretive Statements, published by ASPAN, for issues of nursing care.

* Under extenuating circumstances, the responsible anesthesiologist may waive the requirements marked with an asterisk (*); it is recommended that when this is done, it should be so stated (including the reasons) in a note in the patient's medical record.

STATEMENT ON GRANTING PRIVILEGES FOR ADMINISTRATION OF MODERATE SEDATION TO PRACTITIONERS WHO ARE NOT ANESTHESIA PROFESSIONALS

Committee of Origin: Ad Hoc Committee on Credentialing
Committee of Review: Ambulatory Surgical Care

(Approved by the ASA House of Delegates on October 25, 2005, and reaffirmed on October 26, 2016)

The American Society of Anesthesiologists is vitally interested in the safe administration of anesthesia. As such, it has concern for any system or set of practices, used either by its members or the members of other disciplines that would adversely affect the safety of anesthesia administration. It has genuine concern that individuals, however well intentioned, who are not anesthesia professionals may not recognize that sedation and general anesthesia are on a continuum and thus deliver levels of sedation that are, in fact, general anesthesia without having the training and experience to recognize this state and respond appropriately.

The intent of this statement is to suggest a framework for granting privileges that will help ensure competence of individuals who administer or supervise the administration of moderate sedation. Only physicians, dentists or podiatrists who are qualified by education, training and licensure to administer moderate sedation should supervise the administration of moderate sedation. This statement can be used by any facility—hospital, ambulatory care or physician's, dentist's or podiatrist's office—in which an internal or external credentialing process is required for administration of sedative and analgesic drugs to establish a level of moderate sedation.

REFERENCES

ASA has produced many documents over the years related to the topic addressed by this statement, among them the following:

Guidelines for Delineation of Clinical Privileges in Anesthesiology (Approved by ASA House of Delegates on October 15, 1975, and last amended on October 16, 2013)

Statement on Qualifications of Anesthesia Providers in the Office-Based Setting (Approved by ASA House of Delegates on October 13, 1999; last amended on October 21, 2009; and reaffirmed on October 15, 2014)

Statement on Safe Use of Propofol (Approved by ASA House of Delegates on October 27, 2004, and last amended on October 15, 2014)

Guidelines for Office-Based Anesthesia (Approved by ASA House of Delegates on October 13, 1999; last affirmed on October 15, 2014)

Guidelines for Ambulatory Anesthesia and Surgery (Approved by ASA House of Delegates on October 11, 1973; last amended on October 22, 2008; and reaffirmed on October 16, 2013)

Outcome Indicators for Office-Based and Ambulatory Surgery (ASA Committee on Ambulatory Surgical Care and Task Force on Office-Based Anesthesia, April 2003)

AANA-ASA Joint Statement Regarding Propofol Administration (April 14, 2004)

Practice Guidelines for Sedation and Analgesia by Nonanesthesiologists (Approved by ASA House of Delegates on October 25, 1995, and last amended on October 17, 2001)

Continuum of Depth of Sedation—Definition of General Anesthesia and Levels of Sedation/Analgesia (Approved by ASA House of Delegates on October 13, 1999, and last amended on October 15, 2014)

Practice Guidelines for Preoperative Fasting and the Use of Pharmacologic Agents to Reduce the Risk of Pulmonary Aspiration: Application to Healthy Patients Undergoing Elective Procedures (Approved by ASA House of Delegates on October 21, 1998; effective January 1, 1999; and last amended on October 20, 2010)

The Ad Hoc Committee on Sedation Credentialing Guidelines for Nonanesthesiologists took the contents of the above documents into consideration when developing this statement.

DEFINITIONS

Anesthesia Professional: An anesthesiologist, nurse anesthetist or anesthesiologist assistant (AA).

Nonanesthesiologist Sedation Practitioner: A licensed physician (allopathic or osteopathic), dentist or podiatrist who has not completed postgraduate training in anesthesiology but is specifically trained to personally administer or supervise the administration of moderate sedation.

Supervised Sedation Professional: A licensed registered nurse, advanced practice nurse or physician assistant who is trained to administer medications and monitor patients during moderate sedation under the direct supervision of a nonanesthesiologist sedation practitioner or an anesthesiologist.

Credentialing: The process of documenting and reviewing a practitioner's credentials.

Credentials: The professional qualifications of a practitioner including education, training, experience and performance.

Privileges: The clinical activities within a health care organization that a practitioner is permitted to perform based on the practitioner's credentials.

Guidelines: A set of recommended practices that should be considered but permit discretion by the user as to whether they should be applied under any particular set of circumstances.

* **Moderate Sedation**: "Moderate Sedation/Analgesia ('Conscious Sedation') is a drug-induced depression of consciousness during which patients respond purposefully to verbal commands, either alone or accompanied by light tactile stimulation. No interventions are required to maintain a patent airway, and spontaneous ventilation is adequate. Cardiovascular function is usually maintained."

* **Deep Sedation:** "Deep Sedation/Analgesia is a drug-induced depression of consciousness during which patients cannot be easily aroused but respond purposefully following repeated or painful stimulation. The ability to independently maintain ventilatory function may be impaired. Patients may require assistance in maintaining a patent airway, and spontaneous ventilation may be inadequate. Cardiovascular function is usually maintained."

* **Rescue:** "Rescue of a patient from a deeper level of sedation than intended is an intervention by a practitioner proficient in airway management and advanced life support. The qualified practitioner corrects adverse physiologic consequences of the deeper-than intended level of sedation (such as hypoventilation, hypoxia and hypotension) and returns the patient to the originally intended level of sedation."

* **General Anesthesia**: "General Anesthesia is a drug-induced loss of consciousness during which patients are not arousable, even by painful stimulation. The ability to independently maintain ventilatory function is often impaired. Patients often require assistance in maintaining a patent airway, and positive pressure ventilation may be required because of depressed spontaneous ventilation or drug-induced depression of neuromuscular function. Cardiovascular function may be impaired."

*The definitions marked with an asterisk are extracted verbatim from "Continuum of Depth of Sedation—Definition of General Anesthesia and Levels of Sedation/Analgesia" (Approved by ASA House of Delegates on October 13, 1999, and last amended on October 15, 2014).

STATEMENT

The following statement is designed to assist health care organizations develop a program for the delineation of clinical privileges for practitioners who are not anesthesia professionals to administer sedative and analgesic drugs to establish a level of moderate sedation. (Moderate sedation is also known as "conscious sedation.") The statement is written to apply to every setting in which an internal or external credentialing process is required for granting privileges to administer sedative and analgesic drugs to establish a level of moderate sedation (e.g., hospital, freestanding procedure center, ambulatory surgery center, physician's, dentist's or podiatrist's office, etc.). The statement is not intended nor should it be applied to the granting of privileges to administer deep sedation or general anesthesia.

The granting, reappraisal and revision of clinical privileges should be awarded on a time-limited basis in accordance with rules and regulations of the health care organization, its medical staff, organizations accrediting the health care organization and relevant local, state and federal governmental agencies.

I. Nonanesthesiologist Sedation Practitioners

Only physicians, dentists or podiatrists who are qualified by education, training and licensure to administer moderate sedation should supervise the administration of moderate sedation. Nonanesthesiologist sedation practitioners may directly supervise patient monitoring and the administration of sedative and analgesic medications by a **supervised sedation professional**. Alternatively, they may personally perform these functions, with the proviso that the individual monitoring the patient should be distinct from the individual performing the diagnostic or therapeutic procedure (see *ASA Guidelines for Sedation and Analgesia by Nonanesthesiologists*).

A. EDUCATION AND TRAINING

The nonanesthesiologist sedation practitioner who is to supervise or personally administer medications for moderate sedation should have satisfactorily completed a formal training program in: (1) the safe administration of sedative and analgesic drugs used to establish a level of moderate sedation, and (2) rescue of patients who exhibit adverse physiologic consequences of a deeper-than-intended level of sedation. This training may be a part of a recently completed residency or fellowship training (e.g., within two years), or may be a separate educational program. A knowledge-based test may be used to verify the practitioner's understanding of these concepts.** The following subject areas should be included:

1. Contents of the following ASA documents that should be understood by practitioners who administer sedative and analgesic drugs to establish a level of moderate sedation:
    - *Practice Guidelines for Sedation and Analgesia by Nonanesthesiologists*
    - *Continuum of Depth of Sedation—Definition of General Anesthesia and Levels of Sedation/Analgesia*
2. Appropriate methods for obtaining informed consent through pre-procedure counseling of patients regarding risks, benefits and alternatives to the administration of sedative and analgesic drugs to establish a level of moderate sedation.

3. Skills for obtaining the patient's medical history and performing a physical examination to assess risks and co-morbidities, including assessment of the airway for anatomic and mobility characteristics suggestive of potentially difficult airway management. The nonanesthesiologist sedation practitioner should be able to recognize those patients whose medical condition suggests that sedation should be provided by an anesthesia professional.
4. Assessment of the patient's risk for aspiration of gastric contents as described in the *ASA Practice Guidelines for Preoperative Fasting*: "In urgent, emergent or other situations where gastric emptying is impaired, the potential for pulmonary aspiration of gastric contents must be considered in determining (1) the target level of sedation, (2) whether the procedure should be delayed or (3) whether the trachea should be protected by intubation."
5. The pharmacology of (1) all sedative and analgesic drugs the practitioner requests privileges to administer to establish a level of moderate sedation, (2) pharmacological antagonists to the sedative and analgesic drugs and (3) vasoactive drugs and antiarrhythmics.
6. The benefits and risks of supplemental oxygen.
7. Proficiency of airway management with facemask and positive pressure ventilation. This training should include appropriately supervised experience in managing the airways of patients, or qualified instruction on an airway simulator (or both).
8. Monitoring of physiologic variables, including the following:
    a. Blood pressure
    b. Respiratory rate
    c. Oxygen saturation by pulse oximetry
    d. Electrocardiographic monitoring. Education in electrocardiographic (EKG) monitoring should include instruction in the most common arrhythmias seen during sedation and anesthesia, their causes and their potential clinical implications (e.g., hypercapnia), as well as electrocardiographic signs of cardiac ischemia.
    e. Depth of sedation. The depth of sedation should be based on the ASA definitions of "moderate sedation" and "deep sedation." (See above)
    f. Capnography– During moderate sedation the adequacy of ventilation shall be evaluated by continual observation of qualitative clinical signs and monitoring for the presence of exhaled carbon dioxide unless precluded or invalidated by the nature of the patient, procedure, or equipment.
9. The importance of continuous use of appropriately set audible alarms on physiologic monitoring equipment.
10. Documenting the drugs and fluids administered, the patient's physiologic condition and the depth of sedation at regular intervals throughout the period of sedation and analgesia, using a graphical, tabular or automated record.
11. Regardless of the availability of a "code team" or the equivalent, the non-anesthesiologist sedation practitioner will have advanced life support skills and current certificate such as those required for Advanced Cardiac Life Support (ACLS). When granting privileges to administer moderate sedation to pediatric patients, the non-anesthesiologist practitioner will have advanced life support skills and current certificate such as those required for Pediatric Advanced Life Support (PALS). Initial ACLS and PALS training and subsequent retraining shall be obtained from the American Heart Association or another vendor that includes "hands-on" training and skills demonstration of airway management and automated external defibrillator (AED) use.

When the practitioner is being granted privileges to administer sedative and analgesic drugs to pediatric patients to establish a level of moderate sedation, the education and training requirements enumerated in #1–9 above should be appropriately tailored to qualify the practitioner to administer sedative and analgesic drugs to pediatric patients.

B. LICENSURE

1. The nonanesthesiologist sedation practitioner should have a current active, unrestricted medical, osteopathic, dental or podiatric license in the state, district or territory of practice. (Exception: practitioners employed by the federal government may have a current active license in any U.S. state, district or territory.)
2. The nonanesthesiologist sedation practitioner should have a current unrestricted Drug Enforcement Administration (DEA) registration (schedules II–V).
3. The credentialing process should require disclosure of any disciplinary action (final judgments) against any medical, osteopathic or podiatric license by any state, district or territory of practice and of any sanctions by any federal agency, including Medicare/Medicaid, in the last five years.
4. Before granting or renewing privileges to administer or supervise the administration of sedative and analgesic drugs to establish a level of moderate sedation, the health care organization should search for any disciplinary action recorded in the National Practitioner Data Bank (NPDB) and take appropriate action regarding any Adverse Action Reports.

C. PRACTICE PATTERN

1. Before granting initial privileges to administer or supervise administration of sedative and analgesic drugs to establish a level of moderate sedation, a process should

be developed to evaluate the practitioner's performance. For recent graduates (e.g., within two years), this may be accomplished through letters of recommendation from directors of residency or fellowship training programs which include moderate sedation as part of the curriculum. For those who have been in practice since completion of their training, this may be accomplished through communication with department heads or supervisors at the institution where the individual holds privileges to administer moderate sedation. Alternatively, the nonanesthesiologist sedation practitioner could be proctored or supervised by a physician, dentist or podiatrist who is currently privileged to administer sedative and analgesic agents to provide moderate sedation. The facility should establish an appropriate number of procedures to be supervised.

2. Before granting ongoing privileges to administer or supervise administration of sedative and analgesic drugs to establish a level of moderate sedation, a process should be developed to re-evaluate the practitioner's performance at regular intervals. For example, the practitioner's performance could be reviewed by an anesthesiologist or a nonanesthesiologist sedation practitioner who is currently privileged to administer sedative and analgesic agents to provide moderate sedation. The facility should establish an appropriate number of procedures that will be reviewed.

D. PERFORMANCE IMPROVEMENT

Credentialing in the administration of sedative and analgesic drugs to establish a level of moderate sedation should require active participation in an ongoing process that evaluates the practitioner's clinical performance and patient care outcomes through a formal program of continuous performance improvement.

1. The organization in which the practitioner practices should conduct peer review of its clinicians.
2. The performance improvement process should assess up-to-date knowledge as well as ongoing competence in the skills outlined in the educational and training requirements described above.
3. The performance improvement process should monitor and evaluate patient outcomes and adverse events.

II. Supervised Sedation Professional

A. EDUCATION AND TRAINING

The supervised sedation professional who is granted privileges to administer sedative and analgesic drugs under supervision of a nonanesthesiologist sedation practitioner or anesthesiologist and to monitor patients during moderate sedation can be a registered nurse who has graduated from a qualified school of nursing or a physician assistant who has graduated from an accredited physician assistant program. They may only administer sedative and analgesic medications on the order of an anesthesiologist or nonanesthesiologist sedation practitioner. They should have satisfactorily completed a formal training program in 1) the safe administration of sedative and analgesic drugs used to establish a level of moderate sedation, 2) use of reversal agents for opioids and benzodiazepines, 3) monitoring of patients' physiologic parameters during sedation, and 4) recognition of abnormalities in monitored variables that require intervention by the nonanesthesiologist sedation practitioner or anesthesiologist. Training should include the following:

1. Contents of the following ASA documents:
   - Practice Guidelines for Sedation and Analgesia by Nonanesthesiologists
   - *Continuum of Depth of Sedation—Definition of General Anesthesia and Levels of Sedation/Analgesia*
2. The pharmacology of (1) all sedative and analgesic drugs the practitioner requests privileges to administer to establish a level of moderate sedation, and (2) pharmacological antagonists to the sedative and analgesic drugs.
3. The benefits and risks of supplemental oxygen.
4. Airway management with facemask and positive pressure ventilation.
5. Monitoring and recognizing abnormalities of physiologic variables, including the following:
   a. Blood pressure
   b. Respiratory rate
   c. Oxygen saturation by pulse oximetry
   d. Electrocardiographic monitoring
   e. Depth of sedation. The depth of sedation should be based on the ASA definitions of "moderate sedation" and "deep sedation." (See above)
   f. Capnography–if moderate sedation is to be administered unless precluded or invalidated by the nature of the patient, procedure, or equipment.
6. The importance of continuous use of appropriately set audible alarms on all physiologic monitors.
7. Documenting the drugs administered, the patient's physiologic condition and the depth of sedation at regular intervals throughout the period of sedation and analgesia, using a graphical, tabular or automated record.

B. LICENSURE

1. The supervised sedation professional should have a current active nursing license or physician assistant license or certification, in the U.S. state, district or territory of practice. (Exception: practitioners employed by the federal government may have a current active license in any U.S. state, district or territory.)

2. Before granting or renewing privileges for a supervised sedation professional to administer sedative and analgesic drugs and to monitor patients during moderate sedation, the health care organization should search for any disciplinary action recorded in the National Practitioner Data Bank (NPDB) and take appropriate action regarding any Adverse Action Reports.

C. PRACTICE PATTERN

1. Before granting ongoing privileges to administer sedative and analgesic drugs to establish a level of moderate sedation, a process should be developed to re-evaluate the supervised sedation professional's performance. The facility should establish performance criteria and an appropriate number of procedures to be reviewed.

D. PERFORMANCE IMPROVEMENT

Credentialing of supervised sedation professionals in the administration of sedative and analgesic drugs and monitoring patients during moderate sedation should require active participation in an ongoing process that evaluates the health care professional's clinical performance and patient care outcomes through a formal program of continuous performance improvement.

1. The organization in which the practitioner practices should conduct peer review of its supervised sedation professionals.
2. The performance improvement process should assess up-to-date knowledge as well as ongoing competence in the skills outlined in the educational and training requirements described above.

**The post-test included with the ASA Sedation/Analgesia by Nonanesthesiologists videotape (ASA Document #30503-10PPV) may be considered for this purpose.
1. Contents of the following ASA documents that should be understood by practitioners who administer sedative and analgesic drugs to establish a level of moderate sedation:

STATEMENT ON GRANTING PRIVILEGES FOR DEEP SEDATION TO NON-ANESTHESIOLOGIST SEDATION PRACTITIONERS

Committee of Origin: Ad Hoc on Non-Anesthesiologist Privileging (Approved by the ASA House of Delegates on October 20, 2010)

1. INTRODUCTION

The American Society of Anesthesiologists is vitally interested in the safe administration of all anesthesia services including moderate and deep sedation. As such, it has concern for any system or set of practices, used either by its members or the members of other disciplines that would adversely affect the safety of anesthesia or sedation administration. It has genuine concern that individuals, however well intentioned, who are not anesthesia professionals may not recognize that sedation and general anesthesia are on a continuum, and thus deliver levels of sedation that may, in fact, be general anesthesia without having the training and experience to respond appropriately.

ASA believes that anesthesiologist participation in all deep sedation is the best means to achieve the safest care. ASA acknowledges, however, that Medicare regulations permit some non-anesthesiologists to administer or supervise the administration of deep sedation. This advisory should not be considered as an endorsement, or absolute condemnation, of this practice by ASA but rather to serve as a potential guide to its members who may be called upon by administrators or others to provide input in this process. This document provides a framework to identify those physicians, dentists, oral surgeons or podiatrists who may potentially qualify to administer or supervise the administration of deep sedation.

This document applies only to the care of patients undergoing procedural sedation, and it may not be construed as privileges to intentionally administer general anesthesia. Unrestricted general anesthesia shall only be administered by anesthesia professionals within their scope of practice (anesthesiologists, certified registered nurse anesthetists and anesthesiologist assistants). If the patient loses consciousness and the ability to respond purposefully, the anesthesia care is a general anesthetic, irrespective of whether airway instrumentation is required.

When deep sedation is intended, there is a significant risk that patients may slip into a state of general anesthesia (from which they cannot be aroused by painful or repeated stimulation). Therefore, individuals requesting privileges to administer deep sedation must demonstrate their ability to (1) recognize that a patient has entered a state of general anesthesia and (2) maintain a patient's vital functions until the patient has been returned to an appropriate level of sedation.

Definitions of terms appear at the end of this document. Of special note, for purposes of this document the following definitions are relevant:

1.1 Anesthesia Professional: An anesthesiologist, anesthesiologist assistant (AA), or certified registered nurse anesthetist (CRNA).

1.2 Non-anesthesiologist Sedation Practitioner: A licensed physician (allopathic or osteopathic); or dentist, oral surgeon, or podiatrist who is qualified to administer anesthesia under State law; who has not completed postgraduate training in anesthesiology but is specifically trained to administer personally or to supervise the administration of deep sedation.

2. ADVISORY

This advisory is designed to assist health care facilities in developing a program for the delineation of clinical privileges for practitioners who are not anesthesia professionals to administer sedative and analgesic drugs to establish a level of deep sedation. They are written to apply to every setting in which an internal or external privileging process is required for granting privileges to administer sedative and analgesic drugs to establish a level of deep sedation (e.g., hospital, freestanding procedure center, ambulatory surgery center, physician's or dentist's office, etc.). These recommendations do not lead to the granting of privileges to administer general anesthesia.

The granting, reappraisal and revision of clinical privileges will be awarded on a time-limited basis in accordance with rules and regulations of the health care facility, its medical staff, organizations accrediting the health care facility, and relevant local, state and federal governmental agencies.

NON-ANESTHESIOLOGIST SEDATION PRACTITIONERS

> Note: The *Hospital Anesthesia Services Condition of Participation 42 CFR 482.52(a)* limits the administration of deep sedation to "qualified anesthesia professionals" within their scope of practice. CMS defines these personnel specifically as an anesthesiologist; non-anesthesiologist MD or DO; dentist, oral surgeon, or podiatrist who is qualified to administer anesthesia under State law; CRNA, and AA. See also the *Ambulatory Surgery Center Condition for Coverage 42 CFR 416.42(b).*

Only physicians and other practitioners specifically permitted by CMS, above, who are qualified by education, training and licensure to administer deep sedation may administer deep sedation or supervise the administration of deep sedation when administered by CRNAs. Because training is procedure specific, the type and complexity of procedures for which the practitioner may administer or supervise deep sedation must be specified in the privileges granted.

Any professional who administers and monitors deep sedation must be dedicated to that task. Therefore, the non-anesthesiologist sedation practitioner who administers and monitors deep sedation must be different from the individual performing the diagnostic or therapeutic procedure (see ASA Guidelines for Sedation and Analgesia by Non-anesthesiologists).

3. EDUCATION AND TRAINING

The non-anesthesiologist sedation practitioner will have satisfactorily completed a formal training program in (1) the safe administration of sedative and analgesic drugs used to establish a level of deep sedation, and (2) rescue of patients who exhibit adverse physiologic consequences of a deeper-than-intended level of sedation. This training may be a formally recognized part of a recently completed Accreditation Council for Graduate Medical Education (ACGME) residency or fellowship training (e.g., within two years), or may be a separate deep sedation educational program that is accredited by Accreditation Council for Continuing Medical Education (ACCME) or equivalent providers recognized for dental, oral surgical and podiatric continuing education, and that includes the didactic and performance concepts below. A knowledge-based test is necessary to objectively demonstrate the knowledge of concepts required to obtain privileges. The following subject areas will be included:

3.1 Contents of the following ASA documents (or their more current version if subsequently modified) that will be understood by practitioners who administer sedative and analgesic drugs to establish a level of deep sedation

- 3.1.1 Practice Guidelines for Sedation and Analgesia by Non-Anesthesiologists. Anesthesiology 2002: 96; 1004–1017.
- 3.1.2 Continuum of Depth of Sedation; Definition of General Anesthesia and Levels of Sedation/Analgesia (ASA HOD 2004, amended 2009)
- 3.1.3 Standards for Basic Anesthetic Monitoring (Approved by the ASA House of Delegates on October 21, 1986, and last amended on October 25, 2005)
- 3.1.4 Practice Guidelines for Preoperative Fasting and the Use of Pharmacologic Agents to Reduce the Risk of Pulmonary Aspiration: Application to Healthy Patients Undergoing Elective Procedures (Approved by ASA House of Delegates on October 21, 1998, and effective January 1, 1999)

3.2 Appropriate methods for obtaining informed consent through pre-procedure counseling of patients regarding risks, benefits and alternatives to the administration of sedative and analgesic drugs to establish a level of deep sedation.

3.3 Skills for obtaining the patient's medical history and performing a physical examination to assess risks and co-morbidities, including assessment of the airway for anatomic and mobility characteristics suggestive of potentially difficult airway management. The non-anesthesiologist sedation practitioner will be able to recognize those patients whose medical condition requires that sedation needs to be provided by an anesthesia professional, such as morbidly obese patients, elderly patients, pregnant patients, patients with severe systemic disease, patients with obstructive sleep apnea, or patients with delayed gastric emptying.

3.4 Assessment of the patient's risk for aspiration of gastric contents as described in the ASA Practice Guidelines for Preoperative Fasting. In urgent, emergent or other situations where gastric emptying is impaired, the potential for pulmonary aspiration of gastric contents must be considered in determining

3.4.1 The target level of sedation

3.4.2 Whether the procedure should be delayed

3.4.3 Whether the sedation care should be transferred to an anesthesia professional for the delivery of general anesthesia with endotracheal intubation.

3.5 The pharmacology of

3.5.1 All sedative and analgesic drugs the practitioner requests privileges to administer to establish a level of deep sedation

3.5.2 Pharmacological antagonists to the sedative and analgesic drugs

3.5.3 Vasoactive drugs and antiarrhythmics.

3.6 The benefits and risks of supplemental oxygen.

3.7 Recognition of adequacy of ventilatory function: This will include experience with patients whose ventilatory drive is depressed by sedative and analgesic drugs as well as patients whose airways become obstructed during sedation. This will also include the ability to perform capnography and understand the results of such monitoring. Non-anesthesiologist practitioners will demonstrate competency in managing patients during deep sedation, and understanding of the clinical manifestations of general anesthesia so that they can ascertain when a patient has entered a state of general anesthesia and rescue the patient appropriately.

3.8 Proficiency in advanced airway management for rescue: This training will include appropriately supervised experience to demonstrate competency in managing the airways of patients during deep sedation, and airway management using airway models as well as using high-fidelity patient simulators. The non-anesthesiologist practitioner must demonstrate the ability to reliably perform the following:

3.8.1. Bag-valve-mask ventilation

3.8.2 Insertion and use of oro- and nasopharyngeal airways

3.8.3 Insertion and ventilation through a laryngeal mask airway

3.8.4 Direct laryngoscopy and endotracheal intubation

This will include clinical experience on no less than 35 patients or equivalent simulator experience (See ACGME reference). The facility with oversight by the Director of Anesthesia Services will determine the number of cases needed to demonstrate these competencies, and may increase beyond the minimum recommended.

3.9 Monitoring of physiologic variables, including the following:

3.9.1 Blood pressure.

3.9.2 Respiratory rate.

3.9.3 Oxygen saturation by pulse oximetry with audible variable pitch pulse tone.

3.9.4 Capnographic monitoring. The non-anesthesiologist practitioner shall be familiar with the use and interpretation of capnographic waveforms to determine the adequacy of ventilation during deep sedation.

3.9.5 Electrocardiographic monitoring. Education in electrocardiographic (EKG) monitoring will include instruction in the most common dysrhythmias seen during sedation and anesthesia, their causes and their potential clinical implications (e.g., hypercapnia), as well as electrocardiographic signs of cardiac ischemia.

3.9.6 Depth of sedation. The depth of sedation will be based on the ASA definitions of "deep sedation" and "general anesthesia." (See below).

3.10 The importance of continuous use of appropriately set audible alarms on physiologic monitoring equipment.

3.11 Documenting the drugs administered, the patient's physiologic condition and the depth of sedation at five-minute intervals throughout the period of sedation and analgesia, using a graphical, tabular or automated record which documents all the monitored parameters including capnographic monitoring.

3.12 The importance of monitoring the patient through the recovery period and the inclusion of specific discharge criteria for the patient receiving sedation.

3.13 Regardless of the availability of a "code team" or the equivalent, the non-anesthesiologist practitioner will have advanced life support skills and current certificate such as those required for Advanced Cardiac Life Support (ACLS). When granting privileges to administer deep sedation to pediatric patients, the non-anesthesiologist practitioner will have advanced life support skills and current certificate such as those required for Pediatric Advanced Life Support (PALS). Initial ACLS and PALS training and subsequent retraining shall be obtained from the American Heart Association or another vendor that includes "hands-on" training and skills demonstration of airway management and automated external defibrillator (AED) use.

3.14 Required participation in a quality assurance system to track adverse outcomes and unusual events including respiratory arrests, use of reversal agents, prolonged sedation in recovery process, larger than expected medication doses, and occurrence of general anesthesia, with oversight by the Director of Anesthesia services or their designee.

3.15 Knowledge of the current CMS Conditions of Participation regulations and their interpretive guidelines pertaining to deep sedation, including requirements for the pre-anesthesia evaluation, anesthesia intra-operative record, and post-anesthesia evaluation.

Separate privileging is required for the care of pediatric patients. When the non-anesthesiologist practitioner is granted privileges to administer sedative and analgesic drugs to pediatric patients to establish a level of deep sedation, the education and training requirements enumerated in #1–15 above will be specifically defined to qualify the practitioner to administer sedative and analgesic drugs to pediatric patients.

4. LICENSURE

4.1 The non-anesthesiologist sedation practitioner will have a current active, unrestricted medical, osteopathic, or dental license in the state, district or territory of practice. (Exception: practitioners employed by the federal government may have a current active license in any U.S. state, district or territory.)

4.2 The non-anesthesiologist sedation practitioner will have a current unrestricted Drug Enforcement Administration (DEA) registration (schedules II–V).

4.3 The privileging process will require disclosure of any disciplinary action (final judgments) against any medical, osteopathic or dental license by any state, district or territory of practice and of any sanctions by any federal agency, including Medicare/Medicaid, in the last five years.

4.4 Before granting or renewing privileges to administer or supervise the administration of sedative and analgesic drugs to establish a level of deep sedation, the health care organization shall search for any disciplinary action recorded in the National Practitioner Data Bank (NPDB) and take appropriate action regarding any Adverse Action Reports.

5. PERFORMANCE EVALUATION

5.1 Before granting initial privileges to administer or supervise administration of sedative and analgesic drugs to establish a level of deep sedation, a process will be developed to evaluate the practitioner's performance and competency. For recent graduates (e.g., within two years), this may be accomplished through letters of recommendation from directors of residency or fellowship training programs that include deep sedation as part of the curriculum. For those who have been in practice since completion of their training, performance evaluation may be accomplished through specific documentation of performance evaluation data transmitted from department heads or supervisors at the institution where the individual previously held privileges to administer deep sedation. Alternatively, the non-anesthesiologist sedation practitioner could be proctored or supervised by a physician or dentist who is currently privileged to administer sedative and analgesic agents to provide deep sedation. The Director of Anesthesia Services with oversight by the facility governing body will determine the number of cases that need to be performed in order to determine independent competency in deep sedation.

5.2 Before granting ongoing privileges to administer or supervise administration of sedative and analgesic drugs to establish a level of deep sedation, a process will be developed to re-evaluate the practitioner's performance at regular intervals. Re-evaluation of competency in airway management will be part of this performance evaluation. For example, the practitioner's performance could be reviewed by an anesthesiologist or a non-anesthesiologist sedation practitioner who is currently privileged to administer deep sedation. The facility will establish an appropriate number of procedures that will be reviewed.

6. PERFORMANCE IMPROVEMENT

Privileging in the administration of sedative and analgesic drugs to establish a level of deep sedation will require active participation in an ongoing process that evaluates the practitioner's clinical performance and patient care outcomes through a formal facility program of continuous performance improvement. The facility's deep sedation performance improvement program will be developed with advice from and with outcome review by the Director of Anesthesia Services.

6.1 The organization in which the practitioner practices will conduct peer review of its clinicians.

6.2 The performance improvement program will assess up-to-date knowledge as well as ongoing competence in the skills outlined in the educational and training requirements described above.

6.3 Continuing medical education in the delivery of anesthesia services is required for renewal of privileges.

6.4 The performance improvement program will monitor and evaluate patient outcomes and adverse or unusual events.

6.5 Any of the following events will be referred to the facility quality assurance committee for evaluation and performance evaluation:

- 6.5.1 Unplanned admission
- 6.5.2 Cardiac arrest
- 6.5.3 Use of reversal agents
- 6.5.4 Use of assistance with ventilation requiring bag-valve-mask ventilation or laryngeal or endotracheal airways.
- 6.5.5 Prolonged periods of oxygen desaturation (<85% for 3 minutes)
- 6.5.6 Failure of the patient to return to 20% of pre-procedure vital signs

7. DEFINITIONS

ANESTHESIA PROFESSIONAL–An anesthesiologist, anesthesiologist assistant (AA), or certified registered nurse anesthetist (CRNA).

NON-ANESTHESIOLOGIST SEDATION PRACTITIONER–A licensed physician (allopathic or osteopathic); or dentist, oral surgeon, or podiatrist who is qualified to administer anesthesia under State law; who has not completed postgraduate training in anesthesiology but is specifically trained to administer personally or to supervise the administration of deep sedation.

PRIVILEGES–The clinical activities within a health care organization that a practitioner is permitted to perform.

PRIVILEGING–The process of granting permission to perform certain clinical activities based on credentials, experience, and demonstrated performance

CREDENTIALS–The professional qualifications of a practitioner including education, training, experience and performance

CREDENTIALING–The process of obtaining, verifying, and assessing the qualifications of a practitioner to provide care or services in or for a healthcare organization.

PROCEDURAL SEDATION–The administration of sedative and analgesic drugs for a non-surgical diagnostic or therapeutic procedure.

Definitions of the continuum of sedation:

- ∗ MODERATE SEDATION–"Moderate Sedation/Analgesia ("Conscious Sedation") is a drug-induced depression of consciousness during which patients respond purposefully to verbal commands, either alone or accompanied by light tactile stimulation. No interventions are required to maintain a patent airway, and spontaneous ventilation is adequate. Cardiovascular function is usually maintained."
- ∗ DEEP SEDATION–"Deep Sedation/Analgesia is a drug-induced depression of consciousness during which patients cannot be easily aroused but respond purposefully following repeated or painful stimulation. The ability to independently maintain ventilatory function may be impaired. Patients may require assistance in maintaining a patent airway, and spontaneous ventilation may be inadequate. Cardiovascular function is usually maintained."
- ∗ RESCUE–"Rescue of a patient from a deeper level of sedation than intended is an intervention by a practitioner proficient in airway management and advanced life support. The qualified practitioner corrects adverse physiologic consequences of the deeper-than-intended level of sedation (such as hypoventilation, hypoxia and hypotension) and returns the patient to the originally intended level of sedation. It is not appropriate to continue the procedure at an unintended level of sedation."
- ∗ GENERAL ANESTHESIA–"General Anesthesia is a drug-induced loss of consciousness during which patients are not arousable, even by painful stimulation. The ability to independently maintain ventilatory function is often impaired. Patients often require assistance in maintaining a patent airway, and positive pressure ventilation may be required because of depressed spontaneous ventilation or drug-induced depression of neuromuscular function. Cardiovascular function may be impaired."
- ∗ The definitions marked with an asterisk are extracted verbatim from "Continuum of Depth of Sedation–Definition of General Anesthesia and Levels of Sedation/Analgesia" (Approved by ASA House of Delegates on October 13, 1999, and amended on October 21, 2009).

Expanded definitions of moderate and deep sedation can be found in the CMS Interpretive Guidelines.

8. REFERENCES

The American Society of Anesthesiologists has produced many documents over the years related to the topic addressed by this advisory, among them the following (in alphabetical order):

AANA-ASA Joint Statement Regarding Propofol Administration (April 14, 2004)

Continuum of Depth of Sedation–Definition of General Anesthesia and Levels of Sedation/Analgesia (Approved by ASA House of Delegates on October 13, 1999, and last amended on October 21, 2009).

Distinguishing Monitored Anesthesia Care ("MAC") from Moderate Sedation/Analgesia (Conscious Sedation). (Approved by the ASA House of Delegates on October 27, 2004, and last amended on October 21, 2009)

Guidelines for Ambulatory Anesthesia and Surgery (Approved by ASA House of Delegates on October 11, 1973, and last amended on October 22, 2008)

Guidelines for Delineation of Clinical Privileges in Anesthesiology (Approved by ASA House of Delegates on October 15, 1975, and last amended on October 22, 2008)

Guidelines for Office-Based Anesthesia and Surgery (Approved by ASA House of Delegates on October 13, 1999, and last affirmed on October 21, 2009)

Outcome Indicators for Office-Based and Ambulatory Surgery (ASA Committee on Ambulatory Surgical Care and Task Force on Office-Based Anesthesia, April 2003)

Practice Guidelines for Preoperative Fasting and the Use of Pharmacologic Agents to Reduce the Risk of Pulmonary Aspiration: Application to Healthy Patients Undergoing Elective Procedures. Anesthesiology 1999; 90: 896–905.

Practice Guidelines for Sedation and Analgesia by Non-anesthesiologists. Anesthesiology 2002: 96; 1004–1017.

Standards for Basic Anesthetic Monitoring (Approved by the ASA House of Delegates on October 21, 1986, and last amended on October 20, 2010)

Statement on Granting Privileges for Administration of Moderate Sedation to Practitioners Who Are Not Anesthesia Professionals (Approved by the ASA House of Delegates on October 25, 2005, and last amended on October 18, 2006)

Statement on Qualifications of Anesthesia Providers in the Office-Based Setting (Approved by ASA House of Delegates on October 13, 1999, and last amended on October 21, 2009)

Statement on Safe Use of Propofol (Approved by ASA House of Delegates on October 27, 2004 and amended on October 21, 2009)

In addition the following references may be considered:

ACGME Emergency Medicine residency program guidelines for number of intubations needed: http://www.acgme.org/acWebsite/RRC_110/110_guidelines.asp#res

American Academy of Pediatrics, American Academy of Pediatric Dentistry, Cote CJ, Wilson S, and the Workgroup on Sedation. Guidelines for Monitoring and Management of Pediatric Patients During and After Sedation for Diagnostic and Therapeutic Procedures: An Update. Pediatrics 2006; 118: 2587–2602.

Centers for Medicare and Medicaid Services Revisions to Interpretive Guidelines for Hospital Condition of Participation, December11,2009. http://www.cms.gov/surveycertificationgeninfo/pmsr/itemde-tail.asp?itemid=CMS1231690

Centers for Medicare and Medicaid Services Revisions to Interpretive Guidelines for Ambulatory Surgery Centers Condition for Coverage, Rev 04/01/2015, available at: https://www.cms.gov/Regulations-and-Guidance/Guidance/Manuals/downloads/som107ap_l_ambulatory.pdf. Accessed May 24, 2018.

APPENDIX 4 | BASIC LIFE SUPPORT (BLS) AND ADVANCED CARDIAC LIFE SUPPORT (ACLS)

DANIEL M. MOSELEY, MD, CHRISTOPHER V. MAANI, MD

INTRODUCTION

Moderate and deep sedation occurs in numerous settings, and health care providers may unexpectedly find themselves in situations where emergency resuscitation of patients will be required. A discussion of key concepts found in the latest American Heart Association (AHA) guidelines follows to prepare the provider for these potential emergencies. For more detailed information, the reader is referred to the 2015 AHA guidelines for cardiopulmonary resuscitation and emergency cardiovascular care.[1]

BASIC LIFE SUPPORT

Basic life support (BLS) skills for the health care provider include immediate recognition of sudden cardiac arrest (SCA), early cardiopulmonary resuscitation (CPR), and rapid defibrillation with an automated external defibrillator (AED)[1] (Figure A4.1).

First, assess the patient's responsiveness. The health care provider may check for normal, abnormal, or absent breathing, as well as attempt to elicit a response to stimulus (e.g., voice and touch). Immediate activation of the emergency response system should follow if the patient is unresponsive, and an AED should be obtained if nearby and easily accessible.

It is important to note, however, that the 2015 AHA guidelines "deemphasize" checking for breathing, as well as checking for a pulse, because health care providers may not always be able to accurately do so or may delay prompt intervention. As a result, the provider should take no longer than 10 seconds to check for a pulse, and if no pulse is appreciated in that time, chest compressions should be initiated immediately. However, if the patient suddenly collapses or is not breathing, the provider should assume that SCA has occurred and begin chest compressions without assessing pulses.

An important change in the latest guidelines is this emphasis on early chest compressions. Chest compressions should be initiated before ventilation ("CAB" rather than "ABC," with A for airway, B for breathing, and C for compressions), and this priority shift is a result of growing evidence on the importance of chest compressions to ensure oxygen delivery to the heart and brain.[2]

If a definite pulse is palpable, the health care provider should not initiate chest compressions but give one breath every 5–6 seconds and recheck the patient's pulse every 2 minutes. When respirations normalize, the patient should be placed in a recovery position on his or her side with the lower arm in front of the body.

To start chest compressions, the patient should be placed on a firm surface or a backboard should be placed under the patient if in a hospital bed. The heel of one hand should be placed on the center of the patient's chest, with the heel of the other hand on top of the first. The chest wall should be allowed to completely recoil after each compression to prevent higher intrathoracic pressure, which may inhibit hemodynamics. The new 2015 AHA guidelines recommend the sternum should be depressed 2 inches (5 cm) at a rate of 100–120 compressions per minute (i.e., "push hard and fast"). If two or more providers are present, they should alternate every 2 minutes to prevent fatigue and poor compression quality. It is also important to note that chest compressions should be minimally interrupted to check for a pulse, analyze rhythm, or other activities. If an interruption occurs, it should be limited to less than 10 seconds, except when defibrillating. CPR should continue until an AED arrives, return of systemic circulation (ROSC), or advanced life support personnel arrive.

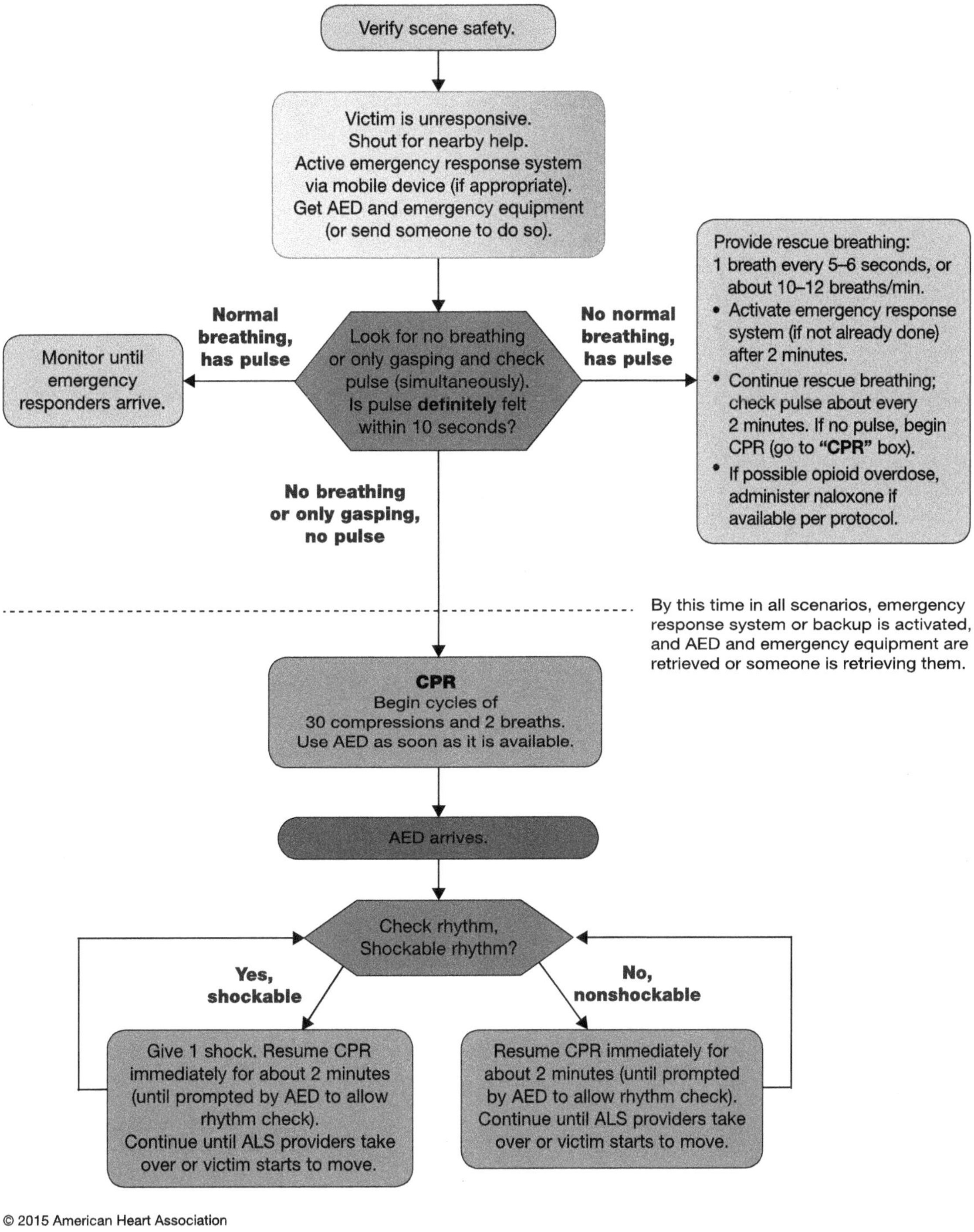

Figure A4.1: *BLS Healthcare ProviderAdult Cardiac Arrest Algorithm—2015 Update.*

After the initiation of chest compressions, ventilation should be attempted. The compression/ventilation ratio is 30:2 if there is no advanced airway (e.g., endotracheal tube). Ventilation can be performed using the head tilt/chin lift maneuver if there is no evidence of head or neck trauma. Each breath is delivered by opening the airway, pinching the patient's nose, and creating an airtight seal, with each breath given over 1 second to produce visible chest rise. Each breath should be a "regular" breath and not a deep breath. Mouth-to-barrier device, mouth-to-nose, mouth-to-stoma breathing are other alternatives, depending on the patient-specific situation. Bag-valve-mask ventilation with room air or oxygen can also be performed when available. A tight seal should be obtained between the face and mask, and the bag should be squeezed two-thirds of its volume for a 1-L bag and one-third for a 2-L bag. For all ventilation methods, the compression/ventilation ratio is still 30:2. Once an advanced airway (endotracheal tube, Combitube, or laryngeal mask airway [LMA]) is placed, one breath should be delivered every 6–8 seconds (8–10 breaths per minute) with no interruption of chest compressions. These recommendations are given to prevent excessive ventilation, which can lead to gastric inflation and complications such as regurgitation and aspiration.

Early defibrillation with an AED is the next key step in the adult BLS sequence and is the treatment of choice for ventricular fibrillation (VF) of short duration. Defibrillation is performed after a 2-minute cycle of CPR in the BLS sequence. However, there is not enough evidence to recommend delaying defibrillation until a cycle of CPR has been done.[3] For in-hospital settings where an AED is available, the defibrillator should be used as soon as possible. If more than one health care provider is present, one provider should initiate compressions while the other activates the emergency response system and obtains an AED. Once the AED has been obtained, the defibrillation sequence is power AED on, follow AED prompts to check rhythm and give one shock if the rhythm is "shockable," and resume CPR immediately after shocking. If the rhythm is "not shockable," CPR should resume immediately, and the rhythm should be checked every 2 minutes. CPR should be continued while the AED is being turned on and pads are being applied to minimize disruptions in chest compressions.

Last, there are special situations that warrant discussion, especially because the healthcare provider can have a significant impact on patient outcome if they are properly recognized. Two of those situations will be discussed here.

Acute coronary syndrome (ACS) is commonly manifested by chest pain, radiation of pain to the upper body, shortness of breath, sweating, nausea, and lightheadedness. Immediate activation of the emergency medical service (EMS) system should follow when these symptoms are present. When appropriate, EMS providers are trained to administer chewable, nonenteric aspirin 160–325 mg, obtain a 12-lead electrocardiogram (ECG), administer oxygen to keep oxygen saturation at 94% or above, administer nitrates (i.e., nitropaste, home dose of nitrate [e.g., Imdur] if available, etc.) in select patients, and administer analgesics such as morphine. Additionally, if an ECG demonstrates ST segment elevation myocardial infarction (STEMI), the patient must then be rapidly transported to a percutaneous coronary intervention (PCI) facility. Prompt PCI has been associated with improved outcomes in STEMI.[4]

Acute ischemic stroke is another situation in which proper recognition and immediate activation of the EMS system can have a significant impact on the patient's outcome. Commonly manifested symptoms of stroke are acute in onset and can include the following: numbness and weakness of the face or upper or lower extremities; confusion; difficulty speaking or understanding; difficulty walking; dizziness; loss of balance or coordination; and severe headache. If fibrinolytic therapy is given within the first 3 hours of symptom onset, neurologic injury is reduced, and patients can have improved outcomes. Patients should be transported directly to a stroke center when possible.

As with any other situation, if the patient is unresponsive, then the BLS sequences, as well as the advanced cardiac life support (ACLS) components discussed next, are critical and should not be delayed, regardless of whether or not the root cause is ACS or acute ischemic stroke.

ADVANCED CARDIAC LIFE SUPPORT

Advanced cardiac life support builds on the BLS sequence to include airway management and ventilation support, management of cardiac arrest, and treatment of bradyarrhythmias and tachyarrhythmias (Figure A4.2).[2]

Advanced airway placement and ventilation support allow for oxygenation and elimination of carbon dioxide. There are insufficient data to recommend when to place an advanced airway in relation to other interventions during resuscitation. However, airway placement should not delay initial CPR and defibrillation, and it is important to note that airway placement can be achieved without interruption of chest compressions. Additionally, only health care providers trained in airway placement should attempt this; the guidelines suggest frequent training for skill maintenance. If advanced airway placement cannot be achieved, bag-valve-mask ventilation can be. Prior to advanced airway placement, cricoid pressure, oropharyngeal airways, and nasopharyngeal airways may be used as adjuncts.

Once an endotracheal tube or supraglottic airway is placed, an immediate assessment for proper placement should follow. Physical examination should reveal bilateral chest rise, bilateral breath sounds, and no breath sounds over the epigastrum. For endotracheal tubes, exhaled CO_2 detectors can be used to confirm correct placement. Additionally, continuous-waveform capnography is now recommended, as it is the most reliable method to confirm and monitor placement of an endotracheal tube. Continuous-waveform capnography also has the advantage of reflecting poor-quality CPR if partial-pressure end-tidal CO_2 ($PETCO_2$) decreases below 10 mm Hg and reflecting ROSC if there is an abrupt and sustained increase in $PETCO_2$ (>40 mm Hg).

After successful placement of an advanced airway, chest compressions should immediately resume with no interruptions for ventilation. Providers should switch roles every 2 minutes to prevent fatigue. There are insufficient data to suggest the goal tidal volume, respiratory rate, and inspired oxygen concentration, but 100% inspired oxygen is often empirically used.

In addition to CPR and ventilation support, management of cardiac arrest involves rhythm-based management with an AED. The adhesive pads or paddles of an AED should be placed in an anterior-lateral position. Other positions are anterior-posterior, anterior–left infrascapular and anterior–right infrascapular. VF, pulseless ventricular tachycardia (VT), pulseless electrical activity (PEA), and asystole are heart rhythms that can lead to cardiac arrest. Only VF and pulseless VT are "shockable" rhythms. If a rhythm check with an AED reveals VF or pulseless VT, the initial shock should be delivered at 120–200 J for a biphasic defibrillator and 360 J for a monophasic defibrillator (Figure A4.2). CPR should immediately resume for 2 minutes, followed by another rhythm check. This cycle of CPR, rhythm check, and shock (if indicated) is repeated every 2 minutes until ROSC is achieved. Following the first shock, epinephrine 1 mg IV/IO can be given and repeated every 3–5 minutes. Following a second shock, a bolus dose of amiodarone 300 mg IV/IO can be given. Subsequent to these initial cycles, epinephrine 1 mg IV/IO and amiodarone 150 mg IV/IO should be alternated. The 2015 AHA guidelines have removed vasopressin use in resuscitation for simplicity.

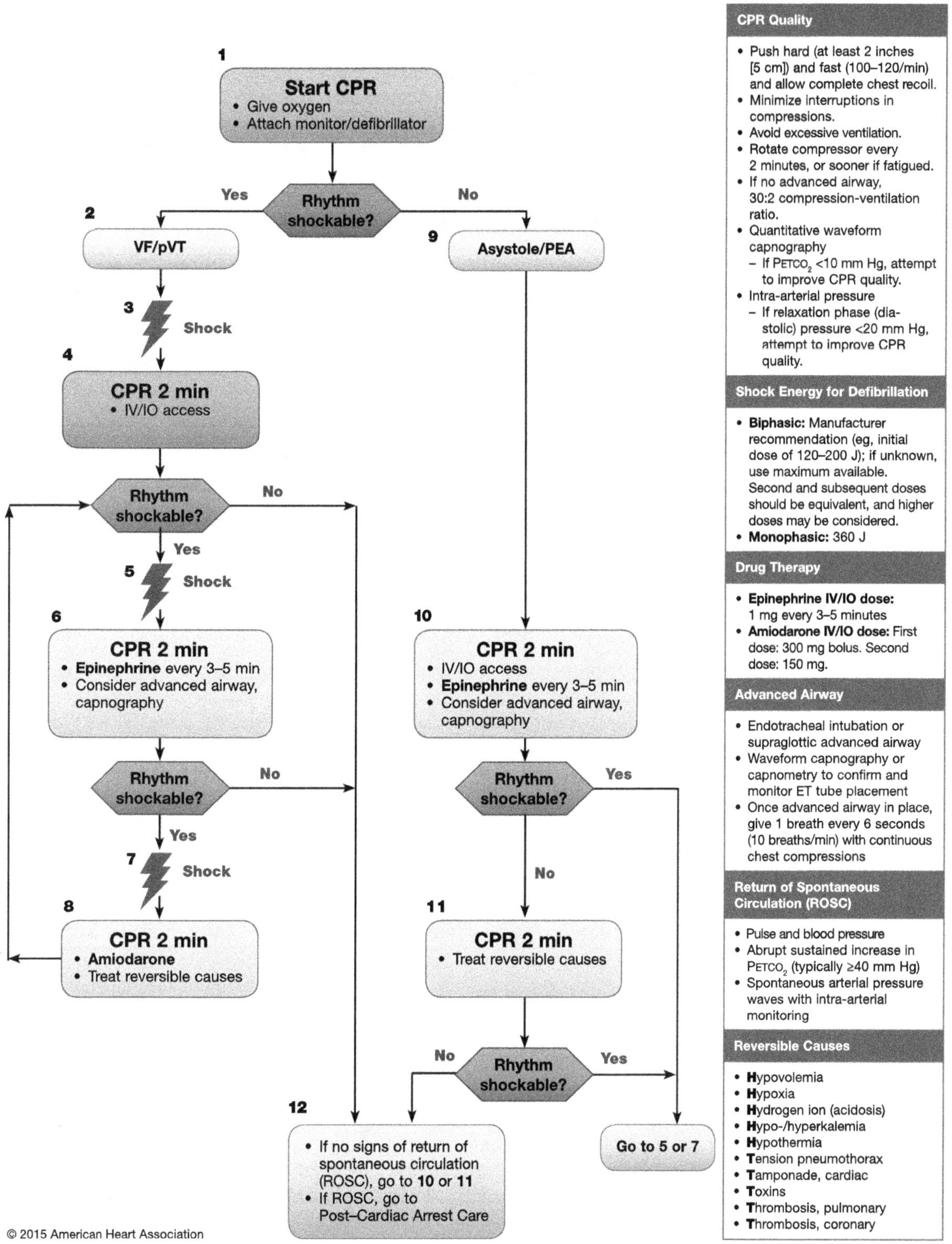

Figure A4.2: Adult Cardiac Arrest Algorithm–2015 Update.

For PEA or asystole, CPR (and not defibrillation) should continue for 2 minutes, followed by another rhythm check. Epinephrine 1 mg IV/IO every 3–5 minutes can be given during this cycle of CPR. If PEA or asystole persists, CPR resumes for 2 minutes. If a rhythm check at any time reveals VF or VT, the preceding sequence for shockable rhythms is initiated. For the treatment of PEA or asystole, atropine is no longer recommended for routine use.

Epinephrine hydrochloride is a vasopressor whose α-adrenergic agonist properties include increasing coronary perfusion pressure and cerebral perfusion pressure. The benefits of epinephrine's β-adrenergic agonist properties are less clear; it may increase myocardial work and reduce subendocardial perfusion. There is evidence that vasopressors may be associated with an increased rate of ROSC, although not necessarily increases in the rate of neurologically intact survival to hospital discharge.

Amiodarone is an antiarrhythmic drug and is preferred for treatment of VF and pulseless VT. It acts at sodium, potassium, and calcium channels, as well as α- and β-adrenergic receptors as an antagonist. There is evidence that amiodarone increases short-term survival to hospital admission compared to lidocaine or placebo, but there has been no evidence suggesting increased survival to discharge.

It is important to note that other ACLS interventions, such as obtaining vascular access, administering drugs, placing an advanced airway, and monitoring continuous-waveform capnography, are recommendations in the AHA guidelines and should not interrupt CPR or defibrillation. Additionally, timely identification and treatment of the underlying cause of cardiac arrest is essential. "The H's and T's" are identified in the guidelines as potentially reversible causes of cardiac arrest and are as follows: hypovolemia, hypoxia, hydrogen ion excess (acidosis), hypoglycemia, hypo-/hyperkalemia, hypothermia, tension pneumothorax, tamponade (cardiac), toxins, thrombosis (pulmonary), and thrombosis (coronary). Examples of interventions that may be critical for effective resuscitation include crystalloid administration for hypovolemia due to sepsis, empiric fibrinolytic therapy for suspected pulmonary embolism, and needle decompression for tension pneumothorax.

Another integral component of ACLS is the timely identification and treatment of unstable bradyarrhythmias and tachyarrhythmias. *Unstable* is defined by the AHA guidelines as "a condition in which vital organ function is acutely impaired or cardiac arrest is ongoing or imminent," and it can be manifested as acute mental status changes, chest pain, acute heart failure, shock, and hypotension. Hypoxemia is a common cause of unstable bradycardia and tachycardia, and as a result each ACLS treatment algorithm begins with an evaluation of the patient's breathing by physical examination and monitors such as pulse oximetry. Patients often require supplemental oxygen and assistance with breathing.

Bradycardia is a heart rate less than 60 beats per minute and should be immediately treated if it is the cause of the patient's instability. The first-line treatment is atropine 0.5 mg IV, which can be repeated every 3–5 minutes up to a maximum dose of 3 mg. If unresponsive to atropine, a dopamine infusion at 2–10 μg/kg per minute, epinephrine at 2–10 μg per minute, or temporary transcutaneous pacing may be utilized. Expert consultation or transvenous pacing may also be required.

There are many types of tachycardia, often classified as narrow complex versus wide complex or regular versus irregular. They may or may not require treatment. However, an unstable tachyarrhythmia should undergo immediate synchronized cardioversion. Intravenous access and patient sedation should be established prior to cardioversion when possible, but should not delay cardioversion if the patient is too unstable.

Cardioversion is synchronized with the QRS complex, and the initial energy dose is adjusted depending on whether unstable atrial fibrillation (120–200 J), atrial flutter (50–100 J), and unstable monomorphic/regular VT (100 J) is detected. If synchronization is not possible, if the QRS complex has a polymorphic appearance, or if the appearance of the QRS complex cannot be determined, then the energy dose should be set as high-energy unsynchronized shocks (i.e., energy doses used for defibrillation). It is important to note that with a heart rate less than 150 beats per minute and the absence of ventricular dysfunction, the tachyarrhythmia is more likely a secondary manifestation of the underlying condition rather than the root cause of the patient's instability. If the patient is not hypotensive, the AHA guidelines suggest a trial of adenosine 6 mg IV with a 12-mg second dose if needed.

In a stable patient with a tachyarrhythmia, further evaluation and intervention can be considered depending on the nature of the QRS complex. If the QRS complex is wide (≥0.12 seconds), the following can be considered: intravenous access, 12-lead ECG, adenosine (if monomorphic), antiarrhythmic infusion, and cardiology consultation. The following antiarrhythmic infusions can be given: procainamide, amiodarone, or sotalol. If heart failure or QT prolongation is absent, procainamide should be administered at 20–50 mg per minute until arrhythmia resolves, hypotension occurs, or QRS increases to greater than 0.18 seconds (50% increase). After this initial dose, the maintenance dose of procainamide is 1–4 mg per minute. Alternatively, amiodarone can be given as 150 mg over 10 minutes and repeated as necessary, followed by a maintenance dose of 1 mg/min for the first 6 hours. If QT prolongation is absent, sotalol can also be considered and administered as 100 mg (1.5 mg/kg) over 5 minutes.

If the QRS complex is narrow (≤0.12 seconds) in a stable patient with a tachyarrhythmia, the following can be considered: intravenous access; 12-lead ECG; vagal maneuvers (i.e., Valsalva maneuver, carotid sinus massage); adenosine (if monomorphic); β-blocker or calcium channel blocker; and cardiology consultation.

There are many pharmacologic treatment options for the various types of tachyarrhythmias, and a discussion of each is beyond the scope of this book. However, the current AHA guidelines provide drug tables that explain indications for use, dosing, common side effects, and contraindications for use.

Once ROSC has been achieved, the guidelines emphasize the need for prompt transition to post–cardiac arrest care. For patients in an outpatient setting, transport to a hospital that can provide coronary intervention, neurologic care, critical care, and hypothermia is the first step. For inpatients, transfer to a critical care unit is the next step. What the best care is for patients after an SCA is an ongoing area of research, but a timely initiation of a multidisciplinary, multisystem approach to patient care is vital, as most deaths occur in the first 24 hours.

REFERENCES

1. Kleiman M, Brenan E, Goldberger Z, et al. Part 5: Adult basic life support and cardiopulmonary resuscitation: 2015 American Heart Association guidelines update for cardiopulmonary resuscitation and emergency cardiovascular care. *Circulation*. 2015;132(18)(suppl 2):S414–S435.
2. Link MS, Berkow LC, Kudenchuk BJ, et al. Part 7: adult advanced cardiovascular life support: 2015 American Heart Association guidelines update for cardiopulmonary resuscitation and emergency cardiovascular care. *Circulation*. 2015;132(18)(suppl 2):S444–S464.
3. O'Connor RE, Al Ali AS, Brady WJ, et al. Part 9: Acute coronary syndromes: 2015 American Heart Association guidelines update for cardiopulmonary resuscitation and emergency cardiovascular care. *Circulation*. 2015;132(18)(suppl 2):S483–S500.
4. Cannon CP, Gibson CM, Lambrew CT, et al. Relationship of symptom-onset- to- balloon time and door- to- balloon time with mortality in patients undergoing angioplasty for acute myocardial infarction. *JAMA*. 2000;283:2941–2947.

APPENDIX 5 | PEDIATRIC EMERGENCY PLANNING AND RESUSCITATION

SHAWN S. JACKSON, MD, PHD, RICHARD D. URMAN, MD, MBA

INTRODUCTION

Anesthesiologists are completing more and more cases outside the operating room (OR), a trend that is true for both pediatric and adult patients. Beyond the OR, anesthesiologists are frequently involved in the endoscopy suite, helping to provide sedation for the placement of peripherally inserted central catheter (PICC) lines or other bedside procedures and helping to ensure safe imaging studies in radiology. As the number of out-of-OR encounters involving the pediatric population increases, a focus on the prevention and management of emergency situations becomes even more important. As resources outside the OR can often be significantly more limited, careful planning and an understanding of resuscitation guidelines are critical for providers taking care of pediatric patients.

The newest American Heart Association (AHA) guidelines for cardiopulmonary resuscitation and emergency cardiovascular care focus on several key areas:

- Prevention of pediatric arrests, including additional team-based training. Development and use of rapid response teams (RRTs) or medical emergency teams (METs).
- A focus on high-quality cardiopulmonary resuscitation (CPR), starting with chest compressions and then including breaths.
- Early access to advanced life support (ALS) care and algorithms

PREVENTION OF PEDIATRIC ARREST

Prevention of pediatric cardiopulmonary arrest has become a focal point of basic life support (BLS) and pediatric advanced life support (PALS) guidelines over the past 5-years.[1,2] While a significant amount of research has focused on high-risk medical and surgical patients who are admitted to the hospital,[3,4] many of these same principals and goals can be applied to the pediatric population outside the OR. Areas of emphasis for the prevention of pediatric arrests can be broadly divided into two main areas: first, stratifying and minimizing risk, especially with the increasing demand of out-of-OR sedation cases[5]; and second, developing and training with pediatric RRTs or METs that may respond to out-of-OR periarrest situations, as opposed to the more typical "anesthesia stat" encountered in the OR.

With regard to the prevention of pediatric arrest situations, several groups, including the American Society of Anesthesiologists (ASA) as well as the American Academy of Pediatrics, have published guidelines for use in establishing out-of-OR anesthesia and sedation practices. Several of the important guidelines include: consistent use of standard ASA monitors, even with minimal sedation cases; use of pre-sedation and pre-anesthesia checklists prior to administration of medications; and the development of algorithms for common periarrest situations (airway obstruction, laryngospasm, bradycardia).

The development of RRTs or METs has also proved to be an important part of addressing periarrest situations and preventing escalation to a full cardiopulmonary arrest.[6] While the size and makeup of such pediatric emergency response teams would vary depending on the caseload and facility size and makeup, it is reasonable to establish a defined team to respond to pediatric out-of-OR emergencies and implement formal team-based training, when possible.

PEDIATRIC BASIC LIFE SUPPORT

The 2015 pediatric BLS algorithm (Figure A5.1) not only shares many similarities with previous versions but also includes some key differences. As in previous versions, the algorithm defines infants as those less than 1 year old and children as those between 1 year old and puberty. A major focus of the updated BLS protocol is to decrease the time between recognition of an emergency event and implementation of high-quality CPR. To decrease this amount of time, the AHA now recommends the CAB approach to CPR, whereby compressions are performed initially and then followed by airway and breathing. In addition, the previous recommendations to "look, listen, and feel" for breathing have also been eliminated, again to decrease the amount of time between recognition of an emergency and implementation of high-quality CPR.

The pediatric BLS algorithm starts with recognition of an emergency situation. After ensuring that the environment is safe for a rescuer to intervene (scene safety), the emergency response system is activated, preferably by a bystander or second rescuer. If an automated external defibrillator (AED) is available on site, the person who activated the emergency response system should also retrieve the AED. After activation of the emergency response system, the patient should be assessed. The rescuer should assess for breathing while simultaneously checking for a pulse. This assessment should last no more than 10 seconds. If the patient is breathing normally and has a pulse, the patient should be closely monitored by the rescuer until additional resources arrive. If the patient has a pulse but is not breathing (or not breathing effectively), rescue breaths should be administered a rate of one breath every 3–5 seconds, or about 12–20 breaths per minute. If the patient is not breathing and does not have a pulse, CPR should begin immediately.

High-quality pediatric CPR begins with chest compressions and follows the CAB approach. While respiratory emergencies are by far the most common reason for cardiopulmonary arrest in the pediatric population, the AHA recommends starting with compressions to decrease the amount of time before effective CPR is initiated. For single-rescuer CPR in the pediatric population, a ratio of 30:2 (30 compressions followed by two breaths) should be utilized. If a second rescuer is available, a ratio of 15:2 should be employed (Table A5.1). Good chest compressions should be at a rate of 100–120 beats per minute. Compressions should take place at the lower half of the sternum, between the nipples, and be of sufficient force to depress the sternum one-third of the anterior-posterior (AP) distance. Adequate recoil of the sternum should be allowed to maximize circulation of blood throughout the body. Rescuers should remember to "push fast and push hard." In infants, the current recommendations are to use the two-finger technique (usually the second and third digits) to provide chest compressions if one rescuer is available and the two-thumb–encircling hands technique if two or more rescuers are available. In children, the heel of one hand should be used with the second hand placed over the first.

Rescue breathing, whether used alone (for patients with a pulse) or as part of CPR, is a critical component of BLS. The pediatric airway differs in several ways from the adult, increasing the risk of obstruction. To help ensure adequate ventilation, rescuers should adopt the head tilt, chin lift maneuver or the jaw thrust, especially useful if there is concern for a traumatic injury to the cervical spine. The delivery of breaths is best accomplished using a bag-valve-mask (when two rescuers are available) connected to an oxygen reservoir. In the event only a single rescuer is available, mouth-to-mask or mouth-to-mouth resuscitation is also appropriate. Breaths should be delivered over the time period of 1 second and should be sufficient to see chest rise. If chest rise is not visualized, the airway should be repositioned as it may indicate signs of an airway obstruction. In an out-of-OR location, end-tidal CO_2 is the gold standard for monitoring ventilation.

If an AED becomes available during CPR, it should be utilized at the earliest opportunity. While continuing appropriate cycles of compressions and breaths, the AED should be opened and the instructions (typically given by voice as soon as the AED is opened or turned on) followed. It is recommended to apply AED pads while compressions and breaths are going. CPR should only be interrupted once prompted by the AED that it is about to analyze the heart rhythm. For children or infants, it is preferable to use appropriate AED pads when they are available. However, the use of adult pads is acceptable if no alternative is available. If the AED analyzes the heart rhythm and determines that a shock is indicated, rescuers should clear the patient and deliver a shock. CPR should immediately begin after shock delivery. A pulse should be checked after approximately 2 minutes, an event that is typically prompted by the AED. If no shock is indicated and the patient still does not have a pulse, CPR should be continued until ALS providers arrive.

PEDIATRIC ADVANCED LIFE SUPPORT

Pediatric advanced life support is a continuation of the principles and guidelines of BLS. In addition to these benefits, PALS adds additional team roles for a multifaceted approach to patient care. Some of these team roles include acting as a team leader, establishing intravenous/intraosseous access, providing chest compressions, administering medications, delivering ventilation and establishing advanced airway access, acting as the code recorder, and managing the defibrillator. These team members come together to deliver care as part of the PALS algorithm. To help achieve team goals, good team members use closed-loop communication, communicate with clear messages, and have clear roles/responsibilities.

The PALS guidelines are broken up into several different algorithms (Figure A5.2). The cardiac arrest algorithm is described in further detail. The most important part of the algorithm is high-quality CPR, discussed previously. While high-quality CPR is ongoing, the patient is attached to a cardiac monitor/defibrillator, and the rhythm is evaluated during a break in CPR (pulse check). The rhythm is categorized into a shockable rhythm, which includes ventricular fibrillation or pulseless ventricular tachycardia, or a nonshockable rhythm, which includes asystole or pulseless electrical activity (PEA).

TABLE A5.1. BLS Rescue Breathing and Chest Compression Guidelines

	RESCUE BREATHING (NO COMPRESSIONS)	CHEST COMPRESSION	SINGLE-RESCUER CPR RATIO	TWO-RESCUER CPR RATIO
Pediatric	12–20/min	One-third the anteroposterior dimension; 100–120 compressions/min	30:2 (compressions to breaths)	15:2 (compressions to breaths)
Adult	10–12/min	At least 2 inches. 100-120 compressions/min	30:2 (compressions to breaths)	30:2 (compressions to breaths)

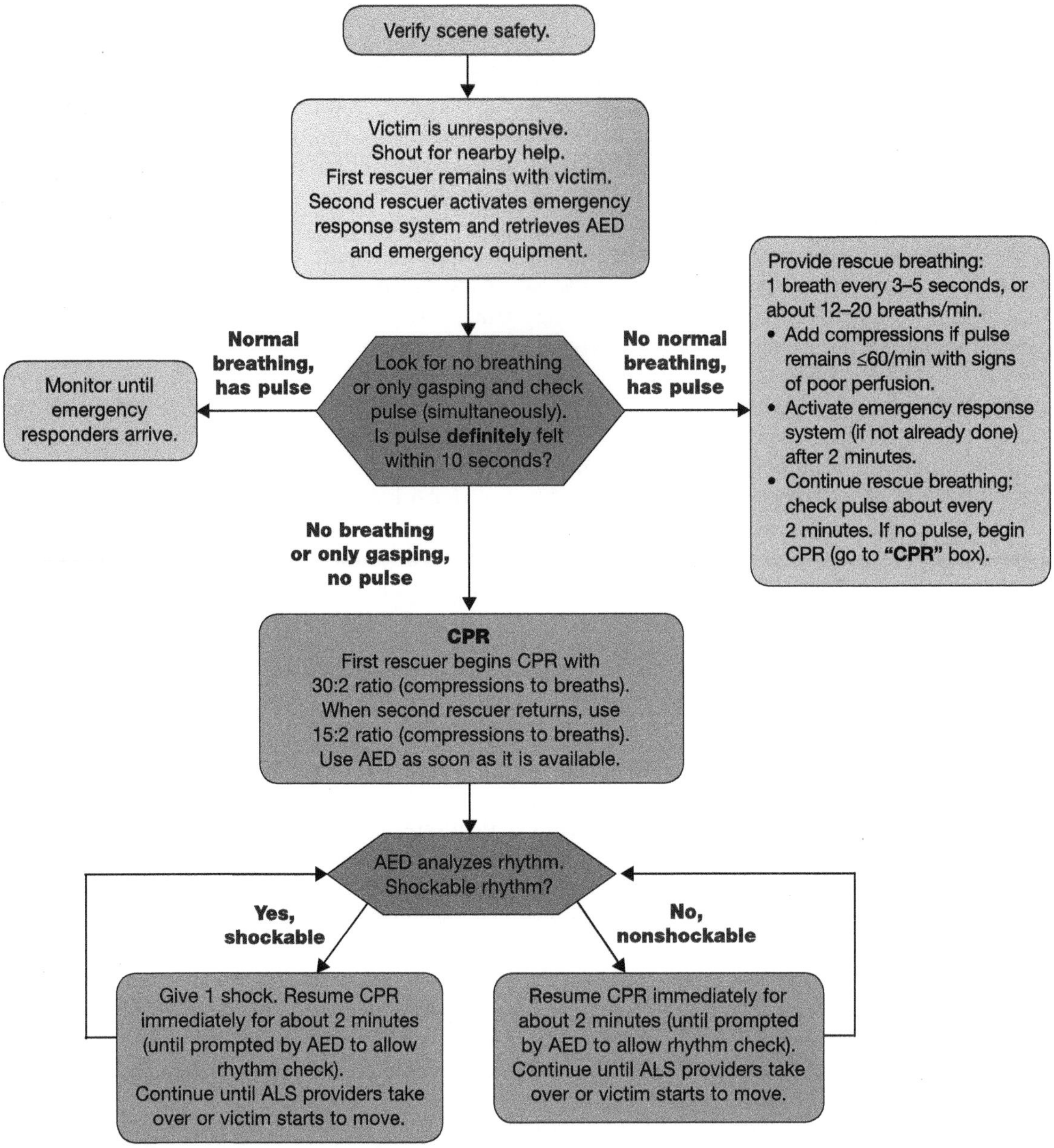

© 2015 American Heart Association

Figure A5.1 *2015 Basic Life Support Algorithm—2015 algorithm as published by the AHA. (reprinted with permission.)*

Shockable rhythms are treated with a combination of high-quality CPR, intravenous/intraosseous medications, and defibrillation. Early defibrillation is a critical component of this pathway. The recommended setting of defibrillation is weight based, with initial shocks at 2–4 J/kg and subsequent doses greater or equal to 4 J/kg. It is recommended not to exceed 10 J/kg (or the adult dose), even with refractory ventricular fibrillation or pulseless ventricular tachycardia. In addition to defibrillation, medications, including epinephrine 0.01 mg/kg every 3–5 minutes, can be administered. For refractory ventricular fibrillation and pulseless ventricular tachycardia, amiodarone 5 mg/kg and lidocaine 1 mg/kg should also be considered. Defibrillation should be repeated every 2 minutes during pulse checks provided the patient is still in a shockable rhythm.

Nonshockable rhythms are treated with a combination of high-quality CPR and intravenous/intraosseous medications. Unlike ventricular fibrillation and pulseless ventricular tachycardia, there is no role for defibrillation for asystole or PEA arrest. Epinephrine 0.01 mg/kg can be repeated every 3–5 minutes, and the patient should continuously be re-evaluated at pulse checks as the patient may develop a shockable rhythm while undergoing CPR.

In addition to high-quality CPR, medications, and defibrillation, PALS highlights the evaluation and treatment of

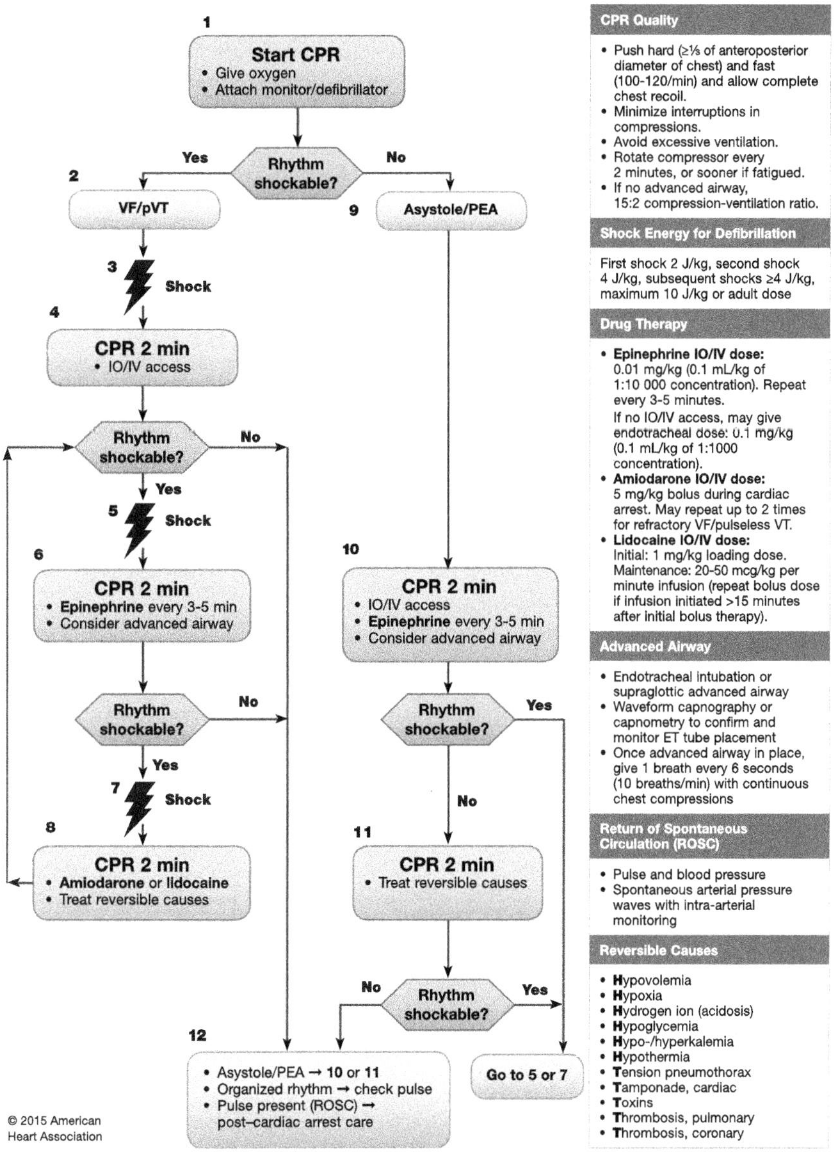

Figure A5.2 *2015 Pediatric Advanced Life Support (PALS) Algorithm—2015 algorithm as published by the AHA. (reprinted with permission.)*

reversible causes that may lead to cardiac arrest. The H's and T's are frequently used to help providers remember these causes and include hypovolemia, hypoxia, hyper- and hypokalemia, hypothermia, hydrogen ion (acidosis), hypoglycemia, toxins, tension pneumothorax, thrombosis (pulmonary or cardiac), and cardiac tamponade. The team leader and other team members should keep these reversible causes in mind and discuss them during code summaries to ensure one of these causes is not missed.

The placement of an advanced airway is also considered in PALS. An endotracheal tube or supraglottic airway is frequently employed during a pediatric arrest. Once an advanced airway has been placed, the 15:2 ratio utilized in CPR is replaced with continuous chest compressions and breaths delivered six gramatically (10 breaths per minute). In addition, an advanced airway provides the opportunity to monitor end-tidal CO_2 ($EtCO_2$). A target $EtCO_2$ during effective CPR should exceed 15 mm Hg, and values less than this should encourage the team to focus on increasing the quality of CPR.

SUMMARY

Pediatric resuscitation guidelines are a key aspect of reducing morbidity and mortality. This is equally, if not more, critical in an out-of-OR environment. The first step is to take measures to reduce and plan for pediatric periarrest situations, including reducing risk and establishing teams or responders who can quickly help in an emergency. Rapid implementation of effective BLS is critical, beginning with chest compressions and then delivering rescue breaths as part of the new emphasis on CAB instead of ABC when performing CPR. Activation of the emergency response and implementation of more advanced PALS protocols, including early defibrillation when indicated, are the next steps to improve outcomes. Overall, when these guidelines are taken together, outcomes can be improved, whether one is practicing in or out of the OR, on an inpatient unit, or outside of the hospital.

REFERENCES

1. de Caen AR, Berg MD, Chameides L, et al. Pediatric advanced life support: 2015 American Heart Association guidelines update for cardiopulmonary resuscitation and emergency cardiovascular care. *Circulation.* 2015;132: S526–S542. doi:10.1161/CIR.0000000000000266.
2. Atkins DL, Berger S, Duff JP, et al. Pediatric basic life support and cardiopulmonary resuscitation quality: 2015 American Heart Association guidelines update for cardiopulmonary resuscitation and emergency cardiovascular care. *Circulation.* 2015;132:S519–S525. doi:10.1161/CIR.0000000000000265.
3. McLellan MC, Gauvreau K, Connor JA. Validation of the Cardiac Children's Hospital Early Warning Score: an early warning scoring tool to prevent cardiopulmonary arrests in children with heart disease. *Congenit Heart Dis.* 2014;9(3):194–202. doi:10.1111/chd.12132.
4. Acker SN, Wathen B, Roosevelt GE, et al. Rapid response team activations in pediatric surgical patients. *Eur J Pediatr Surg.* 2016;(EFirst). doi:10.1055/s-0036-1593384.
5. Coté CJ, Wilson S, American Academy of Pediatrics, American Academy of Pediatric Dentistry. Guidelines for monitoring and management of pediatric patients before, during, and after sedation for diagnostic and therapeutic procedures: update 2016. *Pediatrics.* 2016;138(1):e20161212. doi:10.1542/peds.2016-1212.
6. Sharek PJ, Parast LM, Leong K, et al. Effect of a rapid response team on hospital-wide mortality and code rates outside the ICU in a Children's Hospital. *JAMA.* 2007;298(19):2267–2274. doi:10.1001/jama.298.19.2267.

BLS, basic life support; CPR, cardiopulmonary resuscitation.

INDEX

Tables, figures, and boxes are indicated by an italic *t*, *f*, and *b* following the page number.

Q